Handbook of Speech and Language Disorders

Handbook of Speech and Language Disorders

edited by

Janis M. Costello, Ph.D.
Speech and Hearing Center
University of California, Santa Barbara

and

Audrey L. Holland, Ph.D.
Speech and Hearing Center
University of Pittsburgh

COLLEGE-HILL PRESS, San Diego, California

Library of Congress Cataloging in Publication Data
Main entry under title:

Handbook of speech and language disorders.

Includes indexes.
1. Speech, Disorders of. 2. Speech disorders in children. 3. Language disorders. 4. Language disorders in children. 5. Speech therapy.
I. Costello, Janis M., 1942–   . II. Holland, Audrey L. [DNLM: 1. Language Disorders—in adulthood. 2. Language Disorders—in infancy & childhood. 3. Speech Disorders—in adulthood. 4. Speech Disorders—in infancy & childhood. WL 340 H2365]
RC423.H327   1986   616.85'52   85-26905
ISBN 0-88744-237-4

Contents

Contributors

James Abbs, Ph.D.
Waisman Center, Room 521
Speech Motor Control Laboratories
University of Wisconsin
Madison, WI 53705-2280

Martin Adams, Ph.D.
Program in Communication Disorders
North Office Annex
University of Houston
Houston, TX 77004

Nicholas W. Bankson, Ph.D.
Department of Communicative Disorders
Sargent College of Allied Health Professions
Boston University
48 Cummington Street
Boston, MA 02215

Anthony S. Bashir, Ph.D.
The Children's Hospital Medical Center
Division of Hearing and Speech
300 Longwood Ave.
Boston, MA 02115

Kathryn A. Bayles, Ph.D.
Department of Speech and Hearing Sciences
University of Arizona
Tucson, AZ 85721

John E. Bernthal, Ph.D.
Department of Communication Disorders
University of Nebraska at Lincoln
202 Barkley Memorial Center
Lincoln, NE 68583

Thomas F. Campbell
Department of Speech Pathology
Glenrose Hospital
Edmonton, Alberta, Canada

Marie Capozzi, Ph.D.
Department of Communication
1117 Cathedral of Learning
University of Pittsburgh
Pittsburgh, PA 15260

Robin S. Chapman, Ph.D.
Department of Communicative Disorders
University of Wisconsin-Madison
1975 Willow Drive
Madison, WI 53706

Elizabeth Cole, Ed.D.
School of Human Communication Disorders
McGill University
Montreal, Quebec
Canada, H3G 1A8

Janis M. Costello, Ph.D.
Speech and Hearing Center
University of California—Santa Barbara
Santa Barbara, CA 93106

Richard F. Curlee, Ph.D.
Department of Speech and Hearing Sciences
University of Arizona
Tucson, AZ 85721

G. Albyn Davis, Ph.D.
Department of Communication Disorders
Arnold House
University of Massachussetts
Amherst, MA 01003

Patricia A. Dowden, M.S.
Department of Rehabilitation Medicine
University of Washington
Seattle, WA 98195

Barry Guitar, Ph.D.
Department of Communication Sciences
and Disorders
Allen House
University of Vermont
Burlington, VT 05405

Chris Hagen, Ph.D.
Speech-Language Pathology Department
Speech, Hearing and Neurosensory Center
Children's Hospital and Health Center
Sharp Rehabilitation Hospital
San Diego, CA 92123

M. N. Hegde, Ph.D.
Department of Communicative Disorders
California State University at Fresno
Fresno, CA 93740-0001

Nancy Helm-Estabrooks, D.Sc.
Audiology/Speech Pathology
Boston Veterans Administration
Medical Center
Neurology (Speech Pathology)
Boston University School of Medicine
Boston, MA 02130

Audrey Holland, Ph.D.
Department of Communication
University of Pittsburgh
1117 Cathedral of Learning
Pittsburgh, PA 15260

Jennifer Horner, Ph.D.
Department of Surgery
Duke University Medical Center
Box 3887
Durham, NC 27710

Roger Ingham, Ph.D.
Speech and Hearing Center
University of California—Santa Barbara
Santa Barbara, CA 93106

Mata B. Jaffe, Ph.D.
Rehabilitation Institute of Pittsburgh
6301 North Umberland Street
Pittsburgh, PA 15217

Thomas S. Johnson, Ph.D.
Department of Communication Disorders
Utah State University
UMC 10
Logan, UT 84322

Laurence B. Leonard, Ph.D.
Department of Audiology and Speech
Sciences
Purdue University
West Lafayette, IN 47907

Jacqueline Weis Liebergott, Ph.D.
Emerson College
Division of Communication Disorders
168 Beacon Street
Boston, MA 02116

Craig W. Linebaugh, Ph.D.
Department of Speech and Hearing
George Washington University
2201 G. Street, N.W.
Washington, D.C. 20052

Jeri A. Logemann, Ph.D.
Communication Sciences and Disorders
Frances Searle Building
Northwestern University
2299 Sheridan Road
Evanston, IL 60201

Betty Jane McWilliams, Ph.D.
Division of Speech Pathology-Audiology
Department of Speech and Theater Arts
Cleft Palate Center
University of Pittsburgh
Pittsburgh, PA 15260

Jon F. Miller, Ph.D.
Department of Communicative Disorders
University of Wisconsin—Madison
1975 Willow Drive
Madison, WI 53706

Beth Mineo, Ph.D.
Assistant Director
Bioengineering Program
Association for Retarded Children
2501 Avenue J
Arlington, TX 76006

Penelope Starratt Myers, M.A.
The Speech and Hearing Center
George Washington University
2201 G. Street, N.W.
Washington, CA 20052

Marietta M. Paterson, M.A.
School of Human Communication Disorders
McGill University
Montreal, Quebec, Canada H3G 1A8

William H. Perkins, Ph.D.
Center for the Study of Communication
Disorders
University of Southern California
Los Angeles, CA

Elizabeth M. Prather, Ph.D.
Department of Speech and Hearing Science
Arizona State University
Tempe, AZ 85287

John C. Rosenbek, Ph.D.
Chief, Audiology and Speech Pathology
William S. Middleton Memorial Veteran's
Hospital
2500 Overlook Terrace
Madison, WI 53705

Dennis M. Ruscello, Ph.D.
Department of Speech Pathology and
Audiology
805 Allen Hall
West Virginia University
Morgantown, WV 26506

Martin C. Schultz, Ph.D.
The Children's Hospital Medical Center
Division of Hearing and Speech
300 Longwood Avenue
Boston, MA 02115

Richard G. Schwartz, Ph.D.
Department of Audiology and Speech
Sciences
Purdue University
West Lafayette, IN 47907

Lynn S. Snyder, Ph.D.
Department of Speech Pathology and
Audiology
University Park
University of Denver
Denver, CO 80208

Bernd Weinberg, Ph.D.
Department of Audiology and Speech
Sciences
Purdue University
West Lafayette, IN 47907

Frederick F. Weiner, Ph.D.
Communication Disorders Program
118 Moore Building
Pennsylvania State University
University Park, PA 16802

Susan E. Weismer, Ph.D.
Waisman Center on Mental Retardation
and Human Development
University of Wisconsin—Madison
1500 Highland Avenue
Madison, WI 53706

Robert T. Wertz, Ph.D.
Audiology and Speech Pathology
Veterans Administration Medical Center
150 Muir Road
Martinez, CA 94553

M. Jeanne Wilcox, Ph.D.
School of Speech Pathology and Audiology
Kent State University
Kent, OH 44242

Walter A. Wolfram, Ph.D.
University of the District of Columbia
and Center for Applied Linguistics
Department of Communication Science
College of Liberal and Fine Arts
724 9th Street, N.W.
Washington, D.C. 20001

Kathryn M. Yorkston, Ph.D.
Department of Rehabilitation, RJ-30
School of Medicine
University of Washington
Seattle, WA 98195

Preface

While planning the organization and scope of this volume, the growth of information—paralleled unmercifully by the growth in new questions—taking place today in speech pathology became strikingly clear to me. With the assistance of the series' editor in chief, William H. Perkins, and our publisher, Sadanand Singh, I began to review the progress made in recent years in research and clinical practice. Occasionally, I was dismayed to note that seemingly little action and, therefore, few new developments, had occurred in a given area (hence, some areas are not addressed in this volume). For the most part, however, I was pleased to realize that new developments were taking place at nearly every turn and to observe that many of those advances stemmed directly from an increasing alliance between rigorous scientific method and important clinical pursuits.

The best people to write about recent advances are those who are making them, and this volume is filled by the writings of such persons. Their experiential and experimental knowledge of their topics is obvious in the content of each of these chapters, and I am exceedingly grateful for their willingness to contribute and for the patience they displayed with an everlengthening time line.

This volume is divided into separate sections on recent advances in child phonology and in stuttering. Each section is introduced by a chapter which provides an overview of the major developments in the area in order to set the scene and provide a framework for the description of recent advances in specific areas. Each of the recent advances chapters concentrates on major work, published and unpublished, carried out within the last few years, although the classic studies which often served as the impetus for work being produced now are generally described as well.

It is hoped that this volume and its companions in the *Recent Advances* series will help researchers and clinicians fill a major portion of the gap created by the fast-moving pace of speech pathology today.

Janis M. Costello
Editor

Speech Disorders in Children

Recent Advances

Editor in chief, Speech, Language, and Hearing Disorders Series
William H. Perkins, PhD

Part One

PHONOLOGY AND ARTICULATION

John E. Bernthal
Nicholas W. Bankson

Phonologic Disorders: An Overview

Introduction

Among the communication disorders which speech-language pathologists treat, it is probably safe to say that most clinicians feel more comfortable and competent when dealing with disorders of phonology than with other types of speech and language impairments. There are several factors that may be related to this proposition. First of all, articulatory behavior can be broken down into perceptually identifiable segments and, thus, may be considered more discreet in nature than certain other aspects of communication such as voice, fluency, or language. Second, a hierarchy of linguistic complexity is readily apparent, i.e., isolation, syllables, words, phrases, sentences. Third, clinicians have developed treatment procedures which, at least at an empirical level, have been demonstrated to modify target behaviors, especially with the less severe phonologically disabled individual. It is probable that these factors are related to the observation that clinicians are relatively confident when confronted with articulation impairments. In spite of this confidence, the theoretical constructs and data base supporting clinical decisions have been relatively lacking. Recent developments, however, have begun to bring about changes in this regard.

The past decade witnessed an unprecedented influence of psychology and linguistics on articulation assessment and management. In recent years, some speech scientists have focused their attention on articulatory phenomena. Such influences have served to encourage speech-language clinicians to take a critical look at our knowledge, practice, and research in this area.

The purpose of this chapter is to present an overview of where we have been and where we are going in articulation assessment and management and to identify strands of knowledge that have led to the current state of the art.

It is hoped that the reader will sense that recent advances in the field have led to a better understanding of phonologic disorders, and that such knowledge is establishing a data base that will result in more enlightened clinical decisions.

Functional-Organic Dichotomy

One aspect of articulation of continuing interest among investigators and clinicians is the specific influence of certain etiological factors which have been shown to relate to articulatory events and patterns. Since the early days of speech-language pathology, the terms *functional* and *organic* have often been ascribed to disorders in order to differentiate causal factors. In this book, organically based articulation disorders, such as those associated with neurologic, craniofacial, and hearing impairments, will be discussed in chapters by Jaffe, McWilliams, and Cole and Paterson, respectively. In addition, chapters by Ruscello and Weiner will discuss disorders that have been identified in the literature as nonorganic, functional, and developmental. As a prelude to further discussion of articulation impairments, it may be helpful to consider the background and current status of the functional-organic dichotomy.

In tracing the speech-language pathology literature, the terms "functional" and "organic" have been present for a long time. These terms were originally used in the field of medicine; and since the medical model of diagnosis had such a pervasive effect on the field in the early days, it seems only natural that such usage was adopted by speech-language pathology. As was customary with the medical model, attempts were made to determine the *cause* of the problem or disorder. It was recognized that some problems were related in an obvious way to neurologic, structural, and perceptual factors. It was also recognized, however, that not all disorders were organic in nature, but, rather, some were nonorganic, or to borrow a medical term, "functional." While the term functional was originally synonymous with nonorganic, its meaning was soon broadened to include all disorders of "unknown" causation.

Early writers in the field, such as West, Ansberry, and Carr (1937), cautioned the profession about problems inherent in the use of the term "functional." Such problems, however, are not unique to speech-language pathology. A report from the New York Milbank Medical Conference in 1950 stated the following:

> The semantic difficulty that kept cropping up during the conference was the confusion consequent upon the use of such terms as "organic," "functional," "mental," "physical," and "purely psychological." This confusion was enhanced by the apparently irresistible temptation of even superior scientists to dichotomize phenomena into "organic or functional," "mental or physical."

In spite of the inherent problems with this term, it would appear that practitioners of various disciplines who employ the medical model have a propensity to dichotomize disorders as either functional or organic.

Let us consider the meanings ascribed to the term "functional." The most frequently used definition has focused on an organic/nonorganic dichotomy. Travis (1931) indicated that in the absence of determined or inferred organic pathology, an articulation disorder may be classified as functional. More recently, however, Emerick and Hatten (1974) stated that some children identified as having functional articulation disorders, in which no readily discernible organic basis for the sound errors is found, may "possess subtle neurological impairments." They were especially concerned with children who seem to have difficulty modifying sound productions and who persist in the production of speech sound errors even after instruction. They reported preliminary data which indicate that children who have such persistent articulation disorders show more signs of possible organic impairment, including mild or marginal motoric disability, than either children without articulatory impairment or children who made improvement during the first year of intervention.

Other speech-language pathologists have extended or broadened the definition of "functional" and have indicated that the term should carry no inference of either organic or nonorganic cause, but should simply indicate that there are no obvious signs of structural, perceptual, or neurologic deviations. Some writers have used other labels to replace the term "functional"—such as "developmental errors" or "developmental delay." Powers (1957) has criticized our labeling of functional articulation disorders on the premise that it has constituted "diagnosis by default." Shelton (1978) also pointed out that the term has often served as a "waste basket" category for articulation problems of unknown causation. The lack of etiological and behavioral specificity that characterizes the category has caused some to question whether the term "functional" is even an appropriate or helpful label to be used in identifying articulation disorders.

It would appear that those clients considered to have functional disorders are a very heterogeneous group who might be better labeled as individuals with articulation disorders of *unknown etiology*. Behaviorally, this group varies in severity from those with a single sound in error to those with multiple errors. We would propose that the term "unknown etiology" is a more appropriate descriptor of this population than the term "functional." Not only does "functional" have a variety of meanings, it is also difficult to define on other than a "default" basis.

Factors Related to Phonologic Disorders of Unknown Etiology

Historically, investigators have spent a great deal of effort exploring possible factors related to "functional" articulation disorders. Such variables have included speech sound discrimination, intelligence, dentition, oral sensory perception, laterality, motor skills, personality, educational achievement, and language skills, among others. The types of research designs employed in such studies have typically been either correlational studies of the status of articulation and other variables within individuals or comparisons between nonimpaired subjects and subjects with disorders of articulation on one or more of these variables. As we know, correlational studies do not allow cause-effect statements. Similarly, a functional relationship between variables is not obtained through group comparisons. Thus, studies concerned with disorders of unknown etiology have not, for the most part, been successful in identifying possible causal factors. Shelton and McReynolds (1979) indicated that this may be true because (1) a common factor is not operating across all articulation-impaired individuals, (2) the factors may be too subtle to be identified with the methods used, (3) research methodologies have been inadequate, or (4) the wrong variables have been studied. At best, studies of status relationship have identified only a few variables worthy of further investigation as factors that may contribute to the presence of phonologic disorders. It has been suggested that rather than studying individual variables that relate to disorders of unknown etiology, we might better study a collection of variables simultaneously in order to discover possible relationships between clusters of factors and articulation.

The few studies of this nature (Arndt, Shelton, Johnson, & Furr, 1977; Prins, 1962) that have been done, however, have not been very successful in identifying distinct subgroups of the articulation-impaired population. One such subgroup is children who have been identified as syllable reducers because their speech sound error pattern is characterized by the reduction of CCV or CVC syllables to the CV or VC form. Compared to children whose errors are primarily substitutions, children with syllable reduction errors have a higher total number of articulation errors and make more extensive use of /ʔ/, /h/, and other sounds unlike the "intended" phonemes. Syllable reducers tend to be slower to respond to articulation remediation and have different patterns of transfer and generalization when compared to substituters (Elbert & McReynolds, 1978; Panagos, 1974; Prins, 1962; Renfrew, 1966). They have also been found to have lower IQs, to have more associated neurologic abnormalities, to repeat syllables at slower rates, to be from families rated as lower in socioeconomic status, and to perform more poorly on measures of linguistic ability when compared to substituters (Frisch & Handler, 1974; Prins, 1962). In order to subcategorize a group of children with articulation disorders of unknown etiology, it is necessary to demonstrate in some meaningful fashion that the behaviors seen are reflective of a particular cluster of characteristics. The meaningfulness of such differentiation will be strengthened if a functional relationship can be demonstrated between a change in one or more critical variables and a change in articulatory performance.

Articulation Patterns Associated with Second Language Learning

It seems appropriate in this discussion of factors associated with the presence of articulatory differences to make a statement about the unique problems associated with learning the phonologic system of a second language. Categorically, we must say that phonologic differences associated with second language learning, as well as those associated with geographic or social/dialect, are not appropriately viewed as articulation impairments. It is important to make the point that phonologic differences related to dialect or second language learning are not considered functional or organic impairments.

Etiology and Treatment Models

A wide variety of treatment approaches have been employed with those clients with articulation problems of unknown etiology. Shelton and McReynolds (1979) have delineated the following models:

1. Discrimination model   emphasis on external and internal monitoring, matching one's own productions to a standard model, using auditory,

	proprioceptive, and tactile feedback to control productions automatically.
2. Sensory-motor model	emphasis on production of sounds in various and increasingly complex contexts, with repetition of the motor skills involved in articulation.
3. Operant conditioning model	emphasis on shaping behaviors, programming, contingency management as a means of establishing new behaviors.
4. Phonologic disorders model	emphasis on teaching the phonologic contrasts of a language with efforts to increase the complexity of such contrasts.

All of these models approach articulatory disorders without specific evidence of the cause of the problem, yet there are particular etiologic biases that might be ascribed to the different models (e.g., perceptual deficiency, faulty learning). These models are not mutually exclusive, and, in reality, many clinicians tend to be eclectic in their use of treatment models. It should be pointed out that such models are also used in the treatment of clients whose articulation impairment has an organic base. This observation then raises the whole question of how important etiology is in the treatment of articulation disorders.

While treatment models used in the management of functional and organic articulation disorders are similar, an understanding of the organic basis underlying some articulatory/phonologic impairments is critical for the speech-language clinician. The child without an intact mechanism with which to develop speech and language frequently requires different or even unique assessment and treatment procedures as compared to a child with an intact speech mechanism. For example, the child who is not able to close the velopharyngeal valve adequately—with the result that the nasal cavity is coupled to the oral cavity during production of stops, fricatives, and affricates—may require physical management in order to produce appropriate levels of intraoral air pressure for such consonants. An understanding of which speech errors can be attributed to such a physical impairment and which can be attributed to learning or cognitive factors may be important considerations in management. Likewise, the child whose articulation impairment can be partly attributed to a perceptual deficit caused by a hearing loss will have certain error patterns and problems which can be explained by the hearing loss.

A similar statement can be made relative to the dysarthrias seen in children with neurological impairment in which a child with a moderate to severe motor involvement may display articulation deviations that result not only in unique management procedures but in reduced expectations for change.

The chapters in this book dealing with neurologic speech disorders in children by Jaffee, craniofacial anomalies by McWilliams, and hearing impairment by Cole and Paterson are intended to give the reader current information regarding the types of speech impairments associated with such organic problems. These chapters also discuss why such articulatory characteristics occur and provide management suggestions for individuals with such disorders.

Phonologic Development

The nature of phonologic development has long been of interest to speech scientists, linguists, and speech-language pathologists. For purposes of organization, investigations of phonologic development will be discussed from linguistic and motor-acoustic perspectives.

Schwartz points out in his chapter that child phonologists have not only looked at surface structures (observable phonetic events), but have also made inferences concerning children's underlying representations for sounds produced at the surface level, identified phonologic processes, and discussed the relationship between perception and production. Theories and models of phonologic development from a linguistic perspective have typically focused on phonologic universals (the child's theoretically innate ability to passively acquire a phonologic system). More recently, constructionist theories have emerged in which the child is assumed to take an active role in the construction of his phonologic system.

A second perspective related to phonologic development has been an emphasis on phonetic (surface level) or motor development of speech sounds. This research has focused on the phonetic inventories, coarticulation, and the effects of phonetic context.

The need exists for investigators to study phonologic development from both a linguistic as well as a phonetic perspective in order to obtain a more comprehensive understanding of phonologic development. Such studies require that investigators employ methods typically used in both linguistic and phonetic approaches.

Articulatory-Phonologic Disorders

Research in disordered articulation can also be viewed from motor-acoustic and linguistic perspectives. It has long been recognized that children's misarticulations reflect phonetic and phonemic error types even within the same child. In some instances, speech-language pathologists have viewed articulation errors as motor production problems with remediation focusing on motor practice. The chapter in this volume by Ruscello reflects a bias that remediation of many children's articulation errors can be approached from a motor learning perspective and that motor learning theory can serve as a model for articulatory training. A second type of articulation problem emanates from a linguistic perspective. Sound changes (errors) are described as phonemic or pattern based. The assumption by some speech-language pathologists has been that such phonemic productions reflect factors other than the child's ability to produce a sound at the motor level. In other words, children who substitute /θ/ for /s/ and then substitute /s/ for /ʃ/ are considered to have the necessary phonetic skills in their response repertoires to produce the /s/. Instead, the /θ/ for /s/ substitution probably reflects a phonologic rule operating on a child's phonologic output.

Since the publication of Ingram's monograph *Phonological Disability in Children* (1976), the emphasis on the linguistic aspects of children's speech sounds has been considerable. Weiner makes this observation as well in his chapter in this volume. The emphasis on patterns of sound production and the systematic nature of speech sound errors has resulted in the publication of several evaluation procedures which reflect this linguistic emphasis in the assessment of speech sound errors in children.

Perhaps it is appropriate at this point in the chapter to address the notion of how these disorders which reflect speech sound changes should be labeled. There have been suggestions that individuals with speech sound changes which deviate from the norm for a given age should be identified as having a phonologic disorder rather than an articulation disorder. It is our position that to a considerable extent this argument is a semantic one. There is no doubt that since the publication of Ingram's book in 1976, the focus of what has traditionally been called articulation disorders has been broadened to include a strong phonologic or linguistic emphasis. Some investigators have suggested that the term "articulation disorders" is too restrictive in that it suggests only concern for the motor and acoustic aspects of speech sounds involving just the peripheral aspects of the speech mechanism. On the other hand, it is argued that the term "phonologic disorders" encompasses not only the surface or motor aspects of production but also the underlying adult form, as well as phonologic rules and processes. From this perspective, "phonologic disorders" is a broader, more encompassing, and thus, more appropriate term than articulation disorders. However, some individuals seem to use the term "phonologic disorders" so that it does not include the motor aspects of sound production. When the term "phonologic disorders" is used in such a restrictive sense, it does not encompass the range of problems seen in the children who are the focus of this book. In the chapters which follow, the editor has chosen to employ the term "phonologic disorders" to refer to all children with speech sound errors, thereby using the term in a broad or generic sense to include not only the phonemic aspects of articulation, but also the motor and surface forms of sound productions. When the term articulation appears, it is meant to signify the exclusively perceptual-motoric aspects of phonologic performance.

Trends in Assessment

Since one section of this volume is designed to review recent advances in phonologic disorders, it is appropriate to review past and current practices in assessment of such disorders. Since the 1960s, the traditional assessment battery for articulation status has consisted of the following: (1) a connected speech sample, usually a spontaneous speech sample, (2) a phonetic inventory evoked by a picture-naming task, (3) a measure of articulatory consistency (deep testing), and (4) a measure of imitation or stimulability of segments produced in error. Before discussing the state of the art of each of these aspects of assessment, perhaps it would be helpful to briefly discuss the evolution of the test battery.

Historical Review

It goes without saying that spontaneous or connnected speech samples have always been of critical importance to clinicians, for that is the format in which appropriateness of speech sound production is ultimately judged. Thus, from the beginning of the profession, articulation evaluation has included listening to a talker's connected speech. Reading samples are one method that has often been used in order to obtain a sample of this speech. It should be recognized that reading samples are more artificial than true spontaneous speech, and thus, at the present time, clinicians are more interested in hearing a client produce sounds in a spontaneous situation. As audio tape recorders became widely available, clinicians recorded connected speech samples and used the recordings for more careful analysis than is possible with live online transcription. While the techniques for evoking connected speech samples have been fairly similar throughout the years (e.g., telling stories, answering questions), in recent years published articulation tests have included more formalized methods for obtaining these samples (e.g., pictures designed to evoke story telling responses, repeating a story after the examiner). The use of spontaneous speech samples as a primary data base for analysis has received increased emphasis since the late 1970s due to interest in a more linguistically based assessment of children's phonologic patterns.

As with spontaneous speech samples, phonetic inventories have been used in the assessment of articulatory status almost from the beginning of the profession. Phonetic inventories were developed in order to assess the sounds of the language in a relatively short period of time. In the late 1950s and early 1960s there was a feeling among many speech-language clinicians that since there was a relatively high correlation between overall intelligibility of spontaneous speech samples and the number of errors identified by a phonetic inventory, phonetic inventories could provide an accurate picture of a child's speech sound patterns. Many clinicians even came to use the phonetic inventory as their primary assessment instrument. Since the 1970s, however, there has been increased interest in connected speech samples as a primary sample for analysis, and thus, inventories have come to be used as only one measure in an articulation battery. The shift away from phonetic inventories to connected speech samples as the primary data base was related to the observation that within individuals there is frequently variation in performance between these two measures.

While clinicians have always been interested in clients' abilities to imitate the correct form of their misarticulations, imitative or stimulability testing as a potential prognostic tool was not examined systematically until the late 1950s and early 1960s. Several investigators demonstrated that a child's performance on stimulability tasks was related to the probability for correcting a sound without intervention. This measure continues to be used to determine if clients have the appropriate motor gestures to produce sound segments judged to be in error and to help determine the rate at which remediation can be expected to progress.

A major contribution to the methodology for assessing articulation was the appearance of contextual or "deep testing" of sounds. The prototype for such testing was *The Deep Test of Articulation* (McDonald, 1964). Such instruments allowed for an in-depth analysis of a particular segment by varying the phonetic contexts which preceded and followed a target sound. This addition to the traditional articulation battery provided clinicians with more systematic data regarding variation in sound productions than were typically available through inventories or spontaneous speech samples.

In the following paragraphs each of these elements of a traditional battery will be discussed. The point should be made that interactive variables affect speech samples, since phonologic behaviors are sensitive to linguistic and extralinguistic factors associated with the mode of evocation. However, such factors will not be elaborated in this chapter.

Review of Traditional Test Battery

Connected speech sample

The major advantage of a spontaneous or connected speech sample is its inherent face validity, since correct productions in conversational speech represent the terminal behavior of articulation instruction. In addition, spontaneous samples allow for a judgment of the client's overall intelligibility and may also be used to determine consistency of speech sound productions. Shriberg and Kwiatkowski (1980) suggested that a connected speech sample yields more stable data than alternative measures and recommended its use for their natural phonologic process analysis. The spontaneous speech sample also has the potential to be used for related language analyses, thus enabling an integrated speech-language assessment.

A limitation of spontaneous speech samples is observed in the case of individuals with severe articulation problems when responses are unintelligible and the intent of the message is unknown. Not knowing what a child is attempting to say is a significant problem, not only in transcription, but also in subsequent interpretation of error patterns. Most clinicians recognize this difficulty and use a gloss (an indication by the clinician of what the child attempted to say) in order to insure that the child's intended sounds are part of the data collection procedure.

A second limitation of spontaneous speech samples is the difficulty encountered in obtaining a representative sample of the speech sounds of a language, since the lexicon obtained in a particular sample may not contain an adequate sample of these. However, it may be that if a sample is of sufficient size, the problem of a nonrepresentative sample may not be a critical issue because a child's preference for certain sounds will be revealed, the sounds missing in his repertoire probably reflecting a selective avoidance on his part. Further, since the important sounds will be produced a number of times in such a spontaneous sample, a general picture of a child's phonologic system will be obtained. It is possible that apparent sound preferences may be as much or more a reflection of word preferences as they are of sound preferences. Conversely, the absence of sounds may reflect a selective avoidance or simply a difference in the frequency of occurrence of sounds in the language. Even if the assumption of selective avoidance is valid and a reasonable description of the child's phonology can be inferred from the speech sample, clinicians will typically still desire a more representative and systematic sample of the speech sounds in the language than can be obtained from a spontaneous connected speech sample.

At this time, most investigators and clinicians would agree that a spontaneous speech sample should be included as a routine procedure during the assessment of children with articulation disorders. The issue for which there is still disagreement is the extent to which a spontaneous speech sample should serve as the primary data base of the evaluation. Speech-language clinicians are aware that in the case of many children, the responses obtained from a spontaneous sample may be different from those obtained from other sampling procedures (Shriberg & Kwiatkowski, 1980). With other children, it has been shown that similar results may be obtained in a much shorter time with these alternative methods (DuBois & Bernthal, 1978). In summary, since spontaneous or connected samples have the best face validity, most speech-language pathologists agree that such samples should serve as the primary basis for the assessment and analysis of children's articulation. The second advantage in using continuous speech samples to assess children's articulation/phonologic status is that other language and linguistic analyses can be performed on the same corpus.

Phonetic inventory

The nature of sound inventories has changed little over the past four decades. The number of items, the order of items, vocabulary used, whether or not one or more sound segments are tested in a single item, and size and color of stimulus pictures are some of the minor types of changes seen in these instruments in the past two decades. The major changes have been in the scoring and analysis of such inventories. There has been a definite shift toward more phonetic detail in scoring, and conversely, a moving away from the more traditional scoring system of recording responses as correct or incorrect or even of classifying errors as substitutions, omissions, and distortions. The reason for this change is that clinicians are looking more carefully at error productions so that feature and process errors that may be present are identified. Only through detailed transcriptions do some of these errors surface.

The second major change associated with inventories has been a shift from sound-by-sound analysis to pattern analysis. *The Fisher-Logemann Test of Articulation Competence* (1971) was a notable attempt toward this emphasis on the identification of error patterns across sound segments. A third change which has emerged since 1950 is the collection of normative data which allowed clinicians to compare a child's performance at a particular age to norms for the instrument. These changes have served to increase the versatility of inventories.

Despite the criticism in the literature directed toward picture-naming articulation tests, they continue to enjoy widespread use as a clinical tool. Phonetic inventories allow the clinician to control the sample obtained and thereby assure sampling of all items of interest. In addition, such tests may be administered rather quickly, are convenient to transport, and provide the examiner with an easy-to-analyze sample of speech sound productions.

The most obvious disadvantage of single word inventories is that frequently segments produced in citation form (single words) are produced differently than they are in connected speech samples. It is well known that single word responses do not adequately reflect the effects of coarticulation or the effects of context which in many instances transcend syllable and lexical boundaries. Factors such as syllable structure, stress, and phonetic environment frequently affect production but are not controlled in such tests.

A second criticism is that most speech sound inventories contain only a single utterance of each target sound in each word position. Inconsistency of articulatory productions seen in children during phonological acquisition, as well as in children with articulation disorders, cannot be adequately assessed through such limited sampling. In addition, it is a reasonable speculation that word familiarity may also affect production of individual segments, although we are not aware of data to support this view. Nonetheless, phonetic inventories continue to serve a role in the clinical assessment of the articulation status of children and provide useful information despite their shortcomings.

Stimulability testing

Stimulability testing, advanced by Milisen (1954) in early treatment research, is assessment of the client's ability to imitate at a motor level the adult form of a misarticulated sound but does not provide information about phonemic competence. The unit to be imitated may include isolated sounds, syllables, or words, and usually involves the presentation of visual and auditory cues. The clinician can assume that the subject who is stimulable on an error sound has the motoric skills required to make the articulatory gesture for the target sound. It has been suggested that segments that can be produced via imitation can be corrected more rapidly through intervention than those sounds which cannot be imitated (Winitz, 1975). In recent years, it has been reported that once a sound can be imitated in a syllable or word context, response generalization to nontrained words and syllables begins to occur (McReynolds, 1972). Investigators have also reported that children with the poorest test scores on stimulability tests are most likely to benefit from intervention (Sommers, Leiss, Delp, Gerber, Fundrella, Smith, Revucky, Ellis & Haley, 1967). Other investigators have reported that children aged 5 through 7 who are able to correctly imitate syllables or words containing an error sound have a higher probability for self-correction of those sounds than those who are not stimulable (Carter & Buck, 1958; Farquhar, 1961). A clinical guideline might be that if a child has a mild articulation problem but can imitate the target sound(s) at the syllable level, then remediation may not be indicated. For those with more severe problems, however, sounds that can be imitated may represent a good beginning point for treatment. In summary, stimulability testing provides data that are useful in determining the need for intervention and in making treatment decisions.

Contextual testing

The notion that children's articulation productions are inconsistent (sometimes target sounds are produced correctly, sometimes they are not) is well documented in the literature, and thus some form of contextual or in-depth testing of error sounds has been suggested as part of the traditional articulation test battery. Van Riper (1939) stated long ago that the search for contexts in which an error sound is produced correctly is well worth the investment of time. He suggested that such key words can serve as a place to initiate instruction. Contextual testing is typically done with the *The Deep Test of Articulation* (McDonald, 1964), or the *Sound Production Tasks* (Elbert, Shelton & Arndt, 1967; Shelton, Elbert & Arndt, 1967), or in a connected speech sample. Many clinicians look upon such contextual testing as an initial step in the remediation process. Contextual or deep testing is most important for the clinician who samples the articulation of a given sound only in a limited number of contexts. Such testing can be used to get an idea of consistency of target production or to identify facilitating phonetic contexts. The selection of facilitating contexts also involves other factors (e.g., stress, word position, allophonic variation, frequency of occurrence) in addition to the influence of adjacent sounds. It is a reasonable speculation that the higher the percentage of correct to incorrect utterances identified in contextual testing, the more likely the child will self-correct the error and make progress in remediation. Although Lapko and Bankson (1975) reported a significant correlation between the *The Deep Test of Articulation* for the /s/ sound and the Carter-Buck task for speech sound stimulability for /s/, specific data to support the above speculations are lacking.

Scoring and Analysis

Traditionally, speech-language clinicians have scored responses as substitutions, distortions, omissions, or insertions. While there have been a number of different definitions for sound "omissions," or deletions, this term seems to be a useful concept and has remained in the literature across time, and in recent years omissions have come to be identified with more specificity, e.g., deletion of final consonants, deletion of unstressed syllables, and cluster reductions.

As well, the designation of substitutions and/or additions also seems to be a useful notion, since transcription of such segments is similar across most scoring systems except for the amount of phonetic detail included. On the other hand, use of the term "distortion" is a curious one, since it is really better described as a substitution in which the replacement segment is an incorrect variation within the perceptual boundary of the target sound.

Notation used to transcribe children's utterances will vary with the way the data are to be analyzed. In general, transcription and an analysis of the speech of a child with defective articulation requires use of the International Phonetic Alphabet and some system of diacritics.

The ways in which speech samples have been analyzed are: (1) judgment of overall intelligibility, (2) sound-by-sound analysis, and (3) pattern analysis. In sound-by-sound analysis, the emphasis is on individual segments and the number and type of errors. Typically, such analyses examine the stimulability of individual segments, the consistency of individual segments in a variety of phonetic contexts, comparison with developmental norms of the acquisition data for individual segments, and average number of errors for children of a given age. The third type of error analysis is a pattern analysis in which the examiner focuses on patterns of errors. One error pattern or simplification strategy may account for the sound changes seen across several segments.

The traditional pattern analysis usually consists of reviewing errors for commonalities in terms of place, manner of production, and voicing. The lack of specificity in the manner and place categories have limited their clinical use. The recent trend toward phonologic process analysis partially overcomes this limitation because of its increased specificity. Process labels such as *stopping, gliding for liquids, cluster reduction, final consonant deletion, fronting, backing* all provide specificity to place and manner categories.

We wish to point out that in the paragraph above, these terms only describe errors in the surface structure of the child's phonology and are not intended to make any inference concerning the child's underlying representations of the adult phonemic form. Use of the term "phonologic processes" to refer only to surface structures is not something all speech-language pathologists would agree upon. Authors, in describing procedures for phonologic process analysis, have used the term process differently. Weiner, in his chapter, defines a process by pointing out that the child is assumed to have an underlying phonologic representation nearly equivalent to the adult surface form. Shriberg and Kwiatkowski (1980) selected processes for their natural process analysis procedure that met additional criteria. These criteria specified that a proccess had to meet Stampe's (1973) criteria for a natural process, had to be observed frequently in the speech of young children with delayed speech, and further, had to be scored reliably by speech-language clinicians. In contrast, some investigators use the term "process" only as a label to describe surface patterns without any assumption about underlying representation.

In summary, the appealing notion of using linguistically based analysis procedures is that they facilitate a better understanding of the child's phonologic system and, one hopes, lead to more efficient clinical management. Khan (1982) furnished an example of how a process analysis can provide a better understanding of a child's phonologic system than the more traditional analysis. To describe the common replacement by children of /wawa/ for *water* as a /w/ for /t/ substitution with an omission for the final /ɾ/ does not reveal an accurate picture of the child's phonology. Rather, describing this "error" as an example of syllable reduplication reflects a better understanding of this child's phonology in that the child is repeating a syllable rather than replacing correct sounds with error sounds in the second syllable. Phonologic pattern analysis is not a replacement for traditional assessment procedures but rather, a supplementary tool. Recent recommendations for conducting a complete phonologic assessment include process analysis as but one of several recommended procedures.

Trends in Remediation

For the approximate half century that speech-language pathologists have sought to treat phonologic disorders, clinicians have moved from a point where they had to rely primarily on their own intuitions to the point where a clinical science data base for phonologic disorders has begun to emerge. From a retrospective view, it is possible to trace several trends that appear to reflect a greater sophistication in the management of phonologic disorders. In the following paragraphs we will trace some of the trends and influences in the area of remediation of phonologic disorders.

Historical Review

Traditional treatment

Early approaches to treatment emphasized a phonetic or motor approach to correcting sounds supplemented with perceptual or discrimination training. Sounds were taught one at a time with instruction focusing on "ear training" followed by phonetic placement cueing in order to evoke productions in isolation. Once a sound was established in isolation, production was shifted to increasingly complex contexts (i.e., syllables, words, phrases, sentences). Drill activities formed the heart of the treatment methodology. Such an approach had an inherent logic to it and was supported by early writers in the field.

Sensory-motor influence

In the early 1960s a new thought influenced remediation practices. McDonald (1964) described an approach to remediation that focused less on production of sound segments in isolation and more on syllable productions and the systematic production of sounds embedded in a variety of phonetic contexts. Specifically, McDonald suggested that remediation, based on prior assessment, should focus on sounds being produced in facilitating contexts and on increasing the number of contexts in which a sound was produced correctly. Practice in producing bisyllables and trisyllables with a variety of stress patterns was an integral part of this remediation approach. Thus, the attention of the clinician was directed to the importance of *phonetic facilitation*, which may be defined as improvement in the production of a target sound as a function of phonetic context. While it is probably accurate to say that McDonald's work had a greater impact on assessment procedures than on remediation procedures, nonetheless, his work added an important perspective to the process of making treatment decisions.

Behavioral influence

By the late 1960s and well into the 1970s, concepts from the field of behavioral psychology had a decided influence on the manner in which clinicians approached remediation, both in terms of instruction and the measurement of its effect. Concepts such as pinpointing behaviors, programming stimuli and responses, and controlling behavior by its consequences came into common understanding and application within the profession. In addition, the importance of repeated samplings of target behavior, both before and during treatment, was emphasized. In fact, measurement of responses was an integral part of this behavioral trend and served to foster a number of research studies concerned with articulation treatment (e.g., Bankson, 1974; Elbert & McReynolds, 1978).

It should be pointed out that this behavioral approach to management did not represent a completely novel approach to treatment; rather, in many instances it served as a framework or protocol in which existing intervention methodologies could be utilized. For example, a temporal sequence of clinical events might follow the (1) antecedent event, (2) response, and (3) consequent event paradigm with criterion levels established for progression from one level of instruction to another. Clinicians then inserted traditional as well as novel treatment techniques into this framework. Behavior modification, with its heavy emphasis on programmed instruction and the use of consequating events as a means for changing behaviors (see Costello, 1977) facilitated more sophisticated behavioral routines than had typically been practiced.

As stated above, not only did the behavioral movement serve to influence practices associated with clinical management, but it also served as an impetus for clinical research. Prior to this time there were few investigations which had specifically studied treatment approaches. Lack of interest in treatment research, coupled with the problems inherent in doing group studies (e.g., finding subjects who met similar selection criteria; running large numbers of subjects; and the masking of individual variation within the group mean) served to discourage treatment studies. The functional analysis of behavior, or within-subject experimental design, was perceived by speech-language clinicians as appropriate and convenient for study of the treatment of phonologic impairment (McReynolds & Kearns, 1982).

Behavioral studies have focused on the effect of particular treatment approaches including training sequences and aspects of articulation generalization. While investigations conducted thus far have only scratched the surface of research needed to develop a clinical science of phonologic remediation, efforts to develop a scientific base in the area of remediation have begun.

Linguistic influence

Concurrent with the influence of behavioral psychology on speech-language pathology was the influence which emanated from linguistics. This influence stemmed primarily from work in psycholinguistics, including child phonology, and was related to all aspects of language behavior. Linguists called the attention of speech-language pathologists to the notion that articulation behavior could be described within the framework of language behavior.

The work of Compton (1970) represented one of the early attempts to apply linguistic principles to disordered articulation. He proposed that when a child produced multiple articulation errors, such errors might be related. He demonstrated that a language corpus could be analyzed in such a manner that phonologic rules or patterns that were common across segments could be identified.

Interest in identification of patterns among misarticulations found increased focus through analyzing such errors via a distinctive feature analysis. Such analyses looked for distinctive feature commonalities among sound errors. While various methodologies for doing such analyses were developed, they have not been used widely by clinicians for two reasons: (1) the distinctive features borrowed from linguistic theory were sometimes ill-suited for clinical application and (2) the time required for most feature analysis systems was viewed as too lengthy by clinicians.

A rationale for use of a remediation approach based on distinctive feature analysis is the assumption that training of a feature in one segment will transfer to other segments where the feature is used inappropriately. Investigators have reported preliminary data which demonstrates that feature training in one or more sounds does, on occasion, transfer to other sounds (Costello & Onstine, 1976; McReynolds & Bennett, 1972). The degree of generalization, however, varies across segments, individuals, and linguistic units.

Phonologic process analysis procedures discussed earlier in this chapter were the next type of pattern analysis to emerge in the late 1970s. This type of pattern analysis was based on processes observed in young children developing phonology (Ingram, 1976). Such analyses describe simplification strategies—final consonant deletion, stopping, etc. Remediation that has been suggested for the elimination or suppression of selected processes focuses on targets such as establishing additional sound contrasts including the elimination of homonyms (e.g., [tu] for *two* and *tooth;* [wawa] for *water; waffle; wakeup).* Teaching techniques may also focus on perceptual tasks related to the training of various contrasts. At the present time data regarding the benefits of treatments derived from phonologic process analyses are only of a most preliminary nature, but it may turn out that such analyses lead to novel treatment procedures that are effective for certain clients with multiple errors.

Perhaps the major treatment contribution from linguistics has been in the nature of the target behaviors selected for remediation. For example, instead of treating an individual segment, a clinician may treat several sounds in an affected class or, at least, an exemplar of a class. An approach of this type assumes that generalization across phonemes within the affected class will occur and that the clinician will not have to teach all the segments that reflect the operation of a given phonologic process. If generalization of this type does not occur and a clinician must remediate all affected segments, there may be minimal efficiency in this approach.

When evaluating the current status of remediation, the following statements can be made. While the data base for making treatment decisions is still woefully lacking, nonetheless, the field has moved forward in developing such a base and can at least acknowledge an increase in applied research. Because of the great variability observed among clients, within-subject research designs, including replication with a small number of subjects, have been found particularly useful and have served to advance our data base. A related phenomenon has been the trend toward more precise and thorough measurement of progress in remediation employed by clinicians. Treatment methodologies have expanded in format and sophistication; however, in most instances these expansions have represented adaptations of traditional methodologies. Clinicians have become more interested in children with severe phonologic impairments, and target behaviors selected for treatment with this population have been more often based on pattern analysis, especially phonologic process analysis, than the traditional sound-by-sound analysis. In cases where only a few unrelated sounds are in error, more traditional analyses seem to be adequate.

In terms of those clients with organically based disorders, progress has been made in the identification of particular syndromes and subgroups. It is hoped that identification of such subgroups will lead to more appropriate treatment methodologies for these individuals.

References

Arndt, W., Shelton, R., Johnson, A., & Furr, M. Identification and description of homogeneous subgroups within a sample of misarticulating children. *Journal of Speech and Hearing Research*, 1977, *20*, 263-292.

Bankson, N. Assessment of the effectiveness of articulation therapy. *Journal of National Student Speech and Hearing Association*, 1974, *2*, 13-21.

Carter, E.T., & Buck, M.W. Prognostic testing for functional articulation disorders among children in the first grade. *Journal of Speech and Hearing Disorders*, 1958, *23*, 124-133.

Compton, A. Generative studies of children's phonological disorders. *Journal of Speech and Hearing Disorders*, 1970, *35*, 315-339.

Costello, J.M. Programmed instruction. *Journal of Speech and Hearing Disorders*, 1977, *42*, 3-28.

Costello, J., & Onstine, J. The modification of multiple articulation errors based on distinctive feature theory. *Journal of Speech and Hearing Disorders*, 1976, *41*, 199-215.

DuBois, E., & Bernthal, J. A comparison of three methods for obtaining articulatory responses. *Journal of Speech and Hearing Disorders*, 1978, *43*, 295-305.

Elbert, M., & McReynolds, L.V. An experimental analysis of misarticulating children's generalization. *Journal of Speech and Hearing Research,* 1978, *21,* 136-150.

Elbert, M., Shelton, R.L., & Arndt, W.B. A task for evaluation of articulation change. *Journal of Speech and Hearing Research,* 1967, *10,* 281-288.

Emerick, L., & Hatten, J. *Diagnosis and evaluation in speech pathology.* Englewood Cliffs, N.J.: Prentice-Hall, 1974

Farquhar, M.A. Prognostic value of imitative and auditory discrimination tests. *Journal of Speech and Hearing Disorders,* 1961, *26,* 342-347.

Fisher, H., & Logemann, J. *The Fisher-Logemann Test of Articulation Competence.* Boston: Houghton Mifflin, 1971.

Frisch, G.R., & Handler, L. A neuropsychological investigation of "functional disorders of speech articulation." *Journal of Speech and Hearing Research,* 1974, *17,* 432-445.

Ingram, D. *Phonological disability in children.* New York: American Elsevier, 1976.

Khan, L.M.L. A review of 16 major phonological processes. *Language, Speech, and Hearing Services in Schools,* 1982, *13,* 77-85.

Lapko, L., & Bankson, N. Relationship between auditory discrimination, articulation stimulability and consistency of misarticulation. *Perceptual and Motor Skills,* 1975, *40,* 171-177.

Milisen, R. and Associates. The disorder of articulation: a systematic clinical and experimental approach. *Journal of Speech and Hearing Disorders, Monograph Supplement 4,* 1954.

McDonald, E.T. *Articulation testing and treatment: A sensory-motor approach.* Pittsburgh: Stanwix House, 1964.

McReynolds, L. Articulation generalization during articulation training. *Language and Speech,* 1972, *15,* 149-155.

McReynolds, L., & Bennett, S. Distinctive feature generalization in articulation training. *Journal of Speech and Hearing Disorders,* 1972, *37,* 462-470.

McReynolds, L.V., & Kearns, K. *Single-subject experimental designs.* Baltimore: University Park Press, 1982.

Panagos, J.M. Persistence of the open syllable reinterpreted as a symptom of language disorder. *Journal of Speech and Hearing Disorders,* 1974, *39,* 23-31.

Powers, M.H. Functional disorders of articulation Symptomatology and etiology In L. E. Travis (Ed.), *Handbook of speech pathology.* New York: Appleton-Century-Crofts, 1957.

Prins, D. Analysis of correlations among various articulatory deviation. *Journal of Speech and Hearing Research,* 1962a, *5,* 152-160.

Renfrew, C. The persistence of the open syllable in defective articulation. *Journal of Speech and Hearing Disorders,* 1966, *31,* 370-373.

Report of the 27th Annual Conference of the Milbank Memorial Fund. New York: Hoeber-Harper, 1952.

Shelton, R.L. Disorders of articulation. In P.H. Skinner & R.L. Shelton (Eds.), *Speech, language and hearing.* Reading, Mass.: Addison-Wesley, 1978.

Shelton, R.L., Elbert, M., & Arndt, W.B. A task for evaluation of articulation change: II: Comparison of task scores during baseline and lesson series testing. *Journal of Speech and Hearing Research,* 1967, *10,* 578-585.

Shelton, R.L., & McReynolds, L.V. Functional articulation disorders: Preliminaries to therapy. In *Speech and language: Advances in basic research and practice.* New York: Academic Press, 1979.

Shriberg, L.D., & Kwiatkowski, J. *Natural process analysis.* New York: John Wiley, 1980.

Sommers, R.K., Leiss, R., Delp, M., Gerber, A., Fundrella, O., Smith, R., Revucky, M., Ellis, D., & Haley, V. Factors related to the effectiveness of articulation therapy for kindergarten, first, and second grade children. *Journal of Speech and Hearing Research,* 1967, *10,* 428-437.

Stampe, D. A dissertation on natural phonology. Unpublished doctoral dissertation, University of Chicago, 1973.

Travis, L.E. *Speech pathology.* New York: Appleton, 1931.

Van Riper, C. *Speech correction: Principles and methods.* Englewood Cliffs, N.J.: Prentice-Hall, 1939.

West, R., Ansberry, M., & Carr, A. *The rehabilitation of speech.* New York: Harper & Brothers, 1937.

Winitz, H. *From syllable to conversation.* Baltimore: University Park Press, 1975.

Richard G. Schwartz

The Phonologic System: Normal Acquisition

The translation of Jakobson's 1941 theory in 1968 seems to have been the point from which all recent advances in normal phonologic development emanate. The changes in our views of phonologic acquisition closely parallel the recent changes in our views of other aspects of language acquisition. Rather than viewing acquisition as simply the mastery of inventories of units (i.e., sounds, words, sentences), we have come to think of it as the development of a system in which units are but a single component. In reviewing these recent advances, some theoretical perspective is necessary as a framework for a subsequent discussion of recent issues which have arisen and of the information we have acquired over the last decade concerning phonologic acquisition.

Theoretical Advances

An acceptable theory of child phonology must simultaneously account for a number of aspects of children's speech sound behavior, including both the progression of development and adult phonology, since that is the child's ultimate achievement. Additionally a theory should: (1) account for the acquisition of phonology in any language, (2) be consistent with the amount and type of input received by the child, (3) be consistent with the time typically required for acquisition, and (4) be consistent with the child's abilities in other areas at given points in development (Pinker, 1979).

An ideal theory would also, at least indirectly, account for developmental and acquired disorders of phonology. These represent rather stringent and extensive requirements. Thus, it is not surprising that no current theory of acquisition meets all these requirements. In spite of this, a review seems in order to determine where we currently stand and what may be on the horizon in terms of a theoretical framework for better understanding of phonologic acquisition and disorders.

Structuralists

Jakobson (1968) viewed phonologic acquisition as involving two distinctly different periods, prelinguistic babbling and linguistic production. More recent observations and investigations have indicated that there are differences between these two periods. However, they have also revealed relationships between babbling and linguistic productions contrary to Jakobson's suggestion. It appears that at least in some respects developments in linguistic productions may depend upon developments during the prelinguistic period.

The second aspect of Jakobson's theory concerns what he viewed as the core of phonologic development—the acquisition of a phonemic system. He maintained that the child proceeds through an invariant, universal sequence, governed by a hierarchy of feature oppositions. The developmental sequence is based on a principle of maximum contrast with development moving from an undifferentiated to a differentiated and stratified system of phonemic contrasts. It is extremely important to note that the theory deals with the acquisition of contrasts, not individual sounds. The first contrast throught to be acquired is between what is termed an optimum consonant and an optimum vowel, which contrast maximally (i.e., differ in many features rather than few features). Development proceeds with the acquisition of contrasts that are progressively less distinct in terms of the number of features that differ. Jackobson argued that at any given point in time a child has his own system, distinct from the adult system. However, the child's system is based on an unfolding of the contrast hierarchy rather than active acquisition on the part of the child.

The final aspect of Jakobson's theory involves what is commonly referred to as the regression hypothesis. This entails the notion that in an acquired phonologic disorder, such as in aphasia, the order of loss will be the mirror image of the order of acquisition. Those contrasts acquired latest will be lost first.

Moskowitz (1970, 1973) has added to and modified Jakobson's proposals by considering children's more general recognition of units of speech. She argued that children only gradually recognize and identify smaller units of speech, beginning with the sentence and proceeding to the word-syllable, word and syllable. Recognition of the distinction between word and syllable is a significant attainment and depends upon reduplication (e.g., [wɔwɔ] for *water*). Thus, the child realizes that a syllable is a separable component of a word. Contrary to Jakobson's position, Moskowitz argued that children acquire contrasts between syllables rather than phonemes. This is consistent with more recent views concerning the psychological reality of the syllable in phonologic acquisition (Bell & Hooper, 1978). Finally, Moskowitz observed in diary data reported by Leopold (1947) that some words may be initially acquired independent of a child's phonologic system. For instance, at a time when she was not producing consonant clusters or prevocalic or intervocalic voiceless consonants, Hildegard Leopold first produced the word *pretty* as [prʌti] and then as [prIti]. Over a period of approximately 6 months, her production of the word gradually deteriorated until it was consistent with the way she was producing similar words ([bIdi] for *pretty*). This observation is important for two reasons. It suggests that children have their own phonologic system into which some new words may be only gradually assimilated. Additionally, it demonstrates that the "errors" young children make in producing words are not solely attributable to motoric or perceptual limitations, since at one point in time the child is able to produce the word accurately.

Although these theories have made significant contributions in their focus on the acquisition or loss of a phonologic *system,* they appear to have many weaknesses (Ferguson & Garnica, 1975; Kiparsky & Menn, 1977). First, because of the limited nature of children's early lexicons, there are few minimal pairs (e.g., [kIt vs. bIt]) and many gaps in the sounds produced. Consequently, it is difficult to determine whether or not contrasts are actually present. Second, in spite of Moskowitz's focus on the syllable, the theories are still largely segmental in nature. Thus, they are unable to explain aspects of acquisition and behavior which involve larger units (e.g., words). Finally, since the theories place so much emphasis on the acquisition of contrast, many developmental phenomena such as phonological idioms and developmental error patterns remain unexplained.

Natural Phonology

Natural phonology has led to a somewhat different view of the substance and nature of phonologic acquisition (Stampe, 1973). It has served as the basis for a good deal of recent work concerning normal and disordered development. In the course of these applications, Stampe's theory has been modified and on occasion misrepresented. Consequently, some clarification seems in order.

Several premises form the basis of this theory. First, Stampe maintains that children's perceptions are completely accurate from the outset. Thus, the basis for a child's production is the accurate adult form of the word which is stored as a perceptual representation. All aspects of a child's "errors" are attributable to motor production abilities (e.g., *dog,* child's representation [dɔg], child's production [dɔ]). Second, a set of innate processes which reflect the limitations of the human speech mechanism determine the child's productions. These processes serve to eliminate contrast by leading to the merger of classes of sounds or word forms (e.g., both nasal and oral sounds are produced as oral; forms with and without final consonants are produced as forms without final consonants). Because these processes are supposed to be a natural reflection of the human speech mechanism, they are viewed as universal. This also means that the direction of sound class mergers are predetermined. For example, fricatives may be changed to stops, or obstruents (fricatives, stops, and affricates) may be devoiced, but the reverse of these changes does not typically occur. Evidence for these processes comes from their occurrence across languages, evidence concerning the structure and physiology of the speech mechanism, and inferences regarding ease of articulation.

At the outset of development, processes occur without restrictions of any sort; they are unordered and unlimited. Thus, there are no phonemic distinctions. The child's task in phonologic acquisition is to overcome the limitations caused by these processes by suppression (complete elimination), limitation (allowing them to occur only in certain contexts), or by order ing multiple processes (applying only one of two or more possible processes to a word or words, thereby "blocking" the occurrence of other processes). Individual variations may arise as the result of different courses a child may take in eliminating processes. In doing this, the child is not only overcoming processes, but is also resolving conflicts between processes (e.g., changing all nasal sounds to oral sounds versus changing oral sounds to nasal sounds when nasal sounds precede or follow them). What remains after the child completes acquisition are processes characteristic of that language.

Another important premise of Stampe's proposal concerns the distinction between rules and processes. The basic difference is that rules are learned while processes are innate. In addition, while processes may become limited in the contexts in which they apply, they cannot have formal morphological or lexical restrictions. Rules, though, can have these kinds of limitations, as in the case of velar softening in English which changes words like *electric* to *electricity.* Finally, rules cannot be based on phonetic or physiologic motivations.

Like Jakobson, Stampe maintains that phonologic acquisition is essentially predetermined. According to Jakobson, the phonologic system unfolds. However, according to Stampe, the inborn processes are discarded and the system remains. Neither really credits the child with an active role in constructing a phonologic system.

Stampe's proposal makes an important contribution in its attempt to explain the patterns of children's errors and in proposing a source for such errors. The weakest point in the proposal, however, concerns Stampe's insistence on the accuracy of perception and the use of the adult form as the child's representation. While there is no doubt that by the time the child begins to use language he can discriminate many or most of the speech sounds of English, that does not mean that a given word will be accurately perceived or represented. Additionally, although Stampe's distinction between rules and processes may be theoretically clear (there is some disagreement on this point), in practice it is not always clear. To date, no universally agreed-upon set of natural processes has been constructed. Ease of articulation has always been, and continues to be, an elusive notion. Furthermore, there appear to be patterns of errors in children's speech that are not natural or reflective of the limits of the speech mechanism. It is not clear from Stampe's proposal how such patterns should be regarded. Since they are errors, they would not be regarded as rules. Since they are not natural, the use of the term "processes" as Stampe describes it would seem inappropriate. Finally, other theorists have argued that children play a more active role in constructing a phonologic system.

Constructivists

Several more recent proposals have involved a very different perspective concerning the nature of phonologic acquisition (Ferguson & Macken, 1980; Kiparsky & Menn, 1977; Schwartz & Leonard, 1982; Schwartz & Prelock, 1982; Waterson, 1971; 1981; Menn, Note 1). In contrast to the preceding theories, these proposals all view the child as actively constructing a phonologic system.

Waterson's (1971) prosodic theory differs from previous proposals in its emphasis on individual differences and the role of developing perceptual abilities in determining the nature of children's early productions. According to this proposal, children selectively attend to adult utterances that are in some way highly salient. The focus of the child's perception is on a limited set of salient features of a word. Based on this set, the child constructs a representation, termed a "schema", which serves as the basis for his productions. A given schema may represent more than a single word, thus explaining some of the patterns in children's early speech. For example, the schema for the words *finger* and *window* may involve a palatal or alveolar nasal plus a vowel in a reduplicated form (two identical or nearly identical syllables), such as [ɲẽ:ɲẽ/nɪ:ni:] for *finger* and [ɲe:ɲe:] for *window*. Similarities and differences across children arise as the result of similarities and differences in input to children. More recently, Waterson (1981) has expanded her proposal to include one level of representation involving possible phonetic patterns of the language extracted and synthesized from perceptually salient features. Additionally, a second level of representation involves patterns specific to words along with their meanings. This model links input to these two levels of representation and ultimately to output.

Menn (Note 1) argues for a somewhat different view, emphasizing the role of output or articulatory constraints. Rules also seem to play a role in this model, but serve as a means by which the child can observe an output constraint. For example, a young child may have a constraint such as, "Don't produce any words with more than one consonant, unless the consonants are the same." A number of rules can help to keep the child within this constraint, such as eliminating consonants (e.g., *dog* [dɔ]) or whole syllables *kitty* [kI]), changing one of the consonants so that the consonants are the same (*boat* [boʊbo]), or taking one syllable of a word and duplicating it (*water* [wɔwɔ]). Additionally, this model involves a number of levels of phonologic representation and behavior including output, articulatory instructions, output lexicon (production store), input lexicon (recognition store), and an overall level of abstracted underlying forms. These levels are related by different types of phonologic rules. Similar to Waterson, and in contrast to Stampe, this proposal involves the notion that the child's underlying representation of a word is not necessarily just a copy of correct adult production.

A more recent proposal along the same lines suggests a more balanced view of perception and production in children's phonologic representation and acquisition (Schwartz & Leonard, 1982). Additionally, this proposal considers the role of a child's cognitive abilities in determining the type of representation attributed. The model proposed involves three general levels: phonetic, representational, and organizational. The phonetic level is comprised of two components: perceptual and motoric. The perceptual component involves the basic processes of audition, discrimination, and identification of a signal as speech. The motoric component is responsible for the execution of the motor movements for speech production.

The representational level also includes a perception component and a separate production component. The perception component is comprised of schemas, which are representations of the units of speech that the child has segmented from the adult's speech. While at the outset these may be rather large units, for most children at least some schemas represent words by about the age of 10 months. These, then, are the first words comprehended by the child. During the same period of time, the child is constructing schemes, or plans, for motor action. These also are initially large unstable units as characterized by the child's babbling, but are gradually stabilized and refined so that they, too, are word-like in structure. At both levels, perception and production begin as completely independent systems and maintain some degree of autonomy after acquisition. After the child has constructed a number of schemes and schemas, development proceeds with additions to these repertoires and coordinations between existing schemes and schemas. Once a schema is coordinated with a scheme, the child can both meaningfully produce and comprehend a word. Additionally, this coordination increases the likelihood that a child will attempt a given word.

This is essentially the whole of a child's phonologic representation during the period of sensorimotor intelligence (0-18 months), which roughly corresponds to the period of the first 50 words. During this period, the child, according to Piaget (1962), has limited representational abilities and is lacking any overall representations. Thus, the model is consistent with the child's overall cognitive abilities and with the observations that phonologic behavior during this period is variable, unsystematic, and apparently word-based. Once the child reaches the end of the sensorimotor period, he is able to construct overall representations at the organizational level. This leads to more stable phonologic behavior and more systematic behavior in his simplifications of sounds, syllables, and words. Attempts have been made to describe a number of developmental phenomena such as phonologic idioms and selectivity within the context of this model. Additionally, its implications for differential diagnosis and remediation of speech sound disorders have been specified (Schwartz & Prelock, 1982).

There is clearly a good deal of overlap among these three proposals and others (Ferguson & Macken, 1980; Macken, 1979). While a number of differences remain to be resolved (e.g., number of levels), they seem to represent a significant departure from previous proposals. In general, they are broader in their perspective and, thus, seem better able to deal with a wider range of facts concerning both child and adult phonology. They seem to be more generally consistent with the criteria mentioned earlier, such as time span of acquisition (without falling back on the notion of innateness), the type and nature of input to the child, and consistency with other aspects of development. Also, the last model may have some explanatory value for disordered development. Careful examination of these proposals reveals specific and testable predictions concerning the nature and progression of phonologic acquisition. One general weakness in all of these proposals is their failure to deal with the specific nature and development of motoric and perceptual mechanisms and processes. However, more recently some proposals have begun to address these issues (e.g., Locke, 1979a;

MacNeilage, 1980). Some integration of cognition-oriented and mechanism-oriented proposals may ultimately be required.

These advances in theory are exciting in that they suggest that we are close to having one or more detailed frameworks within which we can examine a wide range of aspects of children's phonologies. The significance of this should not be underestimated. Even though most theories are ultimately proved false, the existence of a theoretical framework can facilitate systematic experimentation (including therapeutic intervention) and consequently, in some cases, a more rapid acquisition of knowledge. While we await the further refinement of these proposals, we can consider the current empirical issues and recent advances in the data available concerning phonologic acquisition.

Current Issues

A number of issues remain unresolved even after many years and, thus, are not new. Others have simply been reformulated because of new information concerning acquisition. Finally, some issues are genuinely new, arising from recent investigations of acquisition. The purpose of this section is to provide a brief listing of those that seem most fundamental and which will consequently be addressed in the subsequent review of phonologic acquisition.

The issues seem to fall into four major areas: the nature of production; the nature of perception; the relationship between production and perception; and the relationships among phonologic acquisition, cognitive development, and other aspects of language acquisition. Issues concerning production include the most appropriate way of describing the nature of children's productions and their relation to the adult target form (features versus sounds versus syllables, versus various types of rules), the description of the course of development, the basis of developmental errors, the nature and sources of variability in production, individual differences in the course of acquisition, and the description and development of contrast. Because of less research activity in the area of perception, the issues have remained more general. Basically, they concern the nature, developmental progression, and description of perceptual abilities. An issue related to both perception and production concerns the roles of input and linguistic perception in phonologic acquisition.

The relationship between perception and production in phonologic acquisition is another topic of interest. The issues center on the developmental sequence in these two components (i.e., whether perception precedes production, follows it, or both) and the reciprocal influence of perception and production (e.g., whether production errors reflect errors in perception).

More recently, we have been increasingly aware of the fact that phonologic acquisition and behavior do not occur in isolation. Instead, other aspects of language (syntax, semantics, pragmatics) and cognitive abilities appear to influence and are influenced by phonologic abilities. Additionally, many aspects of communicative and cognitive development appear to be interrelated. The specific nature and extent of these relationships is an issue of some importance.

Although few if any of these issues have been resolved, recent research has greatly expanded our knowledge in these areas. A review of the current state of our knowledge base follows. Since these issues take somewhat different forms when applied to different levels of development, the remaining portion of the chapter is organized in a developmental sequence.

Prelinguistic Period

The prelinguistic period of development includes the ages from birth to approximately 12 months, when true words first appear. It should be noted that in many children this period may overlap with the beginning of the linguistic period (i.e., babbling may continue when real words emerge).

Perception

Over the last decade, interest in infants' perception of speech has grown at a phenomenally rapid rate. We have gone from a point of having little specific information concerning infant perceptual abilities to a point of having a large body of information concerning these abilities. Most recently, this has led to a shift in issues considered from simply the "what" of prelinguistic perception to examinations of its origins, its developmental progression in this period, the roles of input and experience, and the actual process of perception.

Three types of methodologies have been employed. Two of these procedures are based on some type of orienting response to a novel stimulus. They also depend upon the fact that infants will become habituated with repeated presentations of stimuli they perceive as similar. The first procedure has been termed the high-amplitude sucking procedure. It involves providing the infant with a non-nutritive nipple to be sucked. After a baseline sucking rate is established, the infant is presented with a sound (e.g., "ba") each time sucking occurs. Initially, because of an orienting response, the sucking rate increases to a peak, and then, because of habituation, begins to level off. At this point, infants in an experimental group are presented with a new sound (e.g., "pa") each time they suck, while infants in a control group continue to hear the same sound (i.e., "ba"). If the sucking rate of infants in the experimental group increases (dishabituates) relative to the rate for infants in the control group, this serves as evidence that the infants discriminate the two different sounds. More recently, an alternating pattern of the old and new stimuli has been employed to reduce the memory requirements of the procedure. This has been used with children ranging in age from 0 to 4 months.

The second procedure, the heart rate paradigm, involves presenting a stimulus (e.g., "ba") and measuring the infant's heart rate. In this case the infant does not control the presentation of the stimulus, and orienting is measured by a decrease in the heart rate. The initial stimulus is presented repeatedly in blocks until the child habituates and no longer exhibits an orienting response. Then a new stimulus is presented (e.g., "pa"). If the heart rate decreases, the infant is assumed to discriminate between the two sounds. More recently, Leavitt, Brown, Morse, and Graham (1976) modified this procedure by decreasing the interval between blocks so that memory requirements were reduced. These procedures have been used with infants from about 1 to 8 months of age.

The final procedure, visually reinforced infant speech discrimination, is an adaptation of an audiological procedure used to test children's hearing in a free field. One stimulus (e.g., "ba") is presented repeatedly as a background. Periodically, for a fixed period of time, this sound is changed to a second sound (e.g., "pa"). When this change occurs and the infant's head turns toward the sound, head turning is reinforced by the activation of a toy (e.g., a lit monkey banging cymbals). Subsequently, consistent head turns toward the reinforcer in anticipation of its activation during stimulus change, but not during periods when the change doesn't occur, indicate discrimination. This procedure has been altered to a perceptual constancy paradigm (Kuhl, 1976; 1977; 1980), which allows investigation of the boundaries of sound categories, rather than simply discrimination of two sounds. These procedures have been employed with infants in the 6- to 18-month-age range and may be applicable to somewhat older children as well.

To date, these procedures have yielded a large body of information concerning what infants can and cannot discriminate (Eilers, 1980). They have also been employed in examining a number of issues concerning the perceptual abilities of infants (Eilers, 1980). It appears that, while some aspects of these abilities are innate, other aspects may be dependent on experience or involve a complex interaction of environmental and genetic factors (Aslin & Pisoni, 1980). There also seem to be some rather interesting relationships between characteristics of adult speech to infants and infant perceptual abilities (e.g., Williams, Note 2). For example, infants seem to be able to discriminate differences in place in intervocalic position only when there is a period of silence during closure. Adults seem to make this modification in their speech to young children.

Some findings have been surprising in terms of our prior expectations. It has long been commonplace knowledge that infants may respond differentially to suprasegmental features before they respond in the same way to segmental features. While infants do respond differentially to some varying prosodic cues (Morse, 1972; Spring & Dale, 1977; Kaplan, Note 3), this may not always be the case. It appears that when segmental differences (e.g., /i/ vs. /a/) compete with suprasegmental differences (e.g., pitch differences), children do not evidence discrimination of pitch differences (Kuhl, 1976). Nor is there evidence that stress facilitates segmental discriminations (Jusczyk & Thompson, 1978; Williams & Bush, 1978). Equally surprising is the finding that—contrary to the suggestion that fricatives are among the later acquired sounds in production because they are not discriminated early in development due to late myelination of the auditory (VIII) nerve (Salus & Salus, 1974)—infants are able to discriminate a great many fricatives (Eilers, 1980).

Most investigations of infant speech perception have understandably focused on auditory aspects of these abilities. However, Kuhl and Meltzoff (1982) have employed an infant preference procedure in examining perception as a bimodal phenomenon involving both audition and vision. They found that when infants (18 to 20 weeks of age) are presented simultaneously with film loops of a face producing an /i/ and the same face producing an /a/ along with an auditory presentation of one of these vowels, they spend a longer period of time looking at the face corresponding to the vowel heard. Even more intriguing are their findings that when certain spectral information (i.e., formant frequencies) is removed from the auditory presentation, the infants do not demonstrate a preference for one face over the other. This suggests that, even at this early age, infants are responsive to a relationship between facial configurations or movements and certain auditory spectral characteristics. It also raises the possibility of some general, early link between audition and motor movements for speech. The subsequent translation of this information from infants' perceptions of others to their own motor movements may prove to be an important factor in the development of both speech perception and production.

The exact nature of the relationship between prelinguistic perception and linguistic perception and production remains unclear. However, it seems likely that, given the methods and information currently available, the beginning of an understanding of this relationship is relatively close at hand. For individual children we may ultimately be able to draw some inferences regarding later linguistic abilities from an examination of prelinguistic perception.

Production

We have known for some time that infants' vocalizations start out exclusively as reflexive and vegetative and gradually expand to include nonreflexive and nonvegetative sounds (i.e., speech). Additionally, it has long been known that infants proceed through a series of periods of speech production from cooing (predominantly back vowel-like sounds with some back consonants), to babbling (a wider variety of consonants and vowel strings along with variation in stress and intonation), to jargon (greater control over stress and intonation), to meaningful speech. Finally, as a result of the work of Orvis Irwin and his associates (see Winitz, 1969, for a complete review), we know that, in terms of the specific sounds infants produce, there is a progression from a low proportion of front and high proportion of back consonant-like sounds to a higher proportion of front sounds. Moreover, there is an opposite trend in vowel-like sounds, with a slight increase in back sounds over time.

In the last decade, however, through the use of instrumental analyses in addition to perceptually based examinations (i.e., phonetic transcription), our knowledge of infant vocalization has markedly expanded. The work of several investigators (Stark, 1980; Oller, Note 4; Zlatin, Note 5) seems to generally agree that there are five stages in the development of speech production prior to the emergence of true words or word-like forms.

The first stage begins at birth and lasts from 4 to 6 weeks. Vocalizations during this period are primarily reflexive, including crying, fussing, and primative vegetative sounds. Stark (1980) has characterized some of these sounds as exhibiting the first combination of vocalic and suprasegmental features of crying and consonantal features of vegetative sounds. Nasal and liquid sounds seem to result when the mouth is open during crying, the tongue returns to a position in opposition to the soft palate, and subsequent closure occurs while vocalization continues. There also appear to be some nonreflexive sounds produced during this period. These seem to be predominantly what Oller (Note 4) has termed quasi-resonant nuclei (QRN). Generally, these are vocalizations that involve normal phonation but do not involve clear contrast between an open and closed vocal tract and thus do not reflect the full range of resonance of the vocal cavity. Acoustically, QRNs are identified by a broad range of various low amplitude resonances predominantly below 1200 Hz (Oller, Note 4). Phonetically, these sounds are usually syllabic nasals ([ŋ̩] as in [bʌtn̩]) or high-mid, unrounded (the mouth is usually nearly closed), nasalized vowels (e.g., something like [ɪ̃]). There may also be some seemingly random occurrences of fully resonant nuclei (FRN) which more closely resemble vowels or coos. QRNs, however, seem to predominate even into the next stage and are the most frequent vocalization during the first 4 months (Oller, 1980).

The second stage seems to cover the period from approximately 6 weeks to 4 months and to be generally characterized by cooing and laughter. More nasal consonant elements occur, and voicing may be combined with obstruent (stop, fricative, and affricate) sounds that were previously produced vegetatively without voicing. An important aspect of this is the infant's ability to produce voicing in nondistress states. These "goo" sounds have been observed to be repetitive, and perhaps reflect greater control on the part of the infant. Specifically, at around 3 months, greater control is gained over the tongue and lips which may give rise to some bilabial nasal sounds during play.

Further support for the assumption that infants have at least some control over aspects of their vocalizations during this period comes from early research concerning infant vocal conditioning (Rheingold, Gewirtz, & Ross, 1959; Weisberg, 1963). It has since been recognized that there are some serious weaknesses in this research (Bloom, 1979). However, there is evidence from more recent, better controlled research, that 3-month-old infants do respond differentially (in terms of the pattern or distribution rather than the frequency of vocalization) to contingent and noncontingent stimulation (Bloom, 1977; Bloom & Esposito, 1975). The differential responsiveness takes the form of differing pause times which occur prior to the infants' vocalizations following each type of stimulation. Further research is needed to determine the extent of infants' control over the content of such vocalizations.

Laughter may first appear at around 4 months. It is an important development because it often occurs in the course of interactions. As Stark noted, this involves rapid alteration of voiced and voiceless vocalization as well as a voiced inspiration.

Stage 3 has been referred to as exploratory phonetic behavior (Zlatin, Note 5), vocal play (Stark, 1980), and expansion (Oller, 1980). All three terms describe general characteristics of this period. By this time (4 to 7 months), infants have gained sufficient control over their speech mechanism to allow play with a wide range of speech sounds. Included among the vocalizations of this period are FRNs, vowel-like sounds with resonances above 1200 HZ (Oller, Note 4; Doyle, Note 6), raspberries (Doyle, Note 6), squeaking (Stark, 1980; Zlatin Laufer & Horii, 1977; Doyle, Note 6), growling (Stark, 1980; Zlatin Laufer & Horii, 1977), yelling and sequences of alternating vocalization on egressive and ingressive air (Zlatin Laufer & Horii, 1977; Oller, Note 4). Perhaps the most important aspect of this period is that infants seem to begin to sequence and resequence series of sounds in novel ways and begin to insert pauses into these sequences (Stark, 1980). This development leads to the marginal babbling at the end of this stage. Marginal babbling involves sequences of open vocal tract (FRN) and closed vocal tract sounds. The consistency, repetitiveness, and rigid timing of later babbling is not yet present.

Investigators report a fourth stage, reduplicated or canonical babbling, which lasts from approximately 6 to 10 months. This babbling includes consonant-like sounds and vowel-like sounds (FRNs) arranged in a rather standard timing sequence (e.g., CV or VC). In one sense, the infant seems more limited in this period than the previous period. In concentrated periods, infants seem to produce one specific syllable (e.g., *babababa*). While many vocalizations are in this consonant-vowel reduplicated form, others (e.g., *imi*) may not be (Oller, 1980). As Stark noted, during this period children are increasingly likely to vocalize while looking at an adult rather than while handling objects or performing actions as in previous periods.

The final period is comprised of nonreduplicated or variegated babbling. The same types of timing sequences or alternations of consonant-like and vowel-like sounds are present. However, the sound content of the sequences is no longer restricted to a single sound or syllable. Additionally, other syllable sequences (CVC, VC) may appear. This period is also characterized by the infant's more consistent control over stress and intonation. This leads to what has been traditionally referred to as jargon. Finally, this period may overlap with the beginnings of word-form production (see below).

With these advances, we now know a good deal about the general progression and many specific details concerning what constitutes normal development. Furthermore, the fact that there is at least some relationship between prelinguistic and linguistic productions seems well established (Oller, Wieman, Doyle, & Ross, 1975). These productions share many common characteristics. However, the ability to predict the specific nature of linguistic vocalizations from prelinguistic vocalizations has not yet been achieved. There are a number of other issues which remain unresolved.

While we focus on the surface nature of these vocalizations, there may be more general characteristics (pitch, vocal quality, voicing, resonance, timing, respiration, amplitude) which may provide direct evidence of the infant's motor speech capacity specific to certain components of the speech mechanism (Oller, 1980). The influence of the changing physical characteristics of the infant speech mechanism, linguistic experience and input, and the increasing association of vocalizations with objects and situations all represent issues for further research (Kent, 1981; Netsell, 1981). As we learn more about this period and its relation to linguistic productions, we come closer to understanding the nature of speech production development. Additionally, it may mean that we can evaluate the normalcy of prelinguistic productions.

Transition

The notion that prior to the production of real, recognizable words, children produce vocalizations that only superficially resemble words is not new. A number of diary studies (e.g., Halliday, 1975; Leopold, 1947) have included observations of isolated, segmental vocalizations (vowels, syllables, syllabic consonants) that have some relationship to context (i.e., meaning). More recently, such vocalizations have been described in greater detail (Carter, 1975; 1979; Dore, Franklin, Miller, & Ramer, 1976; Menn, Note 7). They have been referred to varyingly as sensorimotor morphemes, phonetically consistent forms (PCFs), and protowords. In general, these units are unlike babbling in that they are isolable, bounded by pauses, occur with sufficient frequency so as to be recognizable, seem to be related to some recurring aspect of context, and seem to be more phonetically stable than variegated babbling. They are not quite true words in that they are less clearly related to recurring aspects of context (i.e., they are not coherent in their use), and they are less phonetically consistent than true words. Menn employed these two criteria in describing protowords and added the criterion that protowords are less autonomous than true words in that they are tied to an action or a routine.

These forms are perhaps best explained by example. One type of PCF is illustrated by the observation of a child who said [gægi], [gaga], [gagi], [əgagi] on various occasions while chewing crayons, being dressed, and handling a toy (Dore et al., 1976), the common thread here being pleasurable affect on the part of the child. Carter reported the production of an initial [m] followed by a variety of vowels as an apparent request for an object along with a reaching gesture. Protowords, as described by Menn (Note 7), seem somewhat different than most sensorimotor morphemes or PCFs in that they apparently are not based on affect or internal states and they seem to be more object or action specific. Jacob, the one child studied by Menn, produced various versions of [ioio] while watching tape reels go around and while making objects rotate. It is clearly more externally coherent than the first example given above. Protowords have only been observed in one child, who did not exhibit anything more closely resembling PCFs. Consequently, it is unclear whether there is a developmental progression from sensorimotor morphemes or PCFs to protowords to true words. Phonetically consistent forms and protowords may simply prove to be two alternative transitions between babbling and words. Not surprisingly, these preword forms seem to be related both to babbling and to later words. Menn noted that [ioio] appeared first in strings of babble before it was produced as an isolated form. Some true words (e.g., *mine, my, more*) have been traced back to sensorimotor morphemes. There is still a need, however, for more detailed information concerning these relationships.

The most important aspect of these findings is the fact that there are structures which seem to bridge the gap between babbling and true words. Words then develop gradually rather than suddenly. These preword forms may be the child's first linguistic forms used communicatively. The vocalizations which Bates, Camaioni, and Volterra (1975) noted in children's performance of early communicative acts are likely to have been some type of preword form.

The Period of Prerepresentational Phonology

Although the dividing line between preword forms and true words is often somewhat fuzzy, at about 12 months of age children begin to produce their first true words. This represents the beginning of what various investigators have termed the period of the first 50 words (e.g., Nelson, 1973). Although in one study of phonologic development (Ferguson & Farwell, 1975) the decision to focus on children at this level of development was arbitrary, Ingram (1976) has characterized this as a separable period in phonologic acquisition. The basis for this argument is that it is roughly concomitant with the period of sensorimotor intelligence and the period of single word utterances. At around 18 months most children have acquired their 50th word, have begun using two-word utterances and, perhaps more importantly, have attained Stage VI of sensorimotor intelligence. Prior to this stage, children do not have a well-developed representational system according to Piaget (1962). This means that mental representations are isolated, often based on immediate perceptions, and somewhat unstable. Additionally, during this period children do not appear to have any overall representations. One implication for phonologic behavior during this period is that children are likely to be variable in their productions of given words because of unstable representations (e.g., *dog* may be produced on various occasions as [dɔ], [dɔg], [gɔ], [dɔd]). Additionally, because they have no overall representation, children will not exhibit a system of consistently applied rules or processes in their productions, nor will they exhibit a *system* of sound contrasts. In a recent investigation, Schwartz and Folger (1977) compared the phonologies of children who had attained Stage VI of sensorimotor intelligence with those of children who had not yet attained this stage. The pre-Stage VI children evidenced significantly more variability in word production, fewer systematic developmental errors, and fewer systematic contrasts. The authors suggested that prior to attainment of Stage VI of sensorimotor intelligence, it may be inappropriate to credit the child with a set of processes or rules (i.e., mental operations), and a system of sound contrasts. Additionally, rather than equating the boundary of this period with the acquisition of the 50th word (vocabulary size did not explain these differences), it seemed more appropriate to distinguish between representational and prerepresentational phonology.

A number of investigations have revealed some more specific facts regarding phonologic behavior during this general period (see Ingram, 1976 for a review of some early diary studies such as Leopold, 1947; and more recently Leonard, Newhoff, & Mesalam, 1980; Shibamoto & Olmsted, 1978; Menn, Note 7). In general, this period appears to be characterized by individual differences, variability, lack of sound contrasts, and the absence of consistent rules or processes.

Individual differences

One of the more striking observations in light of previous assumptions of universal orders of acquisition has been the seemingly large range of individual differences between children. These differences seem to center on two aspects of phonology: the sounds produced and the characteristics of the adult words attempted. The results of early investigations indicated that such differences were prevalent, but shed little light on their actual range. More recently, Leonard, Newhoff, and Mesalam (1980) examined the word-initial sounds (phones) of 10 children ranging in age from 1;4 to 1;10, for the purpose of specifying the extent of individual differences. In general they found that certain sounds were notably absent across most subjects [ə], [tʃ], [ð], [f], [I], [dʒ], [z], and [r]. Among the sounds produced by all or most subjects were [m], [b], [d], [kʰ], [g], [pʰ], [w]. Five of the children produced [n] and [h]. The remaining consonants were produced by only 2 or 3 children. It should be noted that while some of these represent accurate productions of target sounds, others represent errors. Additionally, in some cases sounds may be freely substituted for one another (see below). Thus, although there is variation in the sounds produced by children during this period, the variation seems to be limited by certain sounds which are produced by most or all children and by sounds that consistently do not appear in young children's productions.

Some investigators have suggested that input may play a major role in determining a child's early phonetic repertoire (e.g., Olmsted, 1971; Waterson, 1971). Although the distributional frequency of sounds may prove to have some general influence in determining the consistencies described above, there is some evidence to suggest that its influence is not absolute. In a second experiment reported by Leonard, Newhoff, and Mesalam (1980), the word-initial sounds produced by a set of twins were examined. These children were no more similar in the sounds produced than any 2 of the 10 children described above. In other words, there were sounds that both children produced, some that neither produced, and some that only one of the twins produced. Since we can assume that these children both received essentially the same input, it seems likely that individual differences are attributable to some other factor. The most logical candidate is the argument by several child phonologists (Kiparsky & Menn, 1977; Schwartz & Leonard, 1982) that each child individually constructs a phonology within some general limitations of the linguistic environment.

Another aspect of phonologic behavior during this period which is also subject to individual differences is selectivity. A number of phonologists have observed that children are selective in the words they attempt. They appear to select words with certain phonologic characteristics and do not attempt words with other characteristics following a variety of individual patterns. These patterns may be based upon the structure or syllable shape of adult words as well as the sounds of which they are comprised. For example, one child reportedly attempted words with an open syllable structure (CV or CVCV), but did not attempt adult words with other syllable shapes (Ingram, 1974). At a similar point in development, Hildegard Leopold (Leopold, 1947) only attempted adult words with initial labial and apical stop and nasal consonants, while another child primarily attempted words with initial fricatives (Ferguson & Farwell, 1975). In general, selectivity appears more likely to influence word-initial sounds (Shibamoto & Olmsted, 1978). It should be noted that Leonard, Newhoff, and Mesalam (1980) reported that, as in the case of production, there are some limitations in the extent of these individual differences. Most, if not all, of the 10 children they studied attempted words beginning with [m], [b], [n], [g], [k], [w], and [p]. None of the children attempted words beginning with [v], [θ], [l], [z], or [r]. Words beginning with other consonants seemed to involve individual differences in terms of whether they were attempted. While these differences might be attributed to differences in input, there is some convincing evidence that this is not a determining factor.

Two types of evidence bear on this issue. The first comes from the twin study reported by Leonard, Newhoff, and Mesalam (1980). In spite of the assumed identical input, these twins did evidence some differences in their pattern of selection of attempted words. Additionally, a series of investigations (Leonard, Schwartz, Chapman, & Morris, 1981; Leonard, Schwartz, Chapman, Rowan, Prelock, Terrell, Weiss, & Messick, 1982; Schwartz & Leonard, 1982) have involved use of a nonsense or unfamiliar word acquisition paradigm. In this general procedure children were presented over a period of time a set of words corresponding to unfamiliar referents (objects or actions), and the acquisition of the words was examined. The words were chosen or constructed individually so that half of the words had phonologic characteristics which were consistent with words the child was producing and attempting (IN), and half of the words had characteristics that were inconsistent with the child's existing phonology (OUT). Across all of these investigations, which collectively involved children with vocabularies between 5 and 75 words, the children consistently acquired more IN than OUT words. Because all of the experimental words were presented an equal number of times, it seems unlikely that input variations are the sole determiners of selectivity.

Two remaining findings concerning this phenomenon should be mentioned. At an early point in this period children are similarly selective in imitative and nonimitative productions (Schwartz & Leonard, 1982). However, toward the end of this period these patterns first begin to disappear. Children stop being selective in imitative productions, while they are still selective in spontaneous productions (Leonard, Schwartz, Folger, & Wilcox, 1978). Regardless of selectivity, the extent of errors in imitative and spontaneous productions is comparable throughout this period. Finally, it has been demonstrated that while selectivity strongly influences production, it has no effect on children's comprehension. Children comprehend words with characteristics that are "out" of their phonologies as readily as words with characteristics that are "in" their phonologies.

The phenomenon of phonological selectivity has both theoretical and clinical import. It provides evidence that children during this period have the perceptual abilities to discriminate between IN and OUT words. Additionally, it provides further evidence for the child's active role in constructing a phonologic system. There have been several suggestions concerning the basis for selectivity. Ferguson (1978) suggested that it serves to simplify the task of phonologic acquisition by allowing the child to focus on a limited number of word types (i.e., sounds and syllable shapes). Alternatively, it has been suggested that selectivity is one of several ways a child may observe certain output constraints or limitations (Menn, Note 1). For example, there may be a constraint in the child's system which "prohibits" the production of final consonants. The limitation may be observed either by omitting final consonants or, more simply, by not attempting to produce adult words with final consonants. Finally, the basis of selectivity may lie in the nature of children's initial perceptual representations (schemas) and their coordination with production representations (schemes) (Schwartz & Leonard, 1982). At the outset and through much of this period, children may only attempt words for which they have an established schema and a coordinated scheme. Other words similar in phonologic composition may also be attempted. These constraints relax gradually as the child's repertoire is expanded to include a greater variety of coordinated schemes and schemas. Ultimately the child may no longer be limited to pre-existing schemes and schemas, and selectivity largely disappears.

Phonologic selectivity may also have some important implications for determining the content of remediation for phonologic disorders. It has been demonstrated that older language-impaired children at this same level of development also exhibit this selectivity (Leonard et al., 1982). Consequently, to insure maximum initial success in a remediation program, one should choose words for training with characteristics that are consistent with the child's phonology.

One final aspect of individual differences during this period, individual learning strategies (Ferguson & Farwell, 1975), warrants consideration. Reduplication is one such strategy which has been observed in children at this point and seems to continue into the next period of phonologic acquisition. Some children frequently produce single syllabic (e.g., *boat*) as well as multisyllabic words (*water*) by producing two or more identical or nearly identical syllables ([boʊbo]; [wɔwɔ]). Other children rarely produce such forms. It appears that a reduplication strategy may be generally related to a child's ability to produce final consonants and more closely to the production of nonreduplicated multisyllabic forms (Fee & Ingram, 1982; Ferguson, 1983; Schwartz, Leonard, Wilcox, & Folger, 1980). Reduplicating a word helps the child avoid final consonant production, but, more importantly, it may be an easier way to produce words with 2 syllables. Other individual learning strategies which may serve similar functions include the use of [j] as a syllable-initial consonant (e.g., *panda* [pa-jan]) across various monosyllabic and multisyllabic words (Priestly, 1977), the production of diminutive forms [i] across a variety of words such as [aʊti] for *out* (Ingram, 1974), and, somewhat later in development, the production of a form *ri-* as a prefix for a variety of multisyllabic words, such as *attack* [ritæk] (Smith, 1973). More recently, Klein (1981) has identified two broader strategies that are related to children's productions of adult multisyllabic words at the end of this period and the beginning of the representational period. She observed that 2 children exhibited various syllable-maintaining strategies in attempting to produce multisyllabic words. The remaining 2 children primarily exhibited various forms of syllable-reducing strategies.

Such "strategies" or patterns in children's phonologic behavior may represent the first instances of their being systematic. However, their identification represents only a first step. We will ultimately need to determine the specific roles of these patterns in phonologic acquisition (see Ferguson, 1983). If this can be accomplished, it should markedly expand our understanding of the process of phonologic acquisition. It might also lead to modification in approaches to altering the phonologic systems of disordered children.

Variability and contrast

As was noted earlier, children seem to be more variable in their productions of words during this period. Specifically, they may produce a given word such as *moon* differently on various occasions (e.g., [bun] [mu] [mun]). Such variability has been measured by calculating a ratio between the total number of different forms produced and the total number of different words produced (Schwartz & Folger, 1977). This ratio was consistently higher, indicating greater variability, in prerepresentational than in representational children. The instability of the child's perceptual and motor representations may be only one source of such variability. During this period, as well as in later periods, variability may also be due to certain contextual factors, motoric factors, and the fact that a child's phonologic system is undergoing rapid change.

Variability has a significant impact on the establishment of contrast between sounds. If a child is producing the word *moon* as described above, he or she clearly does not have a contrast in production between /b/ and /m/ since they may vary without a change in meaning. Such examples are common in children's speech during this period. In fact, it is almost impossible to find what we have traditionally viewed as clear evidence of sound contrast, minimal pairs (e.g., *pit* and *bit*). Consequently, Ferguson and Farwell (1975) have argued that children at this point in development do not have production contrasts between sounds but, rather, between whole words. This has led to an alternate method of evaluating contrasts in children's speech involving the notion of a phone class. A phone class is a sound and all the other sounds with which it may vary in a given position. For example, a child may produce the following: *see* [ti] [di]; *sun* [dʌn] [sʌn] [ʌn]; *feet* [fit]; *play* [beI] peI]. Assuming this is the child's complete production repertoire, the word-initial phone classes would be [s-p-d ø(null)], [f], and [b-p].[1]

The degree of contrast may be measured by the number of phone classes, the number of single-member phone classes, and the mean number of members per class. No age norms are currently available. However, the extent of the child's contrasts may be compared with the adult system in which there would be approximately 24 single-member consonant phone classes. It should be remembered that even though these phone classes contain sounds, the contrast is between words. For example, *see* and *feet* may be considered to contrast because there is no overlap in their word-initial phone classes. Ferguson and Farwell (1975) found no clear evidence of contrast between sounds. Additionally, in an experiment with his son, Braine (1971) tried to teach the child two nonsense words, [ʔi:] and [daI], representing an apparent contrast in his own speech. The words were ultimately produced as [di:] and [da], or [dʌ], suggesting no true contrastive value between the [d] and [ʔ].

An aspect of phonologic behavior observed during this period, which is closely related to the lack of contrast, is homonymy. Homonymy occurs when a child produces two different words in the same way. It has been suggested that normally developing children have a tendency to avoid homonymy by not producing a potentially homonymous word or by altering one of the forms in some way (Ingram, 1975). For example, a child may produce *bow* and *boat* as [boʊ] and [boʊ:], respectively. While some children may avoid homonymy, others may "seek out" or "collect" homonyms to reduce the number of different forms they have to produce for different words (Vihman, 1981). However, even in instances that appear homonymous a child may make imperceptible distinctions between apparently homonymous forms (e.g., less distinct vowel length differences) or distinctions which have no measurable acoustic consequences, such as slight lip rounding versus no lip rounding (Priestly, 1980). Thus, there may not be as many instances of true homonymy as have been reported. One aspect of homonymy for which we have little evidence other than anecdotes is the child's awareness of instances of homonymy. Additionally, the extent of true homonymy (no difference between forms) versus pseudohomonymy (articulatory or acoustic differences between the forms) needs to be determined. Some attempts have already been made to examine the influence of the child's view of whether or not two productions are homonymous and the influence of the hearer's view (Locke, 1979a; 1979b). However, some further research which takes the possibility of pseudohomonymy into account is needed. Another issue concerning homonymy revolves around the possibility that older disordered children might be more "tolerant" of homonymy in their systems (Ingram, 1976). Two recent investigations, one based on diary data from a variety of sources (Ingram, 1981) and one on samples collected in a standardized fashion from normally developing and language-impaired children at the one-word stage, revealed no differences in the extent of homonymy (Leonard, Camarata, Schwartz, Chapman & Messick, Note 8). In both groups there was a wide range of individual variation in the number of homonyms. One final aspect of homonymy which has not been examined in detail concerns a potential relationship with semantic factors (Vihman, 1981). It may prove to be the case that at least some apparent homonyms are actually semantic overextensions. Similarly, some apparent overextensions may prove to be homonyms. Until recently (Smith & Brunette, Note 9) such possibilities have not been considered.

The most consistent observation concerning phonologic behavior during the prerepresentational period is that children's errors do not always follow consistent patterns (Ferguson & Farwell, 1975). Thus, they cannot be readily described in terms of processes or rules (although the notion of variable rules might have some application, cf., Sankoff, 1978). Furthermore, because of the child's cognitive abilities, imputing a system of rules or processes as mental operations may be inappropriate at this stage.

One phenomenon of phonologic behavior described earlier, which further suggests that children at this point in development do not have a rule system into which new words are automatically assimilated, is represented by phonological idioms (Moskowitz, cited in Ferguson & Farwell, 1975). An idiom occurs when a child produces a word accurately, or nearly accurately (as compared with productions of other similar words) when it is first acquired. The accuracy of that production may then "deteriorate" over time. This has also been termed recidivism (Smith, 1973). An example, cited earlier, was Hildegard Leopold's acquisition of the word *pretty* which was initially produced as [prʌti] at 10 months and [prIti] at 11 months. At this point Hildegard did not appear to be producing any other prevocalic or intervocalic voiceless stops. Nor was she producing any consonant clusters in other words. Gradually, the production changed to [pIti] or [pwIti] at 16 months, [pIti] at 21 months, and finally changed to [bIdi] at 22 months. At that point, Hildegard, across all of her words, consistently produced voiceless prevocalic and intervocalic stops as their voiced counterparts and consistently simplified consonant clusters.

Phonological idioms are important for two reasons. First, they indicate that children at this point in development do not have a systematic set of rules into which each newly acquired word is assimilated. Instead, each word seems to be dealt with individually, some being produced more accurately than others. It is only later, when a system of rules develops, that different words with similar characteristics may be treated consistently in the child's phonology (e.g., all pre- and intervocalic stops are produced as voiced; all clusters are simplified). Consequently, a word such as *pretty* may be produced quite accurately at the outset, but as the child develops systematic rules or patterns for simplifying words (errors), its production may deteriorate.

The second important aspect of this phenomenon is that it provides evidence that, at least at one time, the child perceived and produced a word accurately. Thus, later errors (e.g., [bIdi] for *pretty*) may not be attributable to basic perceptual or motoric limitations. Instead, these errors seem more appropriately attributed to some systematic set of patterns or rules for dealing with various characteristics of adult words.

There are two other similar phenomena which also may provide evidence that during the next period of development a phonologic system is operative. They warrant discussion here because of their similarity to phonological idioms. The first has been termed "puzzle phenomena" (Smith, 1973). At a given time a child produced the word *puzzle* as [pʌdl̩], while the word *puddle* was produced as [pʌgl̩]. This demonstrates that the child's inaccurate production of *puddle* was not due to a motor inability to produce this form. It has been argued that this error may be the result of some misperception (cf., Macken, 1980b). However, it might also be taken as evidence that the child's developmental errors are the result of patterns of change applied to the adult forms being attempted regardless of whether they apply to perceptual representations or production representations (e.g., "change voiced fricatives to homorganic stops," "change alveolar stops to velar stops"). A similar point has been made regarding the occurrence of alternation (Dinnsen, Elbert, & Weismer, Note 10). Evidence that a child omits or deletes a final consonant in *dog* [dɔ], yet at the same time produces [dɔgi] has been proposed as evidence that the child has an accurate, perception-based underlying representation of the word *dog* that includes a final /g/.

Thus, given such evidence, Dinnsen et al. argue that final consonant omission ([dɔ] for *dog*) can be assumed to result from the application of some rule. This particular type of evidence should be viewed as less conclusive than the evidence provided by idioms or puzzle phenomena. First, it is not clear that *dog* and *doggie* represent true alternate forms for a child in the same way that an adult recognizes *electric* and *electricity* as alternate forms of a single word. Second, the child's ability to accurately perceive (as well as produce) a [g] in [dɔgi] only ensures that the child can do so in syllable-initial position. The failure to produce this sound in syllable-final position might as readily be attributed to motor or perceptual limitations as to some mental operation or rule without additional evidence.

In summary, this period of phonologic acquisition has proved to be a rich source of observational, anecdotal, and experimental data which support the view of it as a somewhat separable period of development. Children's phonologic behavior during this period may be described as variable, individually different within certain limits, as well as generally unsystematic in terms of rules, patterns, and contrasts, and markedly different from the period to follow. To the extent that much of their behavior seems based exclusively upon individual words without more general patterns, this period could also be termed the period of word-based phonology. Clearly, a good deal of additional research is needed to confirm and further specify the aspects of phonologic behavior described in this section.

The most obvious omission in this discussion has been any information concerning children's perceptual abilities during this period. Some investigations have examined phonetic perception in children at this point in development (Kuhl, 1980). However, to date no investigation has examined phonologic perception (i.e., perception in meaningful units such as words) in these children. The greatest obstacle to such research seems to be methodological. Children of this age are not sufficiently passive to allow the use of heart rate procedures, nor are sucking procedures appropriate. Tasks employed with older children (see the following section) are unlikely to be successful. However, some procedures such as visually reinforced infant speech discrimination (Eilers, 1980) and perceptual constancy (Kuhl, 1980) have the potential for testing perception in meaningful units. The next few years should see some significant advances in our knowledge of perceptual abilities during the prerepresentational period.

The Period of Representational or Systematic Phonology

This period, extending from approximately 18 months to 7 years, incorporates what has been discussed elsewhere (Ingram, 1976) as the period of the simple morpheme and the completion of the phonetic inventory. Since the justifications for viewing these two developments as separable periods in terms of changes in the basic nature of phonologic, cognitive, and general linguistic behavior are significantly weaker than in the case of the preceding period, this division will not be made. The hallmark of the representational period is the apparent systematic nature of children's phonologic behavior. Specifically, children seem to follow fairly systematic patterns in their errors and acquisition. While individual differences may still exist, children appear to be less variable (except in cases where they may vary between correct and previously incorrect productions), become gradually more systematic in their correct or incorrect production of classes of sounds across words and across types of words, and seem to be developing a system of sound contrast in perception and production. In the course of these developments, children also appear to gradually master the phonetic inventory of their language. Finally, during this period the more complex system of rules governing the use of morphophonemics is initially acquired.

Traditionally, we have only considered the general articulatory (production) aspects of speech sounds during this period. Consequently, descriptions of development and clinical applications were limited to information concerning the mastery of the phonetic inventory. Although this is an important aspect of development, it is by no means the whole of phonologic acquisition. The focus of this section will reflect this view.

Production of segments

At the beginning of this period, children's speech can be readily characterized as exhibiting pervasive errors. By the end of the period, errors may be rare or nonexistent. It is what occurs in between these two points that is of interest. With the exception of a few scattered diary studies, until the years between 1930 and 1960, we had little specific information regarding the development of speech production. However, three cross-sectional studies of large numbers of children conducted during that period radically changed that situation (Poole, 1934; Templin, 1957; Wellman, Case, Mengurt, & Bradbury, 1931). The data they provided were almost seductive in their appeal. We were suddenly able to take a given chronological age, look at these data, and determine what sounds should be acquired and what sounds should not yet be acquired. However, while these data have provided some general developmental signposts, their use seems fraught with difficulties.

There are significant weaknesses in both the methods of data collection and data analysis (Bernthal & Bankson, 1981; Schwartz, in press; Shriberg & Kwiatkowski, 1980; Winitz, 1969). Overall, the bases of these norms may be extremely unrepresentative of the speech of individuals and groups. Furthermore, the criteria employed in determining ages of acquisition (e.g., 75% or 100% of the subjects correctly articulating a sound in initial, medial, and final position) may present an extremely distorted picture of development. For example, although the age of acquisition for /t/ is given as 6 years (Templin, 1957), it is likely that most, if not all, children produce this sound accurately in some context at a much earlier age. It is also possible that for a given sound 70% of the children tested were correct in their production at one age, and only a few children caused the age of acquisition to be set at a higher age.

One way in which these latter two difficulties may be partially ameliorated is by considering an average age or age of customary usage rather than an age of mastery. Age of customary usage may be defined as the age at which more than 50% of the children tested correctly produce a given sound in two positions (Sander, 1972). Although this does not compensate for weaknesses in the way such data were collected, it does provide a somewhat better balanced picture of speech sound acquisition. The point remains, however, that these data tell us little about the way in which development proceeds from the point of pervasive errors on a given sound to the points at which customary usage or mastery are reached. What is lacking is a detailed description of children's errors and the nature of their gradual approximation to correct productions. Although it is easy to argue that this is what we need, achieving an agreed-upon description is quite another matter.

Two more recent reports (Ingram, Christensen, Veach, & Webster, 1980; Macken, 1980a) have provided some of these details. Macken described the development of the voicing distinction in stops in 4 English-speaking (1;6 to 2;4) and 7 Spanish-speaking (1;7 to 4;0) children. She found that the ages of acquisition varied considerably, by as much as a year. However, in English there seemed to be 3 general stages: (1) no voicing contrast, (2) a consistent but not audible difference between voiced and voiceless stops, and (3) an approximation of adult VOT distinctions. Additionally, there seems to be a lexical bias in the early stages in favor of words beginning with /b/, /d/, and /k/.

Ingram et al. (1980) studied the acquisition of word-initial fricatives and affricates in 73 English-speaking children ranging in age from 1;10 to 5;11. In general, the order of acquisition was /f/ before /tʃ/, /dʒ/, /ʃ/, before /s/, /v/, /z/, /ɵ/. However, a good deal of individual variation was noted. Additionally, individual children varied in their productions of given sounds across words and also varied in their productions of given words. They also noted some of the more common errors as [s], [p], or [b] for /f/; [b] for /v/; [f] for /ɵ/; [ɵ] for /s/; [x] or [s] for /z/; [s] for /ʃ/; [t], [s], or [ts] for /tʃ/; [d], [ts], or [dz] for /dʒ/. Some allophonic ("distortion") errors were also noted.

Such investigations represent a beginning in obtaining a more complete picture of normal phonetic development. In particular, instrumental analyses and multiple contexts of testing may be critical in establishing the range of normal developmental errors and normal developmental sequences.

It is generally agreed that the most striking characteristic of children's errors during this period is that they appear to be systematic within a given child. Furthermore, although some individual differences exist, these error patterns seem generally consistent across children. Several different approaches have been employed in describing these error patterns. These have included distinctive features, generative phonological rules, and phonological processes. The use of distinctive features involves the application of a set of typically binary (+, −) articulatory and/or acoustic features of speech segments (i.e., consonants and vowels) in describing acquisition and developmental errors. There are a number of such feature systems available (e.g., Chomsky & Halle, 1968; Jakobson, Fant, & Halle, 1963), differing in their relative emphasis on articulatory and phonetic features. Using such a system to describe speech sound development, Menyuk (1968) found evidence for the following order of acquisition: nasal, grave, voice, diffuse, continuant, strident. However, these data are somewhat limited in that it may be difficult to determine precisely when a child acquires an isolated feature.

There are many other limitations in using distinctive features. The binary nature of these features (e.g., ±voicing) may not be an accurate representation of the dimensions of features such as voicing. There may be many values of a feature such as this, rather than simply voiced and unvoiced. Additionally, there is no general agreement as to the specific set of features that should be employed. However, some relatively recent advances in the use of multidimensional scaling procedures (Singh, 1976) or alternative feature values such as markedness (Toombs, Singh, & Hayden, 1981) may help in resolving this problem. Even with this work, questions remain concerning the psychological reality of these features for adults. In paradigms designed to encourage categorizations of sounds according to their features, adults seem unaware of some features commonly included in such systems (LaRiviere, Winitz, Reeds, & Herriman, 1974; Ritterman & Freeman, 1974). The fact that children only gradually acquire a given feature (e.g., voicing) across sounds and words raises further questions about the use of this descriptive device. Finally, the most serious weakness of distinctive features concerns their exclusive focus on segmental aspects of speech. They do not take into account the fact that a given sound may be produced differently in different phonetic contexts and the fact that many developmental errors may be context dependent.

The second major approach to the description of developmental error patterns involves the use of generative rules such as those described by Chomsky and Halle (1968). Such rules involve the assumption that the child has a single underlying form for each word which is then transformed into the surface form (i.e., the production) by the application of these rules. In most cases (Smith, 1973) the assumption is made that the underlying form is based on the child's accurate perception of the adult's production. The rules which are then written formally characterize the relationships between these assumed underlying forms and the child's productions. The rules may be written in terms of sound classes (e.g., consonants, fricatives), individual sounds (e.g., /s/), or features (e.g., $\begin{smallmatrix} + \text{ continuant} \\ + \text{ strident} \end{smallmatrix}$). These rules also can be written to be either context-free (e.g., fricatives → stops, s →t, $\begin{smallmatrix} + \text{ continuant} \\ + \text{ strident} \end{smallmatrix} → \begin{smallmatrix} - \text{ continuant} \\ - \text{ strident} \end{smallmatrix}$) or context-sensitive by using a variety of symbols and conventions (e.g., C → Ø/__#, final consonants are deleted; s → t/__V, /t/ is substituted for /s/ prevocalically). The advantage of such rules is that they can be used to describe errors that are context-specific, unlike distinctive feature descriptions. The disadvantage of such rules is their level of formality and the potentially incorrect assumptions concerning children's underlying forms.

The final method employed in describing patterns of developmental errors involves the use of phonological processes based on Stampe's (1973) proposal. A number of investigators have employed these processes in describing error patterns in normal as well as phonologically impaired children. As mentioned earlier, there is no generally agreed-upon list of processes that can be used to describe these patterns. Investigators have suggested lists of as few as 8 (Shriberg & Kwiatkowski, 1980) up to as many as 40 or more (Ingram 1981; also see Edwards & Shriberg, 1983 for a more complete review). In using few processes, many unified patterns of errors may be overlooked. Using more may divide these patterns so finely that more general patterns may be missed.

Besides the unresolved issue of what specific set of processes should be considered, no resolution concerning the criteria for saying a process exists or quantifying the extent of processes has been reached. For instance, is it a process if a child substitutes /t/ for /s/, but produces other fricatives correctly? Is it a process if a child substitutes a stop for a fricative in only a single word? Is it a process if a child produces all final consonants except for /n/, which is deleted? Within the context of Stampe's theoretical proposal one could argue that all of these are in fact processes. From a more pragmatic standpoint, however, one might argue that these instances are quantitatively different from instances in which a child has an across-sound and an across-word pattern of errors, such as stopping or final consonant deletion. When this kind of distinction is made, it is in part with the intent of differentiating among idiosyncratic productions of words— isolated sound errors which might be attributable to misperceptions or inaccurate motor learning—and patterns of errors which may reflect some organizational aspect of the child's phonology (regardless of whether the origins of these error patterns are perceptual, structural, or motoric). To do this, then, we can require that for a process to exist, the pattern must affect more than a single sound in a sound class (e.g., more than a single fricative for it to be considered stopping) or more than a single sound regardless of class (e.g., more than /n/ deleted in final position). Using more stringent quantitative criteria (a minimum of 4 possible occurrences of a process and a minimum of 20% frequency of occurrence for the process), McReynolds and Elbert (1981) have demonstrated that a process analysis of disordered children's productions with these criteria differs markedly from one without any criteria. If some type of quantitative criteria is not employed, a process, on the surface, does little more than rename an individual error. The only thing it might imply in such instances is that the error is the result of the "natural limitations of the speech mechanism," which may or may not be accurate.

Other, qualitative, distinctions in error patterns may need to be drawn. Not all patterns identified perceptually by transcribers as the same process may be identical. For example, Weismer, Dinnsen, and Elbert (1981) have noted that in disordered children who appear to omit final consonants, the acoustic characteristics of the children's productions may differ significantly. Specifically, some children omit final consonants while maintaining a vowel length distinction between target words with voiced versus voiceless final consonants in the adult forms. Other children do not maintain this distinction. Consequently, it may be inappropriate to group both types of omission under the same process of final consonant deletion. Instead, as Weismer et al. suggest, these qualitatively different types of error patterns may need to be differentially labelled.

Finally, we will ultimately need to make quantitative distinctions among error patterns. Patterns may need to be distinguished in terms of the relative number of sounds affected (e.g., stopping for all fricatives versus stopping for only 3 fricatives). Patterns may also need to be distinguished on the basis of their within-sound, across-word consistency (e.g., stopping for /s/ and /z/ in all productions versus stopping for these sounds in some words, but not others).

The discussion of pattern analysis has thus far tended to focus on rather narrow patterns which, while consistent with the intuitions of some adults (i.e., child phonology researchers), may not have any psychological reality for the child. Instead, children's developmental sound error patterns may simply reflect much more general patterns. Some preliminary evidence for a more general view has recently become available. Menn (Note 1) suggested that in their error patterns, children follow more general constraints such as "don't produce final consonants" in a number of ways (e.g., final consonant deletion, syllable deletion, reduplication, failing to attempt to produce adult words with final consonants). Some diary evidence can be used to support this view. We may have sometimes missed such patterns in other children because our focus has been upon more narrow or isolated rules or processes. Also, in the last several years, evidence for such patterns in the phonologies of disordered children has been reported. Patterns have been observed such as consonant harmony involving the alteration of target words with more than one consonant to forms in which the consonants are similar or identical (Leonard, Miller, & Brown, 1980). Similarly, general patterns of sound preference in which a given consonant is substituted for a variety of consonants following no specific process or rule have been reported (Edwards, Note 11; Weiner, 1981).

While we may simply have missed many such general patterns in the errors of normally developing children, some such patterns have been discussed in terms of individual strategies of phonologic acquisition like those mentioned earlier (e.g., reduplication, syllable-maintaining vs. syllable-reducing). Other individual strategies have been described by Fey and Gandour (1982) and Priestly (1977). Recognition of these apparently individual paths and more general patterns in phonologic acquisition may aid in our understanding of the general process and nature of acquisition as well as in our understanding of phonologic disorders.

Another aspect of production during this period which has received little attention concerns phonetic development. While we have a good deal of information concerning the phonemes children acquire based on the perceptual judgments of transcribers, little information is available concerning aspects of production that are difficult, if not impossible, to perceive (e.g., voice onset time—VOT).

Some limited information has recently become available. Longitudinal data from 4 children suggest that the acquisition of the voicing contrast is gradual, occurring in 3 stages: (1) no contrast, (2) a contrast in VOT which falls within one of the adult categories—usually voiced, and (3) contrast resembling the adult contrast (Macken & Barton, 1980a). In Spanish, where the contrast is between lead voicing and short-lag VOT, the acquisition of this contrast is even more gradual with a mastery occurring after age 4 (Macken & Barton, 1980b). Other features, such as aspiration and spirantization, which add to the voicing contrast in English and Spanish, respectively, also may play a role in this aspect of development. Another such instance involves the earlier mentioned finding that some disordered children maintained a distinction in vowel length (longer vowel length associated with voiced final consonants; shorter vowel length associated with voiceless final consonants) even though the final consonant was not actually produced (Weismer et al., 1981). A similar distinction among children who are not disordered may prove to have some developmental significance. Along the same lines, it was also noted earlier that children's productions of what are perceived to be homonyms may not be truly homonymous (Priestly, 1980). Children may make articulatory distinctions between such words which do not have significant acoustic consequences. There may also be acoustic distinctions that are not perceptible to adult listeners. In all of these cases some instrumental analysis would reveal significant information not apparent in the perceptual judgments of transcription. Thus, the further use of such analyses is critical for more complete understanding of phonetic and phonologic development.

Production of suprasegmentals

Virtually all of the preceding information has focused exclusively on segmental phonology. Until recently, little attention has been directed toward the development of suprasegmentals (intonation, duration, stress, rhythm) and the influence of suprasegmental factors on segmental phonology (see Crystal, 1973; 1975). In a series of studies (Allen, in press; Allen & Hawkins, 1978), the discrimination and production of various aspects of suprasegmentals have been examined in French- , German- , English- and Swedish-speaking children ranging from 2 to 5 years of age. The discrimination and production of lexical stress patterns by these children from differing linguistic environments seems to gradually improve through 4 years of age. The abilities of the children seem to be similar in spite of differences in the stress patterns of the languages they are acquiring. After 4 years of age, however, the children appear to take on patterns characteristic of their native language. In some cases this involved the inability of 5-year-olds to produce and discriminate a pattern of stress that can be produced and discriminated by 4-year-olds.

These findings have been explained in terms of an "attunement" view of language acquisition (Aslin & Pisoni, 1980). Such a view suggests that certain abilities may be "lost" over time because the child only maintains those that are relevant to his or her native language. Further development of stress production and perception occurs through age 12. Atkinson-King (1973) demonstrated that only by age 12 do children accurately discriminate and perceive contrastive stress differentiating compound nouns (*greenhouse*) from noun phrases (*green house*).

Another aspect of suprasegmental phonology that has been examined developmentally is duration. Duration has been examined primarily in terms of the length of individual segments (i.e., vowels and consonants) within words (Gilbert & Purves, 1977; Hawkins, 1979), syllables (Oller & Smith, 1977; Smith, 1978), and larger units (Tingley & Allen, 1975). By 18 months, there is some differential duration of vowels and consonants with vowels reaching adult norms by 4 or 5 years of age. There is greater variability across consonants, with maturity being attained at 10 years of age or later. The relative and absolute duration of two-syllable words appears to approximate adult values by 2 years of age. However, the duration of syllables seems greater than that of adults and decreases only gradually. The results of a more recent investigation (Kubaska & Keating, 1981) suggest that developmental decreases in duration are not related to word familiarity. In fact, when utterance position is controlled, there is no decrease in some cases. The most significant factor in duration appears to be utterance position; nonfinal words are shorter in duration.

There is a need for further research in this area. Specifically, investigations involving greater control of familiarity and experience—perhaps employing nonsense or unfamiliar word/unfamiliar referent paradigms—might yield more conclusive results. A more complete understanding of this aspect of production may provide some clues regarding the child's developing motor control for speech.

A final aspect of suprasegmental phonology which has been considered is the acquisition of intonation. Intonation may be viewed as the prosodic use of tone or changes in fundamental frequency (Allen & Hawkins, 1980). Tone, as it is used in tone languages such as Gã (Kirk, 1973) or Mandarin Chinese (Clumeck, Note 12), functions almost segmentally in contrasting meaning at a word level. However, intonation affects much larger units of speech. Therefore, it should not be surprising that these two types of tone are acquired somewhat differently. In general, it appears that tone contrasts are acquired before rhythmic contrasts and segmental contrasts. The use of pitch for intonational features appears prior to the emergence of language and is gradually used in a systematic fashion (affirmative-negative and falling-rising contrasts). Tone, however, seems tied to the emergence of words; and while some tone characteristics are mastered at a very early age, other characteristics may emerge much later (Clumeck, 1980).

One of the more intriguing aspects of recent research concerning suprasegmental aspects of speech involves the apparent relationships among suprasegmental factors and segmental behavior. For example, unstressed or light syllables are likely to be deleted in initial position and in positions adjacent to another unstressed syllable (Allen & Hawkins, 1980). Similar findings have been reported by Klein (Note 13) regarding the influence of stress as well as serial position of a syllable in determining whether it is produced. She found that final unstressed syllables are most often produced when preceded by another unstressed syllable. In other environments such syllables are more often omitted. A major stress level (primary or secondary) in combination with a later occurring syllable was found to be the most likely situation in which a consonant was retained in multisyllabic words (e.g., *spaghetti* [gɛ]). Such findings represent an important first step in understanding the basis of developmental segmental errors. In the past we have focused largely on segmental aspects of phonology, and suprasegmental aspects were considered separately. Examination of the relationships between segmental and suprasegmental factors may serve to better explain patterns of production in both normally developing and disordered children.

Production of morphemes

The final aspect of speech production which begins to develop during this period is the system of bound morphemes. While such morphemes comprise only a small portion of the child's production, they represent an important advance in the child's phonologic abilities. Ultimately, this is the first clearly generative, rule based aspect of the adult phonologic system acquired by the child. Much of the research has focused on English morphophonology including plural, present progressive, past tense, and third person singular. However, this provides a somewhat limited picture since adjectival (comparative and superlative forms) and adverbial (e.g., *-ly*) inflections also occur in English. Additionally, some other languages (e.g., Hungarian) have extensive inflectional systems that indicate other linguistic information, such as case. In spontaneous speech, inflectional endings may begin to appear as early as 2 years of age, but the first which seems to be acquired (90% correct in obligatory contexts) is the present progressive (Brown, 1973; deVilliers & deVilliers, 1973). This is followed by plurals, possessives, past tense, and third person singular endings. However, even when children master such inflectional endings, we cannot be certain that their use is a reflection of generative rules.

The first evidence we have of the existence of generative morphophonological rules is children's overgeneralizations (e.g., *goed*). Another type of evidence for the generative nature of these rules is provided by studies that have employed Berko's (1958) now classic "Wug" procedure. In this procedure, children are presented with a novel nonsense word in a situation that encourages the use of an inflectional ending (e.g., "Here is a wug. Now there are two _____."). Because such words are novel, if they are inflected in the same way as familiar words, we have evidence for general morphophonological principles or rules. According to Berko's findings many of these rules are acquired by approximately age 5. However, the study did not provide much information concerning the developmental sequence in the acquisition of specific rules.

A subsequent study represented an attempt to provide such information for plural forms (Innes, Note 14). Using a task similar to that used by Berko, the following developmental sequence was found: (1) no extension of a plural rule to novel words, (2) use of rules to pluralize novel words except those ending in fricatives and affricates, (3) use of these rules with all words except those ending with sibilants, (4) use of these rules with all words except those ending in /z/, and (5) complete mastery. This suggests a gradual, phonetically based extension of a morphophonological rule. It remains to be seen whether a similar sequence occurs in the acquisition of rules governing other bound morphemes.

A more recent and extensive experimental study of the relative ease of morpheme acquisition by children between 3 and 9 (Derwing & Baker, 1977) has revealed a pattern similar to the order of acquisition in spontaneous speech mentioned earlier. Children made fewest errors on progressive endings, a greater number of errors on plural and past tense endings, followed by possessive endings and, finally, third person singular endings. The basis for this apparently consistent order and ease of acquisition is still a matter of some debate. In a lengthy disussion of this issue Brown (1973) considered grammatical complexity, semantic complexity, perceptual saliency, and frequency of occurrence. He rejected perceptual saliency and frequency of occurrence as possible determinants and suggested that semantic and grammatical complexity in combination may determine the order of the acquisition.

Still more recently, debate has surfaced concerning the influence of frequency of occurrence on input. When input data are analyzed in certain ways, there appears to be a relationship (Derwing & Baker, 1979; Moerk, 1980; 1981). However, when input data are analyzed differently, there seems to be no relationship between input frequency and the order of morpheme acquisition (Pinker, 1981). The problem centers on the issue of how one compares input with the child's usage of these morphemes in order to infer a causal relationship. To date, there are no satisfactory solutions. New experimental methodologies may be required to resolve this issue.

Further research (Cousins, Note 15) has also raised the possibility that, contrary to Brown's conclusion, perceptual saliency may have a role in determining the order of morpheme acquisition in one aphasic child. While the apparent influence of this factor cannot be generalized to normally developing children, further investigation seems warranted.

An exciting new direction in the study of morpheme acquisition involves the application of information-processing principles to construct a model of morphophonological behavior and acquisition (MacWhinney, 1978). MacWhinney considers three types of abilities as underlying this and other aspects of language acquisition: rote memorization, productive combination, and analogy formation. These are considered to be processes within a more general cyclical process of learning. In learning, acquisition leads to a process of application, which in turn leads to a correction process and then further acquisition. MacWhinney has employed morphophonologic data from various languages and some preliminary computer simulation to explore the nature of these processes. While the simulation is not an exact replication of children's acquisition of bound morphemes, it forces us to think about the specific components and processes that are required. This approach seems to hold a great deal of promise for this and other aspects of language acquisition.

Perception

This section on the representational period of phonologic acquisition has, to this point, focused almost exclusively on production. From the perspective of some child phonologists such an imbalance is perfectly acceptable. Such phonologists might argue that since perception is essentially accurate from the outset of development, no developmental changes would occur during this period (e.g., Smith, 1973; Stampe, 1973). Although data concerning infant speech perception indicate extensive abilities shortly after birth, it must be remembered that this involves perception of segments and acoustic features in the context of nonmeaningful syllables. This does not guarantee that children will accurately perceive aspects of a meaningful word. Nor does it guarantee that, even if "lower level" perception is accurate, the word (or larger unit) will be accurately represented and stored (cf. Braine, 1974). Finally, it has been argued that perception is generally an active rather than a passive process (Bryant, 1974). Many instances of anecdotal evidence can be provided to argue that, in spite of the actual physical characteristics of a stimulus and the actual physical information received by the sensory mechanism, perception involves the interpretation of this information in the context of existing knowledge. It is perhaps a common occurrence for adults to fail to notice or attend to speech errors in conversational speech. In fact, the word in which such an error occurs may be "heard" as a correct production, both because of expectancy and because it is heard and interpreted through the "filter" of the adult's representations and phonologic system. It would not, therefore, be surprising if children's perceptions were altered in some way by their own phonologic representational and organizational systems.

Even though there may be good reason to suspect that young children's perception may only gradually approach that of adults', we still do not have solid empirical evidence to support this view or to describe the actual course of development. A number of studies of phonemic perception in children under 4 years of age have been reported (Edwards, 1974; Garnica, 1971; 1973; Shvachkin, 1973; Strange & Broen, 1980; Barton, Note 16). However, some of these investigations are methodologically or statistically flawed (see Barton, 1975); and others, for pragmatic reasons, have focused on very specific aspects of perception during this period. Thus, we do not yet have a complete picture.

Shvachkin's (1973) investigation of 18 Russian children led to the proposal of an order of acquisition for perception of phonemic contrasts. The method employed involved teaching children nonsense CVC names for objects and then testing their ability to discriminate among these names. In each discrimination item the children were presented with three objects, two of which had names that differed by only one sound (e.g., *bak* and *dak*) and the third differed in all three sounds (e.g., *mup*). A similar procedure employed with English-speaking children yielded a generally comparable order of acquisition (Garnica, 1971). However, in these investigations a criterion of 7 correct out of 10 trials was employed in determining ages of acquisition. Such a criterion is too low because too often it may be reached by chance (Barton, 1975). When a more stringent criterion is employed, these orders of acquisition do not hold true. Apparent differences in ages of acquisition disappear.

More recently, Barton (1975; Note 17) has reported two investigations in which discrimination was examined in children ranging in age from 18 to 24 months in the first, and 27 to 35 months in the second. Minimal pair discriminations were employed using slightly different tasks than those described above. However, the child's response still was to point to a picture or pick up an object when given its name. Most of the younger children were able to discriminate at least *goat/coat* or *bear/pear*. The older children performed far better than Garnica's data indicated, with many instances of errorless discriminations. Consequently, it appears that phonemic discrimination abilities emerge quite early, although some cautionary notes are in order. Barton found that the extent to which the child knew the words being tested had a significant influence on the child's response. Additionally, particularly in the case of the younger children, task difficulty may have impinged on and distorted the results.

A number of earlier investigations examined the accuracy of children's discriminations after age 3 (Graham & House, 1971; Koenigsknecht & Lee, Note 18; Templin, 1957; Wepman, 1958). These investigations have involved a variety of methodologies, including same/different judgments of minimal pairs (real words and nonsense words), word monitoring, and selection of a picture(s) from an array of "minimal pair referents" in response to a word. In general, error rates appear to decrease with age, but children as old as 8 years continue to make some errors. Additionally, it appears that discriminations between stimuli differing by a single feature are more difficult than discriminations between stimuli differing by more than one feature. Few other generalizations are possible because of differences in stimuli and methodologies. The implications of these differences (e.g., real versus nonsense words; relative task difficulty type of response) are not yet fully understood (Barton, 1980).

More recently, some alternate methodologies for examining children's perception have been suggested (Locke, 1980a; 1980b). These alternatives have been drawn from procedures that have been used for some time in examining adult speech perception. They differ significantly in the tasks and types of responses involved from the procedures that have thus far been employed with children. For example, one alternative method involves asking a child if a given stimulus (word or syllable) is more like a second or a third stimulus. Another procedure involves asking a child to judge which one of three stimuli is different from the other two. However, even these tasks may be too difficult for children who are between 2 and 4 years of age. For these children, alternative procedures are needed. Promising sources for such procedures may be conditioning and habituation paradigms used in concept research with infants (e.g., Ross, 1980) as well as the visually reinforced head turn paradigms that have been used with younger children.

A final aspect of perceptual development during this period is the relationship between perception and production. Intuitively, it would seem as though perception and production would be closely related and that, in general, perception abilities at a given point in development would be advanced relative to production. However, these assumptions may not always be accurate. A first indication of their inaccuracy is provided by the somewhat analogous relationship between the production and comprehension of various aspects of language. Although, in general, comprehension is in advance of production, in some aspects of language the reverse appears to be true (Chapman & Miller, 1975). Additionally, very different strategies and processes may be involved in these systems. The same may well be true in the perception and production of speech.

Unfortunately, relatively few investigations have provided conclusive information regarding this relationship. Menyuk and Anderson (1969) found that children identified and categorized /l/, /r/, and /w/ more accurately than they were able to repeat these sounds. However, Zlatin & Koenigsknecht (1976) found comparable levels of behavior in children's identification and production of word-initial voiced and voiceless stops. Using the Schvachkin-Garnica technique, Edwards (1974) found that the phonemic perception of glides precedes their correct production. However, for other sounds, perceptual and productive abilities may appear simultaneously and, in rare instances, production may precede perception. A more recent investigation focusing on the perception and production of approximant consonants (specifically, /r/, /l/, and /w/) supports Edwards' conclusion that both perception and production develop gradually, with perception usually in advance of production (Strange & Broen, 1980). Finally, in findings analogous to those reported by Chapman and Miller (1975), Greenlee (1980) has observed that young children consistently maintain a distinction in vowel duration, but are unable to use this particular cue perceptually in distinguishing voiced from voiceless stops.

The literature concerning the relationship between perception and production seems to be somewhat contradictory, although some general conclusions can be drawn. There are differences as well as similarities in the development of perception and production abilities. Perceptual abilities seem to be generally more advanced than production abilities, with some clear exceptions. This suggests the existence of two separate but related systems. The exact nature of the relationship, however, is still unclear. One of the most important concerns for clinicians and researchers interested in speech sound disorders is the relationship between production errors and perceptual abilities. Such a relationship has yet to be established. Further research is needed involving converging methodologies to clarify these relationships.

Phonology and other aspects of language

Throughout this chapter the phonologic system has been discussed largely in isolation from other language components. This represents a distortion generally accepted for pragmatic reasons. In reality, phonologic behavior and development seem to be intimately related to other aspects of language. The relationship between phonologic and other components may take two forms: (1) the reciprocal influences of phonologic, syntactic, semantic, and pragmatic factors, and (2) the general developmental relationship between phonologies and other linguistic components.

It has long been commonplace knowledge that children make fewer errors producing words in isolation than producing words in sentences. In a series of studies involving children with phonologic and syntactic disorders, Panagos and his colleagues (Panagos & Prelock, 1982; Panagos, Quine, & Klich, 1979; Schmauch, Panagos, & Klich, 1978) have demonstrated that increases in the length and syntactic complexity of utterances led to an increase in speech sound errors. Similarly, they have demonstrated that increases in phonologic complexity (increased numbers of syllables) led to increases in syntactic errors. More recently, Prelock (Note 19) has demonstrated similar effects of increases in complexity on the speech and language of normally developing and disordered children. However, it should be noted that in somewhat younger children, ranging in age from 23 to 34 months, the effects of increases of syntactic complexity on phonologic production are not consistent (Kamhi, Catts, & Davis, Note 20). Kamhi et al. suggest that at some points in development other factors, such as representational abilities, may have a stronger influence on phonologic and phonetic behavior. It may also be true that while phonology is related to other aspects of language, language components remain, to some extent, autonomous. At some point in development there may be a relationship among these components, but not a one-to-one correspondence.

There appear to be other factors which influence speech sound behavior. For instance, Campbell and Shriberg (1982) found fewer instances of phonological processes in words encoding new, as opposed to old or shared, information. The influence of phonologic factors on lexical acquisition was discussed earlier in the chapter in terms of selectivity. Speech perception may be subject to the influence of semantic predictability (e.g., Cole & Jakimik, 1978; Morton & Long, 1976). It has also been demonstrated that in normally developing and language-impaired children at the one-word utterance level, both word type (object vs. action words) and extent of comprehension influence accuracy of production (Camarata & Schwartz, Note 21; Messick & Schwartz, Note 22). Children at this level produce object words more accurately than action words, perhaps because of differences in the conceptual or semantic complexity of these words. Words for which children have demonstrated comprehension tend to be produced less accurately than those for which the child has not demonstrated this degree of understanding. It may be that the child's increased knowledge of a word indicates that the word has been integrated into a phonologic system and is then subject to simplification rules that do not affect it before such integration occurs. Other potentially influencing factors, such as propositional complexity, have yet to be examined.

The other aspect of the relationship between phonology and other components of language is the development of these domains. This issue has been addressed within the context of phonologic disorders and more general linguistic disorders. It appears that, in at least some children, disorders of the phonologic system and disorders of syntax may be concomitant (Menyuk & Looney, 1972; Panagos, 1974; Shriner, Halloway, & Daniloff, 1969; Whitacre, Luper, & Pollio, 1970). Additionally, when language-disordered children are compared with normally developing children at a comparable level of syntactic development, their phonologies are very similar (Schwartz, Leonard, Wilcox, & Folger, 1980). This suggests that, at least during early stages in development, the development of phonology and syntax are closely related. Moreover, when specific disorders of language occur, they may affect phonology as well as other language components. Thus, there appears to be a synergistic relationship among the components of language which needs to be recognized in both discussions and future investigations of phonologic acquisition.

Formal Phonology

By approximately 7 years of age, children appear to be able to produce all the sounds of their language correctly in most, if not all, contexts. Typically, no processes remain other than those that might be characteristic of the child's dialect. However, phonologic acquisition is not yet complete. There are several aspects of phonology, primarily those thought to depend on generative rules, that are not mastered until after age 7. Seven years of age seems to be a landmark of sorts with respect to several aspects of development bearing some relationship to phonologic acquisition. At approximately age 7, children enter what Piaget (1970) has termed "the period of concrete operations." With this attainment, children are able to perform what he has called "mental transformations." A hallmark of this ability is the mental operation of reversibility. Although no direct relationship has been established (cf., Beilin, 1975), it has been suggested that children's understanding and use of active and passive forms of sentences are related to this ability. Similarly, Ingram (1976) has posited that these cognitive abilities may be important to those phonologic developments of this period that require more complex operations.

Another change which takes place during this period involves the child's schooling. By age 7, most children are enrolled in first grade and are beginning to learn to read and spell. The translation of their phonetic system into an orthographic system is likely to have significant effect on the child's whole phonologic system.

In spite of the important changes that occur during this period, we know little about the simultaneous changes in phonologic behavior. This is simply the result of a greater focus on early periods of development in recent research. However, several investigations have provided some preliminary information regarding the developments of this period.

In one study, Moskowitz (1973) examined children's rules concerning vowel shifts (alterations) in different forms of a given word (e.g., *divine-divinity; profane-profanity; serene-serenity*). A nonsense word task required the child to add an *-ity* ending to words that would, and words that would not, require a vowel alteration. Five-year-olds generally made no alterations. The 7-year-old children and some of the children ranging in age from 9 to 12 made alterations, but the correct vowel was not always used. The remaining 9- to 12-year-olds made only the correct vowel change. So the vowel-shift rule appears to be acquired gradually beginning at age 7. Moskowitz suggested that the source of the children's understanding of this shift is their spelling knowledge.

The same source of knowledge may account for another set of findings concerning children's understanding of contrastive stress differentiating nouns from verbs (*'convict* vs. *con'vict*) and compound nouns from noun phrases (e.g., *greenhouse* vs. *green house*). Atkinson-King (1973) found that while 5-year-olds had little or no understanding of this feature, by age 12 children had mastered these distinctions.

The fact that learning to read, learning to spell, and learning a phonology are related is not at all surprising. The specific nature and extent of these relationships are unknown. A study by Read (1971) of preschool children's early spellings suggests that their naive views of spelling are largely influenced by their phonologic knowledge and their rote knowledge of letter names. Other research has indicated that speech processes play an important role in learning to read (Hogaboam & Perfetti, 1978; Lesgold &

Curtis, 1981) but not necessarily in later "skilled" reading (Coltheart, Besner, Jonasson, & Davelaar, 1979). However, a good many issues concerning these relationships remain unresolved (see Lesgold & Perfetti, 1981 for an extensive review). Further research might aid speech-language pathologists in dealing with older impaired children. Additionally, it might enable us to provide reading instructors with more efficacious methods of aiding children in the translation of an oral and auditory phonologic system into an orthographic system (cf., Chomsky, 1970; 1972).

Conclusion

It should now be clear that we have made significant advances in our knowledge of phonologic acquisition since Jakobson's work was first translated in 1968. However, like so many young fields, this geometric expansion of knowledge has led to an exponential increase in the number of questions for which we do not yet have answers. Perhaps in the next decade some research will be conducted within the frameworks of new theories or more refined versions of the theoretical models discussed in this chapter. Such focused research, in conjunction with research conducted outside these frameworks, will provide some of the answers to these questions and, in turn, lead to further refinement of existing theories. Ideally, researchers will also provide clinicians with the specific developmental data they need to plan diagnosis and remediation.

Reference Notes

1. Menn, L. Towards a psychology of phonology: Child phonology as a first step. Paper presented to the Michigan State University Conference on Metatheory: Applications of Linguistic Theory in the Human Sciences, East Lansing, 1978.

2. Williams, L. The effects of phonetic environment and stress placement on infant discrimination of the place of stop consonant articulation. Paper presented to the Boston University Conference on Language Development, 1977.

3. Kaplan, E. The role of intonation in the acquisition of language. Unpublished doctoral dissertation, Cornell University, 1969.

4. Oller, K. Analysis of infant vocalizations: A linguistic and speech science perspective. Miniseminar presented to the American Speech and Hearing Association, Houston, 1976.

5. Zlatin, M. Explorative mapping of the vocal tract and primitive syllabification in infancy: The first six months. Paper presented to the American Speech and Hearing Association, Washington, 1975.

6. Doyle, W. On the verge of meaningful speech. Unpublished master's thesis, University of Washington, 1976.

7. Menn, L. Pattern, control and contrast in beginning speech: A case study in the development of word form and word function. Unpublished doctoral dissertation, University of Illinois, 1976.

8. Leonard, L., Camarata, S., Schwartz, R., Chapman, K. & Messick, C. Homonymy in the speech of children with specific language impairment. Unpublished paper, 1983.

9. Smith, M., & Brunette, D. Homonymy as a strategic conspiracy in phonological and lexical development. Paper presented to the American Speech-Language-Hearing Association, Toronto, 1982.

10. Dinnsen, D., Elbert, M., & Weismer, G. On the characterization of functional misarticulations. Paper presented to the American Speech-Language-Hearing Association, Detroit, 1979.

11. Edwards, M.L. Velar preferences in phonologically disordered children. Paper presented to the American Speech-Language-Hearing Association, Los Angeles, 1981.

12. Clumeck, H. Studies in the acquisition of Mandarin phonology. Unpublished doctoral dissertation, University of California, Berkeley, 1977.

13. Klein, H. The relationship between perceptual strategies and productive strategies in learning the phonology of early lexical items. Unpublished doctoral dissertation, Columbia University, 1978.

14. Innes, S. Developmental aspects of plural formation in English. Unpublished master's thesis, University of Alberta, 1974.

15. Cousins, A. Grammatical morpheme development in an aphasic child: Some problems with the normative model. Paper presented to the Boston University Conference on Language Development, 1979.

16. Barton, D. The role of perception in the acquisition of phonology. Unpublished doctoral dissertation, London, Indiana University Linguistics Club, 1976.

17. Barton, D. The discrimination of minimally different pairs of real words by children 2;3-2;11. Paper presented at the Third International Child Language Symposium, London, 1975.

18. Koenigsknecht, R , & Lee, L. Distinctive feature analysis of speech-sound discrimination in children. Paper presented to the American Speech and Hearing Association, 1968.

19. Prelock, P. Cumulative effects of syntactic and phonological complexity on children's language production. Unpublished doctoral dissertation, University of Pittsburgh, 1983.

20. Kamhi, A., Catts, H., & Davis, M. The effects of increases in language complexity on children's word productions: Evidence for the autonomy of language and phonology. Unpublished paper, 1982.

21. Camarata, S., & Schwartz, R. Phonological production of action words and object words. Paper presented to the American Speech-Language-Hearing Association, Toronto, 1982.

22. Messick, C., & Schwartz, R. Does imitation or comprehension affect phonological production in stage I children? Paper presented to the American Speech-Language-Hearing Association, Toronto, 1982.

References

Allen, G. Linguistic experience modifies lexical stress perception. *Journal of Child Language,* in press.

Allen, G., & Hawkins, S. The development of phonological rhythm. In A. Bell & J. Hooper (Eds.), *Syllables and segments.* Amsterdam: North Holland, 1978.

Allen, G., & Hawkins, S. Phonological rhythm: Definition and development. In G. Yeni-Komshian, J. Kavanaugh, & C. Ferguson (Eds.), *Child phonology Vol. I - Production.* New York: Academic Press, 1980.

Aslin, R., & Pisoni, D. Some developmental processes in speech perception. In G. Yeni-Komshian, J. Kavanaugh, & C. Ferguson (Eds.), *Child phonology. Vol. II. Perception.* New York: Academic Press, 1980.

Atkinson-King, K. Children's acquisition of lexical stress contrasts. *Working Papers in Phonetics,* UCLA Phonetics Laboratory, 1973.

Barton, D. Statistical significance in phonemic perception experiments. *Journal of Child Language,* 1975, *2,* 297–298.

Barton, D. Phonemic perception in children. In G. Yeni-Komshian, J. Kavanaugh, & C. Ferguson (Eds.), *Child phonology. Vol. II. Perception.* New York: Academic Press, 1980.

Bates, E., Camaioni, L., & Volterra, V. The acquisition of performatives prior to speech. *Merrill-Palmer Quarterly,* 1975, *21,* 205–224.

Beilin, H. *Studies in the cognitive basis of language development.* New York: Academic Press, 1975.

Bell, A., & Hooper, J. (Eds.) *Syllables and segments.* Amsterdam: North Holland, 1978.

Berko, J. The child's learning of English morphology. *Word,* 1958, *14,* 150–177.

Bernthal, J., & Bankson, N. *Articulation disorders.* Englewood Cliffs, N.J.: Prentice-Hall, 1981.

Bloom, K. Patterning of infant vocal behavior. *Journal of Experimental Child Psychology,* 1977, *23,* 367–377.

Bloom, K. Evaluation of infant conditioning. *Journal of Experimental Child Psychology,* 1979, *27,* 60–70.

Bloom, K., & Esposito, A. Social conditioning and its proper control procedures. *Journal of Experimental Child Psychology,* 1975, *19,* 209–222.

Braine, M. The acquisition of language in infant and child. In C. Reed (Ed.), *The learning of language.* New York: Appleton-Century-Crofts, 1971.

Braine, M. On what might constitute learnable phonology. *Language.* 1974, *50,* 270–299.

Brown, R. *A first language: The early stages.* Cambridge, Mass.: Harvard University Press, 1973.

Bryant, P. *Perception and understanding in young children: An experimental approach.* New York: Basic Books, 1974.

Campbell, T., & Shriberg, L. Associations among pragmatic function, linguistic stress and natural phonological processes in speech-delayed children. *Journal of Speech and Hearing Research,* 1982, *25,* 547–553.

Carter, A. The transformation of sensorimotor morphemes into words: A case study of the development of "more" and "mine." *Journal of Child Language,* 1975, *2,* 233–250.

Carter, A. The disappearance schema: Case study of a second-year communicative behavior. In E. Ochs & B. Schieffelin (Eds.), *Developmental pragmatics.* New York: Academic Press, 1979.

Chapman, R., & Miller, J. Word order in early two and three word utterances: Does production precede comprehension? *Journal of Speech and Hearing Research,* 1975, *18,* 355–371.

Chomsky, C. Reading, writing and phonology. *Harvard Educational Review,* 1970, *40,* 307–308.

Chomsky, C. Write now, read later. In C. Cazden (Ed.), *Language in early childhood education.* Washington: National Association for the Education of Young Children, 1972.

Chomsky, N., & Halle, M. *The sound pattern of English.* New York: Harper & Row, 1968.

Clumeck, H. The acquisition of tone. In G. Yeni-Komshian, J. Kavanaugh, & C. Ferguson *Child phonology. Vol. I. Production.* New York: Academic Press, 1980.

Cole, R., & Jakimik, J. Understanding speech: How words are heard. In G. Underwood (Ed.), *Strategies of information processing.* London: Academic Press, 1978.

Coltheart, M., Besner, D., Jonasson, J., & Davelaar, E. Phonological encodings in the lexical decision task. *Quarterly Journal of Experimental Psychology,* 1979, *31,* 489–507.

Crystal, D. Non-segmental phonology in language acquisition: A review of the issues. *Lingua,* 1973, *32,* 1–45.

Crystal, D. *The English tone of voice.* London: Edward Arnold, 1975.

deVilliers, J., & deVilliers, P. A cross-sectional study of the acquisition of grammatical morphemes in child speech. *Journal of Psycholinguistic Research,* 1973, *2,* 267-278.

Derwing, B., & Baker, W. The psychological basis for morphological rules. In J. Macnamara (Ed.), *Language learning and thought.* New York: Academic Press, 1977.

Derwing, B., & Baker, W. Recent research on the acquisition of English morphology. In P. Fletcher & M. Garman (Eds.), *Language acquisition.* Cambridge: Cambridge University Press, 1979.

Dore, J., Franklin, M., Miller, R., & Ramer, A. Transitional phenomena in early language acquisition. *Journal of Child Language,* 1976, *3,* 13-28.

Edwards, M. L. Perception and production in child phonology: The testing of four hypotheses. *Journal of Child Language,* 1974, *1,* 205-219.

Edwards, M. L., & Shriberg, L. *Phonology: Applications in communicative disorders.* San Diego: College-Hill Press, 1983.

Eilers, R. Infant speech perception: History and mystery. In G. Yeni-Komshian, J. Kavanaugh, & C. Ferguson (Eds.), *Child phonology. Vol. II. Perception.* New York: Academic Press, 1980.

Fee, J., & Ingram, D. Reduplication as a strategy of phonological development. *Journal of Child Language,* 1982, *9,* 41-54.

Ferguson, C. Learning to pronounce: The earliest stages of phonological development in the child. In F. Minifie & L. Lloyd (Eds.), *Communicative and cognitive abilities—Early behavioral assessment,* Baltimore: University Park Press, 1978.

Ferguson, C. Reduplication in child phonology. *Journal of Child Language,* 1983, *10,* 239-244.

Ferguson, C., & Farwell, C. Words and sounds in early language acquisition: English initial consonants in the first fifty words. *Language,* 1975, *51,* 419-439.

Ferguson, C., & Garnica, O. Theories of phonological development. In E. Lenneberg & E. Lenneberg (Eds.), *Foundations of language development (Vol. I).* New York: Academic Press, 1975.

Ferguson, C., & Macken, M. Phonological development in children: Play and cognition. *Papers and Reports on Child Language Development,* 1980, *18,* 138-177.

Fey, M., & Gandour, J. Rule discovery in phonological acquisition. *Journal of Child Language,* 1982, *9,* 71-81.

Garnica, O. The development of the perception of phonemic differences in initial consonants by English-speaking children. *Papers and Reports on Child Language Development,* 1971, *3,* 1-29.

Garnica, O. The development of phonemic speech perception. In T. Moore (Ed.), *Cognitive development and the acquisition of language.* New York: Academic Press, 1973.

Gilbert, J., & Purves, B. Temporal constraints on consonant clusters in child speech production. *Journal of Child Language,* 1977, *4,* 103-110.

Graham, L., & House, A. Phonological oppositions in children: A perceptual study. *Journal of the Acoustical Society of America,* 1971, *49,* 559-566.

Greenlee, M. Learning the phonetic cues to the voiced/voiceless distinction: A comparison of child and adult speech perception. *Journal of Child Language,* 1980, *7,* 459-468.

Halliday, M. *Learning how to mean: Explorations in the development of knowledge.* London: Edward Arnold, 1975.

Hawkins, S. Temporal coordination of consonants in the speech of children: Further data. *Journal of Phonetics,* 1979, *7,* 235-267.

Hogaboam, T., & Perfetti, C. Reading skill and the role of verbal experience in decoding. *Journal of Educational Psychology,* 1978, *70,* 717-729.

Ingram, D. Phonological rules in young children. *Journal of Child Language,* 1974, *1,* 49–64.

Ingram, D. Surface contrast in phonology: Evidence from children's speech. *Journal of Child Language,* 1975, *2,* 287–292.

Ingram, D. *Phonological disability in children.* New York: Elsevier, 1976.

Ingram, D. *Procedures for the phonological analysis of children's language.* Baltimore: University Park Press, 1981.

Ingram, D., Christensen, L., Veach, S., & Webster, B. The acquisition of word-initial fricatives and affricates by children between 2 and 6 years. In G. Yeni-Komshian, J. Kavanaugh, & C. Ferguson (Eds.), *Child phonology. Vol. I. Production.* New York: Academic Press, 1980.

Jakobson, R. *Child language, aphasia and phonological universals.* The Hague: Mouton, 1968.

Jakobson, R., Fant, G., & Halle, M. *Preliminaries to speech analysis: The distinctive features and their correlations.* Cambridge: MIT Press, 1963.

Jusczyk, P., & Thomson, E. Perception of a phonetic contrast in multi-syllabic utterances by 2-month old infants. *Perception and Psychophysics,* 1978, *23,* 105–109.

Kent, R. Articulatory-acoustic perspectives on speech development. In R. Stark (Ed.), *Language behavior in infancy and early childhood.* New York: Elsevier North Holland, 1981.

Kiparsky, P., & Menn, L. On the acquisition of phonology. In J. Macnamara (Ed.), *Language learning and thought.* New York: Academic Press, 1977.

Kirk, L. An analysis of speech imitations by Gã children. *Anthropological Linguistics,* 1973, *15,* 267–275.

Klein, H. Productive strategies for the pronunciation of early polysyllabic lexical items. *Journal of Speech and Hearing Research.* 1981, *24,* 309–405.

Kubaska, C., & Keating, P. Word duration in early child speech. *Journal of Speech and Hearing Research,* 1981, *24,* 615–621.

Kuhl, P. Speech perception in early infancy: Perceptual constancy for vowel categories. *Journal of the Acoustical Society of America,* 1976, *60,* Supplement 1, S90.

Kuhl, P. Speech perception in early infancy: Perceptual constancy for the vowel categories /a/ and /ɔ/. *Journal of the Acoustical Society of America,* 1977, *61,* Supplement 1, S39.

Kuhl, P. Perceptual constancy for speech-sound categories in early infancy. In G. Yeni-Komshian, J. Kavanaugh, & C. Ferguson (Eds.), *Child phonology. Vol. II. Perception* New York: Academic Press, 1980.

Kuhl, P., & Meltzoff, A. The bimodal perception of speech in infancy. *Science,* 1982, *218,* 1138–1141

LaRiviere, C., Winitz, H., Reeds, J., & Herriman, E. The conceptual reality of selected distinctive features. *Journal of Speech and Hearing Research,* 1974, *17,* 122–133.

Leavitt, L., Brown, J., Morse, P., & Graham, F. Cardiac orienting and auditory discrimination in 6-week-old infants. *Developmental Psychology,* 1976, *12,* 514–523.

Leonard, L., Miller, J., & Brown, H. Consonant and syllable harmony in the speech of language-disordered children. *Journal of Speech and Hearing Disorders,* 1980, *45,* 336–345.

Leonard, L., Newhoff, M., & Mesalam, L. Individual differences in early child phonology. *Applied Psycholinguistics,* 1980, *1,* 7–30.

Leonard, L., Schwartz, R., Chapman, K., & Morris, B. Factors influencing early lexical acquisition. *Child Development* 1981, *52,* 882–887.

Leonard, L., Schwartz, R., Chapman, K., Rowan, L., Prelock, P., Terrell, B., Weiss, A., & Messick, C. Early lexical acquisition in children with specific language impairment. *Journal of Speech and Hearing Research,* 1982, *25,* 554–564.

Leonard, L., Schwartz, R., Folger, M., & Wilcox, M. Some aspects of child phonology in imitative and spontaneous speech. *Journal of Child Language,* 1978, *5,* 403–416.

Leopold, W. *Speech development of a bilingual child: A linguistic record* (4 vols.). Chicago: Northwestern University Press, 1939–1947.

Lesgold, A., & Curtis, M. Learning to read words efficiently. In A. Lesgold & C. Perfetti (Eds.), *Interactive processes in reading.* Hillsdale, N.J.: Lawrence Erlbaum, 1981.

Lesgold, A., & Perfetti, C. Interactive processes in reading. Hillsdale, N.J.: Lawrence Erlbaum, 1981.

Locke, J. The child's processing of phonology. In W. A. Collins (Ed.), *Minnesota symposium on child psychology* (Vol. 12). Hillsdale, N.J.: Lawrence Erlbaum, 1979. (a)

Locke, J. Homonymy and sound change in the child's acquisition of phonology. In N. Lass (Ed.), *Speech and language: Advances in basic research and practice.* New York: Academic Press, 1979. (b)

Locke, J. The inference of speech perception in the phonologically disordered child. Part I: A rationale, some criteria, the conventional tests. *Journal of Speech and Hearing Disorders,* 1980, *45,* 431–444. (a)

Locke, J. The inference of speech perception in the phonologically disordered child. Part II: Some clinically novel procedures, their use, some findings. *Journal of Speech and Hearing Disorders,* 1980, *45,* 445–468. (b)

Macken, M. Developmental reorganization of phonology: A hierarchy of basic units of acquisition. *Linga,* 1979, *49,* 11–49.

Macken, M. Aspects of the acquisition of stop systems: A cross-linguistic perspective. In G. Yeni-Komshian, J. Kavanaugh, & C. Ferguson (Eds.), *Child phonology. Vol. I. Production.* New York: Academic Press, 1980. (a)

Macken, M. The child's lexical representation: The 'puzzle-puddle-pickle' evidence. *Journal of Linguistics* 1980, *16,* 1–17. (b)

Macken, M., & Barton, D. The acquisition of the voicing contrast in English: A study of voice onset time in word-initial stop consonants. *Journal of Child Language,* 1980, *7,* 41–74. (a)

Macken, M., & Barton, D. The acquisition of the voicing contrast in Spanish: A phonetic and phonological study of word-initial stop consonants. *Journal of Child Language,* 1980, *7,* 433–458. (b)

MacNeilage, P. The control of speech production. In G. Yeni-Komshian, J. Kavanaugh, & C. Ferguson (Eds.), *Child phonology. Vol. I. Production.* New York: Academic Press, 1980.

MacWhinney, B. The acquisition of morphophonology. *Monographs of the Society for Research in Child Development,* 1978, *43,* (174), 1–2.

McReynolds, L., & Elbert, M. Criteria for phonological process analysis. *Journal of Speech and Hearing Disorders,* 1981, *46,* 197–204.

Menyuk, P. The role of distinctive features in children's acquisition of phonology. *Journal of Speech and Hearing Research,* 1968, *11,* 138–146.

Menyuk, P., & Anderson, S. Children's identification and reproduction of /w/, /r/ and /l/. *Journal of Speech and Hearing Research,* 1969, *12,* 39–52.

Menyuk, P., & Looney, P. Relationships among components of the grammar in language disorder. *Journal of Speech and Hearing Research,* 1972, *15,* 395–406.

Moerk, E. Relationships between parental input frequencies and children's language acquisition: A reanalysis of Brown's data. *Journal of Child Language,* 1980, *7,* 105–118.

Moerk, E. To attend or not to attend to unwelcome reanalyses? A reply to Pinker. *Journal of Child Language,* 1981, *8,* 627–632.

Morse, P. The discrimination of speech and non-speech stimuli in early infancy. *Journal of Experimental Child Psychology,* 1972, *14,* 718–731.

Morton, J., & Long, J. Effect of word transitional probability on phoneme identification. *Journal of Verbal Learning and Verbal Behavior,* 1976, *15,* 43–51.

Moskowitz, A. The two-year stage in the acquisition of English phonology. *Language,* 1970, *46,* 426–441.

Moskowitz, B. On the status of vowel shift in English. In T. Moore (Ed.), *Cognitive development and the acquisition of language.* New York: Academic Press, 1973.

Nelson, K. Structure and strategy in learning how to talk. *Monographs of the Society for Research in Child Development,* 1973, *38,* (149) 1–2.

Netsell, R. The acquisition of speech motor control: A perspective with directions for research. In R. Stark (Ed.), *Language behavior in infancy and early childhood.* New York: Elsevier North Holland, 1981.

Oller, D. The emergence of speech sounds in infancy. In G. Yeni-Komshian, J. Kavanaugh, & C. Ferguson (Eds.). *Child phonology. Vol. I. Production.* New York: Academic Press, 1980.

Oller, D., & Smith, B. The effect of final-syllable position on vowel duration in infant babbling. *Journal of the Acoustical Society of America,* 1977, *62,* 994–997.

Oller, D., Wieman, L., Doyle, W., & Ross, C. Infant babbling and speech. *Journal of Child Language,* 1975, *3,* 1–11.

Olmsted, D. *Out of the mouths of babes.* The Hague: Mouton, 1971.

Panagos, J. Persistence of the open syllable reinterpreted as a symptom of language disorder. *Journal of Speech and Hearing Disorders,* 1974, *39,* 23–31.

Panagos, J., & Prelock, P. Phonological constraints on the sentence productions of language disordered children. *Journal of Speech and Hearing Research,* 1982, *25,* 171–177.

Panagos, J., Quine, M., & Klich, R. Syntactic and phonological influences on children's articulation. *Journal of Speech and Hearing Research,* 1979, *22,* 841–848.

Piaget, J. *Play, dreams and imitation in childhood.* New York: Norton, 1962.

Piaget, J. Piaget's theory. In P. Mussen (Ed.), *Carmichael's manual of child psychology* (Vol. I). New York: John Wiley, 1970.

Pinker, S. Formal models of language learning. *Cognition,* 1979, *7,* 217–283.

Pinker, S. On the acquisition of grammatical morphemes. *Journal of Child Language,* 1981, *8,* 477–484.

Poole, E. Genetic development of articulation of consonant sounds in speech. *Elementary English Review,* 1934, *11,* 159–161.

Priestly, T. One idiosyncratic strategy in the acquisition of phonology. *Journal of Child Language,* 1977, *4,* 45–65.

Priestly, T. Homonymy in child phonology. *Journal of Child Language,* 1980, *7,* 413–472.

Read, C. Pre-school children's knowledge of English phonology. *Harvard Educational Review,* 1971, *41,* 1–34.

Rheingold, H., Gewirtz, J., & Ross, H. Social conditioning of vocalizations in the infant. *Journal of Comparative and Physiological Psychology,* 1959, *52,* 68–73.

Ritterman, S., & Freeman, N. Distinctive phonetic features as relevant and irrelevant stimulus dimensions in speech-sound discrimination learning. *Journal of Speech and Hearing Research,* 1974, *17,* 417–425.

Ross, G. Categorization in 1- to 2-year-olds. *Developmental Psychology,* 1980, *16,* 391–396.

Salus, P., & Salus, M. Developmental neurophysiology and phonological acquisition order. *Language,* 1974, *50,* 151–160.

Sander, E. When are speech sounds learned? *Journal of Speech and Hearing Disorders,* 1972, *37,* 55–63.

Sankoff, D. *Linguistic variation: Models and methods.* New York: Academic Press, 1978.

Schmauch, V., Panagos, J., & Klich, R. Syntax influences the accuracy of consonant production in language-disordered children. *Journal of Communication Disorders,* 1978, *11,* 315–323.

Schwartz, R. Assessment of speech sound disorders in children. In I. Meitus, & B. Weinberg (Eds.), *Diagnosis in speech-language pathology.* Baltimore: University Park Press, in press.

Schwartz, R., & Folger, M. Sensorimotor development and descriptions of child phonology: A preliminary view of phonological analysis for Stage I speech. *Papers and Reports on Child Language Development,* 1977, *13,* 8–15.

Schwartz, R., & Leonard, L. Do children pick and choose? An examination of phonological selection and avoidance in early lexical acquisition. *Journal of Child Language*, 1982, *9*, 319–336.

Schwartz, R., Leonard, L., Wilcox, M., & Folger, M. Again and again: Reduplication in child phonology. *Journal of Child Language*, 1980, *7*, 75–88.

Schwartz, R., & Prelock, P. Cognition and phonology. In J. Panagos (Ed.), Children's phonological disorders in language contexts. *Seminars in Speech, Language and Hearing*, 1982, *3*, New York: Thieme-Stratton.

Shibamoto, J., & Olmsted, D. Lexical and syllabic patterns in phonological acquisition. *Journal of Child Language*, 1978, *5*, 417–456.

Shriberg, L., & Kwiatkowski, J. *Natural process analysis*. New York: John Wiley, 1980.

Shriner, T., Halloway, M., & Daniloff, R. The relationship between articulatory deficits and syntax in speech defective children. *Journal of Speech and Hearing Research*, 1969, *12*, 319–325.

Shvachkin, N. The development of phonemic speech perception in early childhood. In C. Ferguson & D. Slobin (Eds.), *Studies of child language development*. New York: Holt, Rinehart & Winston, 1973.

Singh, S. *Distinctive features: Theory and validation*. Baltimore: University Park Press, 1976.

Smith, B. Temporal aspects of English speech production: A developmental perspective. *Journal of Phonetics*, 1978, *6*, 37–67.

Smith, N. *The acquisition of phonology: A case study*. London: Cambridge University Press, 1973.

Spring, D., & Dale, P. Discrimination of linguistic stress in early infancy. *Journal of Speech and Hearing Research*, 1977, *20*, 224–231.

Stampe, D. A dissertation on natural phonology. Unpublished doctoral dissertation, University of Chicago, 1973.

Stark, R. Stages of speech development in the first year of life. In G. Yeni-Komshian, J. Kavanaugh, & C. Ferguson, (Eds.), *Child phonology. Vol. I. Production*. New York: Academic Press, 1980.

Strange, W., & Broen, P. Perception and production of approximant consonants by 3-year-olds: A first study. In G. Yeni-Komshian, J. Kavanaugh, & C. Ferguson (Eds.), *Child phonology Vol. II. Perception*. New York: Academic Press, 1980.

Templin, M. Certain language skills in children: Their development and interrelationships. Institute of Child Welfare, Monograph 26, Minneapolis, University of Minnesota Press, 1957.

Tingley, B., & Allen, G. Development of speech timing control in children. *Child Development*, 1975, *46*, 186–194.

Toombs, M., Singh, S., & Hayden, M. Markedness of features in the articulatory substitutions of children. *Journal of Speech and Hearing Disorders*, 1981, *46*, 184–191.

Vihman, M. Phonology and the development of the lexicon: Evidence from children's errors. *Journal of Child Language*, 1981, *8*, 239–264.

Waterson, N. Child phonology: A prosodic view. *Journal of Linguistics*, 1971, *7*, 179–221.

Waterson, N. A tentative model of phonological representation. In T. Myers, J. Laver, & J. Anderson (Eds.), *The cognitive representation of speech*. Amsterdam: North-Holland, 1981.

Weiner, F. Systematic sound preference as a characteristic of phonological disability. *Journal of Speech and Hearing Disorders*, 1981, *46*, 281–286.

Weisberg, P. Social and nonsocial conditioning of infant vocalizations. *Child Development*, 1963, *34*, 377–388.

Weismer, G., Dinnsen, D., & Elbert, M. A study of the voicing distinction associated with omitted, word-final stops. *Journal of Speech and Hearing Disorders*, 1981, *46*, 320–328.

Wellman, B., Case, I., Mengurt, I., & Bradbury, D. Speech sounds of young children. *University of Iowa Studies in Child Welfare*, 1931, *5*.

Wepman, J. *Auditory discrimination test*. Chicago: University of Chicago Press, 1958.

Whitaker, J., Luper, H., & Pollio, H. General language deficits in children with articulation problems. *Language and Speech,* 1970, *13,* 231–239.

Williams, L., & Bush, M. The discrimination of voiced stop consonants by young infants with and without release bursts. *Journal of the Acoustical Society of America,* 1978, *63,* 1223–1225.

Winitz, H. *Articulatory acquisition and behavior.* New York: Appleton-Century-Crofts, 1969.

Zlatin, M., & Koenigsknecht, R. Development of the voicing contrast: A comparison of voice onset time in stop perception and production. *Journal of Speech and Hearing Research,* 1976, *19,* 93–111.

Zlatin Laufer, M., & Horii, Y. Fundamental frequency characteristics of infant non-distress vocalization during the first 24 weeks. *Journal of Child Language,* 1977, *4,* 171–184.

End Note

[1]Leonard, Newhoff, and Mesalam (1980) argued that this method leads to the uncertain assumption that this child would also produce *see* as [si] or[i] and *sun* as [tʌn]. Consequently, they would identify the phone classes as [t-d], [d-s-θ], [f], (b-p]. While this may be more accurate, it may be more difficult to compare with the adult system. The method employed should depend on the purpose of the analysis.

Frederick F. Weiner

A Phonologic Approach to Assessment and Treatment

Since the publication of *Phonological Disability in Children* (Ingram, 1976) the area of articulation disorders has taken a large turn in direction. The focus has broadened to include a phonologic thrust. With this new direction has come an interest in children with multiple misarticulations and unintelligible speech. Researchers and clinicians have viewed the patterns of sound production observed in these children as a separate aspect of language equal in importance to syntax, semantics, or pragmatics. Because of the orderliness of sound errors in these children, researchers have inferred that mentalistic rules must govern surface level sound production. In an attempt to determine the orderliness of sound errors, several evaluation procedures have been published. These include *Assessment of Phonological Processes* (Hodson, 1980), *Procedures for the Phonological Analysis of Children's Language* (Ingram, 1981), *Natural Process Analysis* (Shriberg & Kwiatkowski, 1980), and *Phonological Process Analysis* (Weiner, 1979).

Motivated by the publication of these procedures a great deal of work has been carried out in developing a better understanding of the theory behind a phonologic approach to misarticulation as well as suggestions for assessment and treatment of children who are unintelligible. This new work should certainly be considered as recent advances in the study of phonologic disability and will be summarized and discussed in this chapter. Specifically, the topics to follow will be: What is a Phonologic Process? Perceptual Testing for Phonologic Disorders, Systematic Sound Preference,

Phonologic Development for Unintelligible Speakers, and A Case for Using the Effects of Listener-Speaker Interactions to Facilitate the Treatment of Children with Phonologic Disability.

What is a Phonologic Process?

One of the most prominent characteristics of children with multiple misarticulations is the reduction of phonemic contrasts in comparison to the adult phonemic system. When the reduction in phonemic contrasts appears to be systematic, these patterns of errors have been called phonologic processes.

The term phonologic process, as used in analysis of misarticulation, comes from the theory of Natural Phonology (Donegan & Stampe, 1978). In the most recent version of this theory, it is assumed that the sound patterns of a language are governed by the constraints of the human speech capacity. These constraints include both the limitations of the human vocal tract and the perceptual system. Processes are mental substitutions which unconsciously adapt phonologic intentions to phonetic capacities.

By labeling a phonetic event a phonologic process we are saying that the speaker has subconsciously transformed a phonologic intention in a manner consistent with his phonetic capacity. In children, these phonologic intentions are based on what the child knows about the adult language. In this sense, the child is assumed to have an underlying phonologic representation fairly equivalent to the adult surface form. The phonologic process is a description of how the child subconsciously transforms underlying representations into surface level events. Because the child is in a more language-naive state than the adult, his or her phonetic output is highly subject to natural forces implicit in human vocalization and perception. As a consequence, many phonemic contrasts present in the adult language become obliterated. As children develop and come to know the language function of these phonemic contrasts, they begin to suppress the natural dynamics of vocalization in an attempt to establish these contrasts at the surface level. As a result, their surface level output becomes more like their internal representations.

Unfortunately, the mental events described by phonologic processes are not directly observable. They can only be inferred on the basis of phonetic output and perceptual responses. It is exactly for this reason that the usefulness of phonologic processes has been questioned. Being behaviorally oriented professionals, speech-language pathologists have felt uneasy about the description of events that are not directly observable. This uneasiness has led them to charge that "this kind of analysis appears no more than a relabeling of articulation errors, not a discovery of the operation of processes" (McReynolds & Elbert, 1981, p. 197).

At this time McReynolds and Elbert are correct in making such an assertion. To date there have been few published attempts to verify that phonologic processes are adaptations of internal representations to phonetic output. Furthermore, this concept has been overused by some investigators to the extent that all child misarticulations have been described as processes, whether justified or not. As a result, it is up to those who advocate the use of phonologic processes to justify their existence.

Criteria for the Occurrence of Phonologic Processes

In my view, the major substantiation of a phonologic process is showing that the child "knows" the adult phonemic contrast but does not use it. In this regard Dinnsen, Elbert, and Weismer (Note 1) have proposed three tests. The first is that the process must apply optionally. That is, if a child uses the correct form some of the time, we can infer that the adult form is known and an underlying representation exists. The second is that the adult contrast is expressed in an unconventional manner. An example would be when a child deletes the final consonant in *pig* and *pick*, but still maintains the contrast by lengthening the vowel in *pig*, but not in *pick*. The third test is that the process applies to a very limited class of segments. For example, if a process occurs for only the voiceless members of a class of sounds, the child is demonstrating knowledge of a voiced-voiceless distinction within that class. Assuming that these criteria are valid tests for establishment of processes, there are many examples in the literature and clinical reports of patterns of misarticulation that would qualify as phonologic processes.

As speech-language clinicians, we have all seen children who were inconsistent in their production of certain sounds or classes of sounds. Technically, these would qualify as phonologic processes. But, our assertion that phonologic processes exist would be strengthened if we could describe the conditions surrounding the inconsistency. For example, Dinnsen, Elbert, and Weismer (Note 1) described Jamie, a boy who deleted final consonants. His production of *dog* was /dɔ:/. But when he said the same word with the diminutive suffix added, his production was /dɔgI/. Here we can infer that the child had the underlying representation for /g/ but, because of the process of deletion of final consonants, did not use final /g/.

Another example comes from tests for assimilation. Ordinarily, a child who produces *dog* > /gɔg/ is assumed to assimilate the initial sound with the final /g/. This sound is described as a potential "culprit" which motivated the g/d substitution. To substantiate velar assimilation as a phonologic process, one should observe the child's other attempts to produce /d/ in words without final velar stops. If the child produces the /d/ sound correctly in words like *dish*, *do*, and *date* (words without the culprit /g/), then it might be assumed that the g/d substitution in dog > /gɔg/ was due to the phonologic process called velar assimilation.

A child in our clinic seemed to be using a process in words containing nasals. The following is a short corpus of his responses:

paint /neʔ/	sun /n:ʌʔ/
pig /pI/	soup /tʃup/
tent /nɛk/	swimming /nImI/
toothbrush /tutbʌs/	sweater /tawə\

In each case when the word contained a nasal, the first sound became a nasal. If the word did not have a nasal, then those same sounds were either produced correctly or were replaced by other nonnasal sounds. Here again is an example of a nasal assimilation that would qualify as a phonologic process because the child demonstrated that he had the underlying representation for many of the sounds that were replaced by /n/.

As an example of a child who demonstrated knowledge of an adult phonemic contrast without using that contrast as an adult would, the following short corpus is presented:

ski→/k$^{=}$i/	swimming→/k$^{=}$wImIŋ/
skate→/k$^{=}$et/	sweater→/k$^{=}$wevin/
sleeping→/tlpIn/	snake→/θneæ
sled→/tlek/	snowman→/ønomæ/

Even though this child does not produce these 4 cluster-types (/s/ + stop, /s/ + /l/, /s/ + /w/, and /s/ + nasal) as an adult would, he nevertheless has 4 different cluster-types. One interpretation of this finding could be that the child realizes that at least 4 different /s/ clusters occur in the adult language. From this realization it could be assumed that his underlying representation for the adult form is similar in many respects to that of the adult.

This final example shows the restricted use of a process:

five→/halv/	valentine→/bɑeldlhalm/
thin→/hIn/	this→/jIts/
soup→/hup/	zipper→/dʒlpə/
shoe→/hu/	

In this corpus the child replaces initial voiceless fricatives by /h/ yet other errors occur for initial voiced fricatives. This shows the restricted use of a process and verifies knowledge on the part of the child of a voiced-voiceless phonemic contrast among fricatives.

The above examples are presented to show how one can verify the presence of a process and to provide evidence that mentalistic phonological processes do occur. These examples are important because they demonstrate the role that language plays in sound production.

Perceptual Testing of Phonologic Disorders

In the previous section of this chapter, the point was made that many of a child's misarticulations may be classified as phonologic processes. Such classifications presume that surface speech productions are rule governed and based on an underlying phonemic system. One tool available to the speech-language pathologist to determine the distribution of phonemes in a child's phonologic system would be a description of his perceptual phonemic system. Unfortunately, the major perceptual tests and testing techniques will not provide valid information concerning phonemic perception. Instead, these tests only provide phonetic information. What follows are comments concerning methodological problems with popular perceptual tests and procedures to assess phonemic perception in children with phonologic disability.

By far, the most common form of discrimination testing used by speech clinicians is the same-different paradigm. The two published tests most representative of this paradigm are the *Auditory Discrimination Test* (Wepman, 1973) and a test commonly referred to as the *Templin Speech Sound Discrimination Test* (Templin, 1957). The *Auditory Discrimination Test* has pairs of words in which a single phoneme is contrastive, e.g., *pin - bin*. The *Templin Speech Sound Discrimination Test* has pairs of nonsense syllables. In both tests the child is instructed to say *same* if the paired items are identical, and *different* if the paired items are not identical.

Locke (1980a) presented a critical review of these tests. His review addressed many potential problems in interpretation of test results. First was the problem of the cognitive concept of same versus different. If a child being tested does not know the concept of same and different, incorrect responses may be more a function of this cognitive deficit than difficulty with perception.

Another problem arises when two sounds are allophones of the same phoneme for a child. If /f/ and /θ/ are allophones within a certain child's phonology, this child may respond to a pair of words like /fIn/-/θIn/ with a *same* response. This does not mean that the child does not perceive a difference between /f/ and /θ/. It merely means that the child did not consider the difference to be worth reporting. An analogy would be when an adult hears the words /hɑet⁻/ and /hɑetʰ/. These two words would most likely be reported as the same even though there is a phonetic difference between the two final /t/ sounds. In other words, the adult is capable of perceiving the difference between /t⁻/ and /tʰ/ but, similarly, does not consider this difference worth reporting. Interpretation, then, of the child's *same* response to /fIn/-/θIn/ (using conventional testing) would be that the child cannot hear the difference between /f/ and /θ/ which may, in fact, be an erroneous conclusion.

Another factor is that some people feel that perception testing is useful as an explanation for faulty misarticulation (although this has not been clearly demonstrated empirically). Unfortunately, the items of most of the published discrimination tests have a poor correspondence with the most common misarticulations; i.e., those items which do relate to predictable misarticulations are only a small part of the test. This is further complicated by the two-alternative nature of these tests. This means that a child who is not correctly perceiving has a 50-50 chance of guessing some of these more difficult discriminations.

By far, the most powerful criticism offered by Locke (1980a) was that results of these tests do not help us answer the most important question, which is "whether the child detects a difference between the speech forms he is expected to acquire (that is, adult surface forms) and those already stored (that is, his internal representation)" (p.436). The same-different paradigm asks the child to make decisions concerning two surface forms spoken by the examiner. Locke argued that these decisions may not give us information about the child's phonemic system. For a child whose system held /f/ and /θ/ as allophones of the same phoneme, a /fIn/-/θIn/ item would require him to discriminate between his allophones. If this same child held /f/ and /θ/ as separate phonemes, then the discrimination would be between different phonemes. The problem is that we do not know the relationship between /f/ and /θ/ for the child. In fact, that is exactly the kind of information that our discrimination testing should give us.

On the basis of these criticisms, Locke (1980b) proposed a set of criteria for more efficient assessment of speech perception. These criteria are extremely useful and bear repeating here. The criteria are that the procedure must:

1. examine the child's perception of the replaced sound in relation to the replacing sound, that is, the target phoneme versus its substitution phoneme, or, as in the case of complete omission, silence;
2. observe the same phonemes in identical phoneme environments in production and perception;

3. permit a comparison of the child's performance of target and replacing sounds with his discrimination of target and perceptually similar control sounds;
4. be based on a comparison of an adult's surface form and the child's own internal representation;
5. present repeated opportunities for the child to reveal his perceptual decisions;
6. prevent nonperceptual errors from masquerading as perceptual errors;
7. require a response easily within a young child's conceptual capacities and repertoire of responses; and
8. allow a determination of the direction of misperception (p. 445).

On the basis of these criteria, Locke proposed a new form of discrimination testing called the Speech Production-Perception Task (SP-PT). To perform this test, the clinician first selects a production error such as /θʌm/ → /fʌm/. In this example /θ/ is considered the stimulus phoneme (SP) and /f/ is considered the replacement phoneme (RP). Next the clinician selects a control phoneme (CP). The CP is perceptually similar to the SP, such as /s/ for this example. The tester then selects a picture of *thumb* (the target word) and asks, "Is this /θʌm/? Is this /fʌm/? Is this /sʌm/?" The child is required to answer "Yes" or "No" to each of these questions. Each question is asked 6 times for a total of 18 responses and the order of presentation is randomized.

A child who had perception similar to adults would answer "Yes" to /θʌm/ and "No" to /fʌm/ and /sʌm/. This type of pattern of response would mean that the child's internal representation was the same as the adult's and, therefore, /f/ and /θ/ would be different phonemes in the child's external perceptual system. In the test administration, it is essential that the child answer "No" to the CPs (/sʌm/). Otherwise, the examiner cannot be certain that he is capable of performing to the conceptual requirements of the test. In other words, "No" responses to the CP items establish the validity of the child's responses. Once that is established, we can more readily believe what the child reports about SP and RP.

Some children tested by Locke showed a pattern of response wherein they said "Yes" to /θʌm/, "Yes" to /fʌm/, and "No" to /sʌm/. In this case, these children demonstrated that they were valid perceivers by responding "No" to /sʌm/. But, such children also responded as if /fʌm/ and /θʌm/ were appropriate descriptions of *thumb*. The conclusion to be drawn from this result is that /f/ and /θ/ are both allophones of /θ/ for these children because both, when produced by the adult, matched the children's internal representation for /θ/. In this instance, the children's misarticulation of f/θ was probably motivated by the fact that these two sounds were not contrasted in the children's perceptual phonology.

One other important point brought out by Locke (1980b) was that since different discrimination tests represent different levels of perception, we, as clinicians, should be able to use that information to our advantage in assessing our clients. Consider, for example, the child who answered "Yes" to /θʌm/, "Yes" to /fʌm/, and "No" to /sʌm/. On the basis of SP-PT testing, we know that /f/ and /θ/ are allophones of /θ/ and that the child did not discriminate between them. What we do not know, however, is if this child is capable of discriminating between them. To determine this we should follow up our testing with another form that has the potential to force a child to differentiate between allophones if he is capable. One such test protocol is referred to as an ABX procedure.

In an ABX procedure, the clinician could use two talking puppets, one for each hand. One puppet says "/θʌm/," the other says "/fʌm/," and the clinician asks, "Who said /θʌm/?" In this case, the child is forced to distinguish between his or her allophones. If the child were able to point to the appropriate puppet it would mean that although a distinction between /f/ and /θ/ was not made in the SP-PT test, the child was certainly capable of such a discrimination as was demonstrated by the ABX procedure. Failure to discriminate between /f/ and /θ/ in the ABX would suggest that the child's perceptual errors were not necessarily related to his or her phonemic system. Instead, he may have some form of gross perceptual deficit.

To further elucidate this point, an English-speaking adult with an intact language system can be similarly confronted with an SP-PT and ABX protocol to test perception of /t⁻/ and /tʰ/. For the SP-PT the adult would be shown a picture of a *baseball bat* and asked, "Is this /bæt⁻/?" and "Is this /bætʰ/?" Appropriate responses to both questions would be "Yes" because in English /t⁻/ and /tʰ/ are allophones of the same phoneme. Note that this procedure only tells us that /t⁻/ and /tʰ/ do not change the meaning of the word for the adult. That is, /t⁻/ and /tʰ/ have the same allophonic relationship for the adult as /f/ and /θ/ had for the child who accepted /θʌm/ and /fʌm/. We still do not know from this test whether the adult could distinguish between these allophones. For this, the ABX procedure is administered. In this procedure the examiner would say, "/bæt⁻/, /bætʰ/, which one was /bæt⁻/?" The adult would, no doubt, say that the first word presented was /bæt⁻/. Here the adult was asked to discriminate between the allophones /t⁻/ and /tʰ/ just as the child had been asked to distinguish between the allophones /f/ and /θ/. If the adult was not able to respond correctly in the ABX task we might assume the presence of some form of auditory deficit such as a peripheral hearing loss.

The importance of Locke's contribution was to remind us that there are at least two kinds of perception with which the clinician should be concerned. These types have been periodically referred to as phonetic and phonemic, or power and salience. Phonetic or power perception is most readily assessed when the child is required to make judgments about adult surface forms as in a same-different or ABX paradigm. A phonemic or salience decision is best assessed in a procedure where an internal representation must be compared with one presented by an adult, such as is required in SP-PT testing. In this respect, power decisions are nonlanguage perceptions, and salience decisions are language perceptions. Of course, children must have the ability to make power decisions. But perceptual testing designed to determine the motivation for misarticulation should be salience testing. In this regard, it is not only important for the child to be able to perceive the essential elements of sounds, but it is also important to ignore the nonessential elements. This is entirely different from power testing where children are required to distinguish minimal differences without regard to their function within the language.

Systematic Sound Preference

Whether the speech-language pathologist uses phonologic theory or relies on a more traditional philosophy during assessment, the clinician invariably looks for *patterns of misarticulation*. Sometimes, the patterns are present; other times, the speech-language pathologist describes misarticulation as being *inconsistent*.

Descriptions of inconsistent misarticulation can have at least two interpretations. The first is that the child really is inconsistent. The second is that the child is consistent but the conditions of consistency are not apparent to the clinician. For example, a child who substitutes n/f and p/f may be described as inconsistent. However, if we knew that the n/f substitution was limited to a specific phonetic context, and the p/f substitution was limited to another specific phonetic context, then the child's errors would be more predictable and, therefore, consistent.

Tests for phonologic processes described in the first section of this chapter were recommended when patterns of misarticulation were present. Consequently, before we can even test whether a phonologic process exists, the pattern of misarticulation must be described. To this end, the speech-language pathologist should be aware of some of the unique phonologic processes that potentially can occur in children.

In summarizing unique phonologic processes, Ingram (1976) noted that several children with phonologic disability overused nasalization in their speech. He described this excessive use of nasalization as nasal preference. Ingram also reported an occasional overuse of fricatives, which he similarly termed a fricative preference. Weiner (1981a), in assessing the speech of unintelligible children, found that many demonstrated sound preferences referred to by Ingram. The use of these sounds tended to be predictable. Weiner termed this phenomenon "systematic sound preference." At the same time, and quite independently, Edwards (Note 2) had made very similar observations about sound preference. She termed the phenomenon "favorite sounds" and, like Weiner, found that the occurrence of these sounds was systematic.

One characteristic of the sound preference phenomenon was that no specific favorite sound was seen to occur with any regularity across the children observed. The "choice" of the favorite sound did not seem to be related to sound difficulty, since many children used /k/, /tʃ/, or /θ/, usually acknowledged to be later developing and more difficult to produce. As stated above, the favorite sounds tended to occur systematically so that natural classes of sounds were regularly replaced. The most frequent natural class to be affected was fricatives. Occasionally, sound preference was limited to the voiceless members of a natural class with a further restriction that labials were not affected.

To demonstrate systematic sound preference the following corpus from a child seen in our speech and language clinic is presented:

short → /hɔr/	father → /hadə/
thumb → /hʌm/	this → /dI/
soup → /hup/	zipper → /bIpI/
fire → /faIr/	valentine → /bælɛʔaI/
sugar → /hʊdə/	vacuum → /baʔu/

The first 6 responses are to words beginning with voiceless fricatives. In each case, the voiceless fricative was replaced by /h/, the favorite sound. In the next four responses the words begin with voiced fricatives. For each of these words, the voiced fricative was replaced by a voiced stop. In this example, we see that the sound preference phenomenon affects a natural class of sounds (voiceless fricatives). In doing so, there is justification for considering this to be a phonologic process (see criteria for phonologic processes in the first section of this chapter). Being a phonologic process means that the child's underlying representation for voiceless fricatives is adapted in the above example to be expressed as /h/.

Why and how this happens is uncertain. One plausible explanation would be that for some reason /h/ is perceptually salient for this child. The form /hVC/ or /hVCV/ may be a perceptual structure into which words fall, in the tradition of Waterson (1971). Regardless of the reason, however, this phenomenon represents a neutralization of certain phonemic contrasts and is potentially important to the speech-language pathologists when determining whether a child's misarticulations are consistent or not.

Phonologic Development of Unintelligible Children

The preceding chapter by Richard Schwartz presents a theoretical perspective and discussion of recent issues concerning phonologic acquisition. The focus of his chapter was *normal* phonologic acquisition. The following section is included here because it presents some recent information about phonologic development in children with unintelligible speech. The reader should compare information concerning the normally developing child presented by Schwartz with characteristics of children who do not follow a normal developmental progression. Information concerning unintelligible children was gathered from a longitudinal investigation by Weiner and Wacker (1982).

In this investigation, children were administered the *Phonological Process Analysis* (Weiner, 1979) 3 times at 6 month intervals. The normally speaking children were 3 years of age at the first testing. This age group was selected because they were presumed to have normal developmental articulation errors. The unintelligible children were between 3 and 5 years of age. Results were analyzed in two ways. First, all speech productions were evaluated to determine whether there were patterns of misarticulation. Next, phonetic inventories were determined for each child. Phonetic inventory analysis determined which sounds were used by the children, regardless of target productions.

Results of the pattern analysis were predictable. That is, normally speaking children had too few errors for any patterns to appear. The errors present tended to be sound specific rather than to affect natural classes of sounds. Sound substitutions were generally within the same manner of production resulting in place errors as opposed to manner errors. Certain substitutions appeared over and over again. These were /ð/ → /d/, /θ/ → /f/, /s/ → /θ/, /ʃ/ → /s/, /r/ → /w/ and the replacement of liquids within clusters by /w/.

The unintelligible children, as expected, had many more misarticulations than the normally developing talkers. Substitution errors were patterned and predictable. If a child replaced a nasal by a homorganic stop in one situation, there was a tendency to do it to nasals in other words as well. The nature of substitution errors was also different. Whereas most of the substitution errors for normally developing speakers involved changes in place of articulation, the substitution errors for unintelligible talkers were replacements of one manner of production for another manner of production. In contrast to an f/θ substitution that might be present for an intelligible child, an unintelligible child would more likely replace /θ/ with /t/. Another difference involved the pervasiveness of errors. Normally developing children seemed to have errors for only fricatives and liquids. Unintelligible talkers, on the other hand, demonstrated errors across all manners of production.

In observing the development of phonology in these two groups over a 1-year period there were also other differences. Considering the number of words containing misarticulations in each of the 3 corpora collected from each child, there was greater improvement shown by the normally talking children. That is, they improved 40%, to only 10% for the unintelligible children. This means that sound errors in the children with phonologic disability were persistent, as was predicted by Ingram (1976).

There was also one other major difference in phonologic development between groups. This was the occurrence of *recidivism* among the intelligible children, which was not seen in the unintelligible talkers. Recidivism, as described by Weiner and Wacker (1982), was the correct production of a word at one developmental stage followed by incorrect production at another, later stage. Recidivism is not routinely reported in the literature because most studies of speech development have been cross-sectional. This study, however, was longitudinal, allowing investigators to observe articulation as it developed.

The second form of analysis, the phonetic inventory, yielded even more interesting results. From this analysis it was apparent that many more sounds were used by intelligible than by unintelligible children. Furthermore, sounds missing from the inventories of normally developing speakers seemed to be limited to the fricative-affricate manners, while unintelligible speakers had missing sounds across the whole phonetic spectrum. Another interesting finding was that unintelligible talkers tended to overuse certain sounds. Sometimes this was systematic, wherein an entire class was replaced by one phoneme (cf., Weiner, 1981). Other times, overuse was the result of a combination of phonologic processes. For example, a child who replaced fricatives by homorganic voiced stops would produce /s/, /θ/, /z/, /ð/, /ʃ/, and /ʒ/ as /d/. Therefore, in addition to attempts to use /d/, six fricatives in the child's corpus would appear as /d/, as well as clusters containing the fricative sounds just mentioned.

The greatest difference between groups in the phonetic inventory analysis appeared for clusters. Clusters were almost absent from the corpora of unintelligible children. At the beginning of the investigation, intelligible children used an average of 13.9 different word-initial clusters. Unintelligible children used an average of 4.5. By the end of the study, normally developing talkers used an average of 15.0 to only 5.67 for the unintelligible talkers. Therefore, one of the greatest discrepancies between groups, and a diagnostically significant result, was the frequency of cluster usage.

In summary, the unintelligible children had many patterns of errors. Most involved the replacement of one manner for another across all manners of production. Also, many sounds were completely missing from the phonetic inventories of these children. Sounds present tended to be overused resulting in stereotypic productions. Clusters were rare and slow to develop. And finally, the absolute number of errors seemed to persist over the course of the investigation.

A Case for Using Effects of Speaker-Listener Interactions to Facilitate the Treatment of Children with Phonologic Disability

As you will recall from the first section of this chapter, one of the major assumptions concerning a phonologic explanation for misarticulation is that the disorder is language-based rather than motoric. Given this assumption, the treatment method for unintelligible speech should parallel other methods of language remediation.

In this regard, there is a body of research which provides evidence that pragmatic factors present in the speaker-listener interaction can have a positive effect on communication including improved production of speech. This was demonstrated by Longhurst and Siegel (1973) where subjects were placed in a situation in which they were to provide listeners with instructions necessary to complete a task. The speaker and listener were separated from each other and the message listeners received was periodically distorted. When speakers observed that the listeners were confused, the speakers reduced speaking rates, became more elaborate in their instructions, and supplied more redundant information. Although there were no specific data showing improved articulation, the investigators concluded that the strategies the speakers selected seemed to contribute to improved communication.

This phenomenon was also demonstrated by Gallagher (1977), who intermittently asked the question, "What?" when gathering spontaneous speech samples from children. Results were that revision behaviors including linguistic elaborations, reductions, and sound substitutions occurred frequently. In addition, it was noted that 50% of the phonetic changes were interpreted as closer approximations to the adult model. Although the other 50% were not interpreted as positive changes, they were nevertheless changes. Thus, on the basis of listener responses, children in this investigation altered their phonetic output.

This effect has also been demonstrated in children with misarticulation. In a structured procedure Weiner and Ostrowski (1979) queried children about their misarticulations in three ways. If a child pronounced *fish* as /fIs/, he was asked one of the following 3 questions: (1) "Did you say fish?" (2) "Did you say /fIs/?" or (3) "Did you say /fIθ/?" In the first question, *fish* was produced correctly; in the second, *fish* was produced with the child's error; and in the third *fish* was produced incorrectly with a different error on the target sound than the child used. This procedure was repeated for a number of misarticulated words so that each query occurred an equal number of times for all subjects in the investigation. In response to the queries, children were trained to respond "Yes (or No), I said ____." The number of correct target sounds that occurred for each of the 3 types of queries were then compared to determine whether any or all of these query types had a positive effect on articulation. The results were that type 3 queries had the greatest effect in reducing misarticulation. In fact, a typical response to this type question was, "No!!! I said /fIsss/." The type 3 response was interpreted to convey the greatest amount of listener uncertainty because /fIθ/ was neither the target word nor the child's substitution for the target word. Here again, expressed misunderstanding resulted in changed articulation performance, but this time there was evidence that the change was in a positive direction.

In another investigation, Weiner and Ellis (Note 3) studied children's sound errors resulting in homonymy. An example of such a word pair is *bow* and *boat*, which would both be produced the same for children who delete final consonants. These children were then asked to produce their homonym pairs under 2 conditions. In the first, the words making up the homonym pairs were produced randomly. In the second, the words were presented as minimal pairs, side by side. Results were that children altered their productions of one or both members of the pairs in condition 2. Interpretation was that somehow the children sensed that there would be possible listener confusion in the paired condition and altered their productions to avoid such confusion.

In a discussion of the pragmatics of language, Greenfield and Smith (1976) wrote about the Principle of Informativeness, wherein the selection of elements for encoding by speakers are those perceived to resolve uncertainty. The above investigations provide examples of how this principle also exists at the phonologic level.

In clinical work, speech-language pathologists have also attempted to capitalize on the principle of informativeness. For a child with a w/l substitution, production of the words *white* and *light* would both normally be /waɪt/. If the clinician responded to the child's attempt to say *light* as though the child was saying *white,* the clinician would be sending a listener message similar to listener messages artificially constructed in the experiments described above. On the basis of this information, it would be predicted that the child would change the production of *light* so as to distinguish it from *white.*

This paradigm was used in a clinical investigation by Weiner (1981b). In this investigation, phonologic processes were treated using a minimal contrast paradigm. For the process stopping, word pairs such as *fin-pin, vase-base, zip-dip,* and *sea-tea* were selected. When stopping occurred, the 4 word pairs would be produced as 4 homonym pairs. Children were instructed to play a game where the object was for the clinician to pick up all the pictures of words beginning with fricatives. If the child's word started with a fricative, the clinician would pick it up. If the child pronounced the target sound as a stop, the clinician would pick up the wrong picture. Picking up the wrong picture was a sign of listener misunderstanding. Results of the experiment were that children were able to reduce the number of processes in their speech very rapidly. This was interpreted as support for listener response as a tool in the treatment of phonologic disability.

Of course, this is only one investigation supporting language training principles used to remediate misarticulation. Other investigations need to be conducted to verify effectiveness of some of the recently proposed articulation therapy methods. In fact, many of the methods currently used to treat misarticulation should be tested experimentally.

Conclusions

At this time, I would like to point out that over the past several years many new developments like phonologic theory have found their way into the area of speech-language pathology. Some of these new developments have not stood the test of time because they did not fully explain a particular disorder, nor did they provide useful clinical information. For clinicians to invest the time necessary to understand and use these new concepts, there must be some clinical gain.

In this chapter, I have tried to point out that description of misarticulation by phonologic analysis helps to explain articulation disorders as something more than a new label for an old pattern. But phonologic theory is not always easy to understand and apply. There are tests that must be employed to verify the existence of phonologic processes at both the productive and perceptual level. There are patterns of misarticulation that must be identified as potential phonologic processes. Some may be as unique as those described in the section on systematic sound preference. The point is that an adequate phonologic analysis can be difficult and time consuming. And, as with any new development, the ultimate test should not be the difficulty, but, rather, the clinical usefulness. That is, after having spent a great deal of time learning a new analysis technique, will clinicians be further ahead in treating their clients?

In this regard, I feel that the preliminary treatment data using speaker-listener interactions shows promise of being an effective therapeutic tool. Of course, phonologic theory applied to analysis and treatment of misarticulation is at a fairly early stage. A great deal more information is needed on both theoretical and clinical fronts. Therefore, I anxiously await the next round of "Recent Advances."

Reference Notes

1. Dinnsen, D., Elbert, M., & Weismer, G. On the characteristics of functional misarticulations. Paper presented to the Annual Convention of the American Speech-Language-Hearing Association, Atlanta, 1979.

2. Edwards, M.L. The use of "favorite sounds" by 14 children with phonological disorders. Paper presented at the Language Development Conference, Boston University, 1980.

3. Weiner, F., & Ellis, C. Tolerance for homonymy: A factor in children's misarticulations. Paper presented to the American Speech-Language-Hearing Association, Detroit, 1980.

References

Donegan, P., & Stampe, D. The study of natural phonology. In D. Dinnsen (Ed.), *Current approaches to phonological theory*. Bloomington: Indiana University Press, 1978.

Gallagher, T. Revision behaviors in the speech of normal children developing language. *Journal of Speech and Hearing Research*, 1977, *20*, 303-318.

Greenfield, P., & Smith, J. *Communication and the beginnings of language: The development of semantic structures in one-word speech and beyond*. New York: Academic Press, 1976.

Hodson, B. *The assessment of phonological processes*. Danville, Ill.: Interstate Printers and Publishers, 1980.

Ingram, D. *Phonological disability in children*. New York: American Elsevier Publishing, 1976.

Ingram, D. *Procedures for phonological analysis of children's language*. Baltimore, University Park Press, 1981.

Locke, J. The inference of speech perception in the phonologically disordered child. Part I: A rationale, some criteria, the conventional tests. *Journal of Speech and Hearing Disorders*, 1980, *45*, 431-444. (a)

Locke, J. The inference of speech perception in the phonologically disordered child. Part II: Some clinically novel procedures, their use, some findings. *Journal of Speech and Hearing Disorders*, 1980, *45*, 445-468. (b)

Longhurst, T., & Siegel, G. Effects of communication failure on speaker and listener behavior. *Journal of Speech and Hearing Research,* 1973, *16,* 128-140.

McReynolds, L., & Elbert, M. Criteria for phonological process analysis. *Journal of Speech and Hearing Disorders,* 1981, *46,* 197-204.

Shriberg, L., & Kwiatkowski, J. *Procedure for natural process analysis (NPA) of continuous speech samples: NPA application manual.* New York: John Wiley, 1980.

Templin, M.C. *Certain language skills in children.* Institute of Child Welfare, Monograph Series, No. 26. Minneapolis: University of Minnesota Press, 1957.

Waterson, N. Child phonology: A prosodic view. *Journal of Linguistics,* 1971, *7,* 179-221.

Weiner, F. *Phonological process analysis.* Baltimore: University Park Press, 1979.

Weiner, F. Systematic sound preference as a characteristic of phonological disability. *Journal of Speech and Hearing Disorders,* 1981, *46,* 281-286. (a)

Weiner, F. Treatment of phonological disability using the method of meaningful minimal contrast: Two case studies. *Journal of Speech and Hearing Disorders,* 1981, *46,* 97-103. (b)

Weiner, F., & Ostrowski, A. Effects of listener uncertainty on articulatory inconsistency. *Journal of Speech and Hearing Disorders,* 1979, *44,* 487-503.

Weiner, F., & Wacker, R. The development of phonology in unintelligible speakers. In N. Lass (Ed.), *Speech and language: Advance in Basic Research and Practice, Vol. 8.* New York: Academic Press, 1982.

Wepman, J.M. *Auditory discrimination test.* Chicago: Language Research Associates, 1973.

Elizabeth B. Cole and Marietta M. Paterson

Assessment and Treatment of Phonologic Disorders in the Hearing Impaired

In contemplating contributing yet another treatise on the topic of speech and hearing impairment, one gets a sense of both humility and frustration. The humility is from being in the company of clinicians, researchers, scholars, teachers, and parents who have struggled with the questions and the technology for literally centuries. (See, for example, the review in Ling, 1976, pp. 11-18). The frustration, on the other hand, is from the overwhelming feeling that it has all been said and done before—that there is very little new under the speech-for-the-deaf sun—and that still our overall results are dismal. Few would have been surprised by the statement in the 1979 American Speech-Language-Hearing Association's "Standards for Effective Oral Communication Programs" that "adequate oral communication frequently determines an individual's educational, social, and vocational success" (p. 1002). In view of that, we simply cannot be satisfied with speech intelligibility ratings of "barely intelligible," "not intelligible," and/or "would not speak" for 55.2% of the school-age hearing-impaired population (Jensema, Karchmer, & Trybus, 1978). True, the ratings are somewhat better for that proportion of the children with lesser degrees of hearing loss: 86.2% of those with losses of less than 70 dB were "very intelligible" or "intelligible." But only 54.8% of the children with losses ranging from 71-90 dB (at 500, 1000, 2000 Hz) were rated as "very intelligible" or "intelligible" and only 22.5% with losses greater than 90 dB were in that category.

In presenting speech workshops in the United States, Canada, and Australia, and in teaching graduate student teacher/clinicians, it has become apparent to both authors that the issues which are recurrently problematic regarding development of intelligibility can be divided into the following two broad areas:

Optimizing Input - guaranteeing that as much of the speech signal as possible is put within an accessible range for the child through optimum selection, fitting, and maintenance of amplification; and

Optimizing Instruction - teaching in ways that take into account information about learning, meaningful communication, oral language acquisition, acoustic phonetics, and articulatory phonetics; as well as teaching in ways that employ effective strategies for evoking and practicing motor speech skills, and for making the child's usage of good speech habits automatic in normal spontaneous oral language.

Both of these are areas which we believe require serious improvement in order for more hearing-impaired children to be achieving levels of maximum intelligibility. And, in both areas, there have been recent applications of innovative thought and research which merit widespread consideration and implementation.

Optimizing Input

Hearing Aids

That speech abilities are presently linked to the amount of auditory input available to the child seems undeniable. But reports showing a relationship between the amount of hearing loss and speech intelligibility, such as ones by Jensema, Karchmer, and Trybus (1978); Nickerson (1975); Smith (1975); and Subtelny, Whitehead, and Orlando (1980) tend to be misinterpreted by some professionals as indications of fixed and unchangeable causality. Can it be that the seriousness of the lack of audition (i.e., the simple fact of the hearing loss) makes intelligible speech a nearly unobtainable goal for the majority? Not so! comes the resounding answer from two directions:

1. from those who combine the selection and fitting of auditory prosthetic instruments with information about the acoustic properties of the spoken word; and

2. from competent users of a relatively recent program for teaching speech to hearing-impaired children, which has become popularly known as "The Ling Thing" (Ling, 1976).

When thinking about auditory input to the hearing-impaired child, one must think not only in terms of what the child's unaided thresholds are on the audiogram, but also (more so) in terms of what can become auditorily available to the child through appropriate amplification. It may be useful to employ the model of auditory learning suggested by Hirsh (1970) (detection, discrimination, identification, comprehension) in order to organize the issues surrounding this part of the problem. Detection is the necessary—but not sufficient—prerequisite for the other three abilities to be learned. Consequently, the first consideration is to provide sufficient gain in the child's amplification system to allow the child to detect all of the acoustic cues which he or she is capable of receiving. Recent processes for initial hearing aid selection (e.g., Berger, Hagberg, & Rane, 1977) have attempted to make the procedure a more precise and scientific process, and have consequently included information about speech spectrum characteristics in the calculations. As Byrne (1979), Libby (1980), and Yanick (1980) suggest, gain and output levels can be determined using prescriptive methods that are based on the speech spectrum. Then real ear measurements need to be used for optimizing the fitting by aid adjustments and/or by coupling modifications. In determining the appropriateness of the hearing aid selected and in making adjustments based on real ear (aided) responses, it is obviously critical to employ guidelines which take speech spectrum characteristics into account if the goal is to assure their maximum detectability. One such procedure is that suggested by Ling and Ling (1978). That is, in order for speech to be detected within a normal conversational distance of 2 meters or less, the child's aided responses need to fall within or above the range covered by a banana-shaped area on the audiogram, while maintaining relative proportions adequate for avoiding masking effects. This "speech banana" has approximately a 20 dB intensity range and extends from below 250 Hz through above 6000 Hz in order to account for all of the major acoustic cues in speech. At the present time, hearing aids do not routinely provide large amounts of gain at the upper end of that frequency range (6000 to 8000 Hz). However, there are now a number of aids providing significant amplification (peaks of 50 to 60 dB) at or above 5000 Hz (Rudmin, in press). With regard to amounts of gain possible, Rudmin (1982) found more than 80 models of ear level hearing aids whose (full-on) high frequency average gain was 60 dB or greater. Ling (1981b) offers the clinical observation that children with unaided thresholds down to the following levels can generally be provided gain sufficient to allow the children to detect the essential speech cues:

250	500	1000	2000	4000
85	100	115	115	95 dB

In other words, with a loss of 115 dB at 2000 Hz (for example), it is possible to provide enough real ear gain (65 to 75 dB) in order to expect the child to be evidencing aided responses at approximately 40 to 50 dB. If this were the case, the child could be expected to be able to detect (at a distance of 2 meters), the following acoustic cues which are centered around 2000 Hz ± ½ octave: the second formant of the front vowels, second transition place cues for most consonants, second and third transitions for liquids; turbulence of [ʃ]; [θ]; and [f]; and the third formant for some vowels (Ling, 1976).

In view of the present hearing aid technology, the 54.8% statistic for intelligibility among children with 71-90 dB losses is even more disturbing. Today, a 90 dB threshold at 4000 Hz represents a great deal of residual hearing *potentially* usable for speech cue detection, once optimally aided. However, it should be emphasized that hearing abilities within the speech banana are only potentially usable. That is, the ability to detect these elements auditorily will not automatically guarantee the use of that acoustic information, accessible as it is. A parallel could be drawn here to a normally hearing adult who is physically capable of detecting all of the essential speech sound contrasts in any language which is foreign to him. But the foreign language sounds like just so much verbal noise, unless, or until, the salient speech sound differences are brought to the adult's attention for communicative reasons, and/or through conscious effort on the part of a teacher. And even then, consciously knowing that the differences exist will not guarantee that henceforth the adult will immediately and automatically discriminate among them in listening to the native speaker's oral language. However, in order to even begin this auditory discrimination, identification, and comprehension process, the speech sounds initially must be accessible. Although often further compounded by a lack of normal clarity, the case is similar for a hearing-impaired child: detection is a necessary, but not sufficient, condition in order for auditory learning to occur.

Earmold Coupling Modifications

In addition to advances internal to the aid itself, another area of recent research and innovation is that of earmold coupling systems. (Gastmeier, 1981; Grave & Metzinger, 1981; Killion & Monser, 1980; Libby, 1980, 1981). Modifications can be made in the characteristics of venting, damper elements, and acoustic horns, and done either independently or simultaneously to produce controllable effects on the shape, bandwidth, and fidelity of the system. For example, using a fused mesh damper in the end of the earhook, a detrimental resonance peak at 1000 Hz can be smoothed (Gastmeier, 1981; Libby, 1980, 1981). Additionally, an increasing diameter in the earhook tubing-earmold tip sequence can be maintained producing an acoustic horn effect (Libby, 1980). The acoustic horn has been reported by Libby (1981) as typically producing improvement in sound field warble tone aided thresholds at 3000 to 4000 Hz of 5 to 15 dB (range = 0 to 24 dB). Similarly, Grave and Metzinger (1981) found an average of 13 dB improvement in functional gain at 4000 Hz using an undamped acoustic horn (range = 5 dB to +45 dB). It should be noted that the apparent increase in gain produced by modifications of the earmold coupling system is actually compensating for attenuation which normally occurs using standard earmold coupling procedures. This underlines once again the need to do real ear measurements and the lack of rationale for relying simply on hearing aid manufacturer's specifications in order to estimate amounts of gain being realized by the child. However, it also means that using personal hearing aids,[1] speech information (particularly consonantal) in the 2000 to 4000 Hz range may be more accessible for larger numbers of children who have some residual hearing in that range.

But what about the child who has only low frequency hearing (the frequently seen "corner" audiogram)? Even optimally aided, this child may not be capable of detecting the higher-frequency components of the speech signal. Fortunately, however, if he has aided responses between 30 to 45 dB even at only 250 Hz, he will still be able to detect the fundamental frequency of most female voices; some harmonics of male voices; the nasal murmur for [m, n, ŋ]; the first formant for some vowels; as well as cues for voicing, intonation, intensity, and duration. And, with instruction, these speech cues can make a major contribution toward making his voice sound "normal"—that is, without the hypernasal, monotone, arrhythmic qualities often cited as characterizing "deaf speech" (Nickerson, 1975; Smith, 1975; Subtelny et al., 1980).

Visual and Tactile Devices and Procedures

For the speech sounds with components which are auditorily undetectable, obviously sense modalities other than auditory (i.e., visual, tactile) will have to be employed for bringing the key elements of the sounds within range of the child's attention (Ling, 1976, p. 17, 45-65). Fortunately, spoken communication contains numerous contextual, lexical, semantic, and syntactic redundancies so that even normally hearing people are not utilizing all of the auditory information available to them in order to understand spoken messages (Fry, 1978, pp. 37-39). The underlying assumption seems to be that, using many of the visual and tactile devices, key element(s) can be brought to the child's attention, and then both recognition and production practiced to automaticity in selected linguistic contexts. Then, in normal conversational situations (without the device), the child's linguistic knowledge will allow use of some of those redundancies to comprehend messages and to produce sounds even when lacking acoustic cues. There are a number of workers in this area who have developed visual and tactile devices for recoding the speech signal in order to overcome hearing impairment which precludes auditory detection of the essential acoustic components. (See reviews in Boothroyd, 1975; Oller, Payne, & Gavin, 1980; Strong, 1975.)

When considering the use of visual and tactile devices or procedures for speech training with children, two cautions immediately arise. One concerns the choice of children with whom they are used. It should go without saying that it would be counterproductive to use a visual or tactile device with a child who could actually be detecting the targeted speech component(s) auditorily when optimally aided. (See Ling, 1976, pp. 22-65, for a discussion of the specific advantages of the ear in preference to either vision or taction for detecting speech patterns.)

The other caution particularly concerns those visual and tactile devices that are not portable, such as desk model vibratory devices. The problem with use of these devices is that tasks or abilities developed in using them may remain tied to that training situation and those devices. For example, although it has been possible to train severely-to-profoundly deaf adolescents to discriminate between word pairs based on tactile input alone (Oller et al., 1980), the sense of touch has yet to be successfully employed by itself for understanding speech in normal communication situations. As the Boothroyd (1975), Boothroyd, Archambault, Adams, and Storm (1975), and Strong (1975) results suggest, questions about carry-over from training on isolated parameters to real communication situations have yet to be fully answered.

One other speech recoding procedure should be mentioned at this juncture: the use of Cued Speech (Cornett, 1967). This is a visual system of gestures ("cues") which are used to reduce ambiguity among sounds that appear identical on the lips (e.g., there is a different hand position for signifying [d] versus [t] versus [n] since these three are visually synonymous). The gestures, performed by the speaker in conjunction with talking, are directly tied to the verbal message, and essentially provide a visible recoding of part of the phonetic information. Although use of Cued Speech has been adopted in a number of programs in North America and elsewhere since its introduction in 1967, there have been only three systematic studies of its effectiveness with hearing-impaired children. Results of all three studies have been generally favorable toward the use of cueing, specifically with profoundly hearing-impaired children. It has been shown, for example, that cueing can facilitate speech-reading of isolated sentences, phrases, and words (Clarke & Ling, 1976; Ling & Clarke, 1975). And the extensive study by Nicholls (Note 1) evidenced mean speech reception scores of over 95% for cues used with either lipreading or with lipreading and audition. (Note: "Speech reception" in the Nicholls study refers to prediction of the key word in sentence materials.) However, particularly in view of the need for continued research, the decision to use Cued Speech should be a carefully considered one to avoid some of the following pitfalls of its possible misuse.

As mentioned above, simply being capable of detecting speech features produced by a sender will not necessarily result in the automatic use of available hearing for discrimination and identification of the salient sound patterns, or for comprehension of the sender's message. The child's actual use of his or her auditory capabilities will depend on a variety of factors such as attention, motivation, and knowledge of the fact that verbal-auditory communications have meaning and value, as well as on training and experience with the acoustic elements whose differentiation is salient in the target language. Fortunately, Nicholls's (Note 1) results support the contention that use of cueing does not have a detrimental effect on the child's use of audition for speech reception (in fact, quite the reverse). But promoting the child's optimal use of whatever residual hearing exists will undoubtedly require continued attention and sustained effort on the part of the teacher.

A second possible problem is related to this statement by Cornett (1967):

> The teacher himself will have to spend many hours in practice before he becomes fluent enough to cue his speech . . . without so much preoccupation with the communication process as to impede spontaneity and flexibility of thought in the teaching process. (p. 11)

Along with possibly impeding "spontaneity and flexibility of thought," slow and belabored cueing can distort the normal rhythmic features and pitch variations of the spoken language it is accompanying. When these meaning-loaded components are distorted, several effects are likely:

1. the child may not learn that pitch and rhythm features have meaning and salience in spoken messages; and

2. since the distorted prosodic elements are those which can be auditorily detected by nearly all hearing-impaired children, then the very valuable information that the "corner" audiogram child can

listen to is not presented in a normal fashion. It would, consequently, not be surprising if that child's own speech were similarly arrhythmic and/or distorted in intonational contour.

Finally, having determined that fluency and continued attention to audition are necessary accompaniments to optimal usage of cueing with profoundly hearing-impaired children, the teacher needs to be fully aware that cueing is intended to be an adjunct to spoken language. While the studies cited above suggest that cueing helps the child's reception of oral messages, it should not be expected to simultaneously and automatically teach productive oral language, and/or productive speech skills (Cornett, 1975).

Cochlear Implants

The House Ear Institute (Los Angeles) began investigating the cochlear implant in 1960 with the goal of being able to restore hearing to the deaf by means of the implant (House, Bode, & Berliner, 1981). As of July 1981, a total of 178 persons had received single-electrode cochlear implants either at the Institute or through one of approximately 20 other co-investigators in the United States. Both objective and subjective responses have been generally quite positive in expressions of post-implant improvement (e.g., Campos, 1981; House, Bode, & Berliner, 1981; Luetje, 1981). Results of initial experimentation with multiple electrode implants have been similarly positive (Clark & Tong, 1981). For example, marked improvement in comprehension was obtained by two patients from means of 5% and 11% for a lipreading-alone condition, as compared to 32% and 38% comprehension for the condition when the implant was utilized in addition to lipreading (Martin, Tong, & Clark, 1981). At its present level of development, however, neither single nor multiple electrode implant restores hearing to the extent that it is possible to understand speech through its use alone, and continuing research is focused on developing improved ancillary devices for the processing of speech. What can be detected and used to advantage according to most reports are primarily voicing, nasality, intensity, and durational cues. That this voicing and prosodic information is beneficial is perhaps best attested to by the report that 152 of the 178 implant patients (associated with the House Institute co-investigation) are using the device on a regular basis (House, Bode, & Berliner, 1981). Obviously, selection of candidates for the implant is a crucial issue, and the cochlear implant is still considered an "investigational" procedure by the U.S. Food and Drug Administration (Luetje, 1981). Procedures and criteria for selection have consequently been carefully outlined by the researchers.

However, as Campos states,

> All possible non-invasive alternatives should be pursued
> with each candidate, prior to cochlear implantation.
> However, the cochlear implant. . . should continue to be
> available. . . as a viable means of communication when
> hearing aids are not helpful. (1981, p. 30)

It is possible that, with continued research, cochlear implants may become
an increasingly viable part of the (re)habilitation procedure. It bears mentioning, however, that the rehabilitation problems presented by many post
implant patients at the present time are largely different from those
presented by the majority of hearing-impaired children who are learning
language for the first time and who are doing that with the presence of
some aidable residual hearing.

Summary

The foregoing discussion touches briefly on some of the present
technological and procedural capabilities for optimizing the speech input
to the child, whether auditorily, visually, or tactilely. Unfortunately, for
a variety of reasons, capability is not necessarily accompanied by educational application and implementation.

Optimizing Instruction

The Problem

The problem is, basically, that in spite of all of the existing information
and technology, more than half of our school-age hearing-impaired
children are still rated as less than intelligible. Observations of
characteristics of deaf speech by Hudgins and Numbers (1942) have been
repeatedly and recently verified (see review in Ling, 1976; also, Nickerson,
1975; Smith, 1975; Subtelny et al., 1980). All authors mention such problems as inadequate breath control, excessive and inappropriate pauses,
inappropriate pitch and intonation, hypernasality, excessive tenseness, inappropriate duration of both stressed and unstressed syllables, and omission or misarticulation of some phonemes.

Interestingly, there is not one characteristic of deaf speech mentioned
by those authors that is not also mentioned by Ling (1976) as a remediable,

or preferably, an avoidable problem. In what could be interpreted as an explanation for the continuing poor state of affairs, Ling wrote in 1976:

> Technological advances, emerging knowledge in speech science, and contributions from related areas are having little, or no impact on the speech patterns of many children. . . . It may be concluded that teachers do not have or are not using strategies which integrate current knowledge with compatible, traditional procedures. (pp. 17-18)

This assertion was essentially echoed by Hochberg, Levitt, and Osberger (1980) in a 3-year (U.S.) nationwide project whose long-term goal was to improve speech services to hearing-impaired children. Reasons cited for minimal progress in the area of speech-teaching included limited expectations for the children's speech and inadequate pre-service training in speech teaching. Although 80% of the classroom teachers felt speech-training was important, only 42% of the teachers spent as much as 6 to 20 minutes per day on speech development, and 30% spent between 1 and 15 minutes per day on speech maintenance. Approximately 37% and 45% of the teachers provided no speech development or maintenance (respectively) at all. In view of these numbers, one might wonder how it was ever possible at all for the 54.8% of the children with severe losses and 22.5% of the children with profound losses to achieve speech intelligibility ratings of "very intelligible" and "intelligible." Perhaps this is yet another case of children learning in spite of us, rather than because of us. Of course, some professionals are obtaining intelligibility scores for some hearing-impaired children that are not statistically different from the scores of their normally hearing peers (Ling, 1981a). This certainly lends credibility to the contention that the key to the solution lies in the child's education, and by extension, in the persons responsible for that education. And, in fact, teachers and speech specialists in the Hochberg et al. (1980) survey responded that 80-95% of them would benefit from continuing education in how to improve their competence in speech training. In order to begin to meet some of this need, Hochberg et al. instituted a pilot program of in-service training and a pilot pre-service workshop for faculty members of teacher-training programs. They note that "the magnitude of the problem is even more widespread and far-reaching than was initially supposed, and by and large, the professional personnel most directly involved in the provision of speech services. . . are unprepared to meet [the hearing-impaired children's] needs effectively" (p. 483).

Some Solutions

It would be an ambitious and futile project, indeed, to pretend to fully respond to the needs expressed by teachers and speech specialists by means of anything less than the Hochberg et al. (1980) programs mentioned above. As a partial and potentially very satisfying response, however, the authors would like to refer readers to the speech-teaching program and related ideas described in, for example, Ling (1976, 1978, 1979, 1981a, 1981b) and Ling and Ling (1978). This "Ling Thing," in the opinion of the authors, answers the need for a scientific and systematic program for teaching speech skills to school-age hearing-impaired children. Based on our own experience in using the program and in teaching others to use it, we have observed that there are a number of educational issues and techniques that are recurrently problematic for teachers and clinicians using the program. Space limitations require focusing on a selected few.

The essential concept in working on speech with hearing-impaired children is that the goal is intelligibility in spontaneous use of oral language (Ling, 1979). Somehow this goal often seems to become obscured. One source of the problem may be an over-emphasis on analytic teaching of specific speech segments. A "forest and trees" situation has apparently been created by teachers' desire for and comfort in using techniques primarily designed for simply evoking and rote-practicing speech sounds. Given time and skilled effort, this focus on the elements (albeit co-articulated) is likely to result in the child acquiring great facility in motor speech (articulation) skills. However, the expectation seems to be that intelligible, spontaneous, oral language will also automatically result from motor speech facility. And this is simply not the case. As Ling says, "Motor speech skills are essential but insufficient for the development of spoken communication" (1979, p. 217). A parallel could be drawn to a musician doing tone exercises and practicing memorized scales with the expectation that that would automatically enable him to play Mozart sonatas. Just as the ability to play a Mozart sonata requires a much greater knowledge of music, so does intelligible, spontaneous, oral language require a much greater knowledge of the conventions for communicating and encoding meaning in oral language. In fact, in terms of time allocation, the teacher's primary preoccupation needs to be with facilitating the growth of oral language in meaningful situations. Building speech intelligibility into such a program requires consistent overall expectations for maximum clarity, as well as planned occasions for both incidental and scheduled motor speech practice.

The next two sections of this chapter will offer concrete suggestions aimed at clarifying the intended focus on intelligibility in spontaneous oral language. The suggestions are intended to respond to two sources of misdirection regarding that goal: the overemphasis on speech element minutiae, and the neglect of prosody.

1. Organizing Learning/Teaching

The contention has been made that speech teaching has placed an overemphasis on the evocation and repetitious practice of coarticulated syllables. The question then arises as to how speech learning and teaching can be organized in order to include an appropriate emphasis on motor speech practice within the overall program. It should be noted that some parts of the following discussion could be classified as suggestions for the "transfer to phonology" of phonetic skills. However, the authors would prefer to avoid the exclusively "bottom-up" inference that may be inherent in the idea of phonologic transfer. Our approach is one that attempts to move quickly and recursively from whole to parts to whole (and so on), incorporating facets of "bottom-up" teaching into what is, fundamentally, a "top-down" view of oral language and speech development. Speech learning/teaching following this approach can be discussed in terms of incidental learning/teaching, and scheduled learning/teaching.

Incidental learning/teaching begins with the teacher's consistent expectation for maximum clarity of production of the speech aspects the child has mastered on a phonetic level. It is true that one of the most powerful motivations for children to use clear speech could be expected to be the fact that people understand them better when they speak clearly. However, listeners tend to fill in the gaps and mentally correct distortions from contextual and linguistic redundancy. That is, listeners familiar with the child may be able and willing to adjust their own speech perceptual mechanisms in such a way that they can understand the child even without hearing the level of speech clarity of which the child may be capable. However, unfamiliar listeners are much less likely to be able and willing to make the perceptual adjustments necessary for understanding the child, which has the effect of limiting the number of people with whom communication is possible. Consequently, in order to help the child speak as clearly as possible, as well as learn to automatically implement newly acquired skills, feedback-providing techniques can be consciously employed.

One such technique is positive reinforcement of the child's efforts toward overall clarity and/or of the clarity of specific speech aspects. This can be helpful since it indicates to the child what is being done correctly. Positive reinforcement is also likely to encourage the child's continued efforts, which can be especially important when intelligibility problems are multiple. Reinforcement can be verbal, accompanied or not by a smile, a pat, or a checkmark on the chalkboard.

Another technique for incidental learning/teaching is that of simply reminding the child to attend to speech clarity. This can be accomplished through adoption of a quizzical expression, for example, or by means of a verbal reminder about specific "tricky" words or sounds as they occur. Again, though, this kind of reminding is likely to be most useful for speech aspects that have been mastered on a motor speech level, and is preferably done in a gentle, good-humored fashion. Above all, it should be avoided if there is a chance that it could destroy a communicative event. Often the child's message or a conversational exchange will be judged more important than interrupting to practice a faulty /s/ or /r/. It is suggested that the reminding be accomplished unobtrusively and followed by immediate self-correction on the child's part. If this is not the case, then the teacher can make note of the specific difficulty and incorporate it into later scheduled practice.

The expectation for intelligibility and the techniques mentioned for skillful reinforcement and reminding are, perhaps, obvious to many readers. But these aspects are probably the most difficult ones to employ, as well as the most important ones in terms of actually realizing improvement in the child's intelligibility in spontaneous oral language. Naturally, the effort is likely to be most fruitful if it is a concerted one with all of the child's teachers and family involved to the greatest extent possible.

There is another kind of incidental speech learning/teaching which can occur at various times in the day. This is incidental phonetic practice of targets which a number of children have in common. One example of an activity for this kind of practice is the use of a "Speech Pocket." One could make a pocket out of construction paper and tape it to the back of the classroom door, then jot down a series of targets for the week on cards which fit in the pocket. For example, the group targets could be: (1) bama; (2) bibiBI; (3) fubufubu; (4) 1, 2, 3, 4, 5; (5)∧s_la∧s_la_sla. Each time the class leaves the room, the children line up one by one and produce the target on the card chosen from the pocket as they file out of the room. For variety, the cards could have questions loaded with target sounds written on them, or simple games such as having everyone name a different animal, bird, fruit or state with the /m/ sound in it.

Scheduled learning/teaching can occur in a variety of ways. Ling (1976) recommends providing each child with several practice sessions of 2 to 3 minutes duration at spaced intervals during the day. On the other hand, some teachers have found that as they are becoming familiar with the system, one individual session of 8 to 10 minutes duration is more manageable. Organization of the activities during that individual session can follow a format such as that exemplified in Table 4-1.

Table 4-1
Sample of Individual Teaching Plan for Scheduled Practice

Name:

Date(s):

Target-Stage of Practice	Sense Modality		Techniques	Activities, Materials	Comments
1. /f/ - mutliple redu-plicated syllables, "legato," one breath	Vision Touch →	step 1.	Go from long ʌf and release into vowel ʌf⌣a, slowly with control.	Move hand on table to show how long to hold /ʌf.../, when hand reaches pencil say /a:/.	-Do again, same steps. -Attention to /fi, fu/. Loses frication when coarticulating.
fa fa fa fi fi fi fu⌣fu fu	Audition	step 2.	Remove the crutch of /ʌ/- have child imitate vocali-zation of f ⌣a¹. Check for good coarticu-lation.		
		step 3.	Have child self-monitor, maintain, repeat 3 times for today with /a, i, u/		
2. ba/ma - a. auditory discrimination² b. multiple recursive syllables /ba⌣ma ba⌣ma ba⌣ma/	Audition (free variation)	step 1.	Auditory discrimination - follow-up from last time, build confidence in ability to differentiate ba-ma	2 sets colored blocks	good ✓ -able to discri-minate with confidence -able to do at normal rate

/biꞈmi/,etc.
/buꞈmu/,etc.

Then:
/biꞈma/
/buꞈmi/

step 2.   Syllable practice. Alternate each set 5 times. Student will self-monitor. Do once slowly; then try normal rate.

-encourage more correct productions in meaningful contexts.

3.   /p/ meaningful use
- in initial position only
- look for self correction
- consistent production

Audition
Vision
Touch

step 1.   Quickly review production of /p/ with a range of known vowels.

-good practice,
-not fully automatic at meaningful level

2 pens, 2 pandas,
2 pans, 2 pennies,
2 pears, 2 pigs.

step 2.   Game round the table
a. Name objects.
Q. What's that?
A. It's a _____.

b. Take turns giving and following directions for placing objects in strange places.
Pass me a/the _____ in the _____.
Put a/the _____ a/the _____.

- Trouble with /p/ after the word *The* - practice this context.

¹ The key is to hold the /f/ frication longer than necessary, and then release smoothly into the vowel.
² See Paterson, 1982.

Briefly, the lesson plan format specifies each of the following aspects:

- The stage of practice of each target. Particular targets could be at the stage, for example, of evocation; single, controlled production; multiple repetition (e.g., reduplicated syllables, alternated syllables, recursive or freely varied syllables); or meaningful use in selected words, phrases, expressions, or sentences.
- The appropriate sense modality to be used. This aspect requires knowledge of the child's aided audiogram, as well as some knowledge of acoustic phonetics. If the child has audition that will allow him to hear the salient acoustic elements of the target sound, then use of that auditory capability can be maximized. If, for example, the child has adequately aided hearing at 250 Hz and at 500 Hz, then the acoustic cues[2] distinguishing between /ba/ and /ma/ are available. Thus, the child can be expected to learn to auditorily discriminate between the two sounds. When the hearing loss precludes use of residual hearing, vision and touch will be helpful in evoking and practicing production of a number of sounds. Selective and combined use of sense modalities for speech teaching is described by Ling (1976) and Ling and Ling (1978); and the acoustic characteristics of English are detailed in a number of sources, including Fry (1976), Ling (1978), Minifie (1973), Pickett (1980).
- Techniques for evoking sounds for facilitating practice. Ling (1976) presents a large number of strategies for these purposes.
- Materials, reinforcers, activities. (Self-explanatory)
- The "comments" column is intended for any teacher comments during or after the session which will aid in planning further practice.

The intent of this section has been to describe the overall organization of an approach for speech learning/teaching, the goal of which is the child's use of maximum clarity in meaningful spontaneous productions. The motor speech practice sessions provide an increasing number of productive abilities which can subsequently begin to be required in spontaneous use. However, these scheduled sessions occur for, at most, a total of 15 to 20 minutes per day, and cannot be expected to automatically result in improved intelligibility in spontaneous oral language. Suggestions outlined above for incidental learning/teaching are intended to aid in that process.

2. Strategies for Development of Prosodic Elements

In addition to a need to redirect what appears to be an over-abundance of energy spent in coarticulated syllable practice, the authors perceive a concomitant need to direct more attention to the neglected area of prosody.

The prosodic components of speech in the Ling program are specified as vocalization, duration, intensity, and pitch. "Vocalization" can be interpreted to mean normal quality phonation, or use of an appropriately relaxed and oral voice. Use of normal voicing is important in order to avoid vocal strain, to make pitch and rhythmic changes, and to allow for the oral/nasal contrast. It is also aesthetically more pleasing for the listener. Automatic, controlled flexibility in use of the other three aspects (duration, intensity, and pitch) in speech allows the talker to implement stress, rhythm, and intonation conventions to mark constituent boundaries, as well as to express intent and emotion in ways which the listener will expect and understand. That the prosodic aspects are problem areas for hearing-impaired speakers has been repeatedly noted in the literature (Boone, 1966; Hudgins & Numbers, 1942; Ling, 1976; Nickerson, 1975; Martony, 1968; Smith, 1975; Subtelny et al., 1980). This is particularly distressing in view of the fact that voicing, duration, intensity, and pitch cues are generally available to adequately aided children, even those with only minimal residual hearing (Ling, 1976). The problem seems to be grounded in a lack of information not only about the availability of the acoustic cues, but also about the mechanics of evoking and rehearsing these aspects in speech related ways, and about the necessity of continually and consciously employing and requiring normal variation in developing the segmental aspects.

The aspects of speech selected for separate discussion here include vocal quality, duration, nasality, intensity, and pitch. For each of the selected aspects, the following topics will be addressed: (a) typical problems; (b) physiologic causes; (c) aim of remediation; (d) auditory requirements; and (e) techniques for remediation. The first section to follow will outline techniques for evoking and practicing each aspect on a motor speech level. The final section will suggest activities for getting those practiced abilities to appear in the child's meaningful spoken language.

Vocal Quality and Duration

Typical problems

Hearing-impaired children judged as having an overall voice and breath control problem may evidence one or more of the following: harsh or strident voice quality, abnormal pitch variation, monotone voice, inability to control intensity differences, stop-start vocal production ("machine gun-like" speech), inability to maintain the voiced-voiceless distinction between consonants, talking on residual air, and nasal-sounding vocal production (Boone, 1966, pp. 636; Calvert & Silverman, 1975, pp. 183-190;

Ling, 1976, pp. 12–17; Monsen, 1976, p. 33, 1979, pp. 270–288; Mahashie, Note 2).

Physiologic causes

Hearing-impaired children are born with normal respiratory systems and the capacity for normal laryngeal/pharyngeal function. However, laryngeal abnormalities in the adduction and abduction of the vocal folds and in the production of subglottal pressure can be acquired over time (Pickett, 1980; Mahashie, Note 2). According to Ling (1976), reasons for such abnormality may be several: minimal practice in oral communication, inadequate exploitation of residual audition, a reliance on sensation of tactile vibration for monitoring of articulator placement, and poor voicing habits resulting from uninformed teaching strategies.

Aim of remediation

Remediation goals are to develop controlled vocalizations on well-supported oral breath, to promote correct use of subglottal pressure for controlled durational practice, to remediate improper vocal fold tension in vowel production, and to promote flexibility of tongue movement through coarticulation of vowels and some consonants.

Auditory requirements

Acoustic cues for the detection of the center fundamental frequency of the voice (F_0) for male, female, and child speakers range from approximately 100 to 265 Hertz (Pickett, 1980). As durational variation is one of several factors at least partially carried on the fundamental frequency, children with adequately aided residual audition extending only up to 500 Hz should be able to detect the presence or absence of voicing and subsequently be able to learn to judge durational differences (Ling, 1976, pp. 27–29; Pickett, 1980, pp. 46–47, 61).

Vocal quality work requires use of vowels. Consequently, it is relevant that with adequately aided residual hearing extending only up to 500 Hz, the first formants (F_1) of vowels are perceptible. Residual audition up to 1000 Hz renders F_1 of all vowels and the second formant (F_2) of the low and mid vowels audible. Residual audition up to 2500 Hz would render both formants of all vowels audible and discriminable (Ling, 1976, pp. 227–228; Ling & Ling, 1978, pp. 68–69).

Suggested techniques for remediation

Step 1. Produce a long, strong oral breathstream while holding the sound /a/. The child can feel the release of the teacher's breath with his or her own hand. Then the child could imitate the teacher, attempting to produce the same quality of breathstream while feeling the air flow across his or her own hand. Exaggerated breathiness can be encouraged at this stage with no danger to the child's speech production. Once the child develops flexibility and speed of vocalizations on the breathstream, the exaggerated breathiness will disappear.

Alternative techniques for step 1.

a. Whispering

If the child is unable to produce a breathy flow of air as per Step 1, then a more elemental strategy to evoke the oral breathstream may be required. One could have the child simply blow air from the mouth, making no attempt to voice the vowel /a/ and continue practice until the child is more comfortable with the feeling of the breath flow and is beginning to monitor the strength of the breath with his or her hand. In effect, the child is simply whispering the /h/ phoneme. The result of this is to eliminate vocal fold tension for the present and promote breathiness (Ling, 1976, pp. 204–220, 233). Then the child could make 3 to 5 productions in a row of the same "quality." There should be no harsh or sudden stopping at the end of a breath, but a relaxed cessation. Next, attempt to have the child softly voice /a/ as a syllable is initiated with /h/; the concentration should be on breath flow production. The goal is for the child to coordinate initiation of voicing (based on vocal fold tension) with release of breath (based on adequate subglottal pressure).

b. Panting

It is possible that, on demand, a child may be unable to produce any breathy flow of air at all, even through the whispering technique. To give the child an idea of the required response, it may be helpful to practice panting. The child could imitate short intakes and releases of air as a puppy would in panting and then monitor the resultant breath flow with his or her hand until the sensation of the air passing across the pharyngeal wall and the effect of diaphragmatic excursion feels comfortable. Then, the child could continue to produce multiple repetitions of the short panting but elongate the last breath. This would produce whispered /h/. Production could be stabilized by using the suggestions for whispering (Alternative technique "a").

Step 2. Next the child might produce a very long /a/ sound. The teacher should stop the child's vocalization of the vowel if the sound becomes nasal, harsh, or abnormal in pitch so that learning in error is not promoted. Point out the undesirable change so the child can learn to monitor the quality of his or her own vocalizations. Positively reinforce the child for improved production. Repeat this step until good quality, long duration production is stabilized.

Step 3. Here the child practices initiating, releasing, and re-initiating the vowel /a/, always with the same oral, breath-supported sound. It may be helpful for the teacher to use a hand cue to signal initiation and cessation of syllables and to indicate varying vowel durations. Other ideas for indicating changes in vowel duration include using different lengths of yarn or colored paper, having the child vocalize while tracing 12 inches of /a/ on a ruler, and having the child hold the sound for a given number of seconds.

Step 4. Next, one might move on to syllable practice, continuing to require a relaxed, oral sound, well supported by breath. The teacher could introduce a known consonant and have the child repeat the syllables so that phonation does not cease in-between (i.e., ba͜ba͜ba͜ba). This type of practice is the remedial base for building coarticulation skill and can be likened to "legato" playing of a musical instrument. The object is to go smoothly from one sound to another with a minimal break in phonation. Having the child prolong the vowel prior to beginning the next syllable/consonant is a technique which can be beneficially used in early practice of all phonemes. Once brought to normal rate this technique has the potential of resulting in increased control and fluency of coarticulation.

Step 5. Next one might vary the length and speed of practice so that the child develops confidence and flexibility. "Legato" practice is facilitating at first, but now the child needs to add controlled "staccato" production of sounds to the repertoire. Staccato production occurs when phonation ceases after every syllable and the child must re-initiate with correct vocal-fold tension and subglottal pressure (i.e., ba-ba-ba-ba). The staccato productions shouuld be alternated with the legato (e.g., /ba-ba-ba͜ba/ or /ba͜ba͜ba-ba-ba/) at varying rates of production. By the time the child's accuracy and ease of production have reached the Step 5 level, it is important to recursively integrate the suprasegmentals into the phonetic level practice. For example, as soon as the child has reached this stage of multiple repetitions, practice with stress change could be incorporated. Thus /ba-ba-ba/ becomes /BA-ba-ba/ or /ba-BA-ba/.

Step 6. At this stage of practice, voice and durational control can be generalized to practice of other vowels and diphthongs. Sets or combinations of vowels can be practiced to develop the flexibility in tongue control needed for accuracy, speed, and economical coarticulation in connected speech. That is, once the first 3 vowels /a/, /i/, /u/ have been stabilized in multiple repeated consonant-vowel syllables, combinations of these vowels can be encouraged in free variation with each other. It may be especially helpful to begin this varied vowel practice with one of the high front vowels gliding into one of the back vowels (e.g., /i‿u/). This type of articulatory contrast will produce the greatest amount of obvious tongue movement. It also will highlight the transitions in second formants for the child with adequate hearing. The goal is to obviate the "neutral quality" typical in many hearing-impaired persons' speech (Rothman, 1976, p. 129). Other helpful combinations include: /aI/, /au/, /Ia/, /Iu/. Those combined with /I/ promote the production of the /j/ semivowel which can thus be taught just after the diphthongs in the First Step vowels. (See Ling's [1976] "Phonetic Level Evaluation" form.) For both diphthongs and the /j/ semivowel, the child might initially prolong the first element of the combination until given a hand cue to continue onto the second element (e.g., /a‿i/ or /aʲja/).

Step 7. All subsequently acquired phonemes should be practiced with good voice quality and control of duration as described above.

Nasality

NOTE: Nasality is not a prosodic feature. However, production of nasal-sounding voice is inextricably linked with voice and breath production. Furthermore, it merits separate treatment since it is one of the most commonly cited characteristics of "deaf speech."

Typical problems

The child with hypernasality exhibits speech that is excessively nasal, neutral, or central-sounding rather than oral, clear, forward-sounding.

Physiologic causes

As is well known to speech-language pathologists and audiologists, production of oral or nasal sounds is controlled by the movement of the velum in closing or opening the velopharyngeal port. Hearing-impaired children at birth have the capacity for the development of normal functioning of the velopharynx. However, they often seem to acquire problems making appropriate oral/nasal contrasts. Abnormalities in the opening/closing action of the velum can be acquired through insufficient use of the auditory modality to monitor production of oral sounds, inadequate teaching of the oral/nasal contrast in motor speech production resulting in practiced error on the part of the child, and overall insufficient oral stimulation and practice. (For a more complete discussion of nasality, the reader is directed to Ling, 1976, pp. 249-251.)

Aim of remediation

Remediation goals are to improve auditory awareness of the difference between oral and nasal production of sounds, to develop the oral/nasal contrast in motor speech production, and to remediate faulty velopharyngeal function through practice of facilitative sets of syllables.

Auditory requirements

Children with adequately aided residual audition only up to 500 Hz can detect and discriminate nasality, since the nasal murmur or steady state band of energy which identifies the nasal sounds falls at or below 300 Hz (Ling, 1976, pp. 262-263).

Techniques for remediation

Step 1. The teacher could begin by establishing the ability to auditorily discriminate a nasal from an oral sound. The /ba/ versus /ma/ sounds are suggested initially, since they represent one of the most typical auditory and articulatory confusions. One can simply use two sets of colored blocks and have the child select the color which represents either the /ba/ or the /ma/ as the teacher says one or the other. At first it may be helpful for the teacher to slightly exaggerate the length of the nasal in the syllable [ma] or the plosive burst in the syllable [ba] in order that the child focuses on the salient acoustic properties of the two sounds. After the child has consistently discriminated auditorily between the two syllables, the roles then can be reversed so that the child is producing the /ma/ and /ba/ syllables. More ideas for this and other types of auditory discrimination work are described by Paterson (1982).

Step 2. Reteach phonemes which have already been acquired but which are produced with excessive nasality. Use the steps outlined for remediation of vocal quality and duration to help promote oral sounds.

Step 3. Sets of syllables with adjacent nasal and oral consonants can be practiced in order to facilitate rapid and smooth opening and closing of the velum. All consonant manners of production can be contrasted with all nasal sounds. Initially, however, the voiceless fricatives are especially useful because of their very strong breathstream, which reminds the child of oral production and seems to promote it. The following are examples of various facilitative combinations of syllables:

Condition 1:   (a) /m, n, or ŋ/ versus /f, ʃ, θ/, and later /s/
              e.g., /ʌmʃa‿ʌmʃa‿ʌmʃa‿ʌmʃi/
              /ʌnfa‿ʌnfi‿ʌnfu/

(b) /m, n, or ŋ/ versus any other oral consonant
with free variation.

e.g., /ʌmba͜ʌmba͜ʌmbɒ͜ʌmbi/
/aInda͜ʌnda͜aInda/
and groups of/ omwa; ʌnga; amlav; Imtu/, etc.

Condition 2:   any oral consonant versus /m, n, or ŋ/ with free
variation: e.g., groups of /olna, Iʃma; æbmi;
ɔfno; Isnav/, etc.

Intensity

Typical problems

Intensity problems may be evident from the child's difficulty in producing intensity extremes: that is, a controlled shout versus a whisper. But
it may be even more damaging to conversational fluency and intelligibility
if the child does not use the stress patterns and vowel lengthenings required in spoken language. Since English is a stress-timed language, a
hearing-impaired child's failure to employ expected rhythmic stress pat
terns in sentences can make it difficult for a listener to detect boundaries
among thought groups within a sentence. In addition, the use of stress
indicates a meaning difference between a number of word pairs, such as
the following:

The désert/dessért is hot.

Physiologic causes

Intensity control is linked to the amount and control of subglottal pressure
and is coordinated with vocal fold tension (Ling, 1976; Pickett, 1980, p.87).
Syllables receiving strongest stress in a phrase receive both an increase in
vocal fold tension and in subglottal pressure (Pickett, 1980, p. 88). This
is the reason that hearing-impaired children with poor voice quality and
inadequate breath control often exhibit concomitant problems with both
intensity and pitch. However, the hearing-impaired child has the physiologic
capacity to produce conventional intensity and stress contrasts. With adequate training, the ability can be realized.

Aim of remediation

Remediation goals are to provide children with the ability to monitor
and produce vocalizations varying in intensity over a comfortable range

and to produce controlled and flexible intensity contrasts (in combination with durational aspects) for sentence stress.

Auditory requirements

Acoustic cues for the detection and discrimination of intensity differences should be available to adequately aided children with residual hearing up to 500 Hz (Ling, 1976, p. 27-29).

Techniques for remediation

Step 1. The teacher could begin by initiating teaching with the voice and breath work described under "Vocal Quality" above. Once the child has reached the stage of practice of repetition of multiple reduplicated syllables, the teaching of intensity changes could begin.

Step 2. In order to evoke use of loud voice, our experience has shown it useful to send the child to the other side of the room and speak audibly. Thus, the use of a loud voice performance is logical and meaningful.

Step 3. Intensity steps: Once the child is used to practicing a loud voice from across the room, one can work on decreasing volume in a controlled manner by having the child come toward you in stages. The routine is that the child will start off talking in a very loud voice away from the listener and by the time 5 giant steps have been taken the child should be next to the listener talking in a whisper. Five steps are suggested to coordinate with 5 levels of vocal intensity (very loud, loud, normal, soft, whisper). By reversing the procedure, the child practices going from a whisper to a shout by going away from the listener. Any amount of variety is possible once the child indicates good control. Steps can be jumped so that the child goes straight from normal voice to whisper, or shout to normal voice level. Teachers can invent many individual and group games for this kind of exercise. At this gross level we recommend first working with consonant-vowel combinations, which are the easiest for the child (e.g., ba), and always insisting on the oral supported sound as explained under "Vocal Quality."

Pitch

Typical problems

Difficulties with pitch evidence themselves in monotonous voice quality, incorrect voice register, uncontrolled pitch changes, confusion of pitch for intensity changes, and/or poor use of intonational contours in language.

Physiologic causes

Usually pitch problems are related to too little vocal fold tension, which is realized in a low, monotone voice with little or no sentence intonation. However, occasionally, a child evidences too much vocal fold tension, which results in an abnormally high-pitched voice. In addition to vocal fold tension, insufficient control of subglottal pressure may also be a factor in pitch problems. As mentioned above, differences in subglottal pressure and vocal fold tension also produce intensity contrasts. Consequently, pitch problems and intensity problems are often linked.

Aim of remediation

Remediation goals are to establish controlled and flexible production of pitch contrasts leading to normal intonational contours in running speech.

Auditory requirements

Acoustic cues for the establishment of pitch control necessary for intonation changes are available to children even with residual hearing only up to 500 Hz (Ling, 1976, p. 190).

Techniques for remediation

Step 1. A reasonable starting place would be to initiate breath and voice work as described under "Vocal Quality" above. (Usually pitch would be the last suprasegmental aspect to be specifically remediated.)

Step 2. Once controlled voice and breath production have been accomplished, one can simply ask the child to imitate the teacher's varied pitch production. If this is unsuccessful, hand cues to indicate high, medium, and low pitch might be used. If additional strategies are necessary, Steps 3 and 4 suggested below could be helpful.

Step 3. Lowering pitch:

  a. Yawning relaxes the child and lowers the larynx. As this occurs the only possible type of sound to emerge is an oral one. If the child is instructed to think of a low sound at the same time, it is likely to emerge. The child could do this several times while extending the length of vocalization on /a/ and this might be repeated until the child has developed control. Then the child could vocalize and change pitch on the oral stream of air (think of waves of sound) e.g., /a∿∿a/.
  b. Requesting the child to lower the head to the chest while vocalizing may result in a lowering of the larynx and a change in pitch. The child should listen to the change and feel the movement of the larynx

so that what is happening can be understood. This should be repeated until the child can change pitch without the artificial head movement.

c. The child could begin this activity by continuously voicing /a/ while the teacher walks toward him. Any pitch level would be acceptable to begin with. The longer the child has to hold this sound on one breath, the more effort it will take for him to hold an abnormal pitch placement. Gradually a drop in pitch will usually be noticed as the child releases the faulty placement and allows a more natural, easier placement to occur. The child should be made aware that the lower, more natural voice is the desired one.

Step 4. Raising pitch:

a. This activity could begin by having the child prepare to vocalize, but wait in anticipation of a hand signal to begin. This procedure should have the effect of causing vocal fold adduction in preparation for the emission of a high sound. In essence, one tricks the child into producing the amount of tension required at vocal fold level for a high-pitched sound.

b. The child is then given a mental picture of higher pitch by touching the top of the head gently as the spot to aim for when vocalizing.

c. The vocal folds could then be artificially tensed by having the child push with his or her arms against the table or try to pull upwards while holding firmly to the sides of the chair. When voicing is initiated, the sound produced should be high in pitch.

Step 5. As soon as the child is able to consistently produce pitch change at the gross level with a single vowel, practice with vowel transitions can begin. One could practice gliding downwards and upwards in pitch in a continuous manner. Support this on one breath, i.e.,

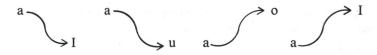

This step is only possible if the child has been progressing well through the vocal quality remediation section.

The preceding section has offered techniques for the remediation and practice of the prosodic elements of speech at the motor speech level. It has also been suggested that work on these minute aspects of motor speech—though necessary to the remediation process—will not automatically result in the child's overall improvement in speech flexibility nor in improved intelligibility to the listener. In order to effect change, elements practiced at the motor speech level must rapidly be used in meaningful situations. The next logical step for a child at this level of remediation is to create and allow for opportunities for meaningful usage of prosodic features in both scheduled and incidental ways.

Scheduled Practice of Prosodic Elements in Limited Meaningful Contexts

> NOTE: As the child is applying the newly acquired prosodic skills to meaningful language, it is important to use linguistic structures and content which are already familiar. (This is an extension of a principle for language learning/teaching cited in Kretschmer & Kretschmer, 1978, p. 257.)

1. Targets:

Parameters of speech production selected for treatment are vocal quality and breath control integrated with stress, intonation, and rhythm.

Requirements:

— Articulation ability at the multiple alternating syllable stage;
— Prior understanding of the linguistic structures involved.

Sample Activities:

a. Children could practice the following common sentences which combine all of the aforementioned elements. It seems useful for the teacher to think of linking each syllable to the next in order to be reminded of how coarticulation might occur. Vowels may be lengthened at first to facilitate movement and joining without destroying intonation and stress.

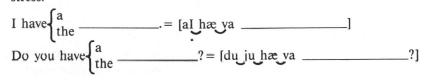

Games can be devised to allow for rapid multi-practice of these variations which are naturally implied (*He has; Do they have?; I don't have; She does*, etc.). Activities should emphasize the conversational/interactional constraints inherent in the sentences and not become a series of rote repetitions of the same sentence. The objective is to allow for scheduled practice and helpful encouragement in using the correct intonational patterns and stress markers, but only to impel growth. Once the child facilitates production through one or two repetitions of a game, responsibility for some aspect of the practice in incidental conversation would be appropriate.

b. Another activity could involve several children and the teacher having one or more objects to toss around, as in the "Hot Potato" game. Whoever is holding the object could say the key sentence or a variation: "Now, I have the ____." That child then passes it on to the next player and says, "Mary, it's yours" or "Catch it, Mary!" "You have it now!", etc.

2. Target: Nasality

Requirements:
— Establishment of the nasal/oral contrast in specific phoneme discrimination;
— Articulation at the multiple syllable level;
— Prior understanding of the linguistic structures involved.
a. Once the child has learned to recognize nasality in a controlled discrimination set, discrimination between oral and nasal sounding production of coarticulated speech in phrases and sentences is appropriate. This highlights again the fact that a difference can be discerned and allows the teacher to begin to pass responsibility on to the child for monitoring of vocal production.

e.g. Oral, Clear, Forward sounding	Nasal, Neutral sounding
May I go out.	May I go out.

The teacher provides both stimuli; the child then simply marks or indicates which was heard. The role reversal technique works well in this instance, with the child attempting to give only the desirable oral production.
b. The following linguistic context can be used for meaningful practice of /d/ versus /n/ after it has been established at the motor speech level.

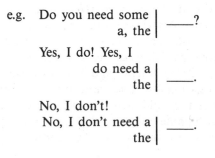

e.g.   Do you need some |
                 a, the | ____?

Yes, I do! Yes, I
         do need a |
             the | ____.

No, I don't!
No, I don't need a |
             the | ____.

Games can be devised which emphasize the interactional/conversational use of those structures. For example, a small group or an individual could prepare a recipe with the teacher. Nonsense or inappropriate objects, utensils, or ingredients could be offered which would create an element of fun, surprise, and spontaneity, as the preparation continued.

c. A game of 20 questions could be played using the same linguistic patterns, while the child or children attempt to guess "how" a task can be completed.

> e.g. Answer: "to build a house." Questions: Do you need some wood? Do you need paint? Do you need many people?

d. Selected phrases from social routines may be chosen for special attention in scheduled practice prior to incidental reminding. Once the nasal/oral contrast has been established, such common phrases as "Hello! Thank you! Good-bye!" should no longer be accepted when produced with nasal-sounding voice.

3. Targets:

Stress (intensity) change in conversation, monitoring of appropriate stress patterns versus monotone or incorrect stress/timing; integrating stress variations with duration and intonation.

Requirements:

— Parameters of speech production selected for treatment are previous establishment of the ability to change intensity production at motor speech level;
— Prior knowledge of the linguistic structures involved.

Sample activities:

a. Through the use of audition and some play-like situations, one could attempt to have the child imitate the production of the modeled loudness of voice. For example, with a young child one can put a doll to bed and say "ssh, ssh" in a whispered voice and then play at waking the doll up by shouting "Boo!" Or games could be arranged so that the children must call out the name of another person very loudly or very softly in order for them to turn around or follow an instruction.

b. Almost all hearing-impaired children shout on the playground. It may be necessary to utilize playground games to practice vocal variety in stress and then remove the work to indoors. The game of "Stop and Go" can be played outside with children taking turns as callers. "Simon Says" is another game that facilitates rapid practice of stress and grosser intensity changes in sentences.

4. Targets:

Parameters of vocal production pinpointed for treatment are intonation (pitch) change in conversation, self-monitoring of intonation pattern versus monotone speaking, and integrating intonational variation with stress and duration.

Requirements:
— Ability to vary pitch grossly at the motor speech level of production;
— Prior understanding of the linguistic structures involved.

Sample activities:
a. Selected phrases from social routines could be chosen for specific, scheduled practice prior to incidental practice. Monotone production should be avoided with attention to correct stress, duration, and overall intonation pattern being most important. Misarticulations could be ignored for the present until flexibility and greater automatic production of prosodic elements is achieved. Some sample phrases are: "Thank you"/"Pardon me!"/"I'm sorry!"/"Excuse me!"

b. Younger children especially enjoy acting out fairy stories, which lend themselves naturally to wide intonational contour variation. This affords children the opportunity to listen closely for intonational change and also to practice production. For example, "Goldilocks" provides the three varied voices of Papa Bear (low voice), Mama Bear (medium voice), and Baby Bear (high voice). Thus, flexibility in use of a consistent specific pitch level is incorporated with the overall intonational contour of the lines of spoken dialogue.

c. Games can be created that specifically encourage practice of the rising intonation patterns associated with Yes/No questions,

   e.g., "Are you big?" "Is this something yellow?"

   Twenty questions is an obvious game for this type of scheduled practice.

d. Each child can be given the task of finding pictures that convey the intent of common expressions of emotion.

e.g., "She's mad/sad/happy/crying."
"You're crazy"/"Don't touch"/"Look out!"
"That's so funny" "Uh – oh" . . .
A quick flashcard game could then be played with the children offering in turn an expression chosen to describe the picture from those currently selected for scheduled practice.

5. Targets:

Speech production parameters selected for treatment are duration variation of syllabic groups in sentences, integration of duration with stress and intonation, continued auditory awareness of durational differences.

Requirements:

— The ability to alternate multiple syllables on one breath;
— The ability to whisper;
— Prior understanding of the specific linguistic structures involved.

Sample activities:

Young, hearing-impaired infants (like their hearing counterparts) can learn durational differences through play by associating certain sounds with a wide range of selected toys. For example: a frog or other jumping animal becomes associated with "hop, hop, hop". An airplane flying can be associated with a long vowel variation a⌒I; short duration can be emphasized in expressive phrases—"He's mad! Stop him! Make him go! No! No!" Similar sorts of strategies can be adapted for work with older children.

Incidental Practice of Prosodic Features

The sample ideas and activities outlined above are intended to show how carry-over of aspects of prosody from scheduled to incidental practice can be achieved. Fundamental to all of these activities is the fact that the teacher must create an environment of high expectations for speech.

The expectations for the child include taking responsibility for:
— Beginning to incorporate into the daily routine the aspects of prosody covered in scheduled practice;
— Using better voice quality and intonational contours in all utterances.
Teacher responsibility then includes:
1. Positive reinforcement for oral-sounding speech. A brief reminder to "begin your talking on your breath" is often sufficient to produce

oral sound. Similarly, the phrase "make your sounds more forward" can help jog the child's memory.

2. Organizing learning/teaching to best facilitate change.
   — Establishing an environment in which children are allowed and encouraged to talk a great deal.
   — Correcting selectively. That is, while establishing improved vocal quality and prosodic skills, many misarticulations probably should be ignored in order to give the child a change to recuperate some of the flexibility in voice use which was not fostered adequately earlier.
   — Keeping in mind that the overall aim is for the child to use spoken language with maximum ease and intelligibility.

Summary

In a recent survey of the school-age hearing-impaired population in the United States, more than half of the children received unacceptable intelligibility ratings (Jensema, Karchmer, & Trybus, 1978). In order for more children to achieve maximum clarity of speech in spontaneous oral conversation, two broad areas require serious improvement: input and instruction. Applications of recent research and innovative thought in each area have been presented in light of the contributions they may make toward achieving the goal of intelligibility. Systematic empirical study of these and other treatment techniques is now needed in order for future advances to be made.

End Notes

[1] A discussion of auditory training systems presently in use (hardwire systems, portable desk trainers, and loop systems, radio frequency direct systems, infared light systems) is outside the scope of this paper. Probably the greatest advantage of these systems is improvement in signal-to-noise ratio, which can be essential in many communication situations both in and out of the classroom. For more information, the reader is directed to (Børrild, 1978; Libby, 1973; Ling, 1978; Ross, 1977; Staab & O'Gara, 1974).

[2] The voiced plosive burst characteristic of the /b/ contrasts greatly with the 200 to 300 Hz nasal murmur of the /m/.

Reference Notes

1. Nicholls, G. Cued speech and the reception of spoken language. Unpublished Master's thesis, McGill University, 1979.

2. Mahashie, J. J. Deaf speakers' laryngeal behavior. Unpublished doctoral dissertation, Syracuse University, 1980.

References

American Speech-Language-Hearing Association. Standards for effective oral communication programs. *ASHA,* 1979, *21,* 198–1002.

Berger, K. W., Hagberg, E. N., & Rane, R. L. *Description of hearing aids: Rationale, procedures and results.* Kent, O: Herald Publishing House, 1977.

Boone, D. Modification of the voices of deaf children. *The Volta Review,* 1966, *68,* 686–692.

Boothroyd, A. Technology and deafness. *The Volta Review,* 1975, *77,* 27–34.

Boothroyd, A., Archambault, P., Adams, R. E., & Storm, R. D. Use of a computer-based system for speech training aids for deaf persons. *The Volta Review,* 1975, *77,* 178–193.

Børrild, K. Classroom acoustics. In M. Ross & T. G. Giolas (Eds.), *Auditory management of hearing-impaired children.* Baltimore: University Park Press, 1978.

Byrne, D. Hearing aid selection: An analysis and point of view. *Archives Otolaryngologica,* 1979, *105,* 519–525.

Calvert, D. R., & Silverman, S. R. *Speech and deafness.* Washington, D. C.: A. G. Bell Association for the Deaf, 1975.

Campos, C. T. Co-investigator experience with the cochlear implant: A report from the Denver Ear Institute. *Hearing Instruments,* 1981, *32,* 26–30.

Clark, G. M., & Tong, Y. C. Multiple-electrode cochlear implant for profound or total hearing loss: A review. *Medical Journal of Australia,* 1981, *1,* 428–429.

Clarke, B. R., & Ling, D. The effects of cued speech: A follow-up study. *The Volta Review,* 1976, *78,* 23–24.

Cornett, R. O. Cued speech. *American Annals of the Deaf,* 1967, *112,* 3–13.

Cornett, R. O. Cued speech and oralism: An analysis. *Audiology and Hearing Education,* 1975, *1,* 26–33.

Fry, D. B. *Acoustic phonetics. A course of basic readings.* Cambridge: Cambridge University Press, 1976.

Fry, D. B. The role and primacy of the auditory channel in speech and language development. In M. Ross & T. G. Giolas (Eds.), *Auditory management of hearing-impaired children.* Baltimore: University Park Press, 1978.

Gastmeier, W. J. The acoustically damped earhook. *Hearing Instruments,* 1981, *32,* 14–15.

Grave, J., & Metzinger, M. The effects of stepped diameter coupling systems on hearing-impaired children. *Hearing Instruments,* 1981, *32,* 27, 66.

Hirsh, I. J. Auditory training. In H. Davis & S. Silverman (Eds.), *Hearing and deafness.* New York: Holt, Rinehart and Winston, 1970.

Hochberg, I., Levitt, H., & Osberger, M. J. Improving speech services to hearing-impaired children. *ASHA,* 1980, *2,* 280–284.

House, W. F., Bode, D. L., & Berliner, K. I. The cochlear implant: Performance of deaf patients. *Hearing Instruments,* 1981, *32,* 13–18.

Hudgins, C. V., & Numbers, C. V. An investigation of intelligibility of speech of the deaf. *General Psychology Monograph,* 1942, *25,* 289–292.

Jensema, C. J., Karchmer, M. A., & Trybus, R. J. The rated speech intelligibility of hearing-impaired children: Basic relationships and a detailed analysis. Office of Demographic Studies, Gallaudet College, Washington, D. C., 1978.

Killion, M. C., & Monser, E. L. CORFIG. In G. A. Studebaker & I. Hochberg (Eds.), *Acoustical factors affecting hearing aid performance.* Baltimore: University Park Press, 1980.

Kretschmer, R. R., & Kretschmer, L. W. *Language development and intervention with the hearing impaired.* Baltimore: University Park Press, 1978.

Libby, E. R., The achievement of optimal amplification for the hearing-impaired child. *The Hearing Dealer,* July, 1973. (reprint).

Libby, E. R. Smooth wideband hearing aid responses: The new frontier. *Hearing Instruments,* 1980, *31,* 12–13, 15, 18, 43.

Libby E. R. Achieving a transparent, smooth, wideband hearing aid response. *Hearing Instruments,* 1981, *32,* 9–12.

Ling, D. *Speech and the hearing-impaired child: Theory and practice.* Washington, D. C.: A. G. Bell Association for the Deaf, 1976.

Ling, D. Auditory coding and recoding: An analysis of auditory training procedures for young children. In M. Ross & T. G. Giolas (Eds.), *Auditory management of hearing-impaired children.* Baltimore: University Park Press, 1978, 181–218.

Ling, D. Principles underlying the development of speech communication skills among hearing-impaired children. *The Volta Review,* 1979, *81,* 211–223.

Ling, D. Early speech development. In S. Gerber & G. Mencher (Eds.), *Early management of hearing loss.* New York: Grune & Stratton, 1981. (a)

Ling, D. Keep your hearing-impaired child within earshot. *Newsounds,* 1981, *6,* 5–6. (b)

Ling, D. & Clarke, B. R. Cued speech: An evaluative study. *American Annals of the Deaf,* 1975, *120,* 480–488.

Ling, D., & Ling, A. H. *Aural habilitation: The foundations of verbal learning in hearing-impaired children.* Washington, D. C.: A. G. Bell Association for the Deaf, 1978.

Luetje, C. M. Single-electrode cochlear implant: Practicality in clinical otologic practice. *Hearing Instruments,* 1981, *39,* 20–23.

Martin, L. F., Tong, Y. C., & Clark, G. M. A multiple-channel cochlear implant: Evaluation using speech tracking. *Archives of Otolaryngology,* 1981, *107,* 157–159.

Martony, J. On the correction of the voice pitch level for severely hard of hearing subjects. *American Annals of the Deaf,* 1968, *119,* 195–202.

Minifie, F. Speech acoustics. In F. Minifie, T. J. Hixon, & F. Williams (Eds.), *Normal aspects of speech, hearing and language.* Englewood Cliffs, N.J.: Prentice-Hall, 1973.

Monsen, R. B. The production of English stop consonants in the speech of deaf children. *Journal of Phonetics,* 1976, *4,* 29–41.

Monsen, R. B. Acoustic qualities of phonation in deaf children. *Journal of Speech and Hearing Research,* 1979, *22,* 270–288.

Nickerson, R.S. Characteristics of the speech of deaf persons. *The Volta Review,* 1975, *77,* 342–362.

Oller, K. D., Payne, S. L., & Gavin, W. J. Tactual speech perception by minimally trained deaf subjects. *Journal of Speech and Hearing Research,* 1980, *23,* 757–768.

Paterson, M. M. Integration of auditory training with speech and spoken language development. In D. G. Sims, G. Walter, & R. Whitehead (Eds.), *Communication training for the severely hearing impaired.* Baltimore: Waverly Press, 1982.

Pickett, J. M. *The sounds of speech communication.* Baltimore: University Park Press, 1980.

Ross, M. Classroom amplification. In W. Hodgson & P. Skinner (Eds.), *Hearing aid assessment and use in audiologic habilitation.* Baltimore: Williams & Wilkins, 1977.

Rothman, H. B. A spectrographic investigation of consonant-vowel transitions in the speech of deaf adults. *Journal of Phonetics,* 1976, *4,* 129-136.

Rudmin, F. R. Letters to the editor: Comment on "Judgments of hearing aid processed music." *Ear and Hearing,* 1982, *3,* 238–239.

Rudmin, F. R. The why and how of hearing /s/. *The Volta Review.* (in press)

Smith, C. R. Residual hearing and speech production in deaf children. *Journal of Speech and Hearing Research,* 1975, *18,* 795–811.

Staab, W. J., & O'Gara, E. J. Auditory training systems for the hearing-impaired: A discussion of types, advantages, and uses. *Hearing Instruments,* September, 1974. (reprint)

Strong, W. J. Speech aids for the profoundly/severely hearing impaired: Requirements, overview, projections. *The Volta Review,* 1975, *77,* 536–556.

Subtelny, J. D., Whitehead, R. L., & Orlando, N. A. Description and evaluation of an instructional program to improve speech and voice diagnosis of the hearing-impaired. *The Volta Review,* 1980, *82,* 85–95.

Yanick, P. Speech processing and hearing rehabilitation. *Hearing Instruments,* 1980, *31,* 24, 26–27.

Dennis M. Ruscello

Motor Learning as a Model for Articulation Instruction

Introduction

Individuals who exhibit articulatory production errors comprise a large segment of speech-language clinicians' caseloads (Weston & Leonard, 1976). In the typical assessment/intervention program, a client's specific production errors are identified, and then a treatment is administered for the purpose of modifying the pattern of misarticulation. There are a number of available treatments that appear to reflect either different theoretical positions (Bernthal & Bankson, 1981) or service delivery models (Costello & Onstine, 1976). Regardless of the clinician's orientation, the productive component of the treatment strategies is directed toward target sound establishment in a variety of training units. The training units can include levels that range from isolated sound practice to spontaneous conversational speech.

If one simply focuses on the training units employed, it appears that two main generalizations become apparent (Ruscello, Note 1). First, the treatment plan proceeds from less complex to more complex units of production training. The initial training level will depend on the client's competence with the target sound, since successful completion of a particular unit facilitates the introduction of more advanced tasks. Second, early treatment sessions involve discrete production such as isolated sound or word practice, while later sessions incorporate usage in continuous discourse. The aforementioned characterization is closely allied with concepts presented in the theoretical constructs of motor skill learning (Ellis, 1972). That is, skilled movements are composed of a series of finely controlled responses which are organized in various sequences. Initially a person practices a motor skill in limited contexts until correct execution of the movement is achieved. As the person continues practice, the movement is carried out in combination with others. Conscious control of the skilled movement eventually shifts to enactment in an automatic, effortless manner.

Salient features in the discussion of motor skill learning include stages of response development and the role of practice in such development. The purpose of this chapter is to present a viewpoint that articulatory training can be conceptualized as a skilled motor learning phenomenon. Literature to be discussed will include the purposes for which practice is used in developing different aspects of motor behavior and the theoretical positions that have been proposed in motor skill learning. In addition, articulatory studies that have investigated various skill learning variables will be reviewed. Finally, clinical implications of theory and research will be presented.

Purposes of Motor Practice

Shelton (1963) presented a position paper that discussed the different purposes of motor practice. Depending on the interests of the learner, practice can be utilized to: increase strength, develop endurance, increase range of motion, or acquire various motor skills. Each of these different purposes requires practice; however, practice techniques will vary as a function of the goal. For example, procedures employed to build strength might include the use of resistance placed against a muscle or muscle group. A person interested in developing strength would carry out practice trials against the resistance. Additional resistance would gradually be introduced as the individual increased strength capabilities.

In contrast to the strength building example, the formation of a motor skill requires the execution of a series of coordinated muscular movements. Initially, the act is novel to a learner; consequently, practice is necessary for the development of the motor skill. The act of throwing a ball involves both arm and general body movement in synchrony. A thrower attempts to achieve some type of target through coordinated movement. The learner who tries to perfect the skilled act practices it under various response conditions. These two examples suggest that practice is an important requisite in both areas; however, the end or terminal behavior dictates the type of practice that is appropriate.

While disciplines such as physical therapy might use motor practice techniques in any of the ways mentioned, the speech-language pathologist is generally involved in skill building (Shelton, Hahn, & Morris, 1968; Shelton, Morris, & McWilliams, 1973).[1] That is, articulatory training may be explained as a process within a framework of motor skill building. In this framework it is necessary to distinguish between a motor pattern and motor skills. Godfrey and Kephart (1969) have stated that a motor pattern consists of a series of skilled motor acts. The acts are performed for the accomplishment of some specific overall purpose. Motor skills, on the other hand, are movements or groups of movements which are components of an overall motor pattern.

In adapting the two-level hierarchy of Godfrey and Kephart to articulatory production, the motor pattern would be analogous to coordinated sequences of movements of the articulators during speech production. The formation of the individual speech sounds would be the skills or subroutines in the overall speech production pattern. The use of this characterization is somewhat of an oversimplification and is not intended to present articulatory production as simply a pattern composed of discrete skilled movements. The author recognizes that production is a dynamic process (Daniloff & Hammarberg, 1973) that defies individual sound segmentation on either acoustic or physiologic bases (Curtis, 1970).

Netsell (1982) has indicated that speech motor production is not a function of stored movement routines or muscle contraction patterns, but a flexible internalized plan that allows for adaptation. The internalized plan of reference is formed through the analysis of afferent information that is available during speech production. In this way modifications may be enacted to insure that motor production goals are realized.

Motor skills have been divided into open and closed categories (Poulton, 1957). In closed skill development an individual learns a movement which is appropriate for a particular goal. Open skill development also involves patterned movement formation; however, the movement is such that it must be executed under varying environmental conditions (Gentile, 1972). Learners must adjust their skilled responses so that they might respond appropriately in different situational contexts. The teaching of articulatory movements would appear more like an open skilled task, since the target behavior must ultimately be used across a variety of phonetic contexts in a number of different speaking environments.

Johnson (1972) has described skilled learning as "the ability to execute a pattern of behavioral elements in proper relation to a certain environment" (p. 10). When evaluating motor skill development, researchers study one or more of the following variables: speed, accuracy, form, and adaptability. Each variable shows some degree of change when a learner develops and eventually perfects a particular skill.

Speed refers to the time in which a skilled movement task is completed. As one perfects a skill, speed will increase to some asymptote which, of course, is dependent on the skill being developed in training. In addition to reduction in execution time, the accurate enactment of a skill also improves through practice. Accurate response is suggestive of stabilization since error rate is minimized. As previously mentioned, motor skill learning involves the proper execution of a movement that is composed of certain behavioral elements. Form refers to the correct sequencing of the behavioral elements to achieve the desired movement. Finally, use of a motor skill across a variety of conditions and situations indicates that the learner has achieved a degree of adaptability. The skill has, in fact, become a part of the learner's repertoire of skilled movements.

In summary, it was stated that there are a number of different purposes for engaging in various motor practice techniques. One purpose which appears relevant to the work of the speech-language pathologist is skill building. Motor skills are coordinated movements organized within a motor pattern. The motor pattern is an organizational hierarchy of a group of related motor skills. It was proposed that speech sounds are skilled movements and the movements are part of the overall motor pattern of speech production. When an individual develops a particular skill through practice, there are measurable components that change as a function of skill refinement.

Theories of Skill Learning

The study of motor skills had undergone a very gradual evolution until the advent of World War II (Schmidt, 1975a). At that time individuals were required to learn complex skills necessary for military occupations, so research efforts in the area were intensified. Following the war, research activities continued and investigators collected data to test various hypotheses. The hypotheses, however, were tied into general learning theory; they did not deal with the question of motor skills exclusively. It was not until the 1960s that theories particular to motor skill were formally introduced. Emergence of theoretical explanations appears related to an increased need for understanding the complexities of motor skill training across many disciplines. Investigators from the fields of industrial engineering, psychology, physical education, special education, and sports medicine were, and are currently, involved in motor skills research and application.

The diversity among disciplines is evident in the various theories that have been formulated.

Fitts (1962) has proposed that a learner passes through certain phases of development when perfecting a skill. The phases indentified by Fitts are cognition, fixation, and automation. Although distinct labels are employed, Fitts has indicated that there is overlap among the stages, and the passage between them is a continuous, rather than a discrete, type of progression.

As Fitts describes it, the cognitive stage is one of mental analysis because the learner is attempting to master the task at hand. The requirements of the task must be determined, and strategies to perform the skill correctly must be formed. During early practice trials the learner continually makes motor adjustments based on the cognitive analysis of previous performance. The adjustments are mediated via internal verbalization and based on the demands of the particular skill.

Following the period of conceptual scrutiny, practice is aimed at fixating the skilled behavior pattern. Continued practice results in enactment at a very low error rate. Gradually, fixation gives way to automation, wherein the execution time required for the skill declines. The motor skill is produced effortlessly and without conscious control under a variety of situations and conditions; it has been automated for inclusion into one's repertoire of skilled motor behavior.

A more physiologic approach in explaining the patterning of skilled movement was proposed by Palliard (1960) through his acquisition-automatization model. In his phase progression, the initial effort or acquisition stage constitutes practice guided via conscious mental control. There is a general tension or stiffness in the musculature that is evident when observing the succession of voluntary movements. The tension gradually dissipates when the person perfects the pattern through practice. Palliard suggested that repetition of the skilled act creates new feedback circuits. For example, early visual reliance might be replaced by other sensory modalities like kinesthetic feedback. The transfer among feedback mechanisms occurs because the movement becomes more automatic to the learner. In addition, voluntary control becomes diminished following automatization; its role becomes delegated to starting and terminating the motor behavior. The desired act is carried out largely on an unconscious basis.

A more recent hypothesis explains skill learning in terms of a problem that necessitates some form of solution (Adams, 1971). During the early period of skill formation a learner executes a movement, but knowledge of results is heavily relied upon. The feedback information is obtained through the learner's own assessment of the performance and that provided by an external source such as an observer. Modifications leading toward correct execution are coded verbally for future trials and the movement pattern is stored in what Adams calls a perceptual trace. The trace is feedback dependent and is frequently modified until the movement pattern becomes stabilized. Since verbal coding strategies are so vital initially, the author refers to this inceptive stage as the Verbal-Motor Stage.

The former stage is gradually replaced by the Motor Stage. The learner has finally altered the perceptual trace so that error is negligible; the process is achieved through practice. Feedback or knowledge of results is no longer vital, since the perceptual trace is stored in a motor memory trace. The learner may recall the movement pattern which is coded into the perceptual trace and stored in a motor memory trace at will. Adams indicates that the perceptual trace is an error dependent or closed loop mechanism, while the memory trace is an open loop phenomenon.

Schmidt (1975b) has presented a theoretical position of skill learning that emphasizes the creation of motor schema. A schema is an internalized rule that allows the application of a particular skilled movement across a variety of contexts. At first a learner tries to form a particular movement pattern through practice; the unsteady movement is eventually transformed into a coordinated, effortless performance. According to Schmidt, when the learner forms the movement pattern, related information is stored was well. The information includes: the existing environmental conditions, the requirements of the motor program, the sensory feedback received following enactment of the skilled pattern, and the outcome of the response. Repetition of the movement results in the abstraction of information regarding the four informational variables and thus a schema is formed.

The novel feature of Schmidt's proposal is his provision of extended use under differing response conditions. A person who perfects a skill with training must generally use it in circumstances that do not clearly parallel practice conditions. For example, a basketball player may learn a shot with practice; however, actual game conditions force him to shoot differently each time. A successful shooter in Schmidt's proposal would have formed a general schema that enables him to carry out the movement without any problem under a variety of circumstances.

Finally, Shelton and McReynolds (1979) reviewed a conceptualization of perceptual-motor performance which was based on the work of Marteniuk (1976). Marteniuk's proposal emphasizes the utilization of information processing by the learner. The central nervous system extracts information that is subject to evaluation, prior to and during a movement sequence. The less familiar the learner is with the movement pattern, the more information there is to consider and, presumably, the slower the patterned-movement time. After the movement pattern is stabilized, the informational load is reduced because the learner need not be concerned with numerous alternatives.

Information processing skills are superimposed on the components of Marteniuk's performance model. The components of perception, decision making, and enactment interplay with incoming information which is available to the learner. Relevant data are perceived and then organized for analysis so that decisions may be made. The importance of perception in initiating the chain of events assumes that perceptually dependent mechanisms of selective attention, short term memory, and long term memory are adequate for task purposes.

According to Marteniuk, following evaluation of the perceptual information, a decision is made concerning a plan of action. As the learner becomes more familiar with the movement task, the decision-making process occurs on an unconscious level. Processing time is then devoted to the actual movement and not to a decision concerning the requirements of the movement. The learner ultimately forms a motor program through continued practice. The motor program operates in an open loop mode and is tied into a general motor schema. The schema is a closed loop process that enables an individual to produce various forms of motor behavior. The hierarchial relation of schema and motor programs permits adaptive regulation of actions requiring skilled motor behavior.

In summary, the theoretical discussions of skill learning use somewhat differing terminology, but they do seem to exhibit a very decided interrelatedness. The authors of these conceptualizations appear to be dealing with skilled learning in much the same way. The salient features among theories center on the variables of: practice, stages of motor skill development, cognitive analysis, and feedback processes.

The use of practice for development, improvement, and subsequent refinement of a particular motor skill is a universal notion. As the learner practices a particular motor skill, modifications from internal or external sources are received and processed for the purpose of establishing performance at a high level of accuracy. Moreover, performance on a motor skill is monitored through observation of practice trials. It is clear that regardless of the hypotheses, practice is the key variable thought necessary for mastery of skilled motor behavior.

Another common feature, stages of motor skill development, is explicitly described by Fitts (1962), Palliard (1960), and Adams (1971) and implicitly mentioned by Schmidt (1975b) and Marteniuk (1976). With the former group, specific stages of skill development through which the learner proceeds are posited. For example, Palliard states that early in skilled learning there is a sluggishness in execution because the learner is acquiring the movement. Following acquisition, further practice strengthens the movement so that it can be used correctly in a variety of contexts. When accurate, effortless use is achieved, automatization has taken place. Schmidt and Marteniuk do not outline distinct stages, but instead discuss the progression of changes which correlate with the learner's competence in performing the movement. Marteniuk suggests that enactment time lessens with proficiency because a correct motor program has been formulated.

In addition, there is a universal provision for some type of cognitive analysis, expecially during the preliminary phase of movement formation. It appears to be a requisite since each theorist states that a prospective learner must evaluate his performance mentally and then incorporate necessary adjustments. Once stabilization has occurred, attention toward mentalistic planning types of activities is minimized. According to Adams (1971), a learner cognitively searches for a solution to the motor problem at hand. Schmidt (1975b) presented the position that correct performance is predicated upon the mental analysis of data during the outset of practice.

The mentalistic notions discussed above appear tied into feedback processes that also figure prominently among theorists. That is, early in the development of a skill, feedback is thought to be of great importance. Incoming sensory information is hypothesized to be employed in guiding movement until it is executed in consistently accurate fashion. When error responses diminish, feedback may be minimized (Adams, 1971; Schmidt, 1975b) or altered in some fashion (Marteniuk, 1976; Palliard, 1960).

Finally, although not a point of similarity, it is interesting to see how the mechanism of general skill developmment has been handled among the various theories. Fitts (1962) and Palliard (1960) did not address the issue; however, Adams (1971) hinted at such a proposal with his introdution of a motor trace. The motor trace is a storage mechanism or collector of motor skills within the learner's repertoire. Schmidt (1975b) further modified the storage idea with his notion of a schema—a generalized motor program for a given class of movement. In Marteniuk's (1976) thinking, a schema is also important for storing general motor routines that can be applied when needed. The generality or inherent flexibility of schema is thought necessary since it would be prohibitive to store a very large number of motor programs. It is obvious that the theorists have progressed from suggested explanations of skill learning to ways in which general motor skills might be organized for utilization.

Each theory has a certain amount of credibility, since various components of each have been submitted to empirical test and supportive data have been obtained (e.g., Carson & Wiegand, 1979); however, the establishment of one theoretical explanation over the others has not occurred. Many of the constructs incorporated into the theories are somewhat difficult to evaluate empirically. Execution of responses can certainly be observed and evaluated, but determination of stages within response development is problematic from a measurement standpoint. For example, Fitts discussed stages of response development but suggested that the skill development process was continuous rather than a series of discrete stages. Similarly, cognitive scrutiny and the role of feedback mechanisms in the establishment of motor skills pose similar measurement problems. Rather than emphasize the above limitations, it should be noted that theory development has greatly expanded and empirical evaluation is continuing (Kelso & Norman, 1978).

Utilization of Skill Development in Articulatory Training

Up to this point, it has been suggested that concepts from motor skill learning be applied to the treatment of articulatory disorders. A direct analogy was suggested between speech production and the motor pattern-motor skills hierarchy that has been discussed. Moreover, a review of motor skill theories indicated a number of parallels between them and certain processes that occur in clinical training. For example, the sluggishness alluded to in early skill acquisition appears to have an articulatory correlate, since some clients initially prolong an articulatory position they are learning. Ruscello and Shelton (1979) conducted an articulatory treatment study that introduced a planning feature prior to the execution of individual practice trials. In their discussion the authors reported the "two subjects indicated they were thinking about what they should do." The observation cited is compatible with the mentalistic analysis outlined in the different motor skill theories. The similarities also have great appeal on an intuitive basis.

Kent and Lybolt (1982) have also proposed that concepts from motor skill learning be used as a basis for treating persons with articulatory disorders. The authors suggest that speakers form motor schema which are codings of intended speech movement targets. The schema are generalized motor routines that allow for flexibility in the achievement of a movement target. That is, a particular target could be realized through various movements that are incorporated into the schema. Since there is so much variability in speech production from factors such as phonetic context, schema could account very nicely for the diversity.

It must be emphasized that the incorporation of motor skill concepts in articulatory training is not meant to imply a direct isomorphic relationship. There is an inherent distortion that one should be aware of when choosing to implement such a model: the model has been adapted from another discipline. Such adaptation, however, is not unusual since training models in speech-language pathology have traditionally been taken from other fields (Schultz, 1972). Schultz summarized his position on models in the following way:

> In summary, then, any rational therapy strategy has an underlying model which provides direction to and constraints on the clinician in his planning and execution. This shaping of therapy occurs even though the clinician may be unaware of the model he is using. The profession should initiate systematic exploration and public discussion of the various theories of therapy and their resultant models upon which clincial interactions are based. (p. 121)

The introduction of a motor skill model in articulation training is not a novel approach since others have also presented training models based on different theoretical underpinnings. (Readers are referred to an excellent discussion of different therapy models that was prepared by Shelton and McReynolds [1979]). It is the position here that the teaching of phonetic production skills may be conceptualized as a motor learning phenomenon. The motor skill model provides an organizational structure and a set of guiding principles applicable to the treatment of persons with articulatory disorders. In line with this conceptualization, articulatory errors are modified through practice in either of two ways. Movements may be taught in place of other movements, or movements may be taught where they were formerly absent. The orientation toward articulatory errors is a reflection of the physiologic nature of motor skill learning; the characterization appears compatible with both the traditional classifications of articulatory errors and the different forms of articulatory pattern analysis (Bernthal & Bankson, 1981).[2]

Studies Employing Motor Skill Model

A number of different theoretical models were described in the previous section of the paper; however, studies to be reviewed below have generally operated under the acquisition-automatization model proposed by Palliard (1960). Nevertheless, issues dealt with are relevant, regardless of the specific model one might use. This section is not meant to be exhaustive but, rather, a selective review of studies pertaining to motor skill learning in articulation.

Measurement of Articulation

In two separate investigations, Shelton and his associates (Elbert, Shelton, & Arndt, 1967; Shelton, Elbert, & Arndt, 1967) developed an articulation assessment procedure from which evolved a methodology for sensitive measurement of articulatory change during articulation instruction. Subjects in both investigations were given lessons based on motor skill-learning principles. Before, during (at beginning or end of every session), and following training, subjects were administered imitative protocols which the authors designated Sound Production Tasks (SPTs). The tasks sampled individually the target phonemes of interest in contexts of isolation, syllables, word pairs, and sentences. The target phonemes occurring in word pairs and sentences were arranged in specific sound environments patterned after the work of McDonald (1964a; 1964b). Subjects in both studies demonstrated statistically significant changes in their SPT scores. Subjects had relatively few correct responses prior to initiation of treatment, but progressed during therapy. In the Shelton, Elbert, and Arndt (1967) study, subjects maintained their SPT production capabilities even after therapy had been terminated for approximately 5 months.

Shelton and his colleagues concluded that SPTs were reliable assessment devices which were sensitive to a subject's change in target sound production. Changes in SPT scores illustrated improvement with training. The authors suggested that the SPT procedure furnished information on the acquisition stage of skill learning but not on automatization. Consequently, Shelton, Elbert and Arndt (1967) stated the following:

> We are currently studying the relationship between task scores and a measure of more spontaneous articulation usage. Measurement of articulation acquisition and of automatization may be expected to contribute to solution of the "carry-over" problem. This solution will probably involve recognition of satisfactory acquisition followed by use of methods to encourage and reinforce correct usage in a variety of speaking situations. (p. 585)

In this statement, Shelton et al. emphasized the need for comparison measures of a target sound production that would be more sensitive to automatization. The inclusion of such a procedure would aid in determining whether a person had transferred target sound production to more spontaneous or conversational-like conditions. Depending on one's theoretical underpinnings, the correct use of a formerly misarticulated sound in novel contexts has been labeled carry-over, generalization, or transfer of training (Mowrer, 1971). In line with a motor skill orientation, generalization is synonymous with the term adaptability.

The final report (Wright, Shelton, & Arndt, 1969) in the series of measurement studies done in Shelton's laboratory introduced more spontaneous measures of articulation production. Talking tasks (TTs) and reading tasks (RTs) were employed in conjunction with SPTs. A TT consisted of 30 samples of the target sound recorded while the subject described various pictures. For RTs, subjects read aloud until 30 tokens of the target sound had been produced. All subjects received treatment based on a motor skills learning model. The findings indicated that subjects showed positive change in TTs and RTs, just as they did with the SPTs; however, the magnitude of the measured change differed among the tasks. SPTs exhibited the greatest improvement followed by the RTs and TTs. The investigators felt that the performance on the sampling tasks suggested subjects had acquired correct articulation of the target sounds; however, automatic usage was not complete. These findings illustrate that differential information concerning acquisition and automatization might be examined by monitoring practice through progressive levels of training material (Ruscello, 1975) and periodic sampling on nontraining types of tasks such as SPTs, TTs, and RTs.

The early treatment studies of Shelton and his colleagues dealt primarily with the methodological consideration of measuring change with treatment based on motor learning principles. Following the development of appropriate measurement tools, additional treatment studies were undertaken so that a number of treatment related issues could be examined.

Acquisition

Chisum, Shelton, Arndt, and Elbert (1969) conducted an articulatory treatment study with subjects who had palatal closure deficits. The authors indicated that their treatment was based on motor skill-learning principles. Training was initiated, when necessary, at the isolated sound level and progressed through nonsense syllables, words, sentences, and conversation. During individual training trials, subjects were instructed to observe and listen while the clinician produced the target item. Following presentation of the target item, the subject attempted to imitate it. The production was evaluated by the clinician and the appropriate feedback given to the subject. Correct responses were verified with verbal affirmation. Incorrect responses were identified. The clinician also furnished placement information thought to be pertinent in assisting the subjects to achieve correct production of the target sound.

The results showed a statistically significant difference between word articulation test scores administered before and after training. Despite the positive treatment change, correlations between articulation difference scores and numbers of practice responses did not demonstrate a significant relationship. In discussing the lack of relationship between articulation change and practice responses, Chisum et al. wrote: "The importance of practice and reinforcement to motor learning is so well established that other factors must be found to account for the relatively low correlations obtained in this study (p. 62)."

They discussed a number of possible reasons including the following:

> Another possible explanation for the low correlations involves the relationship between rate of learning and number of practice responses. For instance, one individual may require 100 practice responses to change an incorrect response to a correct one, whereas another individual may require 200 practice responses to accomplish the same task. The relationship between rate of learning and treatment activities should be studied in future investigations. (p. 63).

The latter explanation seems most plausible in explaining the fact that degree of change on the criterion measure did not correspond with the number of responses that subjects produced in therapy. Individuals require different amounts of practice to attain a specified level of proficiency, and clinicians should be cognizant of this fact. Practice is not synonomous simply with repetition but must be specific to the individual's learning requirements.

One of the more frequent features of the motor skill-learning theories is the emphasis on mentalistic analysis, particulary during the early stages of skill development. Consequently, Ruscello and Shelton (1979) evaluated a treatment that incorporated mental planning and self-assessment features during response acquisition. The authors reasoned that initial practice units should be carried out differently from later practice activities. Utilizing the acquisition-automatization distinction proposed by Palliard (1960), practiced units were dichotomized. Isolated sound, nonsense syllables, and word practice were considered acquisition level activities, and sentences and conversation were automatization. Drill with acquisition level units was done under the conditions of mentalistic focus and self-assessment. That is, subjects in one training group (Group I) were instructed to consider articulatory movements mentally before producing them and then assess their productions. A second group (Group II) also received articulation instruction, but the treatment did not contain mentalistic or self-assessment components. The insertion of the mental focus and self-assessment was prompted by the cognitive participation alluded to by Palliard (1960) and others (Adams, 1971; Schmidt, 1975b). Initially, the experimenter described the movements of the target sound and then presented the actual practice item. The subject was told to "think" about the movement before enactment. Following production, subjects evaluated their responses. The experimenter verified the subjects' assessments or provided other feedback, whichever was necessary. When subjects progressed to sentences and conversation, the mental focus and self-assessment components were withdrawn.

The results indicated a statistically significant advantage for Group I on SPT and TT measures, which were obtained periodically during the instructional period when the planning and self-assessment features were in effect. Group I also required significantly fewer trials in order to complete the acquisition phase of the study. The data suggest that the planning aspect of the experimental treatment was the differentiating feature between the 2 groups because subjects' self-assessments were not generally accurate. They typically identified their correct responses but consistently erred on responses that were misarticulated. Although the authors indicated that the results supported the planning concept, they cautioned against extensive generalization until further study resolved certain experimental issues. In addition, the statistical superiority of Group I was not maintained during sentence and conversational training. It appears that the initial treatment effect which was found did not enhance the performance of Group I subjects during later stages of treatment.

Automatization Treatments

Instead of the usual progression from acquisition to automatization, Johnson, Shelton, Ruscello, and Arndt (1979) evaluated a treatment that was intended to involve simultaneous acquisition-automatization techniques. The investigation was prompted by Diedrich's (1971) observation that some children demonstrated changes in conversational probes even though they had only received instruction directed toward acquisition. In the Johnson et al. investigation a total of 34 preschool subjects were assigned randomly to 1 of 2 treatment groups. Each group practiced similar materials via lessons provided by the experimenters. The difference between groups was that one also had their parents conduct home practice. The home activities, which were carried out in individual practice periods, were introduced when the children demonstrated the ability to articulate correctly their target sound in practice words. At that time, training activities were carried out in both the clinic and home. Prior to beginning home practice, parents received individual instruction on discriminating between correct and incorrect target productions. During the home practice periods, parents monitored the productions of their children. They verbally rewarded correct target phoneme productions and had their children repeat incorrect productions correctly. The number of target sounds evaluated by the parents was gradually increased from 10 to 30 productions each day. Home training advancement was contingent upon the performance of the children during the experimenter-based lessons. Periodic sampling of imitative and conversational skills revealed that both groups improved significantly with training, but there was no statistical difference between the 2 treatment groups. The results indicate that the combined treatment did not result in a decided advantage for those subjects who received it. Since the subjects who also practiced with their parents received even more treatment than the other group, yet showed no superiority in articulation performance, the inclusion of this method of simultaneous acquisition-automatization training is questionable.

Bankson and Byrne (1972) approached automatization through the use of a timed response task. That is, the experimenters speculated that gradual reductions in the time necessary to complete a block of training trials might facilitate automatization. Experimental subjects consisted of five elementary school subjects who had previously acquired correct production of their target sounds but were inconsistent in conversation. For automatization training purposes, subjects read word lists aloud. Each list contained 60 words; lists were read 25 times per day for 10 consecutive days. Reading times were taken with a stopwatch and were gradually required to be decreased as subjects read lists without misarticulating the target sound. Initially, subjects needed approximately 60 seconds to read a list, but with practice and differential reinforcement for decreasing times, times were reduced to a range of 17 to 33 seconds. Conversational probes were obtained in the children's homes, in the clinic, and by an unfamiliar observer on the final day of practice. Despite the fact that accuracy was maintained with increments in speed, performance errors on the conversational probes indicated automatization was not complete. The authors concluded the following:

> The approach we used, based on the concept that articulation is a learned set of motor events, stressed the motor skill. We wanted production of the phoneme to be correct, effortless, and automatic both at the drill level and in spontaneous speech in all of the three settings—at home with a parent, at school with the clinician, and in a new setting with a stranger. In a total of five hours of individual therapy time with each child, a great deal was accomplished, but additional carryover is needed for all of them. Further refinement of this procedure seems warranted. (p. 167).

Shelton, Johnson, and Arndt (1972) evaluated the merits of using exclusive parent participation to produce automatization in the use of formerly misarticulated speech sounds. Before treatment, the 8 school children who served as subjects demonstrated imitative control of their target sounds, but erred inconsistently in conversation. TTs and RTs were measured before treatment, during treatment, and 4 months following the final lesson. The treatment was administered after the parents had received appropriate instruction concerning the identification of correct and incorrect sound productions. The parent-child lessons were carried out daily for a period of 5 weeks. During the first week, parents conducted word drills and monitored target sound productions in conversation. The remaining 4 weeks were devoted to daily conversational monitoring. Parents provided appropriate verbal feedback for correct responses and had the children repeat their errors. Children earned performance points which could be exchanged for small prizes. Statistical analysis showed no significant differences for pre- and post-treatment SPT measures, which was expected since subjects were required to have imitative control of their target sounds prior to treatment and, therefore, produced relatively high pretreatment SPT scores. There were, however, significant differences between pre- and posttreatment TT and RT measures. Comparison of the immediate posttreatment measures with data collected approximately 4 months later showed no significant difference, indicating that the observed treatment change was maintained.

A similar study investigated the development of automatization through parent training activities with preschool children (Shelton, Johnson, Willis, & Arndt, 1975). The 10 children who received the treatment practiced with an experimenter before the parent intervention plan was begun. When the subjects produced a group of training words correctly, practice shifted to the home. The parent program was basically the same as that described in the previous investigation (Shelton, Johnson, & Arndt, 1972). Statistically significant differences were found for pre- and posttreatment comparisons of both imitative and spontaneous measures of articulation. The magnitude of change, however, was greater for the imitative measure (SPT) than the spontaneous measure (TT).

The studies in this particular section have incorporated more spontaneous sampling measures as indices to automatization of target phones. TTs and RTs have been used and gains documented, but the degree of change has been somewhat limited. Overall findings indicate that average posttreatment TT scores are substantially lower than the imitative SPTs scores (Johnson et al., 1979). These data suggest that the teaching strategies were effective in facilitating acquisition when evaluated via SPTs, but limited in the development of automatization as demonstrated in TT scores. Since the goal of articulation training for most individuals is automatic use of target sounds, more effective treatments are still in need of development.

Automatization Measures

The following investigations are not treatment reports but have operated within a motor skill model. Manning and his associates have used auditory masking procedures to estimate the level of automatization achieved by children who had been enrolled in articulatory remediation. The underlying assumption is that reliance on auditory feedback is minimized when target productions are produced on an automatic basis. Manning, Keappock, and Stick (1976) gave the McDonald Deep Test (1964a) to a group of elementary school children who were receiving articulation lessons. Subjects were first given the test under normal test conditions and then in the presence of auditory masking, if they had received a test score of 90% or better on the initial administration. The masking stimulus was 86dB SPL of white noise presented binaurally through head sets. Approximately 4 months after the initial testing, the McDonald test was given again without masking. Subject performance under normal test conditions and masking were compared with results obtained at the end of the 4-month period. Data indicate that performance on the masking condition was more accurate in predicting target sound stability following 4 months with no treatment. While articulation test scores without masking might prove to be an acceptable dismissal criterion for some cases, the masking technique appeared more stringent, thus resulting in a more accurate dismissal procedure.

Manning, Wittstruck, Loyd, and Campbell (1977) categorized a group of misarticulating children into 2 subgroups based on posttreatment McDonald Deep Test scores. Those subjects who scored 80% or higher were placed in the high-acquisition group while those scoring below 80% were placed in a low-acquisition group. After categorization, subjects underwent further McDonald Deep testing with 85dB SPL of competing speech presented binaurally. The children in the low-acquisition group exhibited performance decrements under the masking condition that were significantly greater than those observed for the high-acquisition group. It appears that auditory masking exhibits more disrupting influence for children who have not achieved a high level of sound acquisition/automatization as measured with the McDonald Deep Test.

Summary

To summarize, a number of investigations that have operated within a skill-learning model have been reviewed. Initially, methodological studies were used to develop measurement tools which could substantiate treatment effects. Implementation of the measurement tools across investigations suggest that treatments have been successful in altering patterns of misarticulation. The generalization of target sounds to untaught items has generally been greater on measurement tasks similar to acquisition-type training levels (syllables and words) rather than to more spontaneous or automatic levels. Johnson et al. (1979) stated:

> We have come to consider 33% correct in posttreatment talking tasks (TTs) as a rough comparison point to be surpassed in future articulation research involving subjects who initially make five or fewer correct responses on a sound production task. This presents a challenge to identify or develop a treatment that will better improve conversational speech in a relatively short period of time. (p. 346)

Finally, the response of subjects who were at various levels of response development showed variations in production when responding under auditory masking conditions implying that responses on such a measure might be indicative of one's level of mastery or automatization of an articulatory motor skill.

Treatment Implications

The implications of motor-learning theory and investigative research will be discussed in reference to a number of instructional variables that have been covered in the previous sections. Literature from both skill learning and articulation treatment research will be cited where it appears pertinent.

Practice

The key ingredient in the typical skill-learning paradigm, and also a primary feature in articulation treatment, is practice. An individual is taught to produce a target sound correctly and then it is practiced in various phonetic contexts. An individual executes a particular skill in practice until it has been formed. Jones (1969) has indicated that learning is achieved through various combinations of practice. Practice is intertwined with all aspects of a training program and can be discussed in terms of the scheduling of practice, establishment of performance criteria, and differential practice methods.

In the parlance of motor learning, the issue of scheduling practice is one of distributed versus massed practice (Irion, 1969). Distributed practice consists of periodic responding across some specified time interval. For example, one could practice a particular motor skill a total of 15 times per training session for 5 consecutive days. In a massed practice plan, the motor skill is practiced equally frequently but during a single training session. An example would be a situation wherein the person practices a motor skill during a training session for 75 repetitions once a week. A correspondence in articulatory training would be the clinician's use of either block or intermittent scheduling for clients (Bernthal & Bankson, 1981). The block plan would be analogous to distributed practice, since remediation activities are carried out for short periods over a specific time span. The speech-language pathologist might see a child for 15 minute sessions, 4 times per week, so that opportunities for practice are distributed over a span of 4 sessions. Intermittent scheduling is similar to the massed form of practice; the client responds more frequently over a limited period of time. A child may be seen twice a week for 30 minute articulatory training sessions. Consequently, opportunities for practice must be massed into the allotted time rather than being distributed over a number of sessions.

Bernthal and Bankson (1981) summarized the scheduling data and indicated that block scheduling was slightly superior to intermittent scheduling in terms of dismissal rate. Motor-learning research has supported the employment of distributed practice (Catalano, 1978) in the teaching of motor skills. The agreement from both areas of research suggests that a block schedule would be more amenable to effecting change in articulatory training. However, there is a qualification that needs to be made concerning the issue. Research in motor learning indicates that the difference between massed and distributed practice is one of actual performance, not learning (Dunham, 1976). That is, subjects engaging in massed practice will often show decrements in practice trial performance which have been attributed to factors such as motivation and fatigue. However, comparison between massed and distributed practice groups does not reveal significant differences on adaptability or transfer of training tasks (Schmidt, 1975a).

In consideration of the above factors, we would recommend distributed practice, since this form of responding is more resistant to performance decrements. However, the feasibility of such scheduling is not always a viable option for many speech-language pathologists. Cognizant of the limitation, we would suggest that clinicians utilizing massed practice examine the response records of their clients to determine if performance reductions occur. For example, a client may practice the target sound in word size units during a particular training session. When reviewing the client's practice trials, there might be a drop in response accuracy toward the end of the session. The pattern would be suggestive of a performance drop described earlier. Verification of the performance reduction could be studied through the inclusion of some type of adaptability or transfer of training measure. One would predict stability or improvement in transfer despite transient fluctuations in session performance. If there was also a corresponding decrement in transfer rather than the pattern formerly described, the clinician would need to examine the teaching strategy utilized so that possible modifications might be made.

A common feature of skill-learning research and application is the establishment of performance criteria (Schmidt, 1975b). Similarly, articulatory training procedures that are guided by other theoretical frameworks also incorporate some type of performance criteria in their lesson materials (Costello, 1977; Gerber, 1977). A client must accomplish a training goal under certain conditions that have been set by the clinician. After the conditions have been met, the client is given some different type of practice material. Examples of performance criteria presented by Costello (1977) include: accuracy percentages across a group of trials (e.g., 90% accuracy in a block of 30 training trials); a set number of consecutively correct trials (e.g., 7 correct trials in succession); or some form of time designation (90% accuracy in a 5-minute segment of conversation).

From a skill-learning viewpoint, performance criteria are used because of the tremendous heterogeneity among subjects concerning the amount of practice needed. To illustrate, Ruscello and Shelton (1979) compared 2 groups of children who were receiving different training procedures, but practicing the same materials. The authors set a response achievement criterion of 80% for a block of 10 training trials in each of the levels of isolation, syllables, words, and sentence imitation. The number of responses necessary for individual subjects in either group to reach the imitative sentence condition ranged from 372 to 912 responses. Some subjects required a very limited number of practice trials at each level, while others needed a substantially higher amount of practice across the training levels. The figures reflect individual learning rates that may also be observed in clinical work. In order to allow for individual learning rate differences, one should include response achievement criteria in a training plan.

The final topic in this section concerns differential practice methods that would be suggested from skill learning theory. The various theories that were summarized describe stages of response development. It seems plausible, therefore, that different practice techniques might be beneficial at one stage but discarded eventually in favor of different procedures for subsequent stages. Practice would not simply be sheer repetition, but instead, pursuit of the most economic resolution in the most efficient manner (Bernstein, 1967). Cross (1967) stated that certain practice techniques might be helpful at one stage, but totally inappropriate at some other level of training.

The previously discussed investigation conducted by Ruscello and Shelton (1979) is an example of a treatment plan that incorporated differential practice methods. During the acquisition stage of training, subjects were requested to "think" about the impending movement of their target sound prior to producing it. Following production of the target sound, they judged the accuracy of the sound and received appropriate feedback information from the experimenter. The mentalistic and self-assessment features were eliminated from training when subjects reached sentence and conversational practice levels. By structuring therapy in this way, an effort was made to develop practice methods consistent with Palliard's acquisition-automatization distinction (Palliard, 1960).

The acquisition treatment appeared to influence positively the subjects' misarticulations, and, in particular, the mental participation activity was thought responsible. Nevertheless, there are a number of issues which must be resolved before the treatment is clinically feasible. Mentalistic participation is an abstract concept that must be inferred since it can not be observed or measured directly. Schmidt (1975a) indicated that the mental practice notion has received attention in the skill learning literature, and data suggest that the procedure is of benefit. He believes that mentalistic participation facilitates the formation of execution strategies and other verbal rehearsal features. In addition, the learner probably reviews performance from prior trials so that appropriate adjustments might be implemented in future practice trials (Gallagher & Thomas, 1980). As task familiarity increases, mental participation is of less importance to the learner; it appears to have no effect on performance after the skill has been acquired (Marteniuk, 1976).

Another example of differential practice which might be introduced clinically is the speed drill technique evaluated by Bankson and Byrne (1972). Drill times were gradually reduced while subjects maintained high response accuracy rates. The method was not completely successful; nevertheless, subjects did improve with treatment. Rate drills might enhance the stability of a target response following acquisition, thus assisting with the establishment of effortless, automatic use (Poulton, 1972).

Feedback and Knowledge of Results

The motor learning literature distinguishes between feedback and knowledge of results (Adams, 1971). Feedback is information that learners obtain from evaluation of their own performance. The learner has access to various types of incoming sensory information which function as feedback sources. The incoming information is analyzed internally so that appropriate alterations may be made by the learners. In contrast to feedback, knowledge of results is performance data furnished by an external source. Generally, the speech-language teacher or clinician will evaluate individual responses and provide the learner with information that presumably is useful for future practice. Knowledge of results can be qualitative in nature; for example, a response could be judged either correct or incorrect. Conversely, the experimenter might employ some form of quantitative information which would furnish an accurate index to degree of error. For example, a learner might execute a movement task for the purpose of achieving some specific target. Practice attempts which are not successful in reaching the target could be measured and the off target distances relayed to the learner for future consideration.

Knowledge of results has been systematically studied and a number of generalizations have emerged. Foremost is the fact that knowledge of results is a primary component in facilitating accurate skilled performance, (Newell & Kennedy, 1978). Moreover, the frequency of knowledge of results is directly related to the learning of a motor skill (Bilodeau, 1969). That is, the more frequent the knowledge of results, the better the opportunity for learning to occur. Another generalization is the consistent finding that delays in the dispensation of knowledge of results do not impede, but may aid, in learning (Adams, 1971). Although this might seem to be somewhat in conflict with operant learning principles which emphasize the immediacy of reinforcement following a response (e.g., Costello, 1977), the former statement holds true only when the delay period does not exceed the time between the response that received knowledge of results and the succeeding reponse. It should also be emphasized that delays are in the range of seconds, and there are no intervening activities within the delay period. Presumably, the delay period is an interval wherein response information is stored and later compared with the knowledge of results information that follows. When the learner has firmly established the motor skill, knowledge of results may be withdrawn without adversely affecting performance. According to Schmidt (1975a) feedback takes over when knowledge of results is no longer necessary, and occasional performance problems are identified by an error-detecting mechanism which the learner has constructed internally.

Although the concepts of knowledge of results and feedback have not garnered much attention in articulatory training, the idea of response information or reinforcement has usually been a part of speech treatment discussions (Bernthal & Bankson, 1981; McReynolds, 1970; Van Riper, 1963). The misarticulating client produces a treatment item, then receives information concerning adequacy of the production. Application of the motor skill concepts to articulatory training would be somewhat similar to current practices (Costello, 1977; Gerber, 1977); however, there would be certain procedural differences. The similarity between current practices and the concept of knowledge of results is that the observer evaluates a response and furnishes information to the learner. The proposed differences involve use of delays in providing knowledge of results and frequency of dispensation of knowledge of results. In the typical articulatory treatment, knowledge of results delays in the range of 3 to 15 seconds would be suggested. Delays in excess of the suggested time period have not proven to be effective (Irwin, Nickles, & Hulit, 1973) and such excessive delays would greatly limit opportunities for practice within sessions. In addition, knowledge of results should be given continuously, since establishment of a motor skill is dependent on such initial information to the learner. Once acquisition has been accomplished, knowledge of results might be completely eliminated instead of shifting to some intermittent schedule, as utilized in other learning conceptualizations (Sloane & MacAulay, 1968). It should be noted that the above statements require empirical validation since they have not been studied with articulatory-disordered children.

One of the primary goals of any teaching strategy is that the learner eventually spontaneously uses the taught behaviors in novel encounters. If this did not occur, the speech clinician would be faced with the insurmountable task of teaching a target sound in a seemingly endless number of phonetic contexts and environmental situations. In both motor skills (Carson & Wiegand, 1979) and articulatory research (Elbert, Shelton, & Arndt, 1967), tasks that provide indices to novel usage have been administered before treatment, during treatment, and following the conclusion of treatment. Motor skills investigators obtain information on the adaptability of persons with a motor skill (Johnson, 1972), while proponents of learning theory collect information concerning generalization (Costello & Bosler, 1976). In other descriptions, the term carry-over is employed when discussing this phenomenon (Mowrer, 1971). Shelton, Elbert, and Arndt (1967) advocated the inclusion of adaptability measures, since the measures appear sensitive to changes obtained through training. Diedrich and Bangert (1980) stated that periodic use of adaptability measures supplant the traditional procedures of simply administering an articulation test prior to and following treatment.

In this chapter's earlier reviews of some of the other training implications, concepts from skill learning and other disciplines were presented relative to their similarities and differences; however, such a discussion approach appears unnecessary here. Adaptability and generalization are constructs considered relatively homogeneous by the writer.[3] The classic work of Shelton and his associates (Elbert, Shelton, & Arndt, 1967; Shelton, Elbert, & Arndt, 1967; Wright, Shelton, & Arndt, 1969) has had a great influence in articulatory research and training with their development of SPTs and TTs. Their treatment procedures were carried out under the guise of motor learning theory, and the measures were used to evaluate treatment effects.

If clinicians do not wish to use the standard measures that have been recommended, they can create their own adaptability tasks. However, this writer suggests that the self-made measures reflect Shelton's format. That is, adaptability assessment should incorporate provision for a contrived task and a spontaneous task. The contrived task should contain items that span the usual acquisition regimen and include the target sound in isolation, syllables, words, and phrases. Items used for training purposes should not be presented in the contrived task. The spontaneous task should entail some form of conversational usage by the client and the more natural, the better. Recall that Bankson and Byrne (1972) evaluated spontaneous utilization of target sounds in their clients' homes, in the clinic, and in the presence of an observer unfamiliar to the clients. The clinician should also be sure that an adequate number of tokens have been collected for each task. Bernthal and Bankson (1981) present an excellent account of methods which may be utilized in tabulating adaptability data. In addition, they present very detailed procedures concerning ways in which the clinician may document changes in articulatory behavior.

The sampling format presented above is suggested for two specific reasons: (1) the method is clinically feasible for practicing clinicians; and (2) the tasks provide an estimate of adaptability along the acquisition-automatization continuum. The typical response pattern that has emerged from the employ of SPTs (contrived task) and TTs (spontaneous task) is one that this author refers to as a shadow effect. Generally, the SPTs show an earlier and more rapid departure from pretraining levels than the TTs. The superiority of the SPTs is maintained with the TTs continuing to shadow the short utterance, imitative measurements. Treatment sutdies incorporating these measures (Johnson et al., 1979; Ruscello, 1977) have usually been shorter in duration than actual training intervention and as a consequence have not furnished precise guidelines regarding the measures and terminal performance. However, Diedrich and Bangert (1980) carried out a long-term investigation of /r/ and /s/ misarticulating children who received training from public school speech clinicians. SPTs and TTs were given to the children throughout training and Diedrich and Bangert's recommendations are as follows:

> We believe that children who achieve 75% correct or better on the target phonemes /r/ or /s/ in conversation for two successive probes (one week apart) should be dismissed from therapy. A follow-up probe should be made at four weeks. If the child is still above 75%, but not at 95%, continue with eight-week interval probes. Stop follow-up probes when child is at 95% or better. Reinstate child in therapy if follow-up probes fall below 75% correct. (p. 233).

The masking technique reported by Manning and his group (Manning et al., 1976, 1977) is a somewhat different form of adaptability testing that appears to differentiate between those who have or have not achieved automatic use of their target sounds. The technique does have appeal and could probably be implemented without much difficulty by school speech-language pathologists. It might be particularly helpful in deciding which clients should receive supplementary articulation instruction in the summer months when school is not in session.

The position of this chapter has been that the teaching of articulatory movements could be likened to the teaching of other motor skills. Therefore, theoretical constructs from the discipline of motor learning served as a framework for organizing treatment research and making predictions concerning treatment outcomes. The studies reviewed suggest positive changes have occurred in the production capabilities of experimental subjects when their instruction has been derived from these motor learning constructs, thus adding credence to motor learning theory. We are, however, far from validating a particular motor learning theory; and for that matter, so is the field of motor learning. The constructs applied herein to treatment are more similar to, than different from, constructs from other theoretical proposals because each is directed to one specific end: learning correct articulations. Future studies must explore treatment variables that may result in more efficient teaching strategies. Efficiency in this context is reduced practice time with increased adaptability.

End Notes

[1] Speech-language pathologists have, in certain instances, formulated treatments which focus on one of the other purposes of therapeutic exercise. Interested readers are referred to a paper by Ruscello (1982) for a more detailed discussion.

[2] The physiologic slant is similar to the position of McDonald (1964b), who discussed the overlapping, ballistic movements of the speech articulators.

[3] Generalization in articulatory research has been examined in numerous ways (Costello & Bosler, 1976); however, studies undertaken within a motor learning framework have not explored novel target use in such depth. Consistent with the current discussion, the analogy between adaptability and generalization is limited to that level which Costello and Bosler refer to as intratherapy generalization.

Reference Note

1. Ruscello, D.M. The use of a mental practice feature during the initial stages of phone learning. Unpublished doctoral dissertation, University of Arizona, 1977.

References

Adams, J.A. A closed-loop theory of motor learning. *Journal of Motor Behavior,* 1971, *3,* 111-145.

Bankson. N.W., & Byrne, M.C. The effect of a timed correct sound production task on carryover. *Journal of Speech and Hearing Research,* 1972, *15,* 160-168.

Bernstein, N. *The coordination and regulation of movement.* Englewood Cliffs, N.J.: Prentice-Hall, 1967.

Bernthal, J.E., & Bankson, N.W. *Articulation disorders.* Englewood Cliffs, N.J.: Prentice-Hall, 1981.

Bilodeau, I. McD. Information feedback. In E.A. Bilodeau (Ed.), *Principles of skill acquisition.* New York: Academic Press, 1969.

Carson, L.M., & Wiegand, R.L. Motor schema formation and retention in young children: A test of Schmidt's Schema Theory. *Journal of Motor Behavior,* 1979, *11,* 247-251.

Catalano, J.F. The effect of rest following massed practice of continuous and discrete motor tasks. *Journal of Motor Behavior,* 1978, *10,* 63-67.

Chisum, L. Shelton, R.L., Arndt, W.B., & Elbert, M. The relationship between remedial speech instruction activities and articulation change. *Cleft Palate Journal,* 1969, *6,* 57-64.

Costello, J.M. Programmed instruction. *Journal of Speech and Hearing Disorders,* 1977, *42,* 3-28.

Costello, J., & Bosler, C. Generalization and articulation instruction. *Journal of Speech and Hearing Disorders,* 1976, *41,* 359-373.

Costello, J., & Onstine, J. The modification of multiple articulation errors based on distinctive feature theory. *Journal of Speech and Hearing Disorders,* 1976, *41,* 199-215.

Cross, K.D. Role of practice in perceptual-motor learning. *American Journal of Physical Medicine,* 1967, *46,* 487-510.

Curtis, J.F. Segmenting the stream of speech. In J. Griffith and J.E. Miner (Eds.), *The first Lincolnland conference on dialectology.* Tuscaloosa: University of Alabama Press, 1970.

Daniloff, R.G., & Hammarberg, R.E. On defining coarticulation. *Journal of Phonetics,* 1973, *1,* 239-248.

Diedrich, W.M. Procedures for counting and charting a target phoneme. *Language, Speech, and Hearing Services in Schools,* 1971, 18-32.

Diedrich, W.M., & Bangert, J. *Articulation learning.* Houston, Texas: College-Hill, 1980.

Dunham, P. Distribution of practice as a factor affecting learning and/or performance. *Journal of Motor Behavior,* 1976, *8,* 305-307.

Elbert, M., Shelton, R.L., & Arndt, W.B. A task for evaluation of articulation change: I. Development of methodology. *Journal of Speech and Hearing Research,* 1967, *10,* 281-288.

Ellis, H.C. *Fundamentals of human learning and cognition.* Dubuque, Ia.: W.M.C. Brown, 1972.

Fitts, P. Factors in complex skill training. In R. Glaser (Ed.), *Training research and education.* New York: Wiley, 1962.

Gallagher, J.D., & Thomas, J.R. Effects of varying post-KR intervals upon childrens' motor performance. *Journal of Motor Behavior,* 1980, *12,* 41-46.

Gentile, A.M. A working model of skill acquisition with application to teaching. *Quest,* 1972, *17,* 3-23.

Gerber, A. Programming for articulation modification. *Journal of Speech and Hearing Disorders* 1977, *42,* 29-43.

Godfrey, B.B., & Kephart, N.C. *Movement patterns and motor education.* New York: Appleton-Century-Crofts, 1969.

Irion, A.L. Historical introduction. In E.A. Bilodeau (Ed.), *Principles of skill acquisition.* New York: Academic Press, 1969.

Irwin, R.B., Nickles, A., & Hulit, L.M. Effects of varying latencies in the stimulus-response paradigm of speech therapy. *Perceptual and Motor Skills,* 1973, *37,* 707-713.

Johnson, A.F., Shelton, R.L., Ruscello, D.M., & Arndt, W.B. A comparison of two articulation treatments: Acquisition and acquisition-automatization. *Human Communication,* 1979, *4,* 337-348.

Johnson, H.W. Skill = speed x accuracy x form x adaptability. In R.N. Singer (Ed.), *Readings in motor learning.* Philadelphia: Lea & Febiger, 1972.

Jones, M.B. Differential processes in acquisition. In E.A. Bilodau, (Ed.), *Principles of skill acquisition.* New York: Academic Press, 1969.

Kelso, J.A.S., & Norman, P.E. Motor schema formation in children. *Developmental Psychology,* 1978, *14,* 153-156.

Kent, R.D., & Lybolt, J.T. Techniques of therapy based on motor learning theory. In W.H. Perkins (Ed.), *Current therapy of communication disorders: General principles of therapy.* New York: Thieme-Stratton, 1982.

Manning, W.H., Keappock, N.E., & Stick, S.L. The use of auditory masking to estimate automatization of correct articulatory production. *Journal of Speech and Hearing Disorders,* 1976, *41,* 143-149.

Manning, W.H., Wittstruck, M.L., Loyd, R.R., & Campbell, T.F. Automatization of correct production at two levels of articulatory acquisition. *Journal of Speech and Hearing Disorders,* 1977, *42,* 358-363.

Marteniuk, R.G., *Information processing in motor skills.* New York: Holt, 1976.

McDonald, E.T. *A Deep Test of Articulation.* Pittsburgh: Stanwix House Publications, 1964. (a)

McDonald, E.T. *Articulation testing and treatment: A sensory-motor approach.* Pittsburgh. Stanwix House, 1964. (b)

McReynolds, L.V. Contingencies and consequences in speech therapy. *Journal of Speech and Hearing Disorders,* 1970, *35,* 12-24.

Mower, D.E. Transfer of training in articulation therapy. *Journal of Speech and Hearing Disorders,* 1971, *36,* 427-446.

Netsell, R. Speech motor control: Theoretical issues with clinical impact. In W. Berry (Ed.), *Clinical dysarthria.* San Diego: College-Hill, 1982.

Newell, K.M., & Kennedy, J.A. Knowledge of results and children's motor learning. *Developmental Psychology,* 1978, *14,* 531-536.

Palliard, J. The patterning of skilled movements. In J. Field (Ed.), *Handbook of physiology (Vol. III, Section I) Neurophysiology.* Baltimore: Waverly, 1960.

Poulton, E.C. On prediction in skilled movements. *Psychological Bulletin,* 1957, *54,* 467-473.

Poulton, E.C. Skilled performance. In R.N. Singer (Ed.), *The psychomotor domain: Movement behavior.* Philadelphia: Lea & Febiger, 1972.

Ruscello, D.M. The importance of word position in articulation therapy. *Language, Speech, and Hearing Services in Schools,* 1975, *6,* 190-196.

Ruscello, D.M. A selected review of palatal training procedures. *Cleft Palate Journal,* 1982, *3,* 181-193.

Ruscello, D.M. & Shelton, R.L. Planning and self-assessment in articulatory training. *Journal of Speech and Hearing Disorders,* 1979, *44,* 504-512.

Schmidt, R.A. *Motor Skills.* New York: Harper & Row, 1975. (a)

Schmidt, R.A. A schema theory of discrete motor skill learning. *Psychological Review,* 1975, *82,* 225-260. (b)

Schultz, M.C. The bases of speech pathology and audiology: What are appropriate models. *Journal of Speech and Hearing Disorders,* 1972, *37,* 118-122.

Shelton, R.L. Therapeutic exercise and speech pathology. *Asha.* 1963, *5,* 855-859.

Shelton, R.L., Elbert, M., & Arndt, W.B. A task for evaluation of articulation change: II. Comparison of task scores during baseline and lesson series testing. *Journal of Speech and Hearing Research,* 1967, *10,* 578-586.

Shelton, R.L., Hahn, E., & Morris, H. Diagnosis and therapy. In D.C. Spriestersbach & D. Sherman (Eds.), *Cleft palate and communication.* New York: Academic Press, 1968.

Shelton, R.L., Johnson, A.F., & Arndt, W.B. Monitoring and reinforcement by parents as a means of automating articulatory responses. *Perceptual and Motor Skills,* 1972, *35,* 759-767.

Shelton, R.L., Johnson, A.F., Willis, V., & Arndt, W.B. Monitoring and reinforcement by parents as a means of automating articulatory responses: II. Study of preschool children. *Perceptual and Motor Skills,* 1975, *40,* 599-610.

Shelton, R.L., & McReynolds, L.V. Functional articulation disorders: Preliminaries to treatment. In N.J. Lass (Ed.), *Speech and language: Advances in basic research and practice* (Vol. II). New York: Academic Press, 1979.

Shelton, R.L., Morris, H., & McWilliams, B.J. Nonsurgical management of cleft palate speech problems. In Report from the Committee. *Speech, language, and psychosocial aspects of cleft lip and cleft palate: The state of the art:* ASHA Reports number 9. Washington, D.C.: American Speech and Hearing Association, 1973.

Sloane, H.N. & MacAulay, B.D. Teaching and environmental control of verbal behavior. In H.N. Sloane & B.D. MacAulay (Eds.), *Operant procedures in remedial speech and language training.* New York: Houghton Mifflin, 1968.

Van Riper, C. *Speech correction: Principles and methods* (4th ed.). Englewood Cliffs, N.J.: Prentice-Hall, 1963.

Weston, A.J., & Leonard, L.B. *Articulation disorders: Methods of evaluation and therapy.* Lincoln, Neb.: Cliff Notes, 1976.

Wright, V., Shelton, R.L., & Arndt, W.B. A task for evaluation of articulation change: III. Imitative task scores compared with scores for more spontaneous tasks. *Journal of Speech and Hearing Research,* 1969, *12,* 875-884.

Mata B. Jaffe

Neurological Impairment of Speech Production: Assessment and Treatment

Introduction

Among the neurogenic disorders of communication in children are motor speech disorders: dysarthria and developmental apraxia of speech. Unfortunately, the situation is more complex than that simple statement. These two disorders may coexist and may also accompany a language disorder. Furthermore, some clinicians and researchers feel that there is insufficient evidence to justify the diagnosis of apraxia of speech of a developmental nature. The concept of developmental apraxia of speech is surrounded by controversy, and this chapter will address that controversy.

According to Nicolosi, Harryman, and Kresheck (1978), the term "dysarthria" refers to a collection of motor speech disorders. The impairment originates in the central or peripheral nervous system. Respiration, phonation, resonance, prosody, articulation, chewing and swallowing, and movements of the jaw and tongue may all be affected. The diagnosis of dysarthria excludes apraxia, functional articulation disorders and central language disorders.

Apraxia of speech is defined by Nicolosi et al. (1978) as a nonlinguistic sensorimotor articulation disorder. It is characterized by impairment of the ability to program the positions of the musculature used for speaking and to sequence the movements for producing phonemes. "Dyspraxia" is the term sometimes used to label a less severe form of apraxia. In developmental apraxia of speech (DAS), a congenital condition is assumed. However, as intimated above, even the definition of DAS is somewhat controversial.

These are the two motor speech disorders in children that we will examine: dysarthria and developmental apraxia of speech.

Dysarthria

In the past 10 to 15 years, the role of the speech-language pathologist has changed substantially in relation to neurologically impaired infants and children. These clinicians are working with younger and more severely involved children in an expanded capacity. Some even work with infants in neonatal intensive care units. This shift is due to changes in legislation, earlier identification of neurologically compromised infants or infants at risk for neurologic impairment, evidence from normal infant research concerning the neonate's capacity to learn, and recognition of the efficacy of early identification and intervention with neurologically impaired children and their families.

The Handicapped Children's Early Education Act of 1968 led to establishment of early intervention programs for cerebral palsied and developmentally disabled infants. Some infant stimulation programs use a transdisciplinary approach whereby each team member must have the basic skills needed for total therapeutic interaction with the child and parents. In addition to responsibilities for the development of speech and language, then, the therapist must help the mother in all types of activities that include proper feeding, handling, positioning, and facilitation of gross and fine motor skills. In such settings, the trend has been for therapists to work with very young children (beginning as young as a few months of age) and to demonstrate a wider range of skills than has been the tradition in our field.

Another important legislative act was the Education of All Handicapped Children's Act, PL 94-142, which mandated special education programming for students to 21 years of age regardless of the severity of their handicap. Passage of this law in 1975 made speech and language therapy available to individuals who previously were considered too involved, mentally and/or physically, to benefit from such services. Many of these youngsters were nonverbal, with poor potential for developing serviceable speech. Their needs were part of the incentive for recent advances in nonvocal communication systems and aids and in evaluation and treatment procedures for the feeding and prespeech behaviors which occur during the developmental period that precedes the first word. It is this author's observation and conviction that the clinician who works with younger and/or more severely handicapped children requires knowledge and skills in assessment and treatment in the area of prespeech and feeding.

However, many colleagues, especially university instructors, remain unconvinced that it is the speech-language pathologist's role to feed children or do other nonlanguage-oriented activities. Thus, universities seldom include specific training of this kind in their programs. Their graduates, ill prepared in the areas of prespeech, feeding, and early oral motor development, take jobs in rehabilitation centers, hospitals, and infant-toddler programs where they are expected to have expertise in all that pertains to the oral area.

Augmenting university training programs are training courses in Neuro-Developmental Treatment. This training is particularly useful for clinicians who treat neurologically impaired infants and young children. Such courses are offered in this country and around the world. Guided by the work of Berta Bobath (1967, 1971a, 1971b), Karel Bobath, (1966, 1971), and both together (Bobath & Bobath, 1972), instructors in neuro-developmental treatment (NDT) teach sophisticated assessment and therapy procedures through articles, books, courses, workshops, and conference presentations. Long waiting lists for the basic 8 week NDT course offered to physical, occupational, and speech-language therapists affirm the need for this kind of continuing education. The relatively few speech-language pathologists with NDT training regularly receive letters from programs across the country soliciting their application for jobs that specify an NDT background.

One reason that university programs do not address feeding and oral motor development, assessment, and treatment in more detail is perhaps that the relationship between these early oral motor behaviors and subsequent speech and language development has not been established empirically.

Research in the area of prespeech and feeding with neurologically impaired children is difficult, but not impossible. Morris (1982a) has conducted 2 pilot studies of early feeding and vocal development. The first utilized a screening questionnaire that a paraprofessional or a professional could administer to parents of high risk infants. Questionnaires on 30 infants who failed a prespeech screening and had an abnormal diagnosis at 12 and 24 months were compared with approximately 460 infants with a normal diagnosis at 12 and 24 months. The study attempted to find a cluster of clearly defined problems or prognosticators that would identify children with handicapping conditions associated with a high incidence of speech production problems. There were difficulties inherent in the data collection and analysis. Different diagnostic tools and different criteria for normalcy were used, and there was no consistent follow-up evaluation by a speech-language pathologist. However, the results of this pilot study showed that no single prespeech item or discrete cluster of items clearly separated normal children and children with developmental disabilities.

In a retrospective study, Morris (1982a) sent another set of questionnaires to therapists and parents of infants from 4 to 24 months of age who were in active programs of prespeech and feeding therapy. Diagnostic labels of the 150 infants included cerebral palsy, developmental delay, mental retardation, and chromosomal abnormalities. Preliminary data are currently available on the prenatal history, the children's early feeding history, and the parents' concerns and attempts at finding help. One conclusion was that parents typically identified a feeding problem and looked to the medical community for help, but intervention was regularly postponed. It seemed that pediatricians did not know how to help the parent and infant, probably due to lack of information and lack of standardized tests for identifying infants who should be referred for further evaluation. Parents' reports of feeding problems in their infants were in agreement at least 80% of the time with therapists' descriptions. Recently, a new *Pre-Speech Screening Questionnaire* has been developed to provide a tightly structured study in 2 high-risk-infant follow-up programs. This questionnaire will be available for distribution when field testing with groups of children without unusual birth histories and groups of children at risk has been completed.

Morris (1982a) also conducted a longitudinal study. She observed and filmed the feeding of 6 normally developing infants between birth and 36 months. The infants were studied monthly during the first year, quarterly during the second year, and, finally, at 3 years of age. Morris describes the components of oral movement and their significance in later development of feeding and speech movements, and the parallel relationships between movements and processes described as necessary for both speech production and feeding skills. Major components in the development of both early speech production and feeding skills are the increase in the number and variety of oral movements and positions, differentiation of movements, and more complex coordination ability. Morris suggests that a factor such as gross and/or fine motor development may be involved in the motor skills for both speech and feeding, and thus be responsible for the parallel development of both functions.

Love, Hagerman, and Taimi (1980) examined the relationship between nonspeech oral motor behaviors (biting, sucking, swallowing, and chewing, and 9 infantile oral reflexes) and speech performance in 60 children and young adults with cerebral palsy. They reported a trend, although not completely systematic, for subjects with adequate feeding skills to have better speech. Results generally supported the value of treatment to improve feeding in cerebral palsy, if only to make eating easier and faster and to stimulate gross movement of the oral musculature.

Years ago, in the orientation of Harold Westlake (1951) and Martin Palmer (1947), programs began in which feeding was used as a means of improving oral motor functioning for speech. Then, our profession rejected the concept of the interrelationship of oral movements for speech and for eating. However, clinicians today have been using the feeding process as part of their treatment programs with the working hypothesis that it may improve sensorimotor patterns for better speech and communicative interactions, as well as the child's feeding skills. If we are to meet the challenge of assessing and treating neurologically impaired infants and very young children, we must gather research data to verify the activities that we hypothesize as being clinically appropriate. Morris (1982a) suggests that the group of children with severe gastrointestinal problems, but intact nervous systems, who have not been fed by mouth may offer the opportunity to explore the interrelationship issues.

The following sections will discuss assessment and treatment. The most recent advances in the area of dysarthria in children are in prespeech behaviors.

Assessment

Representing a significant contribution for evaluating speech disorders in neurologically impaired children is the Pre-Speech Assessment Scale (PSAS), a rating scale for the measurement of prespeech behaviors from birth through 2 years (Morris, 1982b). Standardized tools to measure articulation and other speech and language parameters of the older, verbal child have been available, but none were capable of evaluating the prespeech development of the child with sensorimotor impairment. The PSAS can be used with a wide variety of children with delayed or disordered development, including children with cerebral palsy, apraxia of speech, mental retardation, sensory-integrative dysfunction, and other developmental disabilities. Any child functioning below the 2-year level in prespeech development can be appropriately tested.

The PSAS systematically examines feeding, respiration-phonation, and sound play—sensorimotor skills considered to be important for the later development of the more complex act of speech production. The clinician is encouraged to make extensive clinical observations of overall postural tone and movement, head and trunk control, response to sensory stimulation, and response to specific treatment techniques.

Both gross motor and prespeech behaviors of the neurologically impaired child can be divided into abnormal movement patterns, primitive movement patterns, and higher developmental movement patterns. The PSAS provides a way of simultaneously observing and scoring behaviors within the normal developmental ranges of 1 to 24 months on an equal interval scale, and pathological or abnormal behaviors on an ordinal scale. A double-scaling system takes into account the normal/abnormal contrast for prespeech development by measuring the child's performance in each area against specific behavioral descriptions in a section on normal development and a section on abnormal development. The PSAS attempts to place the child's behavior in a specific performance area according to a developmental age range while acknowledging that performance may still be somewhat different qualitatively from that of a normal infant at that age.

The scores are transferred to a graph which allows the therapist to compare the child's levels and problems within each area, to compare developmental abilities across categories, to assign or revise treatment goals and priorities, and to note progress or lack of progress from one evaluation period to the next.

Scoring protocols for the PSAS were based on the above-referenced longitudinal study of 6 normal infants who were filmed from birth to 36 months, and on the scored profiles of approximately 800 developmentally disabled children. Over 200 therapists who have undergone training in the use of the PSAS have provided extensive clinical input into its development and into its content, format, and organization. Studies of interexaminer reliability for behavioral observations and for scoring have indicated that therapists trained in a 4-day workshop can use the PSAS with a clinically acceptable level of reliability.

In addition to its use as an evaluation tool, the PSAS can be recommended because it provides probably the most definitive and complete information on normal sequential development and abnormal deviations of the precursors of speech available in one volume.

Another recent assessment tool was developed by Mysak (1980), who has long been interested in cerebral palsy and dysarthria. Central to Mysak's approach is the concept of neuroevolution of speech viewed as "the progressive integration and elaboration of lower sensorimotor integration centers by higher ones until the ultimate integration of integration centers results in bipedal standing, walking, and talking behavior" (Mysak, 1980, p. 19). He traces this evolution phylogenetically and ontogenetically. Mysak's (1980) *Neurophysiological Speech Index* (NSI) is a clinical tool for evaluating the development of a child relative to a "neurophysiological speaking age". It includes behaviors that children normally achieve by 18 to 24+ months of age. The NSI has ratings based on expected reflexes in infants and ratings based on the presence of persisting infantile reflexes in older infants and children. It is a composite of the Basic Movements

Index and the Skilled Movements Index. The author suggests using the *Neurophysiological Speech Index* primarily as a guide for planning therapy and judging progress and, secondarily, as an index of the child's neurophysiological speech age.

In this author's opinion, Mysak's recent work continues to be difficult reading, hampered by use of idiosyncratic terminology such as "face talk." Furthermore, the NSI lacks standardization, validity, and reliability information. Developmental milestones are based on normative data which are not referenced. Speech-language pathologists would probably find the *Neurophysiological Speech Index* difficult to use.

Treatment

Treatment of dysarthria in children is not researched in the most recent literature. However, corresponding to the interest in prespeech and feeding assessment and the development of assessment tools is an interest in early intervention and in the principles and strategies for treating prespeech and feeding problems of the young and/or severely neurologically impaired child. Much of the current sensorimotor programming for neurologically impaired children is based on the writings of Mueller (1972, 1975) and based on the NDT approach. A review of recent writings on treatment, emphasizing feeding, follows.

Perske, Clifton, McLean, and Stein (1977) have collected contributions by "knowledgeable persons" about their programs and handicapped persons at mealtimes. While this is not a how-to-do-it handbook, it does attempt to increase the sensitivities and skills of those who feed seriously handicapped persons. The editors point to a movement toward making mealtimes as important for handicapped persons as for the rest of us. Contrasting in style, Gallender (1979) presents the anatomic and physiologic aspects of eating handicaps and relates and illustrates specific techniques and instructional materials on particular eating handicaps.

Campbell (1982) developed a problem-oriented approach to make the therapist, teacher, or parent "the expert" in identifying problems and creating solutions to help the child with feeding difficulties acquire basic feeding skills. The material is divided into 3 major parts. The first section introduces approaches to feeding problems and general methods for handling specific concerns. Five major feeding problems are presented in the second section in a flow chart format so the reader can identify the child's specific difficulties, develop appropriate goals, select possible solutions, and evaluate their effectiveness. The last section includes some common techniques for the management of the feeding problems identified.

Morris (1977) developed a manual primarily for use with young children with mild to severe degrees of neurologic impairment with or without mental retardation. It is designed to instruct teachers, therapists, and parents how to help children develop better control for eating. Program guidelines, many illustrated with photographs, are suggested according to the probable causes of the child's feeding difficulties. Morris points out that often the solution to the problem of feeding depends on physically handling and positioning the cerebral palsied child to decrease spasticity or involuntary movements of the total body as well as the mouth, face, and throat. She also emphasizes the critical importance of involving the parents or parent substitutes as active participants in the treatment program. They must understand the goals, underlying rationales, and the steps in the program, and learn the specific procedures. Further, the therapist must understand the family situation and routine and the difficulty parents and child may have in changing their ways of feeding.

Davis (1978) describes prespeech development in normal and atypical children. Early intervention is advocated with the major goal of establishing muscle tone and neuromuscular patterns–which are as normal as possible–in respiration and feeding, as a foundation for achieving more normal speech development. Davis describes intervention and specific activities.

Unfortunately, there are many excellent clinicians, especially those trained in neuro-developmental treatment, who have the most to offer in the area of prespeech treatment and who present workshops and courses of exceptional quality, but who have not published their work. Morris (1982a), however, has written about prespeech and speech therapy with neurologically impaired children, emphasizing early intervention and a physiologic and neurologic orientation toward treatment. Morris considers the following as important concepts:

1. Abnormal postural tone and movement patterns interfere with speech (and feeding) patterns. Abnormal tone reduces the options for normal movement and normal sensory feedback.
2. Hypersensitivity and hyposensitivity to sensory stimulation can reduce the opportunities for learning.
3. Motor learning is predominantly motor-sensory-motor learning. There is a need to prevent the establishment of abnormal patterns and to provide a spontaneous option for the child to feel and sense a different, more normal way of moving.
4. Early automatic patterns of oral movement provide a model for similar movements to be incorporated later into speech production.
5. Treatment is an ongoing process and way of life to be incorporated throughout the day.

With these assumptions, Morris offers the following basic goals for a communication skills program for children with neurologic deficits:
1. normalization of the child's postural tone through inhibition of abnormal and strong postural reflexes;
2. simultaneous stimulation and facilitation of normal postural reactions and automatic responses;
3. feedback to the child's system of correct tone and performance; and
4. constant awareness of the communication dynamics between the child and others in the environment.

In the assessment section of this chapter Mysak's assessment procedure, the *Neurophysiological Speech Index,* was discussed. Mysak (1980) chooses the term "neurospeech therapy" to designate his treatment approach to emphasize the overall neurologic focus in speech therapy with the cerebral palsied child. His theory is based on "the progressive and successive integration of lower sensorimotor integration centers by higher centers and, finally, the integration of the right hemisphere by the left hemisphere" (p.184). He, too, advocates beginning therapy with children below 1 year of age, during the prespeech period, because the plasticity of the infant brain could prevent fixation of abnormal movement patterns, deformities, and contractures.

Mysak considers the stimulation of basic listening movements, speech postures, hand movements, and basic speech movements to be fundamental to neurospeech therapy. He describes preparatory physical maneuvers to enrich sensorimotor experiences, to induce relaxation, to normalize tone, posture, and movement, and to facilitate integration and elaboration of reflexes. His suggestions for normalizing facial and oral area sensitivity and facilitation of drinking and eating movements are similar to those suggested by aforementioned authors (Campbell (1982); Davis (1978); Gallender (1979); Morris (1977, 1982a); Mueller (1972, 1975).)

Mysak facilitates speech postures through various postures of the body, head, and parts of the oral mechanism, and through isolation of body parts and movements. He combines these with appropriately timed speech sound stimulation. He suggests neuro-facilitation techniques, such as resisted movement maneuvers or reversed movement maneuvers, to counteract limitations in direction and range of articulatory movement. To increase sensory awareness, he recommends exercises such as increased pressure for bilabial sounds, longer contacts for stop and continuant sounds, and elongated vowel sounds. Symbolic facial and hand gestural communications are viewed as facilitators of speech and enhancers of communication.

Treatment programs for young children with dysarthria can successfully include simultaneous goals and treatment to improve prespeech, feeding, phonation-respiration, and language functions. Successful treatment of the child with central nervous system dysfunction requires an integrated approach. Therapy will be effective if the therapist does not rely on specific techniques but observes thoughtfully, reevaluates continually, and modifies treatment according to the responses of the child.

In summary, our profession is faced with the reality of assessing and treating younger and more severely involved children with neurologic impairment. The recent trend, clinically if not academically, is to approach this challenge by working in transdisciplinary and interdisciplinary teams toward common goals for the child and family. Such an integrated approach generally includes the area of prespeech and feeding as well as the more traditional speech-language assessment and therapy for dysarthria. To be effective, the therapist needs to understand and treat the child's entire system, not just the mechanisms directly involved in speech. There are many unanswered questions about the efficacy of this kind of treatment. Though difficult, research in this area is sorely needed.

Developmental Apraxia of Speech

Known by a variety of labels such as "developmental motor aphasia", "articulatory apraxia or dyspraxia", and "childhood verbal apraxia", a motor programming disorder in children was first described by Hadden in 1891. Currently the most common term is developmental apraxia of speech (DAS). This speech disorder is characterized by impaired ability to program, combine, and sequence the elements of speech. It is considered to be a neurologic, sensorimotor speech disorder and is differentiated from dysarthria and functional articulation disorders in children (Nicolosi et al., 1978). The apraxic child demonstrates impairment, in varying degrees, in the ability to position the articulators consistently to produce speech and sound combinations.

There is confusion in the literature as to the behaviors that are important for the diagnosis of DAS. Thus, the practicing clinician often does not feel confident in labeling a given child's speech pattern as developmental apraxia of speech. Table 6-1 illustrates the wide range of characteristics that have been suggested to be part of DAS. Some of the problem is due to assumptions based on the adult literature on verbal apraxia, even though the differences between children and adults are great enough that perhaps the terminology should not be the same. Rosenbek (Note 1) pointed out differences in apraxia of speech between adults and children and suggested reasons for these differences.

Apraxia is defined by a symptom cluster—another source of confusion. Not *all* symptoms must be present; no *one* characteristic or symptom *must*

TABLE 6-1
Reported characteristics of developmental apraxia of speech

CHARACTERISTICS	AUTHORS
Early History	
History of feeding problems; noninformative crying; little distinguishable vocal play, babbling, imitation, or self-imitation during infancy	Aram & Glasson, Note 2 Eisenson, 1966
Family History	
Strong family history of speech, language, and learning disorders	Aram & Glasson, Note 2 Morley, 1972 Saleeby, Hadjian, Martinkosky, & Swift, Note 3
Neurological Findings	
High incidence of "soft" neurological findings; generalized dyspraxia	Crary, Note 4 Eisenson, 1966 McClumpha & Logue, Note 5 Yoss & Darley, 1974a
Nonspeech Findings	
Deficits in oral perception	Loevner, Note 6 Prichard, Tekieli, & Kozup, 1979
Oral nonverbal apraxia co-occuring	Aram & Glasson, Note 2 Chappell, 1973 Eisenson, 1966 Rosenbek & Wertz, 1972 Yoss & Darley, 1974a
Poor self monitoring	Edwards, 1973 Fawcus, 1971 Morley, 1972 Morley & Fox, 1969 Yoss & Darley, 1974a
Gross motor incoordination	Aram & Glasson, Note 2
Speech	
Markedly reduced repertoire of phonemes	Aram & Glasson, Note 2 Chappell, 1973 Edwards, 1973 Fawcus, 1971 Morley, 1972
Extraordinarily poor imitative skills for articulation	Chappell, 1973 McClumpha & Logue, Note 5 Rosenbek, Hansen, Baughman, & Lemme, 1974

TABLE 6-1 (cont.)
Reported characteristics of developmental apraxia of speech

CHARACTERISTICS	AUTHORS
Speech (cont.)	
Significant problems in phonetic synthesis for speech	McClumpha & Logue, Note 5
Highly inconsistent errors	Nicolosi et al., 1978 Rosenbek & Wertz, 1972
Misarticulations that are grossly inconsistent at the imitative level and generally consistent (primarily simplifications) in spontaneous speech	McClumpha & Logue, Note 5 Rosenbek, Note 1
Delayed and deviant speech development	Aram & Glasson, Note 2 Rosenbek & Wertz, 1972
Prominent phonemic errors: omissions (errors are more often omissions than substitutions of sounds and syllables), distortions, additions, repetitions, prolongations	Rosenbek & Wertz, 1972
Frequent methathetic errors, sequential sound production difficulties	Aram & Glasson, Note 2 Edwards, 1973 Morley, 1972 Rosenbek & Wertz, 1972
Misarticulations of vowels as well as consonants	Rosenbek & Wertz, 1972
Adequate repetitions of sounds in isolation; connected speech more unintelligible than would be expected on the basis of single word articulation tests results	Rosenbek & Wertz, 1972
Errors varying with the complexity of articulatory adjustment; most frequent errors on fricatives, affricates, and consonant clusters	Crary, Note 4 Rosenbek & Wertz, 1972
Groping trial-and-error behavior manifested as sound prolongations, repetitions, or silent posturing which may precede or interrupt imitative utterances	Rosenbek & Wertz, 1972
Oral diadochokinetic rates, especially for /pʌ tʌ kʌ/, slower than normal and often incorrectly sequenced	Aram & Glasson, Note 2 Crary, Note 4 Yoss & Darley, 1974a
More voicing errors than by children with functional articulation disorder	Yoss & Darley, 1974a
2- and 3-feature errors, prolongations and repetitions of sounds and syllables, additions, and distortions present in repetition speech tasks	Yoss & Darley, 1974a

CHARACTERISTICS	AUTHORS
Speech (cont.)	
Distortions, 1- place feature errors, additions, and omissions in spontaneous speech	Yoss & Darley, 1974a
Prosodic disturbances, such as slower rate and equalized stress	Edwards, 1973 Glasson, Note 7 Rosenbek & Wertz, 1972 Yoss & Darley, 1974a
Difficulty sequencing sounds and larger speech units, with the complexity and length of the utterance governing the degree of verbal apraxia evidenced; greater difficulty on polysyllabic words	Aram & Glasson, Note 2 Chappell, 1973 Edwards, 1973 Eisenson, 1966 Glasson, Note 7 Morley, 1972 Rosenbek & Wertz, 1972 Yoss & Darley, 1974a
Oral-nasal resonance confusions	Glasson, Note 7 Yoss & Darley, 1974a
More omission errors than in functional articulation disorder	Smartt, LaLance, Gray, and Hibbett, 1976
Breakdown in the spatial and temporal coordination of speech	Crary, Note 4; Note 8 Glasson, Note 7
Language	
Receptive abilities inordinately superior to expressive abilities	Aram & Glasson, Note 2 Rosenbek & Wertz, 1972 McClumpha & Logue, Note 5
Pervasive expressive language disorder	Aram & Glasson, Note 2 Ekelman, Note 9 Ekelman & Aram, 1983 Rosenbek, Note 1
Co-occurrence with aphasia, dysarthria, specific learning disability	Aram & Glasson, Note 2 Rosenbek & Wertz, 1972 Yoss & Darley, 1974a
Disordered basic language processes	Aram & Glasson, Note 2 Ekelman, Note 9 Ekelman & Aram, 1983 Loevner, Note 6 Rosenbek, Note 1
Prognosis	
Very slow in improving speech; typically poor response to "traditional" speech therapy	Chappell, 1973 Court & Harris, 1965 Daly, Cantrell, Cantrell & Aman, 1972 Fawcus, 1971 Rosenbek et al., 1974

be present; and the typically reported symptoms are not *exclusive* to developmental apraxia of speech. Compounding the problem is the observation that children change over time. For example, one client was diagnosed as apraxic at 3 years of age when he was essentially nonverbal. Without knowing his history, it is doubtful that a speech pathologist first meeting this child when he was 5½ years old would consider the label "developmental apraxia of speech". By this time he displayed a mild to moderate expressive language disorder and misarticulations characterized by a frontal lisp, distorted /l/ and /r/, and productions such as "whipskers" for whiskers and "ephalant" for elephant.

It is also extremely difficult to conduct research on a disorder for which identification of subjects is a problem. Many clinicians feel that this is a heterogeneous, rather than homogeneous population. Logue (Note 10) believes that single subject research is the most promising way to study DAS. In research to date, subjects represent a wide range of age, IQ, severity of communication disorder, concomitant disabilities, and organic signs. While there are children for whom neurologists have designated a neurologic basis for their speech disorder, it is currently debated whether the children under discussion actually have neurologic disorders. There is a small body of literature about developmental apraxia of speech: probably the major works have yet to be written.

American journal articles describing apraxic children began to appear in the 1970s with Rosenbek and Wertz in 1972, then Yoss and Darley (1974a), and Rosenbek et al., in 1974. Presentations at national, regional, and state conventions addressing verbal apraxia in children have been particularly popular in the last 10 years. There is a strong clinical interest in the disorder, even though a relatively small percentage of children receive this diagnostic label. Clinicians have found the diagnosis of developmental apraxia of speech useful for a number of children whose speech is particularly resistant to change, and many clinicians diagnose apraxia by first eliminating all else. Now it appears that the pendulum has swung again with writers who are challenging the existence of developmental apraxia of speech as a clinical entity. There are those who believe that we have embraced the area of apraxia without proper evidence—either empirical or clinical.

Behavioral Descriptions of the Symptomatology of Developmental Apraxia of Speech

Various authors have described the behavioral characteristics of apraxia. As indicated above, Table 6-1 lists these characteristics and includes earlier as well as recent authors. Perusal of this table may provide insight for the reader regarding the problems that arise in pinpointing the defining characteristics of this disorder.

A recent critical review of the literature written about developmental apraxia of speech by Guyette and Diedrich (1981) has spurred the controversy, which is likely to continue. In their survey of over 100 publications on adult and childhood apraxia and on principles of diagnosis, they conclude that there are as yet no convincing empirical bases to support assumptions regarding the existence of a readily differentiated DAS clinical population. Regarding nonspeech symptoms sometimes reported to characterize DAS (neurological "soft" signs; poor oral motor and diadochokinetic skills; the presence of concurrent language, sensory and/or intellectual deficits; positive family histories for speech disorders; the imbalanced distribution of the disorder between males and females; and the wide range of prognoses that have been claimed for DAS), Guyette and Diedrich illustrate the myriad of contradictory findings reported in that literature, leaving none of those characteristics to be reliable indicators of DAS. Further, they draw the same conclusions when they report the literature's findings on the speech symptoms various writers have attributed to DAS children. They discuss supposed symptoms such as articulatory inconsistency; inability to imitate; the display of particular articulatory error patterns related to sound omissions, vowel productions, or errors on consonant clusters, fricatives, and affricates; increasing errors with increasing lengths of utterances; and problems of prosody (including the classic groping behaviors of adult apraxia), sequencing, voicing, and oral-nasal differentiation. They suggest that most of these reported speech symptoms have been based on clinical impressions, and the few that have been studied empirically either have been shown not to occur in the speech of supposed DAS subjects or not to differentiate that speech from the speech of children with functional disorders of articulation.

Further, Guyette and Diedrich suggest that it is no wonder the literature is so diverse and inconclusive where the behavioral description of DAS children is concerned, considering the ways in which subjects have been selected for the studies that have produced these inconsistent findings. It is exceedingly circular to select subjects on the basis of behavioral characteristics that the study itself is designed to discover. So, their observation that subjects have been selected on the basis of defective oral movement skills (Smartt et al., 1976; Yoss & Darley, 1974a), or because someone has previously diagnosed them as apraxic by some unknown criteria (Prichard, Tekieli, & Kozup, 1979; Rosenbek & Wertz, 1972), or because they've made insignificant progress in therapy (Ferry, Hall & Hicks, 1975; Prichard et al., 1979; Aram and Glasson, Note 2), would almost necessarily produce a highly heterogeneous population. And that is, in fact, what has been shown in comparative reviews of the literature.

Guyette and Diedrich (1981; in press) make one further observation regarding the ways in which DAS children have been studied in the literature. They point out the absence of treatment studies demonstrating such children to be positively affected by certain treatments and not by others. In fact, treatment research in general is quite sparse with this population, so one has to wonder about the value of providing a diagnostic label from which no specific treatment has yet evolved.

More doubt regarding the likelihood of reliably identifying subgroups of DAS children is raised in an empirical study conducted by Williams, Ingham, and Rosenthal (1981). This study was, in fact, a direct replication of the Yoss and Darley (1974a) study that was essentially the first experimental attempt to determine whether a group of misarticulating children could be realistically described as DAS and shown to be different from other misarticulating children. In both studies essentially the same battery of speech and nonspeech tasks was given to 30 children with moderately to severely defective articulation but normal intelligence, hearing, and language development, and no apparent primary organic etiology. In both studies the same battery was also administered to an age- and sex-matched control group.

While Yoss and Darley found several characteristics that appeared to distinguish between children with apparently functional misarticulations and those whom they suggest could be called DAS children (separated arbitrarily on the basis of their isolated volitional oral movement—IVOM—scores), the findings of Williams et al. were at variance with almost every Yoss and Darley conclusion. Whereas Yoss and Darley's 2 groups of misarticulating subjects were significantly different on nonspeech IVOM scores, SVOM (sequenced volitional oral movements), and neurologic findings, in the Williams et al. study the 2 groups of misarticulators differed only on the variable used to divide the groups originally—IVOM scores. The 3 measures mentioned above might be assumed to be hallmarks of DAS, but they were not differentiating for the Williams et al. subjects. By conducting a discriminant function analysis on 14 speech variables, both studies pinpointed 6 variables that significantly discriminated the 2 speech disordered groups on the basis of the repeated speech tasks in the test battery, but only 2 variables overlapped: the sum of 2-feature errors and the sum of addition errors. Yoss and Darley's groups were differentiated primarily by neurologic findings which were uninfluential variables for the Williams et al. subjects. For spontaneous speech tasks, Yoss and Darley's analysis pinpointed 5 variables that could reliably separate the 2 groups of speech disordered subjects, with neurologic findings leading the way once again; but the Williams et al. analysis found no variables that could reliably separate the 2 groups of subjects. Essentially the only variable upon which the 2 studies agreed was a finding that diadochokinetic rates for the production of /kʌ/ were significantly slower for the potentially DAS group of subjects. Although Williams et al. appropriately suggest differences between the 2 studies that might account for differences in their findings (severity differences between the 2 potential DAS groups, differences in referral sources and, therefore, in the likelihood of the presence of neurologic "soft" signs, etc.), one is again left wondering whether it is currently possible to unambiguously differentiate DAS children from other misarticulating children.

Apparently there are those who believe it is, because work continues in relation to this disorder. Recent investigations which hold promise for a better understanding of this disorder are by Crary (Note 4; Note 8), Comeau & Crary (Note 12), and Towne and Crary (Note 13). They suggest a neurolinguistic perspective, and take the position that DAS usually encompasses both phonology and syntax. They state that the underlying deficit in phonologic development is limitation in the control of the spatial and temporal properties of articulation. Glasson's (Note 7) spectrographic analysis also suggested temporal coordination difficulties in DAS. The studies by Crary and his colleagues describe phonologic process profiles and investigate phonologic influence on syntactic performance. The authors suggest that the expansion of syntactic skills may depend on a certain level of proficiency in production of closed-syllable shapes. These studies, in general, support the studies by Aram and Glasson (Note 2), Ekelman (Note 9), Ekelman & Aram (1983) and Loevner (Note 6), as well as observations by many clinicians, that language processes may also be disordered in DAS.

Clearly, most investigators who are interested in DAS do not doubt its existence, but do feel a need for further delineation and exploration. It is anticipated that the many questions surrounding differential diagnosis will be addressed over the next few years. Some clinicians suggest that the advantages of making such a diagnosis are that it can provide a rationale for intensifying therapy, may prevent mismanagement, may direct family and patient counseling, may lower the expectancy for articulation proficiency, and may support a decision to introduce an augmentative system. With this in mind, as well as the general topic of symptomatology of DAS, the following is a review of the available measurement and assessment tools.

Measurement and Assessment Tools

As the reader has no doubt assumed from the previous section, a differential diagnosis of DAS is complicated and continues to elude many diagnosticians. There are very few tests specific to the assessment of DAS, and none have sufficient norms, standardization, validity, and reliability findings to be considered more than tentative measures which may hold potential. They await empirical data as to their ultimate value.

One such assessment is an unpublished protocol, *Motor Speech Examination* (Logue, Note 10; Note 14), which attempts to identify deficits in a child's motor speech planning. The examination assesses these motor skills and behaviors: (1) nonvolitional oral behaviors, (2) indices of dominance and laterality, (3) cranial nerve function, (4) diadochokinesis or multiple cranial nerve integration, (5) competitive articulatory posturing, (6) motor speech integration, and (7) imitative and spontaneous articulatory production skills.

Another test is the *Screening Test for Developmental Apraxia of Speech* (Blakeley, 1980), developed to aid in differential diagnosis and to suggest when further speech and language assessment and neurologic evaluation is needed. A cluster of symptoms, selected on the basis of the work of authors referred to in this chapter, is thought by Blakeley to have implications for a diagnosis of verbal apraxia. The following 8 subtests make up the test: I. Expressive Language Discrepancy, II. Vowels and Diphthongs, III. Oral-Motor Movement, IV. Verbal Sequencing, V. Articulation, VI. Motorically Complex Words, VII. Transpositions, and VIII. Prosody. A raw score is converted to a total weighted score and applied to a probability graph to determine exclusion from or inclusion into an apraxia group. The test takes approximately 10 minutes to administer.

Guyette and Diedrich (in press) reviewed the *Screening Test for Developmental Apraxia* to point out their concerns over the use of this instrument. Their review explored the literature Blakeley cited as support for the symptomatology which the test is designed to sample, examined the standard parameters of test construction, and presented data summarizing the author's use of this instrument. The review suggested that the references cited by Blakeley offered little empirical support for his claim that the symptoms of developmental apraxia of speech are those sampled in this test, and they concluded that a test to diagnose developmental apraxia of speech is premature and unjustified because there is still no agreement on the symptomatology of the disorder. Guyette and Diedrich further point out that the *Screening Test for Developmental Apraxia of Speech* has yet to be validated and that no test/retest reliability data are reported for the children or the examiners.

Treatment

The literature regarding developmental verbal apraxia addresses symptomatology and differential diagnosis more than it deals with therapy. Therapy is often described as a slow and difficult process, and many clinicians base a diagnosis of developmental apraxia on the lengthy and arduous course of treatment as well as on supposedly characteristically deviant articulatory patterns.

Most early work in the treatment area contained case studies (Dabul, 1971; Daly et al., 1972; Hadden, 1891; Rosenbek et al., 1974; Rosenthal, 1971; Logue & McClumpha, Note 15) or suggestions based on clinical experience (Chappell, 1973; Edwards, 1973; Eisenson, 1972; Morley, Court, Miller, & Garside, 1955; Morley & Fox, 1969; Yoss & Darley, 1974b; McClumpha & Logue, Note 5). They emphasized primarily: capitalizing on the visual modality and reading; association of correct sound production with visual, motor, and auditory cues; introduction of highly contrasted sounds; gradual increase in length and complexity of linguistic units; backward chaining; stimulation for syllable shapes and movement patterns rather than single phonemes; use of intonation and rhythm; decrease in speaking rate by clinician and child; and sensorimotor stimulation or oral motor facilitation. Truly needed are investigations to systematically evaluate the therapeutic effectiveness of a variety of treatment approaches.

Rosenbek (Note 1) suggests that the best current treatment methods for both apraxic children and adults are very similar except for obvious differences such as the selection of therapy material. He lists these methods as Total Communication; Melodic Intonation Therapy; the motokinesthetic approach; contrastive stress drills to exploit the effects of meaning; and pacing methods with intersystemic or gestural reorganization, utilizing movement via pacing boards, syllabic tapping, and the like.

Total Communication

Total Communication, speech combined with all modes of communication, but primarily manual communication, may be a viable treatment approach with some apraxic children. This would probably be because: (1) the child has not experienced a history of failure; (2) the visual channel, which may be a stronger input channel than the auditory one, is utilized, (3) the child can watch his or her own hands for feedback; (4) the fine motor competence required of speech is absent; (5) the hands are easier for the clinician to mold and shape than the mouth; (6) the signs can be extended in time without distortion, while speech is transitory; (7) a degree of iconicity in sign language facilitates language growth, and (8) the sign can help the child's speech by the association of a meaningful gross motor movement with units of speech. An effective Total Communication program emphasizes meaning, spontaneous communication, and consequences of communicative acts rather than imitation, repetition, and drill.

For these reasons, Jaffe (Note 16; Note 17) proposes extensive use of manual sign language and the manual alphabet in a treatment program

for young children who are considered to be moderately to severely apraxic. In the early stages of therapy, sign language can be the major communication system, and in the later stages, signs and finger spelling can
augment verbal communication. Total Communication is introduced at
the onset, not as a last resort. By repeated association, it appears that
signs may help the child recall and correctly articulate sound patterns and
produce correct syntactic sequences. The use of signs with speech can
help the clinician slow the rate of presentation and help the child reduce
rate of utterance. The manual alphabet is introduced to establish a meaningful, visual-motor and kinesthetic movement pattern to cue production
of the target phonemes and to facilitate blending and sequencing of
phonemes.

Over a 9-month period, preliminary data were collected on 4 young
apraxic children in individual and group therapy situations and parent-
child interactions. All of the children showed a decrease in gestures and
unintelligible vocalizations with an increase in signs and intelligible verbalizations, combinations of signs and speech, and total communicative
output.

Melodic Intonation Therapy

The recent application of Melodic Intonation Therapy (MIT) with
developmentally apraxic children (Doszak, McNeil, & Jancosek, Note 18;
Helfrich-Miller, Note 19; in press) may also prove to be an important
treatment approach. Melodic Intonation Therapy has been used successfully with adult apraxic patients (Berlin, 1976; Sparks, Helm, &
Albert, 1974; Sparks & Holland, 1976). This technique focuses on the formulation of propositional expressive language through use of intoned
sequences. Its original intent was to place emphasis on recovery of propositional language (Albert, Sparks, & Helm, 1973) rather than on the motor
aspects of speech production. Sparks and Holland (1976), however, noted
that while MIT is directed toward language, some clinicians have also
reported success adapting it to improve slurred articulation and to reduce
the frequency of phonemic errors in some apraxic patients.

The following are suggested as rationales for using this approach with
apraxic children: (1) alterations in prosody—rhythm, stress, and
intonation—may improve speech production, (2) the emphasis on movement may improve phonemic and linguistic sequencing through intersystemic organization, and (3) the reduced rate of verbal input and verbal
output may facilitate correct articulatory placement and inclusion.

Helfrich-Miller (Note 19; in press) adapted procedures, previously
described in the literature with adult aphasics, for a treatment program
with developmentally apraxic children. In place of tapping out a rhythm,

manual sign language was substituted in the MIT hierarchy to facilitate sequencing and language structure. Three levels were hierarchically arranged to move the child in small graded steps toward achieving normal speech prosody. The progression from the first to the third level entailed 4 principles: (1) increased length of unit, (2) increased phonemic, morphologic, and syntactic complexity, (3) decreased dependency on the clinician, and (4) diminished reliance on intoning and signing. It was essentially an imitative program.

Helfrich-Miller has treated children as young as 2 years of age with less formalized adaptations of MIT. The ideal candidate for a formalized program, however, is a 7- to 8-year old, with moderate to marked verbal apraxia, demonstrating poor repetition skills. Such a child would need an MLU of at least 3 to 4 words and an attention span of at least 15 to 20 minutes. Children with accompanying dysarthria are not candidates for this technique.

Data presented on 2 children reported convincing gains in articulation, sequencing abilities, and expressive language. Both children took 11 months to finish the program. Once the formalized program was completed, the use of MIT principles continued throughout therapy. The children were taught to self-cue through intonation and signing to facilitate linguistic sequencing. When the program is used appropriately, Level III is not the end of MIT but the beginning of an internalized cueing system which seeks to normalize sequencing abilities in apraxic children.

Doszak et al. (Note 18) evaluated the effectiveness of MIT in improving prosodic and articulatory features in a single subject, a 10-year-old male diagnosed as having developmental apraxia of speech. A time series withdrawal design (ABAB) was used to determine the effects of MIT versus nontreatment. Data were analyzed by 2 objective and 1 subjective measure: vowel duration (on all CVC productions) and percentage of duration of final contour compared to the entire sentence duration (on sentence productions), and listener judgments (on the same recurrent sentence production during the picture description), respectively. Duration measures were made on a 4-channel oscillograph and a Visipitch. The 2 objective measures revealed significant ANOVA results for the vowel duration measures and no significant change in the duration of the final contour between any test sessions. Listeners judged the later speech samples as "better sounding." The authors concluded that MIT was effective in improving this subject's speech, inferred that MIT or some component of MIT reduced vowel durations, and suggested further research on the efficacy of MIT with developmentally apraxic children and on the relationship between perceptual changes and acoustic or physiologic changes in speech.

Motokinesthetic and motor learning approaches

Emphasizing motokinesthetic techniques is the moto-sequential tactile therapy, or "touch-cue" approach (Bashir, Jones, & Bostwick, Note 20; Jones, Note 21). This is a systematic approach to teaching individual speech sounds and enhancing sound-sequencing abilities. The clinician presents auditory and visual stimuli along with touch-cue points that are designated points on the face which the child touches during production of consonant, consonant-vowel, CVC and VC drills. Therapy is divided into 3 stages, each stage establishing basic skills that will be elaborated in subsequent stages of therapy. Stage I is a collection of articulation drills, arranged in order of difficulty. These drills are to develop self-monitoring and to teach association of auditory, visual, and touch cues. Stage II incorporates the learned sequences from Stage I into the production of real and nonsense words. The phonemic chains increase in complexity to form multisyllabic chains and words. Stage III is concerned with carry-over of these skills into controlled and spontaneous speech. The program depends on the family for cooperation and has a parent-teaching component. Undoubtedly, many therapists are employing such techniques with children who have poor articulation apparently due to a motor planning deficit or hearing impairment, so the approach should be put to empirical test. Motokinesthetic approaches may hold promise for treating developmentally apraxic children.

Another speech-motor training program is the *Monitoring Articulatory Postures* (MAP), developed and refined by Logue (1978; Note 10). The MAP is designed for the child whose breakdown in the programming system seems to occur when integrated movements of phonation, respiration, and articulation are superimposed on nonspeech oral-motor movements.

The premise of MAP is that the apraxic child needs to develop a reliable motor command before concentrating on sound production. The program is in 3 phases. Phase I, Articulatory Posture Training, intends to teach the child to establish and to maintain vowel and consonant associated postures. In Phase II, Speech Shadow Imitation, the clinician first presents a visual model only, then gradually fades the visual emphasis and introduces the auditory model for the first time. Phase III, Competitive Articulatory Posturing, is the most critical phase of the MAP program. It requires considerable anticipatory and reprogramming capability which the author believes is an important prerequisite for articulate speech. The clinician instructs the child to position the articulators to produce a particular vowel, consonant, or word, and then instructs the child to produce a competing vowel, consonant, or word, instead. Thus, the program progresses from simple imitation of vowel postures to the reprogramming necessary to produce a word after assuming the anticipatory posture of a contrasted word. Logue has not yet reported data on the effects of this treatment strategy, including the necessity or helpfulness of each of the stages in the treatment. (One might wonder if the first 2 steps requiring imitation might not be inordinately difficult for an apraxic child, if the inability to voluntarily imitate motor movements is, in fact, a hallmark of the disorder.)

Rate control

One investigation provides an excellent empirical therapy evaluation method which serves as a rare model for the kind of treatment research needed in this confused area of DAS. Rosenthal, Williams, and Ingham (Note 22) conducted an experimental therapy program, the intent of which was to systematically evaluate the effectiveness of certain treatment procedures with 1 female and 3 male apraxic subjects who ranged in age from 10 to 14 years. Subjects were labeled apraxic on the basis of 2 independent diagnoses from qualified speech-language clinicians and on the observation of a history of very slow response to therapy. The treatment program was designed to successively establish correct articulation during slowed oral reading, gradually increase reading rates to a normal level, and then transfer this skill to "monologue" speech.

In Stage I, 6 experimental procedures were sequentially introduced and assessed for each subject. First, the rate of a reading machine was adjusted to approximately 50% of each child's baseline reading rate, established in 6 to 12 5-minute "sessions." The percentage of words correctly articulated was calculated on-line for each subject during alternating 5-minute intervals requiring rate change or returning to baseline conditions. All subjects showed an increase in the percentage of words read correctly under the condition of slowed rate, and this was therefore incorporated into the remaining 5 procedures of Stage I.

Subsequent experimental conditions were introduced in the same fashion and evaluated according to their effect on the percentage of words correctly articulated. Condition 2 introduced response contingent reinforcement wherein subjects earned 1 cent for every 10 correctly articulated words. In Condition 3, following incorrectly articulated words, the experimenter provided the correct production while the subject listened but did not repeat the word. During Condition 4, the clinician again provided a model following incorrectly articulated words and the subject was required to imitate the word immediately. (It is interesting to note that this was ineffective at producing improved articulation for 3 of the 4 subjects.) Because certain subjects had retained particular phonemes in error at this stage of the treatment, in Condition 5 the experimenters implemented phoneme instruction wherein the experimenter demonstrated and described placement and manner of production of the relevant error phonemes and gave the subjects the opportunity to practice words containing those typically misarticulated phonemes. Then Condition 4 was reintroduced so that the effects of specific phoneme instruction could be evaluated. The last experimental treatment procedure introduced during this stage of the treatment—designed to establish correct articulation at slowed reading rates—was to highlight each subject's remaining incorrect phoneme occurrences by contingently providing an explanation of the error; e.g., if the subject read "beat" instead of "beach", the experimenter said, "/tʃ/ at the end: beach"; and the child read the word again.

Following the establishment of 85% correct articulation during slowed oral reading by the end of Condition 6 for all subjects, the next phase gradually moved the reading rate to the subject's normal rate, concurrently providing contingent feedback (a beep) for each incorrectly articulated word. This was followed by a similar progression from slowed to normal speaking rates requiring maintenance of the 85% correct articulation performance in monologue speech. Subsequently, 95% correct production in monologue was required. The final evaluation of the treatment effects occurred when the subjects were required to talk in monologue with no experimenter-controlled feedback of any kind. The data showed maintenance of 95% correct articulation for each subject at that subject's normal speaking rate.

The authors report that 3 procedures appeared to be effective for all 4 subjects: rate control, phoneme production instruction, and the highlighting of error phonemes. They also recommended including reinforcement for correct responding in a therapy program for apraxic children because it produced positive change for all of the subjects (although only marginally for 2), and they believed its presence helped the children persevere in the therapy program. They also pointed out that each condition proved effective for at least 1 of the 4 subjects, so that each might be considered and individually examined with future subjects.

Even though it is, obviously, valuable to know that rate control procedures have been demonstrated to be an effective component of successful treatment for DAS, this study was reported in greater detail than others because it also serves as an example of the careful, systematic, and empirical way in which treatment can be conducted. More research of this nature is required before much of value can be written about the treatment of children diagnosed as DAS.

Final Comments

It was stated earlier that the major works about developmental apraxia of speech have probably yet to be written. These are some of the issues that remain unanswered, with suggestions for further research.

1. Empirical evidence is needed to support all of the clinically defined characteristics of apraxia. Critics have raised the question of whether subjects designated as "apraxic" by one researcher would be "apraxic" by another researcher's criteria. More rigorously designed descriptive studies with larger sample sizes are required to develop an agreed-upon definition of developmental apraxia of speech and to generate hypotheses for careful exploration in experimental studies.

2. Information regarding early developmental nonspeech, prespeech, and speech behaviors that may be indicators of later-appearing DAS would clearly lead to earlier diagnosis and treatment. Kron (1970) found that some infants showed unexplained irregularities of the sucking response and hypothesized that disorganized sucking activities may be related to brain dysfunction. It would be helpful to discover whether verbal apraxia could be predicted in the hospital nursery by studying the earliest infant oral behavior. Eisenson (1972); and Aram and Glasson (Note 2) have suggested other items in supposed apraxic children's histories that may be early signs of DAS and should be systematically investigated.

3. Whether or not neurologic dysfunction can be reliably measured or should be included as a necessary component in the diagnosis of DAS must be resolved.

4. The question of whether verbal apraxia is a motor sequential disturbance which is free from the symbolic aspects of language or whether developmental apraxia in children exists as part of a language disorder remains unanswered.

5. Production of connected speech has been reported and analyzed in a few existing studies (Crary, Note 4; Ekelman, Note 9; Ekelman & Aram, 1983). Analysis of connected speech samples may reveal more and/or different information about the articulatory and linguistic aspects of DAS.

6. There is a need for longitudinal and follow-up studies to help in differential diagnosis, to describe changes over time, and to document the effects of treatment.

7. The aspect of oral perception and sensation and its hypothesized relationship to developmental verbal apraxia needs to be explored further. Some studies (Prichard et al., 1979; Loevner, Note 6) showed

that apraxic children performed significantly more poorly than normal children and articulation-disordered children on tests of oral stereognosis. Are measurements of oral sensory perception of primary importance in etiology and/or differential diagnosis of developmental apraxia of speech?

8. Rosenbek, Wertz, and Darley (1973) noted that certain adult apraxics had a low tolerance for 2-point discrimination tasks. It has been observed clinically that many apraxic children do not tolerate touch well and are especially hypersensitive to touch in and around the mouth. Supporting these clinical reports were the striking differences observed in test-taking behavior between normally speaking and developmentally apraxic children on tests of oral sensory processing (Loevner, Note 6). What is the explanation and significance of these findings?

9. If children with developmental apraxia of speech demonstrate poor tactile/kinesthetic/proprioceptive functioning, could a therapy program based on improving these functions be effective in improving the child's motor programming for speech? Ayres (1973) feels that the tactile system is primarily concerned with the ability to program a skilled motor act, and that dysfunction of the vestibular and other proprioceptive mechanisms may also contribute to the state of generalized apraxia in children. Ayres explains it as a problem in sensory integration. While results of sensory-integrative therapy with children demonstrating overall or verbal apraxia are not well documented, it is an intriguing concept worthy of study that tactile and even vestibular stimulation may improve oral motor and speech programming on a neurologic basis.

10. Sonderman (Note 23) showed that performance on various volitional oral movement tasks was unrelated to articulatory performance but was related to age. We need more studies on normal growth and development of children's ability to perform nonverbal oral motor tasks upon which to base comparisons of children with disordered speech.

11. Finally, there is a need for careful studies comparing a variety of treatment approaches and techniques with this population of children.

Currently, the state of the art relative to verbal apraxia in children is similar to that of acquired apraxia in adults 10 years ago. The writings and investigations of the 1970s, upon which we have based our understanding of developmental apraxia of speech, are being challenged. Speech and language pathologists have an unprecedented opportunity to ask pertinent questions, to share their clinical experiences in evaluation and treatment, and to conduct research in this area. Increased interest in developmental apraxia of speech should generate even more accelerated advances within the next 10 years.

Reference Notes

1. Rosenbek, J.C. Treating apraxia of speech in children and adults. A short course presented at the 4th Annual Three Rivers Conference of Communicative Disorders, Pittsburgh, 1982.

2. Aram, D.M., & Glasson, C. Developmental apraxia of speech. Paper presented at the Annual Convention of the American Speech –Language– Hearing Association, Atlanta, 1979.

3. Saleeby, N.C., Hadjian, S., Martinkosky, S.J., & Swift, M.R. Familial verbal dyspraxia: A clinical study. Paper presented at the Annual Convention of the American Speech and Hearing Association, San Francisco, 1978.

4. Crary, M.A. Developmental verbal dyspraxia: A phonological research perspective. Paper presented at the Annual Convention of the American Speech-Language-Hearing Association, Toronto, 1982.

5. McClumpha, S.L., & Logue, R.D. Approaches to children with motor programming disorders of speech. Paper presented at the Annual Convention of the American Speech and Hearing Association, San Francisco, 1972.

6. Loevner, M.B. An investigation of perceptual abilities in developmental apraxia of speech and comparison with functional articulation disorders. Unpublished doctoral dissertation, University of Pittsburgh, 1979.

7. Glasson, C. Spectrographic analysis of developmental apraxia: Temporal coordination difficulties. Paper presented at the Annual Convention of the American Speech-Language-Hearing Association, Los Angeles, 1981.

8. Crary, M.A. Phonological process analysis of developmental verbal dyspraxia: A descriptive study. Paper presented at the Annual Convention of the American Speech-Language-Hearing Association, Los Angeles, 1981.

9. Ekelman, B.L. Syntactic and semantic findings in developmental verbal apraxia. Paper presented at the Annual Convention of the American Speech-Language-Hearing Association, Los Angeles, 1981.

10. Logue, R.D. Apraxia revisited. Short course presented at the Annual Convention of the Pennsylvania Speech –Language– Hearing Association. King of Prussia, 1983.

11. Aram, D.M. Sequential and nonspeech practic abilities in children with developmental verbal apraxia. Paper presented at the Annual Convention of the American Speech-Language-Hearing Association, Los Angeles, 1981.

12. Comeau, B.S., & Crary, M.A. Developmental verbal dyspraxia: A morphophonemic analysis. Paper presented at the Annual Convention of the American Speech-Language-Hearing Association, Toronto, 1982.

13. Towne, R.L., & Crary, M.A. Syntagmatic distance as a phonological variable in developmental verbal dyspraxia. Paper presented at the Annual Convention of the American Speech-Language-Hearing Association, Toronto, 1982.

14. Logue, R.D. Assessing speech motor behavior: An examination protocol. Presented at the Annual Convention of the American Speech and Hearing Association, Houston, 1976.

15. Logue, R.D., & McClumpha, S.L. Apraxia of speech in children: A case description. Paper presented at the Annual Convention of the American Speech and Hearing Association, New York, 1970.

16. Jaffe, M.B. Treatment approaches with developmentally apraxic children. Paper presented at the Annual Convention of the American Speech-Language-Hearing Association, Detroit, 1980.

17. Jaffe, M.B. Developmental apraxia of speech: Updating clinical skills. Short course presented at the North-East Regional Conference of the American Speech-Language-Hearing Association, Philadelphia, 1981.

18. Doszak, A.L., McNeil, M.R., & Jancosek, E. Efficacy of Melodic Intonation Therapy with developmental apraxia of speech. Paper presented at the Annual Convention of the American Speech-Language-Hearing Association, Los Angeles, 1981.

19. Helfrich-Miller, K.R. The use of Melodic Intonation Therapy with developmentally apraxic children. Paper presented at the Annual Convention of the American Speech-Language-Hearing Association, Detroit, 1980.

20. Bashir, A.S., Jones, F., & Bostwick, R.Y. A touch cue method of therapy with developmentally apraxic children. Paper presented at the Annual Convention of the American Speech-Language-Hearing Association, Detroit, 1980.

21. Jones, F. Moto-sequential tactile therapy. A paper written for Emerson College, 1975.

22. Rosenthal, J., Williams, R., & Ingham, R.J. An experimental therapy programme for developmental articulatory dyspraxia. Paper presented at the Annual Convention of the Australian Association of Speech and Hearing, Launceston, Tasmania, 1978.

23. Sonderman, J.C. The relationship between volitional oral movement production and articulation competence. Unpublished doctoral dissertation, University of Pittsburgh, 1978.

References

Albert, M., Sparks, R., & Helm, N.   Melodic Intonation Therapy for aphasia. *Archives of Neurology*, 1973, *29*, 130-131.

Ayres, A.J.   *Sensory integration and learning disorders*. Los Angeles: Western Psychological Services, 1973.

Berlin, C.I. On: Melodic Intonation Therapy for Aphasia by R.W. Sparks and A.L. Holland. *Journal of Speech and Hearing Disorders,* 1976, *41,* 298-300.

Blakeley, R.W.   *Screening Test for Developmental Apraxia of Speech*. Tigard, Ore.: C.C. Publications, 1980.

Bobath, B.   The very early treatment of cerebral palsy. *Developmental Medicine and Child Neurology*, 1967, *9*, 373-391.

Bobath, B.   *Abnormal postural reflex activity caused by brain lesions* (2nd ed.). London: William Heinemann Medical Books, 1971. (a)

Bobath, B.   Motor development: Its effect on general development and application to the treatment of cerebral palsy. *Physiotherapy*, 1971, *57*, 526-532. (b)

Bobath, K.   *The motor deficit in patients with cerebral palsy*. London: Little Club Clinics in Developmental Medicine #23, William Heinemann Medical Books, 1966.

Bobath, K.   The normal postural reflex mechanism and its deviation in children with cerebral palsy. *Physiotherapy,* 1971, *57,* 515-525.

Bobath, K., & Bobath, B.   Cerebral palsy. Part 1. Diagnosis and assessment of cerebral palsy. Part 2. The neurodevelopmental approach to treatment. In P.H. Pearson & C.E. Williams (Eds.), *Physical therapy services in the developmental disabilities*. Springfield, Ill.: Charles C. Thomas, 1972.

Campbell, P.H.   *Problem-oriented approaches to feeding the handicapped child*. Akron, O.: The Children's Hospital Medical Center of Akron, 1982.

Chappell, G.E.   Childhood verbal apraxia and its treatment. *Journal of Speech and Hearing Research,* 1973, *16,* 362-368.

Court, D., & Harris, M.   Speech disorders in children. Part II. *British Medical Journal,* 1965, *2,* 409-411.

Dabul, B.L. Lingual incoordination-language delay: A case of a lazy tongue? *California Journal of Communication Disorders,* 1971, *2,* 30-33.

Daly, D.A., Cantrell, R.P., Cantrell, M.L., & Aman, L.A. Structuring speech therapy contingencies with an oral apraxic child. *Journal of Speech and Hearing Disorders,* 1972, *37,* 22-32.

Davis, L. Pre-speech. In F.P. Connor, G.G. Williamson, & J.M. Siepp (Eds.). *Program guide for infants and toddlers with neuromotor and other developmental disabilities.* New York: Teachers College Press, Columbia University, 1978.

Edwards, M. Developmental verbal dyspraxia. *British Journal of Disorders of Communication,* 1973, *8,* 64-70.

Eisenson, J. *Aphasia in children.* New York: Harper & Row, 1972.

Eisenson, J. Developmental patterns of non-verbal children and some therapeutic implications. *Journal of Neurological Science,* 1966, *3,* 313-320.

Ekelman, B.L., & Aram, D.M. Syntactic findings in developmental verbal apraxia. *Journal of Communication Disorders,* 1983, *16,* 237-250.

Fawcus, R. Features of a psychological and physiological study of articulatory performance. *British Journal of Disorders of Communication,* 1971, *6,* 99-106.

Ferry, P.C., Hall, S.M., & Hicks, J.L. 'Dilapidated speech': Developmental verbal apraxia. *Developmental Medicine and Child Neurology,* 1975, *17,* 749-756.

Gallender, D. *Eating handicaps.* Springfield, Ill.: Charles C. Thomas, 1979.

Guyette, T.W., & Diedrich, W.M. A critical review of developmental apraxia of speech. In N.J. Lass (Ed.), *Speech and language: Advances in basic research and practice* (Vol.5). New York: Academic Press, 1981.

Guyette, T.W., & Diedrich, W.M. A review of the Screening Test for Developmental Apraxia of Speech. *Language, Speech, and Hearing Services in Schools,* in press.

Hadden, W.B. On certain defects of articulation in children, with cases illustrating the results of education of the oral system. *Journal of Mental Science,* 1891, *37,* 96-105.

Helfrich-Miller, K.R. Melodic Intonation Therapy with developmentally apraxia children. In Aram, D.M. (Ed.) Seminars in Speech and Language: *Developmental Verbal Apraxia.* In press.

Kron, R.E. Prognostic significance of sucking dysrhythmias. In J.F. Bosma (Ed.), *Symposium on oral sensation and perception.* Springfield, Ill.: Charles C. Thomas, 1970.

Logue, R.D. Disorders of motor-speech planning in children: Evaluation and treatment. *Communicative Disorders: An Audio Journal for Continuing Education, Vol. 3.* New York: Grune & Stratton, 1978.

Love, R.J., Hagerman, E.L., & Taimi, E.G. Speech performance, dysphagia and oral reflexes in cerebral palsy. *Journal of Speech and Hearing Disorders,* 1980, *45,* 59-75.

Morley, M.E. *Development and disorders of speech in childhood (3rd ed).* London: E. & S. Livingstone, 1972.

Morley, M., Court, D., Miller, H., & Garside, R. Delayed speech and developmental aphasia. *British Medical Journal,* 1955, *2,* 463-467.

Morley, M.E., & Fox, J. Disorders of articulation: Theory and therapy. *British Journal of Disorders of Communication,* 1969, *4,* 151-165.

Morris, S.E. *Program guidelines for children with feeding problems.* Edison, N.J.: Childcraft Education Corp., 1977.

Morris, S.E. *The normal acquisition of oral feeding skills: Implications for assessment and treatment.* Boston: Therapeutic Media, 1982. (a)

Morris, S.E. *The Pre-Speech Assessment Scale.* Clifton, N.J.: J.A. Preston, 1982. (b)

Mueller, H.A. Facilitating feeding and prespeech. In P.H. Pearson & C.E. Williams (Eds.), *Physical therapy services in the developmental disabilities.* Springfield, Ill.: Charles C. Thomas, 1972.

Mueller, H.A. *Feeding, speech.* In N.R. Finnie (Ed.), *Handling the young cerebral palsied child at home* (2nd ed.), New York: Dutton, 1975.

Mysak, E.D. *Neurospeech therapy for the cerebral palsied* (3rd ed.). New York: Teachers College Press, Columbia University, 1980.

Nicolosi, L., Harryman, E., & Kresheck, J. *Terminology of communication disorders: Speech, language, hearing.* Baltimore: Williams & Wilkins, 1978.

Palmer, M. Studies in clinical techniques. II. Normalization of chewing, sucking and swallowing reflexes in cerebral palsy: A home program. *Journal of Speech Disorders,* 1947, *12,* 415-418.

Perske, R., Clifton, A., McLean, B., & Stein, J. (Eds.). *Mealtimes for severely and profoundly handicapped persons.* Baltimore: University Park Press, 1977.

Prichard, C.L., Tekieli, M.E., & Kozup, J.M. Developmental apraxia: Diagnostic considerations. *Journal of Communication Disorders,* 1979,*12,*337-348.

Rosenbek, J.C., Hansen, R., Baughman, C.H., & Lemme, M. Treatment of developmental apraxia of speech: A case study. *Language, Speech, and Hearing Services in Schools,* 1974, *5,* 13-22.

Rosenbek, J.C., & Wertz, R.T. A review of fifty cases of developmental apraxia of speech. *Language, Speech, and Hearing Services in Schools,* 1972, *3,* 23-33.

Rosenbek, J.C., Wertz, R.T., & Darley, F.L. Oral sensation and perception in apraxia of speech and aphasia. *Journal of Speech and Hearing Disorders,* 1973, *16,* 22-36.

Rosenthal, J. A token reinforcement programme used in the treatment of articulatory dyspraxia in a nine-year-old boy. *Journal of the Australian College of Speech Therapists,* 1971, *21,* 45-48.

Smartt, J., LaLance, L., Gray, J., & Hibbett, P. Developmental apraxia of speech: A Tennessee Speech and Hearing Association subcommitte report. *Journal of the Tennessee Speech and Hearing Association,* 1976, *20,* 21-31.

Sparks, R.W., Helm, N., & Albert, M. Aphasia rehabilitation resulting from Melodic Intonation Therapy. *Cortex,* 1974, *10,* 303-316.

Sparks, R.W., & Holland, A.L. Method: Melodic Intonation Therapy for aphasia. *Journal of Speech and Hearing Disorders,* 1976, *41,* 287-297.

Westlake, H. *A system for developing speech with cerebral palsied children.* Chicago: The National Society for Crippled Children and Adults, 1951.

Williams, R., Ingham, R.J., & Rosenthal, J. A further analysis of developmental apraxia of speech in children with defective articulation. *Journal of Speech and Hearing Research,* 1981, *24,* 496-505.

Yoss, K.A., & Darley, F.L. Developmental apraxia of speech in children with defective articulation. *Journal of Speech and Hearing Research,* 1974, *17,* 399-416. (a).

Yoss, K.A., & Darley, F.L. Therapy in developmental apraxia of speech. *Language, Speech, and Hearing Services in Schools,* 1974, *1,* 23-31. (b)

Betty Jane McWilliams

Speech Problems Associated with Craniofacial Anomalies

Introduction

Craniofacial malformations, while rare, constitute a major group of handicaps in children. They are usually complex and far-reaching in their life implications. Many are obviously genetically determined, while others occur sporadically. Until recent years, such conditions were considered to be untreatable. Individuals suffering from these problems were often shunted to the margins of society or were institutionalized with the result that speech-language pathologists had only limited experience in the diagnosis and treatment of their communicative deficits. That situation is changing, and speech-language pathologists are now being confronted with new challanges and opportunities in relation to the treatment of the wide variety of craniofacial malformations which have been identified.

Definition

The term "craniofacial malformation" has grown increasingly popular since 1971, when Paul Tessier described the surgical treatment of the severe facial deformities associated with craniofacial synostosis. *Cranio* refers to any skeletal deformity of the head at or above the lower eyelids, and *facial* to any abnormality below that level. *Synostosis* means that there is premature osseous union of bones that are normally distinct. Thus, theoretically, craniofacial malformations are those that affect both the cranium and the face. However, there has been a recent trend to include in the definition malformations affecting any part of the craniofacial complex. The reason for this is that these defects, whether severe or less complicated, are often treated in the same interdisciplinary facilities that once were concerned primarily with cleft lip, cleft palate, or both.

Figure 7-1 shows an infant with Pierre Robin Syndrome, an anomaly that involves only the face. Note the small chin, or *retrognathic mandible*. This is usually associated with a cleft of the soft palate, but the cranium is unaffected. The syndrome is complicated by *glossoptosis*, or retraction of the tongue into the pharyngeal space, rendering normal breathing impossible in many cases. About one-third of these children have learning disabilities ranging from mild to severe (McWilliams, Note 1). The origin of these problems is unclear. They may be logically related to early oxygen deprivation, or there may be prior neurological problems, which also contribute to the infant's inability to manage the tongue in the restricted oral space (Mallory & Paradise, 1979). In addition, the symptoms of Pierre Robin are sometimes just one part of a complex group of disorders comprising at least a dozen other syndromes, some of which do include the cranium (Cohen, 1976). Figure 7-2 shows an open palatal cleft, again a defect involving only the oral structures.

Figures 7-3A and 7-3B present a patient with Crouzon disease, or craniofacial *dysostosis*, which includes an abnormally shaped head, maxillary hypoplasia (midfacial deficiency), prognathism (prominent mandible), hypertelorism (wide-set eyes), exopthalmos (protruding eyes caused by shallow orbits), and low-set ears. These children are not usually mentally retarded. Crouzon is clearly a craniofacial abnormality as is Apert Syndrome (Figures 7-4A and 7-4B). This latter syndrome has many characteristics similar to Crouzon, but they are more severe. In addition, palatal deformities are common. *Syndactly* (webbing or union) of the fingers and toes is always present. While overt palatal clefts are sometimes seen, a more frequent deformity is a very high-arched narrow palate with excessive pile-up of tissue on the maxillary arch. While this often looks like a true cleft, it is not. Mental retardation is more common in Apert Syndrome than in Crouzon and may occur in as many as 50% of those affected.

These examples of representative craniofacial abnormalities should make the reader aware of the wide variety of forms, severity, and life implications of these birth defects. They should also suggest the possibility that similar variations in structure might be acquired as the result of surgical intervention or injury. Figures 7-5A and 7-5B show a young woman with

FIGURE 7-1
An infant with Pierre Robin Syndrome.

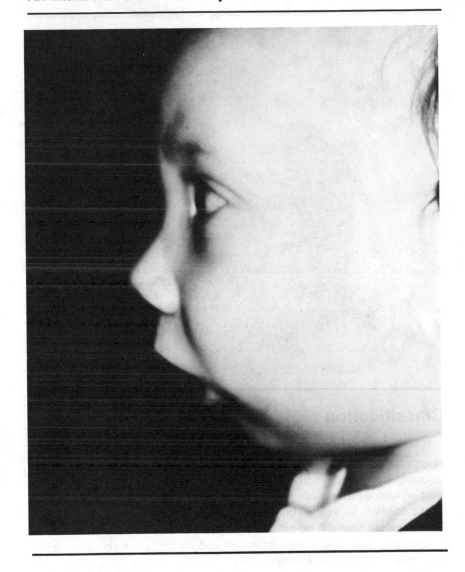

a prognathic mandible and marked open bite, which resulted from a fall from a second-story window at the age of 2½. She is an example of an *acquired* facial defect.

FIGURE 7-2
An open palatal cleft.

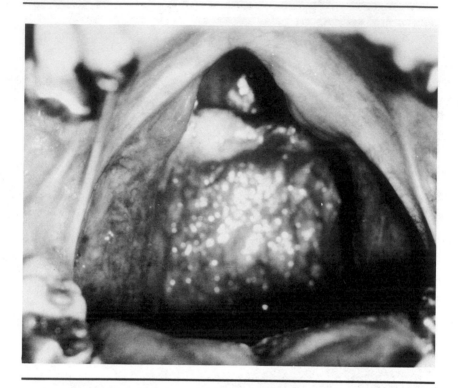

Classification

Whitaker, Pashayan, and Richman (1981) proposed a classification system for these kinds of defects. It takes into account the variations found in craniofacial malformations as described above and permits the inclusion of various forms of clefts and other deficits involving just the face or the cranium, as well as those in which both are malformed in some way. They suggest that all craniofacial anomalies may be classified into 5 categories based on etiology, anatomy, and current treatment principles. The basic system is as follows:

I. Clefts
    Centric (Midline)
    Acentric (Lateral)

II. Synostoses
    Symmetric
    Asymmetric

III.   Atrophy – hypoplasia   V.   Unclassified

IV.   Neoplasia – hyperplasia

The authors point out that any of the malformations may vary from subtle to extreme. The reader is referred to the article for more details on this and other systems of classification (Whitaker et al., 1981).

Occurrence

Extensive malformations of the craniofacial structures are relatively rare. It is estimated that approximately 1,200 babies with profound defects are born each year in the United States. Yet, as better discernment techniques become available, heretofore undiagnosed problems, particularly those with mild degrees of expressivity, are being appropriately described, diagnosed, treated, and studied. The sad designation of "funny looking kid," or "f.l.k.," has now taken its place with other historically used terms that are both cruel and inaccurate. When the speech-language pathologist sees an unusual looking child, however, it is incumbent upon him or her to investigate and learn as much as possible about the condition. Referral to a center for appropriate evaluation may make the difference between a marginal life and a fruitful one.

Syndromes

Many craniofacial deformities can be recognized as discrete syndromes manifested by groups of symptoms regularly occurring together, so that affected children and adults look much alike even though there is no family relationship. This is true of Crouzon (Figures 7-3A and 7-3B) and of Apert (Figures 7-4A and 7-4B), as well as of many other syndromes. There are literally hundreds of such syndromes, not all of which include craniofacial abnormalities, that have already been described, and Gorlin (Note 2) suggested that several new ones were being identified each month. Sparks and Millard (1981) have provided brief descriptions of the speech problems associated with some of these syndromes. Speech pathologists are becoming more and more involved in both the identification and treatment of syndromes, and there are increasing numbers specializing in the communicative disorders of such patients. This represents a new frontier that is expanding slowly but surely.

FIGURE 7-3A
A patient with Crouzon's disease (craniofacial dysostosis).

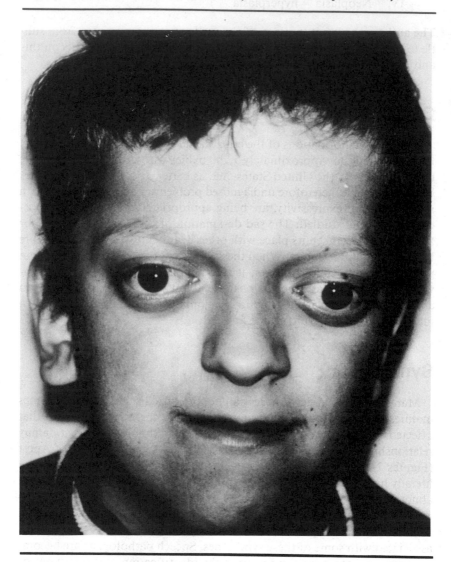

Associated Problems

Syndromes involving craniofacial abnormalities and craniofacial defects not identified as syndromes often include malformations that will affect

FIGURE 7-3B
A patient with Crouzon's disease (craniofacial dysostosis).

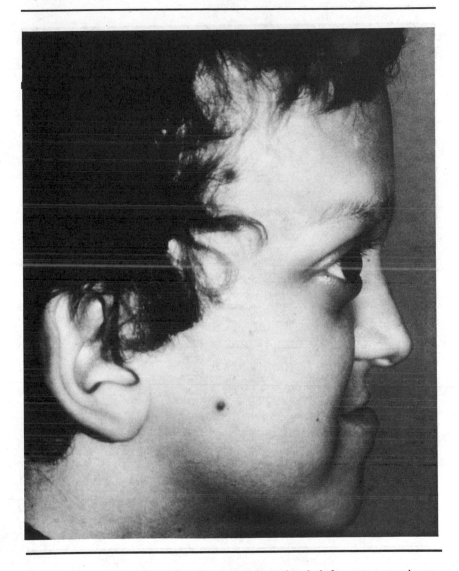

function in some major ways. For example, palatal clefts may occur in approximately 154 syndromes (Cohen, 1978). Smith (1976) includes 55 of these. Thus, children so affected may have all the speech problems that occur if palatal repair does not result in the ability to achieve velopharyngeal

FIGURE 7-4A
A patient with Apert's Syndrome.

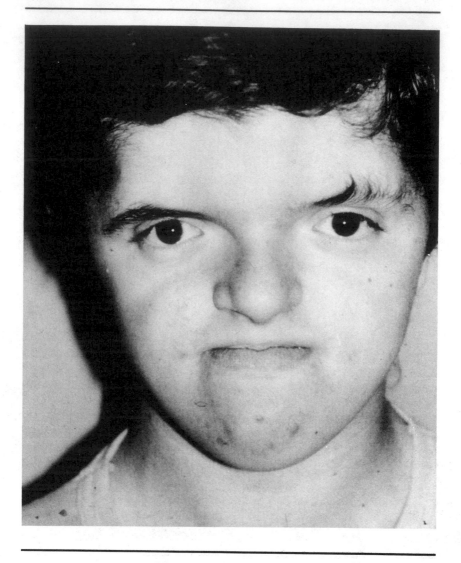

closure. In addition, the other structural deviations may complicate their speech disorders and make them difficult to diagnose and treat. Velopharyngeal incompetency *per se* will not be discussed in this chapter. However, Figures 7-6A and 7-6B show such a patient. This man has

FIGURE 7-4B
Syndactly of Apert's Syndrome.

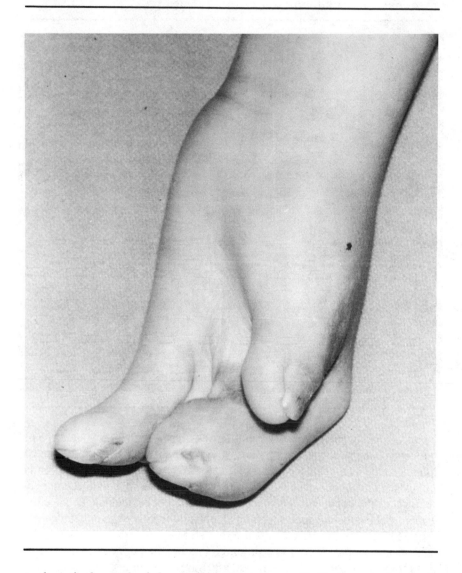

oculoauriculovertebral dysplasia, known also as Goldenhar syndrome. It
is thought by some that this may be a variant of hemifacial microsomia
(Gorlin, Pindborg, & Cohen, 1976). Birth defects in this patient include
scoliokyphosis (lateral and posterior curvature of the spine), right upper

FIGURE 7-5A
A patient with a prognathic mandible and marked open bite acquired
as a result of childhood injury.

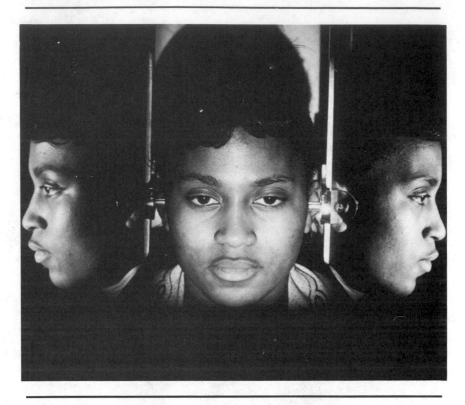

lid ptosis, right auricular tags and microtia, nasal deformities, relative or
real macroglossia, and cleft palate. The problems occurring because of
questionable management of the cleft, and now complicating his already
involved condition, are an oronasal fistula in the soft palate, surgical
removal of the premaxilla, increasing his midfacial deficiency, and a short
upper lip. He also has mild mental retardation but is seen as educable even
though he has spent most of his life in a state institution. Hearing in the
left ear is normal. Speech is unintelligible since he cannot get a lip seal,
cannot produce tongue tip elements, and cannot maneuver his tongue for
consonant production in the limited space available. This man has no consonants that are accurately produced, and he is a poor candidate for therapy
prior to massive facial reconstruction. He is an example of a person who
was probably destined to have disordered speech because of his basic struc-

FIGURE 7-5B
A patient with a prognathic mandible and marked open bite acquired as a result of childhood injury.

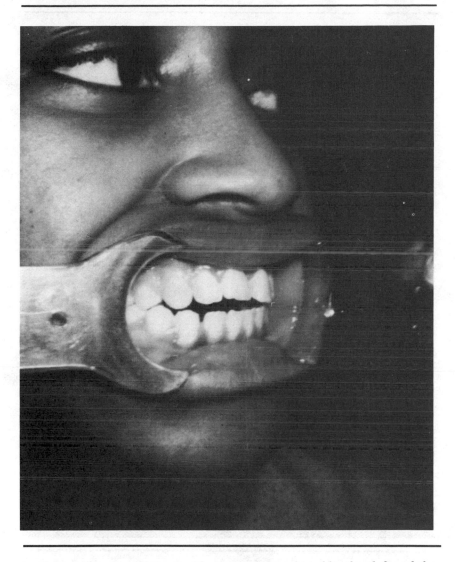

tural deviations but whose problems were exacerbated by the cleft and the way in which it was treated.

Smith (1976) lists various conditions that are associated with specific syndromes. The informed speech-language pathologist should be alerted

FIGURE 7-6A
A patient with Goldenhar Syndrome (oculoauriculovertebral dysplasia).

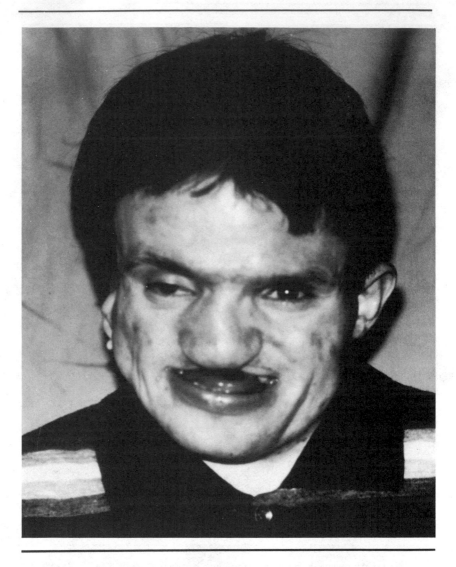

to these symptoms and be ready to investigate them thoroughly. You will note that 36 disorders are associated with "deafness," which includes all degrees of hearing impairment, 73 with some form of ear deformity, and

FIGURE 7-6B
A patient with Goldenhar Syndrome (oculoauriculovertebral
dysplasia).

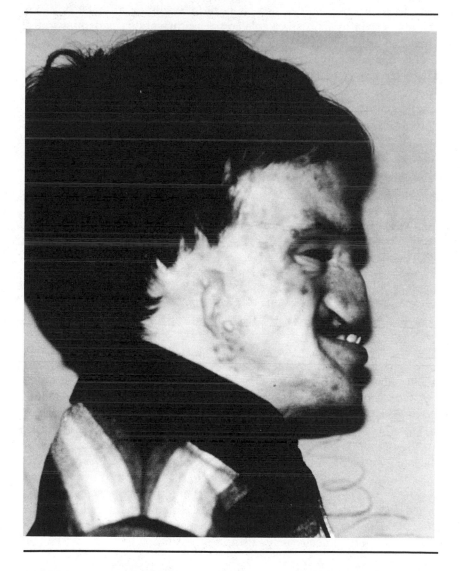

38 with frequent or occasional maxillary hypoplasia, often with a narrow
or high-arched palate. Fifty are associated with micrognathia, 6 with prognathism, 4 with *microstomia* (small mouth), 8 with *macrostomia* (greatly

exaggerated mouth width), 7 with cleft or irregular tongue, and 7 with *macroglossia* (excessively large tongue, sometimes filling the oral cavity). Any of these deficits, separately or in combination, may be responsible for communicative defects, especially those involving articulation, even though, within limits, remarkable compensatory ability is demonstrated again and again, clinically. Specifying the exact nature of resulting speech problems is impossible at this time because of the wide range of expressivity seen from one patient to another and, quite simply, because there are a sparsity of published data.

Mental Retardation

The risk of mental retardation in association with craniofacial malformations can be extremely high. Within any given syndrome the degree of retardation may be highly variable, so it is dangerous to make predictions about the intelligence of specific children since they may not be representative of the population trends. However, in Rubinstein-Taybi Syndrome, an IQ range of 17 to 86 suggests that some reduction in intelligence is almost invariable (Smith, 1976) and that the range is from profound retardation through the borderline classification. DeMeyer, Zemon, and Palmer (1964) go so far as to say that "the face predicts the brain." For example, in the median cleft face syndrome, a major characteristic is *hypotelorism* (close-set eyes), and this is almost always associated with brain damage and mental retardation, as is hypertelorism when it is extreme and is the only facial anomaly (DeMeyer, 1967). On the other hand, Russell-Silver syndrome is associated with slow motor development and so may easily be misdiagnosed as mental retardation even though intelligence is almost always normal as, indeed, it is in a number of other syndromes.

When mental retardation is a factor, articulation and language development are likely to reflect the reduced level of functioning, and that aspect of the problem must be weighed against the purely structural components. In view of the hundreds of problems that exist and the high degree of variability present in the expression of these disorders, it is wise to read about the syndrome or anomaly under consideration in order to derive a general picture of the nature of the defect and then to *examine the child* who has it. There is no substitute for that. It is simply inaccurate to assume that *any* disorder is perfectly equated with mental retardation, but it must not be ignored clinically if it exists.

Hearing Impairment

All children who have palatal clefts, whether other abnormalities are present or not, will suffer from otitis media or middle-ear effusions

(Paradise & Bluestone, 1969). Ear deformities are quite common in children with craniofacial variations, and these may result in severe conductive losses or, in some instances, in sensorineural losses. For example, Treacher Collins syndrome, or mandibulofacial dysostosis, is associated with malformation of the auricles, often including atresia, and with defects of the external ear canal. These defects result in conductive hearing losses. Wardenburg syndrome, on the other hand, includes severe bilateral sensorineural hearing loss in about 20% of the cases. When these profound losses are present, the hearing becomes the major problem and tends to diminish the relevance of other abnormalities such as cleft palate or other structural deviations in the oral cavity. Speech and language problems of all kinds will be associated with these syndromes, but they will have multiple causation.

Psychosocial Factors

Communication is an interactional phenomenon and assumes an exchange between and among people. When human relationships are disrupted, communicative skills suffer in some way. A child born with massive defects to which society responds is always at increased risk for psychosocial problems. Society itself may reject him or her in subtle or not-so-subtle ways. If this occurs, the person with the craniofacial malformation may seek partial relief by entering into conversations as infrequently as possible and may refuse to talk at all in some especially threatening situations. The "practice" necessary to perfect speech patterns may not occur if basic human relationships are disrupted. Thus, language delay and articulatory immaturities *may* be accounted for in part by psychosocial immaturity, a sense of worthlessness and loneliness, and inability to handle the social attitudes encountered in day-to-day living. MacGregor (1951) conducted in-depth interviews of 115 patients who required plastic surgery for the correction of varying degrees of facial disfigurement. She concluded that the majority of these patients were dismayed by their own mirror images and that they "saw their handicaps reflected in the reaction of others toward them." They were aware of staring, remarks, curiosity, questioning, pity, rejection, ridicule, whispering, nicknames, and discrimination, all of which made them unhappy and self-conscious. Whether these feelings were based on reality or not is not at issue. They represented the social perceptions of facially disfigured human beings. As such, they cannot be discounted, especially since the majority were viewed also as having adjustment difficulties including feelings of inferiority, self-consciousness, frustration, preoccupation with the deformity, hypersensitivity, anxiety, hostility, paranoia, withdrawal, antisocial states, and psychosis. MacGregor pointed out that the problems of these patients are at least partially traceable to the negative attitudes and prejudices that help both to create and to perpetuate special difficulties for the facially disfigured. Obviously, this is not the most fertile soil in which to nurture communicative skills.

Rusk (1963) also observed that the face is the focus of attention in interpersonal relationships and is the area most closely identified with the intimate, personal entity that one calls "self." He added that people with facial disfigurement encounter countless human and social indignities and deprivations. The literature abounds in similar statements from many other authors (MacGregor, 1951). Nonverbal aspects of communication are also undoubtedly influential since alterations in facial expression may be impaired, and general communicative behavior may be adversely affected.

The speech-language pathologist has a big responsibility to help children with craniofacial deficits find a place in the world and to work with that world to become more caring and accepting. A big job! But perhaps far more relevant than therapy for faulty articulation—important as that is.

Nature of Disordered Speech

Morrees, Burstone, Christiansen, Hixon, and Weinstein (1971) stated that the likelihood of defective speech increases as the number of structural deviations increases. This remains a reasonable statement of the relationship between structure and speech, although that relationship is not a perfect one. Many authors attest to the remarkable ability of speakers to compensate within limits for major structural abnormalities in the vocal tract (Bloomer, 1971; Peterson, 1973). Witzel (Note 3) recognized these compensatory abilities but suggested that there are probably limits beyond which speech will invariably be defective. While these limits are yet to be specified, we recognize the virtual impossibility of normal speech for the young man pictured in Figures 7-6A and 7-6B and previously described.

As noted earlier, one of the barriers to using solid data upon which to make precise determinations is that there is only very limited literature available. Both craniofacial and orthognathic problems (those involving the malpositioning of the bones of the maxilla, mandible, or both) have been incompletely studied, and it has been almost impossible to conduct well-designed prospective studies. Much that has been written is quite general and is plagued by the probability that certain of the patients reported on have been misdiagnosed. This is not surprising when the similarities and subtle differences among many of the syndromes are taken into account (Peterson, 1973). Information about speech has lagged behind that in almost all other areas. In the Smith (1976) work, the word *speech* does not even appear in the index. In Gorlin et al. (1976), the index carries only 2 references under speech and 9 under voice.

Diagnosis

It is clear that the individual suffering from any one of hundreds of craniofacial anomalies associated with speech problems must have a thorough diagnostic evaluation in order to determine as accurately as possible why the speech is in some way defective and if the craniofacial anomaly can be held responsible in whole or in part. Peterson-Falzone (1976) has wisely advised us to keep looking even after we think we have found the answer. In order to decide that the speech is defective because of the structural differences that exist, the speech defect or defects must stand in functional relationship to structure. For example, the protrusion of the tongue during /s/ production in a patient with a marked anterior open bite is reasonable, and the structure and function can logically be related to each other. However, if the same patient had an f/θ substitution, structure would not provide a reasonable explanation for the error, since the tongue is physically capable of articulating with the anterior teeth.

The diagnostic process is essential, too, because given syndromes show wide variations, and the only valid approach to treating resulting speech problems is on an individual basis relating structure and function to the speech pattern that exists. Even if it were possible to describe the speech commonly associated with specific syndromes, a full-length textbook would be necessary to cover the hundreds of variations that would have to be included. In addition, the data are too sparse to make that practical. Instead, the speech-language pathologist is urged to acquire a standard reference on syndromes (Cohen, 1978; Gorlin et al., 1976; Smith, 1981) and to use it diligently as an index of structural variations encountered clinically. Only by very careful case documentation can we ever hope to have more useful data than we have today.

A helpful reference in learning to make significant observations is a 1980 article by Salinas. He points out in the introduction to his systematic examination format that orofacial abnormalities occur in approximately 25% of Mendelian syndromes, in virtually all of the chromosomal disorders, and in several multifactoral disorders. This is an impressive array of disorders that can affect speech, but speech pathologists are only now becoming active in recognizing these important structural variations and in participating on and cooperating with management teams.

Appropriate to this attitude regarding diagnosis is the work of Bloomer and Hawk (1973). They describe the speech mechanism as a tube extending from the laryngopharynx to a bifurcation at the nasopharynx and proceeding via its oral and nasal pathways. Within this simple tubal system, musculoskeletal valves close, constrict, and open to regulate the breathstream and the laryngeally generated sound. These valves influence air pressure, modify and direct energy and airflow, and modify vocal resonance for the production of vowels and consonants. Impairment of the ability to achieve adequate valving anyplace in the system may be responsible for defective speech. Writing about ablative surgery of the face and of the oral and pharyngeal cavities, Bloomer and Hawk (1973) stress the importance of knowing (1) the sites and types of lesions which may impair speech, (2) the nature of the disturbed speech which may follow, and (3) the means for modifying the speech. These same three necessities sum up what is required to understand speech deviations standing in functional relationship to structural deviations. In speech disorders resulting from craniofacial problems, the structures that will be responsible are those to which the important speech pathway is related.

These structures may include the face; the oral, pharyngeal, and nasal cavities; dentition; palate; and tongue. Bloomer (1971), the first to write comprehensively about such problems, refers to them as *orofacial abnormalities*. He includes in his description all the tissues of the orofacial complex—supporting structures of cartilage and bone, teeth, muscles, tendons, motor and sensory nerves, glandular and soft tissue, and skin.

Articulation Errors Associated with Severe Malocclusions

Most of the major craniofacial abnormalities involve some type of serious malocclusion, and it is the malocclusion that appears to be most intimately related to the articulatory problems which occur. These dental and skeletal relationships have been variously classified, often according to Angle (1899). In a Class I occlusion, the mesiobuccal cusp of the maxillary first molar rides comfortably in the buccal groove of the mandibular first molar, and the maxilla is just slightly larger than the mandible. This type of dental relationship is unremarkable and is not usually directly or indirectly responsible for speech problems. The exception to this is when missing or malplaced individual teeth interfere with tongue movement or placement, or when there is an open bite. Angle's Class II occlusion is represented by the mesiobuccal cusp of the maxillary first molar being anterior to the buccal groove of the mandibular first molar. Thus, the maxillary teeth are seen as protrusive to the mandibular. In a Class III relationship, the reverse occurs, and the mandibular teeth are anterior to the maxillary. When there is an opening between the maxillary and mandibular incisors, an *open bite* results. These occlusal patterns may relate only to teeth or to their underlying bony support as well. For example, in mandibular retrognathia the mandible is too small in relation to the maxilla, while in prognathia the mandible is too large to relate well to the maxilla. These problems may also occur as the maxilla interacts with the mandible. Visual examination without cephalometric measurements may be quite misleading. A mandible that appears to be prognathic may actually be of normal size, while a maxilla that is too small is responsible for the "pseudoprognathism." Figures 7-7A (Sassouni, Note 4) and 7-7B (Sassouni, 1969) show variations found in many craniofacial disorders and in orthognathic problems.

It is clear that occlusal variations of minor degree cannot usually be held responsible for speech problems. Many studies have failed to find a relationship (Bernstein, 1956; VanThal, 1935). Others (Bloomer, 1971; Van Riper, 1972) have observed that there is an amazing human ability to compensate even for severe malocclusions.

However, in severe Class II or Class III malocclusions, either with or without open bite, there may be difficulty with lip approximation in connected speech and even with the production of labiodental phonemes. Bilabials may be produced labiodentally if that maneuver can be executed, or /f/ and /v/ may sometimes be produced by action of the lower teeth against the upper lip. In extreme cases, the tongue articulating with the upper teeth may be a substitute gesture. There is a tendency for compensatory efforts to become more bizarre and less successful as the deformities become more and more severe (Bloomer, 1971).

Sibilant phonemes may also be adversely affected in Class II and Class III occlusions and in open bites. The tongue may be carried too low, it may be retruded (Guay, Maxwell, & Beecher, 1978), or the oral port opening may be too large (Klechak, Bradley, & Warren, 1976). Sibilant articulation will obviously be the most sensitive to these occlusal problems as the tongue seeks an appropriate intraoral target that is too far forward, too far back, or altered by an open-bite relationship which destroys the vertical directional behavior of the tongue as well as the horizontal. Bilabial and labiodental consonants appear to have much greater tolerance for these variations than have sibilants.

The majority of orthodontic problems can be treated successfully by the orthodontist without the necessity of extraordinary measures. A small group of such patients, however, and these include those with craniofacial and severe facial anomalies, must be managed surgically, if at all. Witzel (Note 3) reported on 111 such patients prior to and following surgery for

FIGURE 7-7A
Variations found in craniofacial disorders and orthognathic problems.

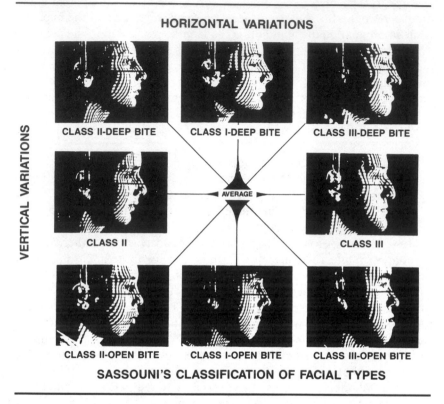

SASSOUNI'S CLASSIFICATION OF FACIAL TYPES

their orthognathic problems of a skeletal nature. None of these was identified as having particular syndromes. She administered the 141-item Templin-Darley Test of Articulation (1969) and, based on the literature indicating most difficulty with sibilants, labiodentals and bilabials, used 3 subtests of 39, 10, and 21 items, respectively. Prior to surgery, 54% of 41 subjects in Group A (patients who did not require Le Fort I osteotomies) had articulation errors of some type. This percentage was reduced to 20% following surgery with no speech therapeutic intervention. Prior to surgery, 46% of the subjects had sibilant errors (most on /s/ and /z/), and this became 17% after surgery, again without speech therapy. Only 15% of the subjects had bilabial errors before their operations and only 3% afterward. Five percent had labiodental errors at the start of treatment and none at its completion.

FIGURE 7-7B
Variations found in craniofacial disorders and orthognathic problems.

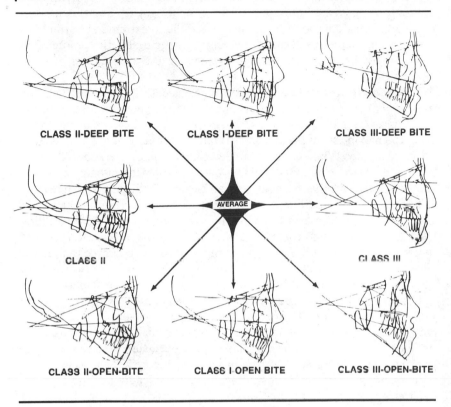

The 70 subjects in Group B required the more complex Le Fort I procedure, which is designed to reposition the maxilla by moving it forward and tilting it appropriately to correct for midfacial deficiency. Seventy-four percent of these subjects had articulation errors prior to surgery, and 36% retained errors following surgery. Sibilants were disordered in 70% before surgery and in 30% afterward. Again labiodental and bilabial errors were infrequent, both occurring in 8.6% of the sample. These latter errors were reduced to 2.7% and 4.3% after surgery.

Forty-two of these 70 subjects also had palatal clefts. It is interesting that 71% of the subjects with clefts had sibilant errors before their Le Fort I procedures and that 43% retained their errors following surgery, as opposed to 21% of the 69% of noncleft subjects with sibilant distortions.

On the other hand, neither labiodental nor bilabial errors occurred either before or following surgery in the cleft subjects.

It is apparent from this study that sibilant articulation, occurring as it does at a valve created normally between the tongue tip and the midportion of the maxillary arch, is highly vulnerable to extreme abnormalities which require surgery and that correcting the structural deficits more often than not results in significant improvement in the articulation of these phonemes.

In certain of the craniofacial malformations described in the literature, maxillary or mandibular deviations, or both, are important aspects of the syndrome. Apert syndrome and Crouzon disease are both associated with midfacial hypoplasia and with Class III malocclusions, often with a reduced oronasal airway. While there are no developmental, or even good descriptive studies of these patients available, clinical evidence presented by Peterson (1973) suggests that both physical and speech findings may range from mild to severe. She describes one patient with Apert who produced /f/ as a lingualabial, /v/ as a bilabial fricative, and /t/ and /d/ by holding the anterior portion of the tongue blade against the lower border of the upper incisors. I would suspect, from the picture incorporated in the article and from the articulation errors described, that he would also have had distorted sibilants caused by the anterior tongue blade articulating with the upper incisors. She also describes a second patient with more severe manifestations of the syndrome and a more serious speech problem, including distortion of all sibilants and affricates, which could be considered obligatory because of the severe Class III malocclusion with the resulting unavoidable aberrations in tongue placement. Figure 7-2 shows a patient with Apert syndrome and the midfacial retrusion leading to these errors.

Crouzon syndrome (Figure 7-3) is a disorder akin to Apert, but is less severe in its manifestations. These patients do not have the syndactyly of hands and feet associated with Apert. They do have similar, but less severe, craniofacial features, however. They may have essentially normal speech, mild disorders with little or no relationship to their abnormal oral features, or defective speech that seems to be directly related to their structural variations. Peterson (1973) describes 2 mildly involved children and 1 severely impaired child who was required to carry his head in an extended position in order to maintain an airway for breathing. He demonstrated oral distortions of sibilants, both fricatives and affricates, and inconsistent distortions of /r/ and /I/—most of which appeared to be related to abnormal tongue placement necessitated by faulty mandible-tongue-maxilla relationships.

We support Peterson's findings from observations of our own cases. A brother and sister and twin brothers all demonstrated anteriorly distorted sibilants. Figures 7-3A and 7-3B show one of the twin boys. Our cases all had denasalized /m/, /n/, and /ŋ/ in association with mouth breathing, necessitated by the reduction in size of the pharyngeal space.

Elfenbein, Waziri, and Morris (1981) reported on the speech characteristics of 6 children, 4 with Apert, 1 with Crouzon, and 1 with Saethre-Chotzen syndrome. One of the subjects with Apert had no speech and appeared to be severely retarded. All of the others had sibilant distortions, and all but 1 had affricate problems. The authors conclude that these articulatory deviations are the logical result of the oral-structural anomalies. It would be difficult to argue otherwise.

The midfacial deficiency seen in both Apert and Crouzon and the forward-riding tongue associated with the poorly related maxilla and mandible, lead almost universally to sibilant errors. While other errors may also be present as previously described, they are far overshadowed by these marked sibilant, which appear to respond minimally to speech therapy as long as the oral structures remain poorly related. Research is needed before we will be able to do more than rely on clinical experience, which can sometimes be misleading.

Two brothers with otopalatodigital syndrome (Figures 7-8A and B and 7-9A and B) serve to highlight the articulation errors associated with this x-linked, recessively inherited disorder. The usual patient is male with a prominent, overhanging forehead, prominent supraorbital ridges, antimongoloid slant, ocular hypertelorism, broad depressed nasal bridge, midfacial flattening, mild retardation, retarded skeletal maturation, malformed fingers and toes with variable curvatures, cleft palate, small oral cavity, and conductive hearing loss. The older of the 2 cases presented here is 18 years old. He demonstrates a severe open bite with malocclusion, midfacial deficiency, incomplete cleft of the secondary palate, small oral opening and oral cavity, and moderate retardation requiring special education. His speech is of low volume and somewhat monotonous, and sibilants are palatalized with the anterior tongue protruding into the space created by the open bite. He is intelligible, but the speech problem is noticeable.

The younger brother is 10 years of age. His physical characteristics are similar to his brother's, but less severe. He retains minor immaturities in his speech pattern, notably f/θ. Aside from those problems, his speech mirrors that of his brother with the addition of "muffling," seemingly a result of the small oral port and cavity. Once again, the relevance of oral structures is emphasized.

It is appropriate to point out here that children born with cleft palates, with or without one of the 154 syndromes which may include some form of clefting, are also prime candidates for these highly complex occlusal

FIGURE 7-8A
Patient, age 18, with otopalatodigital syndrome.

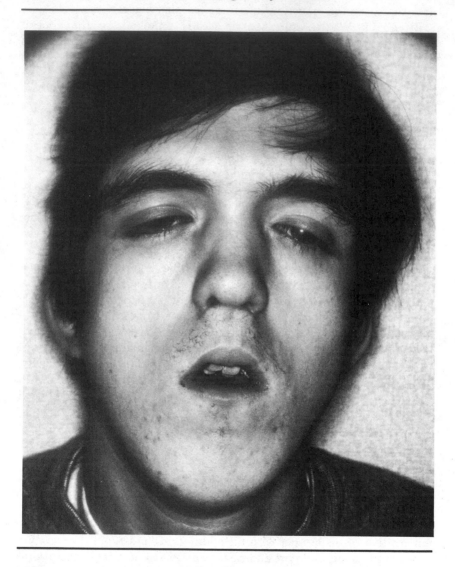

problems, and their speech will have the potential to be similarly affected. It will be necessary in those cases for the clinician to make the distinction between distortions caused by velopharyngeal incompetency and those

FIGURE 7-8B
Patient, age 18, with otopalatodigital syndrome.

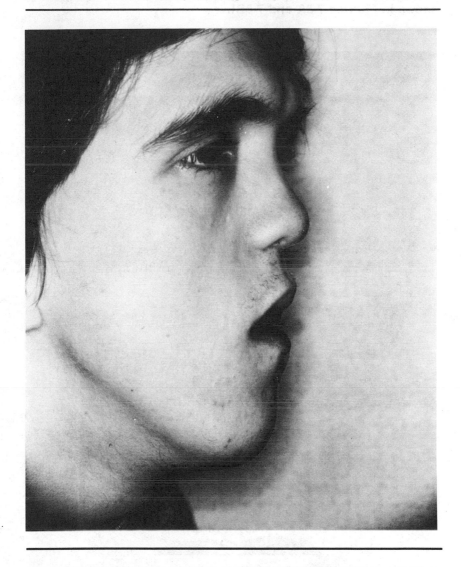

related at least in part to maxillary-mandibular relationships. Complicating the diagnosis and management of such children will also by the high occurrence of cross bite and mising teeth as is seen in Figure 7-10. These dental

FIGURE 7-9A
Patient, age 10, with otopalatodigital syndrome (brother of patient shown in Figures 7-8A and 7-8B).

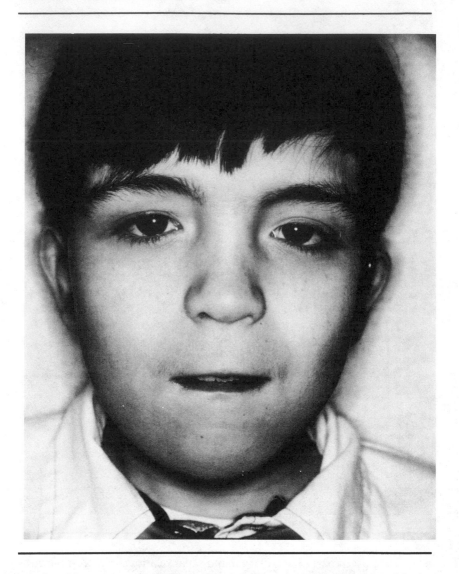

relationships may contribute to frontal distortions of sibilants with the tongue finding its way primarily into the large space on the right and secondarily into the smaller space on the left.

FIGURE 7-9B
Patient, age 10, with otopalatodigital syndrome (brother of patient
shown in Figures 8A and 8B).

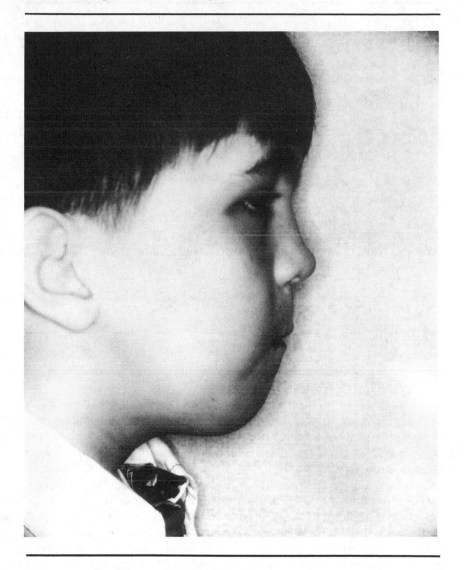

It is important for the student to be aware that any craniofacial or orthognathic abnormality that results in a marked discrepancy between the
maxilla and the mandible or in an open bite has the potential for creating

FIGURE 7-10
An example of cross bite and missing teeth.

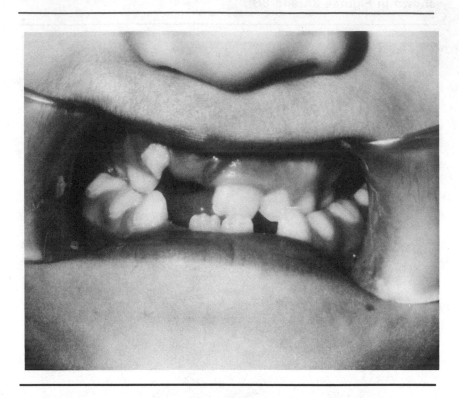

a relationship between the tongue and the aberrant structures that can result in faulty anterior articulation, particularly of sibilant phonemes. These defects are usually of the distortion type. Bloomer (1971) has proposed that such distortions be referred to as "malphones," since the phonologic system is usually not faulty. He also makes the critical observation that it is necessary to know the form of abnormal lingual valving and how the distortion or malphone is related to the dimensions and configuration of the articulatory structures. This requires, of course, careful study and diagnosis; and there is a margin of error even when such instruments as videofluoroscopy are used. However, it is necessary for the speech pathologist to think in far more precise terms than has been true with traditional articulation testing. It is not enough to recognize that there are articulatory distortions in these cases. It is necessary to know as much as possible about the how and why of the deviations under consideration.

Articulation Errors Associated with Lingual Anomalies

Certain of the craniofacial disorders include variations in the structure of the tongue. These are considerably less likely to occur than are the structural deformities discussed in the previous section, and even less is understood about their relationship to speech and how they should be treated.

There is considerable evidence that an absent or rudimentary tongue may have only minimal effects on speech (Bloomer, 1971; Gorlin et al., 1976; Peterson-Falzone, 1976). However, Bloomer notes the distortion of sibilants in a 13-year-old girl with a small tongue. Amazing compensatory behaviors have been described for a tongueless speaker by Eskew and Shepard (1949). Smith (1976) lists no syndromes associated with aglossia or microglossia, while Gorlin et al. (1976) describe two cases of Moebius syndrome, one with a "small tongue" and the other with "atrophy of the tongue" from birth. Since these patients have bilateral facial paralysis, their speech is usually disordered and can be described as dysarthric. It would be difficult to determine the role of the size of the tongue in these cases.

Hemiatrophy of the tongue is usually seen in hemifacial atrophy (Gorlin et al., 1976). This disorder, progressive in nature, also includes atrophy of the face on the affected side with resulting severe malocclusion. These cases are complex and usually are complicated by Jacksonian epilepsy. Speech problems have not been described, but they are likely to relate both to dysarthria and to the often severe occlusal manifestations.

Macroglossia, or an enlarged tongue, appears to pose a greater threat to speech than does a rudimentary or small tongue. Beckwith-Wiedmann syndrome (Gorlin et al., 1976) is characterized by macroglossia as a major symptom which often leads to respiratory and feeding difficulties in infancy. The syndrome is also marked by omphalocele, enlargement of the viscera, cytomegaly of the adrenal cortex, accelerated skeletal maturation, prominent eyes and occiput, mandibular prognathism and open bite (may be secondary to large tongue), hypoglycemia in early infancy, among others. Growth of the oral cavity is sometimes enough to accommodate the tongue, but partial glossectomy may be necessary. In this and other conditions where the tongue fills the oral cavity, speech may be seriously impaired because there is no space for articulation to occur. In addition, the oral cavity may be so constricted that voice will be muffled. Children with macroglossia may be intelligent and have excellent language development. One case known to the writer, however, had unintelligible speech with articulatory variations on all consonants. The tongue filled the entire available space so that the lips could not be approximated for labial consonants, which were produced by action between the upper lip and the massive blade of the tongue. No compensation was possible because of the enormity of the tongue. Surgery is required in these extreme cases.

Certain syndromes with enlarged tongue may be complicated by a high incidence of mental retardation as in several of the mucopolysaccharidoses, mucolipidoses, and related disorders (Gorlin et al., 1976). Hurler syndrome is an example.

Summary

Speech defects emerging out of the complicated craniofacial disabilities now receiving increasing clinical attention may be explained partially on the basis of associated hearing losses, mental retardation, and psychosocial factors including societal responses to the disorders. Speech problems may be related also to the malformation of oral structures, which may be too seriously impaired to permit normal speech.

Articulation disorders associated with congenital malformations of the craniofacial complex tend to be distortions of sibilants related to dental or skeletal malocclusions, particularly when open bit is present. Labials may be affected when the lips cannot be approximated, and nasals may be essentially eliminated when the size of the pharyngeal space is significantly diminished. An excessively large tongue will usually be more of a hazard to speech than will a very small or rudimentary tongue and may seriously reduce intelligibility.

While the human organism is unquestionably capable of amazing feats of compensation, there are physical limitations beyond which speech therapy is not a useful mode of treatment in the absence of surgical alteration of the impaired structures. On the other hand, there is evidence to show speech improvement following such surgery without intervention by the speech pathologist. Thus the speech pathologist must know when to recommend speech therapy, when to refer for consultation and other forms of intervention including surgical and orthodontic, and how to work in concert with specialized clinics providing the necessary care.

Speech Therapy

Introduction

As we have already suggested, speech therapy in the presence of these massive oral deformities is almost never effective. Correction of the defect, insofar as that is possible, is the first stage of treatment. As we have also shown, these alterations are sometimes followed by spontaneous changes of a positive nature in speech. However, such improvement does not occur universally, and speech therapy may be required. Unfortunately, there are almost no data available about speech therapy for communication deficits associated with craniofacial or orofacial anomalies.

Social-Interactional Therapy

Long and Dalson (1982) found that 1-year-old infants with cleft palates, a group not specifically addressed in this chapter, were significantly less likely to pair gestural and vocal behaviors than were noncleft children. The authors speculated that there may be a stage in development when nonspecific vocalizations become attached to gestures of communicative value to the child and that children with clefts are deficient in this regard.

The failure of these children to make transitions of this type could point to early disruption in social interaction. While there is only limited research in relation to children with clefts, and none concerning children with craniofacial problems, the information that is available supports our view that infant stimulation and socialization programs of various sorts are highly desirable for most children with facial disfigurement.

Parent Training

It is our philosophy that therapy should emerge out of a careful diagnostic evaluation and that it should be planned so that the desired goals can be accomplished as simply and quickly as possible. Formal therapy should never be undertaken if informal techniques and encouragement will enable a child to function at his or her maximum capacity. Thus, it is logical to educate parents so that they can help to modify the child's interactive environment, if that is necessary, and can capitalize on opportunities in daily living to enhance communication. Parent training of this type can result in parents who read to their children, understand the advantages of listening and responding when their children "read" or talk to them, parallel talk as their children play, increase life experiences, encourage peer interaction, foster independence, and reinforce and expand on communicative attempts. In short, the child must learn about, and be rewarded for, interacting verbally with others. This *learning* is of both a cognitive and a pragmatic nature and encompasses the child's feeling system.

We know of no formal approaches that have been suggested for the parents of children with craniofacial problems. Hahn (1979) recommended a 4-session series for the parents of children with clefts, and this system has elements in it that can be modified for children with other facial anomalies.

The first session occurs when the child is an infant and is designed to acquaint the parents with the normal speech mechanism and its function and the way in which their child's structure differs. They are helped to understand normal speech and language development and are taught by the speech pathologist to interact and to enter into vocal play with their infant. They are encouraged to allow the child time for response and to reinforce responses when they occur. The parents are taught to use single words strongly, clearly, and repetitiously quite early in the child's life, as the situation determines their appropriateness. The parents are expected to begin verbal stimulation immediately after the first session, and they are informed that the speech pathologist will provide additional help in future sessions.

The second session occurs when the child is 12 months old. The clinician again demonstrates procedures, this time incorporating single key words presented and stressed in the context of simple statements and questions. At this time the parents are encouraged to widen the child's experiences and to describe them in simple terms. Since infants with clefts often have palatal surgery at about 1 year of age, the surgery and its effects on speech development are also discussed.

The third session is 6 to 8 weeks after surgery, and it stresses the child's imitation of initial consonants. The parents stimulate single words until the baby uses a few words spontaneously. Then they are instructed to stimulate 2-word combinations. The parents are taught to use reinforcers such as words of approval, candy, or kisses. We prefer social reinforcers since communication is a social function.

The fourth session is planned when the child is about 3½, at which time the importance of a peer group is emphasized along with planning to help the child understand the nature of his or her physical impairment. (We prefer both of these latter activities to be ongoing from birth.) If formal speech therapy is required, it is implemented at this time.

The important aspects of this program for those with craniofacial anomalies lie in its stress on the normal developmental patterns of children. The program can be modified for children according to their needs and extended for parents who cannot manage without regular support from the speech pathologist. On the other hand, extreme care must be exercised to avoid conditioning parents to respond to their children as if speech problems are inevitable. This attitude can be detrimental rather than helpful. In reality, the goal is to assist parents to do well what all parents should be doing with young children. If the parents are doing well on their own, reinforce their efforts! Avoid intervention that may lead them to think they are not handling the situation satisfactorily.

Other detailed programs of this type have been described by Philips (1979) and Brookshire, Lynch, and Fox (1980). All of these systems of therapy relate to the developmental landmarks seen in normal children. It is essential that undue anxiety not be triggered in parents whose children are developing slowly. Thus, any activities undertaken should begin at the child's own developmental level and should not be too demanding too early. For this reason, it is necessary to provide for a complete developmental assessment before deciding to undertake any therapy. In addition, the goal is always to help the child derive satisfaction out of communicative experiences so that he or she will be comfortable and at ease in any situation. Avoid any activity which the parents and child do not enjoy!

Play Groups

Irwin and McWilliams (1974) and Tisza, Irwin, and Scheide (1973) used various types of play therapy, including a great deal of creative dramatics with cleft children. They learned that the children had initial difficulty with expression of feelings but that they were finally able to reveal unconscious conflicts, which could then be treated or controlled in a make-believe world so that helplessness was minimized. This approach to improving communicative skills and to increasing verbal output can and should be incorporated into the techniques regularly used by speech pathologists.

Preschool Programs

Preschools of various sorts are highly desirable for children with facial disfigurement provided the teachers are informed, understanding people who will encourage and provide opportunities for children to relate to each other and who understand the semantics of disfigurement and the subtle ways in which children who are different can be rejected completely or maneuvered into marginal positions within the group. A skillful teacher assisted by informed parents and insightful speech pathologists can minimize the negative potential that is always present and create, instead, a warm, understanding environment in which communicative skills are nurtured and fostered.

Articulation Therapy

When articulation errors remain 3 months postoperatively, diagnostic evaluation should be carried out to be certain that the structure, often falling short of the ideal, is compatible with improved articulation. If it is, then articulation therapy, usually stressing placement, is indicated. Postoperatively, articulation therapy for these patients does not differ from articulation therapy for any other group, with the possible exception of the stress on placement. This emphasis is essential since the original speech pattern was acquired in an abnormal oral environment to which the speaker had to adapt as well as he or she was able. With the change in the oral environment, it is not unusual for the individual to maintain, sometimes with difficulty, the preoperative pattern. Thus, the old habits must be eliminated and replaced by new articulatory behaviors—a far-from-easy task, especially in children over the age of 8 and in adults.

A word of caution is necessary relative to the outcome of articulation therapy for individuals with defects of oral structures. Prognosis is always dependent on anatomy and physiology, and it is often necessary to accept less than perfect speech as the best that can be achieved. It is incumbent on the speech pathologist, therefore, to understand the relationship of function to structure and to learn early to make valid judgments. Otherwise, people who are doing as well as they can will be subjected to useless therapy, or those who can improve may be denied the help they require.

Therapy for Resonance Disorders

Hyponasality

Hyponasality is usually caused by resistance in the nasal airway or at its entrance. When this occurs in association with such problems as a shallow pharynx and midfacial deficiency, it is often eliminated when the airway is opened up by maxillary advancement, adenoidectomy, or any other procedure designed to enlarge the space. Speech therapy is not the solution prior to surgery, and it is not usually required after surgery. If, in rare cases, an individual has a patent airway but continues to close off the airway during the production of nasals in an effort to maintain speech as it was preoperatively, articulation therapy may be safely undertaken. The warning here is that the speech pathologist must be secure in the knowledge that the airway *is* open.

Hypernasality

After midfacial advancement, some patients may develop hypernasality as the result of the deepening of the pharyngeal space. When this occurs, it is necessary that there be a complete assessment of the velopharyngeal valve. This can best be done in a multidisciplinary cleft palate clinic equipped to evaluate the valve during function. If incompetence is present, surgical correction will be required. If speech was normal prior to the maxillary advancement, the prognosis is favorable.

Sometimes, following a pharyngeal flap, residual incompetence remains. If it is unequivocal, there is very little that can be accomplished by speech therapy, and a secondary surgical procedure may be required. If closure is inconsistent, that is, if the valve is successful in separating the oral from the nasal cavity on some speech tasks but not on others, or if closure can be obtained during blowing or whistling as observed on multiview videofluoroscopy or through a transnasal endoscope, speech therapy can *sometimes* be helpful. The therapy procedures described by Shprintzen, McCall, and Skolnick (1975) are recommended. This is a detailed therapy program which makes use of operant procedures performed systematically, moving from the task on which closure is achieved to speech activities at increasing levels of difficulty, until the hypernasality has been eliminated and the inconsistent valving has become consistent. This therapy is suitable only for those subjects who meet the criteria and may be unsuccessful even for some of them. However, it is worth trying under the proper circumstances.

Speech pathologists should understand that speech therapy should probably not be undertaken at all for at least 3 months following a pharyngeal flap procedure and that spontaneous speech improvement may continue for about 1 year after surgery.

Concluding Remarks

Individuals with craniofacial and orofacial malformations are often not candidates for speech therapy either before or after corrective surgery. Therapy, when it is indicated, must be based on evidence that the structure is compatible with better speech than is being produced. If that is the case, therapy for these patients does not differ in any remarkable way from speech therapy in general.

Reference Notes

1. McWilliams, B. J. Learning disorders in children with Pierre Robin syndrome. In preparation.

2. Gorlin, R. J. Clefts in syndromes. Paper presented at the Annual Convention of the American Cleft Palate Association, Phoenix, 1972.

3. Witzel, M. A. Orthognathic defects and surgical corrections: The effects on speech and velopharyngeal function. Unpublished doctoral dissertation. The University of Pittsburgh, 1981.

4. Sassouni, V. Sassouni's classification of facial types, University of Pittsburgh, Unpublished.

References

Angle, E. H. Classification of malocclusion. *Dental Cosmos,* 1899, *41,* 248–264.

Bernstein, M. Relation of speech defects and malocclusion. *Alpha Omegan,* 1956, *50,* 90–97.

Bloomer, H. H. Speech defects associated with dental malocclusions and related abnormalities. In L. E. Travis (Ed.), *Handbook of speech pathology and audiology.* New York: Appleton-Century-Crofts, 1971.

Bloomer, H. H., & Hawk, A. M. Speech considerations: Speech disorders associated with ablative surgery of the face, mouth, and pharynx—Ablative approaches to learning. *ASHA Reports No. 8.* Washington, D. C.: American Speech and Hearing Association, 1973.

Brookshire, B. L., Lynch, J. I., & Fox, D. R. *A parent-child cleft palate curriculum: Developing speech and language.* Tigard, Ore.: C. C. Publications, 1980.

Cohen, M. M. The Robin Anomalad—Its nonspecificity and associated syndromes. *Oral Surgery,* 1976, *34,* 587–593.

Cohen, M. M. Syndromes with cleft lip and cleft palate. *Cleft Palate Journal,* 1978, *15,* 306–328.

DeMeyer, W. The median cleft face syndrome: Differential diagnosis of cranium bifidum occultum, hypertelorism and median cleft nose, lip and palate. *Neurology,* 1967, *17,* 961–971.

DeMeyer, W., Zeman, W., & Palmer, C. O. The face predicts the brain: Diagnostic significance of median face anomalies for holoprosencephaly (arrhinencephaly). *Pediatrics,* 1964, *34,* 256–263.

Elfenbein, J. L., Waziri, M., & Morris, H. L. Verbal communication skills of six children with craniofacial anomalies. *Cleft Palate Journal,* 1981, *18,* 59–64.

Eskew, H. A., & Shepard, E. E. Congenital aglossia. *American Journal of Orthodontia,* 1949, *35,* 116–119.

Gorlin, R. J., Pindborg, J. J., & Cohen, M. M. *Syndromes of the head and neck* (2nd ed.). New York: McGraw-Hill, 1976.

Guay, A. H., Maxwell, D. L., & Beecher, R. A radiographic study of tongue posture at rest and during phonation of /s/ in Class III malocclusion. *Angle Orthodontia,* 1978, *48,* 10–22.

Hahn, E. Directed home training program for infants with cleft lip and palate. In E. R. Bzoch (Ed.), *Communicative disorders related to cleft lip and cleft palate.* Boston: Little, Brown, 1979.

Irwin, E., & McWilliams, B. J. Play therapy for children with cleft palates. *Children Today,* 1974, *3,* 18–22.

Klechak, T. L., Bradley, D. P., & Warren, D. W. Anterior open bite and nasal port constriction. *Angle Orthodontia,* 1976, *46,* 232–242.

Long, N. V., & Dalston, R. M. Paired gestural and vocal behavior in one-year-old cleft lip and palate children. *Journal of Speech and Hearing Disorders,* 1982, *47,* 403–406.

MacGregor, F. C. Some psychosocial problems associated with facial deformities. *American Sociological Review,* 1951, *16,* 629–638.

Mallory, S. B., & Paradise, J. L. Glossoptosis revisited: On the development and resolution of airway obstruction in the Pierre Robin syndrome. *Pediatrics,* 1979, *64,* 946–948.

Morrees, C. F., Burstone, C. J., Christiansen, R. L., Hixon, E. H., & Weinstein, S. Research related to malocclusion, A state-of-the-art workshop, the oral-facial growth and development program, N.I.D.R. *American Journal of Orthodontia,* 1971, *59,* 1–18.

Paradise, J. L., & Bluestone, C. D. Diagnosis and management of ear disease in cleft palate infants. *Transactions of the American Academy of Ophthalmology and Otolaryngology,* 1969, *73,* 709–714.

Peterson, S. J. Speech pathology in craniofacial malformations other than cleft lip and palate. *Asha Reports No. 8.* Washington D. C.: American Speech and Hearing Association, 1973.

Peterson-Falzone, S. J. Speech and language problems in selected craniofacial anomalies. *Communicative disorders: An audio journal for continuing education.* New York: Grune and Stratton, 1976.

Philips, B. J. Stimulating syntactic and phonological development in infants with cleft palate. In K. R. Bzoch (Ed.), *Communicative disorders related to cleft lip and palate* (2nd ed.). Boston: Little, Brown, 1979.

Rusk, H. A. *Conference on facial disfigurement: A rehabilitation problem.* U. S. Department of Health, Education, and Welfare, V. R. A., 1963.

Salinas, C. F. An approach to an objective evaluation of the craniofacies, birth defects: *Original Article Series,* Volume XVI, 1980, *5,* 47–74. March of Dimes Birth Defects Foundation.

Sassouni, V. A classification of skeletal facial types. *American Journal of Orthodontia,* 1969, *55,* 109–123.

Shprintzen, R. J., McCall, G. N., & Skolnick, M. L. A new therapeutic technique for the treatment of velopharyngeal incompetence. *Journal of Speech and Hearing Disorders,* 1975, *40,* 69–83.

Smith, D. W. *Recognizable patterns of human malformation* (2nd ed.) *(Vol. VII): Major problems in clinical pediatrics.* Philadelphia: W. B. Saunders, 1976.

Smith, D. W. *Recognizable patterns of human deformation: Identification and management of mechanical effects on morphogenesis (Vol. XXI): Major problems in clinical pediatrics.* Philadelphia: W. B. Saunders, 1981.

Sparks, S. N., & Millard, S. Speech and language characteristics of genetic syndromes. *Journal of Communication Disorders,* 1981, *14,* 411–419.

Templin, M. C., & Darley, F. L. *Templin-Darley Tests of Articulation.* Seattle: University of Washington Press, 1969.

Tessier, P. The definitive plastic surgical treatment of the severe facial deformities of craniofacial synostosis. *Plastic Reconstructive Surgery,* 1971, *48,* 419–442.

Tisza, V. B., Irwin, E., & Scheide, E. Children with oral-facial clefts: A study of the psychological development of handicapped children. *Journal of the American Academy of Child Psychiatry,* 1973, *12,* 292–313.

Van Riper, C. *Speech Correction: Principles and methods* (5th ed.). Englewood Cliffs, N.J.: Prentice-Hall, 1972.

VanThal, J. H. The relationship between faults of dentition and defects of speech. *Proceedings of the Second International Congress of Phonetic Science.* Cambridge: Cambridge Press, 1935.

Whitaker, L. A., Pashayan, H., & Richman, J. A proposed new classification of craniofacial anomalies. *Cleft Palate Journal,* 1981, *18,* 161–176.

Part Two

STUTTERING

STUTTERING

Richard F. Curlee

Stuttering Disorders: An Overview

An extraordinary amount of information about stuttering and stutterers has been published in the past several decades. Recent research has significantly advanced our understanding of the nature of stuttering and of its treatment. Nevertheless, much of what we know comes from isolated studies, many of which have lacked satisfactory experimental controls or have employed small, perhaps unrepresentative, samples. Such methodological limitations particularly characterize the studies on children who stutter. Consequently, our information about stuttering is somewhat fragmentary and rarely will support unqualified conclusions. This chapter will summarize current information on stuttering in children and will attempt to evaluate its scientific credibility. Tentative conclusions will be drawn when warranted, and potential areas of fruitful inquiry will be suggested.

The Nature of Stuttering

Objective standards of fluency are not available, and there is still substantial uncertainty regarding the specific nature of the types of disruptions in speech that should be considered as stuttering. For the most part, fluent speech has been defined as the absence of disfluencies, and data on the perceptual or acoustic characteristics of fluency are extremely limited. In contrast, there have been many studies of stutterers' and nonstutterers' speech disruptions and of listeners' reactions to such disfluencies. As a result, information on the nature of stuttering must be synthesized from many different studies that have posed a variety of questions. For example: What types of speech disruptions, if any, distinguish stutterers' speech? Which disfluencies are listeners most likely to judge as stuttering? How consistent are listeners in identifying stuttering? Are behavioral and perceptual definitions of stuttering similarly useful? How comparable are the fluent portions of stutterers' and nonstutterers' speech? Succeeding paragraphs will briefly summarize the findings from a number of such studies as we consider characteristics which differentiate the speech of stutterers from that of nonstutterers.

It is apparent from casual observation and data from a number of controlled studies that stutterers evidence more speech disruptions than nonstutterers. Still, nonstutterers have many of the same types of disfluencies as stutterers, and some nonstuttering talkers are more disfluent than some stutterers. Such overlap may best be illustrated by Johnson's (1961a) comparisons of 100 stutterers with 100 nonstutterers. There was some overlap between the two groups on each of 8 types of disfluency. For example, 30% of the nonstutterers uttered more phrase repetitions than 30% of the stutterers, while 20% of the stutterers had fewer word repetitions than 30%-40% of the nonstuttering group. Nevertheless, overlap in the two groups' part-word repetitions approximated only 10%, and few nonstuttering talkers evidenced any sound prolongations or broken words. Johnson concluded that interjections, revisions, and phrase repetitions are likely to be considered by listeners as normal disfluencies, while part-word repetitions have the highest probability of being classified as stuttering. These conclusions were supported by Young's (1961) findings that ratings of stuttering severity increased with slowed speech rate and the frequency of part-word repetitions, sound prolongations, and broken words. Similarly, Schiavetti (1975) reported that severity ratings of feigned part-word repetitions ranked higher than sound prolongations, followed by interjections and word repetitions. The overlap in disfluency types observed among nonstuttering and stuttering adults has also been found in several empirical studies with children (Johnson & Associates, 1959; Yairi, 1972; F.H. Silverman, 1974). In addition, differences in the relative frequency of children's disfluency types have also been reported. For example, Voelker (1944) found that children who stuttered evidenced significantly more sound prolongations, syllable repetitions, and word repetitions than did their nonstuttering peers. Similarly, Floyd and Perkins (1974) found no overlap in the frequency of syllable disfluencies of preschool stutterers and nonstutterers.

Speech disruptions that occur within words are more likely to be judged by listeners as stuttering than are other types of disfluencies.

Williams and Kent (1958) compared a variety of feigned disfluencies and found that listeners judged syllable repetitions and sound prolongations as instances of stuttering more consistently than they did revisions, interjections, or word and phrase repetitions. Using recorded speech samples of stutterers and nonstutterers, Boehmler (1958) obtained similar findings with both naive and experienced listeners. More recently, Huffman and Perkins (1974) studied the reactions of school teachers to audio recordings of various types of disfluencies that were simulated with and without tension. They found that part-word repetitions, sound prolongations, and hesitations were identified as stuttering more often than were other disfluency types. In addition, those disfluencies produced with audible stress or tension were judged as stuttering more often than were the same types of disfluencies without simulated effort. It also seems noteworthy that judges without special training or instruction appear to classify speech disfluencies similarly to expert professional judges. Because school-age children evidence similar perceptual standards when listening to adult speakers (Giolas & Williams, 1958), it is unlikely that such standards result from either training or personal experiences. Comparable studies with child speakers have not been completed, but it seems likely that similar results would be found. Thus, the types of disfluencies that listeners most often identify as stuttering are the same types that occur more frequently in stutterers' speech than in that of nonstuttering talkers.

Much of what we know about the nature of stuttering relies heavily on listeners' judgments, and listeners are often inconsistent in their judgments. Boehmler (1958) reported that listeners classified part-word repetitions of nonstuttering talkers as instances of stuttering about as often as they did those of stutterers. It may also be noteworthy that listeners readily identify nonstutterers' feigned disfluencies as stutterings or as having been spoken by a stutterer (William & Kent, 1958; Huffman & Perkins, 1974). Such findings are consistent with the view that normal disfluencies and instances of stuttering occupy the same perceptual continuum, with the speech disruptions judged consistently as stutterings or as normal disfluencies at the opposite extremes of the continuum. If so, people may be classified as stutterers as the frequency of their unambiguous instances of stuttering increases or becomes a substantial proportion of all their disfluencies. Although MacDonald and Martin (1973) concluded that stuttering and disfluency were separate, unambiguous response classes that can be differentiated reliably by listeners, a follow-up study (Curlee, 1981) that controlled for independence of listener judgments could not replicate their findings. Indeed, the latter study found overlap in listeners' judgments on more than 70% of all the disfluencies and stutterings identified. Thus, a substantial proportion of the speech disruptions observed in the utterances of chronic adult stutterers are likely to be judged inconsistently by listeners and may reflect, in part, the instructions, the context, and the conditions under which such judgments are made. The extent to which these findings can be generalized to children who stutter is not known, but it seems plausible that a large proportion of children's speech disruptions would be judged ambiguously as stuttering or as normal disfluencies. These speculations, and others, may have important practical and theoretical implications and warrant systematic study.

There is ample evidence from a number of different studies that listener agreement on frequency of stuttering is high. It usually exceeds .80 and often averages above .90 (Young, 1969; Young & Downs, 1968; Curlee, Perkins, & Michael, Note 1). Such agreement has been demonstrated consistently among both naive and experienced listeners (interjudge agreement) and between different judging sessions with the same listeners (intrajudge) agreement). There is substantially less agreement, however, on the specific words or the loci of speech disruptions that are identified as disfluencies or as instances of stuttering, an issue that warrants further discussion. In an early study of listener agreement, Tuthill (1946) remarked that only 37% of all words judged as stuttered had been marked by all listeners. Likewise, Williams and Kent (1958) noted that there was considerable disagreement about which words were stuttered among listeners judging taped utterances of simulated disfluencies. Young (1975a) described a systematic study of interjudge agreement across a variety of listening conditions. He found high agreement among judges ($r \geq .90$) for frequency of stuttering; however, listener agreement on which words were stuttered was substantially lower, approximating .50 regardless of practice, training, or instructions. Similarly low levels of listener agreement were reported recently by Martin and Haroldson (1981) when the words judges had identified as stuttered were compared on a word-by-word basis.

Young suggested that having listeners mark only words and not allowing them to identify stuttering on intervals between words could affect agreement adversely. This possibility was explored as part of a study in which listeners' ability to differentiate between instances of stuttering and disfluencies was studied (Curlee, 1981). As in previous investigations, interjudge agreement on frequency of stuttering during speaking and reading tasks yielded correlation coefficients in the .90s. These same listener judgments, when analyzed in terms of specific words and intervals marked as stuttered, yielded interjudge agreements which averaged less than .30. Intrajudge agreement on specific units marked as stuttered, though somewhat higher, still averaged only in the .50s. Instead of improving agreement, allowing listeners to select both words and intervals between words resulted in less consistent judgments of stuttering. Thus, data from several studies yield relatively high estimates of reliability when analyzed in terms of agreement on frequency of stuttering; however, when agreement is evaluated on a unit-by-unit basis, listeners' uncertainty about specific instances of stuttering becomes apparent.

Studies of listener agreement usually instructed judges to use one of two basic ways of defining stuttering. One type of definition asks listeners to count specific types of behaviors, such as part-word repetitions and audible or silent prolongations, as stuttering. The other type asks listeners to count any type of speech disruption which they personally perceive to be an instance of stuttering. The former instructions can be considered as a behavioral definition of stuttering, the latter as a perceptual definition. Two recent studies have compared listener agreement using each type of definition (Curlee, 1981; Martin & Haroldson, 1981). Both studies asked listeners to use Wingate's (1964) definition and their own personal perceptual standards of stuttering during alternate listening sessions. Both studies found unit-by-unit agreement comparably low for both types of definitions. Apparently, a substantial proportion of judged instances of stuttering are not agreed on by most judges, or by the same judge on different occcasions, when satisfactory controls assure that judgments are made independently.

Frequent, repeated judgments by the same listener of the same speech sample, or by several listeners working collaboratively, likely violate requirements of observational independence, and the reliability of such judgments cannot be estimated satisfactorily. Since behavioral and perceptual definitions are comparable in identifying frequency of stuttering, both can be used satisfactorily as an index of severity or of change. Indeed, it is an enormous practical advantage to clinicians that frequency counts of stuttering are relatively stable and reliable across a variety of listening conditions for both naive and experienced listeners. Unfortunately, the observed disagreement among independent observers regarding specific instances of disfluencies poses a significant methodological problem for researchers interested in behavioral, physiological, or acoustical correlates of stuttering or other speech disruptions. Moreover, such disagreements suggest that the isolation of specific disruptions in the flow of stutterers' speech may also be of questionable validity.

In view of listeners' apparent difficulty in distinguishing between normal disfluencies and stuttering and in identifying specific instances of stuttering reliably, it may be surprising that stutterers' and nonstutterers' fluent utterances can be differentiated. Wendahl and Cole (1961) compared the fluent portions of 8 stutterers' aloud readings with comparably edited recordings of the same passage read aloud by 8 nonstutterers who had been matched for age and reading proficiency. Groups of unsophisticated judges who listened to these matched utterances rated stutterers' speech as less normal in rate and rhythm and as evidencing more force or strain. Moreover, the fluent samples of each stutterer were identified as those of a stutterer significantly more often than those of the nonstutterer with whom the subject was matched. Using the same matched recordings, Young (1964) asked different listeners to identify which samples were those of stutterers; however, their judgments about a talker's utterances were made without benefit of a comparison to those of the talker's matched control. Young found that 3 of the 16 talkers were identified as stutterers by a significant majority of listeners, although 1 of the 3 was a nonstutterer. Similarly, of the 8 talkers who were identified by listeners as nonstutterers, 2 were stutterers. The remaining 5 speakers, all of whom were stutterers, were not consistently classified by listeners as either stutterers or nonstutterers. These findings led Young to conclude that stutterers' fluent speech cannot be readily differentiated from that of nonstutterers. Methodological and analytical differences between these two studies likely account for the differences in their outcomes. Paired-stimulus presentations of stutterers with nonstutterers often provide listeners with sufficient cues to distinguish nonstuttering from stuttering talkers. For example, even when the fluent utterances of treated, adult stutterers and nonstutterers are paired, listeners are usually able to differentiate most stutterers reliably (Ingham & Packman, 1978; Runyan & Adams, 1978, 1979). In contrast, recent studies with children who stutter indicate that most cannot be reliably differentiated from their matched, nonstuttering peers, even when paired presentations of fluent utterances are employed (Colcord & Gregory, Note 2; MacIndoe & Runyan, Note 3). Additional studies are needed to determine if these findings can be replicated.

What, then, should be concluded from the literature we have just reviewed? It is obvious that most of what we know about stutterers' speech comes from studies of chronic adult stutterers. These studies indicate that there are quantitative and qualitative differences in the speech disruptions of stutterers when compared to those of persons who are not stutterers. Listeners count the frequency of stuttering in adults in a reliable manner, even though there may be considerable disagreement regarding which interruptions in speech are instances of stuttering. In addition, listeners are comparably reliable using a perceptual or a behavioral definition of stuttering. While there may be substantial overlap between groups of stutterers and nonstutterers, stutterers typically evidence more frequent speech disruptions, particularly part-word repetitions, prolongations, and, possibly, hesitations. The latter type of disfluency has not been investigated as thoroughly as other speech disruptions, however. Evidence is also accumulating regarding differences in the perceptually fluent utterances of adult stutterers. Such differences have been demonstrated perceptually in several paired-stimulus studies, although the acoustic bases of such differences are uncertain. In any event, it seems clear that most listeners can reliably identify who is a stutterer and how often he stutters; considerable difficulty is encountered, however, in determining exactly when each instance of stuttering occurs.

Comparable objective studies of children's speech are not available. We do not know how reliable listeners are in assessing children's disfluencies because empirical studies are lacking. Based on clinical reports about the difficulty involved in determining whether some young children have begun to stutter or not, it seems doubtful that listeners would evidence better agreement on the speech disruptions of young children. Intuitively, it seems more likely that perceptual distinctions between children's normal disfluencies and stuttering may be more ambiguous than between those of adults. Recent comparisons of the fluent speech of stuttering and nonstuttering children suggest that only a small proportion of young stutterers may evidence perceptually distinctive fluency, and follow-up longitudinal studies are warranted to determine if such differences are related to severity or to subsequent remissions. Much of what has been written about stuttering in children has been based on reports of clinical observations or brief studies of small groups of children who stutter. Consequently, the empirical foundation of our information on the speech of children who stutter is not secure, particularly with regard to younger children who have not been stuttering long.

In view of the apparent perceptual ambiguity between stutterers' normal disfluencies and instances of stuttering and the apparent distinctiveness of the "fluent" segments of their utterances, it is of questionable validity to view adult stutterers' speech as consisting of intermittent instances of stuttering which occur during the flow of ongoing, normal speech. If the perceptual boundaries of instances of stuttering are uncertain, and if stutterers' fluent utterances are distinctive from those of nonstutterers, classifying stutterers' speech into discrete segments of stuttered, disfluent, or fluent speech may distort the inherent continuity of their speech characteristics or of disordered dimensions that should be studied. While instances of stuttering can serve as a reliable index of stuttering severity, and may have many practical clinical applications, its use as a unit of study in research that is directed at understanding the nature of stuttered speech clearly limits the perspective of such research. Indeed, different perspectives may yield more fruitful insights.

Speech Characteristics of Young Stutterers

Data Obtained by Direct Observation

Much of the data on how stuttering begins has been obtained retrospectively through questionnaires or interviews with parents and with older stutterers. Data based on direct observations made by trained observers have usually involved cross-sectional studies of children who have been stuttering for some time; ascertainment of children shortly after they begin to stutter is probably biased by severity of onset, with the more severe being seen sooner. In addition, there have been few empirical studies of the fluency characteristics of nonstuttering children during the course of speech and language development. Indeed, adequate normative data on the fluency or disfluency of normally developing children, of children with suspected fluency problems, or of confirmed young stutterers do not exist. Systematic longitudinal studies are needed to resolve many important questions concerning stuttering onset.

Two longitudinal studies pertinent to the onset of stuttering are available. Epidemiological data from a study of 1,000 families in England have been summarized by Andrews and Harris (1964), and the findings of a larger, more recent study completed in the United States have been reported by LaBenz and LaBenz (1980). Unfortunately, both of these studies provided only limited information on speech characteristics, accessory behaviors, and associated features of beginning stutterers. As a result, it is not clear how the speech of those children who were identified as having fluency problems specifically differed from that of other children in the studies. Moreover, neither study provided the type of data needed to identify patterns of progression or remission of stuttering among the children studied. Consequently, the findings from these studies cannot help us identify the empirical bases on which beginning stutterers may be differentiated from their normally disfluent peers.

What is known about the disfluencies of normally developing young children comes mainly from a few cross-sectional investigations. The number of children observed at different age levels has been relatively small, thereby severely restricting our appreciation of how the characteristics studied vary within the population. Limitations in our data base hinder clinicians trying to identify children who are beginning to stutter, and perpetuate theoretical disagreements about the nature of stuttering. In spite of the paucity of normative data, there is substantial agreement among independent reviewers about a number of findings (Adams, 1980; Bloodstein, 1981; Curlee, 1980a; Johnson, 1980; Van Riper, 1982). Unfortunately, such agreement among authors of disparate theoretical persuasions may generate more confidence in the available information than the data warrant, and probably, does not encourage additional research that is needed.

Repetitions are common characteristics of preschoolers' speech. Winitz (1961) observed infants' vocalizations during 30 consecutive breaths at 12 age levels from birth to age 2. The number of infants observed at each age level varied from 31 to 80. He reported that infants' prelinguistic repetitions seemed to peak at around 1 year of age, then to decrease steadily during their second year of life as words began to occur more frequently in utterances. These findings are consistent with those of several other studies with older preschoolers. Metraux's (1950) cross-sectional investigation, involving 207 children between 18 and 54 months of age, developed qualitative speech profiles for six age groups ranging in size from 16 to 42 children. Her descriptions indicated that "developmental stuttering" was evidenced for the first time among 2½-year-olds, even though part-word, word, or phrase repetitions were common characteristics of the 1½- and 2-year-old age groups. How developmental stuttering was differentiated from other disfluencies is not clear; however, it is implied that the frequency and apparent effort associated with a child's speech disruptions may have been involved. In an earlier study of preschoolers' repetitions and language development, Davis (1939, 1940) observed 1-hour speech samples of 62 children from 24 to 60 months of age. She found that word and phrase repetitions decreased with age, but syllable repetitions did not. Based on personal observations of several active and former stutterers in her sample, Davis concluded that syllable repetitions differentiated stutterers from nonstutterers. Correlations between measures of children's language acquisition and their speech repetitions were generally low, and, according to Davis, lacked either theoretical or practical importance. Finally, Yairi's (1981) study of 33 normally talking 2-year-olds found that single-syllable word and part-word repetitions constituted about 39% of all their disfluencies. There was a substantial range in the frequency of disfluency across children, but all types of disfluencies were observed, even tense pauses and sound prolongations. Whole-word repetitions and revisions were the most frequently occurring disfluency types for these 2-year-olds, each accounting for slightly more than 21% of all disfluencies.

In another recent study, Bjerkan (1980) observed essentially no sound prolongations, blocks, or part-word repetitions in the speech samples of 108 nursery school children between 2 and 6 years of age. In contrasting these findings with observations of two preschool children who stutter, Bjerkan concluded that early stuttering typically involves disruptions within word boundaries. This conclusion supports an earlier finding of Floyd and Perkins (1974), who found no overlap in the frequency of syllable disfluencies (which included repetitions, prolongations, and interjections of syllables) between four preschool stutterers and 20 normally speaking peers. Although Yairi (1981) found a relatively high proportion of syllable repetitions among his group of nonstuttering 2-year-olds, he did not, unfortunately, have a comparison group of young stutterers with whom to contrast the frequency of part-word disfluencies.

It is important to note that only a few stutterers have been involved in these studies, and generalizing these findings to other children who may be starting to stutter may not be warranted. Indeed, Bloodstein's (1974; 1981) observations of young stutterers have convinced him that whole-word repetitions characterize the speech disruptions of beginning stutterers more than any other type of disfluency. He has argued that much of the data from other studies reflect the tension and fragmentation which he believes comes to characterize more and more of stutterers' speech the longer they stutter. Still, Van Riper (1982) has reported data on 61 clients, all of whom were seen within 3 weeks of stuttering onset, and in whom he observed more part-word than whole-word repetitions. Obviously, the severity of these onsets may have biased Van Riper's findings, and additional data are needed from better controlled longitudinal studies to resolve these issues. Supporting Van Riper, however, Yairi's (1983) study of 22 2- and 3-year-old children found that syllable repetitions were all but a universal characteristic of stuttering onset reported by parents and that 3 or more units per repetition typified such speech disruptions of 90% of the children studied.

A number of studies report considerable overlap in the type and frequency of disfluencies that are observed among stuttering and nonstuttering children. The most extensive accumulation of such data involved a series of studies by Johnson and Associates (1959). One study compared the disfluencies of 68 boys and 21 girls who stuttered with those of a matched group of nonstutterers. Both groups averaged 5 years of age, ranging from 2½ to slightly above age 8. According to parents' reports, stuttering had begun, on the average, 18 months prior to observation in the study. Thus, speech findings may not be representative of children who are just beginning to stutter. Although Johnson emphasized the overlap between the two groups' speech characteristics, there were a number of reliable group differences found. Stuttering children were disfluent significantly more often than nonstuttering children, with part-word repetitions and sound prolongations showing the least overlap between the 2 groups. In addition, the children who stuttered evidenced substantially more units per repetition than did nonstutterers. Subsequent studies of elementary school-aged children have reported similar patterns of overlap and distinction between stuttering and nonstuttering children (F.H. Silverman, 1974; Yairi, 1972). Likewise, Westby (1979) compared the speech of 10 stutterers, 10 highly disfluent nonstutterers, and 10 typically disfluent nonstuttering children. She found that the highly disfluent nonstutterers' speech disruptions were more similar to those of stutterers than to those of the typically disfluent nonstutterers. Similarly, E.M. Silverman's study (1972) of 10 4-year-old nonstutterers reported frequent observations of the types of disfluencies often identified as stuttering. Apparently, objective differentiation of young stutterers cannot be as straightforward as we would like.

There is considerable evidence that groups of stuttering and nonstuttering children produce the same types of disfluencies. While there is disagreement about how much overlap is found in the frequency of disfluencies, expecially part-word repetitions and sound prolongations, it is apparent that the frequency and pattern of disfluencies evidenced by *some* stuttering children can be quite similar to that of *some* children usually regarded not to be stutterers. For the most part, however, the data indicate that there is little overlap among *most* nonstutterers and *most* stutterers. Moreover, it can also be noted that few studies have included hard articulatory or glottal attacks or hesitations as disfluencies, therby ignoring disruptions in fluency that are commonly observed in many stutterers. Some of the disagreement found in the literature may reflect differences in authors' theoretical perspectives and interpretations of findings rather than differences in data. Furthermore, Westby's study indicates that stutterers can be differentiated from highly disfluent nonstutterers even though the basis for such differentiation may not be apparent.

Data Obtained from Parent Interviews

Information on the speech characteristics of beginning stutterers obtained from parent interviews agrees substantially with the observational studies just summarized. As might be anticipated, there have been similar disagreements about how such data should be interpreted. There seems to be general agreement that repetitions constitute the most frequent types of disfluency observed in children when they first begin to stutter (Glasner & Rosenthal, 1957; Johnson & Associates, 1959; Van Riper, 1982). The largest and most comprehensive of these studies compared reports from parents of 150 stutterers with those from parents of 150 nonstutterers (Johnson & Associates, 1959). The authors emphasized the similarities found in parents' descriptions of their children's speech and argued that the two parent groups had reacted in strikingly different ways to essentially the same types of childhood disfluencies. In short, parents of children who began to stutter were believed to have misdiagnosed their children's normal nonfluencies, thereby initiating the problem of stuttering. Subsequently, however, these interpretations of the study's findings have been challenged by several authors (Curlee, 1980a; McDearmon, 1968; Van Riper, 1982). For example, it has been pointed out that only half of the parents of nonstutterers were able to describe their child as having any speech disruptions, and most of these descriptions consisted of such disfluencies as pauses between words, interjections, difficulties expressing ideas, or repetitions of words or phrases. Thus, approximately 95% of the parents of normally developing children apparently had not noticed any disruptions in their child's speech or reported only those types of disruptions commonly considered to be normal disfluencies. Approximately 4% of nonstutterers' parents indicated they had observed part-word repetitions or prolongations on occasion, and less than 1% reported ever having observed their child hesitate in the middle of a word, block, or not finish sentences. On the other hand, approximately 75% of the parents of stuttering children indicated that sound prolongations, part-word repetitions, blocks, and signs of tension or struggle had characterized their child's speech at the time of their initial concerns. As with studies involving direct observations of stutterers' and nonstutterers' speech, parent reports suggest that overlap in stuttering and nonstuttering children's disfluencies does not involve a majority of either group once a problem is suspected. Nevertheless, accurate identification of some beginning stutterers may present a diagnostic challenge to clinicians, and extensive observations and evaluations of some children's speech in different speaking circumstances may be necessary.

Loci

The speech disruptions of stutterers do not occur randomly and, with few exceptions, are distributed similarly to those of nonstutterers. It has been shown that the disfluencies of adult stutterers and nonstutterers tend to occur on the same words across repeated utterances, and so do those of stuttering and nonstuttering children (Bloodstein, 1960; Bloodstein, Alper, & Zisk, 1965; Neelley & Timmons, 1967; Williams, Silverman, & Kools, 1969). For both stutterers and nonstutterers of school-age and older, speech disruptions occur more frequently, and thereby more consistently, on longer words, content words, words beginning with consonants, and words of lower predictability, but only stutterers have substantially more speech disruptions at the beginning of sentences (Blankenship, 1964; Chaney, 1969; Mann, 1955; F.H. Silverman, 1972; Silverman & Williams, 1967; Williams, Silverman, & Kools, 1969). Preschool-age children, stutterers and nonstutterers alike, also evidence speech disruptions more often while initiating utterances and, in contrast to older age groups, on such function words as pronouns and conjunctions (Bloodstein & Gantwerk, 1967; Helmreich & Bloodstein, 1973; F.H. Silverman, 1974). Recently,

Bloodstein and Grossman (1981) reported that young stutterers' whole-word repetitions occur almost exclusively at the beginning of syntactic units. Obviously, such characteristics represent different ways of classifying linguistic phenomena in a convenient manner, and different characteristics that are related statistically to speech disruptions can also share other common attributes. For example, longer words are more likely to be content words as well as words of lower predictability than are shorter words. Longer words may also differ from shorter words in terms of suprasegmental stress or may require greater motor or linguistic planning. In any event, stuttering appears to be sensitive to the same factors or constraints that affect the speech disruptions of nonstuttering talkers.

Variability

One of stuttering's more puzzling attributes is its seeming variability. Even casual observation indicates that stuttering varies in form, frequency, and severity from situation to situation, listener to listener, or from one moment to another during the same conversation. Yet, groups of stutterers evidence similar reactions to a number of speaking conditions. Unfortunately, we have little empirical information about how groups of children who stutter respond to different conditions, even though it is possible that much of what we know about adult stutterers may apply to children, especially those who are older. Empirical studies of adults have shown, for example, that stuttering is substantially decreased while speaking or reading in time to rhythmical stimuli (Brady, 1969; Fransella & Beech, 1965; Martin & Haroldson, 1979), reading aloud in unison with another (Adams & Ramig, 1980; Ingham & Packman, 1979; Johnson & Rosen, 1937), singing (Bloodstein, 1950; Colcord & Adams, 1979; Healey, Mallard, & Adams, 1976), speaking slowly in a prolonged manner with or without DAF (Curlee & Perkins, 1969; Johnson & Rosen, 1937; Soderberg, 1969b), talking while alone (Bloodstein, 1950; Hood, 1975) speaking during auditory masking (Adams & Hutchinson, 1974; Cherry & Sayers, 1956; Perkins & Curlee, 1969), or talking during response-contingent stimulation of stuttering (Ingham & Andrews, 1973; Martin & Haroldson, 1979; Siegel, 1970). Experimentation has demonstrated that reduction of stuttering with reduced syllable rate depends on prolongation of phones within the syllable (Perkins, Bell, Johnson, & Stocks, 1979). Another experimentally demonstrated relationship, which appears to be invariant and must, therefore, be accounted for in any adequate understanding of abnormal dysfluency, is the reduction of stuttering with whispering, and its elimination with voiceless lipped speech (Perkins, Rudas, Johnson, & Bell, 1976). Conversely, stuttering usually has been found to increase in frequency or severity as audience size increases (Bloodstein, 1950; Siegel & Haugen, 1964), when stuttering is anticipated (Johnson & Sinn, 1937; Milisen, 1938) or in circumstances in which communicative stress or general tension or anxiety appear to be elevated (Bloodstein, 1950; Gray & Brutten, 1965). There is some evidence that the frequency of nonstutterers' disfluency varies similarly. For example, disfluencies of nonstutters are reduced while speaking in time to rhythmical stimulus (F.H. Silverman, 1971), under auditory masking (Silverman & Goodban, 1972), and during repeated readings of the same passage (Soderberg, 1969a; Williams, Silverman, & Kools, 1968).

Although there are numerous clinical reports suggesting that preschool stutterers' speech disruptions vary noticeably across speaking conditions, adequately controlled empirical studies are lacking. There is evidence that preschoolers' stuttering decreases with response-contingent stimulation (Martin, Kuhl, & Haroldson, 1972; Reed & Godden, 1977) or while speaking in time to rhythmical stimulus (Coppola & Yairi, Note 4). Because few empirical studies have been completed with children, especially preschoolers, substantial gaps in our knowledge remain. The weight of available evidence suggests that speech disruptions of stutterers follow patterns of occurrence similar to those observed among persons who do not stutter. An apparent exception is the substantially greater percentage of stuttering among adult stutterers that occurs at the beginning of utterances and syntactic units. Although substantially fewer data are available for children, the disfluencies of young stutterers and nonstutterers appear to vary in loci and in frequency as a function of the same variables, and there are no demonstrably reliable findings to the contrary. Thus, a theory which accounts for the relationships between stuttering and various speaking conditions or psycholinguistic variables may also account for the speech disruptions of nonstutterers.

Onset

Stuttering can be viewed as a developmental problem that begins most often during the course of a child's speech and language development. Onset is usually insidious; both Morley (1957) and Van Riper (1982) found abrupt onsets of stuttering in only a small percentage of clients, even those examined soon after parents had become concerned about fluency. Their observations are supported by most parent reports (Bloodstein, 1981). Indeed, Bloodstein has hypothesized that mild tension and fragmentations are common features of all preschoolers' speech, which can worsen with communicative stress for some and lead to chronic stuttering. Most stutterers are identified during their preschool years (Andrews & Harris, 1964;

Dickson, 1971; Johnson & Associates, 1959), and there are relatively few onsets after age 9 (Young, 1975b). Although some children may start stuttering around the time they begin to speak in short utterances, most have been using sentences a year or more before they begin (Johnson & Associates, 1959). Andrews and Harris (1964) estimated that the risk of stuttering onset is highest between ages 2 and 5 and gradually decreases thereafter until age 12, when future risk approximates zero. Reports of stuttering beginning during adolescence or adulthood are sparse and essentially anecdotal. Van Riper (1982) noted that such reports often describe abrupt onsets that are associated with an emotional shock or physical injury. It is possible that some late onsets may involve recurrences of early stuttering problems that have been forgotten or that some fluency problems, though similar in many ways to stuttering, may differ from developmental stuttering upon more careful observation. As with other areas of uncertainty, additional research is needed.

Stutterer-Nonstutterer Differences

In recent years, increasing importance has been placed on relatively small but consistent differences found in empirical comparisons of groups of stutterers and nonstutterers. Recent reviews of such findings have been presented by Andrews, Craig, Feyer, Hoddinott, Howie & Neilson (1983) and Bloodstein (1981). As might be expected, there is considerable disagreement concerning which differences, if any, result in stuttering, which result from stuttering, and which covary with stuttering or stutterers but are not causally related. For the most part, differences between stutterers and nonstutterers appear to fall within the range of normal variation, and there is extensive overlap between the two groups. It can also be noted that the variability among groups of stutterers is usually substantially greater than that found among comparison groups. The greater heterogeneity of stutterers' data appears to reflect greater variability in performance across different stutterers as well as less consistent performance of individual stutterers on the same task than is found among nonstutterers. Consequently, it should be remembered throughout subsequent paragraphs that generalizations from studies of groups of stutterers are not valid when applied to many individual stutterers.

Cognition

Cognitive abilities or functions of stutterers differ from those of nonstutterers in a number of ways. Stutterers' average performance on intelligence tests falls about one-half a standard deviation below the mean of normal speakers (Andrews & Harris, 1964; Okasha, Bishry, Kamel & Hossan, 1974; Schindler, 1955). Stutterers are also somewhat slower in speech and language development (Andrews & Harris, 1964; Berry, 1938; Darley, 1955) and evidence other speech and language impairments more often (Blood & Seider, 1981; Schindler, 1955; Williams & Silverman, 1968; Winitz & Darley, 1980). As would be anticipated, there is also consistent evidence that stutterers' educational placement and academic achievement, on the whole, lags behind that of nonstuttering children (Darley, 1955; Schindler, 1955; Williams, Melrose, & Woods, 1969). Several well-controlled EEG studies have found differences between stutterers and nonstutterers across a number of different tasks (Moore & Haynes, 1980; Moore & Lang, 1977; Sayles, 1971; Zimmerman & Knott, 1974). Such differences in EEG activities may reflect different cerebral processing activities as well as cerebral dysfunctions. Tests of stutterers' central auditory abilities (Hall & Jerger, 1978; Molt & Guilford, 1979; Toscher & Rupp, 1978), ear preference for meaningful stimuli on dichotic listening tasks (Curry & Gregory, 1969; Sommers, Brady, & Moore, 1975) and auditory tracking skills (Sussman & MacNeilage, 1975) have found, though somewhat less consistently, differences between groups of stutterers and nonstutterers. As might be expected, it is not clear to what extent many of these findings can be applied to children who stutter, particularly those who ultimately recover.

Motor Abilities

Investigations of stutterers' overall motor abilities have found relatively few differences in motor coordination or dexterity. In general, the data are sufficiently inconclusive that one can neither eliminate the possibility of subtle differences between stutterers' and nonstutterers' nonspeech motor abilities nor clearly implicate any specific differences with confidence. Studies of the speed and accuracy with which stutterers use their speech mechanisms have yielded similarly inconsistent results for the most part. Within the past few years, however, a number of different investigators have found reliable differences in voice reaction times. In 1976, Adams and Hayden reported that adult stutterers were significantly slower initiating and terminating phonation of an isolated vowel. Starkweather, Hirshman, and Tannenbaum (1976) found adult stutterers to be similarly slow initiating phonation across a variety of different syllables. Comparable findings have been reported subsequently for both adults and children in a number of different studies (Cross & Luper, 1979; Cullinan & Springer, 1980; Reich, Till, & Goldsmith, 1981; Starkweather, Franklin, & Smigo, Note 5). Several of these studies have also included observations of stutterers' nonspeech vocal and manual reaction times. While all of these studies have found the average reaction times of stutterers slower on speech tasks than that of nonstutterers, nonspeech vocal and manual latencies have differed in some studies but not in others. In addition, Cullinan and Springer (1980) found that when their 20 stuttering children were divided into a group of 11 who had concomitant language or articulation problems and a group of 9 whose only problem was stuttering, only the children with concomitant speech-language problems differed significantly from the nonstuttering comparison group. Since most studies have used fewer than 15 subjects per group, inconsistent reports of statistical reliability should be expected. Some discrepancies among studies are not easily accounted for, however. For example, while Cross and Luper (1979) found a high positive correlation between voice and finger reaction times, Starkweather, Franklin, and Smigo (1981) found a moderate negative correlation.

Such findings are intriguing and clearly warrant further investigation; nevertheless, their significance to stuttering is not clear. Apparently, stutterers' reaction times may be slower for speech and some nonspeech tasks, with speech task latencies differentially slower. Because differences have been found even in relatively young stutterers, it seems unlikely that slower reaction times are a consequence of stuttering. If slower reaction times reflect some type of motor dysfuntion common to stutterers, such problems likely extend beyond the larynx, perhaps even the speech mechanism. It is obvious that longer response latencies do not necessarily result in stuttering, since most people with motor speech impairments do not stutter and since there is considerable overlap in stutterers' and nonstutterers' reaction times. Indeed, it seems more plausible that stutterers' slower reaction times and speech disruptions result from their inability to execute rapid, precise complex motor responses. Data from these studies and those involving fiberoptic (Conture, McCall, & Brewer, 1977) and EMG (Freeman & Ushijima, 1978) investigations of stutterers' laryngeal behavior during stuttering have been used to support the hypothesis that the larynx plays a primary role in stutterers' speech disruptions. Such arguments must be carefully constrained to be credible. Clearly, the larynx is not essential to stuttering. If it were, stuttering could not persist following laryngectomy, and, yet, occasionally it does. Whether or not subsystems of the speech mechanism are hierarchically arranged is debatable. If they are, then it is not clear how one subsystem of the mechanism could be more involved or more responsible for stuttering than other subsystems of the same mechanism. At best, these findings may represent critical keys to our future understanding of stuttering. Only further research can tell.

Personal Adjustment

Several relatively complete reviews of information about stutterers' personal adjustment are available, and specific investigations will not be covered here (Bloch & Goodstein, 1971; Bloodstein, 1981; Goodstein, 1958; Sheehan, 1958; Van Riper, 1982). However, there is general agreement among these reviews that: stutterers fall within the normal range on tests of personality and are more similar to normal persons than to psychiatric comparison groups; that personalities of severe stutterers do not differ reliably from those whose stuttering is mild; that older stutterers' personalities do not differ in significant ways from those of younger stutterers; that parents of stutterers are not substantially more maladjusted than parents of children who do not stutter. Even though many people apparently have a negative stereotype of stutterers' personalities (Turnbaugh, Guitar, & Hoffman, 1979; Woods & Williams, 1976), standardized tests do not reveal a reliable pattern of traits or characteristics for groups of stutterers. The few consistent reports of differences between stutterers' and nonstuttering persons' self-confidence or anxiety usually have been attributed to normal, secondary reactions to a communication disability. It is interesting to note in this regard, however, that Prins (1972) found more prevalent signs of maladjustment among subjects with other communication disorders than among a matched group of stutterers. It is possible, of course, that studies of heterogeneous groups of stutterers have obscured distinctive personality patterns of several different subgroups or that current measures of personal adjustment are not able to differentiate stutterers' abnormal adaptations from normal variations in personality. Because most of what we know comes from studies of adults, such information may not be pertinent to factors which precipitate stuttering onset or which lead to recovery. Nevertheless, it is clear that there is no credible body of evidence which indicates that stutterers' personal adjustments are of significance to either the etiology or the maintenance of stuttering.

Incidence and Prevalence

It has been estimated that about 4% to 5% of the population stutter for some period during their lives (Andrews & Harris, 1964; Bloodstein, 1981; Curlee, 1980a; Van Riper, 1982). In contrast, the prevalence of stuttering, among school-age children approximates 1% or less (Bloodstein, 1981; Brady & Hall, 1976; Hull, Mielke, Williford, & Timmons, 1976; Winitz & Darley, 1980; Young, 1975b). Stuttering may be somewhat less prevalent during high school years than elementary school and is probably more prevalent during preschool years, but adequate documentation is lacking.

Data from several more recent studies (Brady & Hall, 1976; Winitz & Darley, 1980) suggest that stuttering may be less prevalent than was indicated by previous studies; however, different ascertainment procedures and criteria for identifying stutterers do not permit direct comparisons across studies. Although all studies reporting prevalence or incidence estimates can be challenged on the basis of several methodological limitations (Curlee, 1980a; Ingham, 1976; Young, 1975b), their data are relatively consistent. Indeed, even prevalence and incidence differences among different cultures or socioeconomic groups are relatively small and have often been interpreted to accommodate authors' differing theoretical biases.

One of the few findings for which there is complete agreement across studies is that more males than females stutter. While the proportion of male to female stutterers has varied somewhat from study to study, most findings cluster around a 3:1 male-to-female ratio (Bloodstein, 1981; Van Riper, 1982). Males also manifest such other problems as asthma, epilepsy, chorea, spina bifida, or cleft palate more frequently than females and differ from females in terms of stature, longevity, baldness, and education. Bloodstein (1981) believes that the sex ratio may be positively related to age, with the proportion of males to females increasing in older age groups. Recent data reported by Yairi (1983) on stuttering onset among 2- and 3-year-olds indicate an equal sex distribution for children who begin to stutter this young. The data available on this issue are limited, however, and may only reflect sampling errors across studies. If further studies confirm this finding, it would be important to determine if there is a differential recovery rate between males and females or if males begin to stutter at somewhat older ages than females.

The prevalence of stuttering is substantially higher among persons with cerebral damage (Bloodstein, 1981; Bohme, 1968; Van Riper, 1982). For example, among the mentally retarded, prevalence appears to increase with severity of cognitive deficits, and may be even higher among those whose retardation has resulted from organic etiology (Bloodstein, 1981; Boberg, Ewert, Mason, Lindsay, & Wynn, 1978; Brady & Hall, 1976; Van Riper, 1982). These data suggest that incidence may be higher and recovery lower among people with cerebral dysfunction. There have also been a number of reports in the past decade describing fluency impairments that result from cerebral lesions (Farmer, 1975; Helm, Butler, & Benson, 1978; Quinn & Andrews, 1977; Rosenbek, Messert, Collins, & Wertz, 1978). Apparently these stutter-like speech impairments may or may not be accompanied by apraxia, dysarthria, or aphasia, and are often transient, but may persist if cerebral lesions are bilateral (Helm, Butler, & Benson, 1978). Similar types of speech disruptions have also been reported as an early sign of a patient's progressive neurological deterioration following long-term, chronic dialysis (Rosenbek, McNeil, Lemme, Prescott, & Alfrey, 1975). While such patients' speech disruptions obviously resemble stuttering in many ways, systematic studies of their patterns of occurrence or of patients' response to masking, rhythm, or response-contingent stimulation have not been reported. It is still not clear, therefore, to what extent these acquired fluency impairments are identical to stuttering or reflect a distinctive type of motor speech disorder.

Interest in the familial incidence of stuttering has been renewed in recent years, and several current reviews of these findings are available (Bloodstein, 1981; Shechan & Costlcy, 1977). The recent work of Kidd (1977), Kidd, Kidd, and Records (1978), Kidd, Oehlert, Heimbuch, Records, & Webster (1980), Gladstein, Seider, and Kidd (1981), and Howie (1981) have extended the findings of earlier studies and strongly implicate the role of genetic factors in stuttering. The evidence can be summarized as follows: The risk of stuttering is at least three times higher among first-degree relatives of active or recovered stutterers than in the general population. Incidence is higher among the offspring of stutterers than among their siblings, while first-degree male relatives of female stutterers are four times more likely to stutter than first-degree female relatives of male stutterers. Concordance of stuttering among monozygotic twin pairs is substantially higher than among dizygotic pairs controlled for age, sex, and independence of classification. Nevertheless, about 25% of monozygotic twin pairs are discordant for stuttering, and both stuttering severity and recovery from stuttering appear to be independent of familial incidence. Consequently, while the evidence for stuttering's genetic transmission is growing steadily, it is also clear that environmental factors play a role in some, if not all, onsets of stuttering. It is important to remember that the contributions of genetic factors to behavioral differences or dysfunctions are likely to be indirect. The structural or organic characteristics transmitted genetically to individuals probably impose only certain limits on behavior. If so, genetically inherited traits or abilities may best be viewed as predisposing conditions in which a given behavior may be manifested. It is also likely that genetically based predispositions limit behavior differently as a function of different environmental factors. Our present state of knowledge, therefore, does not permit us to identify the critical predispositions that may be transmitted genetically or to describe how such predisposing limitations interact with the environment to bring about stuttering. Recent research may help us to ask more important, more critical questions, but much remains to be answered.

Etiological Considerations

Again, there are compelling, albeit indirect, data supporting the hypothesis that a predisposition to stutter is transmitted genetically. An individual's level of susceptibility could result from a single gene or from a number of genes acting in combination (Kidd, 1977). It is tempting to speculate that a polygenic model of inheritance may account for the high variability usually found among groups of stutterers. Regardless, it is apparent that a number of environmental factors may influence whether an individual's predisposition to stutter will, in fact, be manifested in the development of a stuttering problem. This perspective hypothesizes that predispositions to stutter are continuously distributed across all speakers with a developmental threshold dividing the distribution into two discontinuous groups, stutterers and nonstutterers. Current data suggest that one's liability for exceeding this threshold is highest after connected speech begins during the preschool years and decreases with age thereafter. As noted previously, however, many critical questions remain to be answered. For example, what cognitive, motor, or affective functions or abilities are involved in one's predisposition to stutter, what environmental factors increase or decrease one's susceptibility to stutter, and how do predispositional and environmental factors interact to precipitate the onset of stuttering? It should also be acknowledged that factors that precipitate stuttering onset may differ from those that affect stuttering severity or recovery. It has been argued that those characteristics associated with the persistence of chronic stuttering, as well as many of the differences found between adult stutterers and nonstutterers, probably reflect attributes that have functioned as barriers to recovery (Curlee, 1980a). Thus, much of the information available about stutterers may not be representative of most children who stutter. At the present time, all etiological explanations are unsatisfactory, a circumstance which will likely continue until a better understanding of the genetic-neurophysiological bases of fluency and disfluency are available and described in specific operational terms.

Clinical Management of Stuttering Children

It should be apparent from the information reviewed pertaining to the overlap in speech and language characteristics across stutterers and nonstutterers that reliable identification of those children who are just beginning to stutter can be difficult, particularly if the frequency or severity of their speech disruptions is relatively low. For the most part, evaluation strategies and procedures employed with children who are suspected of being incipient stutterers have evolved through the experiences of clinicians rather than through controlled empirical studies. The types of observations made and the characteristics assessed may often reflect practitioners' beliefs regarding the etiology of stuttering. Several recent publications have recommended guidelines for distinguishing beginning stutterers from normally nonfluent children (Adams, 1977; Curlee, 1980a; Gregory & Hill, 1980; Johnson, 1980). For the most part, the guidelines presented by these authors were strikingly similar with part-word repetitions, prolongations, difficulties initiating utterances, and signs of struggle proposed as distinguishing signs of incipient stuttering. While the rationales of these authors have some empirical support, the reliability and validity of the clinical evaluation procedures now used to differentiate normally speaking children from beginning stutterers are essentially unknown.

Prognosis

Information on prognosis comes from two types of studies: investigations of treatment outcomes and of the spontaneous remission of stuttering. Neither type of study will support many conclusions that cannot be challenged. A number of different treatment procedures seem beneficial, at least for adult stutterers (Andrews, Guitar, & Howie, 1980). Few chronic adult stutterers appear to experience complete recoveries, however. Because most remission studies have involved interviews or questionnaire surveys, there is always some uncertainty that those who claim recovery ever really stuttered or that all recoveries from early episodes of stuttering were identified. Second, it is doubtful that the samples studied are representative of the general population of all stutterers. Futhermore, the bases for claiming recovery are not clear, since a substantial proportion of those who claim to have recovered also report occasional recurrences of stuttering. The role of treatment in most studies is also unclear. Ingham (1983) has argued convincingly, for example, that common-sense speech modification practices (e.g., slowing down) used by parents or older stutterers probably account for many of the "spontaneous remissions" reported in the literature. Finally, there is no accepted standard of how long one must be free of stuttering to claim recovery. Despite such limitations, a number of inferences are viable until further research indicates otherwise.

People report recoveries from stuttering at all ages, whether associated with formal treatment or not, but more remissions occur before or during puberty (Andrews & Harris, 1964; Dickson, 1971; Glasner & Rosenthal, 1957; Shearer & Williams, 1965; Sheehan & Martyn, 1970). It is not clear to what extent the duration of subjects' stuttering problems may contribute to these findings, but the chance of either beginning to stutter or of recovering from stuttering are substantially reduced among older adolescents and adults. It has been suggested that these findings may reflect neurophysiological changes that accompany maturation of stutterers' nervous systems during the course of years of severe chronic stuttering which, after a certain age, becomes more resistant to change and to remission of stuttering (Curlee, 1980a). There may also be fewer complete recoveries that occur at older ages. Shearer and Williams (1965) noted less frequent reports of residual stuttering episodes among those subjects whose remissions had occurred by 13 years of age. This finding needs to be replicated with larger, more representative samples, and large scale studies of both active and recovered stutterers are needed to explore stuttering's persistence and its remission past young adulthood. Such studies are essential if we are to determine the conditions under which stutterers recover or if we are to gain a better understanding of the circumstances in which systematic formal treatment procedures are necessary to effect recovery, in contrast to those remissions associated with common-sense practices adopted by parents and older stutterers.

A substantial proportion of people who begin to stutter recover, perhaps as high as 80% (Andrews & Harris, 1964; Cooper, 1972; Dickson, 1971; Glasner & Rosenthal, 1957; Sheehan & Martyn, 1970). Recovery rates of 80% or higher would account for the differences in current estimates of stuttering prevalence and incidence. Wingate's (1976) compilation of remission studies clearly shows that older, recovered stutterers report substantially fewer remissions during their childhood years than might be anticipated from studies of younger recovered stutterers. Such discrepancies could reflect poor ascertainment of recovered stutterers among older age groups or frequent recurrences of stuttering after early reports of remission. The questionable reliability and validity of subjects' reports cannot be discounted, either. For example, approximately two-thirds of the parents of the high school students who had identified themselves as recovered stutterers in Lankford and Cooper's (1974) study denied that their children had ever stuttered. The only longitudinal study in which both stuttering onsets and remissions were determined by direct observation rather than report found a recovery rate of 79% by age 16 (Andrews & Harris, 1964). It seems safe to conclude, therefore, that chances for complete recovery, whether associated with treatment or not, are relatively high, especially among children.

It is believed that most stuttering remissions, whether associated with formal treatment or not, occur gradually (Johnson & Associates, 1959; Shearer & Williams, 1965; Wingate, 1964). These beliefs are based largely on the recollections of self-identified, recovered stutterers. Consequently, the information now available to us is of uncertain reliability and validity.

If stuttering becomes more intermittent and less severe over an extended period of time during recovery, which seems to be the case, it may not be possible to identify subjects' specific ages at remission, and it may be more appropriate to conceive of recovery as representing a continuum of behaviors. If so, there are at least three groups who warrant careful study—completely recovered stutterers, partially recovered stutterers, and active stutterers. Systematic longitudinal investigations of such groups may provide valuable insights for our understanding of both the recovery process and of relapse, two crucial areas of information that are of great practical importance.

Findings from several studies indicate that recovery may be inversely related to severity of stuttering. Sheehan and Martyn (1970) estimated the recovery rates of college students who had rated their stuttering as mild, moderate, or severe at 87%, 75%, and 50%, respectively. In addition, they found that stutterers who reported blockings as their initial symptoms had recovered less frequently than those whose initial problems involved only repetitions. This finding was replicated among elementary and junior high school students by Dickson (1971). Similarly, Glasner and Rosenthal (1975) found that remission was related to the number of disfluency types reported by parents of entering first graders. More than half of the children whose stuttering was limited to one type of disfluency (repetition, prolongation, or hesitation) had stopped stuttering at the time of the study; but only a third of those with two or three disfluency types had stopped. More recently, Panelli, McFarlane, and Shipley (1978) examined 15 preschoolers at onset of stuttering and again several years later. During this time, 12 stopped stuttering. The children who recovered had evidenced substantially fewer speech disruptions and accessory features during their initial evaluation than the 3 whose stuttering had persisted. The notion that less severe stutterers are more likely to recover is intuitively appealing; such is the case for other types of problems and disorders. Still, we could place more confidence in these findings if they were not based largely on self-ratings, parent reports, or recollections of long-passed events. Such measures are of questionable reliability.

Remission of stuttering has not been found to be related to age of onset (Andrews & Harris, 1964; Sheehan & Martyn, 1970), familial incidence (Sheehan & Martyn, 1970), or therapy (Andrews & Harris, 1964; Glasner & Rosenthal, 1957; Shearer & Williams, 1965; Sheehan & Martyn, 1970; Wingate, 1964). It should be noted that the lack of statistical relationship between treatment and recovery may be biased by differences in which severe and mild stutterers are seen for therapy. It is also plausible that these findings could reflect the use of less effective treatment methods than those currently employed. The finding that neither stuttering severity nor recovery are related to familial incidence of stuttering suggests that both severity and remission of stuttering may be determined substantially by environmental factors. Thus, most stutterers recover regardless of severity, family background, or treatment history. These findings, if reliable, have important implications for genetic counseling, counseling of parents of beginning stutterers, and clinical management strategies.

While the odds for recovery clearly favor most young stutterers, it is not possible to determine the prognosis of an individual child with confidence. One of the few prospective empirical studies of prognostic factors was reported by Stromsta in 1965. As part of an initial evaluation, sound spectograms were made of the disfluencies of 63 children who were suspected of stuttering. A follow-up questionnaire 10 years later found that most of the children who continued to stutter had evidenced abnormal formant transitions and abrupt terminations of phonation on the spectographic recordings of their disfluencies made during their initial evaluations. Conversely, most of those who recovered had not. Operational criteria for analyzing these spectograms were not described, and it is not known how many of the children received therapy. Consequently, additional study is needed to determine if these findings are replicable and clinically useful for prognostic purposes.

Treatment of Children Who Stutter

There have been few well-controlled studies of therapy for children who stutter. As a consequence, adequate empirical support for treatment approaches used with young stutterers is lacking. The present discussion will provide only a general overview of current habilitative practices, since following chapters will cover these issues in detail. As might be expected, a variety of techniques have been advocated for stuttering children and their parents. Many seem to reflect authors' etiological biases; most have evolved during trial-and-error experiences of clinical practice; and a few have been developed through preliminary clinical research.

Indirect treatment approaches have been used most often with young stutterers, particularly those who are just beginning to stutter and who are not evidencing accessory or associated features of stuttering (Curlee, 1980b). Intervention under these circumstances can be viewed as an attempt to prevent the development of a chronic stuttering problem. These approaches presume that modifying a child's environment can affect speech and usually involve parent counseling that is intended to reduce environmental pressures or communicative stress experienced by a young stutterer. Some authors (Bar, 1973; Curlee, 1980a; Johnson, 1980) have also advocated that parents deliberately reinforce fluent speech or model slower speech rates (Johnson, 1980). Others have modified more general parent-child interaction patterns (Shames and Egolf, 1976). Thus, some indirect approaches directly manipulate circumstances seemingly associated with more fluent speech. Although indirect approaches seem to be widely accepted and used with young stutterers, their effectiveness is essentially unknown. There have been few single-subject studies completed, and matched treatment groups of untreated young stutterers have not been used to control for spontaneous recoveries which may occur in group studies.

Once a child has begun to evidence accessory and associated features of stuttering with some consistency and is viewed as a confirmed stutterer, direct treatment approaches are used more frequently (Curlee, 1980b). This strategy appears to reflect the belief that a substantial proportion of these children will become chronic stutterers if left untreated and that direct intervention will not be harmful. A number of techniques have been utilized, and most studies report decreases in stuttering. Certainly, most provide sufficient evidence to justify further, more systematic investigation, and there is no evidence that such approaches may be detrimental to young stutterers. Direct approaches have involved contingency management procedures for both instances of stuttering (Costello, 1980; Martin, Kuhl, & Haroldson, 1972; Reed & Godden, 1977) and fluent utterances (Costello, 1983; Leach, 1969; Manning, Trutna, & Shaw, 1976; Peters, 1977; Rickard & Mundy, 1965; Shaw & Shrum, 1972), training of fluency-maintaining speaking behaviors (Ryan, 1971; Shine, 1980; Coppolo & Yairi, Note 3), and teaching of how to stutter with less effort (Gregory & Hill, 1980; Van Riper, 1973; Williams, 1979). In addition, some clinicians also advocate use of an indirect approach with parents and teachers in order to optimize the child's environment for achieving more fluent speech, thereby supplementing direct procedures intended to improve speech (Johnson, 1961b; Van Riper, 1973; Zwitman, 1978). The effectiveness of direct approaches used alone or in combination with counseling is also largely unknown.

The available data indicate that a wide variety of techniques may produce marked decreases in stuttering; however, untreated comparison groups have not been used. Moreover, stuttering may also covary with other behavior, at least in some children. For example, Wahler, Sperling, Thomas, Teeter, and Luper (1970) reported that two children with mild behavior problems, who also stuttered, received contingency management procedures designed to reduce their respective behavior problems. In single-subject ABAB experimental designs, the frequency of each child's problem behavior *and* stuttering decreased concurrently, although there was no evidence that inadvertent contingencies had occurred on stuttering. In this study, stuttering appeared to change in association with the modification of other behaviors, even though the mechanism for such changes is not understood.

In most instances, the permanence of reported decreases or the extent to which stuttering is improved in everyday speaking situations is not known. There are several reports, however, that changes observed in therapy often appear to generalize spontaneously for many young stutterers (Ryan, 1971; Martin, Kuhl, & Haroldson, 1972; Reed & Godden, 1977; Shaw & Shrum, 1972; Shine, 1980). These observations have involved a relatively small number of children, without matched controls for spontaneous recovery. Such findings need replication and more systematic study, since generalization of treatment effects is a major problem for many adult stutterers. While the data are not conclusive, there is reason to suspect that treatment of children who stutter may result in better, longer-lasting results than we can achieve with adults. Consequently, many important advances in our ability to facilitate children's recovery from stuttering seem within reach, awaiting further study and exploration.

Reference Notes

1. Curlee, R., Perkins, W., & Michael, W. Reliability of judgments of instances of stuttering. Paper presented at the Annual Convention of the American Speech and Hearing Association, New York, 1970.
2. Colcord, R., & Gregory, H. A perceptual analysis of fluency in stuttering and nonstuttering children. Paper presented at the Annual Convention of the American Speech-Language-Hearing Association, Los Angeles, 1981.
3. MacIndoe, C.A., & Runyon, C.M. A perceptual comparison of stuttering and nonstuttering children's nonstuttered speech. Paper presented at the Annual Convention of the American Speech-Language-Hearing Association, Los Angeles, 1981.
4. Coppola, V., & Yairi, E. Rhythmic speech training with preschool stuttering children. Paper presented at the Annual Convention of the American Speech and Hearing Association, Atlanta, 1979.
5. Starkweather, C.W., Franklin, S., & Smigo, T. Voice-finger reaction-time difference: Correlation with severity. A paper presented at the Annual Convention of the American Speech-Language-Hearing Association, Los Angeles, 1981.

References

Adams, M. A clinical strategy for differentiating the normally nonfluent child and the incipient stutterer. *Journal of Fluency Disorders,* 1977, *2,* 141-148.

Adams, M. The young stutterer: Diagnosis, treatment and assessment of progress. *Seminars in Speech, Language, and Hearing,* 1980, *1,* 289-299.

Adams, M.R., & Hayden, P. The ability of stutterers and nonstutterers to initiate and terminate phonation during production of an isolated vowel. *Journal of Speech and Hearing Research,* 1976, *19,* 290-296.

Adams, M.R., & Hutchinson, J. The effects of three levels of auditory masking on selected vocal characteristics and the frequency of disfluency of adult stutterers. *Journal of Speech and Hearing Research,* 1974, *17,* 682-688.

Adams, M.R., & Ramig, P. Vocal characteristics of normal speakers and stutterers during choral reading. *Journal of Speech and Hearing Research,* 1980, *23,* 457-469.

Andrews, G., Craig, A., Feyer, A. M., Hoddinott, S., Howie, P., & Neilson, M. Stuttering: A review of research findings and theories circa 1982. *Journal of Speech and Hearing Disorders,* 1983, *48,* 226-246.

Andrews, G., Guitar, B., & Howie, P. Meta-analysis of the effects of stuttering treatment. *Journal of Speech and Hearing Disorders,* 1980, *45,* 287-307.

Andrews, G., & Harris, M. *The syndrome of stuttering.* Clinics in Developmental Medicine, No. 17. London: Spastics Society of Medical Education and Information Unit in association with Wm. Heinemann Medical Books, 1964.

Bar, A. Increasing fluency in young stutterers vs. decreasing stuttering: A clinical approach. *Journal of Communication Disorders,* 1973, *6,* 247-258.

Berry, M.F. The developmental history of stuttering children. *Journal of Pediatrics,* 1938, *12,* 209-217.

Bjerkan, B. Word fragmentations and repetitions in the spontaneous speech of 2-6-year-old children. *Journal of Fluency Disorders,* 1980, *5,* 137-148.

Blankenship. J. "Stuttering" in normal speech. *Journal of Speech and Hearing Research,* 1964, *7,* 95-96.

Bloch, E.L., & Goodstein, L.D. Functional speech disorders and personality: A decade of research. *Journal of Speech and Hearing Disorders,* 1971, *36,* 295-314.

Blood, G.W. & Seider, R. The concomitant problems of young stutterers. *Journal of Speech and Hearing Disorders,* 1981, *46,* 31-33.

Bloodstein, O. A rating scale study of conditions under which stuttering is reduced or absent. *Journal of Speech and Hearing Disorders,* 1950, *15,* 29-36.

Bloodstein, O. The development of stuttering: I. Changes in nine basic features. *Journal of Speech and Hearing Disorders,* 1960, *25,* 219-237.

Bloodstein, O. The rules of early stuttering. *Journal of Speech and Hearing Disorders,* 1974, *39,* 379-394.

Bloodstein, O. *A handbook on stuttering* (3rd ed.) Chicago, Ill.: National Easter Seal Society, 1981.

Bloodstein, O., Alper, J., & Zisk, P.K. Stuttering as an outgrowth of normal disfluency. In D.A. Barbara (Ed.), *New directions in stuttering.* Springfield, Ill.: Charles C. Thomas, 1965.

Bloodstein, O., & Gantwerk, B.F. Grammatical function in relation to stuttering in young children. *Journal of Speech and Hearing Research,* 1967, *10,* 786-789.

Bloodstein, O., & Grossman, M. Early stutterings: Some aspects of their form and distribution. *Journal of Speech and Hearing Research,* 1981, *24,* 298-302.

Boberg, E., Ewart, B., Mason, G., Lindsay, K., & Wynn, S. Stuttering in the retarded: II. Prevalence of stuttering in EMR and TMR children. *Mental Retardation Bulletin,* 1978, *6,* 67-76.

Boehmler, R.M. Listener responses to non-fluencies. *Journal of Speech and Hearing Research,* 1958, *1,* 132-141.

Bohme, G. Stammering and cerebral lesions in early childhood. Examinations of 802 children and adults with cerebral lesions. *Folia Phoniatrica,* 1968, *20,* 239-249.

Brady, J.P. Studies on the metronome effect on stuttering. *Behavior Research and Therapy,* 1969, *7,* 197-204.

Brady, W.A., & Hall, D.E. The prevalence of stuttering among school-age children. *Language, Speech, and Hearing Services in Schools,* 1976, *7,* 75-81.

Chaney, C.F. Loci of disfluencies in the speech of nonstutterers. *Journal of Speech and Hearing Research,* 1969, *12,* 667-668.

Cherry, C. & Sayers, B. Experiments upon the total inhibition of stammering by external control, and some clinical results. *Journal of Psychosomatic Research,* 1956, *1,* 233-246.

Colcord, R.D., & Adams, M.R. Voicing duration and vocal SPL changes associated with stuttering reduction during singing. *Journal of Speech and Hearing Research*, 1979, *22*, 468-479.

Conture, E.G., McCall, G.N., & Brewer, D.W. Laryngeal behavior during stuttering. *Journal of Speech and Hearing Research*, 1977, *20*, 661-668.

Cooper, E.B. Recovery from stuttering in a junior and senior high school population. *Journal of Speech and Hearing Research*, 1972, *15*, 632-638.

Costello. J. Operant conditioning and the treatment of stuttering. *Seminars in Speech, Language, and Hearing*, 1980, *1*, 311-325.

Costello, J.M. Current behavioral treatments for children. In D. Prins & R.J. Ingham (Eds.), *Treatment of stuttering in early childhood: Methods and issues.* San Diego: College-Hill, 1983.

Cross, D.E., & Luper, H.L. Voice reaction time of stuttering and nonstuttering children and adults. *Journal of Fluency Disorders*, 1979, *4*, 59-77.

Cullinan, W.L., & Springer, M.T. Voice initiation and termination times in stuttering and nonstuttering children. *Journal of Speech and Hearing Research*, 1980, *23*, 344-360.

Curlee, R. A case selection strategy for young disfluent children. *Seminars in Speech, Language, and Hearing*, 1980, *1*, 277-287.(a)

Curlee, R. Assessment and treatment strategies for young stutterers. *Communicative Disorders*, 1980, *5*, 11. (b)

Curlee, R. Observer agreement on disfluency and stuttering. *Journal of Speech and Hearing Research*, 1981, *24*, 595-600.

Curlee, R., & Perkins, W.H. Conversational rate control therapy for stuttering. *Journal of Speech and Hearing Disorders*, 1969, *34*, 245-250.

Curry, F.K.W., & Gregory, H.H. The performance of stutterers on dichotic listening tasks thought to reflect cerebral dominance. *Journal of Speech and Hearing Research*, 1969, *12*, 73-82.

Darley, F.L. The relationship of parental attitudes and adjustments to the development of stuttering. In W. Johnson & R.R. Leutenegger (Eds.), *Stuttering in children and adults.* Minneapolis: University of Minnesota Press, 1955.

Davis, D.M. The relation of repetitions in the speech of young children to certain measures of language maturity and situational factors: Part I. *Journal of Speech Disorders*, 1939, *4*, 303-318.

Davis, D.M. The relation of repetitions in the speech of young children to certain measures of language maturity and situational factors: Part II and III. *Journal of Speech Disorders*, 1940, *5*, 235-246.

Dickson, S. Incipient stuttering and spontaneous remission of stuttered speech. *Journal of Communication Disorders*, 1971, *4*, 99-110.

Farmer, A. Stuttering repetitions in aphasic and nonaphasic brain damaged adults. *Cortex*, 1975, *11*, 391-396.

Floyd, S., & Perkins, W.H. Early syllable dysfluency in stutterers and nonstutterers: A preliminary report. *Journal of Communication Disorders*, 1974, *7*, 279-282.

Fransella, F., & Beech, H.R. An experimental analysis of the effect of rhythm on the speech of stutterers. *Behavior Research and Therapy*, 1965, *3*, 195-201.

Freeman, F.J., & Ushijima, T. Laryngeal muscle activity during stuttering. *Journal of Speech and Hearing Research*, 1978, *21*, 538-562.

Giolas, T.G., & Williams, D.E. Children's reactions to nonfluencies in adult speech. *Journal of Speech and Hearing Research*, 1958, *1*, 86-93.

Gladstein, K., Seider, R., & Kidd, K. Analysis of the sibship patterns of stutterers. *Journal of Speech and Hearing Research*, 1981, *24*, 460-462.

Glasner, P.J., & Rosenthal, D. Parental diagnosis of stuttering in young children. *Journal of Speech and Hearing Disorders*, 1957, *22*, 288-295.

Goodstein, L.D. Functional speech disorders and personality: A survey of the research. *Journal of Speech and Hearing Research,* 1958, *1,* 359-376.

Gray, B.B., & Brutten, E.J. The relationship between anxiety, fatigue and spontaneous recovery in stuttering. *Behavior Research and Therapy,* 1965, *2,* 251-259.

Gregory, H., & Hill, D. Stuttering therapy for children. *Seminars in Speech, Language and Hearing,* 1980, *1,* 351-363.

Hall, J.W., & Jerger, J. Central auditory function in stutterers. *Journal of Speech and Hearing Research,* 1978, *21,* 324-337.

Healey, E.C., Mallard, A.R., & Adams, M. Factors contributing to the reduction of stuttering during singing. *Journal of Speech and Hearing Research,* 1976, *19,* 475-480.

Helm, N.A., Butler, R.B., & Benson, D.F. Acquired stuttering. *Neurology,* 1978, *28,* 1159-1165.

Helmreich, H.G., & Bloodstein, O. The grammatical factor in childhood disfluency in relation to the continuity hypothesis. *Journal of Speech and Hearing Research,* 1973, *16,* 731-738.

Hood, S.B. Effect of communicative stress on the frequency and form-types of disfluent behavior in adult stutterers. *Journal of Fluency Disorders,* 1975, *1,* 36-47.

Howie, P.M. Concordance for stuttering in monozygotic and dizygotic twin pairs. *Journal of Speech and Hearing Research,* 1981, *24,* 317-321.

Huffman, E.S., & Perkins, W.H. Dysfluency characteristics identified by listeners as "stuttering" and "stutterer." *Journal of Communication Disorders,* 1974, *7,* 89-96.

Hull, F.M., Mielke, P.N. Williford, J.A., & Timmons, R.J. National Speech and Hearing Survey, Final report. Project No. 50978, Office of Education, Bureau of Education for the Handicapped, U.S. Department of Health, Education and Welfare, 1976.

Ingham, R.J. "Onset, prevalence, and recovery from stuttering": A reassessment of findings from the Andrews and Harris study. *Journal of Speech and Hearing Disorders,* 1976, *41,* 280-281.

Ingham, R. Spontaneous remission of stuttering: When will the emperor realize he has no clothes on? In D. Prins & R. Ingham (Eds.), *Treatment of stuttering in early childhood: Methods and issues.* San Diego: College-Hill, 1983.

Ingham, R.J., & Andrews, G. Behavior therapy and stuttering: A review. *Journal of Speech and Hearing Disorders,* 1973, *38,* 405-441.

Ingham, R.J., & Packman, A.C. Perceptual assessment of normalcy of speech following stuttering therapy. *Journal of Speech and Hearing Research,* 1978, *21,* 63-73.

Ingham R.J., & Packman, A. A further evaluation of the speech of stutterers during chorus- and nonchorus-reading conditions. *Journal of Speech and Hearing Research,* 1979, *22,* 784-793.

Johnson, L. Facilitating parental involvement in therapy of the disfluent child. *Seminars in Speech, Language, and Hearing,* 1980, *1,* 301-309.

Johnson, W. Measurements of oral reading and speaking rate and disfluency of adult male and female stutterers and nonstutterers. *Journal of Speech and Hearing Disorders, Monograph Supplement No. 7,* 1961, 1-20. (a)

Johnson, W. *Stuttering and what you can do about it.* Minneapolis: University of Minnesota Press, 1961. (b)

Johnson, W., & Associates. *The onset of stuttering.* Minneapolis: Univeristy of Minnesota Press, 1959.

Johnson, W., & Rosen, L. Studies in the psychology of stuttering: VII. Effect of certain changes in speech pattern upon frequency of stuttering. *Journal of Speech Disorders,* 1937, *2,* 105-109.

Johnson, W., and Sinn, A. Studies in the psychology of stuttering: V. Frequency of stuttering with expectation of stuttering controlled. *Journal of Speech Disorders,* 1937, *2,* 98-100.

Kidd, K.K. A genetic perspective on stuttering. *Journal of Fluency Disorders,* 1977, *2,* 259-269.

Kidd, K.K., Kidd, J.R., & Records, M.A. The possible causes of the sex ratio in stuttering and its implications. *Journal of Fluency Disorders,* 1978, *3,* 13-23.

Kidd, K.K., Oehlert, G., Heimbuch, R.C., Records, M.A., & Webster, R.L. Familial stuttering patterns are not related to one measure of severity. *Journal of Speech and Hearing Research*, 1980, *23*, 539-545.

LaBenz, P., & LaBenz, E.S. *Early correlates of speech, language, and hearing.* Littleton, Mass.: PSG Publishing, 1980.

Lankford, S.D., & Cooper, E.B. Recovery from stuttering as viewed by parents of self-diagnosed recovered stutterers. *Journal of Communication Disorders*, 1974, *7*, 171-180.

Leach, E. Stuttering: Clinical application of response-contingent procedures. In B.B. Gray & G. England (Eds.), *Stuttering and the conditioning therapies.* Monterey, California: Monterey Institute of Speech and Hearing, 1969.

MacDonald, J.D., & Martin, R.R. Stuttering and disfluency as two reliable and unambiguous response classes. *Journal of Speech and Hearing Research*, 1973, *16*, 691-699.

Mann, M.B. Nonfluencies in the oral reading of stutterers and nonstutterers of elementary school age. In W. Johnson & R.R. Leutenegger (Eds.), *Stuttering in children and adults.* Minneapolis: University of Minnesota Press, 1955.

Manning, W.H., Trutna, P.A. & Shaw, C.K. Verbal versus tangible reward for children who stutter. *Journal of Speech and Hearing Disorders*, 1976, *41*, 52-62.

Martin, R., & Haroldson, S.K. Effects of five experimental treatments on stuttering. *Journal of Speech and Hearing Research*, 1979, *22*, 132-146.

Martin, R., & Haroldson, S.K. Stuttering identification: Standard definitions and moment of stuttering. *Journal of Speech and Hearing Research*, 1981, *24*, 59-63.

Martin, R.R., Kuhl, P., & Haroldson, S. An experimental treatment with two preschool stuttering children. *Journal of Speech and Hearing Research*, 1972, *15*, 743-752.

McDearmon, J.R. Primary stuttering at the onset of stuttering: A re-examination of data. *Journal of Speech and Hearing Research*, 1968, *11*, 631-637.

Metraux, R.W. Speech profiles of the pre-school child 18 to 54 months. *Journal of Speech and Hearing Disorders*, 1950, *15*, 37-53.

Milisen, R. Frequency of stuttering with anticipation of stuttering controlled. *Journal of Speech Disorders*, 1938, *3*, 207-214.

Molt, L.F., & Guilford, A.M. Auditory processing and anxiety in stutterers. *Journal of Fluency Disorders*, 1979, *4*, 255-267.

Moore, W.H., Jr., & Haynes, W.O. Alpha hemispheric asymmetry and stuttering: Some support for a segmentation dysfunction hypothesis. *Journal of Speech and Hearing Research*, 1980, *23*, 229-247.

Moore, W.H., Jr., & Lang, M.K. Alpha asymmetry over the right and left hemispheres of stutterers and control subjects preceding massed oral readings: A preliminary investigation. *Perceptual Motor Skills*, 1977, *44*, 223-230.

Morley, M.E. *The development and disorders of speech in childhood,* Edinburgh: Livingstone, 1957.

Neelley, J.N., & Timmons, R.J. Adaptation and consistency in the disfluent speech behavior of young stutterers and nonstutterers. *Journal of Speech and Hearing Research*, 1967, *10*, 250-256.

Okasha, A., Bishry, Z., Kamel, M., & Hassan, A.H. Psychosocial study of stammering in Egyptian children. *British Journal of Psychiatry*, 1974, *124*, 531-533.

Panelli, C.A., McFarlane, S.C., and Shipley, K.G. Implications of evaluating and intervening with incipient stutterers. *Journal of Fluency Disorders*, 1978, *3*, 41-50.

Perkins, W.H., Bell, J., Johnson, L., & Stocks, J. Phone rate and the effective planning time hypothesis of stuttering.. *Journal of Speech and Hearing Research*, 1979, *22*, 747-755.

Perkins, W.H., & Curlee, R.F. Clinical impressions of portable masking unit effects in stuttering. *Journal of Speech and Hearing Disorders*, 1969, *34*, 360-362.

Perkins, W.H., Rudas, J., Johnson, L., & Bell, J. Stuttering: discoordination of phonation with articulation and respiration. *Journal of Speech and Hearing Research,* 1976, *19,* 509-522.

Peters, A.D. The effect of positive reinforcement on fluency: two case studies. *Language, Speech, and Hearing Services in Schools,* 1977, *8,* 15-22.

Prins, D. Personality, stuttering severity and age. *Journal of Speech and Hearing Research,* 1972, *15,* 148-154.

Quinn, P.T., & Andrews, G. Neurological stuttering—a clinical entity? *Journal of Neurology, Neurosurgery and Psychiatry,* 1977, *40,* 699-701.

Reed, C.G., & Godden, A.L. An experimental treatment using verbal punishment with two preschool stutterers. *Journal of Fluency Disorders,* 1977, *2,* 225-233.

Reich, A., Till, J., & Goldsmith, H. Laryngeal and manual reaction times of stuttering and nonstuttering adults. *Journal of Speech and Hearing Research,* 1981, *24,* 192-196.

Rickard, H.C., & Mundy, M.B. Direct manipulation of stuttering behavior: An experimental-clinical approach. In L.P. Ullmann & L. Krasner (Eds.), *Case studies in behavior modification.* New York: Holt, Rinehart, & Winston, 1965.

Rosenbek, J.C., McNeil, M.R., Lemme, M.L., Prescott, T.E., & Alfrey, A.C. Speech and language findings in a chronic hemodialysis patient: A case report. *Journal of Speech and Hearing Disorders,* 1975, *40,* 245-252.

Rosenbek, J., Messert, B., Collins, M., & Wertz, R.T. Stuttering following brain damage. *Brain and Language,* 1978, *6,* 82-96.

Runyan, C.M., & Adams, M.R. Perceptual study of the speech of "successfully therapeutized" stutterers. *Journal of Fluency Disorders,* 1978, *3,* 25-39.

Runyan, C.M., & Adams, M.R. Unsophisticated judges' perceptual evaluations of the speech of "successfully treated" stutterers. *Journal of Fluency Disorders,* 1979, *4,* 29-38.

Ryan, B.P. Operant procedures applied to stuttering therapy for children. *Journal of Speech and Hearing Disorders,* 1971, *36,* 264-280.

Sayles, D.G. Cortical excitability, perseveration, and stuttering. *Journal of Speech and Hearing Research,* 1971, *14,* 462-475.

Schiavetti, N. Judgments of stuttering severity as a function of type and locus of disfluency. *Folia Phoniatrica,* 1975, *27,* 26-37.

Schindler, M.D. A study of educational adjustments of stuttering and nonstuttering children. In W. Johnson, & R.R. Leutenegger (Eds.), *Stuttering in children and adults.* Minneapolis: University of Minnesota Press, 1955.

Shames, G., & Egolf, D. *Operant conditioning and the management of stuttering.* Englewood Cliffs, N.J.: Prentice-Hall, 1976.

Shaw, C.K., & Shrum, W.F. The effects of response-contingent reward on the connected speech of children who stutter. *Journal of Speech and Hearing Disorders,* 1972, *37,* 75-88.

Shearer, W.M., & Williams, J.D. Self-recovery from stuttering. *Journal of Speech and Hearing Disorders,* 1965, *30,* 288-290.

Sheehan, J.G. Projective studies of stuttering. *Journal of Speech and Hearing Disorders,* 1958, *23,* 18-25.

Sheehan, J.G., & Costley, M.S. A reexamination of the role of heredity in stuttering. *Journal of Speech and Hearing Disorders,* 1977, *42,* 47-59.

Sheehan, J.G., & Martyn, M.M. Stuttering and its disappearance. *Journal of Speech and Hearing Research,* 1970, *13,* 279-289.

Shine, R.E. Direct management of the beginning stutterer. *Seminars in Speech, Language, and Hearing,* 1980, *1,* 339-350.

Siegel, G.M. Punishment, stuttering, and disfluency. *Journal of Speech and Hearing Research,* 1970, *13,* 677-714.

Siegel, G.M., & Haugen, D. Audience size and variations in stuttering behavior. *Journal of Speech and Hearing Research,* 1964, *7,* 381-388.

Silverman, E. -M. Preschoolers' speech disfluency: Single syllable word repetition. *Perceptual Motor Skills,* 1972, *35,* 1002.

Silverman, E. -M. Word position and grammatical function in relation to preschoolers' speech disfluency. *Perceptual Motor Skills,* 1974, *39,* 267-272.

Silverman, F.H. The effect of rhythmic auditory stimulation on the disfluency of nonstutterers. *Journal of Speech and Hearing Research,* 1971, *14,* 350-355.

Silverman, F.H. Disfluency and word length. *Journal of Speech and Hearing Research,* 1972, *15,* 788-791.

Silverman, F.H. Disfluency behavior of elementary-school stutterers and nonstutterers. *Language, Speech, and Hearing Services in Schools,* 1974, *5,* 32-37.

Silverman, F.H. & Goodban, M.T. The effect of auditory masking on the fluency of normal speakers. *Journal of Speech and Hearing Research,* 1972, *15,* 543-546.

Silverman F., & Williams, D. Loci of disfluencies in the speech of stutterers. *Perceptual Motor Skills,* 1967, *24,* 1085-1086.

Soderberg, G.A. A comparison of adaptation trends in the oral reading of stutterers, inferior speakers and superior speakers. *Journal of Communication Disorders,* 1969, *2,* 99-108. (a)

Soderberg, G.A. Delayed auditory feedback and the speech of stutterers: A review of studies *Journal of Speech and Hearing Disorders,* 1969, *34,* 20-29. (b)

Sommers, R.K., Brady, W.A., & Moore, W.H., Jr. Dichotic ear preferences of stuttering children and adults. *Perceptual Motor Skills,* 1975, *41,* 931-938.

Starkweather, C.W., Hirschman, P., & Tannenbaum, R.S. Latency of vocalization onset: Stutterers versus nonstutterers. *Journal of Speech and Hearing Research,* 1976, *19,* 481 492.

Stromsta, C. A spectrographic study of dysfluencies labeled as stuttering by parents. *De Therapia Vocis et Loquelae, Vol. I,* XIII Congress, International Society of Logopedics and Phoniatrics, 1965.

Sussman, H.M. & MacNeilage, P.F. Hemispheric specialization for speech production and perception in stutterers. *Neuropsychologia,* 1975, *13,* 19-26.

Toscher, M.M., & Rupp, R.R A study of the central auditory processes in stutterers using the Synthetic Sentence Identification (SSI) test battery. *Journal of Speech and Hearing Research,* 1978, *21,* 779-792.

Turnbaugh, K.R., Guitar, B.E., & Hoffman, P.R. Speech clinicians' attribution of personality traits as a function of stuttering severity. *Journal of Speech and Hearing Research,* 1979, *22,* 37-45.

Tuthill, C. A quantitative study of extensional meaning with special reference to stuttering. *Speech Monographs,* 1946, *13,* 81-98.

Van Riper, C. *The treatment of stuttering.* Englewood Cliffs N.J.: Prentice-Hall, 1973.

Van Riper, C. *The nature of stuttering* (2nd ed.). Englewood Cliffs, N.J.: Prentice-Hall, 1982.

Voelker, C.H. A preliminary investigation for a normative study of fluency: A clinical index to the severity of stuttering. *American Journal of Orthopsychiatry,* 1944, *14,* 285-294.

Wahler, R., Sperling, K., Thomas, M., Teeter, N. & Luper, H. The modification of childhood stuttering: Some response-response relationships. *Journal of Experimental Child Psychology,* 1970, *9,* 411-428.

Wendahl, R.W., & Cole, J. Identification of stuttering during relatively fluent speech.. *Journal of Speech and Hearing Research,* 1961, *4,* 281-286.

Westby, C.E. Language performance of stuttering and nonstuttering children. *Journal of Communication Disorders,* 1979, *12,* 133-145.

Williams, D. A perspective on approaches to stuttering therapy. In H. Gregory (Ed.), *Controversies about stuttering therapy.* Baltimore: University Park Press, 1979.

Williams, D.E., & Kent, L.R. Listener evaluations of speech interruptions. *Journal of Speech and Hearing Research,* 1958, *1,* 124-131.

Williams, D.E., Melrose, B.M., & Woods, C.L. The relationship between stuttering and academic achievement in children. *Journal of Communication Disorders,* 1969, *2,* 87-98.

Williams, D.E., & Silverman, F.H. Note concerning articulation of school-age stutterers. *Perceptual Motor Skills,* 1968, *27,* 713-714.

Williams, D.E., Silverman, F.H., & Kools, J.A. Disfluency behavior of elementary-school stutterers and nonstutterers: The adaptation effect. *Journal of Speech and Hearing Research,* 1968, *11,* 622-630.

Williams, D.E., Silverman, F.H., & Kools, J.A. Disfluency behavior of elementary-school stutterers and nonstutterers: Loci of instances of disfluency. *Journal of Speech and Hearing Research,* 1969, *12,* 308-318.

Wingate, M.E. A standard definition of stuttering. *Journal of Speech and Hearing Disorders,* 1964, *29,* 484-489.

Wingate M.E. *Stuttering: Theory and treatment.* New York: Irvington, 1976.

Winitz, H. Repetitions in the vocalizations of children in the first two years of life. *Journal of Speech and Hearing Disorders, Monograph Supplement No. 7,* 1961, 55-62.

Winitz, H. & Darley, F.L. Speech production. In P.J. La Benz & E.S. La Benz (Eds.), *Early correlates of speech, language, and hearing.* Littleton, Mass.: PSG Publishing Company, 1980.

Woods, C.L., & Williams, D.E. Traits attributed to stuttering and normally fluent males. *Journal of Speech and Hearing Research,* 1976, *19,* 267-278.

Yairi, E. Disfluency rates and patterns of stutterers and nonstutterers. *Journal of Communication Disorders,* 1972, *5,* 225-231.

Yairi, E. Disfluencies of normally speaking two-year-old children. *Journal of Speech and Hearing Research,* 1981, *24,* 490-495.

Yairi, E. The onset of stuttering in two- and three-year-old children: A preliminary report. *Journal of Speech and Hearing Disorders,* 1983, *48,* 171-177.

Young, M.A. Predicting ratings of severity of stuttering. *Journal of Speech and Hearing Disorders, Monograph Supplement, No. 7,* 1961, 31-54.

Young, M.A. Identification of stutterers from recorded samples of their "fluent" speech. *Journal of Speech and Hearing Research,* 1964, *7,* 302-303.

Young, M.A. Observer agreement: Cumulative effects of repeated ratings of the same samples and of knowledge of group results. *Journal of Speech and Hearing Research,* 1969, *12,* 144-155.

Young, M.A. Observer agreement for marking moments of stuttering. *Journal of Speech and Hearing Research,* 1975, *18,* 530-540 (a)

Young, M.A. Onset, prevalence, and recovery from stuttering. *Journal of Speech and Hearing Disorders,* 1975, *40,* 49-58. (b)

Young, M.A., & Downs, T.D. Testing the significance of the agreement among observers. *Journal of Speech and Hearing Research,* 1968, *11,* 5-17.

Zimmerman, G.N., & Knott, J.R. Slow potentials of the brain related to speech processing in normal speakers and stutterers. *Electroencephalographic Clinical Neurophysiology,* 1974, *37,* 599-607.

Zwitman, D.H. *The disfluent child: A management program.* Baltimore: University Park Press, 1978.

Martin R. Adams

The Differential Assessment and Direct Treatment of Stuttering

During the past 10 to 12 years, there have been several significant developments in the assessment and treatment of children who stutter. We have seen emergence of behavioral criteria that can be used for the purpose of discriminating between the incipient or beginning stutterer and the normally disfluent child. Furthermore, findings have shown that speech and other behavioral problems associated with the stuttering of one youngster may differ appreciably from the behavioral deviations evident in another. Mindful of the existence of these disparities, some clinicians have developed differential assessment procedures to probe for them. The responses of a young stutterer tested in this way are then used as a basis for planning therapy. Since children will present diverse assessment profiles, it follows that a treatment regimen constructed for one patient might be quite unlike the remediation program established for another. Whatever form the therapy takes, the chances are good that a direct approach to clinical intervention will be employed. This direct involvement of youngsters in treatment surely represents the most profound change in our orientation to the management of stuttering in children. It hardly need be said that for years there was a strong preference for indirect methods such as parent counseling and play therapy. While these techniques are still viable treatment options, they are less popular today.

Here then, summarized, are the 3 key developments cited thus far: (1) the formulation of behavioral criteria for discriminating between the incipient stutterer and the normally disfluent child; (2) the generation of differential assessment techniques to probe for dimensions of stuttering in children; and (3) the construction and application of direct approaches to the treatment of young stutterers. In the next sections of this chapter, we shall take a rather detailed look at each.

Behavioral Criteria for Discriminating Between the Incipient Stutterer and the Normally Disfluent Child

One of the most intimidating problems that confronts the speech-language pathologist involves making clinical discriminations between the incipient stutterer and the normally disfluent child. This differentiation is made formidable by what is at stake: If a child is inappropriately identified as a beginning stutterer, then he or she would presumably be inserted into a treatment program. At the least, his time and that of the clinician would be wasted because therapy is simply not needed; and some believe that such unnecessary treatment might serve to create a problem where one does not in fact exist. Of course, clinicians would not want to mistakenly identify an incipient stutterer as being normally disfluent since such an error would lead to the withholding of remediation where it was actually needed. In the absence of this treatment, there would be a greater opportunity for various aspects of the stuttering pattern to become habituated. That would make the problem more difficult to modify in the future when a correct evaluation was finally rendered. Obviously, there are serious potential consequences associated with mistakenly viewing a normally disfluent child as an incipient stutterer, or with the faulty evaluation of an incipient stutterer as a normally disfluent youngster.

Less than 20 years ago, little had been done to delineate guidelines that might be used to make this crucial differentiation. Thus, clinicians were forced to rely mainly on their intuitions and past experiences when confronted with a child suspected of being an incipient stutterer. If, on those occasions, these workers paled before the task of differentially evaluating the youngster, we can understand why. Fortunately, this situation has now taken a decided turn for the better. Reference is made here to the fact that during the last 5 years, several attempts have been made to identify and describe behavioral criteria that might be used to accurately discriminate between the incipient stutterer and the normally disfluent child. Pertinent are the efforts of such individuals as Adams (1977; 1980), Curlee (1980), Gregory and Hill (1980), Johnson (1980) and Conture (1982). The differential evaluation profiles formed by these workers were developed from their clinical experience and research efforts, and those of still other professionals.

What is remarkable about these profiles is how similar they all are. Granted that the speech-language pathologists who developed the profiles have been influenced by one another. Yet, to a significant extent, these clinicians established their profiles independently. This is a matter of some import because it means that without biasing each other, these professionals have come to similar conclusions about what characteristics to associate with early stuttering and normal disfluency. This high degree of agreement gives some credence to the profiles themselves.

Since the profiles are so much alike, it would be wasteful to examine each of them separately. Instead, descriptions of the fluency behavior characteristics that are common to the profiles that have been developed are presented.

Common Profile Characteristics

In judging a child to be an incipient stutterer, it is now believed that the presence of the following signs or symptoms is crucial: (1) Part-word repetitions and prolongations make up in excess of 7% of all words spoken; (2) the part-word repetitions are marked by at least 3 unit repetitions (e.g., "bee-bee-bee-beet" vs. "bee-bee-beet"); (3) the part word repetitions are also perceived as containing the schwa in place of the vowel normally found in the syllable that is being repeated (e.g., "buh-buh-buh-beet" vs. "bee-bee-beet"); (4) the prolongations last longer than 1 second; and (5) difficulty in starting and/or sustaining voicing or air flow is heard in association with the part-word repetitions and prolongations. As more and more of these 5 signs are noted in a child's speech, a clinician can be increasingly confident that he or she is dealing with an incipient stutterer. Contrariwise, the fewer of these symptoms that are noted, the more likely that the youngster is normally disfluent. Whichever choice is made, it ought to be based on the foregoing and other behavioral data, be compatible with case history information that bears on the incidence of stuttering in the child's family, take into account any current trends in the frequency of occurrence of the youngster's disfluency (i.e., has it been steadily increasing or decreasing?), and address such other considerations as the presence or absence of emotional and behavioral reactions to the fluency failures by the child, as well as parental attitudes toward their offspring and his fluency irregularities. A final differential evaluation would then be based on the sum of the behavioral evidence and case history information just cited.

Acting on the Outcomes of Differential Evaluations

Based on the foregoing review, there would appear to be 3 possible outcomes of the differential evaluation process. First, a child may present an unequivocal picture of *normal disfluency.* That is, he exhibits none or just one of the signs of incipient stuttering mentioned in the previous section. Or, a youngster might evince what Adams (1980) has referred to as an *ambiguous clinical picture,* or what Gregory and Hill (1980) have described as *borderline atypical disfluency.* That is, the youngster exhibits just 2 or perhaps 3 of the 5 signs of incipient stuttering cited earlier. Finally, the child could reveal a clear pattern of *incipient stuttering.* That is, a clinical picture that includes 4 or all 5 of the symptoms of beginning stuttering could be presented. In this section we shall examine the approaches that have been recommended for dealing with members of each of these 3 groups.

The Normally Disfluent Child

Youngsters identified as being normally disfluent are certainly not candidates for therapy, even in some indirect form. Instead, it is widely agreed that parental counseling is the essential next step to take once a clinician is confident that the child in question is normally disfluent. Within counseling, parents are provided with the assessment of normal disfluency and are given general information about the development of dimensions of speech and language in children. The danger signs of incipient stuttering are identified so that the parents can monitor any hints of these behaviors that might later appear in their child's utterances. In addition, the parents are offered guidance designed to neutralize any lingering concerns they might have over their offspring's development of fully normal speech and are assured of the clinician's ongoing willingness to be of help should the child's fluency development take a negative turn. Lastly, a recheck of the child is usually scheduled for some future date.

Typically, all of the foregoing steps can be accomplished in a brief period of time after the youngster's evaluation. On occasion, however, parents may exhibit such an excess of anxiety about their child's speech development that one or more return visits to the clinic for further counseling will be required. The completion of counseling, however long it might take, marks the end of the clinician's involvement with the child and parents. Nothing else need be done unless a future reevaluation has been set up or is requested.

The Child with an Ambiguous Clinical Picture or Borderline Atypical Disfluency

If there is consensus over how to deal with the normally disfluent child, there is some disagreement over the approach to take with the youngster who presents an ambiguous clinical picture (Adams, 1980) or borderline atypical disfluency (Gregory & Hill, 1980).

As was noted earlier, Adams (1980) has suggested that when a youngster evinces an ambiguous clinical picture, it is best to be cautious and conservative. Direct therapy is bypassed in favor of indirect methods. These take the form of parental counseling if it is needed, and a program for monitoring the child's speech. Specifically, the parents observe their offspring's fluency on a day-by-day basis and then report to the clinician at a prearranged time each week. This tack is taken for up to 6 months. During that period it is expected that the child's speech pattern will change, either for better or worse. Whatever the case, the alterations that do occur should make the youngster easier to evaluate *unequivocally*. If a clear picture of incipient stuttering does materialize, then a direct treatment program is immediately set into motion. In contrast, if the child has gravitated into a clear pattern of normal disfluency, then that assessment is made and the parental monitoring regimen is gradually phased out. On rare occasions, a youngster's ambiguous clinical picture will not change within the 6 months allotted for the counseling and monitoring program. When that happens it should be assumed that the negative features of the child's ambiguous pattern are starting to become habituated and thus require direct and immediate treatment.

Gregory and Hill (1980) are far more prompt and direct in their dealings with the child who they refer to as exhibiting borderline atypical disfluency. To begin with, they will conduct a comprehensive evaluation of this youngster to see if he exhibits other behavioral irregularities and/or disorders of speech and language. Even if the results of this far-reaching assessment show the child to be free of other defects, the borderline atypical disfluency is subject to a combined direct and indirect treatment program. The specifics of this dual approach will be presented in a subsequent section. For the present it suffices to say that this regimen involves interactions between the clinician and the youngster, between the clinician and the parents, and between the parents and their offspring. Upon completion of therapy, procedures for monitoring the child's fluency are set up and reevaluations are scheduled for the future. Even more elaborate rehabilitative measures are taken with the youngster who evinces borderline atypical disfluency *and* other disturbances in speech and language behavior. Again, we shall defer comment on Gregory and Hill's specific rehabilitative tactics until later.

The Incipient Stutterer

There is now wide agreement that once a firm evaluation has been made, therapy should be routinely recommended for the incipient stutterer. Yet, before treatment can begin, the clinician must decide whether intervention should be direct or indirect, and what should be included in a child's rehabilitative program. However, before we can develop answers to these inquiries it is necessary to come to some understanding of what the terms "indirect" and "direct" therapy mean. In this chapter, and elsewhere in this book (see Guitar, Chapter 10), a relatively narrow meaning has been applied to the label "indirect therapy." That is, we shall consider as "indirect" any therapy in which a professional strives to enhance a client's fluency by means *other* than stimulating speech responses and applying consequences to them. Within the boundaries of this definition, indirect treatment does not require that the child be placed in a formal treatment setting or even be dealt with at all for that matter. For example, parent counseling is a form of indirect therapy wherein the child is excluded from the rehabilitative process. Anxiety deconditioning through systematic desensitization, play therapy, and drug tranquilization are also types of indirect treatment. In these latter 3 cases, the client is involved, being seen by a speech-language pathologist, psychologist, or physician. However, the youngster's speech responses are not actively evoked for the purpose of manipulating them through orderly application of consequences.

In sharp contrast to this definitional posture, we shall attach a very broad meaning to the term "direct therapy." That is, we will refer to as "direct" any regimen that, at the least, places a child in a treatment setting with a qualified speech-language clinician who actively evokes speech responses and then applies consequences to one or more aspects of the client's ensuing utterances, all for the purpose of augmenting fluency. Within this framework, a clinician could work directly on stuttering in an effort to reduce or eliminate it. Of course, neither stuttering nor fluency need be the focus of therapeutic stimulation. Rather, fluency might be increased (and stuttering decreased) as a by-product of the clinician's direct modification of other dimensions of communication such as speaking rate, or the length and complexity of the child's utterances.

Starting several years ago, and continuing until about 1970, it was commonplace for clinicians to employ indirect therapy in the form of parent counseling as the *sole* means of treating young stutterers. By the 1970s some speech-language pathologists (Ryan, 1971) began to deviate from this approach and make *exclusive* use of a rather circumscribed set of direct operant methods in their work with child stutterers. Questions have been raised, however, about this pattern of making exclusive use of a single indirect or direct rehabilitative approach with most, if not all, clients. It has been pointed out that to employ just one treatment tactic, and no other, requires the assumptions that the form of therapy being used is superior to other methods, and that this one treatment program is well suited to essentially all young stutterers. As an alternative to the "single method" view, several clinicians have suggested that differences between young stutterers must be identified and taken into account when planning and conducting therapy. The process by which disparities among stutterers may be uncovered is herein referred to as a "differential assessment."

Differential Assessment of the Incipient Stutterer

The idea that differential assessment was even necessary grew out of a view that is 25 years old; namely, that stuttering may be a multidimensional disorder (Van Riper, 1958). Conceiving of stuttering in this way raises the possibility that dimensions of the problem may differ from stutterer to stutterer. In turn, this would mean that persons who stutter could be segregated into subgroups on the bases of different background characteristics and/or behaviors. With the notable exception of studies by Berlin (Note 1) and Andrews and Harris (1964), this line of thinking received scant attention until the 1970s. At that point a steady increase in efforts to identify and describe dimensions of stuttering began (cf., Canter, 1971; Prins & Lohr, 1972; Van Riper, 1971). The most recent contributors to this work have been Glyndon and Jeanna Riley, and Aaron Smith and David Daly.

The Rileys hypothesized that problems in attending, perceiving, comprehending, encoding, and executing a speech response could function separately, together, or in combination with various environmental factors to promote stuttering. To look into this possibility, they started to collect data from young stutterers through formal tests, informal probes, and longitudinal observations. They also have taken extensive case histories, interviewed parents, and observed parent-child interactions. Occasionally, as this work progressed, these researchers reported on their findings (Riley & Riley, Notes 2 and 3). Then in 1979, the Rileys published a compilation of results they culled from a much larger pool of data drawn from 176 children who stuttered. Portions of the data presented in this article came from 76 young stutterers between the ages of 3 and 12 years. Using factor analysis [1], they were able to identify 4 factors that they believed represented "neurologic components" (Riley & Riley, 1979, p. 283) of stuttering. They also described 2 "intrapersonal components" and 3 "interpersonal components" (Riley & Riley, 1979, p. 282). Subsequently, each member of this total of 9 components was studied among 54 stuttering children who ranged in age from 3 to 11 years. This subset of the larger groups of 176 and 76 youngsters was singled out for study because of the availability of more complete and analyzable test results and other forms of pertinent information. Table 9-1 contains a distillation of some of the major findings provided by the Rileys in their 1979 publication. The table includes the identification and the more prominent behavioral characteristics of each of the 9 components. Also found in Table 9-1 are figures showing the percentages of the 54 children that exhibited clinically significant levels of each component.

Several additional comments need to be made regarding the distribution of components across the 54 children studied. First, all of these youngsters exhibited as least 1 of the 9 components. However, 9.2% of these stutterers were free of neurologic components. Slightly more than 90% of the children evinced at least 1 neurologic component, with over 18% of them showing 3 or all 4 of these components. Seventy-four percent of the children were considered to have neurologic components, the behavioral indices of which were judged to be significant enough to warrant therapeutic attention.

What is missing from the Rileys' 1979 report is some indication of the various ways in which the components might cluster together. This matter was dealt with in a more recent investigation. In this follow-up study (1980), they applied factor analysis to the data gathered from the larger subgroup of 76 stutterers. The results of this study provide insights into the interrelationships that appear to exist among the neurologic components. The more important of these findings indicated that: (1) Stutterers who exhibited reduced linguistic ability were also likely to possess relatively poor auditory perceptual skills and motor problems, as well; (2) children with poor scores on the motor component were good candidates to exhibit some of the characteristics of the attending component (i.e., hyperactivity, perseveration, and/or distractibility), though the motor difficulties of these same children could exist independent of linguistic and auditory perceptual deficits; and (3) youngsters exhibiting auditory processing problems could nonetheless present better-than-average overall language, oral, and fine motor abilities.

As was noted in Table 9-1, the Rileys identified what they believe are four components of a more general neurologic dimension of stuttering. Striking support for this view has evolved out of the experimental work of Smith and Daly (Note 4). During the summers of each year from 1973 to 1980, they have had the opportunity to conduct extensive tests and behavioral observations on youngsters who were attending a residential stuttering therapy program.

During their summers of data collection, Smith and Daly screened 128 stutterers. Twenty-eight of these children exhibited cluttering, cleft palate, cerebral palsy, epilepsy, mental retardation, hearing loss, aphasia, or

TABLE 9-1
Nine components of stuttering identified by Riley and Riley (1979).

Component/Key Behavioral Correlates	Percentages of 54 Children Exhibiting Each Component
Neurologic Components	
Attending problems as evidenced by distractibility, perseveration, hyperactivity, irability to concentrate on tasks, and low frustration tolerance.	36%
Auditory processing problems as evidenced by delayed responses to tasks, need to have directions repeated, clarified, or presented in some other way; self-corrections by the child after he has started to respond.	27%
Sentence formulation problems as evidenced by inability to formulate a sentence from a stimulus word; utterances made up of short, fragmented phrases; utterances marked by word reversals and transpositions; use of verbs and other grammatic elements that lack appropriate complexity; poor sentence repetition ability.	31%
Oral-motor problems as evidenced by poor performance on diadochokinetic tasks; errors during syllable repetition; anywhere from mild to severe articulatory inaccuracy.	69%
Intrapersonal Components	
High self-expectations on the part of the child as evidenced by the youngster's apparent difficulty in accepting anything other than "top" performance from himself; child spontaneously makes unfavorable comments about himself to peers.	38%
Manipulative stuttering as evidenced by the child's ability to direct parental behavior and/or gain parental attention with stuttering.	25%
Interpersonal Components	
Disruptive communicative environment as evidenced by adult-child conversations that are too rapidly paced; pressure on the child for prompt responding, thus denying him the chance to organize his thoughts; interruptions of the child as he speaks; and adults acting rushed as they wait for the child to speak.	53%
High expectations of the child by his elders as evidenced by adults' expressions of perfectionistic attitudes; adults' fostering of competitiveness; adults' unrealistically high assessment of child's true ability.	51%
Abnormal parental need for the child to stutter as evidenced by their demonstrable rejection of the child because of the stuttering; parental rejection of several other aspects of child's behavior.	5%

emotional difficulties in addition to their stuttering. These individuals were excluded from further testing on the grounds that they were not typical members of the stuttering population. The remaining 100 youngsters, ranging in age from 8 to 19 years, and with a mean age of 13 years, were exposed to a wide-ranging battery of tests that included the entire Wechsler Intelligence Scale, the Benton Visual Retention and Design Copy Test, Raven's Progressive Matrices, the Purdue Pegboard, the Smith Symbol Digits Written and Oral Substitutions, the Memory for Unrelated Sentences, and tests for articulation, language, and stuttering severity.

Based on test results, 12 youngsters were identified as possessing both stuttering and an articulation defect. Another 14 children were identified as being stutterers and learning disabled. The third and largest group contained 74 youngsters, whose stuttering was not attended by either errors of articulation or learning disabilities.

Having identified these 3 subgroups of stutterers, Smith and Daly probed within each subject's test data for indications of "neuropsychological deficits" (Smith & Daly, Note 4). Among the largest group of 74 youngsters, 32 of them (43%) presented evidence of anywhere from 3 to 9 signs indicating organic cerebral dysfunction. Twenty of the 74 stutterers evinced 2 signs. Another 12 of the 74 exhibited 1 sign. That left just 10 youngsters who were free of any signs of organic cerebral dysfunction. In the stuttering + defective articulation subgroup, 9 of the 12 children (75%) provided 3 or more signs of organic cerebral dysfunction. One individual showed 2 signs, another child revealed 1 sign, and the twelfth youngster exhibited no signs. Even more skewed was the incidence of signs in the stuttering + learning disability subgroup. Therein, 13 of the 14 youngsters (93%) evinced 3 or more signs. The remaining stutterer presented 2 signs. Thus, when the findings for the 3 subgroups are taken together, 54 of the 100 children exhibited what Smith and Daly refer to as a "strong indication" of organic cerebral dysfunction; that is, 3 or more signs. Twenty-two of the 100 youngsters evinced 2 signs; that is, what Smith and Daly label as "equivocal" signs of cerebral involvement. Twenty-four of the 100 young stutterers revealed "no compelling evidence of organicity" (Smith & Daly, Note 4); that is, 1 or no signs.

The findings of the Rileys (1979; 1980) and Smith and Daly (Note 4) could well be the strongest evidence that stutterers may have multiple disorders, and that the total clinical picture of one individual may differ from that of another. Still, we must recognize that the work of these two teams of researchers was descriptive of correlations among the variables they chose to study. These sorts of results do not allow us to draw inferences or implications regarding causality. Nonetheless, within their frame of reference the Rileys, Smith and Daly, and other workers

Table 9-2
Recommended Minimum Contents of a Differential Assessment Battery for Children Diagnosed as Incipient Stutterers.

1. Observation of the child's ability to direct, focus, and sustain attention on diagnostic materials and tasks.
2. Observation of the child's verbal and nonverbal activity levels.
3. Observation of any perseverative tendencies.
4. Formal testing of auditory retention span.
5. Formal testing of auditory discrimination ability.
6. Formal testing of auditory verbal comprehension.
7. Formal or informal testing of object naming.
8. Elicitation of story telling from the child in order to estimate (a) mean length of utterance; (b) level of grammar and syntax; (c) word retrieval ability; (d) vocabulary development and usage.
9. Formal language testing.
10. Testing of the motor speech mechanism with tasks that include (a) simple syllable repetition; (b) syllable sequence repetition; (c) alternating lateralization of the tongue; (d) articulatory accuracy during connected speech; (e) sustained phonation; and (f) measurement of voice onset time.
11. Case history taking including inquiries into parents' attitudes towards the child and his stuttering.
12. Observation of any behaviors reflecting the child's awareness of his stuttering.
13. Observation of any behaviors reflecting negative reactions by the child to the stuttering.
14. Testing of the child's ability to effectively increase his fluency.
15. Observation of verbal and nonverbal interactions between parent(s) and child.

(Adams, 1980; Gregory & Hill, 1980) have stressed that, clinically, children who exhibit incipient stuttering should be exposed to a differential assessment. Gregory and Hill have even extended this position to include youngsters who evince borderline atypical disfluency. Recommendations as to the minimum contents of a differential assessment "package" are presented in itemized form in Table 9-2. The tasks and techniques suggested for use are modeled after many of those used by the Rileys (1979, 1980) and, to a lesser extent, by Gregory and Hill (1980).

The contents of Table 9-2 do not represent an all-encompassing statement on what functions to test or what behaviors should be specially noted in the differential assessment of young stutterers. Nonetheless, what has been offered should provide clinicians with a good general idea of the depth and breadth of this sort of evaluation. If sufficient in scope, the differential assessment can produce data that will guide the clinician in forming answers to the questions, "Should therapy be indirect or direct?" and "What should be included in a child's rehabilitative program?" In the next 2 sections we shall address these inquiries and show in each how key results from the differential assessment can be used to make clinical decisions that pertain to the planning and implementation of treatment.

Indirect or Direct Therapy?

In the view of some, this author included, the choice between indirect and direct therapy can be made on the basis of 4 bits of differential assessment data. They are: (1) The clinician's judgment of the child's degree of awareness of stuttering; (2) the apparent extent of the youngster's negative reaction(s) to the problem; (3) the presence of other complicating behavioral problems; and (4) the existence of disturbances in the parent-child relationship. Two guidelines, loosely applied, fit here. First, one might give serious consideration to indirect therapy when the child exhibits little awareness of his stuttering, no negative reactions to it, and no other behavioral problems. Here, indirect rehabilitation might well be preferred because it ought to minimize the chances of focusing the patient's attention on the speech production process and drawing attention to stuttering. The second guideline provides for indirect therapy in circumstances where an hypothesized immediate cause[2] of the stuttering seems to involve an agent *external* to the youngster's speech system; for example, a breakdown in the parent-child relationship, anxiety, or psychological difficulties in some other form. In cases fitting these descriptions, indirect treatment in the forms of parent counseling, anxiety deconditioning, drug tranquilization, and/or psychotherapy would seem wise choices.

In opposition, some sort of direct therapy strategy could be recommended when a child demonstrates negative reactions to the stuttering or, at least, acknowledges its existence. Many children who respond in these ways feel relief and support when a helping adult deals with the stuttering in a calm and open manner. Moreover, some sort of straightforward approach is almost obligatory because the child's demonstrable awareness of the problem makes it pointless to try to avoid focusing on the speech production process as indirect methods do.

Others might suggest that a direct approach should also be selected in cases where the immediate cause of the stuttering seems attributable to an agent operating within the child's speech system. Remember, tests of auditory retention, auditory discrimination, language, and the like were included in the differential assessment because of the possibility that disorders of these functions could promote stuttering. If such does seem to be a possibility, then the deficient function might be treated directly with the view that fluency may improve as a by-product of this intervention.

Up to this point, we have talked as though clinicians must employ either some indirect tactic or a direct methodology on an exclusive basis. In actuality, the vast majority of contemporary therapies for children who stutter include both indirect and direct manipulations, with a decided emphasis on the latter. As was noted early in this chapter, the trend toward use of more direct treatments can be viewed as perhaps the most significant change in our orientation to the management of stuttering in children. We turn now to a description of these primarily direct protocols.

Direct Therapy Programs for Young Stutterers Group Studies

The Gregory and Hill Program

Gregory and Hill view children's disfluencies as falling at various points along a continuum that ranges from typical or usual disfluencies through borderline atypical disfluencies to the most atypical disfluencies. Here, we shall concentrate on the primarily direct treatment regimen that Gregory and Hill (1980) recommend for the child who exhibits the most atypical disfluencies. Once a youngster is observed exhibiting the most unusual disfluencies, Gregory and Hill proceed with a differential assessment. Their purpose here is to uncover any variables that are impeding, or could hamper, a child's development of normal fluency. Results of the differential assessment are then used to construct an individualized therapy program that deals with the salient factors identified in the assessment. This specially tailored regimen involves 2 hours of one-to-one contact and a half hour in a therapy group each week. The program is designed to meet 5 key objectives.

The first objective is to "avoid creating or increasing the child's awareness of a speech problem or stuttering" (1980, p. 357). This is accomplished by describing the treatment as having children attend "school" instead of therapy. In school they will have their own "teacher" who will engage them in enjoyable talking and listening games and other sorts of activities. By proceeding in this way, the focus of therapy is allowed to fall on fluency and behaviors that facilitate fluent speech. With youngsters who exhibit high levels of awareness of their speech disturbance, a more pointed approach can be taken. Specifically, Gregory and Hill follow Williams's lead and recommend talking with the child about "bumpy and smooth speech," and "talking hard and talking easy" (Williams, 1971, pp. 1073-1093; 1979, pp. 241-268).

The second objective is "to increase the amount of fluency that the child experiences" (1980, p. 358). Principally, this is accomplished by having the clinician model for the child an effortless, comfortable, flowing speech pattern that also involves smooth and gradual articulatory transitions into a word, through it, and then onto the following word.[3] Several steps can be taken to facilitate the child's acquisition of the target speech pattern that the clinician has modeled. Smooth, flowing speech can be exemplified by rolling a ball or small car across a table. Articulatory gestures can be slowed to an even greater extent. An edible or tangible reward for proper speech patterning can be introduced to heighten motivation. If bodily tension seems to be interfering with the child's success, then the role playing of such effortless activities as walking in space or floating on water can be interjected into treatment. The target speech pattern is to be used by the youngster as he responds to a series of verbal tasks that have been arranged from the nonpropositional to the propositional. It is considered to be stabilized if the youngster produces the pattern on 90% of the responses across 20 trials in each of 4 consecutive treatment sessions. When this high level of proper response has been achieved, opportunities can be contrived for the child to use the target pattern on propositional single-word responses outside the therapy room and with the parents. For instance, the clinician might offhandedly prompt the child to "tell Mommy one thing you would like for dinner tonight."

Generalization of fluent single-word, target speech responses to settings outside the clinic marks the point where work can begin on utterances of somewhat longer length. This advancement in the Gregory and Hill program could be to 2-, 3-, or even 4-word utterances. The length of responses, their degree of propositionality, and the types of cues introduced to prompt a child are not rigidly fixed. Rather, clinicians are encouraged to use data from the differential assessment and from the phases of treatment already completed to determine the next level in the child's program. For example, imagine a young child who, in spite of his stuttering, presents an otherwise normal differential assessment profile and has responded promptly and positively in the first stage of rehabilitation. With such a child it might well be appropriate to skip the 2-word level and imitative responding and go immediately to 3-word responses that would be evoked with questions posed by the clinician. In contrast, consider a stutterer with an identified deficit in auditory verbal comprehension who first responded slowly and erratically at the 1-word level. To accelerate this child's program by omitting 2-word imitative responding might be risky. Gregory and Hill's obvious thrust here is toward flexibly tailoring steps in treatment to each patient's abilities. This approach to increasing the length of the child's utterances and then transferring them to extraclinical speech situations can be pursued until the mean length of the youngster's responses are within normal limits.

Work on transfer and generalization at each stage of a child's regimen is accompanied by the introduction of techniques for "building tolerance toward fluency disrupting influences" (Gregory & Hill, 1980, p. 359). The establishment of this "tolerance" is Gregory and Hill's third objective. To achieve it the clinician reviews the stutterer's case history and observes the child in the therapy setting and in interactions with the parents. This is done for the purpose of forming a list of factors that appear to be associated with the disruption of fluency. The factors identified on the list are then arranged in a rank order from seemingly least to apparently most disruptive of fluency. To increase a youngster's tolerance for these disruptive stimuli, the clinician systematically introduces them into treatment, starting with the least fluency-disrupting cue and gradually working up to the most disorganizing influence. For example, suppose that a loss of listener attention and being interrupted in midsentence have been identified as the cues that are least and most disruptive of fluency, respectively. Once fluent use of the target speech pattern is well established, the clinician could start to occasionally shift attention away while the child is speaking. If the youngster starts to stutter, then the clinician returns the attention and encourages resumption of the target speech pattern. As fluency stabilizes at a high level once more, the clinician's inattention is introduced again. This process of interjecting, removing, and then reinserting the fluency disrupter is sustained until the child's vulnerability to that stimulus has been lowered. At that point, the clinician would move on to the next disruptive stimulus on the rank-ordered list and proceed in the same way until the most disruptive influence (being interrupted, in our example) had been dealt with effectively.

The fourth objective is to help the child "gain competence in all areas judged to be potential hazards to fluency" (Gregory and Hill, 1980, p. 359). From the contents of Table 9-2 we can see that this might involve weaving into the fabric of treatment procedures for dealing with problems such as a short attention span, reduced auditory verbal comprehension, and slow and inaccurate word retrieval.

We come now to the fifth and final objective, that being "to increase a child's self-confidence or self-acceptance in areas judged to have a potential impact on fluency" (Gregory and Hill, 1980, p. 360). Here, Gregory and Hill endeavor to deal with personality variables and attitudes that could affect fluency. Thus, inappropriate behaviors such as perfectionism, withdrawal, aggressiveness and irrational fears, identified in the case history and/or during the child's presence in the clinic, would become targets for modification.

At this juncture, one other aspect of the Gregory and Hill program needs to be mentioned. That involves 1 hour per week of parent counseling that is run in parallel with the child's therapy. Often, this counseling is conducted as the parents observe their child in treatment. The goals of the counseling regimen are to help parents: (1) identify and discriminate between the various types of disfluency; (2) observe and make accurate written records of their offspring's episodes of atypical disfluency; (3) develop the ability to identify and appropriately modify environmental forces that are disrupting their child's fluency; (4) acquire good models of those behaviors that promote the development of normal fluency; (5) form reasonable expectations for their child and the child's behavior; and (6) comprehend features of their youngster's behavior that may intrude on the generalization of fluency to extraclinical settings, or interfere with the maintenance of higher levels of generalized fluency.

Gregory and Hill (Note 5) provided individual data for a group of 20 children who completed their therapy program. These youngsters ranged in age from 3;6 to 6;3 years. All of them had been given a differential assessment. Deficits identified in some of these youngsters included trouble in attending, learning disabilities, language disorders, combined language-learning disabilities, errors of articulation, voice pathology, and psychological difficulties. Thus, whenever possible, treatment was planned so as to deal not only with fluency, but with these other problems as well. Duration of treatment ranged from 24 to 64 weeks with an average duration of approximately 40 weeks. All of the subjects were tested in 2 conditions both prior to treatment and then immediately after the therapy period ended. The 2 conditions were speaking in a dialogue with a clinician, and speaking during a play activity as the clinician applied various sorts of "pressure" to the child.

From the foregoing description it is clear that the Gregory and Hill regimen contains many parts. Therefore, the assignment of improvement of fluency or any other aspect of performance to any particular aspect of the therapy is virtually impossible. Treatment effects are so intermixed that we cannot decide with any certainty what caused what. With that constraint in mind, Table 9-3 shows that as a group, the 20 children treated

TABLE 9-3

Pre- and posttherapy mean percentage and range of disfluency values across 2 conditions for children treated in Gregory and Hill's program.

	Dialogue		Speech During Play With Clinician Applying Pressure on Patient	
	Pretherapy	Posttherapy	Pretherapy	Posttherapy
Less typical disfluencies*				
Mean % disfluencies:	12.34	1.51	10.45	1.62
Range:	.60–40.7	0.00–7.1	1.60–32.0	0.00–7.0
More typical disfluencies +				
Mean % disfluencies:	9.30	4.85	8.51	4.41
Range:	1.90–19.2	0.00–12.5	.53–21.3	0.00–13.6
Total disfluency				
Mean % disfluencies:	10.82	3.18	9.48	3.02
Range:	5.80–48.0	0.00–19.0	2.13–37.3	0.00–14.7

*Sound-syllable repetitions and prolongations included here.

+ Word and phrase repetitions, sound-syllable interjections, and revisions included here.

in the Gregory and Hill program experienced sizable pre- to posttherapy reductions in less typical disfluencies, more typical disfluencies, and, quite naturally, total disfluencies across the 2 test conditions. For a group of patients averaging 4.29 years to exhibit means of 3.18% and 3.02% of words disfluent is encouraging. Readers must remember that *normal* children of this age are still exhibiting somewhere between 1% and 5% of words disfluent in their speech (Davis, 1939). Unquestionably, the posttherapy mean percentage disfluency scores of Gregory and Hill's group fall within this acceptable range. Moreover, Gregory and Hill (1980) report that their subjects' progress was maintained when measured anywhere from 9 to 18 months following the end of treatment. In 6 cases, maintenance was rated as "poor" or "uncertain" (Gregory & Hill, Note 5). These less-than-desirable outcomes were attributed to psychological disturbances in the child and/or poor parental involvement and follow-up in the counseling program.

Riley and Riley's Component Program

In view of their work on differential assessment, it is not surprising that Riley and Riley have assembled a multidimensional treatment regimen for young stutterers. Recall that, based on the differential assessment data they gathered, Riley and Riley (1979) identified 9 components of stuttering (Table 9-1). Youngsters exhibiting various combinations of these components along with their stuttering are placed in individualized rehabilitation programs that contain techniques specifically designed to deal with whatever components are present.

Whenever necessary, attending disorders are treated first, primarily by means of behavior modification (e.g., positive reinforcement for sustaining eye contact for progressively longer periods of time). Second, intra- and interpersonal components are targeted for management. Parent counseling is used to reduce disruptive influences in the child's communicative environment, to help the parents develop more realistic expectations of their offspring, and to alter the consequences attached to any stuttering that is thought to be manipulative in nature. Parents who evince a need for their child to stutter are referred for longer term and more systematic psychotherapy. Coincidentally, the stuttering children are guided into adopting more reasonable expectations of themselves and their behavior and are provided with opportunities to build self-esteem.

The neurologic components of auditory processing, sentence formulation, and oral-motor problems are dealt with third. To manage auditory processing deficits, patients are trained to follow directions of increasing length and complexity. Then, children are instructed to postpone responding for progressively longer intervals so as to develop some tolerance for these delays. Also, youngsters are rewarded for suppressing their urges to respond impulsively. Sentence formulation deficiencies are handled by showing a child a word and then guiding him through the generation of increasingly longer and grammatically more complex sentences that include the stimulus word. Further, patients are encouraged to develop a general sense of sentence length and syntax prior to the execution of an utterance. Oral-motor problems are managed in a variety of ways. There are drills on the accuracy of vowel and consonant posturing and on the production of single and then bi- and trisyllabic sequences. Accuracy in all these productions is achieved initially at a reduced rate of speaking. Then, rate is increased progressively through the systematic application of reinforcement. Fourth, starter, postponement, and avoidance behaviors attendant to a child's stuttering are removed by having the child actively engage in their inhibition. This is done prior to the management of stuttering behaviors per se.

The manipulation of stuttering itself is the last step taken in therapy. Techniques used here include teaching a patient the easy onset of voicing or air flow for vowel or consonant production and instruction on how to sustain the breathstream for speech-making purposes. Additionally, the child is taught to "bounce" and "slide" (Riley & Riley, 1979, p. 289), so as to first attain less effortful stuttering and, eventually, normal disfluency.

Readers will remember from the section on differential assessment that the Rileys studied the distribution of their components in a sample of 54 stutterers. Subsequently, these youngsters were inserted into individualized treatment regimens tailored to fit their differential assessment profiles. Forty-four of these children completed therapy and were accessible for re-evaluation as much as 48 months later. Riley and Riley (Note 6) have provided treatment outcome and maintenance data for this group of children.

As a general rule, treatment took less time if the patient entered therapy before age 6. Youngsters aged 3 to 4 years required fewer hours of remediation than did stutterers 6 years old and older. In part, this difference can be accounted for by the fact that 75% of the children who were enrolled in clinic prior to their sixth birthday *"did not need any direct stuttering behavior treatment"*[4] (Riley & Riley, 1979, p. 289). In other words, the successful modification of a child's components was associated with significant spontaneous improvement in stuttering such that it never became the direct target of therapy. The problem here is that we cannot determine how much of this improvement to attribute to spontaneous recovery that would have occurred without treatment, and how much to the treatment itself. Without a no-treatment control group, this issue cannot be settled. Whatever the case, it is interesting that, in contrast to the younger group of stutterers, 91% of the patients 6 years old and older did need direct modification of their stuttering. These older children were also more likely to need management of starter, postponement, and avoidance behaviors. Since these latter responses and stuttering required clinical attention, the older patients were in treatment longer than their younger counterparts.

These across-age-group differences aside, 36 (82%) of the 44 youngsters were reported as exhibiting either no stuttering or mild residual stuttering in clinic, home, and school at the end of rehabilitation. Twelve months later, all but one of the 36 individuals had either maintained their clinical gains or had improved even further. During the 12-to-24-month interval after therapy ended, 2 children who had made major gains in treatment returned to the clinic for additional maintenance work. One had regressed slightly but was able to regain the improvement previously made. The other patient suffered a rather serious relapse and was not able to recoup this lost ground.

In mild contrast to these results, just 8 (18%) of the 44 stutterers reached the end of therapy with significant residual stuttering or only slight improvement. One of these individuals did progress during the 12 months leading to the first follow-up. The remaining 7 stutterers still exhibited their disappointing end-of-treatment status.

In the 24-to-48-month interval since treatment was terminated, the foregoing patterns have remained essentially unchanged. While complete data are not yet available on all 44 patients, about 80% of these children remain significantly improved, while approximately 20% of them show little change from the picture they presented when therapy started. It is also worth mentioning that the parents of the youngsters who made major progress in therapy expressed great satisfaction over their offsprings' improvement. These parents reported that their children's speech "sounded normal with regard to rate, loudness, stress and pitch" (Riley & Riley, Note 6) except during infrequent moments of stuttering.

Bruce Ryan's GILCU Approach

GILCU is an acronym for "Gradual Increase in Length and Complexity of Utterance." This label very accurately describes the basic strategy in Ryan's program (1974). That is, fluency is instated at the single-word level and then at levels of increasing length and linguistic complexity. As conceived by Ryan, the GILCU program is administered across 3 modes of responding: oral reading, monologue, and conversation. To begin, a clinician instructs the child to "speak more slowly and easily" (Ryan, 1974, p. 88), and then to read a list of simple words (e.g., "ball...car...man"). When the child achieves the criterion level of fluency on this task, a list of 2-word responses is introduced. Attainment of the criterion level of fluency at the 2-word level allows for advancement of the stutterer to the oral reading of 3-word phrases. This basic tactic is followed through the reading of 4- , 5- , and 6-word responses, then to a single sentence, and on to 2, 3, and 4 consecutive sentences. After that, response length is determined by unit of time, starting with utterances that are 30 seconds in length, then 1 minute, 1½ minutes, 2, 2½, 3, 4, and, finally, 5 minutes. There are 18 steps altogether in the oral-reading response mode. As soon as the youngster completes the eighteenth step, the treatment is recycled back to Step 1, but now in the monologue mode of responding. When the next 17 steps are finished in monologue, treatment is recycled back to Step 1 in the conversational mode. Through the thoughtful selection and preparation of speech-evoking stimuli (e.g., word lists, two-word phrases, pictures, etc.), a clinician can exercise anywhere from a strict to a modicum of control over the length and complexity of the client's responses.

For Ryan, transfer involves the child's production of fluent speech "in a wide variety of settings and with many different people" (1974, p. 94). This part of treatment is organized and conducted just as carefully and systematically as the establishment phase. Specifically, transfer can start with the clinician and child conversing in the therapy room, but with the door open. To transfer the youngster's fluency beyond the realm of one-to-one conversations, additional people are introduced, one at a time, into the therapy room. Then, to generalize the child's fluency to strangers and new situations in the natural environment, the patient is taken away from the clinic to locales such as neighborhood stores, shops, and the library. The last step in transfer involves the carry-over of fluency to settings in which the child participates routinely (i.e., home and school).

When the client has achieved a specified criterion level of fluency throughout this multi-step transfer program, the time has come for the transition into maintenance. The goal of maintenance is "fluent speech in a wide variety of settings, with many different people over a long period of time" (Ryan, 1974, p. 105). In Ryan's approach, maintenance involves 3 major steps. They are: (1) self-regulation of one's own fluency through careful monitoring; (2) intermittent home practice; and (3) periodic return visits to the clinic for rechecks and any such reinstruction as might be needed.

It can be seen from Table 9-4 that the patients in the GILCU program experienced major reductions in their stuttering. The mean scores shown testify to the efficacy of the GILCU approach with the youngsters treated. It is also worth mentioning that very recently, Ryan, Rustin, and Ryan (Note 7) have reported similar results for the GILCU methodology following its application in England. Finally, there is one other bit of information that

TABLE 9-4
Pretherapy, posttherapy, and follow-up stuttered words-per-minute range and mean values for 6 elementary-age patients treated in Ryan's GILCU program.

	Stuttered Words Per Minute	
	Range	*Mean*
Pretherapy:	2.85–13.35	7.81
End of establishment phase of therapy:	0.00–0.5	.06
Follow-up*:	0.00–0.5	0.2

Note: After B. Ryan, *Programmed Therapy for Stuttering in Children and Adults*. Springfield, Ill.: Charles Thomas, 1974, pp. 89 and 109.

The values shown here were excerpted from a larger data pool published by Ryan. Ryan's data were not offered in their entirety because some of the scores pertained to adult stutterers and obviously do not belong in the chapter.

*Follow-up measures were made an average of 10.4 months after the child had reached the end of the GILCU program. Follow-up data not available on 1 of the original 6 children.

also gives a measure of indirect support to the use of GILCU with children who stutter. That is, the basic GILCU strategy has been integrated into virtually every demonstrably successful stuttering therapy program for children. We found it in the approaches advocated by Gregory and Hill and by the Rileys. It will appear again in the next regimen to be presented, that being the one developed by Richard Shine.

Richard Shine's Treatment

Richard Shine is yet another therapist for stutterers who advocates the administration of a differential assessment prior to the start of treatment (1980). The assessment includes formal testing, observations of parent-child interactions, the taking of a case history, the measurement of stuttering severity, an analysis of the stuttering itself, and an examination of the physiologic and aerodynamic processes that are integral to speech production.

Apropos of the last 2 parts of the assessment, Shine measures stuttering frequency and describes the topography of all observable symptoms.

Note is taken of any struggle behavior the child might be exhibiting. As regards the evaluation of physiologic and aerodynamic processes, it focuses on any abnormal respiratory, phonatory, or articulatory behaviors that are present. Then, Shine attempts to ascertain the locus of speech breathing (e.g., clavicular, thoracic, abdominal), the regularity and timing of respiratory cycles, and the arrangement of breath groups. Phonation is evaluated for the presence or absence of hard glottal attacks and the child's ability to maintain continuous flow throughout an utterance. Vocal sound pressure level, fundamental frequency, the tension and force in articulatory posturing, and the rate of articulatory movement are all assessed. A judgment is rendered on the appropriateness of the youngster's resonance patterns and estimates are made of stress and intonation use. Finally, attention is devoted to studying the effectiveness with which the youngster coordinates respiration, phonation, and articulation while speaking. The findings of the extensive analysis of stuttering and the physiology and aerodynamics of the child's speech behavior play a central role in shaping Shine's fluency-building program. This regimen is rounded out by the insertion of additional techniques suitable for dealing with any problems other than stuttering that were identified during the differential assessment.

Once the differential assessment has been completed, Shine initiates a 5-phase treatment program. He refers to the first phase as the "picture identification prestep" (1980, p. 344). Shine's goal is to identify, in a collection of pictures, about 50 that the youngster can name quickly and with reliable fluency. These pictures and the words that go with them are used as the first set of stimuli in the next 2 phases of treatment. In the second phase, the clinician attempts to establish speaking variables that are compatible with fluency. Initially, this entails developing in the young stutterer a basic understanding of the concept of an "easy speaking voice" (p. 345). The third part provides the child with fluency training during highly structured activities. One crucial aspect of this structure requires that the clinician select stimulus materials and response modes for the child that will strictly control the length and complexity of the youngster's utterances.[5] The fourth phase involves fluency training during conversation in a host of real-life speech situations.[6] The final phase uses procedures that are designed to ease the patient out of therapy, make provision for assessing the stability of progress after treatment has ended, and help the child maintain improved fluency.

As we look back over Shine's methods, we can see that they begin with a differential assessment and are followed by a direct approach to therapy. Although this treatment is presumably based on the differential assessment, what is not evident is the way in which that evaluation's results are used to determine the phases of therapy through which a child must pass.

This would seem to be an instance in which a differential assessment, to be clinically useful, should lead to differential treatment. There is nothing in Shine's writing to indicate that it does, or that a differential assessment is even needed.

One of Shine's students undertook a comprehensive examination of the effectiveness of her mentor's therapy program (Mason, Note 8). At the start of treatment, the 14 children studied ranged in age from 2;9 to 8;0. Therapy for these youngsters lasted from 1 to 28 months. The mean duration of treatment was approximately 10½ months and involved an average of 56.7 sessions, each of which was 40-50 minutes in length. The 14 children were assessed at the start of treatment, at treatment's end, and then at some point following that termination date, but no sooner than 14 months after therapy had been completed. One child was tested 5 years after his treatment program was concluded. The average time lapse between the end of treatment and the follow-up examination was 3 years, 2 months.

Portions of the testing of the 14 children included the gathering of a 200-word sample of their conversational speech, a rating of their stuttering severity, and qualitative ratings by parents of changes in their offspring's speech. The data collected in these ways were first scrutinized on a subject-by-subject basis. From this initial examination, Mason reported that one stutterer's follow-up test results indicated that a significant relapse had occurred. Individual scores for this youngster were presented and discussed, but then removed from the data pool for the larger sample. Results for the remaining 13 children are presented in Table 9-5. As can be seen, they experienced a substantial reduction in their disfluency by the end of treatment. Moreover, this improvement was sustained at least through the date of the follow-up assessment. Consistent with these findings, it is not surprising that estimates of stuttering severity at follow-up ranged from zero (no stuttering) to mild, with 11 youngsters being rated as very mild. Comparable judgments by parents also were reported. Specifically, before treatment, the speech of all 13 children was rated by their parents as either fair or poor. By the end of therapy, four children had speech that was rated as very good. Nine youngsters were rated as good. When follow-up testing was undertaken, nine children were rated as having very good speech, and four were believed to have good speech. Obviously, several of the youngsters had continued to progress in their parents' eyes months after therapy had ended.

Single Case Studies

Dating back to 1965 and continuing to the present, clinically oriented operant researchers have sought to manipulate the stuttering and/or

TABLE 9-5
Pretherapy, posttherapy, and follow-up range and mean values for 14 child stutterers on measures of stuttered words per minute, words spoken per minute, and struggle behaviors.

		Pretherapy	*Posttherapy*	*Follow-Up*
Stuttered words per minute				
	Mean:	13.90	1.70	1.30
	Range:	4.00–22.0	0.00–8.40	0.6–2.60
Words spoken per minute				
	Mean:	*	*	129.80
	Range:	*	*	118.0–143.0
Frequency of struggle behaviors				
	Mean:	*	*	0.00
	Range:	*	*	0.00

Note: After D. Mason. Unpublished Master's thesis, East Carolina University, 1981.

*Pre- and posttherapy measures of words spoken per minute and the frequency of occurrence of struggle behaviors were unavailable to Mason.

fluency of young stutterers through the simple expedient of applying various consequences to these behaviors. Experiments of this type number about 20 now (c.f., Rickard & Mundy, 1965, Shaw & Shrum, 1972; Martin, Kuhl, & Haroldson, 1972), rendering a review of each of them far beyond the scope of this chapter; however, the philosophy underlying the view of stuttering and fluency as operant behaviors and some of the treatment procedures that can emerge from that view are described by Costello (1980). These reports are important to us because they fit our definition of "direct" therapy (see p. 8). Therefore, a summary or overview of them is in order.

The studies in question have all attempted to test the hypotheses that stuttering and/or fluency are operant behaviors—responses whose frequencies of occurrence are controlled by the consequences attached to them. Generally, reinforcers are consequences that we associate with an increase in response frequency while punishers are consequences associated with a decrease in the frequency of responding.

In the conduct of operant studies of stuttering and fluency, the researchers have relied heavily on what has been referred to as the ABA design or some variation thereof. In this type of experiment, which is well suited for the detailed analysis of individual subjects' behavior, the first "A" is used to designate a "baserate" time period. During this segment, the subject under test is simply instructed to speak in monologue or conversation, or perhaps to read aloud. The investigator withholds the reinforcer or punisher and does nothing but carefully count the frequency of occurrence of all behaviors of interest; for example, part-word repetitions, interjections, and/or words spoken fluently. During the "B" (treatment) segment, the experimenter arranges for certain consequences to be applied to a specific aspect of the child's speech behavior. For example, the youngster may receive a token for nonstuttered utterances of a predetermined length, with a certain number of tokens later exchanged for the privilege of bringing a friend along to the treatment sessions (Peters, 1977). Or, points earned for fluent utterances might be removed following moments of stuttering (Ryan, 1971). In some instances, these contingencies are explained to the child beforehand (Shaw & Shrum, 1972)—sometimes the child is even pointedly told, "Try not to stutter"— but explanations and instructions are not typical or mandatory for the success of the treatment. Whatever the case, the child is *not* given instructions such as "talk slowly" or "let some air out" that could aid in speaking more fluently or reducing stuttering by requiring the use of altered speech patterns. The child simply begins talking or reading and the experimenter starts to apply the consequence(s), at the same time noting the frequency of occurrence of the target behavior. If that response is an operant, then it will increase in frequency with the application of the reinforcer, or decrease in frequency with the delivery of a punisher.

In the "A" segment that follows "B," the reinforcer or punisher is removed. This provides the researchers with a chance to observe whether the elimination of the consequence is associated with a reversal of whatever behavior change was noted in "B." Specifically, the experimenter watches to see if the target response returns to its baseline frequency of occurrence. Subsequently, the investigation can be terminated or the consequence reintroduced to see if that step is again associated with some change in the frequency of occurrence of the response of interest. This re-presentation of the consequence creates what has been labeled an ABAB withdrawal design (Herson & Barlow, 1976), which is nothing more than an elaboration on the basic ABA model we have been talking about, but is more rigorous because it requires a replication of the treatment effect and is more appropriate for clinical research because it terminates the experiment in the treatment condition.

The operant studies that have just been described produced two extraordinarily interesting findings. First, neither the application of reinforcers for fluency nor punishers for stuttering has been reported to be associated with any obvious unpleasant emotional reactions among the children tested. Second, in one experiment after another, introduction of reinforcement and/or punishment contingencies has been associated with clinically significant increases in nonstuttered speech and decreases in the frequency of occurrence of stuttering. Taken together, these results demonstrated that direct approaches to the manipulation of fluency and stuttering could be given the most serious consideration rather than rejected out of fear that such straightforward tactics would surely exacerbate the young stutterer's problem (Costello, 1983).

Before concluding this summary, there is one other aspect of the operant research that needs to be mentioned. Specifically, it is noteworthy that the youngsters who served as subjects had not been exposed to a differential assessment prior to their participation in the studies. Therefore, we cannot be sure if these youngsters were in possession of the neurologic, interpersonal, and intrapersonal problems identified by such workers as the Rileys (see p. 9). But let us assume for the moment that any number of these difficulties were present in at least a few of the children. The point to be made here is that it didn't seem to matter. That is to say, in spite of the presumed coexistence of these various complicating conditions and stuttering, the simple process of applying consequences was sufficient to modify the behavior of the children tested. Granted that in some cases this improvement was transient, lasting only until the end of the experiment or shortly thereafter, in most cases treatment effects with young children have been shown to be pervasive and lasting (e.g., Martin, Kuhl, & Haroldson, 1972; Reed & Godden, 1977). Nonetheless, the results of the operant research raise a question that is likely to be hotly debated in the years ahead. That is, is a differential assessment even necessary and must the results from it be used in planning therapy? Costello (1983) embraces the view that stuttering treatment with children should begin with "the basics"—contingent positive feedback for nonstuttered utterances combined with contingent negative feedback for each moment of stuttering—and that only if performance data indicate this simple, direct treatment to be ineffective should "additives" such as rate control, easy onset, or modifications in the language required of the child be introduced into the treatment regimen. She suggests that information gathered during a pretreatment differential assessment would be a good source for pointing the clinician toward potentially facilitating additives, but that ABAB manipulations within the treatment should serve as tests of the actual effectiveness of the selected additive.

Conclusion

It hardly seems arguable that we have made very significant advances in the direct treatment of stuttering in children. Where clinically we used to move with great caution and insecurity, we are now able to proceed with more optimism. Where we once felt lucky if solid fluency was achieved in a minority of our young stutterers, we can now anticipate a much larger number of successful treatment outcomes. This is certainly a happy state of affairs because among stutterers of all ages, it is the afflicted child who possesses the best prognosis for improvement. Indeed, it is the stuttering child who has the best chance of attaining fully normal speech. If that goal once seemed unrealistic, it is now most decidedly within reach.

End Notes

[1] Briefly put, a factor analysis makes it possible to discover commonalities that may exist between 2 or more variables. Such a discovery then "reduces" the set of variables to a single factor. For example, the tasks of following spoken directions and responding appropriately to spoken questions, both tap a common factor—auditory verbal comprehension. The same 2 tasks and the task of repeating a sequence of numbers share the common factor of auditory retention. Once a factor is identified, it is then possible to statistically estimate the extent to which it can account for the variability in a group's responses to tasks.

[2] The term "immediate cause" refers to those forces in the here and now that appear to be triggering the stuttering. Immediate causes are to be contrasted to distal causes (Freeman, 1979). The latter refers to the original instigators of the disorder. Thus, we might say that the immediate cause of a patient's stuttering is difficulty in starting and sustaining voicing. Inquires about the origin of this phonatory defect would direct us toward the distal cause.

[3] This implied slight reduction in the rate of articulation would surely create a modest drop in the number of syllables or words spoken per minute. This point is made because of the growing importance being placed upon decrements in speaking rate as an integral part of stuttering therapy.

[4] The present author has added italics for emphasis.

[5] Ryan's influence here is obvious as Shine clearly notes in his writing (1980).

[6] Shine (1980) has noted that these sorts of formal transfer activities are not needed with many preschool stutterers. Their fluency seems to generalize spontaneously from formal activities like language lotto to more typical verbal exchanges away from the clinic. The present author has made similar observations (Adams, 1980), as have others (Martin, Kuhl, & Haroldson, 1972; Shaw & Shrum, 1972).

Reference Notes

1. Berlin, A. An exploratory attempt to isolate types of stuttering. Unpublished doctoral dissertation. Northwestern University, 1954.

2. Riley, G., & Riley, J. Clinical subtypes of stuttering among 100 children. A paper presented at the Annual Convention of the American Speech and Hearing Association. San Francisco, 1972.

3. Riley, G., & Riley, J. Differential strategies for diagnosing and treating children who stutter. A short course presented at the Regional Convention of the American Speech and Hearing Association, Portland, Ore., 1976.

4. Smith, A., & Daly, D. Neuropsychological assessment: Implications for the treatment of aphasic and stuttering clients. Unpublished manuscript of a paper included within a miniseminar presented at the Annual Convention of the American Speech-Language and Hearing Association. Detroit, 1980.

5. Gregory, H., & Hill, D. Personal communication, 1981.

6. Riley, G., & Riley, J. Personal communication, 1981.

7. Ryan, B., Rustin, L., & Ryan, B. Comparison of speech and therapy of English and American stutterers. A paper presented at the Annual Convention of the American Speech-Language and Hearing Association. Los Angeles, 1981.

8. Mason, D. A follow-up study of fluency training with the young stutterer (ages 2-9 to 8-0 years). Unpublished Master's thesis, East Carolina University, 1981.

References

Adams, M. A clinical strategy for differentiating the normally nonfluent child and the incipient stutterer. *Journal of Fluency Disorders*, 1977, *2*, 141-148.

Adams, M. The young stutterer: Diagnosis, treatment, and assessment of progress. In W. Perkins (Ed.), *Seminars in Speech, Language, and Hearing*, *1*(4), 289-300. New York: Thieme-Stratton, 1980.

Andrews, G., & Harris, M. *The syndrome of stuttering*. London: Heinemann Medical Books, 1964.

Canter, G. Observations of neurogenic stuttering: A contribution to differential diagnosis. *British Journal of Disorders of Communication*, 1971, *6*, 139-143.

Conture, E. *Stuttering*. Englewood Cliffs, N.J.: Prentice-Hall, 1982.

Costello, J. M. Operant conditioning and the treatment of stuttering. In W. H. Perkins (Ed.), Strategies in stuttering therapy. *Seminars in Speech, Language, and Hearing*, 1980, *1*, 311-327. New York: Thieme-Stratton.

Costello, J. M. Current behavioral treatments for children. In D. Prins & R. J. Ingham (Eds.), *Stuttering in early childhood: Treatment methods and issues*. San Diego: College-Hill, 1983.

Curlee, R. A case selection strategy for young disfluent children. In W. Perkins (Ed.), *Seminars in Speech, Language, and Hearing*, *1*(4), 277-288. New York: Thieme-Stratton, 1980.

Davis, D. The relation of repetitions in the speech of young children to certain measures of language maturity and situational factors. *Journal of Speech Disorders*, 1939, *4*, 303-318.

Freeman, F. Phonation in stuttering: A review of current research. *Journal of Fluency Disorders*, 1979, *4*, 79-90.

Gregory H., & Hill, D. Stuttering therapy for children. In W. Perkins (Ed.), *Seminars in Speech, Language, and Hearing*, *1*(4), 351-364. New York: Thieme-Stratton, 1980.

Herson, M., & Barlow, D. *Single case experimental designs*. New York: Pergamon, 1976.

Johnson, L. Facilitating parental involvement in therapy for the disfluent child. In W. Perkins (Ed.), *Seminars in Speech, Language, and Hearing*, *1*(4), 301-310. New York: Thieme-Stratton, 1980.

Martin, R., Kuhl, P., & Haroldson, S. An experimental treatment with two preschool stuttering children. *Journal of Speech and Hearing Research*, 1972, *15*, 743-752.

Peters, A. D. The effect of positive reinforcement on fluency: Two case studies. *Language, Speech, and Hearing Services in Schools*, 1977, *8*, 15-22.

Prins, D., & Lohr, F. Behavioral dimensions of stuttered speech. *Journal of Speech and Hearing Research*, 1972, *15*, 61-71.

Reed, C. G., & Godden, A. L. An experimental treatment using verbal punishment with two preschool stutterers. *Journal of Fluency Disorders*, 1977, *2*, 225-233.

Rickard, H., & Mundy, M. Direct manipulation of stuttering behavior: An experimental-clinical approach. In L. Ullmann & L. Krasner (Eds.), *Case studies in behavior modification*. New York: Holt, Rinehart, 1966.

Riley, G., & Riley, J. A component model for diagnosing and treating children who stutter. *Journal of Fluency Disorders*, 1979, *4*, 279-294.

Riley, G., & Riley, J. Motor and linguistic variables among children who stutter. *Journal of Speech and Hearing Disorders*, 1980, *45*, 504-514.

Ryan, B. Operant procedures applied to stuttering therapy for children. *Journal of Speech and Hearing Disorders*, 1971, *36*, 264-280.

Ryan, B. *Programmed therapy for stuttering in children and adults*. Springfield, Ill.: Charles C. Thomas, 1974.

Shaw, C., & Shrum, W. The effects of response-contingent reward on the connected speech of children who stutter. *Journal of Speech and Hearing Disorders*, 1972, *37*, 75-88.

Shine, R. Direct management of the beginning stutterer. In W. Perkins (Ed.), *Seminars in Speech, Language, and Hearing*, *1*(4), 339-350. New York: Thieme-Stratton, 1980.

Van Riper, C. Experiments in stuttering therapy. In J. Eisenson (Ed.), *Stuttering: A symposium*. New York: Harper & Brothers, 1958.

Van Riper, C. *The nature of stuttering*. Englewood Cliffs, N.J.: Prentice-Hall, 1971.

Williams, D. Stuttering therapy for children. In L. Travis (Ed.), *Handbook of speech pathology*. New York: Appleton-Century-Crofts, 1971.

Williams, D. A perspective on approaches to stuttering therapy. In H. Gregory (Ed.), *Controversies about stuttering therapy*. Baltimore: University Park Press, 1979.

Barry Guitar

Indirect Treatment of Stuttering

Indirect stuttering therapies are those approaches which try to ameliorate a child's stuttering by working on some other aspect of his behavior or environment. An indirect therapy may, for example, work on the child's interactions with parents, on command of language, or on behavior at school. Whatever the focus of treatment, the goal is to decrease the stuttering. The organization of this review is in terms of where the emphasis of the indirect treatment is placed. These include: parent counseling, psychotherapy, drug therapy, control of nonspeech behavior, language-oriented approaches, parent-child interaction, and psychomotor therapy.

There are a variety of reasons for the clinician to select one of these indirect approaches instead of working directly on the child's stuttering. There may be, for example, a reluctance to let the child become aware of his stuttering, for fear it will become worse (Van Riper, 1973). In this case, parent counseling to change the child's environment is typically employed. In other cases, however, a different rationale determines the choice. The clinician may believe that a significant cause of the child's stuttering lies beyond speech production and the child's attitude about speech difficulty. Thus, the nature of the problem may be thought to be beyond the reach of direct therapy. In these cases, an indirect approach—for example, psychotherapy—is chosen according to the clinician's theoretical bent, in accord with what he or she believes to be the significant cause. Still another rationale is both theoretical and empirical. A broad theoretical orientation may lead the clinician to select several variables for experimentation;

then, those that are demonstrated to influence the child's stuttering, empirically, are selected for use in treatment. Parent-child interaction approaches use this rationale.

In this review each of the indirect approaches is described as though it were used as a total treatment package for the child. This is not usually true in practice, however. Sometimes, one indirect approach, such as a language-oriented treatment, may be combined with another indirect approach, such as parent counseling. In other instances, an indirect approach may be combined with a direct approach. Another way in which this review may slightly distort reality is in not including all available indirect approaches. The most readily available published and orally presented reports of indirect treatments have been included, but some worthwhile approaches have undoubtedly been overlooked. Having acknowledged some of the inadequacies of this attempt to present the state of the art, we shall begin with parent counseling.

Parent Counseling

By far the most common indirect approach to treatment is for the speech-language pathologist to counsel the parents of the stuttering child. The goal of this counseling is to help the parent identify and change behaviors which increase the child's stuttering. Inherent in most of the approaches in this category is the assumption that parental feelings and consequent behaviors, while not necessarily the original cause of the stuttering, can worsen the child's stuttering and make it chronic. Thus, in distinction to psychotherapy, parent counseling usually focuses on those behaviors that can be observed to influence the child's stuttering. Feelings are dealt with in the context of how they lead to overt behaviors that aggravate stuttering.

In his book, *Treatment of Stuttering*, Van Riper (1973) describes his own strategies for parent counseling. His approach, taken from several sources and borrowed by many others, aims at reducing parents' feelings of guilt, inadequacy, and ignorance. Another of Van Riper's aims is to help parents manipulate environmental variables influencing their child's stuttering. He advocates that the clinician: (1) maintain a highly accepting attitude toward the parents; (2) help the parents understand what might be influencing the child's stuttering; and (3) create, in the counseling session, a supportive and objective environment in which the parents can discover for themselves which changes in their behavior will reduce the child's stuttering. Specific activities include having the parents keep a daily log of situations in which their child is most fluent and situations in which stuttering occurs a great deal. In addition, Van Riper gradually involves parents in the direct treatment of the child. For Van Riper, parent counseling is usually only an adjunct to direct stuttering therapy for the child. Unfortunately, he has not reported data on the outcome of his combined approach.

Another version of parent counseling is provided by Ainsworth and Gruss (1981) in the most recent edition of *If Your Child Stutters—A Guide for Parents*. This book serves as a paperbound parent counselor by itself. It is probably best used, however, as a supplement to counseling by a speech-language pathologist. Ainsworth and Gruss share the assumption that environmental factors may exacerbate mild disfluency so that it becomes chronic stuttering. The most critical variables, in their estimate, are related to the child's feelings of security and acceptance. Consequently, the book emphasizes ways in which parents can increase their sensitivity to the child's emotional needs. Specific guidelines for parents are given in extended discussions of ways of meeting children's needs. The following suggestions are abstracted from some of the authors' guidelines:

1. decrease criticism;
2. decrease over-control;
3. help the child to release feelings constructively;
4. give the child more attention and support in a crisis;
5. discipline without decreasing the child's sense of security;
6. accept the fact that as other skills are developing, fluency may suffer; and
7. accept disfluencies by realizing that the child is doing the best he can.

Another approach to parent counseling is described in *Understanding Stuttering* by Cooper (1979). This booklet provides information regarding the nature of stuttering and gives parents several suggestions for helping their child. The information section appears to be designed to allay parents' fears that they may have caused the child's stuttering problem, but may also help them realize that their child's stuttering is within the range of normal disfluency (if such is the case). The section on suggestions for parents helps parents to identify their negative feelings toward their child's stuttering and to understand how these feelings may be transmitted to the child. Helpful feelings and responses are suggested. Cooper briefly describes how the child may benefit when parents make responses which:

1. indicate the parent is not angry with the child because of the stuttering;
2. convey that the parent is not blaming the child for the stuttering; and

3.   help the child identify and express personal feelings.

Booklets such as those by Ainsworth and Gruss, Cooper, and others offer several advantages for parent counseling. Among them are: (1) Parents can digest this material at their own pace rather than being required to process it during counseling sessions. (2) The material can be carefully prepared by experienced clinicians to carry a message of acceptance as well as information. (Despite the best intentions, a neophyte counselor may lack a little of both.) (3) The material is always available although a counselor might not be. For small relapses after treatment has terminated, a handy and good booklet may serve as a Band-Aid in place of a major operation involving many trips to a speech pathologist.

Unfortunately, despite the fact that over 100,000 copies of *If Your Child Stutters* and 12,000 copies of *Understand Stuttering* have been distributed, there appears to be little data on their effectiveness. Experimental studies involving counseling with and without a particular booklet are feasible, although control of clinician bias may be difficult. It may also be informative to study parent-child interactions before, during, and after the provision of reading material for parents. Measures of the child's stuttering and parent interactions may reveal what the parents can change via written materials, and to what extent those changes are related to the child's stuttering. In these experiments, clinician counseling of the parents can be administered (and assessed) following a trial of written materials to ensure that parents and child are not deprived of adequate treatment.

Another approach to parent counseling is presented in workshop format for clinicians by Bailey and Bailey (1977; 1982). They advocate modeling of slow, easy, simple speech in a low "time-pressure" context. They also teach Adlerian principles of child rearing that parents can use to help their child feel more competent, more free, and more independent. The Baileys' backgrounds in both speech pathology and counseling place a strong emphasis on parent-child interactions apart from speech. Specific suggestions for parents include:

1.   Tune into the child's feelings as much as possible, encouraging their expression through such techniques as active listening and reflection of the feelings back to the child.

2.   Train the child in those skills you think are important, rather than expecting them to be learned without instruction.

3.   Don't continually teach the child. Allow some things to be learned independently.

4.   Let the child take on as much responsibility—do as much for himself or herself—as possible.

5. Instead of rewards, use encouragement, which implies faith in the child.

The approach described by Bailey and Bailey has not been studied systematically. It would be particularly useful to have data on whether indirect stuttering treatment is any more effective when parents are counseled about child-rearing practices apart from issues regarding their child's speech.

Conture's (1981) indirect treatment approach is specifically designed for cases in which the parents, but not the child, are concerned about the child's stuttering. Conture suggests parent counseling combined with play therapy or general language stimulation for the child. Parent counseling is aimed at helping the parents change environmental influences on the child's speech so that fluency may be increased. Play therapy and/or general language stimulation by the clinician is used as a model from which the parent can learn new styles of interaction. Among the things which are modeled and encouraged are:

1. treating the child with "unconditional positive regard";
2. listening to the content rather than the form of the child's speech;
3. setting down firm rules for the child's behavior;
4. giving the child clear instructions on those tasks that are expected of him or her; and
5. reading slowly and calmly to the child, and allowing the child freedom to interrupt.

Conture implies that once these skills are learned by the parents, they can then proceed on their own to change the child's environment. Conture's implicit position is that if the child is not concerned about stuttering, stuttering will probably be outgrown, so long as environmental conditions are right. Thus, with parents who are concerned about their child's mild disfluencies, a major thrust of treatment is allaying their fears, decreasing unduly high expectations, and increasing the child's sense of security and self worth. Such an approach, like those of Van Riper, Bailey and Bailey, and Ainsworth and Gruss, may or may not be effective. As we have said before, without data it is difficult to estimate which components of these indirect treatments are most effective; without data, it is not clear how many of the children treated with these indirect treatments would not have recovered "spontaneously"; without data, it is not even possible to state how many of the children treated with these indirect treatments recovered at all.

Psychotherapy

Almost all approaches to stuttering therapy with children, direct and indirect, contain a degree of psychotherapy. This section will deal with those that seem to be more psychotherapy than anything else.

In a recent *Smithsonian* (May, 1981), Michael Kernan described the work of Philip Glasner, a psychotherapist who treats stuttering children. Glasner's work, depicted as well outside the mainstream of today's stuttering therapy, appears to be similar to the psychotherapy or play therapy for stuttering advocated by several speech pathologists over the last 25 years (Murphy & FitzSimmons, 1960; Van Riper, 1973; Wyatt & Herzan, 1962). The *Smithsonian* article, however, emphasizes differences between Glasner's approach and any other speech therapy. Glasner apparently sees stuttering as "not a speech disorder at all, but a symptom of far-reaching emotional disturbances" (p. 109). Consequently, his treatment is aimed at reversing the emotional disturbances through parent counseling and, one assumes, play therapy. The example of treatment given in the article suggests Glasner seeks to have the child find understanding and emotional support in the therapist. The same example also suggests that Glasner teaches the child to use loose, easy speech movements. If this is typical of Glasner's approach, it is not pure psychotherapy, but traditional play therapy for stuttering with direct intervention added for good measure. The author of the article quotes Glasner as indicating that "every child patient he has discharged after treatment has not only stopped stuttering but has developed into a far more integrated and better-adjusted person. " No data are available to confirm or deny this optimistic claim.

Van Riper's treatment of the "garden variety" beginning stutterer is another version of psychotherapy combined with direct speech therapy. Van Riper (1973) describes his approach as involving "free and directed play since young children are already experts in this activity" (p. 400). Free play is used to create an emotionally supportive relationship into which a hierarchy of more and more direct speech therapy activities is introduced. Van Riper uses a more truly psychotherapeutic treatment, however, for certain children. This is an approach that has no direct speech therapy, but uses only permissive play activity. Some stutterers with deep emotional conflicts need, in his view, this type of therapy which allows them to "express unacceptable feelings...to utter the unspeakable...to recreate and master many of the stresses that formerly disrupted their lives" (p. 398). Although Van Riper gives few specific guidelines for doing psychotherapy with stuttering children who need it, he excerpts several interesting case examples to illustrate how play therapy might be done.

Van Riper's general approach to psychotherapy with children is similar to the play therapy for young stutterers detailed by Murphy and FitzSimmons (1960). Murphy and FitzSimmons shun the goals of directive speech therapy. Instead, "the clinician is truly nondemanding and nonjudgmental. He respects the child's 'right to stutter, ' his right to express previously forbidden attitudes, his right to resist the therapeutic plan... " (p. 236). Using "permissiveness within realistic limits, " the clinician builds a relationship which allows the child to feel secure and learn to express feelings. This, in turn, is expected to lead to a significant lessening of the stuttering symptoms. Once again, however, we are not given evidence of the effectiveness of treatment, for either Van Riper's or Murphy and FitzSimmons' approaches.

In contrast to the above, Wyatt and Herzan (1962) do report outcome data on their approach to psychotherapy with stuttering children. While not rigorous by today's standards, the data-oriented approach is impressive for its time. Wyatt and Herzan's treatment was based on their belief that stuttering is the product of a child's conflict between anger at his mother (for the inevitable separation between mother and child) and fear of further separation. The child's anger is supposedly suppressed because of this fear. Wyatt and Herzan's treatment was carried out by speech pathologists under the advice of a child psychotherapist. The aims were to foster free expression of feeling. While the child was learning to cope with previously unexpressed feelings, impulses, and wishes, the mother was undergoing counseling. She was learning to be aware of, and accept, her feelings. The expression of feelings and acceptance of them was then transferred to the mother-child relationship. The goal of treatment was achieved when the child could feel safe in expressing anger, as the mother learned to accept the anger without feeling threatened.

As additional tools of therapy, Wyatt (1969) also encouraged (a) use of short, simple sentences in talking to the child, (b) setting aside time each day for the mother and child to be alone, and (c) a passive style of interaction on the part of the therapist or mother so that time pressure on the child would be reduced. These latter three aspects of Wyatt's therapy are not uncommon in other indirect therapy strategies. Two of them, the use of short sentences and reduction in time pressure, do not appear to derive directly from the stated goals of psychotherapy. It is problematic, therefore, to attribute improvement in Wyatt's clients simply to psychotherapy. Wyatt's treatment outcome data are difficult to interpret, even apart from contamination by other treatment effects besides psychotherapy.

In their report of treatment outcome, Wyatt and Herzan (1962) present the results of the above treatment for 20 children, discussed as a younger group (12 children, ages 2-6) and an older group (8 children, ages 8-15). The younger children received from 4 to 14 treatment sessions, whereas the older, more confirmed stuttering children received from 10 to 33 sessions. Children were dismissed from treatment "whenever the child had shown normal speech over a period of several months" (p. 650). Evaluation was done at the end of the school year in which the child was treated and again in October of the following school year. Of the 12 children in the younger group, 10 showed marked improvement or spoke with normal fluency. Of the 8 children in the older group, 5 showed marked improvement or a return to normal speech. Elsewhere, Wyatt (1969) has reported that children who were unimproved (in this case, 5 of the 20 children) seemed to be living in family situations which were "emotionally unhealthy" or had high, long-standing stress.

Despite the relatively good success rate (15 markedly improved out of 20), no further study of these techniques has been reported. This apparent lack of interest may be due to the relatively demanding nature of this type of treatment. Few school therapists have the training or time to carry out psychotherapy with both parent and child for 45 minute sessions. Moreover, there is no hard evidence that Wyatt's aggression-anxiety hypothesis about stuttering is valid and that psychotherapy is, therefore, needed.

Drug Therapy

Essentially, there have been no major advances recently in the use of drugs to treat stuttering. An earlier report (Gattuso & Leocata, 1962) on the use of drug *haloperidol* with children had held out some hope. These workers suggested that 80% of the stuttering children treated had completely recovered after a month of treatment. After this optimistic assessment, other workers (Cozzo & Gabrielli, 1965; Prins, Mandelkorn, & Cerf, 1974; Rantala & Petri-Larmi, 1976; Tapia, 1969) followed with studies which examined the effects of haloperidol on both children and adults. This second wave of studies cautiously suggested that some patients showed marked improvement, while many did not. Bloodstein's (1981) summary table of the results of treatment highlights the fact that of all therapy categories, drug therapy has the fewest follow-up measures. Long term benefits after haloperidol treatment is terminated are a particularly valid concern because extended use of the drug is contraindicated by its unpleasant side effects.[1]

Control of Nonspeech Behavior

A relatively recent approach to indirect stuttering treatment is aimed at deviant nonspeech behaviors. Wahler, Sperling, Thomas, Teeter, and Luper (1970) demonstrated that when two sets of parents were taught to control undesirable nonspeech behaviors of their children, the children's stuttering decreased both in the clinic and at home. For one child the target of treatment was "oppositional behavior. " (The child regularly would not follow parental instructions and requests.) For the other child, the targets of modification were constant shifts of activity from one enterprise to another. The researchers point out that although the stuttering decreased concomitantly with the decreases in deviant behaviors, analysis did not show stuttering and deviant behaviors to be linked by stimulus control. Moments of stuttering were not inadvertently directly manipulated by the contingencies delivered for the deviant behaviors. Thus, some third set of variables seems to have been common to both. Luper (Note 1) suggests that the decrease in stuttering may have resulted from the more relaxed, cooperative atmosphere that developed between parent and child once the parents felt they could control their child's behavior. It would be interesting to find out if the behavioral change would work in the other direction. If aspects of the parental behavior critical to maintaining stuttering could be isolated and changed, would the undesirable nonspeech behaviors change as well?

This focus on nonspeech behaviors in stuttering initiated by Wahler et al. has been incorporated into a treatment plan for mild stutterers by Zwitman (1978). The overall aim of Zwitman's approach is to develop consistency in the day-to-day parent-child interaction. Such consistency would seem to do much toward influencing that "third set of variables" alluded to above, which may control both misbehavior and stuttering. The steps in this treatment plan include teaching the parent ways to (1) react to disfluency, (2) improve the child's self-concept and security, and (3) react to misbehavior.

Zwitman's book is designed to be used by clinicians who meet with parents in a group over a period of several weeks. Parents learn new ways of behaving by completing questionnaires and checklists and discussing these in the group. Traditional "parent counseling" suggestions (improving listening skills, structuring conversation in the home to lessen verbal competition, being generous with praise and reassurance) are combined with behavioral management. Parents are taught to respond to misbehaviors by expressing their feelings promptly and using time-out when necessary. Parents are encouraged to give the child clear-cut responsibilities in the home, and to reinforce desirable behavior consistently. Such a broad-spectrum approach, well-structured for step-wise learning, appears to have a good chance of succeeding. Unfortunately, this approach has yet to be systematically researched. Obviously, it is likely that some aspects of this approach are more effective than others. The meetings between parents and clinicians, where feelings are identified and accepted, may be the most powerful aspect of this program. Or, the imposition of a consistent approach to parent-child interactions may be the key. It is also possible that none of this treatment has any positive effect on the speech of the stuttering child. As yet, we don't know.

Language Oriented Approaches

Several studies have suggested that the language development of stuttering or highly disfluent children may be delayed (Andrews & Harris, 1974; Berry, 1938; Kline & Starkweather, 1979; Morley, 1957; Muma, 1971; Murray & Reed, 1977; Wall, 1980; Westby, 1979). There is also evidence that as nonstuttering children are learning new linguistic forms, normal disfluency tends to increase (Colburn, Note 2; Hall, 1977). In light of these findings, a case could be made that stuttering is an outgrowth of difficulty in language acquisition. There are also reports in the literature suggesting that a specific subgroup of stutterers is characterized by language disability (Riley & Riley, 1979; Van Riper, 1982). As evidence of language problems in stutterers accumulates, clinicians are naturally becoming interested in indirect approaches to stuttering which focus on language. There are as yet, however, few published accounts of language-oriented therapy for young stutterers.

Meryl Wall and her colleague Florence Meyers have initiated some language-oriented treatment, following the lead provided by Wall's (1980) finding that a group of stuttering children showed delayed syntax development, compared to their normal peers. Their recent work (Meyers & Wall, 1982; Wall & Meyers, Note 3) has explored ways in which psycholinguistic, psychosocial, and physiological influences on stuttering can be explored in diagnosis and treatment. The psychosocial aspect of their approach employs parent counseling and modeling to help parents reduce social pressures on the child. The physiologic component is used especially when direct treatment is indicated. This component teaches the child loose articulatory contacts, gentle phonatory onsets, and other aspects of "easier talking" similar to Williams (1971) and Dell (1979).

Wall and Meyers combine psycholinguistic information with parent counseling to teach parents ways in which their use of language can facilitate their child's fluency. Slower speaking rate, simpler syntax and semantics, use of open-ended questions, and verbal facilitation of story telling are some of the changes in parent speech and language which may be taught. Meyers and Wall also make use of psycholinguistic principles in their play therapy. They advocate a low-structure situation in which the clinician begins by evoking only brief and syntactially simple responses from the child, gradually working up to more complex responses. As they point out, it is as though the GILCU program (Ryan, 1974) were applied to spontaneous speech. Wall and Meyers' approach combines many techniques from a variety of sources, but is unique in the authors' strong linguistic orientation.

No measurement of treatment effectiveness is yet available, but they have begun to collect data on outcome. Although Meyers and Wall's multifaceted approach may prove beneficial to many children, analysis of the effects of the various components may turn out to be ticklish, if not unmanageable. Analysis of the component contributions is an issue on which all clinical researchers may not agree. Some may be content to know how effective a broad-spectrum approach can be, while others may not be content until they know the relative contributions to successful outcome of each subcomponent. Contributions to knowledge regarding theoretical and treatment issues on the role of language variables in the genesis and management of stuttering, however, cannot accrue from this work unless the effect of the language component of treatment is sorted out from the psychological counseling and motor learning treatments that are occurring concurrently.

The indirect treatment strategies used by Riley and Riley (1983) contain a substantial linguistic/cognitive component (although other aspects are addressed, also). At intake, the Rileys evaluate stuttering children in 4 disability categories: (1) attending, (2) oral motor discoordination, (3) auditory processing, and (4) sentence formulation. The children's home environments are examined for 2 potential stressors: (5) communicative stress, and (6) unrealistic parental expectations. A portion of treatment focuses on improving the child's abilities in any of the first 4 disability categories in which the child is found to be weak. Some commercially available materials (e.g., Semel, 1976) are available for some of these categories; others are remediated with the Rileys' own programs. Parent counseling, with the help of *If Your Child Stutters: A Guide for Parents* (Ainsworth & Gruss, 1981) is used to reduce stresses in the environment. In many cases, these indirect strategies are supplemented with direct stuttering modification (using, for example, response contingent stimulation).

Results from the Rileys' treatment (Note 4) have been evaluated for 16 of 19 children, ages 3-9, who were treated using both the Rileys' indirect and direct treatments. Data indicate that for the entire group of 19 children, Stuttering Severity Instrument (SSI) (Riley, 1972) scores were reduced by

57% using the indirect approaches described above to modify contributing and maintaining factors. SSI scores were then reduced an additional 30% using direct stuttering modification. Sixteen of the 19 children were assessed at least 24 months after treatment. Seven were "entirely free" of stuttering, 7 were "almost free" of stuttering, and 2 had regressed. If the "almost free" stutterers are counted as successes, the Riley's combined direct and indirect approach was successful with 88% of the children in the group studied.

Nelson's (Note 5) approach to indirect stuttering treatment also contains a strong psycholinguistic component. In her initial conference with parents, Nelson encourages them to become aware of how their child's fluency varies with a number of psycholinguistic factors. These factors include:

1. abstractness of the topic talked about;
2. immediacy of the event discussed;
3. complexity and familiarity of the language used; and
4. communicative intent of the child's utterances.

Two other nonlinguistic factors which may affect the child's fluency are also brought to the parents' attention:

1. excitement level of the speaking situation;
2. competitiveness of the speaking situation.

In addition to engaging the parents in keeping a log of potential influences on their child's fluency, Nelson also observes the parent-child interaction herself. She notes that the following communicative and psycholinguistic pressures are apt to be placed on the child by the parents via their speech: (a) directing the child's activity, (b) trying to evoke display of child's knowledge, (c) speaking rapidly, (d) using long, complex sentences, and (e) asking about an earlier event.

Nelson's treatment approach is to help the parents—through advising them, modeling for them, and having them practice—decrease some of the above-mentioned communicative pressures on the child. Since this treatment focuses on the nature of the parents' speech and language which is directed toward the child, it can be considered a language-oriented treatment, but it also rings of the earlier-described parent counseling treatment philosophies. The following items are a sample of the ways in which parents would be encouraged to change their own speech and language:

1. slow speech rate—to give the child extra language formulation time as the child's speech rate is developed;
2. no demands for display speech—to lessen demands on memory and language formulation;

3. reduce questions—to reduce social and linguistic pressure on the child;

4. talk in the "here and now" (rather than discussing the past, the future, or abstractions)—to reduce syntactic and conceptual demands;

5. use echo speech (judiciously)—to let the child know his or her message was received;

6. increase attention when the child is talking—to reduce the child's ambivalence about being heard; and

7. speak in simple sentences with many pauses between them (as well as periods of silence during play)—to reduce language comprehension and formulation pressure.

Nelson's treatment approach is to begin with this indirect strategy. If the child does not show some decrease in stuttering in response to 3 weeks of indirect treatment, Nelson uses direct treatment as well (see Nelson, Note 5). Nelson's data indicate that for 7 children (average age, 3; 7), treated with her indirect approach alone and followed up for longer than 6 months postdiagnosis, the outcomes were as follows: 4 children (2 severe, 1 moderate, and 1 mild at diagnosis) were 100% fluent; 1 child (mild) was 90% fluent; 1 child (mild) was 75% fluent; 1 child (mild) was 50% fluent. Of the 7 children, 4 were evaluated at follow-up by the clinician and 3 by parents.

It appears that psycholinguistic approaches are now being explored by an increasing number of clinicians. This may be a particularly productive area, especially in relation to the onset of stuttering. There are, however, many complexities involved in accounting for cause-effect relationships among these variables. Changing one environmental variable (such as parent speech rate, complexity of utterance, or extent of questioning) can affect the child's stuttering in many ways. Changing these variables can physically relax the child, can give a slow mechanism more time to coordinate, and can unburden an overtaxed cognitive capacity. The research-minded clinician, while pleased if such a treatment promotes change in stuttering clients, may be dismayed at the difficulty of knowing which variables are related to success with which children. The contribution of language treatment to therapy outcome may be best assessed when conventional language therapy appropriate to the child is administered alone for a period with a serious effort given to limiting the effects of other treatment variables. Alternatively, a conventional language therapy component may be delivered to a group of child stutterers in the context of another (stuttering) treatment approach, and the long-term outcome compared to that of a similar group who get essentially the same treatment without language therapy. This would assume that both of these groups of children would be assessed as needing some language oriented remediation.

Parent-Child Interaction

First described by Egolf, Shames, Johnson, and Kasprisin-Burelli (1972), parent-child interaction therapy for stuttering seeks to train parents in new ways of talking to their children. This treatment examines parent-child interactions in the clinic. Treatment then focuses on changing neither responses to stuttering, nor management of behavior, but the content and style of the parent-child interaction on the part of the parent. Egolf and his coworkers (Kasprisin-Burelli, Egolf, & Shames, 1972) first demonstrated that parents of stuttering children talked more "negatively" to their children than parents of nonstutterers. Clinicians then modeled for parents a positive, accepting way of interacting. This style produced a greatly reduced frequency of stuttering in the child. Parents then adopted this style of interaction themselves and it was found (in 5 of 9 cases) that their children maintained reduced frequency and severity of stuttering several months after treatment was over. Unfortunately, no data were available to demonstrate the extent to which each parent and clinician changed his or her behavior.

In this study, a relatively large range of positive interactions were modeled for parents. These included: (a) reward and praise for verbal output, (b) attentive listening, (c) open discussion of feelings, especially about stuttering, and (d) noninterruption, among others. Although most of the interactions modeled for the parents were generally more positive and accepting, clinicians tailored their responses to the individual parent-child dyad. That is, the clinicians assessed the parents' style of interacting and modeled an opposite style. This approach probably allowed for individual variations in children's needs to be met more specifically.

Following the lead of Egolf and his associates, Guitar, Kopff, Kilburg, and Conway (Note 6) have also experimented with treatment focused on parent-child interactions. In a single case study, they explored the use of videotaped parent-child play sessions as a stimulus for treatment. The child in this study was a 5-year-old girl whose stuttering frequency at diagnosis was 9.4% syllables stuttered and whose speech rate was 74 syllables per minute. Her blocks were accompanied by eye blinks, facial tension, sighing, head movements, and momentarily stopped articulatory postures. In each therapy session, one of the girl's parents would view new tapes of his or her previous play session with the child. The other parent would experiment with new styles of interaction while being videotaped in play with the child. After several weeks the child became normally fluent and has stayed fluent for 5 years. Posttreatment analysis of the parent-child interactions reveal that as the child gradually became fluent, the parents were changing many aspects of their behavior.

Initial analysis of the tapes indicated that decreases in the mother's speech rate were highly correlated with decreases in the child's stuttering. An analysis of the child's stuttering, which considered primary stuttering separately from secondary stuttering, indicated that primary stuttering appeared more highly correlated with speech rate changes, but secondary stuttering (tension, awareness, avoidance behaviors) was more highly correlated with the proportion of positive, accepting statements in the mother's conversation.

Although this type of treatment and analysis appear to have promise for evaluating and changing factors related to the child's stuttering, a finer-grained examination of the relevant variables should be undertaken. The gross categories of parent speech rate or parental acceptance need to be broken down further. Speech rate includes not only the rate at which sounds are spoken, but also the lengths of pauses between words and phrases (Nelson, Note 5; Starkweather, Note 7, Williams, Note 8). Moreover, as speech rate slows, other aspects of parent behavior may change. Parents may slow their general movements, as well. They may speak with a different voice quality and lower fundamental frequency. There are also myriad changes that may accompany increases in the proportion of parents' positive, accepting statements. They may include changes in body language and vocal inflection. Clinicians are only just beginning careful analysis of those aspects of parent behavior that influence their children's fluency. Perhaps a better understanding of them will lead to better indirect approaches to treatment. Future case studies of this type should also explore the use of single subject designs (e.g., McReynolds & Kearns, 1982) which may permit us to understand the cause-effect relationships between parent behavior and stuttering changes.

Psychomotor Therapy

This review of indirect stuttering therapies leaves out many treatments used abroad because English translations of treatment descriptions are not generally available. Recently, however, a description of some psychomotor strategies used in Europe has become available in English (Versteegh-Vermeij, Note 9). A number of therapists for stutterers in Europe, particularly in the Low Countries, have been experimenting with treatment focused on awareness of body posture, movement, and other aspects of the physical self. This work is an extension of a number of psychomotor therapies which view psychosomatic disorders as the result of emotional blockages. Elizabeth Versteegh-Vermeij, a well known therapist in The Netherlands, has pioneered the use of body-oriented therapy with stuttering children and their parents. In her treatment, parents and children are taught to become aware of the physical feelings of their bodies in isolated movements and then in movements which involve physical touching with others. Versteegh-Vermeij encourages children to develop physical confidence and free, full physical movement in parent-child groups. Her observation is that children (and adults) who gained acceptance and awareness of their physical selves were able not only to make substantial changes in their stuttering, but maintained their fluency after treatment. European therapists do not tend to collect pre- and posttreatment data; consequently, there appears to be little substantiation of the benefit of psychomotor or body-oriented therapies. Clinical researchers in some European stuttering treatment centers are now working to remedy this.

Summary and Conclusions

It is evident, even in this brief account, that the indirect approaches described have much in common. Of the 17 approaches reviewed, 9 advocate encouraging free expression of feeling by the child. Five suggest slowed speech rates by parents and 5 advise parents to increase their attentiveness when their child is speaking. Four encourage clear, firm disciplinary rules, and 3 indicate that parents' use of simple language in their conversation would be helpful. These are timeless remedies; they have probably been suggested for parents for decades. It is noteworthy, though, that all of the suggestions would probably be very beneficial to the nonstuttering as well as to the stuttering child. Thus, most of these approaches are not likely to make a stutterer worse or hurt a misdiagnosed nonstuttering talker. It is our impression, however, that these suggestions (as well as others) are not easy for parents to follow. Busy parents with many more immediate concerns are likely to need a great deal more than suggestions. Hence, programs like those of Zwitman (1978) and of Egolf and his coworkers (1972), which specifically train parents in desired behaviors, seem, on the face of it, more likely to succeed.

But how are we to know which programs do succeed? Recent contributions by Ingham (Ingham & Costello, Chapter 11, this volume; Ingham, Note 10) describe a system of measurement that will allow us to learn a little more about how effective a treatment is. Ingham suggests measuring a child's stuttering (percentage of syllables stuttered and syllables spoken per minute) several times, both in clinic and out, prior to treatment. This provides a baseline of the child's behavior. This measurement, so Ingham advocates, should continue repeatedly during treatment and repeatedly afterwards, for long-term follow-ups, both overt and covert. Although this thoroughness may not be possible for every clinician, careful measurement before and repeated careful measurement after treatment seems a minimum if we are to understand how effective various therapies or their components are.

However, assessment of stuttering frequency and speech rate may not provide enough to determine appropriate treatment. Curlee (1980), in his review of therapy for children, suggests use of direct treatment for those stutterers who show 3 "danger signs, " and an indirect approach for those who don't. Thus, if we are to follow Curlee's advice, we need to find ways of assessing these 3 danger signs: (1) struggling during disfluencies, (2) fear of stuttering, and (3) perceiving speech as a handicap. If these danger signs are related to potential for recovery, a treatment, direct or indirect, which reduced or eliminated these signs might help substantially. Hence, the need for finding reliable measures of "accessory behaviors, " including fear and avoidance of speech. These measures will help us determine which treatments to use for each client, as well as how effective each treatment is.

Effectiveness of treatment is a particularly difficult issue when indirect treatment is being assessed because of the potential for spontaneous recovery. In his review, Curlee points out that spontaneous recovery data show that 75% to 80% of those individuals who ever stuttered recover without treatment. Thus, a tough-minded view would be that if an indirect treatment is doing anything at all, more than 75% of all stutterers treated should recover. Of the 17 treatments described in our review, only 6 provided data on outcome. Two of these, Wahler et al. (1970) and Guitar et al. (Note 6), were essentially single subject studies. They cannot be evaluated as recommended general treatment strategies or considered tests of treatment effectiveness until they have been replicated on more subjects. The Rileys' approach showed a 57% decrease in symptoms via indirect treatment. However, since these children were severe enough to be given direct in addition to indirect treatment, a comparison of their overall outcome (88% of the children appear to have substantially recovered) with other indirect treatments is inappropriate here.

A comparison of the remaining treatments with the spontaneous recovery data must take into account Curlee's (1980) observation that some of the recovered stutterers in the spontaneous recovery literature still stutter in some situations. When we evaluate the reports of Wyatt and Herzan (1962), Egolf et al. (1972), and Nelson (Note 5), we might assume that "substantially improved" stutterers in 2 of these reports are comparable to the "recovered stutterers" in Curlee's figures. In Nelson's report it is a moot point as to whether both the 90% fluent and the 75% fluent (measured at follow-up) children should be called "recovered stutterers." So we would ask, then, how do these 3 remaining reports stack up against a 75% spontaneous recovery rate? Wyatt and Herzan's data indicate that 75% of their clients recovered. In the Egolf et al. study, only enough data were available to show that 55% recovered. Nelson's data can be interpreted to suggest that either 86% or 71% of her clients recovered. The tough-minded critic would wonder if most of these treatments are accomplishing anything at all.

In our view, this comparison of treatment outcome with 75% spontaneous recovery is unduly harsh on indirect therapies. After all, indirect therapies usually treat stutterers who are severe enough to be of concern to their parents. Many of the spontaneously recovered stutterers probably were not that severe. Moreover, some of the 75% spontaneously recovered stutterers may have been unwitting benefactors of indirect treatments. They may have never known it, because their parents never told them. Recent reviews of the spontaneous recovery literature have also lowered this figure of 75%. Ingham (1983), for example, suggests that for younger children, spontaneous recovery rates may be closer to 50%. Even this 50% recovery is suspected by Ingham to be contaminated by the effects of formal and informal treatment attempts, making recovery not truly "spontaneous."

Despite these doubts, the point must still be made that advocates of indirect treatment have not yet provided data showing that most indirect treatments are more effective than no treatment at all. This conclusion makes a strong case for multiple pretreatment measures (to show that stutterers are not rapidly recovering on their own) and/or control groups of children who are not treated. These control measures are invaluable in showing treatment effectiveness. To be effective, treatments need only demonstrate that treated children improve substantially more than if they were untreated for the same period of time. Even if the untreated children would eventually spontaneously recover, they may be needlessly undergoing years of stuttering. Many adults who have recovered spontaneously in their teen-age years speak with fear and loathing of their childhood stuttering traumas.

How are we to improve treatments? Clinician-researchers are becoming curious about what components of a treatment approach are helpful. This curiosity may lead directly to more effective, more focused treatments. Clinicians are exploring such things as which child-speech variables change when parent behaviors are manipulated. One aspect of this research is analysis of clinician-child or parent-child interactions in natural therapy environments. This will lead toward understanding which particular adult variables seem to be related (directly or indirectly) to a child's stuttering.

This can suggest which, if any, adult variables might be changed to decrease stuttering. Williams (Note 8) discusses some work which deals in this way with rate variables. This work is difficult because it may take considerable training for an adult to change, for example, one speech rate variable (e.g., pause time) without changing another (e.g., articulation rate). But the payoff for this difficult work is great. Only by such experimental manipulation of discrete variables can we really understand what are the more direct antecedents of improvements in a stuttering child's speech.

In summary, the advances we are seeing in indirect approaches have been a quiet whisper amid the tumult of the same old treatments for stuttering children. But it is hoped, as we see an increase in the cries for accountability, the calls for more data by journal editors, and the availability of funding for treatment research, that clinicians will be examining the subcomponents of their treatments and measuring relevant variables, intent on improving treatment outcome.

End Note

[1] The author once took haloperidol over several weeks, in the interest of science. Fluency improved slightly, but he developed the annoying side effect that the upper half of his body was usually falling asleep, while much of the lower half was in continual, agitated movement.

Reference Notes

1. Luper, H. Personal communication, 1982.

2. Colburn, N. Disfluency behavior and emerging linguistic structures in preschool children. Unpublished doctoral dissertation, Columbia University, 1979.

3. Wall, M., & Meyers, F. *Clinical management of childhood stuttering*. Baltimore: University Park Press, in preparation.

4. Riley, G., & Riley, J. Personal communication, 1982.

5. Nelson, L. Language formulation related to disfluency and stuttering. Paper presented at the Conference on Evaluation of Disfluency, Prevention of Stuttering, and Management of Fluency Problems in Children, Northwestern University, Evanston, Illinois, 1982.

6. Guitar, B., Kopff, B., Kilburg, H., & Conway, P. Parent verbal interaction and speech rate: A case study in stuttering. Paper presented at the Convention of the American Speech-Language-Hearing Association, Los Angeles, 1981.

7. Starkweather, C. W. The development of speech fluency and the definition of a fluency problem. Paper presented at the Conference on Evaluation of Disfluency, Prevention of Stuttering, and Management of Fluency Problems in Children, Northwestern University, Evanston, Illinois, 1982.

8. Williams, D. Emotional and environmental problems in stuttering. Paper presented at the Conference on Evaluation of Disfluency, Prevention of Stuttering, and Management of Fluency Problems in Children, Northwestern University, Evanston, Illinois, 1982.

9. Versteegh-Vermeij, E. Stress and body-oriented therapy. Paper presented at the Speech Foundation of America Conference, St. Petersburg, Florida, 1983.

10. Ingham, R. Evaluation and assessment procedures. Paper presented at the Conference on Evaluation of Disfluency, Prevention of Stuttering, and Management of Fluency Problems in Children, Northwestern University, Evanston, Illinois, 1982.

References

Ainsworth, S., & Gruss, J. F. *If your child stutters—A guide for parents.* Memphis: Speech Foundation of America, 1981.

Andrews, G., & Harris, M. *The syndrome of stuttering.* Clinics in Developmental Medicine, No. 17, London: Spastics Society Medical Education and Information Unit in association with Wm. Heinemann Medical Books, 1964.

Bailey, A. A., & Bailey, W. Workshop on childhood stuttering. Georgia and Tennessee Speech and Hearing Associations Convention, Chattanooga, Tenn., 1977.

Bailey, A. A., & Bailey, W. Workshop on childhood stuttering. Collier County Public Schools, Naples, Florida, 1982.

Berry, M. Developmental history of stuttering children. *Journal of Pediatrics, 1938, 12,* 209-17.

Bloodstein, O. *A handbook on stuttering* (3rd ed.). Chicago: National Easter Seal Society, 1981.

Conture, E. *Stuttering.* Englewood Cliffs, N.J.: Prentice-Hall, 1981.

Cooper, E. *Understanding stuttering.* Chicago: National Easter Seal Society, 1979.

Cozzo, G., & Gabrielli, L. La therapie du begayement avec les butyrophenones. *De Therapia Vocis et Loguelae,* Vol. I. XIII Congress of the International Society of Logopedics and Phoniatry, 1965.

Curlee, R. Assessment and treatment strategies for young stutterers. In L. Bradford & R. Wertz (Eds.), *Communicative disorders: An audio journal for continuing education.* New York: Grune & Stratton, 1980.

Dell, C. *Treating the school-age stutterer: A guide for clinicians.* Memphis: Speech Foundation of America, 1979.

Egolf, D., Shames, G., Johnson, P., & Kasprisin-Burelli, A. The use of parent-child interaction patterns in therapy for young stutterers. *Journal of Speech and Hearing Disorders, 1972, 37,* 222-232.

Gattuso, R., & Leocata, A. L'Haloperidol nella terapia della balbuzie. *Clinical Otorhinolaryngology, 1962, 14,* 227-234.

Hall, P. The occurrence of disfluencies in language-disordered school-age children. *Journal of Speech and Hearing Disorders,* 1977, *42,* 364-369.

Ingham, R. Spontaneous remission of stuttering: When will the emperor realize he has no clothes on? In D. Prins & R. J. Ingham (Eds.), *Treatment of stuttering in early childhood: Methods and issues.* San Diego: College-Hill, 1983.

Kasprisin-Burelli, A., Egolf, D., & Shames, G. A comparison of parental verbal behavior with stuttering and nonstuttering children. *Journal of Communication Disorders,* 1972, *5,* 335-346.

Kernan, M. Starting young is a key to working with stutterers. *Smithsonian,* 1981, *12,* 108-116.

Kline, M., & Starkweather, C. Receptive and expressive language performance in young stutterers. *Asha,* 1979, *21,* 797.

Meyers, F., & Wall, M. Toward an integrated approach to early childhood stuttering. *Journal of Fluency Disorders,* 1982, *7,* 47-54.

Morley, M. *The development and disorders of speech in childhood.* Edinburgh: Livingstone, 1957.

Muma, J. Syntax of preschool fluent and disfluent speech: A transformational analysis. *Journal of Speech and Hearing Research,* 1971, *14,* 428-41.

Murphy, A., & FitzSimmons, R. *Stuttering and personality dynamics*. New York: Ronald Press, 1960.

Murray, H., & Reed, C. Language abilities of preschool stuttering children. *Journal of Fluency Disorders*, 1977, *2*, 171-176,

Prins, D., Mandelkorn, T., & Cerf, A. Effects of haloperidol upon stuttering. *Asha*, 1974, *17*, 508.

McReynolds, L., & Kearns, K. *Single-subject experimental designs*. Baltimore: University Park, 1982.

Rantala, S. - L., & Petri-Larmi, M. Haloperidol (Serenase) in the treatment of stuttering. *Folia Phoniatrica,* 1976, *28,* 354-361.

Riley, G. A stuttering severity instrument for children and adults. *Journal of Speech and Hearing Disorders*, 1972, *37*, 314-321.

Riley, G., & Riley, J. A component model for diagnosing and treating children who stutter. *Journal of Fluency Disorders*, 1979, *4*, 279-293.

Riley, G., & Riley, J. Evaluation as a basis for intervention. In D. Prins and R. Ingham (Eds.), *Treatment of stuttering in early childhood*, San Diego, CA: College-Hill, 1983.

Ryan, B. *Programmed therapy for stuttering in children and adults*. Springfield, Ill: Charles C. Thomas, 1974.

Semel, E. *Semel Auditory Processing Program*. Chicago: Follet Educational Publishing, 1976.

Tapia, F. Haldol in the treatment of children with tics and stutterers—and an incidental finding. *Psychiatry Quarterly*, 1969, *43*, 647-649.

Van Riper, C. *The treatment of stuttering*. Englewood Cliffs, N.J.: Prentice-Hall, 1973.

Van Riper, C. *The nature of stuttering* (2nd ed.). Englewood Cliffs, N.J.: Prentice-Hall, 1982.

Wahler, R., Sperling, K., Thomas, M., Teeter, N., & Luper, H. The modification of childhood stuttering: Some response-response relationships. *Journal of Experimental Child Psychology*, 1970, *9*, 411-428.

Wall, M. A comparison of syntax in young stutterers and nonstutterers. *Journal of Fluency Disorders*, 1980, *5*, 321-326.

Westby, C. Language performance of stuttering and nonstuttering children. *Journal of Communication Disorders*, 1979, *12*, 133-145.

Williams, D. Stuttering therapy for children. In L. E. Travis (Ed.), *Handbook of speech pathology*. New York: Appleton-Century-Crofts, 1971.

Wyatt, G. *Language learning and communication disorders in children*. New York: Free Press, 1969.

Wyatt, G., & Herzan, H. Therapy with stuttering children and their mothers. *American Journal of Orthopsychiatry, 1962, 23*, 645-59.

Zwitman, D. *The disfluent child*. Baltimore: University Park Press, 1978.

Roger J. Ingham
Janis M. Costello*

Stuttering Treatment Outcome Evaluation

Although researchers in stuttering find few areas of agreement, it would seem that today all agree about the importance of systematic measurement in the evaluation of stuttering treatment outcomes. And they would probably agree that over the past decade the management and evaluation of stuttering therapy has been improved by increasing use of measurement methodology. Much of the methodology that has begun to emerge in reports on stuttering therapy is almost wholly attributable to the pervasive influence of behavior therapy principles on stuttering treatment research (Costello, 1982; Ingham, 1983). What researchers still do not agree upon, however, would appear to be the certainty with which current measurement methods adequately account for the constructs implicated in the notion of therapy success or failure. Further, there is no evidence that the measurement methodology described in stuttering research reports has yet invaded the realm of clinical practice (Costello, 1979). The general purpose of this chapter, therefore, will be to offer some considerations on the problems of stuttering treatment outcome evaluation. These considerations will be in two parts: (1) a review of the principal issues in stuttering treatment evaluation, and (2) derivation of a viable clinical format that will assist clinicians and researchers to identify effects of treatment. Both parts will endeavor to identify some of the more important recent developments in the evaluation of stuttering treatment outcome.

*This chapter was prepared while Dr. Costello was Foundation Fellow at Cumberland College of Health Sciences, Sydney.

Stuttering Treatment Evaluation Issues

The clinical validity of the measures and treatment evaluation strategies used in stuttering treatment reports continues to concern researchers and clinicians alike (Gregory, 1978; Sheehan, 1980). Much of this concern can be traced to the absence of agreed upon criteria for evaluating therapy. Some attempts have been made to resolve this problem (Andrews & Ingham, 1972; Ingham, 1981; Ryan, 1974; Silverman, 1981), but none has produced commonly accepted methods for determining the clinical merit of stuttering therapy. Some of the issues that need to be resolved before acceptance is likely were recently summarized by Bloodstein (1981, pp. 386-390). He presented 11 criteria that he believes need to be considered when evaluating stuttering therapy. In what follows, these criteria will be presented (mainly in abridged form) and reviewed for their contribution to the search for clinically suitable measurement methods [2]. This will also provide a useful vehicle for reviewing some recent developments in therapy outcome evaluation.

> *1.   The method must be shown to be effective with an ample and representative group of stutterers. The single-subject design has a place in scientific research. It has been widely misused, however, in the area of research on stuttering therapy, where most single cases written up for publication are apparently chosen for the precise reason that they were successes. This practice produces a distorted picture. In the end we learn little from it beyond what we already know—that somewhere, at sometime almost any therapy can achieve a remarkable result for some stutterers.*

This is not only a criterion, but a recommendation that therapy evaluation should not depend on single-subject research. This is an important recommendation since it challenges the worth of single-subject therapy research designs. Actually the point at issue is the external validity of these designs. Single-subject research designs entered therapy research for a variety of reasons; foremost was the failure of group designs to identify critical aspects of the clinical process (Hersen & Barlow, 1976). Since group trends usually fail to reflect individual treatment response patterns, they also fail to discern the treatment's differential effects on certain individuals and, hence, themselves do not answer Bloodstein's first criterion. Quite obviously, single-subject studies can only show that a treatment has produced some profitable (or unprofitable) results for some stutterers; but that is far from a trivial finding, particularly if the study is internally valid and clearly specifies the treatment's effects. Furthermore, when such findings are replicated on additional subjects, then they not only increase the generality of the findings as Bloodstein would wish, but also strengthen our knowledge about a treatment and highlight relevant considerations for the design of subsequent group studies.

Regarding the concern about reporting only successful treatments, it is worth noting that this tradition probably permeates group research as much as single-subject research.

In the continuing struggle to find reliable treatments, there is increasing evidence that carefully managed time-series investigations are markedly improving clinical knowledge. Bloodstein's claim that a method must be effective across "representative" stutterers may, unwittingly, subscribe to the "uniformity assumption myth" (Kiesler, 1966)—the notion that there should be a uniform treatment suitable for a uniform client. Even treatment techniques promoted as useful for most stutterers, notably the prolonged speech procedures (Andrews, Guitar, & Howie, 1980), have benefited from controlled single-subject investigations (Ingham, 1983).

> 2. *Results must be demonstrated by objective measures of speech behavior such as frequency of stuttering or rate of speech, and by judges' ratings of severity. Such measurements should be made before, during, and after treatment by observers other than the experimenters themselves or without knowledge that might influence their judgment, and due account must be taken of the observers' reliability.*

There are two aspects to this criterion: the types of measures and their reliability. The first refers mainly to the construct validity of measures currently used to assess stuttering behavior. Frequency counts of stuttering and, to a lesser extent, ratings of stuttering severity have become almost *the* descriptive datum for this disorder. Significantly, Bloodstein recommends counts of stutterings, rather than measures of *disfluencies* or *dysfluencies*. Also of interest is the absence of reference to different disfluency categories, a method of measuring stuttering that seems to have faded in its use in treatment. Severity ratings present a number of problems, mainly because there is no agreed-upon method for rating severity. The principal purpose of severity ratings during treatment is to ensure that frequency reduction is not offset by worsening severity. One common method for determining severity is to measure the duration of individual moments of stuttering (Costello, 1981; Costello & Ingham, in press). The difficulty with this measure is that it, too, may lack construct validity, for duration may not be the feature that clinicians or clients regard as stuttering's severity. Speech rate measures, though essential to show that treatment benefits are not simply due to reduced rate, are questionable for similar reasons. At best, syllables per minute (Andrews & Ingham, 1972) or articulation rate scores (Perkins, 1975) only broadly indicate whether the subject is speaking unnaturally fast or slow. And for this reason, there may also be merit in supplementing this measure with perceptual judgments of the naturalness of the subject's speech (see below).

The importance of observer reliability is seemingly self-evident—yet that does not seem to be true for many researchers. A staggering number of treatment reports and experimental studies fail to report relevant reliability data (Ingham, 1983)—a fact that destroys the credibility of much of the current treatment literature. Even when reliability data are provided, they are rarely reported in a way which makes it possible to determine whether a study's reported data trends are also reliable (Hawkins & Dotson, 1975; McReynolds & Kearns, 1982).

One other issue concerns the methods used to obtain stuttering counts and speech rate. There is now a growing body of evidence that clinicians can capably count both of these variables "on line" and reliably (Ingham, 1983).

> *3. Reports of therapeutic success must be based on repeated evaluations and adequate samples of speech. The great variability of stuttering from time to time and under different conditions is liable to result in assessments that are unrepresentative.*

This criterion is simple to justify, but less simple to prescribe. It is unclear how frequently such evaluations should be made, or what represent adequate samples of speech. Repeated evaluation helps determine whether the variability within and between speaking situations has been unambiguously and significantly modified by treatment. This means that the duration of evaluation cannot always be standardized across individuals—a source of difficulty for the use of group designs in therapy research. The same issue applies to sample size, although there is increasing acceptance of a method used by Ryan (1971; 1974)—that is, 5-minute samples of conversation, monologue, and oral reading. However, the sufficiency and representativeness of this, or any other arbitrarily determined sampling interval, is currently undocumented.

One attempt to derive a methodology that prescribes minimal frequency and sample size parameters will be outlined below. But this attempt is also hindered by the impoverished amount of research into stuttering variability across situations—a surprising circumstance in view of developments in recording technology. The problems involved in recording stuttering in "natural" circumstances have also received insufficient attention (Ingham, 1981). However, the advent of portable microcassette recorders should make it possible to obtain adequate speech samples in representative speaking situations.

The method of choosing "representative" speaking situations has also received very little attention in the treatment literature. One obvious method is to derive these situations from speaking log books prepared by the subject in advance of the treatment study; this would help identify situations that can be regularly used for assessment.

Most treatment research presumes that stuttering variability is largely affected by situational factors. Those may not be the only factors involved. Another feature of variability can be a tendency for time factors to influence variability (Ingham, 1981). The duration of time the subject spends speaking in certain situations, or even the time of day assessments are made, might be worthy areas of investigation.

4. Improvement must be shown to carry over to
speaking situations outside the clinical setting.

This is much related to Criterion 3. Most clinicians are aware that vast differences may occur between clinic and extraclinic speech performance, but evidence showing this difference is surprisingly small. Studies by Ingham and Packman (1977), Resick, Wendiggensen, Ames, and Meyer (1978), and Ingham (1982) go some way towards illustrating this criterion's importance.

Another interesting consideration is the boundary of the "clinical setting." The mere presence of a tape recorder or an assessor in the subject's nonclinic setting may evoke clinic-related speech performance (Ingham, 1981). For example, subjects may be assessed via telephone conversations from home or elsewhere, but the accompanying "assessment variables" may make these telephone conversations atypical (see Ingham, 1981; 1982). The only available solution to this problem would seem to be some form of occasional covert assessment.

5. The stability of the results must be demonstrated
by long-term follow-up investigations. Any number
of methods for making stuttering disappear have been

*known for many years: the great and persistent prob-
lem of stuttering therapy is how to keep the stutterer
from relapsing. Relatively little is known about the
subject of relapse.*

Long-term therapy investigations are becoming more common, despite
their technical and conceptual difficulties; not the least of these is the length
of time needed to prove that treatment has produced a durable improvement. Some of the issues associated with maintenance of treatment effects
have been discussed elsewhere (Ingham, 1981) and will be taken up again
later in this chapter.

Bloodstein (1981) suggests that "perhaps eighteen months to two years
is the shortest interval after which most experienced clinicians would not
feel unduly optimistic in hoping that the improvement was lasting" (p. 387).
But their optimism should be tempered by information on what has transpired
in that period. Many current treatment programs incorporate strategies for
preventing relapse. These include speech practice, routine clinic visits, and
continuing interaction with previously treated patients. These may be useful
and even crucial techniques for sustaining improvement, but they may also
confound the most clinically desirable effect—sustained improvement with
the same level of attention to speech that is used by normal speakers. That
is not to deny the advantages of "aided" maintenance; it simply suggests
that clinicians should recognize that there are different types of sustained
improvement. Needless to say, this topic is in dire need of investigation.

Increasing attention is being devoted to both the measurement and management of maintenance (Boberg, 1981). There may be some value in "booster"
treatments, and in treatment schedules designed to sustain treatment gains
for increasingly longer intervals. Another interesting area of treatment research
concerns the use of self-management techniques. There are also numerous
suggested approaches to maintenance that need investigation (Boberg, Howie,
& Woods, 1979; Hanna & Owen, 1977; Ingham, 1981; Shames, 1981). These
mainly include self-help groups, regular speech practice schedules, and the
assistance of "significant others. " A large number of other, ostensibly useful,
approaches have been reviewed by Stokes and Baer (1977).

One aspect of relapse that has attracted attention is the stutterer's attitude
towards communication at the end of treatment. The problem of devising
valid measures of attitudes and the shaky foundations of research claiming that poor communication attitudes influence long-term outcome are
current concerns (Guitar, 1979, 1981; Guitar & Bass, 1978; Ingham, 1979,
1981; Ulliana & Ingham, in press). Nevertheless, it is highly likely that persons
who show little interest in sustaining speech practice or fulfilling treatment
requirements will be strong candidates for posttreatment relapse. The complex

factors that enjoin patients to seek treatment, wait lengthy periods for treatment to begin, and then complete its often demanding requirements deserve much more research attention. It may well emerge that these are among the most important variables in the success, or otherwise, of the treatment process.

> 6. *Suitable control groups or control conditions must be used to show that reductions in stuttering are the result of treatment.*

This criterion highlights the need for treatment designs that overcome threats to their internal validity. The advantage of the within-subject time-series designs (Hersen & Barlow, 1976) is that the effect of most nontreatment-related variables can be identified by the judicious choice of a baserate(s) duration and measurement conditions. The difficulty is to be certain that all validity threats have been controlled before, during, or even after treatment. For instance, one important nontreatment factor that is rarely controlled is the amount and nature of influence that the client is able to exert over stuttering frequency or severity prior to treatment. Certainly a treatment's effects should be independent of the extent and/or duration of such factors.

Group designs as a control procedure can only partially avoid some of the problems of assessing treatment effects since, as was previously mentioned, most fail to identify individual treatment responses. One compromise is a multiple baseline across subjects design wherein treatment is introduced for each subject following nontreatment baselines of differing lengths. Another difficulty with group designs is the choice of an appropriate control group. The best designed group studies presume that roughly matched group mean stuttering frequency, group mean speech rate, and perhaps age and sex, will ensure that the groups have potentially equivalent reactions to the treatment condition. There are literally no data that justify this assumption of uniformity. Even less defensible is the notion that meaningful findings can be derived by merging the differences between subject groups, treatment management techniques, measurement quality, assessment procedures, and treatment time from different therapy studies; but such are the assumptions beneath the use of the "meta-analysis" (Smith & Glass, 1977) technique that Andrews, Guitar, and Howie (1980) used to draw comparisons between different stuttering treatment techniques.

The inherent weakness of meta-analysis for evaluating the effects of a stuttering therapy should be almost self-evident, but it is clearly revealed by examining the foundations of one of the main conclusions reached by Andrews et al. They concluded "that treatments based on training a stutterer in prolonged speech and gentle onset techniques are superior to other types of treatment" (p. 305). While there is evidence to indicate that prolonged speech treatments are indeed successful for many stutterers, the basis for this claim hinges on an investigation that virtually excluded reference to certain treatment techniques and relied upon extremely questionable post-treatment data from others. By necessity, the meta-analysis technique cannot deal with single-subject studies and so almost all reports on response contingent procedures were excluded from their comparison. (The exception was a study by Martin and Haroldson (1969) which was not designed to evaluate therapy outcome). Also, out of the 12 "prolonged speech" studies included for investigation only two reported using beyond-clinic data, and one of these used an extensive uncontrolled maintenance program in the interval when outcome data were collected (Ingham, 1983). It is little wonder that Eysenck (1978) described this method's concern for data quantity rather than quality as an "exercise in mega-silliness" (p. 517), a concern echoed by Sheehan (1980).

Along with suitable designs for discerning stuttering treatment effects there is also a need for clinically viable designs that determine when treatments are impotent, or are no longer needed because their effects have generalized. These phenomena have been identified in some studies through the use of within-session ABA designs, such as that reported by Costello (1975), or multiple baselines (Martin, Kuhl, & Haroldson, 1972). There is also a need to determine the time required to decide when treatment is *not* effective or, conversely, the changes in performance that indicate clinically significant treatment effects.

> 7. *The subjects' speech must sound natural and spontaneous to listeners, and the subjects must be free from the need to monitor their speech.*

This criterion has grown in importance in recent years because of therapies that rely on changing the client's speech pattern. Some investigators have measured naturalness by using listeners to rate speech samples either for normalcy or naturalness (Jones & Azrin, 1969; Perkins, Rudas, Johnson, Michael, & Curlee, 1974). Others have tested whether listeners are able to distinguish the stutterer's posttreatment speech from speech samples of normally fluent speakers (Ingham & Packman, 1978; Runyan & Adams, 1978, 1979). Another approach measures aspects of speech, such as vowel duration or rate, in order to relate the subject's speech to normal speech (Metz, Onufrak, & Ogburn, 1979). A different approach to this task is emerging from research by Martin (1981; Martin, Haroldson, & Triden, in press), who found that listeners could rate short speech samples for naturalness on a 9-point scale with high levels of reliability. In consequence, Martin and Ingham are investigating the effects on stuttering and speech quality of feeding back to subjects every 30 seconds a listener's speech naturalness rating of the subject's speech. Preliminary results show that clinicians perform this task with high reliability, and that for some stutterers, providing on-line feedback regarding the naturalness of their speech may positively influence their observed speech quality. Similar endeavors have not been made to measure for "spontaneity" but, in principle, there is no reason why listener judgments could not be used for the same purpose.

Regarding the issue of monitoring, Shames and Florance (1980) reported measuring "monitored" and "unmonitored" speech during their treatment program. Their procedure requires speakers to nominate speaking intervals in which either type of speech will be used. Unfortunately, without independent measures of this variable(s), it is difficult to determine whether speakers can manipulate speech monitoring. But, more importantly, it is not clear how much, or what form of monitoring is desirable for normal speech behavior. Related to this is Webster's (1974) attempt to partially evaluate outcome from the Hollins program by asking listeners on follow-up questionnaires to indicate "how much attention must you pay to the task of speaking fluently?" This may help determine whether posttreatment effects oblige speakers to concentrate excessively on their "fluency." These preliminary efforts at measuring for monitoring of speech may have some problems, but, at present, no efforts have been made to measure the spontaneity that Bloodstein believes is necessary for normally fluent speech.

> *8. Treatment must remove not only stuttering, but also the sense of handicap and the person's self concept as a stutterer.*

This type of criterion is often presumed to present a special challenge to treatments that are mainly concerned with modifying or removing stuttering. It is assumed that a "sense of handicap," or a stutterer's "self-concept" are constructs that either retain the problem or are the essence of the problem. And, more significantly, it is assumed that their removal or alteration is necessary to the treatment's success. However, no data have ever shown that changes in stuttering do *not* also influence the "sense of handicap," or change the talker's concept of himself as a talker. That is not to suggest that patterns of behavior associated with stuttering will readily and immediately change when the disorder is modified. It would be rather surprising, for example, if embarrassing or constantly avoided circumstances were suddenly of no concern when stuttering ceases. Again, no data have shown that the persistence of such reactions is essentially abnormal or prevents normal fluency.

Surprisingly, Bloodstein (1981) partly justifies this criterion by referring to Andrews and Cutler's (1974) claim that the removal of stuttering in one situation was not sufficient to change stutterers' attitudes towards speaking. In fact, Andrews and Cutler's data actually show that when treatment was extended to other situations (in the course of a transfer procedure), the attitude scores showed concomitant and favorable changes. This aligns with findings from a subsequent investigation by Ulliana and Ingham (in press) on the attitude scale (S24) used in Andrews and Cutler's study which shows that the scale's scores are probably strongly influenced by the frequency of stuttering that occurs in situations referenced in the scale's items. In other words, it is highly likely that the "attitudinal factors" measured by the S24 are simply correlates of stuttering frequency. There is no reason to expect that a "sense of handicap," or "self-concept," might not also be related to actual stuttering frequency. In short, there is no evidence (to date) that such variables need particular attention within treatment in order to ensure therapy success.

> *9. The success of a program of therapy should not be inflated by ignoring dropouts.*

Numerous examples of this problem exist in the stuttering treatment literature (Ingham, 1983). This is a problem in almost all areas of treatment research and, when excessive, prevents any meaningful conclusions from a study. The problem may well be much greater than is evident from studies in which large scale dropouts have been reported. For example, in single-subject studies it is very rarely indicated that the treated subjects were the *only* subjects on whom the procedure was tried. This information can be exceedingly important, as is demonstrated by numerous subjects who have dropped out of haloperidol treatment programs (Ingham, 1983). Their response probably reflects the less savory effects of this treatment, and serves to contraindicate haloperidol as a preferred treatment for suttering (Guitar, Chapter 10, this volume). Obviously the true clinical value of many treatments can only emerge when clinical researchers carefully ascertain the reasons for dropouts, and also report on nonresponders in the course of single-subject research.

> *10. The method must be shown to be effective in the hands of essentially any qualified clinician, including those without unusual status, prestige, or force of personality.*

and

> *11. The method must continue to be successful when*
> *it is no longer new and the initial wave of enthusiasm*
> *over it has died away.*

These are much related criteria that refer to the treatment's replicability and clinical viability. Actually, these criteria appear to have been met by many of the current therapy procedures, although most "replication" studies invariably highlight the contribution of additional treatment factors or therapy variations and are probably conducted by particularly enthusiastic clinicians. At the same time, an increasing number of treatment reports are now being written to reveal both the strengths and weaknesses of certain procedures, especially those using prolonged speech and its variants (Ingham, 1983). This is a vital shift in much stuttering therapy research and meets the spirit of Bloodstein's criterion. At the same time, many of the response contingent and prolonged speech treatment programs are continuing to produce benefits even now that the "initial wave of enthusiasm" has receded.

Bloodstein's (1981) criteria highlight most of the critical issues that need consideration in evaluating stuttering therapy. Some of the criteria seem questionable, most notably Criteria 1 and 8, but in general they are useful guides to stuttering therapy evaluation. Their limitation is that they are relatively nonspecific guides and provide insufficient information to help clinicians evaluate their own therapy endeavors. The purpose of clinical research is not only to design and evaluate treatments but also to improve therapy practice. So, in what follows, an attempt will be made to develop a set of guidelines for measuring treatment efficacy in therapy management. These guidelines will embrace most of Bloodstein's criteria and include a distillation of pertinent findings from recent clinical research.

Towards a Therapy Evaluation System

Introduction

The purpose here is to develop a therapy evaluation system suitable for most stuttering therapy procedures. It is not posed as a "final solution," but draws on the current treatment literature to derive some necessary operations that should accompany therapy. Actually, any search for an all-purpose treatment evaluation design seems to have about as much chance of succeeding as the search for the Holy Grail. Indeed, the problem in such a search is to be able to recognize treatment success. For, if the object of stuttering therapy is to produce normally fluent speech, then that objective continues to be hindered by the absence of measures (or sets of measures) that can be used to describe normal fluency (Starkweather, 1980). But if clinicians are prepared to settle for an assessment strategy that shows when stuttering is changing as a function of treatment, and when some of the presumed relevant features of normal fluency are evident, then perhaps the search will not be fruitless.

One potential impediment to the search is the differing therapy formats among stuttering treatments. There are obvious differences between treatments concerned with directly modifying stuttering and those that treat stuttering by modifying other behaviors. That is not a major impediment, however, since all ultimately aim to modify stuttering, and so their efficacy can probably be related to various speech performance measures. More problematic is whether treatment is delivered intensively or intermittently. Since intensive treatment should produce improved speech more rapidly, the format will need sufficient flexibility to accommodate different expected rates of change. Thus within- and beyond-clinic assessments may need to be made relatively more frequently for intensive programs. Nevertheless, even this problem is surmountable provided the format's principal components and the guidelines for indentifying therapy effects are suitable for both methods. Another difficulty might be the age of clients; there is some indication (Ingham, 1983) that children may be more responsive to certain treatments than adolescents or adults. It is possible that this difference might extend to rates of change, plus any criteria for determining clinically significant improvement. The same arguments could apply to differences in the intellectual level of clients, for there is also some indication that retardates respond more slowly to treatment (Ingham, 1983). The resolution to each of these difficulties is reasonably straightforward if the format is derived empirically. In other words, where data exist that demand exceptional formats, then such formats should be formulated.

Formulating the Evaluation System

The most significant lesson learned from the checkered history of stuttering therapy is that a useful treatment evaluation system should be designed so that it can embrace the known and anticipated variability of stuttering. It must be a system that is capable of demonstrating that therapy progress or outcome is not confounded by the known untreated variability of the subject's stuttering. Treatment evaluation formats that are suitable for this purpose are beginning to emerge from the time-series quasi-experimental designs (Hersen & Barlow, 1976) typically used in within-subject research. They are especially suitable because they not only identify variability, but also help deal with concerns such as accountability, decision making, and outcome evaluation. Furthermore, they are not only the most powerful designs available for determining sources of within-subject variability, but they are also the only ones that will enable the clinician to discern whether therapy is responsible for generalization.

The strength, or internal and external validity, of these designs in a therapy evaluation system depends on data collection within and beyond the therapy setting at clinically relevant intervals before, during, and after treatment. In short, the foundation of the recommended system is an integration of the now familiar multiple baseline and ABA designs. But the clinical viability of this system depends on finding some basis for determining clinically significant frequency, duration, and content of measurement within the system's design. The rationale for one such determination will now be outlined.

The Data Base, or What to Measure

There is probably little argument that an appropriate evaluation system requires access to audio-recorded speech within relevant speaking situations. Perhaps these recordings could be supplemented by video recordings to ensure that the visual aspects of stuttering (especially for severity measurement) are taken into account. In the absence of this facility, there is value in utilizing directly observed performance data.

Perhaps the minimal clinical data would be stuttering frequency counts and syllables (or words) spoken during talking time. They provide the bases for calculating percentages of syllables (or words) stuttered and syllables (or words) per minute—two of the most commonly used indices for recording the speech behavior of stutterers. These measures in turn assist clinicians in gauging changes in stuttering, and the contribution that the amount and rate of speaking make to stuttering variability.

Stuttering counts

The frequency of "moments of stuttering" may not fully depict the extent of disability caused by stuttering. However, this measure has certainly passed the test of time. The virtue of stuttering frequency counts is that they can be integrated with treatment via on-line measurement, while assessing the treatment's success (or otherwise) in removing the crux of the disorder. Most current therapies aim to remove all instances of stuttering, so it is becoming less important that those instances be described as more or less "severe" or as "part-word repetitions," etc. It also makes little sense now to confound stuttering counts with counts of normal disfluencies. There is increasing acceptance that clinicians (and certainly lay observers) are able to distinguish between disfluencies and stutterings (MacDonald & Martin, 1973).[3] This is an important point since there is no obvious advantage in a treatment that removes normal disfluencies but is less successful in removing stutterings. Conversely, a treatment that removes all disfluencies, normal and abnormal, may actually succeed in producing unusual fluency.

There are at least two dangers in relying on frequency counts of stuttering alone in order to evaluate treatment. The first relates to severity. Occasionally, a very low frequency of stuttering may contain exceptionally long moments of stuttering (Ingham, 1981). For this reason, there is good cause to record the duration or visible features of low frequency stuttering. The second reason concerns the role of word avoidance. This must be the least researched stuttering phenomenon, yet one of the best known features of the disorder—especially in adults. Perhaps the only way of measuring its presence is the subject's report and instructional tests for its influence. The latter may be ascertained by asking the subject to try to minimize stuttering for an interval, possibly by "avoiding stutterings" during spontaneous speech, and then comparing this interval with another in which the reverse instruction is given.

Speech rate

The primary reason for measuring speech rate is that it is generally accepted that reduced speech rate may be sufficient to produce reduced stuttering. Of course, reduced speaking as such would have the same effect. Less publicized is the possibility that abnormally fast speech rate may also reduce stuttering (Ingham, Martin, & Kuhl, 1974). However, there is no accepted method for measuring speech rate. One stumbling block is the relationship between existing rate measures and normally fluent speech rate. Speech rate measurement, as Starkweather (1980) has recently pointed out, needs to be much more complex than simple counts of words or syllables per minute. For what is a perceived as "fast" or "slow" turns out to be partially relative, but also dependent upon variables such as sound durations, pause durations, coarticulation, and rate of syllable production. Consequently, the currently used clinical measures of speech rate only approximate what is a perceived rate, or what might be normal rate. In light of this, what options are available?

For some years the senior author and colleagues have used 170 to 210 syllables per minute as a target normal speech rate (Ingham, 1981). But this measure (allowing for its imperfections) is based on a relatively unusual speaking condition: a monologue that is not interrupted by the conversational exchanges typical of most speech behavior; plus it is the speech rate of young adults. Furthermore, these overall syllable-per-minute scores are neither as useful nor, probably, as valid as Perkins's (1975) measure of articulation rate which excludes pauses and occurrences of stuttering. However, in the absence of pertinent speech rate data, both measures probably provide different, but clinically useful, measures of rate during therapy (Costello, 1981; Costello & Ingham, in press).

Another reflection of the need for research in this area is that there is little information on the relevant target speech rates that should pertain to the subject's age. There are some data from school children which indicate that the average syllables-per-minute rates in normal speech progressively increase throughout childhood. Kowal, O'Connell, and Sabin (1975) have shown that in kindergarten years this rate is about 50% of adult rates and rises to near adult rates by around 12 years. At present, those data might provide the best guide for estimating the expected syllable-per-minute rates for different age groups at the end of treatment. Perhaps a better alternative, certainly one worthy of investigation, is the subject's natural speech rate during stutter-free intervals. Admittedly, these intervals (depending on their length) may be influenced by stuttering frequency, but they may also be more appropriate bases for determining the talker's "normally" fluent rate. Actually, the clinician's perceptual judgment of what is an acceptable and normal rate may ultimately translate into the most clinically suitable syllable-per-minute scores for the individual case—especially if speech normalcy or naturalness ultimately emerges as a reliable basis for determining this measure.

There are numerous reasons why speech rate and stuttering frequency measures are necessary, yet incomplete, for assessing speech performance in treatment. The most important is the imperfect connection between zero stuttering at "normal" speech rate and speech that is perceived as normally fluent (Ingham, 1981; Perkins,1981). The need to improve this connection largely stems from the proliferation of treatments that procure "fluency" via unusual speech patterns, such as the variants of prolonged speech. Adams (1982), for example, has been particularly concerned about the need to gain much more information on the indices needed to identify normally fluent speech. Starkweather (1980) also explored these issues and concluded that fluent speech "is the quality of speech that includes rapid and easy, as well smooth production" (p. 195). But, as yet, no known combination of measurement operations quantifies that speech quality.

Speech quality

A number of approaches to the task of measuring speech quality have already been mentioned. These include ratings of naturalness, prosody, rate, and fluency, plus perceptual analyses of differences between speech samples from nonstutterers and treated stutterers. These measures may evaluate the results of treatment but, unfortunately, they cannot be readily integrated with the treatment process in the same fashion as stuttering counts and rate. However, one promising development, as was previously described, is the use of on-line ratings of naturalness, provided it is possible to establish the reliability and validity of such ratings.

In general terms, therefore, measures that have maximum utility in a therapy context are those that yield dual-function data: (1) they provide bases for establishing within- and beyond-clinic treatment effects, and (2) they contribute to treatment operations (i.e., can be used on-line during treatment). Such dual function measures may not aid all therapies, but for most current therapies they should serve the first function. In passing, it is interesting to note the increasing recognition of the value of measures that do more than passively chart the subject's progress through therapy. Indeed, measures that permit decisions about the efficacy of therapy may have an integral role as treatment agents. It is this latter function which is being used lately to assist the transfer and maintenance of therapy effects (Ingham, 1980; 1982).

Where to Collect Data

The crux of the system described herein is the establishment of multiple "standard" measures of the client's speech performance within and beyond the treatment setting. The conditions of such measures should be determined individually for each client so that they provide representative samples to tap the variability inherent in speaking performance within and beyond the clinic. These standard measures would, then, be administered regularly and repeatedly throughout the course of the clinician's (or clinical researcher's) clinical relationship with the client.

Within-clinic measures

It is well known (but not well documented) that stuttering may vary considerably across different speaking tasks and situations (Bloodstein, 1981; Guitar, 1975; Ingham & Packman, 1977; Resick, Wendiggensen, Ames, & Meyer, 1978; Ryan, 1974). A variety of within-clinic measures have been used rather arbitrarily in the literature, their usefulness being determined partly by the information they give regarding relevant parameters of the client's speech performance and, partly, by the convenience they offer to the clinician. What should be regarded as necessary? The most obvious contenders are converstional speech, monologues, and oral reading, since they are useful not only for assessment but are typically treatment activities as well. Oral reading is included mainly because of its utility in certain therapies; otherwise, it seems strange that so many stuttering assessment procedures recommend a task that is rarely performed in the natural environment (except occasionally in the school setting). Nevertheless, it does have the presumed advantage of controlling for word avoidance. Clinician-client conversations and telephone conversations, both heavily laced with questions, are obviously good choices. The latter task is especially useful because of its suitability for beyond-clinic treatment and assessment as well. The ideal duration for each task is yet another "unknown," but in the context of demands on clinician time, perhaps each should be three minutes.

Beyond-clinic measures

The choice of the situations in which the subject's speech should be measured will be conditioned by the recordability of the situation as much as its validity. The recording process has been greatly assisted by the availability of exceedingly small, good quality microcassette recorders that should be within the resources of a clinic or a client. They can be worn comfortably and equipped with remote hand controls that simplify recording in most situations.

The choice of recordable assessment situations presents some complicated, but not unsolvable, difficulties. There are some logical choices: parents or spouse, peers, and significant others, and a reasonable cross-section of regularly occurring occasions where the client talks. The frequency and variety of talking situations occurring for individual stutterers could be derived with reasonable precision from logs kept by the client (or the client's parent) previous to enrollment in the treatment program (Darley & Spriestersbach, 1978). The number of beyond-clinic measures regularly obtained for each client will differ according to the breadth and frequency of a given client's talking occasions. The goal is that the clinician's (or experimenter's) beyond-clinic samples reflect the variability that would be found were it possible to have data on all of the client's speech throughout every day. (See Ingham & Packman, 1977, for an example of such continuous and complete measurement.) Typical beyond-clinic measures for children might contain standard samples of talking with the family during dinner, with a sibling during playtime, with the mother while riding in the car, and at school during "show and tell," and reading group.

The typical adult client might provide recordings of speech from typical work situations, frequently occurring social situations, and conversations with his or her spouse at home.

The validity of the selected situations may be aided by two other considerations: use of the client's self-judged "difficult" (but recordable) situations, and the relative frequency with which these situations occur. These additional considerations should certainly be included within the decision base for choosing samples from the client's environment. A logical starting point for deciding the length each sample should be is that it reflects the client's typical talking time in similar settings. For example, if a child's speech with a parent occupies, say, 50% of his or her estimated talking time, then recordings of similar talking should account for about 50% of the beyond-clinic data collected for that client.

When to Collect Data

Reaching an agreeable decision about the frequency and duration of samples in a repeated measures assessment design involves at least three considerations: identifying variability, establishing that a treatment is "working," and managing data. However, taking account of these considerations in a generally acceptable therapy format is like putting together a jigsaw puzzle that has its pieces shaped by special interest groups whose members can never agree—arguably one common characteristic in this field. Nevertheless, there may be some parts of the puzzle that can be solved using compromise pieces.

Perhaps the first puzzle piece—identifying variability—should come from the ranks of clinical researchers. The difficulty is that these persons also offer little guidance on the minimum number of data points needed to reflect variability. For compromise purposes, therefore, perhaps the much-referenced text by Hersen and Barlow (1976) should be a guide. They recommend at least three "data points" in any phase of an evaluation design employing data trend comparisons, although many of their text's examples use four or more data points for this purpose. Perhaps, therefore, the seemingly small number of four is an acceptable starting point. But does this translate into measuring relevant behavior for four consecutive days, once every four weeks, or perhaps, once every four months? This piece of the puzzle should probably come from two interest groups: practicing clinicians and the editors of journals reporting treatment studies, for it relates to the frequency with which treatment is offered, and the interval of time needed to convince peers that treatment efficacy has been established. The factors involved in constructing this piece will be deferred for the moment.

The third, and most overlooked factor, is the sheer task of data collecting from audio recordings, and the subject's ability to obtain such recordings.

Determining a Treatment Effect

Once a suitable measurement schedule has been determined and introduced during the pretreatment period, it is continued throughout the instatement and transfer phases of the program. The next task is to find a suitable time frame that can be used to decide whether or not the therapy procedures are beneficial. This could lead to a veritable Pandora's Box— comparing different therapies and their effects. Fortunately, the interior of the box is not as daunting as might be expected. We can at least take advantage of a body of therapy literature to gain some idea of the rate of change in target behaviors from successfully treated clients. Indeed, if that literature cannot be used for this purpose, then it has virtually no external validity (Birnbrauer, 1981). At the very least, it should show the expected rate of change in stuttering if a client responds to a particular treatment. For example, if the chosen treatment was one of the response contingent procedures, then perhaps a less dramatic decline in stuttering frequency should be expected when compared with rhythm or any of the numerous variants of prolonged speech. On the other hand, the relevant target behavior for these speech pattern techniques is usually eventual restoration of normal speech rate , thus extending the time needed ultimately to determine treatment responsiveness.

There is no reason to skirt the "treatment effect time" issue with generalities since much of the reviewed treatment literature—at least that which provides single-subject data—is able to be summarized for this purpose. Tables 11-1 and 11-2 provide summaries of the treatment studies that permit estimates of the treatment time required for stuttering or disfluencies (sometimes "dysfluencies") to decrease by at least 50% relative to baserate. The term "successful outcome" is used in a very broad sense. It refers to those subjects who were reported, at the end of their treatment, to have reduced stuttering by at least 50% without decreased speech rate (when these data are reported). A 50% reduction in stuttering is certainly far from absolute treatment success, but, in the spirit of compromise, it is regarded as evidence that a substantial change in performance has been achieved by the treatment. The successfully treated subjects have been divided into children, those 12 years of age or younger (see Table 11-1), and adults (see Table 11-2). This is for no special reason, other than the recurring suggestion in the literature that children appear to respond more rapidly to some treatments than adults. Generally the tables confirm that children do respond a shade more rapidly to most treatment procedures, particularly the response

TABLE 11-1

This table summarizes the results of a survey of stuttering treatments involving children 12 years of age or younger. The survey was designed to identify studies in which it was possible to discern the treatment time needed for individual subjects to reduce stuttering or disfluencies by more than 50% relative to pretreatment performance. That point was established when the target behavior reached the 50% reduction level on two assessment occasions. In the case of the "Gradual Increase in Length and Complexity of Utterance" (GILCU), the 50% reduction level was regarded as equivalent to half the time required to achieve the designated treatment target. For the speech pattern procedures, the 50% reduction level was regarded as equivalent to half the time required to complete the treatment's instatement phase.

METHOD	PROCEDURE	STUDY	HOURS REQUIRED FOR 50% REDUCTION IN TARGET BEHAVIOR	NUMBER OF SUBJECTS/AGE RANGE
Response Contingent	GILCU	Costello (1980)	15.50	1/11
		Johnson, Coleman, & Rasmussen (1978)	10.50	1/6
		Ryan (1974)	3.30–30.05	6/7–9
		Mowrer (1975)	5.00	1/10
	Positive Reinforcement	Peters (1977)	0.60	2/8
		Shaw & Shrum (1972)	0.67	3/9–10
	Combined Punishment and Reinforcement	Ryan (1974)	1.00–6.00	2/9

Category	Subcategory	Reference		
Punishment		Martin & Berndt (1970)	0.67	1/12
		Martin, Kuhl, & Haroldson (1972)	1.33-2.00	2/3-4
		McDermott (1971)	1.20	1/9
		Reed & Godden (1977)	1.33-1.67	2/3-5
Masking	Continuous	MacCulloch, Eaton, & Long (1970)	6.00	4/11.9
Speech Pattern	Rhythmic Stimulation	Herscovitch & Le Bow (1973)	2.00	2/12
	MCSR	Brady (1971)	4.00	1/12
	DAF/ Prolonged Speech	Ryan (1971)	2.00	1/8
		Ryan (1974)	5.65-20.25	2/8-12
		Turnbaugh & Guitar (1981)	4.50	1/12
Speech Pattern	Regulated Breathing	Hee & Holmes (1976)	1.50	1/10
	Shadowing	Ottoni (1974)	1.30	1/9
Traditional	Programmed	Ryan (1974)	2.30	1/10

TABLE 11-2
Table incorporates the same information as Table 11-1 but for subjects older than 12 years.

METHOD	PROCEDURE	STUDY	HOURS REQUIRED FOR 50% REDUCTION IN TARGET BEHAVIOR	NUMBER OF SUBJECTS/ AGE RANGE
Response Contingent	GILCU	Mowrer (1975) Ryan (1974)	5.00–9.75 5.25–19.30	2/23,31 3/16–35
	Punishment	Costello (1975) Ryan (1974)	1.83 3.05–5.15	1/18 2/15,20
	Self-management	James (1981) La Croix (1973)	23.00 1.00	1/18 2/?
Anxiety Reduction	Reciprocal Inhibition	Boudreau & Jeffrey (1973)	12.00	4/16–22

Speech Pattern	Rhythmic Stimulation	Brady (1971)	5.00–31.00	17/14–53
	Prolonged Speech	Andrews (1973)	5.00	1/?
	DAF/ Prolonged Speech	Boberg & Fong (1930)	15.00	1/19
		Goldiamond (1965)	3.08	2/40,?
		Ingham & Andrews (1973)	1.63–4.60	11/18–56
		Ryan (1974)	1.00–88.60	23/14–45
		Webster (1970)	5.00–20.00	8/15–47
Biofeedback	EMG	Guitar (1975)	2.67	1/32
Traditional	Programmed	Ryan (1974)	1.45–12.05	9/14–43

contingent techniques. The rate of response to the GILCU and speech pattern techniques are more difficult to translate since there is no clear indication of the time taken to reach 50% improvement. For this reason, half the treatment time, or talking time, required to reach the final target behavior was judged equivalent to 50% improvement. This is probably the main reason why these treatments appear to take longer to reach the "treatment effect" criterion.

Resolving the Treatment Design Puzzle

The next task is to translate the preceding information into solution pieces for the treatment design puzzle. The first issue must be the frequency with which baseline and subsequent measures during and after treatment should be made. Andrews and Harvey (1981) have gathered data that they suggest show that pretreatment speech measures from adult stutterers do not show improvement over a 6-week nontreatment period. Thus, the most conservative treatment design might incorporate up to 6 weeks of weekly recordings of the subject's speech within and beyond the clinic prior to the initiation of treatment. The least conservative, though possibly the most practical, approach might utilize the 4-data point principle, with a minimum of, say, once weekly recordings of all selected within- and beyond-clinic speech samples. This would seem to provide adequate sampling of the existing variability in the client's stuttering across settings and time.

Clinicians should be aware that this recommended 4-week base rate data collection interval is not necessarily a period of clinical inactivity. It is during this period that the clinician might train the client's spouse or parents not only to collect appropriate beyond-clinic recordings but also to score these recordings reliably. Also, in some instances the authors have found that the base rate recording procedure, per se, appears to have produced "treatment effects", thus influencing subsequent intervention decisions. Finally, the base rate period can be used to organize the format of treatment procedures. The methods for choosing these procedures are considered in more detail by Costello and Ingham (in press).

Tables 11-1 and 11-2 suggest that the treatment phase for almost all current data-based treatments should not exceed about 12 treatment hours for children or 23 hours of treatment for adults, before a decision is made as to whether the chosen treatment should be continued or changed. Actually, quite discernible trends in relevant data should be expected by the fifth hour if some treatments are likely to be beneficial. Of course, this does not mean the treatment will be ultimately successful, since it is likely that many treatment failures showed evidence of responsiveness within the suggested time frames. On the other hand, relatively few successful treatments demonstrated responsiveness over longer intervals.

If treatment is progressing appropriately, at some point within-clinic and beyond-clinic data will begin to converge until speech performance under all conditions has reached criterion. At this point, the clinician will need to make some decision about the number of data collection occasions that are needed to verify that change and thus indicate the appropriateness of termination of the establishment-transfer phase of treatment. The simple fact is that there are almost no data that can be used to address this issue. Perhaps the sole exception occurs in a single-subject study by Ingham and Packman (1977). Obviously, more data are needed to address this issue, one research area in which group data would be useful. In the absence of those data, the clinician might be best advised to rely on the data collection intervals used thus far throughout baseline and treatment. These will provide at least one source for determining whether clinically significant changes have resulted from treatment. Perhaps, therefore, the client's performance pattern over four beyond- and within-clinic data collection points, while treatment has ceased, might be one rational basis for deciding whether maintenance procedures should be introduced to the therapy process. However, there are more complex issues associated with assessing treatment outcome that will be discussed later.

Dismantling Therapy

It may well be that a number of treatments are tried before a therapy strategy is found that will achieve within- and beyond-clinic treatment gains. These will be strategies that establish and transfer treatment gains. It is, therefore, necessary for the assessment process to incorporate strategies that will indicate when the initial phase of treatment (i.e., establishment and, if necessary, transfer) should be replaced by maintenance strategies.

There is general agreement that active maintenance strategies are necessary components of the therapy process, although that is often difficult to believe considering the slight amount of research they have attracted. There are some very limited data available that demonstrate the efficacy of some maintenance techniques (Boberg, 1981; Boberg, Howie, & Woods, 1977; Ingham, 1980, 1981, 1982), though they give no guidance on how to choose assessment procedures for this phase. To some extent, that task has been eased by some useful data that suggest that when beyond-clinic generalization occurs in the treatment of preschool children, then unassisted maintenance will follow (Ingham, 1983; Prins & Ingham, 1983). But the evidence is certainly not so persuasive in the case of older-aged children.

As mentioned earlier, repeated beyond- and within-clinic assessments at the end of treatment should continue over at least four data collection points. This should provide a reasonable basis for estimating the initial stability of these gains. However, the dismantling of the therapy process may also blend with treatment and assessment procedures. One internally valid method of establishing when treatment should be withdrawn is to use a period when the beyond/within-clinic data collection scores (i.e., nontreatment scores) and therapy-controlled measures of speech performance begin to merge. Martin, Kuhl, and Haroldson (1972) demonstrated the prospects of this strategy when they compared treatment and nontreatment setting performance of two preschool stutterers treated by contingency arrangements. Costello (1975) used this strategy during therapy sessions by comparing nontreatment and treatment intervals over contingency-managed therapy sessions.

A strategy used by the senior author in recent years (Ingham, 1980; 1981; 1982) involves systematic withdrawal of regular assessment sessions contingent upon sustained performance, plus comparisons with intermittent covert assessments. This is also an example of how beyond-clinic (or within-clinic) assessments can serve dual functions; that is, they decrease the contact frequency with the client but remain a useful source of speech control.

The above-mentioned method for continuing maintenance and evaluation illustrates how maintenance and outcome evaluation strategies may be gradually integrated. In this procedure the subject is required to return to the clinic initially for two once-weekly assessments, and if the target behavior (0% syllables stuttered at between 170 and 210 SPM) is maintained in all within- and beyond-clinic assessments, then the subject "earns" a 2-week rest from assessments. If these 2-week-apart assessments achieve the target behavior, then the subject earns a 4-week rest from assessments. This systematic and performance-contingent withdrawal of assessment continues until two 32-week-apart assessments are passed successfully. If the subject fails on any assessment (that is, has one stuttering or departs from the target speech rate on any task), then the weekly assessments are reinstated. Recently this procedure was successfully used in conjunction with a self-management technique (specifically, self-evaluation training) in order to shift the responsibility for conducting this performance-contingent assessment strategy to the subject (Ingham, 1982). These procedures have been mainly used with adults, but they have also been useful with older-aged children (Ingham, 1980). Of most relevance here is the fact that the data from these studies have been supplemented by nonperformance-contingent assessments made in beyond-clinic conditions, thereby establishing the point when the data from the nontreatment-related assessments blend with those from the treatment-related assessments. They have also been supplemented by a wide variety of covert assessments that have shown, in some cases, that data gained from overt and covert assessments differ markedly. Generally, these concurrent assessments indicate that the maintenance strategy may be phased out well before the 32-week-apart assessment point.

Covert assessment

Undoubtedly, covert assessment procedures are among the most contentious assessment techniques used in stuttering therapy. Some recent group studies (Howie, Woods, & Andrews, 1982; Andrews & Craig, 1982) have questioned their worth by finding that covert and overt group data are not significantly different 6 months or more after treatment. But studies on individuals (Ingham, 1980; 1982) have shown that the data from both sources may be quite different well after the initial phase of treatment has ceased. In consequence, covert assessments certainly have the potential of providing the most clinically valid treatment assessment data, particularly when used in conjunction with relevant overt assessment data. Their claim to validity, however, is only as strong as their claims to be unobtrusive—and these claims are often difficult to defend. There are various types of covert and perhaps not-so-covert assessment techniques that might be relatively free of the reactive features of overt assessment, features that many clinicians suspect produce "artificial" posttreatment data. Perhaps the most useful is the "unplanned telephone call," made, ideally, by a person not associated with the treatment. Other relevant information may be obtained from the subject's associates, and can then be validated by carefully arranged recordings. Admittedly, this all sounds uncomfortably unethical, but it need not be. In the case of older-aged children, adolescents, and adults, it is unlikely that the assessment's validity will be threatened if, before treatment, the client agrees that such assessments will only be used to test the treatment's worth. The authors have often used this procedure over the past decade, and have yet to meet one client who found it to be unacceptable. More importantly, it has often provided an immensely useful clinical service. For instance, if repeated unobtrusive assessments yield evidence of poorer performance compared to other, more directly obtained measures, then the consequent trend of performance scores can be used to determine the merit of continuing an extraclinic treatment procedure. When the extraclinic covert data fail to show improvement, then it may be necessary to integrate such data with treatment. For example, in the current applications of the above-described maintenance schedule, clinicians intermittently telephone subjects. If the clinician detects stuttering, then, regardless of whether the subject "passed" the previous assessment, the subject automatically fails that assessment and returns to the initial step in the maintenance schedule.

How should covert assessments be organized within an assessment schedule? Like all other assessment decisions, the decision to use covert assessment should be guided, where possible, by treatment and evaluation considerations. However, the difficulty with this form of assessment is that its "cover" is vulnerable if it is used too frequently. This type of assessment probably carries adequate treatment and assessment value if it occurs on at least four occasions during the transfer phase and on another four occasions during the immediate posttreatment assessment phase. This allows the clinician to decide whether the subject's assessed speech performance is reflected in less stimulus-bound conditions. Probably the most practical procedure for this purpose is an unannounced telephone conversation with a person unconnected with the treatment. It is up to the clinician to decide how the data should be obtained, but there is no reason why it cannot be assessed on-line by a trained clinician. The frequency with which covert assessments should be made during the maintenance phase largely depends on the duration of that phase. Of course, in turn, this raises the issue of time spans for posttreatment assessments, the final phase of this suggested format.

Follow-up Assessment

To date, our literature has little information that could be used to justify the use of certain prescribed follow-up intervals or follow-up assessments. The typical recommendations are that posttreatment assessments should occur at intervals ranging from a few weeks to five years (Silverman, 1981). What this reflects is yet another area of confusion, this time about the function of posttreatment evaluation. The primary purpose of the follow-up evaluation is surely to establish whether the client is unimproved, improved, or free of his or her problem after a period in which variables likely to influence the problem have had every opportunity to occur. The fact that a subject shows improvement, or otherwise, at follow-up may have very little to do with treatment. Quite clearly, the longer the interval between cessation of treatment and follow-up evaluation, the more likely it is that this interval will be filled with variables of far more relevance to current performance than the original treatment. Unfortunately, there is also little information available on the nature of these variables, but there are some logical contenders: practice regimes, "significant others," self-control of speech performance, and even additional treatment are good prospects for consideration.

At best, it would appear that follow-up evaluation may give the clinician and client knowledge about the current state of the disorder and some useful hypotheses about the durability of the treatment's effects. For this reason, perhaps the most practical guideline for follow-up evaluation is to schedule intermittent assessments over the following year. This will probably accommodate a clinic's annual time-tabling arrangements, and is consistent with the intervals used in many clinical studies.

The frequency of follow-up assessments presents another imponderable. Perhaps the logical solution is to use the "four-data-point" principle from the previously mentioned therapy assessment format. This means that follow-up assessments should occur at 3-month intervals. And in order to determine the validity of this trend, perhaps these assessments should be interspersed with another four covert assessments.

The content of these posttreatment assessments deserves additional comment. The logical contenders are the within- and beyond-clinic assessments used over the initial therapy phases. Perhaps the most practical option for covert assessment is a 3-to-5 minute surprise telephone call involving a question-answer conversation with a stranger. But at least two other assessments may be important: some form of assessment of the subject's speech quality (discussed above) and a questionnaire similar to those devised by Webster (1974) and Perkins (1981). The main value of Webster's questionnaire, for instance, is that it solicits the subject's judgment on the extent of attentiveness or self-monitoring required to continue to speak fluently. At present, no other means are available for determining the extent to which therapy gains are sustained at the cost of unusual levels of attention to speaking. Once again, there are no available norms for this part of Webster's questionnaire, but it might be expected that over the follow-up period there should be some evidence that the subject's level of attention to his speech declines in concert with sustained improvements. That would seem to be one final clinically valid indication of treatment success.

Conclusions

Let us now try to put together all the pieces of our therapy assessment puzzle. It begins when we have established the subject's suitability for therapy. This followed by a base rate period containing repeated within- and beyond-clinic recorded assessments. There should be at least four once-weekly within- and beyond-clinic assessments over the base rate period which would, therefore, extend for four weeks. These assessments continue at this frequency during the establishment and transfer phases of therapy. When data from all within- and beyond-clinic measures show criterion performance for four consecutive assessments, formal treatment could be terminated. Thus, at the end of the establishment or transfer phase, beyond-

and within-clinic assessments should continue for the same duration as the base rate in order to establish performance stability, or otherwise. The subsequent maintenance phase may include decreasingly frequent assessments that might also be tied to the treatment process. The pattern of maintenance assessments should continue until they occur at 3-month intervals. At this point, they should fade into follow-up assessments made at 3-month intervals over a year.

The overt within- and beyond-clinic assessment procedure throughout the preceding format should be supplemented by at least four unobtrusive or covert assessments made during both the treatment and transfer phases, plus another four assessments during the immediate posttreatment phase. In addition, perhaps covert assessments (of one form or another) should be made at regular intervals over the maintenance and follow-up periods. The content of the overt assessments should include representative speech samples from the client's natural environment, plus oral readings, monologues, and telephone conversations within the clinic.

The minimum data used in assessments should be syllables per minute and/or articulation rate, and percentage of syllables (or words) stuttered. These data should be supplemented by ratings of speech quality, especially during the final part of the treatment phase. The posttreatment phase of therapy might also include a questionnaire which solicits the subject's estimate of the extent to which it is necessary to "control" speech performance.

We hope that this suggested therapy management system will be given serious consideration as one means of shifting stuttering therapy towards a reasonably common pattern of assessment. This might help achieve a clearer understanding of the therapy process—an understanding that will be of immense benefit to all concerned with this disorder. There is an almost desperate need for a data base from field clinicians on the outcome of current stuttering therapy procedures. If clinicians could be encouraged to gather and report data within the suggested system, then the profession should be considerably advanced in solving that need, for only clinicians can show the strengths and weaknesses of these treatments in the field, rather than in the research laboratory. At the same time, the use of this system would go some distance towards meeting Bloodstein's (1981) therapy evaluation criteria. Finally, it should be mentioned that the suggested therapy management system has already been used successfully in clinical conditions. Ingham and Onslow (1983) have prepared a Stuttering Treatment Evaluation Manual which incorporates guidelines on the use of the previously described procedures. There is every indication from the trial use of this manual with various clinicians in diverse settings that the procedures can be easily implemented.

End Notes

[1] The content of this chapter takes as a starting point some ideas about stuttering treatment outcome evaluation that were first presented in Ingham (Note 1) and further developed in Ingham (1983).

[2] The interested reader is urged to read Bloodstein's justification for each criterion.

[3] Less decisive findings have been reported by Curlee (1981).

Reference Note

1. Ingham, R. J. Towards a therapy assessment procedure for treating stuttering in children. Paper presented at the Conference on Evaluation of Disfluency, Prevention of Stuttering, and Management of Fluency Problems in Children. Northwestern University, Evanston, IL 1982.

References

Adams, M. R. Fluency, nonfluency, and stuttering in children. *Journal of Fluency Disorders,* 1982, *7,* 171–185.

Andrews, G. Stuttering therapy: How simple can an effective treatment programme become? *Australian Journal of Human Communication Disorders,* 1973, *1,* 44–46.

Andrews, G., & Craig, A. Stuttering: Overt and covert measurement of the speech of treated subjects. *Journal of Speech and Hearing Disorders,* 1982, *47,* 96–99.

Andrews, G., & Cutler, J. Stuttering therapy: The relation between changes in symptom level and attitudes. *Journal of Speech and Hearing Disorders,* 1974, *39,* 312–319.

Andrews, G., Guitar, B., & Howie, P. Meta-analysis of the effects of stuttering treatment. *Journal of Speech and Hearing Disorders,* 1980, *45,* 287–307.

Andrews, G., & Harvey, R. Regression to the mean in pretreatment measures of stuttering. *Journal of Speech and Hearing Disorders,* 1981, *46,* 204–207.

Andrews, G., & Ingham, R. J. An approach to the evaluation of stuttering therapy. *Journal of Speech and Hearing Research,* 1972, *15,* 296–302.

Birnbrauer, J. S. External validity and experimental investigation of individual behavior. *Analysis and Intervention in Developmental Disabilities,* 1981, *1,* 117–132.

Bloodstein, O. *A handbook on stuttering* (3rd ed.). Chicago: National Easter Seal Society, 1981.

Boberg, E. *Maintenance of fluency.* New York: Elsevier, 1981.

Boberg, E., & Fong, L. Therapy program for young retarded stutterers. *Human Communication,* 1980, *2,* 95–102.

Boberg, E., Howie, P., & Woods, L. Maintenance of fluency: A review. *Journal of Fluency Disorders,* 1979, *4,* 93–116.

Boudreau, L.A., & Jeffrey, C.J. Stuttering treated by desensitization. *Journal of Behavior Therapy and Experimental Psychiatry,* 1973, *4,* 209–212.

Brady, J. P. Metronome-conditioned speech retraining for stuttering. *Behavior Therapy,* 1971, *2,* 129–150.

Costello, J. M. The establishment of fluency with time-out procedures: Three case studies. *Journal of Speech and Hearing Disorders,* 1975, *40,* 216–231.

Costello, J. M. Clinicians and researchers: A necessary dichotomy? *Journal of the National Student Speech and Hearing Association,* 1979, *7,* 6–26.

Costello, J. M. Operant conditioning and the treatment of stuttering. In W. H. Perkins (Ed.), *Strategies in stuttering therapy. Seminars in Speech, Language and Hearing, 1,* New York: Decker, 1980.

Costello, J. M. Pretreatment assessment of stuttering in young children. *Communicative Disorders: An Audio Journal for Continuing Education.* New York: Grune & Stratton, 1981.

Costello, J. M. Techniques of therapy based on operant theory. In W.H. Perkins (Ed.), *Current therapy of communication disorders.* New York: Thieme-Stratton, 1982.

Costello, J. M., & Ingham, R. J. Assessment strategies for child and adult stutterers. In W. Perkins & R. Curlee (Eds.), *Nature and treatment of stuttering: New directions.* San Diego: College-Hill, in press.

Curlee, R. F. Observer agreement on disfluency and stuttering. *Journal of Speech and Hearing Research,* 1981, *24,* 595–600.

Darley, F. L., & Spriestersbach, D. C. *Diagnostic methods in speech pathology.* New York: Harper & Row, 1978.

Eysenck, H. J. An exercise in mega-silliness. *American Psychologist,* 1978, *33,* 517.

Goldiamond, I. Stuttering and fluency as manipulatable operant response classes. In L. Krasner & L. P. Ullmann (Eds.), *Research in behavior modification.* New York: Holt, Rinehart, & Winston, 1965.

Gregory, H. H. (Ed.) *Controversies about stuttering therapy.* Baltimore: University Park Press, 1978.

Guitar, B. Reduction of stuttering frequency using analog electromyographic feedback. *Journal of Speech and Hearing Research,* 1975, *18,* 672–685.

Guitar, B. E. A response to Ingham's critique. *Journal of Speech and Hearing Disorders,* 1979, *44,* 400–403.

Guitar, B. E. A correction to "A response to Ingham's critique." *Journal of Speech and Hearing Disorders,* 1981, *46,* 440.

Guitar, B., & Bass, C. Stuttering therapy: The relationship between attitude change and long term outcome. *Journal of Speech and Hearing Disorders,* 1978, *43,* 392–400.

Hanna, R., & Owen, N. Facilitating transfer and maintenance of fluency in stuttering therapy. *Journal of Speech and Hearing Disorders,* 1977, *42,* 65–76.

Hawkins, R. P., & Dotson, V. A. Reliability scores that delude: An Alice in Wonderland trip through the misleading characteristics of interobserver agreement scores in interval recording. In E. Ramp & G. Semb (Eds.), *Behavior analysis: Areas of research and application.* Englewood Cliffs, NJ: Prentice-Hall, 1975.

Hee, J. C., & Holmes, P. A. Elimination of stuttering by a regulated breathing approach. *Journal of Communication Pathology,* 1976, *8,* 40–44.

Herscovitch, A., & LeBow, M. D. Imaginal pacing in the treatment of stuttering. *Journal of Behavior Therapy and Experimental Psychiatry,* 1973, *4,* 357–360.

Hersen, M., & Barlow, D. H. *Single-case experimental designs.* New York: Pergamon, 1976.

Howie, P. M., Woods, C. L., & Andrews, G. Relationship between covert and overt speech measures immediately before and immediately after stuttering treatment. *Journal of Speech and Hearing Disorders,* 1982, *47,* 419–422.

Ingham, R. J. Comment on "Stuttering therapy: The relation between attitude change and long-term outcome." *Journal of Speech and Hearing Disorders,* 1979, *44,* 397–400.

Ingham, R. J. Modification of maintenance and generalization in stuttering treatment. *Journal of Speech and Hearing Research,* 1980, *23,* 732–745.

Ingham, R. J. Evaluation and maintenance in stuttering treatment: A search for ecstasy with nothing but agony. In E. Boberg (Ed.), *Maintenance of fluency.* New York: Elsevier, 1981.

Ingham, R. J. The effects of self-evaluation training on maintenance and generalization during stuttering treatment. *Journal of Speech and Hearing Disorders,* 1982, *47,* 271–280.

Ingham, R. J. *Stuttering and behavior therapy: Current status and experimental foundations.* San Diego: College-Hill, 1983.

Ingham, R. J. & Andrews, G. An analysis of a token economy in stuttering therapy. *Journal of Applied Behavior Analysis,* 1973, *6,* 219–229.

Ingham, R. J., Martin, R. R., & Kuhl, P. Modification and control of rate of speaking by stutterers. *Journal of Speech and Hearing Research,* 1974, *17,* 489–496.

Ingham, R. J., & Onslow, M. *Stuttering treatment evaluation manual.* Sydney: Cumberland College of Health Sciences, 1983.

Ingham, R. J., & Packman, A. Treatment and generalization effects in an experimental treatment for a stutterer using contingency management and speech rate control. *Journal of Speech and Hearing Disorders,* 1977, *42,* 394–407.

Ingham, R. J., & Packman, A. Perceptual assessment of normalcy of speech following stuttering therapy. *Journal of Speech and Hearing Research,* 1978, *21,* 63–73.

James, J. E. Behavioral self-control of stuttering using time-out from speaking. *Journal of Applied Behavior Analysis,* 1981, *14,* 25–37.

Johnson, G. F., Coleman, K., & Rasmussen, K. Multidays: Multidimensional approach for the young stutterer. *Language, Speech, and Hearing Services in Schools,* 1978, *9,* 129–132.

Jones, R. J., & Azrin, N. H. Behavioral engineering: Stuttering as a function of stimulus duration during speech synchronization. *Journal of Applied Behavior Analysis,* 1969, *2,* 223–229.

Kiesler, D. J. Some myths of psychotherapy research and the search for a paradigm. *Psychological Bulletin,* 1966, *65,* 110–136.

Kowal, S., O'Connell, D. C., & Sabin, E. F. Development of temporal patterning and vocal hesitations in spontaneous narratives. *Journal of Psycholinguistic Research,* 1975, *4,* 195–207.

LaCroix, Z.E. Management of disfluent speech through self-recording procedures. *Journal of Speech and Hearing Disorders.* 1973, *38,* 272-274.

MacCulloch, M. J., Eaton, R., & Long, E. The long term effect of auditory masking on young stutterers. *British Journal of Disorders of Communication,* 1970, *5,* 165–173.

MacDonald, J. D., & Martin, R. R. Stuttering and disfluency as two reliable and unambiguous response classes. *Journal of Speech and Hearing Research,* 1973, *16,* 691-699.

Martin, R. R. Appercus. In E. Boberg (Ed.), *Maintenance of fluency.* New York: Elsevier, 1981.

Martin, R. R., & Berndt, L. A. The effects of time out on stuttering in a 12 year old boy. *Exceptional Children.* 1970, *36,* 303-304.

Martin, R. R., & Haroldson, S. K. The effects of two treatment procedures on stuttering. *Journal of Communication Disorders,* 1969, *2,* 115–125.

Martin, R. R., Haroldson, S. K., & Triden, K. A. Stuttering and speech naturalness. *Journal of Speech and Hearing Disorders,* in press.

Martin, R. R., Kuhl, P., & Haroldson, S. K. An experimental treatment with two preschool stuttering children. *Journal of Speech and Hearing Research,* 1972, *15,* 743–752.

McDermott, L. D. Clinical management of stuttering behavior: A case study. *Feedback,* 1971, *1,* 6–7.

McReynolds, L. V., & Kearns, K. P. *Single-subject experimental designs in communicative disorders.* Baltimore: University Park Press, 1982.

Metz, D. E., Onufrak, J. A., & Ogburn, R. S. An acoustical analysis of stutterer's speech prior to and at the termination of therapy. *Journal of Fluency Disorders,* 1979, *4,* 249–254.

Mowrer, D. An instructional program to increase fluent speech of stutterers. *Journal of Fluency Disorders,* 1975, *1,* 25–35.

Ottoni, T. M. Uso de la tecnica delineamento del habla para cambiar la conducta verbal. *Revista Interamericana de Psicologia,* 1974, *8,* 3-4.

Perkins, W. H. Articulatory rate in the evaluation of stuttering treatments. *Journal of Speech and Hearing Disorders,* 1975, *40,* 277-278.

Perkins, W. H. Measurement and maintenance of fluency. In E. Boberg (Ed.), *Maintenance of fluency.* New York: Elsevier, 1981.

Perkins, W. H., Rudas, J., Johnson, L., Michael, W. B., & Curlee, R. F. Replacement of stuttering with normal speech: III. Clinical effectiveness. *Journal of Speech and Hearing Disorders,* 1974, *39,* 416-428.

Peters, A. D. The effect of positive reinforcement on fluency: Two case studies. *Language, Speech, and Hearing Services in Schools,* 1977, *8,* 15-22.

Prins, D., & Ingham, R. J. *Treatment of stuttering in early childhood: Methods and issues.* San Diego: College-Hill, 1983.

Reed, C. G., & Godden, A. L. An experimental treatment using verbal punishment with two preschool stutterers. *Journal of Fluency Disorders,* 1977, *2,* 225-233.

Resick, P. A., Wendiggensen, P., Ames, S., & Meyer, V. Systematic slowed speech: A new treatment for stuttering. *Behaviour Research and Therapy,* 1978, *16,* 161-167.

Runyan, C. M., & Adams, M. R. Perceptual study of the speech of "successfully therapeutized" stutterers. *Journal of Fluency Disorders,* 1978, *3,* 25-39.

Runyan, C. M., & Adams, M. R. Unsophisticated judges' perceptual evaluations of the speech of "successfully treated" stutterers. *Journal of Fluency Disorders,* 1979, *4,* 29-38.

Ryan, B. P. Operant procedures applied to stuttering therapy for children. *Journal of Speech and Hearing Disorders,* 1971, *36,* 264-280.

Ryan, B. P. *Programmed therapy for stuttering in children and adults.* Springfield, IL: Charles C. Thomas, 1974.

Shames, G. H. Relapse in stuttering. In E. Boberg (Ed.), *Maintenance of fluency.* New York: Elsevier, 1981.

Shames, G. H., & Florance, C. L. *Stutter-free speech: A goal for therapy.* Columbus: Charles E. Merrill, 1980.

Shaw, C. K., & Shrum, W. F. The effects of response-contingent reward on the connected speech of children who stutter. *Journal of Speech and Hearing Disorders,* in W. H. Perkins (Ed.), *Strategies in Stuttering Therapy.* 1972, *37,* 75-88.

Sheehan. J. G. Problems in the evaluation of progress and outcome. *Seminars in Speech, Language, and Hearing, 1,* New York: Decker, 1980.

Silverman, F. H. Relapse following stuttering therapy. In N.J. Lass (Ed.), *Speech and language: Advances in basic research and practice* (Vol. 5). New York: Academic Press, 1981.

Smith, L. M., & Glass, G. Meta-analysis of psychotherapy outcome studies. *American Psychologist,* 1977, *32,* 752-760.

Starkweather, C. W. Speech fluency and its development in normal children. In N.J. Lass (Ed.), *Speech and language: Advances in basic research and practice* (Vol. 4). New York: Academic Press, 1980.

Stokes, T. F., & Baer, D. M. An implicit technology of generalization. *Journal of Applied Behavior Analysis,* 1977, *10,* 349-367.

Turnbaugh, K. R. & Guitar, B. E. Short-term intensive stuttering treatment in a public school setting. *Language, Speech, and Hearing Services in Schools,* 1981, *12,* 107-114.

Ulliana, L., & Ingham, R. J. Behavioral and nonbehavioral variables in the measurement of stutterers' communication attitudes. *Journal of Speech and Hearing Disorders,* in press.

Webster, R. L. Stuttering: A way to eliminate it and a way to explain it. In R. Ulrich, T. Stachnik, & J. Mabry (Eds.), *Control of human behavior* (Vol.2). Glenview, IL: Scott Foresman, 1970.

Webster, R. L. *The Precision Fluency Shaping Program: Speech reconstruction for stutterers.* Roanoke, VA: Hollins Communication Research Institute, 1974.

Speech Disorders in Adults

Recent Advances

Editor in chief, Speech, Language, and Hearing Disorders Series
William H. Perkins, PhD

Preface

As was true of our efforts in the earlier volume, *Speech Disorders in Children: Recent Advances,* this volume on the assessment and management of speech disorders among adult populations is a compilation, authored by the best qualified researcher-clinicians, of recent research and critical thought regarding articulatory disorders, second language (phonology) acquisition, voice disorders, and stuttering. These chapters illustrate in an eloquent fashion the rapid increase in knowledge that is occurring, seemingly daily, in each of these areas, and they provide a framework for weaving this new information into the fabric of our current knowledge. For those of us who find ourselves increasingly unable to keep up with new developments, these authors give us a chance to catch up, at least for a time.

This volume is divided into separate sections on recent advances in adult articulation and phonology, voice disorders, and stuttering. Each section is introduced by a chapter that provides an overview of the major developments in the area in order to set the scene for the description of recent advances in specific areas. Each of the chapters on recent advances concentrates on major work carried out within the last few years, although the classic studies that often served as the impetus for work being produced now are generally described as well.

It is a healthy sign for our discipline and profession that a series of *Recent Advances* volumes is needed. Let's hope that our health continues to blossom and that this injection of new knowledge will serve to stimulate still more in the future, thus providing a sturdy base for continued growth and enhanced clinical services to speech disordered adults.

Janis M. Costello
Editor

Part One

ARTICULATION AND PHONOLOGY

Jeri A. Logemann

Assessment and Treatment of Articulatory Disorders in Adults: State of the Art

Adult articulation disorders are typically neurologically or anatomically based. They result from damage to neurologic control of the vocal tract (as in stroke, head trauma, and neurologic disease), to the muscles that produce changes in vocal tract shape for speech (as in muscular dystrophy), or to the structures of the vocal tract themselves (as in surgical or traumatic ablation) (Canter, 1964; Darley, Aronson, and Brown, 1968; Joanette and Dudley, 1980; Nakano, Zubick, and Tyler, 1973; Summers, 1974). In the main, these disorders are acquired well after the adult has attained a normal receptive and expressive phonologic system.

Figure 1-1 presents a schema for an optimal knowledge base in the area of acquired adult articulation disorders, against which currently available data can be compared. As a basis for all diagnosis and treatment planning, the exact nature of each disorder should be understood, beginning with the anatomic and physiologic changes created in the structures of the vocal tract and their movement patterns during speech. This information should be available in order to interpret the acoustic and perceptual characteristics of the disorder, because it has become apparent that more than one vocal tract gesture can produce the same acoustic or perceptual result.

In addition to a basic understanding of the nature of each disorder, its natural course must be documented in order for clinicians to diagnose and treat it optimally. Many of these acquired disorders result from trauma (e.g., stroke, head trauma, injury) or surgery, from which some recovery can be anticipated. Others are related to progressive neurologic disease (e.g.,

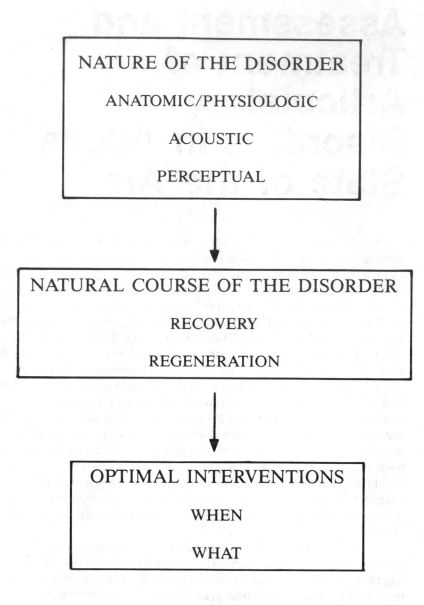

Figure 1–1. An optimal data base for the understanding, diagnosis, and management of acquired adult articulation disorders.

amyotrophic lateral sclerosis, multiple sclerosis, Parkinson's disease) which will cause increasing decrement in function. Thus, data on the nature of the disorder must be collected longitudinally to determine the anatomic and physiologic changes that can be anticipated with recovery or with degeneration.

Finally, with detailed information on the nature of the disorder and its natural course, clinical investigators can design and evaluate optimal treatment strategies and can determine the best time for their introduction in the recovery or degenerative process.

Disorders of Neurologic Origin

Neurogenic disorders affecting the articulation patterns of adults are often the most complex because they can affect the function of the entire vocal tract—including the oral cavity, pharynx, larynx, and respiratory system—rather than the movement of a single articulator. These acquired neurogenic articulation disorders in adults must be considered, then, in the broadest sense, as movement disorders of the entire speech production mechanism (Kent and Netsell, 1975; Netsell, Daniel, and Celesia, 1975).

In the case of *apraxia*, the disorder results from cortical damage to the areas controlling motor programming, but is manifested as a disturbance in the normal movement patterns of the vocal tract to produce phonemic sequences (La Pointe and Johns, 1975; Trost and Canter, 1974; Wertz, La Pointe, and Rosenbek, 1984).

In the *dysarthrias*, the neuromotor behaviors involved in reaching a sequence of articulatory targets in connected speech are no longer executed normally. The locations and nature of the damage to the controls of these behaviors are not entirely understood, nor is the way in which damage to the neuromotor system translates into muscle function for vocal tract movement during speech production.

Evaluation of Articulatory Disorders of Neurologic Origin

Many of the early studies of the nature of apraxia and dysarthrias required trained listeners to analyze the error articulations and describe the voice disorders produced by each patient (Berry, Darley, Aronson, and Goldstein, 1973; Brown, Darley, and Aronson, 1970; Burns and Canter,

1977; Critchley, 1981; Darley, Aronson, and Brown, 1968, 1969, 1975; Farmakides and Boone, 1970; Linebaugh, 1979; Logemann, Boshes, Blonsky, and Fisher, 1977; Logemann and Fisher, 1981; Mawdesley, 1973; Peacher, 1947, 1950). The goal of these attempts was to construct a list of descriptive terms to be used diagnostically to distinguish apraxia and the various dysarthrias from each other and from other acquired articulation problems. Most of these investigators were also seeking to define the nature of the disorders as they affected some or all of the vocal tract. In reality, the descriptive terminology was often imprecise and usually overlapped across the various disorders, making discrimination among them difficult.

In examining the nature of apraxia, many investigators have concentrated on phonetic analyses of the patients' productions (Johns and Darley, 1970; La Pointe and Johns, 1975; Trost and Canter, 1974). Other investigators have quantified the changes in vocal tract control in apraxia and the dysarthrias through assessment of specific acoustic parameters (Blumstein, Cooper, Goodglass, Statlender, and Gottleib, 1980; Kent and Netsell, 1975; Kent, Netsell, and Abbs, 1979; Lehiste, 1968; Ludlow and Bassich, 1982). For example, Kent and colleagues (1979) conducted an acoustic study of the dysarthria associated with cerebellar disease. They examined the speech of five persons with ataxic dysarthria, including an acoustic analysis of consonant-vowel-consonant (CVC) words, words of varying syllabic structure, simple sentences, the Rainbow passage, and conversation. The most consistent and marked abnormalities observed in the spectrograms were alterations of normal timing patterns with prolongation of several speech segments and a tendency toward equalizing the duration of the syllables. The formant structure of vowels in the CVC words was judged to be essentially normal except for the transitions into and away from the segments. The more severe the dysarthria, the larger the number of segments lengthened and the greater the degree of lengthening. This strengthens the concept of cerebellar control of rate of movement by the maintenance of normal targeting behavior. In discussing the results of their work, the authors suggest that the effects of speech therapy, medication, surgery, or other intervention strategies for patients may be more accurately and simply measured through these acoustic techniques.

Some investigators have attempted to relate acoustic measures to the perceptual judgments of listeners. In 1982, Ludlow and Bassich conducted a study of two types of dysarthric patients: parkinsonian patients and those with Shy-Drager syndrome. The purpose of this study was to determine whether acoustic measures of the speech of dysarthric patients differentiated their impairment from normal as well as perceptual ratings. The results indicated that, in fact, the two types of dysarthria could be distinguished from normal by both the acoustic measures and the perceptual ratings of speech. However, to distinguish the two types of dysarthria from each other, a composite score of several measures was necessary, indicating that a pattern of impairment rather than the degree of impairment is important in characterizing the patient's speech disorder.

Currently, several new, relatively noninvasive instrumentation techniques are being applied to the physiologic study of the nature of vocal tract movement patterns in neurologically impaired patients (Hirose, Kiritani, Ushijima, and Sawashima, 1978; Itoh, Sasanuma, Hirose, Yoshioka, and Ushijima, 1980; Kiritani, Ito, and Fujimura, 1975; Sonies, 1982; Sonies, Shauker, and Stowe, 1982). X-ray microbeam study of pellet movement during speech permits assessment of movement patterns of preselected points in the vocal tract as well as simultaneous acoustic and other physiologic measures. Ultrasound techniques may add to our understanding of the function of specific tongue musculature during speech production. Studies utilizing these procedures will add to our knowledge of speech movement patterns in apraxic and dysarthric patients— information previously collected through more traditional methods (Blonsky, Logemann, Boshes, and Fisher, 1975; Canter, 1963, 1965a, 1965b; Hardy, 1965; Hirose, 1971; Iwata, von Leden, and Williams, 1972; Kent and Netsell, 1975; Leanderson, Meyerson, and Persson, 1972; Meyerson, 1973).

Other noninvasive techniques for more accurate *clinical* assessment of vocal tract physiology are being developed and refined for application to the study of adults with acquired articulation disorders. For example, Netsell and Hixon (1978) have developed a noninvasive method for clinically estimating subglottal air pressure. This technique permits estimation of the driving pressure to the larynx and upper airway delivered by the respiratory system during speech production. This kind of examination can help the clinician to determine whether respiratory drive is sufficient to produce good laryngeal tone in the neurologically impaired patient, and thus can determine whether reduced respiratory control is a significant aspect of the patient's speech disorder. Barlow and Abbs (1983) have developed force transducers for the evaluation of labial, lingual, and mandibular motion impairments. This instrument will permit assessment of the motor control integrity of each motor subsystem independently. As other physiologic assessment procedures are simplified for clinical use, a routine battery of tests may be developed for use in diagnosis and management of neurologically impaired patients with speech motor control disturbances. Such a battery is sorely needed.

From this brief review of research on the nature of apraxia and the dysarthrias, it is evident that our current data base contains a large number of perceptual studies of the speech output of patients with these disorders, a moderate number of acoustic analyses of their speech productions, fewer studies of the physiologic nature of these movement disorders for speech, and very few investigations that assess and relate all three aspects of vocal tract dysfunctions.

Very few of the studies of dysarthria and apraxia have examined patients longitudinally to assess predictability of recovery or deterioration in neuromotor control of the vocal tract (Dworkin and Hartman, 1979; Logemann, Boshes, and Fisher, 1973; Mackay, 1963; Rigrodsky and Morrison, 1970). Nor have many investigations systematically assessed the effects of medication on movement disorders of the vocal tract (Birkmayer and Hornykiewicz, 1961). Often, any systematic changes with time have been obliterated by heterogeneous populations of patients, differing either in diagnosis, stage of disease, current medications, or time after onset.

When an adult is initially seen by a speech pathologist for evaluation and treatment of an articulation disorder, the first issue to be addressed is differential diagnosis. Since articulatory disorders in adults can signal the onset of degenerative neurologic diseases of various types, the clinician should be able to compare results of neuromotor testing of the patient's vocal tract control with an information base on typical patterns of change over time on selected measures in patients with specific neurologic diseases. Unfortunately, such a data base is not available. Very few studies have followed up patients longitudinally or have classified patients according to the stage of disease or the time after onset of symptoms. Dworkin and Hartman (1979) followed up a patient with amyotrophic lateral sclerosis to assess the progression in speech deterioration and swallowing. They found a relatively rapid deterioration, including reduction in tongue strength and rate of tongue movement, rate and strength of velopharyngeal function, and laryngeal disturbance.

Logemann and Fisher (1981) and Logemann, Fisher, Boshes, and Blonsky (1978) examined parkinsonian patients at various stages of the disease and found a systematic increase in the phonemes (and vocal tract structures) involved as the disease stage worsened. Unfortunately, few of these studies have included acoustic, physiologic, and perceptual analyses, so that firm conclusions regarding changes in vocal tract movement patterns over time could not be made.

Intervention Strategies for Articulatory Disorders of Neurologic Origin

Development of effective intervention strategies suffers from the lack of basic information on the nature of the disorders and their progression over time (recovery or deterioration). However, in the past ten years, clear trends in management have emerged. First, some clinical investigators are using physiologic and acoustic measures to analyze the patient's movement disorder(s) and to identify those components contributing most significantly to overall intelligibility (e.g., respiratory control, velopharyngeal incompetence) and are then focusing intervention strategies on the parameters so identified (Netsell and Daniel, 1979). These investigators and others are then applying the physiologic or acoustic measures to the evaluation of the interventions as they are implemented.

Second, several techniques to enhance the patient's feedback or awareness of specific vocal tract movements are being evaluated (Daniel and Guitar, 1978; Hanson and Metter, 1980; Netsell and Cleeland, 1973; Rubow, Rosenbek, Collins, and Celesia, 1984). In several reports, lip function has been improved with electromyographic (EMG) biofeedback. In a study by Hand, Burns, and Ireland (1979), a patient with lip hypertonia and retraction was treated with EMG biofeedback in order to demonstrate a reduction in postural lip hypertonicity and to demonstrate that reduction during a number of complex speech activities. The patient's hypertonicity decreased over six biofeedback sessions. It was hypothesized that the hypertonicity decreased because of reduced anisometric contraction, a reduction of isometric contraction, or a relearning of agonist and antagonist muscle balance. Several other authors have demonstrated ability to reduce lip hypertonia in parkinson patients by use of EMG biofeedback (Netsell and Cleeland, 1973).

Third, prosthetic techniques are being increasingly used as intervention strategies in these patients, including bite block prostheses (Lybolt, Netsell, and Farrage, 1982), palatal lift prostheses (Netsell and Daniel, 1979; Schweiger, Netsell, and Sommerfield, 1970), and palatal reshaping prostheses. In each case, the prosthesis is designed to increase functional capacity of particular articulators within the vocal tract. For example, the palatal lift prosthesis elevates the palate to facilitate velopharyngeal closure. A palatal augmentation reshaping prosthesis lowers the palate to meet the tongue that does not elevate sufficiently.

Adults with Speech Disorders Resulting From Ablation of Vocal Tract Structures

As in adults with neurologically based articulation disorders, the earliest studies, and the greatest number of investigations on the nature of speech changes in patients after ablation of vocal tract structures, have examined perceptual and acoustic differences.

Peacher (1947), Herberman (1958), and Brodnitz (1960) described the postoperative speech patterns of their glossectomized subjects by noting the particular phonemes that proved to be the most difficult to produce. Skelly and associates (Donaldson, Skelly, and Paletta, 1968; Skelly, Donaldson, Fust, and Townsend, 1972; Skelly, Donaldson, and Fust, 1973; Skelly, Spector, Donaldson, Brodeur, and Paletta, 1971) have reported some information concerning the intelligibility scores of their glossectomized patients. In an unpublished paper presented at the 1972 American Speech and Hearing Association convention, Seilo, La Riviere, and Dimmick (1972) reported intelligibility scores of a glossectomy patient as determined by listener response to the reading of two word lists from the Rhyme Test (Fairbanks, 1958) and to the production of five vowels and three diphthongs in an [h] CVC context. In addition, they provided a confusion matrix for initial consonants as assessed by three "experienced listeners."

In any attempt to assess the relationship between structure and speech function in the patient after ablation of vocal tract structures, it is not sufficient to merely specify acoustic and perceptual changes or residual tissue structure and mobility. It is necessary to define accurately and objectively the characteristics of vocal tract movement during speech. Radiographic studies of articulatory gestures completed by Logemann and Bytell (1979), Logemann, Fisher, and Bytell (1982), Georgian, Logemann, and Fisher (1982), and Lazarus and Logemann (1982), have defined specific changes in vocal tract movement patterns after ablative surgery. The relationship between listener preception, acoustic features, and these productions has also been explored (Georgian, Logemann, and Fisher, 1982; Lazarus and Logemann, 1982).

Several investigators have found there is a minimal inter- and intrasubject variability in speech and swallowing measures when patients are carefully categorized according to the extent and nature of their ablative and reconstructive procedures. When functional changes in speech articulation patterns were compared across groups by Logemann and Bytell (1978), Logemann, Fisher, and Bytell (1977), and McConnell (1982), it was clear that each group of patients categorized by data on their resection-reconstruction procedures had a distinct profile of functioning that was different in the detailed characteristics of speech articulation and in the resultant acoustic and perceptual parameters. When Logemann and Bytell (1978) and McConnell (1982) categorized surgically treated oral cancer patients by extent of resection and nature of reconstruction, it became apparent that the severity of changes in speech articulation patterns after surgery related to the extent of the lingual resection and the nature of the reconstruction, *nature of the reconstruction* being the most important predictor of function in patients with less that one half of the tongue included in the resection, and *extent of resection* the most important predictor of function when more than 50 per cent of the tongue was resected. This research has clarified the role of surgical reconstruction as the foremost rehabilitation strategy. A number of surgeons are attempting improvements in oral reconstruction. Unfortunately, their results often are not examined in a careful, detailed, and systematic way in terms of their effect on speech movement patterns, acoustic characteristics, or listener perceptions.

Only a small amount of physiologic, acoustic, and perceptual data on recovery of more normal speech articulations by postoperative oral cancer patients, with and without therapeutic interventions, is available (Brodnitz, 1960; Duguay, 1964; Georgian, Logemann, and Fisher, 1982; Herberman, 1958; Seilo et al., 1972; Lazarus and Logemann, 1982). Although it is clear that the same acoustic and perceptual result can be created by more than one vocal tract gesture, our knowledge of which specific articulatory strategies produce the same perceptual judgments by the listener is minimal and is insufficient to apply in teaching patients optimal compensatory articulation strategies. The most frequent intervention described in the clinical literature involves development of intraoral prostheses to compensate for the loss of range of movement in vocal tract structures (Cantor, Curtis, Shipp, Beumer, and Vogel, 1969; Lehman, Hulicka, and Mehringer, 1966; Leonard and Gillis, 1982; Logemann, Sisson, and Wheeler, 1980; Moore, 1972; Wheeler, Logemann, and Rosen, 1980). Two basic approaches have been utilized in prosthetic rehabilitation of the oral cancer patient: maxillary prostheses designed to lower and reshape the palatal vault and thus facilitate contact of the residual tongue to the palate (Cantor et al. 1969; Logemann et al., 1980; Wheeler et al., 1980), and mandibular prosthetics with some attempt made to create a "prosthetic tongue" to improve intelligibility after essentially total glossectomy (Leonard and Gillis, 1982; Moore, 1972).

The timing of introduction of these prosthetic devices is currently open to question, with some investigators advocating early implementation with redesign as function recovers (Logemann et al., 1980), and other clinicians suggesting introduction of prostheses once the patient's function has reached a plateau, some time after the ablative incident (Drane, 1973).

Augmentative Communication Strategies

Over the past ten years, speech-language pathologists have increasingly recognized the need to offer communication aids to patients whose speech is unintelligible (Coleman, Cook, and Meyers, 1980; Copeland, 1974, Skelly, Schinsky, Smith, and Fust, 1974; Vanderheiden and Grilley, 1976). Much of the attention in the area of alternative communication has focused on development and application of communication aids and systems for multiply handicapped children whose cognitive and language skills are just developing or are impaired (McDonald and Schultz, 1973; Montgomery, 1983; Shane and Bashir, 1980; Vanderheiden, Kelso, Holt, and Raitzer, 1977). In contrast to the special needs of these multiply handicapped children, most of the adults with acquired articulation disorders have normal receptive and expressive language, can solve problems, and can see relationships. They merely lack adequate intelligible speech to meet all of their communication needs (Beukelman and Yorkston, 1977; Silverman, 1983).

Initially, the alternative communication systems used by these speech impaired adults were manual (signing, gesturing, writing) or varieties of communication boards (Calculator and Dollaghan, 1982; Skelly et al., 1974). More recently, electronic devices, including computer systems producing digitized speech output, have been developed (Linebaugh, Baird, and Baird, 1983). Several authors have described the devices currently available, and many hospitals have now organized laboratories or centers for alternative communication as resources to speech-language and hearing professionals and patients in their communities (Linebaugh, Baird, Baird and Armour, 1983; Vanderheiden and Grilley, 1976). These centers purchase and maintain samples of a wide variety of alternative communication systems, which patients can see and use on a trial basis. Since many of these devices are quite expensive and cannot be purchased by each hospital or clinic for trial use by patients, the concept of the alternative communication center as a community resource is an excellent one. Many of the centers offer consultation and evaluation services to speech-language pathologists and their patients in the community regarding selection of the best system for a particular patient.

Several major problems currently face clinicians in selection of an instrument with and for a patient: maintaining a working knowledge of the advantages and disadvantages of the ever-increasing number and types of prosthetic devices available, and identifying the relevant criteria for selection of a device with and for a patient. The first problem is partially solved by the alternative communication centers just described. Unfortunately, however, very few of the available alternative communication systems have been evaluated in controlled studies of their utility, listener acceptance, patient acceptance, and effect on recovering oral communication with various types of patients.

Criteria for selection of a particular instrument by and for a particular patient have not been uniformly agreed upon. Several models for decision making have been offered in the literature (Coleman et al., 1980; Owens and House, 1984; Shane and Bashir, 1980). Each author has attempted to construct a type of decision tree or logic diagram to parallel the questions the clinician should answer or ask about the patient's capabilities in the process of selecting an instrument for a particular patient. Few studies have described the typical length of use of various systems or problems encountered, including the need to change systems as any of the patient's neuromotor, linguistic, or cognitive abilities or communication needs change.

The counseling process for patients and families when the speech-language pathologist believes alternative methods of communications are needed has received little attention. Yet, this recommendation by the clinician may arouse strong feelings of failure, inadequacy, and lack of acceptance in the patient and family if the information on the patient's need for such aids is not carefully introduced and reinforced. In some cases, the patient and family may believe the clinician is abandoning them or giving up on the goal of recovering or maintaining intelligible speech. In other cases, the move to an alternative communication system may signal one more loss in function in the face of progressive neurologic disease or malignancy. The role of the speech-language pathologist in counseling, reinforcement, and support, in conjunction with other professionals, deserves greater attention.

Though the number and electronic complexity of available electronic augmentation communication systems are increasing, several limitations still exist. First, the devices that produce digitized speech are not always easily intelligible to naive listeners, and often sound mechanical. Second, the size of many devices makes them less mobile than is desired by many patients, especially those who are ambulatory. Third, the cost of many of the better instruments makes them unavailable to many patients, particularly many older persons with limited resources that have already been strained by long illness, hospitalizations, and the like.

Thus, many advances have been made in the use of alternative communication systems by adults with acquired articulation disorders. However, much additional research and development are needed before optimal devices and procedures for their selection and introduction to patients are available.

Summary

Many of the discrepancies between the ideal information base illustrated in Figure 1-1, and the current state of the art in adult articulation disorders as described here, relate to the difficulties in implementation of the research needed to expand our information base.

First, physiologic techniques that permit easy, relatively noninvasive study of movement patterns of vocal tract structures during speech in a large number of subjects are just beginning to be developed and used to study disorder groups (Hirose et al., 1978; Kiritani et al., 1975; Sonies, 1982). Simultaneous studies of movement patterns, air flows and pressures, EMG in select muscle groups, and other physiologic and acoustic measures are needed but require complex instrumentation not widely available. In place of these physiologic studies, many investigators have substituted acoustic and perceptual evaluations of various types of adult patients with acquired articulation disorders, recognizing the limitations of their results in extrapolating the underlying anatomic or physiologic nature of the disorder. To date, the majority of physiologic studies that have been completed examined only a small number of patients. How and where these individual patients fit into the continuum of recovery or degeneration of the disease entity they represent is often difficult for the reader to know.

Few studies have followed up specific homogeneous patient groups longitudinally to define patterns of recovery or degeneration. Availability of large homogeneous groups of patients early in their diagnosis is a problem for many investigators not located in major medical or population centers.

On these bases, it is easy to understand why therapy for acquired adult articulation disorders is in its infancy. Without a clear understanding of the nature and natural course of these disorders, systematic design and evaluation of therapy interventions, including the optimal time to introduce them in the process of recovery or deterioration, is impossible. With the latest breakthroughs in instrumentation, and greater attention given to these disorders, the optimal data base defined in Figure 1-1 should be rapidly achieved, with a resultant improvement in accurate and early diagnosis and in the ultimate effectiveness of speech management.

References

Barlow, S., and Abbs, J. (1983). Force transducers for the evaluation of labial, lingual, and mandibular motor impairments. *Journal of Speech and Hearing Research, 26,* 616-621.

Berry, W., Darley, F., Aronson, A., and Goldstein, N. (1973). Dysarthria in Wilson's disease. *Journal of Speech and Hearing Research, 17,* 169-183.

Beukelman, D., and Yorkston, K. (1977). A communication system for the severely dysarthric speaker with an intact language system. *Journal of Speech and Hearing Disorders, 42,* 265-270.

Birkmayer, W., and Hornykiewicz, O. (1961). Der L-3, 4-Dioxyohenylalanin (Dopa) effect bei der Parkinson akinese. *Wiener Klinische Wochenschrift, 73,* 787-799.

Blonsky, E., Logemann, J., Boshes, B., and Fisher, H. (1975). Comparison of speech and swallowing function in patients with tremor disorders and In normal geriatric patients. A cineradiographic study. *Journal of Gerontology, 30,* 299-303.

Blumstein, S., Cooper, W., Goodglass, H., Statlender, S., and Gottlieb, J. (1980). Production deficits in aphasia: A voice onset time analysis. *Brain and Language, 9,* 153-170.

Brodnitz, F. S. (1960). Speech after glossectomy. *Current Problems in Phoniatry and Logopedics, 1,* 68-72.

Brown, J., Darley, F., and Aronson, E. (1970). Ataxic dysarthria. *International Journal of Neurology, 7,* 302-318.

Burns, M., and Canter, G. (1977). Phonemic behavior of aphasic patients with posterior cerebral lesions. *Brain and Language, 4,* 492-507.

Calculator, S., and Dollaghan, C. (1982). The use of communication boards in residential setting: An evaluation. *Journal of Speech and Hearing Disorders, 47,* 281-287.

Canter, G. (1963). Speech characteristics of patients with Parkinson's disease: I. Intensity, pitch and duration. *Journal of Speech and Hearing Disorders, 28,* 221-229.

Canter, G. (1965a). Speech characteristics of patients with Parkinson's disease: II. Physiological support for speech. *Journal of Speech and Hearing Disorders, 30,* 44-49. (a)

Canter, G. (1965b). Speech characteristics of patients with Parkinson's disease: III. Articulation, diadochokinesis and overall speech adequacy. *Journal of Speech and Hearing Disorders, 30,* 217-224. (b)

Canter, G. (1964). Neuromotor pathologies of speech. *American Journal of Physical Medicine, 46,* 659-666.

Cantor, R., Curtis, T., Shipp, T., Beumer, J., and Vogel, B. (1969). Maxillary speech prostheses for mandibular surgical defects. *Journal of Prosthetic Dentistry, 22,* 253-257.

Coleman, C., Cook, A., and Meyers, L. (1980). Assessing nonoral clients for assistive communication devices. *Journal of Speech and Hearing Disorders, 45,* 515-526.

Copeland, K. (1974). *Aids for the severely handicapped.* New York: Grune & Stratton.

Critchley, E. (1981). Speech disorders of parkinsonism: A review. *Journal of Neurology, Neurosurgery, and Psychiatry, 44,* 751-758.

Daniel, B., and Guitar, B. (1978). EMG feedback and recovery of facial and speech gestures following neural anastomosis. *Journal of Speech and Hearing Disorders, 43,* 9-20.

Darley, F., Aronson, A., and Brown, J. (1968). Motor speech signs in neurologic disease. *Medical Clinics of North America, 52,* 840-844.

Darley, F., Aronson, A., and Brown, J. (1969). Differential diagnostic patterns of dysarthria. *Journal of Speech and Hearing Research, 12,* 462-496.

Darley, F., Aronson, A., and Brown, J. (1975). *Motor speech disorders.* Philadelphia: W. B. Saunders.

Donaldson, R. C., Skelly, M., and Paletta, F. X. (1968). Total glossectomy for cancer. *American Journal of Surgery, 116,* 585-590.

Drane, J. B. (1973). Prosthetic considerations in oral ablative surgery. *ASHA Reports, 8,* 39-41.

Duguay, M. J. (1964). Speech after glossectomy. *New York Journal of Medicine, 64,* 1836-1838.

Dworkin, J., and Hartman, D. (1979). Progressive speech deterioration and dysphagia in amyotrophic lateral sclerosis: Case report. *Archives of Physical Medicine and Rehabilitation, 60,* 423-425.

Fairbanks, G. (1958). *Voice and articulation drillbook.* New York: Harper.

Farmakides, M., and Boone, D. (1970). Speech problems of patients with multiple sclerosis. *Journal of Speech and Hearing Disorders, 25,* 385-390.

Georgian, D., Logemann, J., and Fisher, H. (1982). Compensatory articulation patterns of a patient after 20% glossectomy. *Journal of Speech and Hearing Disorders, 47,* 77-82.

Hand, C., Burns, M., and Ireland, E. (1979). Treatment of hypertonicity in muscles of lip retraction. *Biofeedback and Self Regulation, 4,* 171-181.

Hanson, W., and Metter, E. (1980). DAF as instrumental treatment for dysarthria in progressive supranuclear palsy: A case report. *Journal of Speech and Hearing Disorders, 45,* 268-276.

Hardy, J. (1965). Air flow and air pressure studies. *ASHA Reports, No. 1,* 141-152.

Herberman, M. A. (1958). Rehabilitation of patients following glossectomy. *Archives of Otolaryngology, 67,* 182-183.

Hirose, H. (1978). Electromyography of the articulatory muscles: Current instrumentation and technique. *Haskins Laboratory Status Reports on Speech Research, SR 25/26,* 73-85.

Hirose, H., Kiritani, S., Ushijima, T., and Sawashima, M. (1978). Analysis of abnormal articulatory dynamics in two dysarthric patients. *Journal of Speech and Hearing Disorders, 43,* 96-105.

Itoh, M., Sasanuma, S., Hirose, H., Yoshioka, H., and Ushijima, T. (1980). Abnormal articulatory dynamics in a patient with apraxia of speech: X-ray microbeam observation. *Brain and Language, 11,* 66-75.

Iwata, S., von Leden, H., and Williams, D. (1972). Air flow measurement during phonation. *Journal of Communication Disorders, 5,* 67-69.

Joanette, Y., and Dudley, J. (1980). Dysarthric symptomatology of Friedreich's ataxia. *Brain and Language, 10,* 39-50.

Johns, D., and Darley, F. (1970). Phonemic variability in apraxia of speech. *Journal of Speech and Hearing Research, 14,* 131-143.

Kent, R., and Netsell, R. (1975). A case study of an ataxic dysarthric: Cineradiographic and spectrographic observation. *Journal of Speech and Hearing Disorders, 40,* 115-134.

Kent, R., Netsell, R., and Abbs, J. (1979). Acoustic characteristics of dysarthria associated with cerebellar disease. *Journal of Speech and Hearing Research, 22,* 627-648.

Kiritani, S., Ito, K., and Fujimura, O. (1975). Tongue-pellet tracking by a computer controlled x-ray microbeam system. *Journal of the Acoustic Society of America, 57,* 1516-1520.

La Pointe, L., and Johns, D. (1975). Some phonemic characteristics in apraxia of speech. *Journal of Communication Disorders, 8,* 259-269.

Lazarus, C., and Logemann, J. (1982, November). *Compensatory articulation patterns in a 70% glossectomee.* Paper presented at the Annual Convention of the American Speech-Language-Hearing Association, Toronto.

Leanderson, R., Meyerson, B., and Persson, A. (1972). Lip muscle function in parkinsonian dysarthria. *Acta Otolaryngologica, 74,* 271-278.

Lehiste, I. (1968). *Some acoustic characteristics of dysarthria.* Basel: S. Karger.

Lehman, W., Hulicka, I., and Mehringer, E. (1966). Prosthetic treatment following complete glossectomy. *Journal of Prosthetic Dentistry, 16,* 344-350.

Leonard, R., and Gillis, R. (1982). Effects of a prosthetic tongue on vowel intelligibility and food management in a patient with total glossectomy. *Journal of Speech and Hearing Disorders, 47,* 25-30.

Linebaugh, C. (1979). The dysarthrias of Shy-Drager syndrome. *Journal of Speech and Hearing Disorders, 44,* 55-60.

Linebaugh, C., Baird, J., Baird, C., and Armour, R. (1983). Special considerations for the development of microcomputer based augmentative communication systems. In W. Berry (Ed.), *Clinical dysarthria.* San Diego: College-Hill Press.

Logemann, J., Boshes, B., Blonsky, E., and Fisher, H. (1977). Speech and swallowing evaluation in the differential diagnosis of neurologic disease. *Neurologia, Neurochirigia, Psychiatria, 18,* 71-78.

Logemann, J., Boshes, B., and Fisher, H. (1973). The steps in the degeneration of speech and voice control in Parkinson's disease. In J. Siegried (Ed.), *Parkinson's disease.* Vienna: Hans Huber.

Logemann, J., and Bytell, D. (1978, November). *Articulation patterns of five groups of head and neck surgical patients.* Paper presented at the Annual Convention of the American Speech and Hearing Association, San Francisco.

Logemann, J., and Bytell, D. (1979). Swallowing disorders in three types of head and neck surgical patients. *Cancer, 44,* 1095-1105.

Logemann, J., and Fisher, H. (1981). Vocal tract control in Parkinson's disease: Phonetic feature analysis of misarticulations. *Journal of Speech and Hearing Disorders, 46,* 348-352.

Logemann, J. A., Fisher, H., Boshes, B., and Blonsky, E. (1978). Frequency and cooccurrence of vocal tract dysfunctions in the speech of a large sample of Parkinson patients. *Journal of Speech and Hearing Disorders, 43,* 47-57.

Logemann, J., Fisher, H., and Bytell, D. (1977, November). *Functional effects of reconstruction in partially glossectomized patients.* Paper presented at the Annual Convention of the American Speech and Hearing Association, Chicago.

Logemann, J., Sisson, G., and Wheeler, R. (1980). The team approach to rehabilitation of surgically treated oral cancer patients. *Proceedings of the National Forum on Cancer Rehabilitation, 222-227,* Williamsburg, VA, November 13-15.

Ludlow, C., and Bassich, C. (1982). The results of acoustic and perceptual assessment of two types of dysarthria. In W. Berry (Ed.), *Clinical dysarthria.* San Diego: College-Hill Press.

Lybolt, J., Netsell, R., and Farrage, J. (1982, November). *A bite-block prosthesis in the treatment of dysarthria.* Paper presented at the Annual Convention of the American Speech-Language-Hearing Association, Toronto.

Mackay, R. (1963). Course and prognosis in amyotrophic lateral sclerosis. *Archives of Neurology, 8,* 117–127.

Mawdesley, C. (1973). Speech in parkinsonism. In D. Calne (Ed.), *Advances in neurology 3: Progress in the treatment of parkinsonism.* London: Raven.

McConnell, F. (1982, April). *Effects of surgical reconstruction on speech after oral ablative surgery.* Paper presented at the American Academy of Head and Neck Surgery, New Orleans.

McDonald, E., and Schultz, A. (1973). Communication boards for cerebral palsied children. *Journal of Speech and Hearing Disorders, 38,* 73–88.

Meyerson, B. (1973). EMG characteristics of labial articulatory muscles in parkinsonism. In J. Siegfried (Ed.), *Parkinson's disease.* Vienna: Hans Huber.

Montgomery, J. (1983). Communication systems for the child without speech. In W. Perkins (Ed.), *Dysarthria and apraxia.* New York: Thieme Stratton.

Moore, D. (1972). Glossectomy rehabilitation by mandibular tongue prosthesis. *Journal of Prosthetic Dentistry, 28,* 429–434.

Nakano, K., Zubick, H., and Tyler, H. (1973). Speech defects in parkinsonian patients. *Neurology, 23,* 865–870.

Netsell, R., and Cleeland, C. (1973). Modification of lip hypertonia in dysarthria using EMG feedback. *Journal of Speech and Hearing Disorders, 38,* 131–140.

Netsell, R., and Daniel, B. (1979). Dysarthria in adults: Physiologic approach to rehabilitation. *Archives of Physical Medicine and Rehabilitation, 60,* 502–508.

Netsell, R., Daniel, B., and Celesia, C. (1975). Acceleration and weakness in parkinsonian dysarthrias. *Journal of Speech and Hearing Disorders, 40,* 467–480.

Netsell, R., and Hixon, T. (1978). Noninvasive method for clinically estimating subglottal air pressure. *Journal of Speech and Hearing Disorders, 43,* 326–330.

Owens, R., and House, L. (1984). Decision-making processes in augmentative communication. *Journal of Speech and Hearing Disorders, 49,* 18–45.

Peacher, W. (1947). Speech disorders in World War II: VII. Treatment of dysarthrias. *Journal of Nervous and Mental Diseases, 106,* 66–76.

Peacher, W. (1950). The etiology and differential diagnosis of dysarthria. *Journal of Speech and Hearing Disorders, 15,* 252–265.

Rigrodsky, S., and Morrison, E. (1970). Speech changes in parkinsonism during L-Dopa therapy: Preliminary findings. *Journal of the American Geriatric Society, 18,* 142–151.

Rubow, R., Rosenbek, J., Collins, M., and Celesia, G. (1984). Reduction of hemifacial spasm and dysarthria following EMG biofeedback. *Journal of Speech and Hearing Disorders, 49,* 26–33.

Schweiger, J., Netsell, R., and Sommerfield, R. (1970). Prosthetic management and speech improvement in individuals with dysarthria of the palate. *Journal of the American Dental Association, 80,* 1348–1353.

Seilo, M. T., LaRiviere, C., and Dommick, K. C. (1972). *Report on the speech intelligibility of a glossectomee: Perceptual and acoustic observations.* Paper presented at the Annual Convention of the American Speech and Hearing Association, San Francisco.

Shane, H., and Bashir, A. (1980). Election criteria for the adoption of an augmentative communication system: Preliminary considerations. *Journal of Speech and Hearing Disorders, 45,* 408–414.

Silverman, F. (1983). Dysarthria: Communication-augmentation systems for adults without speech. In W. Perkins (Ed.), *Dysarthria and apraxia.* New York: Thieme-Stratton.

Skelly, M., Donaldson, R., and Fust, R. (1973). Glossectomee speech rehabilitation, Springfield, IL: Charles C Thomas.

Skelly, M., Donaldson, R., Fust, R., and Townsend, D. (1972). Changes in phonatory aspects of glossectomee intelligibility through vocal parameter manipulation. *Journal of Speech and Hearing Disorders, 37,* 379-389.

Skelly, M., Schinsky, L., Smith, R., and Fust, R. (1974). American Indian sign (Amerind) as a facilitator of verbalization for the oral verbal apraxic. *Journal of Speech and Hearing Disorders, 39,* 445-456.

Skelly, M., Spector, D., Donaldson, R., Brodeur, and Paletta, F. (1971). Compensatory physiologic phonetics for the glossectomee. *Journal of Speech and Hearing Disorders, 35,* 101-114.

Sonies, B. (1982). Oral imaging systems: A review and clinical applications. The *Journal of the National Student Speech Language Hearing Association, 10,* 30-43.

Sonies, B., Shauker, T., and Stowe, M. (1982, November). *Frontiers in oral imaging: Instrumentation and clinical application.* Paper presented at the Annual Convention of the American Speech-Language-Hearing Association, Toronto.

Summers, G. W. (1974). Physiologic problems following ablative surgery of the head and neck. *Otolaryngologic Clinics of North America, 7,* 217-250.

Trost, J., and Canter, G. (1974). Apraxia of speech in patients with Broca's aphasia: A study of phoneme production accuracy and error patterns. *Brain and Language, 1,* 63-80.

Vanderheiden, G., and Grilley, K. (Eds.) (1976). *Nonvocal communication techniques and aids for the severely physically handicapped,* Baltimore: University Park Press.

Vanderheiden, G., Kelso, D., Holt, C., and Raitzer, G. (1977). Development of flexible teacher-modifiable communication aids for the severely and extremely motor impaired. *Proceedings of the 4th Annual Conference on Systems and Devices for the Disabled* (pp. 86-91). Seattle: University of Washington.

Wertz, R., LaPointe, L., and Rosenbek, J. (1984). *Apraxia of speech in adults.* Orlando, FL: Grune & Stratton.

Wheeler, R., Logemann, J., and Rosen, M. (1980). Maxillary reshaping prostheses: Effectiveness in improving speech and swallowing of post-surgical oral cancer patients. *Journal of Prosthetic Dentistry, 43,* 313-319.

James H. Abbs
John C. Rosenbek

Some Motor Control Perspectives on Apraxia of Speech and Dysarthria

In our approaches to speech neuropathologies over the last 30 years, we have acquired certain methods, concepts, and definitions. For example, speech errors in dysarthria and apraxia of speech populations have been classified with the same schemes used for distinguishing the languages of the world. Likewise, descriptive techniques from experimental phonetics (e.g., perceptual, acoustic, and aerodynamic analyses) have been applied. Speech pathologists have also become involved in a number of theoretic issues, such as the "level" of these neural dysfunctions in relation to the phonetician's classic, multilayer analogy of the the speech production process. One example of such an issue is whether apraxia of speech is a disorder at the linguistic or the motor level. Many of these particular lines of description and theory appear, in part, to be historical accidents; current approaches to speech neuropathologies emerged from linguistics, experimental phonetics, and the educational and behavioral sciences. Accident or not, they have influenced the profession's perspective on theoretic and practical issues.

While some of the inheritance from these traditional antecedents has been useful, there is a danger of being misguided like the proverbial blind men in their exploration of the elephant. That is, if the attempt is to understand and treat human speech problems as breakdowns in social interaction or as loss of abstract symbol systems used for communication, such behavioral and linguistic approaches may, by themselves, be adequate. However, if by contrast the attempt is to understand the causal relations between certain brain dysfunctions and the programming, execution, and control of speech movements, equal emphasis must be placed upon the neurophysiology of motor control. The inclusion of current knowledge from motor control (as this area currently is defined [cf. Brooks, 1981]) requires careful consideration of the complex and flexible nature of motorsensory processes. As a bonus, the investigator becomes sensitive to the limitations of traditional concepts and analyses developed originally in experimental phonetics for other purposes.

The degree of imbalance in current approaches to speech neuropathologies is reflected in the nearly exclusive use of acoustic, aerodynamic, or perceptual analyses to discern the movement patterns of the vocal organs, seemingly as a basis upon which to make subsequent inferences regarding function and dysfunction of the nervous system. For example, acoustic signals are interpreted via models of vocal tract resonance that assume a general linear relation between vocal behavior and certain signal parameters. Paradoxically, little or no parallel consideration is given to the even more complex and nonlinear properties of muscle contraction, biomechanics, motor unit recruitment, and so on. This omission is particularly striking because neurophysiologic data indicate that determining moment-to-moment nervous system actions is exceedingly difficult even when the motor behaviors (movement and muscle activity) are observed directly (cf. Alexander, 1981; Partridge and Benton, 1981). Hence, as noted, these neurophysiologic considerations bring into sharp focus the parallel ambiguity in discerning motor-sensory operation from the far less direct acoustic, aerodynamic, or auditory-perceptual analyses. For these and other reasons to be discussed, a neuromotor control approach is needed to augment and verify traditional analyses and to provide a more rational perspective for considering these disorders in both the laboratory and the clinic. That is, while traditional methods from experimental phonetics are accepted within speech pathology, and many practitioners are "comfortable" with their use, a broader approach to dysarthria and apraxia is likely, in the long run, to provide a fundamental basis for sustaining future progress.

In this context, the purpose of this chapter is to offer some alternative interpretations on the nature, evaluation, and management of dysarthria and apraxia of speech from a state-of-the-art neuroscience perspective. Throughout this presentation, it is our hope to raise questions and offer information that will stimulate future research and new ideas on these particular disorders. Some of our notions are speculative, but they are included to provoke debate and to illustrate the equally speculative nature of some of the current "plausible" hypotheses. It should be noted that this chapter is not intended to be a review of all recent research on dysarthria and apraxia of speech. Nor is our goal to provide specific information that can be translated immediately into clinical activities; we will be encouraged if that happens. Rather, the primary objective is to provide a catalyst for a more direct focus upon the actual functions and dysfunctions of the nervous system. In parallel, we hope to retain those aspects of our earlier knowledge that remain useful, while discarding baggage we have acquired in traveling on some dead end roads.

Rationale for a Motor Control Approach

In attempting to study, diagnose, or treat dysarthria and apraxia of speech, our fundamental objective is to address problems in the nervous system programming and execution of speech movements. While we admit to the general accuracy of the platitudes suggesting that speech is one of the human's most "complex" motor behaviors, it is undeniable that speech production is nevertheless a *motor act* with commonalities to other voluntary motor behavior in terms of muscle contractions, movements, biomechanics, motoneuron recruitment, and so on. As such, in the attempt to decipher nervous system function for speech production, it is useful to acknowledge and understand these common elements, thereby giving us at least an initial perspective on the complexities involved.

Table 2–1 is a list of the probable components of speech neuromotor programming and control, drawn from both contemporary neurophysiology and parallel knowledge of speech production processes. In the sequence from the acoustic signal output of the speech production system (level 1) to successively "deeper" levels of motor-sensory function (levels 3, 4, 5, etc.), it is apparent that several critical processes have not been considered carefully in analyses of speech motor control. For example, the way that motoneuron signals activate muscle actions (level 2) has alone been the subject of an estimated 100,000 reported investigations. Without knowledge of this critical link, inferences from peripheral to higher levels is fraught with potential error. Seldom, however, are any of the potential influences of muscle, the neuromotor end organ of the speech production system, considered even implicitly in interpretations of speech neuropathologies. It might be argued that the process of translating motoneuron signals to muscle contraction is a simple one, and hence a linear relation can be assumed. However, as noted recently by Partridge and Benton (1981) in their extensive review of muscle biomechanics research, "a number of

Table 2–1. Probable Biologic Processes Underlying "Significant" Speech Production Features

1. *Acoustic and aerodynamic properties of the vocal conduit,* including physical discontinuities or nonlinearities

2. *Biomechanical properties,* e.g., muscle mechanics, load dynamics, geometric nonlinearities, boundary conditions

3. *Lower level reflexive actions,* via lower brainstem or spinal cord pathways

4. *Modifiable, long-loop reactions* (transcortical cerebellar-cerebral, etc.), possibly developed or refined with experience

5. *Internal CNS refinement and predictive correction processes,* variably dependent on moment-to-moment ascending afferents

6. *Sets of general, prelearned motor goals,* as a basis for overall guidance of CNS execution and programming

7. *Linguistic specification of "segmental" or suprasegmental goals,* as currently hypothesized or as yet undefined

   or, most likely,

8. *Variable and awesomely complex interactions among all levels of this biolinguistic process*

models exist that approximate parts of muscle function, but all of the models inescapably have appreciable defects. Deficiencies lie in both the formal models available and in defects in our understanding of the rules of the biological muscle as it responds to mechanical and neural actions" (p. 47). In short, Partridge and Benton indicate that our current knowledge does not, except under restricted circumstances, allow us to understand the seemingly simple relation between motoneuron firing patterns and movement, to say nothing of inferring in the opposite direction (i.e., from movement to nervous system actions).

Similarly, in noting the potential role of the primary sensory and motor cortices to the control of movement, Evarts (1981), while documenting the involvement of a transcortical feedback pathway, offers a number of plausible, yet tentative, hypotheses concerning the actual function of that pathway and its peripheral sensory motor correlates. Given the complex, multiple levels of motor programming and control (see Table 2–1), it is critical to consider the undeniable contributions of these various processes to the relatively superficial events we are able to observe at the speech production periphery. In other words, for any apparently significant normal or abnormal feature of the speech production output, be it perceptually, acoustically, aerodynamically, or electromyographically detected, we cannot, without being extremely careful, talk about the nervous system origins of that feature. What should be apparent from these comments is that the surface analysis procedures we are able to apply to neurologically impaired speech production systems are likely to yield indices of dysfunction that are "an awesomely complex and variable combination of all levels of this biolinguistic process" (see Table 2–1). However, despite this caution, it is possible, based upon the substantial and largely ignored literature on motor neurophysiology, to extend and critically examine our current notions concerning the nature, assessment, and treatment of speech neuropathologies.

Also of particular value in this effort is the emergence in the last ten years of clinical neurophysiology. Clinical neurophysiology (as a subspecialty of neurology) has the following goals: (1) to provide a quantitative profile of the neurologic signs and performance deficits with which to diagnose, prescribe, and evaluate treatment; (2) to relate these disease associated indices to working models of the normal and neurologically impaired nervous system; and (3) to examine these profiles of the nervous system to identify and test hypotheses that might point to improved programs of assessment and treatment (cf. Stalberg and Young, 1981). From this effort, the size of which is illustrated by several volumes of clinical neurophysiology research edited by one scholar (Desmedt, 1973–1982), has come a data base upon which to consider current approaches to the nervous system dysfunctions underlying apraxia of speech and dysarthria. While consideration of all the potential implications of clinical neurophysiology and motor control for speech neuropathologies is outside the scope of this chapter, the data and sources cited should provided a basis for parallel review and synthesis efforts by most readers.

From the standpoint of what might be gained from acknowledging the limitations of certain current perspectives on speech neuropathologies, we should like to borrow a quote from motor neurophysiologist and Nobel Laureate Ragnar Granit (1977): "In dealing with objects of our research whose explanation from the standpoint of present-day science is insufficient, greater scientific clarity is achieved by fully realizing what cannot be explained than by stealing a march on science with suppositions. We cannot reach further than to understand what can be understood and realize what we cannot understand" (p. 1). To paraphrase, if we don't know where we really are now, how can we make intelligent decisions on how to get where we want to go?

The Distinction Between Diagnosis and Assessment: The Critical Use of Descriptive Terms

In the discussions that follow, at least an implicit emphasis will be placed upon examining the current semantics of dysarthria and apraxia of speech, and the degree to which these terms, in and of themselves, become issues, often without a substantive foundation. In this vein, it appears important to consider the categorizing processes involved in accomplishing our clinical objectives and ask what the conventional labels and terms do and do not provide.

It has been common to distinguish the different neuropathologies of speech via contrastive profiles of descriptive behaviors. One common difficulty, in neurology as well as speech pathology, has been the assumption that these diagnostic indicators of a particular neuropathologic syndrome are coincident with or underlie the debilitating performance deficits associated with the disease. For example, in the person with spastic dysarthria, it has been assumed that some of the diagnostically distinct speech signs can be ascribed to hypertonicity in the form of muscle spasms. The so-called "strained-strangled voice" observed in these dysarthric persons is thought to be due to antagonistic or spastic co-contraction of the intrinsic laryngeal muscles. In this example, the term spasticity has been borrowed from neurology, and further assumptions have been made that this manifestation of the motor disorder in the limbs is present also in the laryngeal muscles, and that "spasticity," per se, is a causal factor in the speech disorder. To the knowledge of the present authors, muscle activity in the intrinsic laryngeal muscles has not been observed in a classic case of spastic dysarthria; that is, the suggestion of spastic hypertonicity is conjecture. Additionally, it is not clear, even to the clinical neurophysiologists who have spent their careers attempting to quantify and treat spasticity, how best to define it (cf. Lance, 1980; Landau, 1980). For example, is spasticity exclusively a velocity-dependent increase in stretch reflexes, causing a pathophysiologic increase in resistance to a neurologic examiner's externally imposed movement? Or, as suggested by some, is it synonymous with the so-called upper motoneuron syndrome involving decreased dexterity, loss of strength, increased tendon jerks, increased resistance to passive stretch, and hyperactive flexion reflexes? It is apparent that spasticity is not a unidimensional phenomenon. Perhaps most critical to this example is the current consensus among experimental and clinical neurologists that while spasticity, per se, is an excellent diagnostic sign, the increased hypertonus-hyperactive stretch reflex-flexor spasms seen in these patients are largely independent from the actual motor performance deficits present in parallel. Landau (1980) was particularly candid and clear in reviewing several lines of evidence (Denny-Brown, 1980; Duncan, Shahani, and Young, 1976; Landau, 1974, 1980; Sahrman and Norton, 1977) concerning the relation between hypertonic signs and motor performance impairments in spastic patients. He noted, "However useful to clinical diagnosis may be the increase of excitability at anterior horn cells and to some extent muscle spindles, these phenomena have little more relation to the patient's disability than does the insertion of the rectal thermometer in pneumonia" (p. 20). In this context, one must seriously question the assertion that so-called strained-strangled voice is the result of antagonistic muscle "spastic" hypertonus in the larynx.

There is obviously a very important message in this example for the distinction between diagnosis and assessment. That is, while it is logical and intuitively appealing to make the inference that hypertonus and spasms are the *major underlying cause* of motor disabilities in persons with spasticity or upper motoneuron syndrome, this inference does not stand up to empirical scrutiny. Indeed, this unfounded assumption was made by both clinical and research neurophysiologists over the years, and millions of dollars were spent on attempts to eliminate hypertonus with the expectation that the motor deficit associated with this disorder would be improved in parallel. As noted by Landau (1980), these results have been disappointing.

It is also likely that some of the most salient distinguishing indicators for differential diagnosis of these speech neuropathologies may not be related causally to the speech performance deficits that are present in parallel. That is, in the use of traditional techniques from experimental phonetics, or even so-called physiologic measures, examination must be made of the extent to which certain acoustic, aerodynamic, auditory-perceptual, or electromyographic features of speech "abnormality" are related *causally* to deficits in functional communication or speech movement coordination and control. Certainly, it would seem a minimal scientific requirement that such descriptive analyses focus upon measures that are correlated to the degree of functional speech disturbance. Correlational analyses, without analytic models or explicit hypotheses for verifying causality, are highly subject to misinterpretation. However, these data, at the least, would assist us in determining what aspects of performance aberration are epiphenomena, and hence of minor significance, and at the same time identify those aberrant features that might reflect overall performance deficits. If we adhere to these requirements in our research and treatment, we might avoid repeating the errors made in the attempted treatment of spasticity and also enhance the rational basis for focusing our programs of rehabilitation. To return to the example of limb spasticity discussed earlier, it is apparent that reducing or eliminating flexor spasms or hyperactive stretch reflexes through various treatments was not of particular benefit in improving motor function. Treating certain superficial aberrations (e.g., acoustic segment durations) may be similarly futile unless such aberrations have been demonstrated as negative neurologic manifestations and not simply epiphenomena. The message is clear. The seemingly compelling causal relations that might be observed in clinical populations may not be valid; the nervous system often does not function in intuitively obvious ways, and the requirement for formal testing of unquantified assertions, no matter how appealing they may be, cannot be relaxed. The penalty for an absence of seemingly harsh empiricism in clinical endeavors is ineffective treatment.

Conceptualization of the Speech Motor Control Process

As noted at the outset of this chapter, certain extant models of the speech production process appear to have had considerable impact upon our conceptualization of speech neuropathologies, and thus upon the way in which these disorders are assessed, treated, and studied. One such "model," either implicitly or explicitly incorporated in most thinking about normal and disordered speech production systems, portrays the speech production process as a succession of independent levels proceeding from semantic, to syntactic, to phonologic formulations. Phonetic goals are achieved via the seemingly mechanical operation of motor programming and execution. Such representations may be quite functional if the issues addressed are in the domain of psycholinguistics. However, this representation carries with it certain simplifying assumptions, which may be counterproductive in our approaches to dysarthria and apraxia of speech. One of these assumptions is that intended phonologic-phonetic goals yield stereotyped and consistent muscle activities, movements, and vocal tract shapes at the periphery. More specifically, this model implies that once a string of phonetic goals is specified, the "lower levels" of this process involve the more or less direct activation of a set of muscle actions. Further, it is implied that the set of muscle actions is essentially the same every time a particular phonetic string is produced. This conceptualization implies a single, isolated level of motor programming, and hence the execution process is conceived primarily as the transmission of temporally-spatially correct signals to the periphery.

In the context of numerous recent experiments on these motor programming, coordination, and execution processes, this view (or the subtle variations on it presented in many accounts of speech production) is simply not tenable. That is, in the last decade we have seen an exponential increase in the research efforts on voluntary motor control; it has been estimated that 500 papers per month are published in this area (Partridge, 1976). Hence, on the basis of this intensive application of new techniques to discern the character of nervous system function in movement control (cf. Desmedt, 1978 [1973–1982]; Houk and Rymer, 1981; Rack, 1981, for reviews), extensive evidence indicates that speech motor programming and execution cannot be characterized in this traditional manner. As Marsden (1982) noted recently in regard to motor execution:

> in the real world, such admittedly central motor programs are never isolated from peripheral feedback which must operate at all stages in the sequence of a motor act. Computing technology has introduced the concept of hierarchic schemes that greatly simplify and shorten the programming of robot manipulations. Such systems, remarkably reminiscent of the various levels of Hughlings Jackson, utilize different levels of control, each one of which regulates its own particular function or parameter. The levels of control are arranged in hierarchic order, the more general subordinating and modulating the more specific. Each level receives information about the state of the other levels. In practice, the entire hierarchical system operates as a whole to produce an integrated, smooth performance. (p. 523)

While this observation is based upon experiments conducted on limb motor behavior in man and waking animals, parallel observations in the speech production system suggest qualitatively similar principles of motor programming and execution. For example, inasmuch as programming and associated descending signals appear to be under continual modulation and updating via ascending afferent information, it is apparent that the generation of a given articulatory movement or vocal tract shape is not prespecified stereotypically, but rather varies from one production of a given utterance to a repeated production of that same utterance. This is indeed what has been observed empirically. Hughes and Abbs (1976) transduced the movements of the upper lip, lower lip, and jaw during repeated productions of a particular utterance. The classic model discussed earlier would predict, within certain system noise limits, that these articulators would move essentially in the same way for these repeated productions. However, when the actual movements were observed for multiple repetitions of the same utterance, there was not a stereotypic pattern. For a given repetition, when the jaw moved a large distance in producing an oral opening for a vowel, the upper and lower lips moved a small distance; for another repetition, the relative magnitude of movement between these coordinated structures was reversed. More specifically, the normal motor control of the oral opening was not achieved in a stereotypic manner, but rather involved a considerable degree of repetition-to-repetition trade-off between movements of these three contributing articulators. Similar trade-offs have been reported between the tongue and the jaw (Fujimura, 1981) and the rib cage and abdomen (Hunker and Abbs, 1982). Further observations have been made indicating that two synergistic muscles that contribute to the movement of a given structure likewise trade off in their contributions from one generation of that movement to another, both in the limbs (Lacquaniti and Soechting, 1982) and in the speech production system (Abbs, 1979; Abbs and Gracco, 1984; Gentil, Gracco, and Abbs, 1983; Sussman, MacNeilage, and Hanson, 1973). Specifically, these latter observations indicate that two synergistic muscles that contribute to movement of a given structure (e.g., orbicularis oris inferior and mentalis in their conjoint contribution to lower lip elevation) are not activated stereotypically but trade off in the repetition-to-repetition generation of the same movement (Abbs, 1979; Abbs and Gracco, 1984).

Figure 2-1 provides a concrete, albeit simplified, example of these variations for three productions of the utterance /aba/ that were equivalent in terms of their phonologic, aerodynamic, acoustic, and auditory-perceptual characteristics. The upper and lower lip movements for these productions are shown, illustrating three different patterns of movement. Obviously, the muscle activity underlying these productions is different as well; essentially, this example illustrates complementary variation between upper and lower lip gestures to carry out an equivalent phonologic plan of action.

These observations on normal speech motor programming and execution are consistent with the comments made by Marsden and may require certain modifications in the traditional model presented earlier and in terms of the way speech pathologists have conceptualized the neuropathologies of speech. Initially, it is apparent that the motor execution and programming of speech is not a single operation, but a hierarchical process with considerable variation in the ways objectives and subobjectives are accomplished. That is, while the overall goals of the system output (e.g., oral opening, degree of oral constriction, subglottal pressure) might be considered part of the general phonologic plan of action, the temporal-spatial implementation of these goals via multiple movements is apparently programmed at another level of the system. Indeed, it is apparent that there

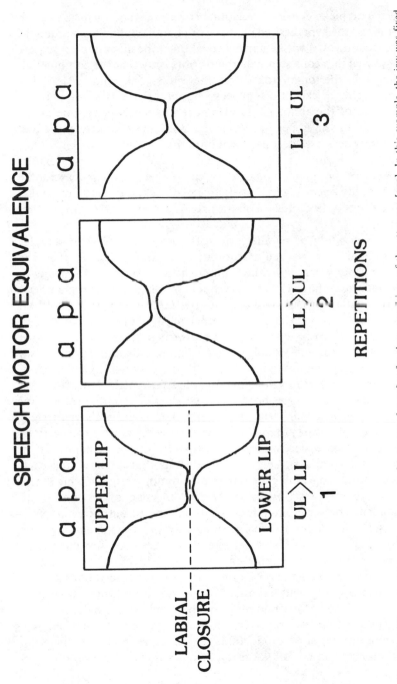

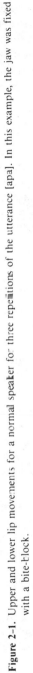

Figure 2-1. Upper and lower lip movements for a normal speaker for three repetitions of the utterance [apa]. In this example, the jaw was fixed with a bite-block.

is not a stereotypic or consistent relation between the movements of a given articulator and the hypothesized phonetic or phonologic goals. For example, production of a vowel with a narrow vocal tract opening does not require that the jaw be in a consistently high position, only that the combination of the jaw and the tongue together achieve this goal. Similar flexibility in the peripheral execution process apparently exists for relative contributions of the abdomen and rib cage to total lung volume or for contributions of the upper lip, lower lip, and jaw to oral opening and closing. Recent observations involving the introduction of small, unanticipated errors in lip movements suggest that this flexible, multimovement coordination process is accomplished via afferent ascending signals, possibly operating in a predictive manner (Abbs and Cole, 1982; Abbs and Gracco, 1982, 1984; Folkins and Abbs, 1975, 1976; Gracco and Abbs, 1982).

The observation of parallel trade-offs between synergistic muscles acting to achieve a particular movement further suggests that the neuromotor level where individual muscle actions are programmed is in turn separate from the level where individual movements are programmed. That is, the action of a particular muscle is not stereotyped for a given movement, but rather covaries, with other muscles also contributing to that movement from one repetition of the movement to another. Therefore, it is apparent that individual muscle contractions are at least two programming steps removed from the level of the nervous system where the so-called phonetic or overall goals are predetermined. Hence, the level of the nervous system where the so-called concept of action or the general motor plan is determined, perhaps involving phonologic goals, is different from the levels of motor programming where specific muscle contractions and movements are determined. In terms of our considerations of dysarthria and apraxia of speech, it is obvious that a useful approach involves questions concerning the possible neuromotor levels at which these problems are manifest. Because of the absence of a one-to-one correspondence between phonologic goals and motor outputs, it appears far less useful to attempt to separate motor dysfunctions from linguistic ones, especially with superficial peripheral measures. An intriguing issue regarding levels of programming concerns the distinction between oral, nonverbal apraxia, and apraxia of speech. Physiologic observations in these populations may reveal some additional distinctions concerning differences in the levels of motor programming for these behavioral deficits.

In addition to variations in individual movements and muscle contractions for repeated productions of the same utterance, there are parallel variations in overall vocal tract shapes for multiple productions of the same acoustic end product (Ladefoged, DeClark, Lindau, and Papcun, 1972; Lindau, Jacobson, and Ladefoged, 1972). All of these variations in movements, muscle contractions, and vocal tract shapes operate under the general principle of motor equivalence (cf. Bernstein, 1967; Hebb, 1949; Lacquaniti and Soechting, 1982; Lashley, 1930; Morasso, 1981). Motor equivalence is generally defined as a nervous system operation in which the same intended motor objective is accomplished with variation in the individual movements and muscle contractions that combine to produce that intended goal. This principle of motor control has particular implications for traditional experimental phonetic measures of speech neuropathologies. Initially, it is apparent that utterance productions judged equivalent by more global measures are likely to be very different in terms of underlying patterns of muscle activity, movement, or specific vocal tract configuration. The power of inferences made from these global measures to patterns of movement, muscle contraction, or nervous system activity in any but the most general terms is, therefore, very limited. For example, if the vocal tract acoustic transfer function underlying a particular vowel formant pattern requires certain vocal tract length characteristics or relative volumes of front and back cavities, these apparently are *not* produced in a stereotyped manner. Rather, they are produced through combinations of lip protrusion and laryngeal height for vocal tract length, and combinations of pharyngeal constriction–tongue body forwarding for front cavity–back cavity dimensions (Ladefoged et al., 1972; Lindau et al., 1972). Indeed, we have known for some time the substantial degrees of freedom available in the production of vowels (cf. Stevens and House, 1955, 1961, concerning covariable contributions of upper airway articulators). Similar variability is obviously available in the production of air pressures and air flow rates for speech, where manipulations in the upper airway size, shape, and cavity wall impedance, along with temporal-spatial variations in glottal abduction-adduction, allow for substantial degrees of freedom in the production of aerodynamically equivalent patterns (Muller and Brown, 1980).

In the same way, and perhaps to a greater extent, auditory-perceptual analyses, whether involving broad or narrow phonetic transcription, are subject to very serious limitations in the making of inferences to underlying movements and muscle contractions or specific moment-to-moment patterns of nervous system operation. We know from perceptual studies the degree to which speech acoustic signal cues can be varied and still remain acceptable in relation to phonetic categorization or from the standpoint of intelligibility. For example, the perceptual domain in /i/-ness is obviously not simply an absolute or relative formant frequency pattern; rather, it has perceptually significant acoustic features of duration, intensity, and fundamental frequency that have been shown to influence its identification. Inasmuch as these features apparently can be weighted relatively, especially in contextual speech, there appears to be a substantial possibility that perceptual equivalence is achieved, despite considerable idiosyncratic or compensatory acoustic variations (cf. Lindblom, 1982).

Given these potential sources of variation in the manner in which apparently equivalent productions (based upon acoustic, aerodynamic, or auditory-perceptual observations, or a combination thereof) are generated, it seems that in populations of disordered speakers known to invoke idiosyncratic compensatory adjustments, no single measure is adequate for inferences regarding underlying nervous system function or dysfunction. That is, these single measure analyses are, by definition, insensitive to the motor control equivalence variations. Moreover, that insensitivity is probably greatest where motor equivalence adjustments and maladjustments are employed with varying degrees of success in attempts to minimize the effects of nervous system abnormalities (Gracco and Muller, 1981; Nashner and Grimm, 1978).

This argument is supported, in part, by the general difficulty where global analyses have been employed in distinguishing among dysarthric subpopulations or between certain dysarthric and verbal apraxic groups. Practically every published analysis of the acoustic characteristics of dysarthric speech includes certain common features (e.g., increased vowel durations, inappropriate or lengthened pauses or both), despite known differences in the underlying neuropathophysiology. Similarly, when subjected to quantitative analyses, the numerous and long-standing attempts at auditory-perceptual distinctions between the speech of athetoid and spastic dysarthric persons reflect limited success, at best. The limited distinguishing capabilities of these global measures might be due to the fact that the nervous system has a finite set of compensation–motor equivalence adjustments. For example, some of these compensatory processes are likely to be invoked similarly by speakers with such conditions as cerebellar disease or apraxia of speech. Slowing of speech rate could be one such common strategy, despite rather substantial differences in the underlying neuropathophysiology. Further, when one is able, via global analyses, to distinguish the speech of two populations of patients with motor disorders, interpretations are further clouded. That is, the distinguishing features could reflect differences in compensatory capabilities and could be related only indirectly to primary motor performance deficits. In general, the implications of these considerations are that clinically we must attempt to observe the motor behavior of the speech production system under conditions where the complex and semiunpredictable normal and abnormal motor equivalence compensatory strategies are minimized.

Given the limitations of observing the movements of all the speech structures during normal productions, this consideration, by necessity, translates to an argument for evaluations based upon simpler nonspeech gestures in parallel with our more traditional analyses. Most clinicians, of course, recognize this, at least implicitly, as is reflected in their use of the oral peripheral examination. Attempting to assess speech neuropathologies on the basis of speech behavior alone is comparable to asking our automobile mechanic to assess a malfunction in our automobile engine as we drive by on the interstate highway. Perhaps if we simplify our analyses, we can begin to focus rehabilitation on specific, less global motor malfunctions, and hence refine our approaches to these disorders. This argument, however, implies that nonspeech motor impairments are of value in assessing and managing motor speech disorders. This raises the classic issue of whether speech and nonspeech motor functions share a common underlying neural substrate.

How Special is Speech?

A long-standing question in the assessment and treatment of motor speech disorders is related to two other questions. Do impairments in the motor control of nonspeech activities such as chewing and swallowing, or volitional nonspeech maneuvers (as observed in the oral peripheral examination), correlate with, or are they indicative of, parallel impairments in speech motor function? Further, does rehabilitation focused upon either feeding or nonspeech "voluntary" control of speech motor subsystems carry over, in its benefits, to improved speech control? Initially, it seems apparent that in lower motoneuron damage the carryover is likely to be high. That is, rehabilitation in the form of strengthening, if successful for nonspeech tasks, should yield improvements in speech as well. This issue, however, has been debated more intensely regarding speech motor problems resulting from supranuclear damage, either congenital or acquired.

Several lines of old and recent evidence are of particular relevance to this issue. Initially, it is important that speech and nonspeech motor tasks be defined from a current neurophysiologic perspective. Chewing, swallowing, and other orofacial vegetative functions are known to be neurophysiologically distinct from nonspeech tasks performed voluntarily. That is, it is documented that these vegetative functions are largely controlled via certain subcortical pattern generators, networks of brainstem reflexes, or both (cf. Dubner, Sessle, and Storey, 1978; Wyke, 1974). For example, Hoffman and Luschei (1980) demonstrated that while motor cortical activity was not involved in moment-to-moment control of chewing in rhesus monkeys, operantly conditioned biting (a "more voluntary" task using the same jaw muscles) was clearly under cortical influence. They noted, "a likely explanation for this observation is that the reciprocal action of the jaw closing and opening muscles during chewing is patterned elsewhere in the brain" (p. 342). Other recent work in the differential control of "automatic" and learned movements suggests a parallel dichotomy for the muscles of the respiratory system (Phillips and Porter, 1977) and the facial muscles (Denny-Brown, 1960). As noted recently by Evarts (1981):

> It might at first seem odd that corticospinal neurons controlling precise skilled movements terminate on motoneurons controlling intercostal muscles that participate in an act as automatic and primative as respiration, but Phillips and Porter point out that these terminations are probably related to the use of respiratory muscles in speech and song rather than in breathing. . . . Destroying the corticospinal projection to thoracic motoneurons does not impair the use of respiratory muscles for respiration, though these same muscles may be useless for speech. (p. 1113)

These considerations offer a new perspective on this long-standing controversy. That is, on the basis of current neurophysiologic observations, this issue does not appear to be one of speech versus nonspeech motor control. Rather, the critical distinction may be whether the nonspeech movements are controlled in a conscious, voluntary manner, as in speech, in contrast to vegetative movements that are more or less automatic. This interpretation appears to square with the data, both old and recent, that are available to address this issue. Perhaps the most concentrated effort in this area came in a series of master's theses conducted under the direction of James Hardy in the 1960s (Hixon, 1963; Murphy, 1966; Smit, 1969; Smith, 1964).

In these studies the relationship between several different orofacial speech tasks was examined in dysarthric subjects, and the results were interpreted with remarkable uniformity to indicate that speech "may well be dissimilar to other neuromuscular processes involving identical muscle groups" (Hardy, 1970, p. 60). In evaluation of these classic studies in light of the modified interpretation just offered, the motor task comparisons and correlations made must be examined carefully. The investigation reported by Hixon and Hardy (1964) is exemplary. Essentially, in this study independent indices were obtained for degree of speech severity, diadochokinetic rates for several different stop sounds, and rates of nonspeech voluntary movements such as lateral movements of the tongue. Degree of impairment in nonspeech vegetative movements such as chewing and swallowing was not reported. The results suggest fairly high correlations (0.70 to 0.75) between severity of speech and syllable diadochokinetic rates, and somewhat lower correlations between speech severity and rates of nonspeech movements (0.41 to 0.56).

The fundamental problem with Hixon and Hardy's study (1964) is that the comparison of these correlations does not support the interpretation of speech versus nonspeech control differences. The speech and the CV syllable diadochokinetic tasks obviously involved the respiratory system, larynx, and pharynx, as well as the tongue, lips, and jaw. By contrast, the tongue, lip, and jaw movements were sampled individually in the nonspeech movement tasks. Because the subject populations observed were probably variable in the degree of respiratory, laryngeal, and pharyngeal motor impairment, this would have the effect of reducing the correlations between severity of speech disorders and the rates of either lip, jaw, or tongue nonspeech movements. Recent data argue for ubiquitous differential speech subsystem impairment in patients with cerebral palsy and Parkinson's disease (cf. Abbs, Hunker, and Barlow, 1983; Barlow and Abbs, 1982; Hunker, Abbs, and Barlow, 1982). Indeed, given the near certainty of this contaminating factor, the correlations reported between individual articulator nonspeech movement rates and speech severity are relatively high; one of the present authors has actually cited these observations as support of an overlap between control processes for speech and nonspeech control (Abbs, Sutton, Larson, and Eilenberg, 1973). Another factor supporting an alternate interpretation for the Hixon and Hardy (1964) results was that the correlation between the degree of judged speech severity and the diadochokinetic rates for pVtVkV syllables (0.53) was in the same range as the correlations between judged speech severity and nonspeech movement rates. Additionally, the nonspeech movement that had the poorest correlation to speech severity (0.28) was raising the tongue to the aveolar ridge and lowering it, a maneuver that required a larger range of movement than for rapid production of diadochokinetic [da]s. By way of reinterpretation, the comparisons made in these often cited studies offer support, indirectly and directly, for a *common neuromuscular substrate* underlying control of speech and nonspeech *voluntary* tasks.

Direct evidence supporting a common neural substrate for the control of voluntary, nonspeech movements and speech are provided by instrumental observations of nonspeech control impairments of the tongue, lips, and jaw, and comparison of these measures with impairments in the movements of the same structures during speech (Barlow and Abbs, 1984; Hunker et al., 1982; Hunker and Abbs, 1984). Figure 2-2 shows a profile of nonspeech control impairment in a subject with congenital spasticity

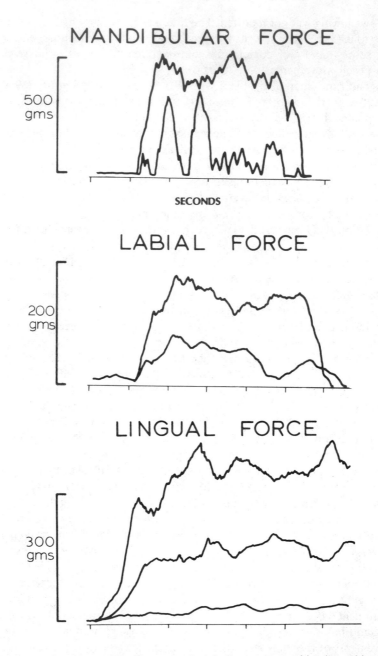

Figure 2–2. Comparison of fine force control of the lips, tongue, and jaw in a subject with congenital spasticity.

and dysarthria. As is apparent, the greatest degree of control impairment (with respect to normal performance) for this static force task was in the jaw; the lips and tongue were far less impaired. In this subject, a bite-block was placed between the teeth, effectively eliminating the need to control movement in the disproportionately impaired jaw. The result of the bite-block upon speech is shown in Figure 2-3, which contrasts the upper lip, lower lip, and jaw movements for conditions with the jaw free to vary and with the jaw fixed. Substantial improvements are apparent in the regularity of the upper and lower lip movements, intraoral air pressure (both magnitude and duration), and the durations and amplitudes of the vowels as reflected in the audio signal. These data are representative of those from a larger study, which demonstrated a high correlation (0.89) between degree of impairment in the voluntary, nonspeech control of the lips, jaw, and tongue, and measures of speech severity (Barlow and Abbs, 1984). Similarly, in a group of parkinsonian dysarthric subjects, Hunker and colleagues (1982) found a positive correlation between degree of labial rigidity, range of lip movement, and severity of dysarthria. In summary, these latter data and the previously considered neurophysiologic and neuroanatomic findings suggest that nonspeech control of precise, voluntary activities is likely to be impaired in the same manner as speech motor behavior.

The implications for assessment and rehabilitation from this working hypothesis are several. Initially, on the basis of the data shown in Figure 2-3, it is obvious that assessment of impairments solely on the basis of spontaneous speech behavior, whether movement observations, acoustic analyses, or simply a sage clinical ear is used, may not permit differentiation of a jaw control impairment from a lip or tongue impairment. These data from spastic and hypokinetic dysarthric subjects address an important point made previously regarding the relative insensitivity of more global indices provided by acoustic or aerodynamic analyses. Specifically, it is unlikely that without use of a bite-block the critical jaw control impairment in the spastic dysarthric subject would have been discernible from such measures as formant frequencies, vowel durations, and air pressure measures. Similarly, conventional global measures would not be sensitive to the differential degree of upper and lower lip rigidity in the parkinsonian dysarthric patients. Hence, observations of voluntary nonspeech control tasks obviously are useful to separate potential subsystem motor impairments. This logic carries over to rehabilitation as well. That is, if impairments of voluntary nonspeech control are parallel to those for speech, improvements on selected, voluntary nonspeech tasks could be expected to enhance speech control as well, depending of course on the site of the lesion and neural tissue remaining to support voluntary and learned behaviors. Thus, for the rehabilitation of the spastic dysarthric subject

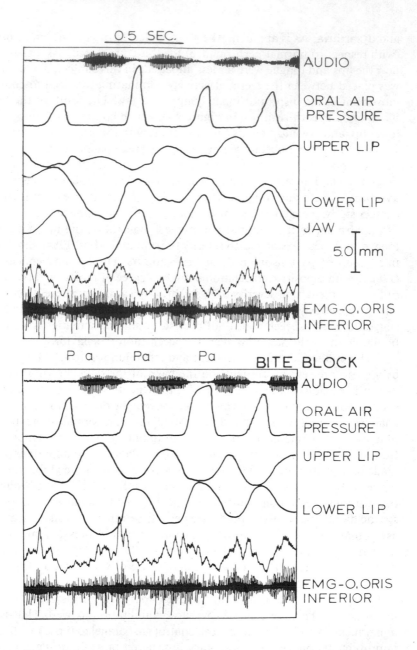

Figure 2–3. Comparison of labial-mandibular movements for a subject with congenital spasticity without (upper panel) and with (lower panel) a bite-block.

shown in Figure 2–3, a logical step would be improvement of voluntary jaw control. Even helping this patient to position the jaw at a neutral height would be an improvement, because such a position would allow for more regular, smooth movement of other articulators, as was observed with the jaw fixed. These observations should not be interpreted as a suggestion that this dysarthric subject will ever regain control of the speech mechanism in a "normal" manner (e.g., conscious concentration upon careful positioning of the jaw may always be necessary) or as an argument for exclusive or primary use of nonspeech activities in therapy.

These interpretations have interesting implications for other forms of rehabilitation as well. For example, some treatments used in cerebral palsy have emphasized the facilitation of chewing and swallowing as a means for improving speech function. Despite the considerable zeal with which these programs are sometimes pursued, there is little direct evidence to support their value for speech improvement. The apparent difference in neural substrate for control of vegetative orofacial function and control of speech and nonspeech voluntary behavior argues against the utility of these therapies for speech. This argument appears to be supported by the recent observations of Love, Hagerman, and Taimi (1980), who found no consistent relation between severity of speech impairment in 60 children with cerebral palsy and the presence of dysphagia. Love and colleagues likewise reported the absence of a correlation between aberrations in oromotor reflexes and severity of speech impairment. This latter finding is consistent with interpretations suggesting that brainstem-mediated reflexes, posited earlier to be involved in speech motor control (McLean, Folkins, and Larson, 1979; Netsell and Abbs, 1975, 1977), subserve vegetative and protective functions; these brainstem reflex pathways appear to be largely inactive during the execution of normal speech production (Abbs and Cole, 1982; Abbs and Gracco, 1984; Gracco and Abbs, 1982). In particular, these observations emphasize the more direct role of cerebellar and cortical pathways in the normal speech motor control process, an interpretation that is consistent with that of Evarts (1981, 1982), as noted previously.

While these considerations offer a supporting basis for assessment and treatment of dysarthria via nonspeech voluntary control tasks, the details of this approach need to be considered in light of current "state-of-the-art" assessment procedures and their underlying neurophysiologic rationale. Regarding apraxia of speech, instrumental analyses of voluntary control of nonspeech behaviors in this population have not been conducted, to the knowledge of the authors of this chapter. Given the controversy surrounding this disorder, such analyses appear critical.

Theoretical Evaluation of Current Assessment and Treatment Procedures

The treatment of dysarthria has increasingly involved emphasis upon more focused physical intervention, including biofeedback, palatal lifts, posturing, and abdominal binding (cf. Hixon, 1975; Netsell and Daniel, 1979; Rosenbek and LaPointe, 1978; Rubow, 1981; Rubow and Netsell, 1979). These physically oriented treatments, while often experimental, can be contrasted to earlier, more global approaches, in that optimal success may require detailed assessment of information concerning each patient's speech mechanism pathophysiology (Netsell and Daniel, 1979). To be more specific, it may not be optimal to utilize relaxation biofeedback to reduce muscle tone if the nature, degree, and distribution of that increased tone and its causal relation to speech performance deficits are not documented. Indeed, it is obvious that the long-term advancement of treatment intervention in both dysarthria and apraxia of speech depends as much upon the quality of the assessment in revealing the motor pathophysiology as upon the cleverness of the techniques themselves. Unfortunately, the effectiveness of current clinical assessment procedures in determining actual neuropathophysiology has not been evaluated systematically. Indeed, many assessment procedures for dysarthria are idiosyncratic to particular clinicians, making evaluation of their effectiveness difficult. To avoid imposing our own idiosyncracies, we will focus on assessment techniques that have been based upon published data.

As noted recently (cf. Abbs et al., 1983), assessment procedures, as they are advocated for use in many clinical settings, involve several serial steps if the diagnostician's purpose is to localize the lesion and to specify the apparent speech system neuropathophysiology. Initially, auditory-perceptual evaluation of the dysarthric speech is made, with attempts via speech task manipulations, to identify the nature of impairments in the major components of the speech production system (i.e., respiratory, phonatory, articulatory). This evaluation is augmented by a more or less standard oral-peripheral examination. Second, on the basis of formal or informal auditory-perceptual classification procedures (e.g., Darley, Aronson, and Brown, 1969a, 1969b, 1975) and knowledge of the parallel neurologic findings, differential categorization of the apparent neurologic syndrome is often considered. Many speech pathologists are extremely skilled at identifying certain disease clusters via auditory-perceptual analyses. Identification of the neurologic syndrome offers some insight into potential pathophysiology. However, despite the appeal of this step, inferences as to the "associated" movement and muscle contraction impairment manifestations in the speech production system are difficult. These inferences are commonly based on concurrent neurologic observations of the limb motor system and on classic, stereotypic descriptions of the syndrome-associated limb pathophysiology as provided in the limb movement disorders literature. For example, if the differential diagnosis yields the identification of hypokinetic dysarthria (for example, in Parkinson's disease), it is inferred (or assumed) that the speech motor impairment is a manifestation of rigidity, hypokinesia or bradykinesia, resting tremor, or a combination of these features in the muscles and movements of the speech production system. This pathophysiologic profile is, of course, a classic neurologic description of motor disorder signs in the limbs (Delong and Georgopoulos, 1981; Marsden, 1982). Aside from the difficulties with auditory-perceptual analyses of motor equivalence compensation discussed earlier, this assessment approach is based on two fundamental and related assumptions. The first assumption is that limb pathophysiology provides a valid basis for making inferences regarding associated speech motor problems. That is, there is an explicit assertion that the neuropathophysiology of movement disorders is manifest uniformly across limb and speech motor subsystems. This leads to a second assumption that the motor subsystems of the speech production system similarly are impaired uniformly as a result of a particular suprabulbar or supraspinal injury. In other words, the lips, tongue, jaw, larynx, pharynx, velopharynx, and respiratory system will show similar patterns of motor deficit. It is apparent that the validity of these two assumptions determines the degree to which these particular assessment procedures provide directions for treatment of the speech system pathophysiology.

These issues are perhaps most important if one considers the physiologic perspective of Hardy (1967) and the multicomponent representation of the speech production system that Netsell (1979) proposed as a guiding framework for physiologic assessment and treatment of motor speech disorders. As noted, this multicomponent orientation evolved from the argument that assessment of different speech motor subsystems is necessary to develop an optimal program of component-focused rehabilitation. This approach is particularly appealing in evaluating potential lower motoneuron disorders where differences in subsystem impairments might be present because of selective damage in some cranial nerves and not others. At issue, however, is whether it is necessary to conduct multiple subsystem assessment in dysarthrias of suprabulbar origin. While many experienced speech pathologists know the answer to this question, there is considerable value in offering a more detailed analysis with specific hypotheses. Hypothetically, if suprabulbar lesions uniformly impair all the motor subsystems of speech production system, evaluation of only one speech motor subsystem may be necessary. It could be possible to evaluate the control impairments in the most accessible speech motor subsystems (e.g., the lips) and infer the control impairments in the jaw, tongue, larynx, velum, and respiratory structures. However, if a suprabulbar lesion results in a nonuniform control impairment across the speech motor subsystems, determinations of speech motor impairment cannot be made from observations of a single motor subcomponent. Similarly, it would be difficult to make parallel inferences from limb motor impairments, as classically defined, to presumed pathophysiology in the orofacial system (cf. Darley et al., 1975). From the standpoint of motor neurophysiology (in determining the general validity of either the multiple speech component or the auditory-perceptual inferential assessment approaches), the question is whether the suprabulbar structures provide a uniform function in control of the body's motor subsystems. In short, *is the movement control required by the CNS uniform in nature for the limbs, abdomen, rib cage, larynx, pharynx, jaw, tongue and lips?* If the answer to the question is negative and the control requirements are substantially different, then damage at suprabulbar levels should yield nonuniform impairments among cranial and spinal motor subsystems.

There are several ways to approach these issues, the major avenues being analytic and empirical. To illustrate the value of a motor control approach as advocated previously, we should like to review the analytic considerations (i.e., examination of underlying limb and speech production subsystem motor neurophysiology), and, in parallel, note some recent physiologic observations of speech motor subsystem dysfunctions in subjects with "pure" suprabulbar impairments. A priori, the analytic approach offered by *systems physiology* is useful in evaluating the potential central nervous system control of different speech and spinal motor subsystems (cf. Milhorn, 1966; Partridge, 1976; Robinson, 1981a; Talbot and Gessner, 1973). This systems approach analysis requires that the major functional subsystem properties be identified and evaluated. As such, this evaluation, based upon current knowledge of motor physiology, yields the minimal subset of critical motor subsystem characteristics that must be considered for central nervous system control (cf. Muller, Abbs, and Kennedy, 1981). If these critical properties are functionally similar for different motor subsystems, we have reason to argue for CNS control uniformity. In addition to addressing the issue of speech-motor-subsystem-differential control and impairment, these considerations offer numerous testable hypotheses for focused research in speech motor disorders. For example, it is not very satisfying to simply acknowledge differential impairment. Rational therapy will flourish if we know, in pathophysiologic terms, why certain systems are differentially impaired.

The major components of a typical systems physiology–based neuromuscular model that are known to influence control can be readily identified (cf. Houk and Henneman, 1967; Houk and Rymer, 1981; Rack, 1981). These components include *system movement characteristics* (acceleration, velocity, and range of movement); *system biomechanics* (multimuscle geometry, muscle force generation characteristics, and passive mechanics including inertial, elastic, and viscous properties); *efferent activation of the muscles* (such as motoneuron innervation ratio, muscle fiber mechanical properties, and histochemical properties); *sensory innervation* (density and presence of muscle spindles, tendon organs, joint receptors, and cutaneous or mucosal mechanoreceptors); and *the pattern of efferent and afferent influences on the lower motoneuron pool*, including the distribution and nature of peripheral afferent influences, reciprocal or recurrent inhibition processes, and inputs from descending cortical pathways. These system physiology properties are of major significance in discerning how particular motor systems are controlled by the nervous system, as is reflected in a substantial body of evidence from experimental and mathematical analyses of motor systems in animals and human beings (cf. Houk, 1972; Houk and Rymer, 1981; Neilson, Andrews, Guitar, and Quinn, 1979; Rack, 1981; Robinson, 1981b).

On the basis of a neuromuscular subsystem evaluation of the properties of speech and limb motor subsystems, it is apparent that there are several critical physiologic and neurophysiologic differences. An illustration of the basis for this conclusion is the neuromuscular system profiles for a few speech and upper limb motor subsystems. These differences are evident even at the most peripheral level in the movement and biomechanical characteristics of these subsystems. The biomechanical properties of motor systems dictate the muscle contraction patterns (and hence CNS control signals) required to produce certain patterns of movement (cf. Abbs and Eilenberg, 1976; Houk, 1972; Houk and Henneman, 1967). For example, mass (inertial) properties impose an undeniable newtonian requirement upon the force necessary to movement up to a certain velocity. Likewise, "fluid friction" (viscosity) found in most biologic tissue requires proportional increases in muscle force as greater movement velocities are necessary. Thus, while slow movements of two motor subsystems can be activated in a comparable manner (with respect to the muscle contraction–CNS control signals), differences in acceleration or velocity for one system will require major control signal reorganization, depending upon their relative magnitudes of inherent inertia and viscosity (cf. Abbs and Muller, 1980; Pedotti, Krishnan, and Stark, 1978). From these data, one could predict with some confidence that the motor reorganization for changes in speech rate would require different processes for each speech motor subsystem, with further implications for the neurologically impaired. In relation to biomechanical comparisons of the lips, jaw, and upper limbs, we know that the lips do not have a significant inertial (mass) component, while these other movement systems require inclusion of inertia in their biomechanical profile (Abbs and Muller, 1980). It may be significant that the movements of the lips are generally more rapid than those of these other structures. Indeed, for slower speech movements, the lips can be controlled in a manner that is relatively more direct than comparable motor systems with significant inertial properties. Perhaps with certain forms of nervous system damage, control of lip movements would be less impaired than movements of other motor subsystems.

The potential influence of these movement and biomechanical characteristics upon control requirements is apparent when one considers the control of eye movements where different central nervous system mechanisms have been determined for rapid movements (saccadic), slow movements (smooth pursuit), and static positioning (fixation). That is, within the ocular motor system, there are documented neuroanatomic differences in the control network that vary as a function of movement demands (Robinson, 1981b). These different eye movements are selectively impaired by lesions of the nervous system (Phillips and Porter, 1977). On the basis of clinical observations, movement-dependent neural control differences have also been suggested by Kornhuber (1975), who proposed that postural movements are highly dependent upon the basal ganglia, while fast, "ballistic" movements are more dependent upon the cerebellar circuits. Obviously, if Kornhuber's distinction is useful, basal ganglia lesions should cause differential impairment among the various speech or limb motor subsystems, depending upon whether their movements are slow or fast.

As noted previously, recent investigations in both in limb and speech motor control document the moment-to-moment contributions of ascending afferent signals, operating at all levels of the motor programming process. Additionally, afferent control aberrations have played a prominent role in many theoretic models of movement disorders. Thus, in this context of potential control differences, it is useful to compare the nature of sensory innervation among motor subsystems. While the jaw and upper limbs have muscle spindle, joint, and tendon receptors (Harrison and Corbin, 1942;

Kubota, Masegi, and Osani, 1974; Lund, Richmond, Touloumis, Patry, and Lamarre, 1978), the lips have none of them (Folkins and Larson, 1978; Lovell, Sutton, and Lindeman, 1977), and the tongue has only muscle spindles (Bowman, 1968; Cooper, 1953; Fitzgerald and Sachithanandan, 1979). The larynx, like the jaw, apparently has each of these receptors (Baken, 1971; Larson, Sutton, and Lindeman, 1974; Lucas Keene, 1961). Clearly, if we assume, on the basis of current evidence, a role for these afferent systems in the control of movement, their differential distribution across motor subsystems indicates parallel differences in the required CNS control signals (cf. Houk and Rymer, 1981; Muller et al., 1981). Regarding motor impairments, it might be hypothesized that the hypertonus associated with spasticity would be greatest in motor subsystems where spindle afferents are abundant (cf. Landau, 1980).

Yet another important factor in the control required of the CNS is the nature of the neural influences (peripheral, central, and local) impinging upon the lower motoneuron pool. By definition, these influences must determine the final pattern of motoneuron signals to the muscle. Additionally, several prominent notions concerning pathophysiology implicate aberrant integration of influences impinging on these lower motoneurons. With regard to afferent influences on motoneurons, it is notable that while spindles in the jaw and upper limbs make monosynaptic connections, spindle afferents from the larynx and tongue are not so configured (Bowman and Combs, 1968; Bratzlavsky and vander Eecken, 1974; Neilson et al., 1979). For example, labial and lingual mechanoreceptor influences on motoneurons are known to be polysynaptic. However, it appears doubtful that lingual muscle spindles have any direct autogenic influence on the lingual motoneurons. Further, while spindle primary (IA) afferents in the limbs make connections to all motoneurons in a muscle, in the jaw, spindles appear to make connections only to smaller motoneurons (Appenteng, O'Donovan, Somjen, Stephens, and Taylor, 1978).

The nervous system control implications of these subsystem-dependent, afferent influences upon the lower motoneuron pool appear particularly significant, especially with regard to such phenomena as the size principle of motoneuron recruitment (cf. Burke, 1981; Henneman, Somjen, and Carpenter, 1965). The differential influences of spindle feedback on jaw motoneurons may influence their recruitment order. Inasmuch as the lips do not have spindles influencing the lower motoneuron pool, these muscles also are likely to show differences in motoneuron recruitment patterns in comparison to the limbs and jaw. A number of reports suggest motor neuropathologies have associated aberrations in motoneuron recruitment patterns (Milner-Brown, Stein, Lee, and Brown, 1980; Petajan, Jarcho, and Thurman, 1969). Finally, while patterns of recurrent and reciprocal inhibition are manifest for the upper limbs via lower motoneuron interactions with collaterals to inhibitory interneurons and spindle afferents, parallel processes do not appear to be operating for the cranial nerves. Rather, it appears that control of these important inhibitory patterns is regulated more centrally in the orofacial system (Dubner et al., 1978; Penders and Delwaide, 1973; Shahani and Young, 1973). Of major importance may be the potentially related fact that in primates (including human beings) motoneurons of the lips, jaw, tongue, and respiratory muscles receive monosynaptic inputs from corticomotor sites (Kuypers, 1958; Watson, 1973), while the motoneurons of the trunk and upper and lower limbs (independent of the digits) do not (Carpenter, 1976).

These neurophysiologic and neuroanatomic differences are almost irrefutable evidence that the central nervous system (CNS) does not control the limbs or the individual speech motor subsystems in the same manner. Indeed, a differential neuromuscular substrate appears to be the rule rather than the exception; the nature and size of motor-sensory and sensorimotor cortical representations make this conclusion painfully obvious. The inescapable prediction from these considerations, based upon specific and available evidence in the motor neurophysiology literature, is that damage to the CNS at a suprabulbar or supraspinal level will result in motor control impairments that are different among the speech production subsystems and the limbs. This conclusion is supported indirectly by even a casual perusal of the clinical neurophysiology literature. That is, hypogamma and hypergamma motor drive to muscle spindles, loss or aberrations in recurrent inhibition, and selective impairment of influences upon motoneuron pool recruitment patterns have all enjoyed some popularity as partial pathogenic explanations for spasticity, rigidity, tremor, ataxia, hypotonia, dysmetria, and asthenia. If some of these explanations are even partially correct, and because the implicated physiologic processes (e.g., presence of spindles, operation of recurrent inhibition) differ from one motor subsystem to another, then the neuropathophysiology must differ as well. This hypothesis has some support in observations of differential muscle contraction impairments between the upper and lower limbs (e.g., degrees of spasticity, rigidity, and tremor).

By way of direct support, several recent physiologic observations in parkinsonian ataxic, and spastic dysarthric patients indicate that such differential impairment among the motor subsystems of the speech production mechanism is the rule rather than the exception (Abbs et al., 1983; Barlow and Abbs, 1982; Hunker et al., 1982).

The implications of this ubiquitous nonuniformity of speech motor subsystem impairments are several. Initially, because global measures of the speech motor system may not in general permit one to discern impairments of individual articulators, determination of speech motor subsystem pathophysiology is enhanced by use of direct observations using voluntary, nonspeech tasks. In this manner, it may be possible to identify those speech motor subsystems manifesting the greatest degree of impairment and to focus treatment for maximum effectiveness. Improvements in speech motor function could possibly be enhanced by initial emphasis upon those subsystems that are either most severely impaired or allow for the most direct and effective intervention. This focused approach is thus contrasted to conventional, more globally oriented treatments. With these global treatments, it is assumed (or hoped) that if the dysarthric talker is given an overall behavioral target, inherent compensatory processes that are indiscernible to the therapist will allow for achievement of that objective. It may be, however, that optimal therapy must be focused in such a manner as to aid in those compensatory strategies. Perhaps without direct focus on the impairments in specific subsystems, the necessary compensatory adjustments may be indiscernible to the dysarthric talker as well. A particularly useful example of the importance of multimotor system evaluation offered by Abbs and colleagues (1983) was that of an adult with congenital spastic dysarthria. This person's condition was evaluated by a neurologist and a speech pathologist, both of whom observed the classic signs of spasticity and spastic dysarthria. Given this diagnosis, a uniform pattern of motor control impairment across the speech motor subsystems might be predicted. However, what was revealed from instrumental observation of the lip, tongue, and jaw control for nonspeech tasks was substantial weakness in the lips and tongue; control instability was present only in the jaw. Given this observation, it is likely that optimal treatment would involve some attempts at increasing strength in the lips and tongue, but a very different approach is necessary for improving jaw control. If a global strategy (e.g., general relaxation or positioning) had been used, these treatments might have been ineffective for the labial and lingual weakness that had gone undetected by the conventional speech or neurologic assessments. What is unfortunate about the phenomenon of differential speech motor subsystem impairments is that it has not been recognized and exploited earlier; the supporting data, the underlying motor control rationale, and the technology utilized have been available for over 20 years from work in motor neurophysiology and systems bioengineering.

Conclusion and Summary

While the foregoing discussions have dealt with some apparently important issues in the assessment and treatment of speech neuropathologies, these considerations represent only the tip of the proverbial iceberg. There are numerous examples of similarly significant questions that are addressed by current work in neurophysiology and motor disorders; for example, it was not possible, given the scope of this discussion, to also discuss (1) the demonstration that normal and disordered *cognitive* processes are a significant factor in motor programming and control (cf. Abbs and Kennedy, 1982; Marsden, 1982); (2) potential neurophysiologic mechanisms of compensatory patterns in individuals with motor disorders (Grimm and Nashner, 1978); (3) predictions of lesion sites in particular dysarthric populations and subpopulations based upon recent somatotopic investigations of orofacial and laryngeal representation in the basal ganglia, cerebellum, and cerebral cortex; (4) data-based definitions of movement and muscle contraction aberrations in patients with Parkinson's disease, congenital and acquired spasticity, or cerebellar impairment that replace and refine qualitative, semantically ambiguous terms such as akinesia, asthenia, and spasticity; or (5) a neurophysiologic rationale and specific methodology for the meaningful assessment of sensorimotor integrity as a potential factor in many speech motor neuropathologies. However, what is apparent from the issues discussed and this fundamental perspective is that some of the arguments occupying the energy of clinical scientists working on the speech neuropathologies become nonissues if all the available data are incorporated. From the standpoint of scientific integrity and underlying humanitarian objectives, speech neuropathologists cannot afford to be generalists, and hence they miss the substantial advances that have been made in the last ten years in the understanding of motor control and disorders thereof. Our clinical and research activities in this area must reflect the most relevant and recent information that the neurosciences have to offer. This wealth of information provides the basis from which we can further choose and refine those measures that provide the best insights into nervous system function and dysfunction. Professionally, adopting this approach may be critical, especially as new developments in areas such as clinical neurophysiology offer increasingly focused measures to discern specific aspects of nervous system function and dysfunction. That is, one danger of continuing traditional approaches (using borrowed measures that may yield ambiguous, albeit conventional data) is that the neurologist and physiologist will develop techniques for assessment of speech motor system function and dysfunction without the participation of individuals with primary education in the speech neuropathologies. Some work in this area is already under way, especially in Europe, where medically educated professionals conduct motor-sensory evaluations of the orofacial system in the neurologically impaired (cf. Bennett and Jannetta, 1980; Bratzlavsky, 1976; Dengler and Struppler, 1981; Schonle, 1982; Shahani and Young, 1973; Thumfart, 1981).

References

Abbs, J. H. (1979). Speech motor equivalence: A need for a multilevel control model. In E. Fischer-Jorgenson, J. Rischel, and N. Thorsen (Eds.), *Proceedings of the Ninth International Congress of Phonetics* (pp. 318-324). Denmark: Institute of Phonetics.

Abbs, J. H., and Cole, K. J. (1982). Consideration of bulbar and suprabulbar afferent influences upon speech motor coordination and programming. In S. Grillner, B. Lindblom, J. Lubker, and A. Persson (Eds.), *Speech motor control* (pp. 159-186). New York: Pergamon Press.

Abbs, J. H., and Eilenberg, G. R. (1976). Peripheral mechanisms of speech motor control. In N. J. Lass (Ed.), *Contemporary issues in experimental phonetics* (pp. 139-168). New York: Academic Press.

Abbs, J. H., and Gracco, V. L. (1982). Motor control of multi-movement behaviors. Orofacial muscle responses to load perturbations of the lips during speech. *Society for Neuroscience, 8,* 282 (Abstract).

Abbs, J. H., and Gracco, V. L. (1984). Control of complex motor gestures: Orofacial muscle responses to load perturbations of the lip during speech. *Journal of Neurophysiology, 51*(4), 705-723.

Abbs, J. H., Hunker, C. J., and Barlow, S. M. (1983). Differential speech motor subsystem impairments in subjects with suprabulbar lesions: Neurophysiological framework and supporting data. In W. Berry (Ed.), *Clinical dysarthria* (pp. 21-56). San Diego: College-Hill Press.

Abbs, J. H., and Kennedy, J. G. (1982). Neurophysiological processes of speech movement control. In N. J. Lass, L. V. McReynolds, J. L. Northern, and D. E. Yoder (Eds.), *Speech, language and hearing* (pp. 84-108). Philadelphia: W. B. Saunders.

Abbs, J. H., and Muller, E. M. (1980). *Neurophysiological and biomechanical factors in articulatory movement.* Paper presented at the Conference on the Production of Speech, Austin, Texas.

Abbs, J. H., Sutton, D., Larson, C., and Eilenberg, G. R. (1973). *Neuromuscular mechanisms underlying speech production (Program Project NINCDS NS11780).* Seattle: University of Washington.

Alexander, R. M. (1981). Biomechanics of skeleton and tendons. In V. B. Brooks (Ed.), *Handbook of physiology, Section 1 (Vol. II: Motor control, Part 1)* (pp. 17–42). Bethesda, MD: American Physiological Society.

Appenteng, K., O'Donovan, M. J., Somjen, G., Stephens, J. A., and Taylor, A. (1978.) The projection of jaw elevator muscle spindle afferents to fifth nerve motoneurons in the cat. *Journal of Physiology, 279,* 409–423.

Baken, R. J. (1971). Neuromuscular spindles in the intrinsic muscles of the human larynx. *Folia Phoniatrica, 23,* 204–210.

Barlow, S. M., and Abbs, J. H. (1982). Impairment control of orofacial muscle force in congenital spastics. *Society for Neuroscience, 8* (Part 2), 953 (Abstract).

Barlow, S. M., and Abbs, J. H. (1984). Orofacial fine motor control impairments in congenital spastics: Evidence against muscle spindle-related performance deficits. *Neurology, 34,* 145–150.

Bennett, M. H., and Jannetta, P. H. (1980). Trigeminal evoked potentials in humans. *EEG Clinical Neurophysiology, 48,* 517–526.

Bernstein, N. (1967). *The co-ordination and regulation of movements.* Oxford: Pergamon Press.

Bowman, J. P. (1968). Muscle spindles in the intrinsic and extrinsic muscles of the Rhesus monkey's (*Macaca mulatta*) tongue. *Anatomical Record, 161,* 483–488.

Bowman, J. P., and Combs, C. M. (1968). Discharge patterns of lingual spindle afferent fibers in the hypoglossal nerve of the Rhesus monkey. *Experimental Neurology, 21,* 105–119.

Bratzlavsky, M. (1976). The connections between muscle afferents and motoneurons of the muscles of mastication. In D. J. Anderson and B. Matthews (Eds.), *Mastication* (pp. 147–151). Bristol: Wright.

Bratzlavsky, M., and vander Eecken, H. (1974). Afferent influences on human genioglossus muscle. *Journal of Neurology, 207,* 19–25.

Brooks, V. B. (1981). *Handbook of physiology, Section 1 (Vols. I and II: Motor control, Parts 1 and 2).* Bethesda, MD: American Physiological Society.

Burke, R. E. (1981). Motor units: anatomy, physiology and functional organization. In V. B. Brooks (Ed.), *Handbook of physiology, Section 1 (Vol. II: Motor control, Part 1)* (pp. 345–422). Bethesda, MD: American Physiological Society.

Carpenter, M. B. (1976). *Human neuroanatomy.* Baltimore: Williams & Wilkins.

Cooper, S. (1953). Muscle spindles in the intrinsic muscles of the human tongue. *Journal of Physiology, 122,* 193–202.

Darley, F. L., Aronson, A. E., and Brown, J. R. (1969a). Differential diagnostic patterns of dysarthria. *Journal of Speech and Hearing Research, 12,* 246–269.

Darley, F. L., Aronson, A. E., and Brown, J. R. (1969b). Cluster of deviant speech dimensions in the dysarthrias. *Journal of Speech and Hearing Research, 12,* 462–496.

Darley, F. L., Aronson, A. E., and Brown, J. R. (1975). *Motor speech disorders.* Philadelphia: W. B. Saunders.

DeLong, M., and Georgopoulos, A. P. (1981). Motor functions of the basal ganglia. In V. B. Brooks (Ed.), *Handbook of physiology, Section 1 (Vol. II: Motor control, Part 2)* (pp. 1017–1062). Bethesda, MD: American Physiological Society.

Dengler, R., and Struppler, A. (1981). Neurophysiological diagnosis of trigeminal nerve function. In M. Sammii and P. Jannetta (Eds.), *The cranial nerves* (pp. 302–311). Berlin: Springer-Verlag.

Denny-Brown, D. (1960). Motor mechanisms—Introduction: The general principles of motor integration. In H. W. Magoun (Ed.), *Handbook of physiology, Section 1* (pp. 781–796). Washington, DC: American Physiological Society.

Denny-Brown, D. (1980). Preface: Historical aspects of the relation of spasticity to movement. In R. G. Feldman, R. R. Young, and W. P. Koella (Eds.), *Spasticity: Disordered motor control* (pp. 1-16). Chicago: Year Book Medical Publishers.

Desmedt, J. E. (Ed.) (1973-1982). *Progress in clinical neurophysiology (10 vols.).* Basel: S. Karger.

Dubner, R., Sessle, B. J., and Storey, A. T. (1978). *The neural basis of oral and facial function.* New York: Plenum.

Duncan, G. W., Shahani, B. T., and Young, R. R. (1976). An evaluation of baclofen treatment for certain symptoms in patients with spinal cord lesions. A double cross-over study. *Neurology, 26,* 441-446.

Evarts, E. V. (1981). Role of motor cortex in voluntary movements in primates. In V. B. Brooks (Ed.), *Handbook of physiology, Section 1 (Vol. II: Motor control, Part 2)* (pp. 1083-1120). Bethesda, MD: American Physiological Society.

Evarts, E. V. (1982). Analogies between central motor programs for speech and limb movements. In S. Grillner, B. Lindblom, J. Lubker, and A. Persson (Eds.), *Speech motor control* (pp. 19-42). London: Pergamon Press.

Fitzgerald, M. J. T., and Sachithanandan, S. R. (1979). The structure and source of lingual proprioceptors in the monkey. *Journal of Anatomy, 128*(3), 523-552.

Folkins, J. W., and Abbs, J. H. (1975). Lip and jaw motor control during speech: Responses to resistive loading of the jaw. *Journal of Speech and Hearing Research, 18,* 207-220.

Folkins, J. W., and Abbs, J. H. (1976). Additional observations on responses to resistive loading of the jaw. *Journal of Speech and Hearing Research, 19,* 820-821.

Folkins, J. W., and Larson, C. R. (1978). In search of a tonic vibration reflex in the human lip. *Brain Research, 151,* 409-412.

Fujimura, O. (1981). Temporal organization of articulatory movements as a multi-dimensional phrasal structure. *Phonetica, 38,* 66-83.

Gentil, M., Gracco, V. L., and Abbs, J. H. (1983). Multiple muscle contributions to labial closure during speech: Evidence for inter-muscle motor equivalence. *Proceedings of the 11th International Congress of Acoustics,* pp. 11-14 (Abstract).

Gracco, V. L., and Abbs, J. H. (1982). Temporal response characteristics of the perioral system to load perturbations. *Society for Neuroscience, 8,* (Part 2), 282 (Abstract).

Gracco, V. L., and Muller, E. M. (1981, November). *Analysis of supraglottal air pressure variations in spastic dysarthria.* Paper presented at the American Speech, Language, and Hearing Association, Los Angeles.

Granit, R. (1977). *The purposive brain.* Cambridge, MA: MIT Press.

Grimm, R. J., and Nashner, L. M. (1978). Long loop dyscontrol. In J. E. Desmedt (Ed.), *Cerebral motor control in man: Long loop mechanisms* (Vol. 4) (pp. 70-84). Basel: S. Karger.

Hardy, J. C. (1967). Suggestions for physiological research in dysarthria. *Cortex, 3,* 128-156.

Hardy, J. C. (1970). Development of neuromuscular systems underlying speech production. *ASHA Reports: Speech and the Dentofacial Complex: The State of the Art, Proceedings of the Workshop, 5,* 49-68.

Harrison, F., and Corbin, K. B. (1942). The central pathway for the jaw-jerk. *American Journal of Physiology, 135,* 439-445.

Hebb, D. O. (1949). *The organization of behavior.* New York: John Wiley and Sons.

Henneman, E., Somjen, G., and Carpenter, D. O. (1965). Excitability and inhibitability of motoneurons of different sizes. *Journal of Neurophysiology, 28,* 599-620.

Hixon, T. J. (1963). *Restricted motility of the speech articulators in cerebral palsy.* Unpublished master's thesis, University of Iowa.

Hixon, T. J. (1975). *Respiratory-laryngeal evaluation.* Paper presented at the Veterans Administration Workshop on Motor Speech Disorders, Madison, Wisconsin.

Hixon, T. J., and Hardy, J. C. (1964). Restricted mobility of the speech articulators in cerebral palsy. *Journal of Speech and Hearing Disorders, 29,* 293-306.

Hoffman, D. S., and Luschei, E. S. (1980). Responses of monkey precentral cortical cells during a controlled jaw bite task. *Journal of Neurophysiology, 44,* 333-348.

Houk, J. C. (1972). On the significance of various command signals during voluntary control. *Brain Research, 40,* 49-53.

Houk, J. C., and Henneman, E. (1967). The feedback control of skeletal muscles. *Brain Research, 5,* 433-451.

Houk, J. C. and Rymer, W. Z. (1981). Neural control of muscle length and tension. In V. B. Brooks (Ed.), *Handbook of physiology, Section 1 (Vol. II: Motor control, Part 1)* (pp. 257-323). Bethesda, MD: American Physiological Society.

Hughes, O. M., and Abbs, J. H. (1976). Labial-mandibular coordination in the production of speech: Implications for the operation of motor equivalence. *Phonetica, 44,* 199-221.

Hunker, C. J., and Abbs, J. H. (1982). Respiratory movement control during speech: Evidence for motor equivalence. *Society for Neuroscience, 8* (Part 2), 946 (Abstract).

Hunker, C. J., and Abbs, J. H. (1984). Physiological analyses of parkinsonian tremors in the orofacial system. In M. R. McNeil, J. C. Rosenbek, and A. E. Aronson (Eds.), *The dysarthrias: Physiology-acoustics-perception-management* (pp. 69-100). San Diego: College-Hill Press.

Hunker, C. J., Abbs, J. H., and Barlow, S. M. (1982). The relationship between Parkinson rigidity and hypokinesia in the orofacial system: A quantitative analysis. *Neurology, 32*(7), 749-754.

Kornhuber, H. H. (1975). Cerebral cortex, cerebellum, and basal ganglia: An introduction to their motor function. In E. V. Evarts (Ed.), *Central processing of sensory input leading to motor output.* Cambridge, MA: MIT Press.

Kubota, K., Masegi, T., and Osani, K. (1974). Muscle spindle in masticatory muscle and its trigeminal mesencephalic nucleus. *Bulletin of the Tokyo Medical and Dental University* (Suppl. 21), 3-6.

Kuypers, H. G. J. M. (1958). Corticobulbar connections to the pons and lower brainstem in man: An anatomical study. *Brain, 81,* 364-388.

Lacquaniti, F., and Soechting, J. F. (1982). Coordination of arm and wrist motion during a reaching task. *Journal of Neuroscience, 2,* 399-408.

Ladefoged, P., DeClark, J., Lindau, M., and Papcun, G. (1972). An auditory-motor theory of speech production. *UCLA Working Papers in Phonetics, 22,* 48-75.

Lance, J. W. (1980). Pathophysiology of spasticity and clinical experience with baclofen. In R. G. Feldman, R. R. Young, and W. P. Koella (Eds.), *Spasticity: Disordered motor control* (pp. 185-203). Chicago: Year Book Medical Publishers.

Landau, W. M. (1974). Spasticity: The fable of a neurological demon and the emperor's new therapy. *Archives of Neurology, 31,* 217-219.

Landau, W. M. (1980). Spasticity: What is it? What is it not? In R. G. Feldman, R. R. Young, and W. P. Koella (Eds.), *Spasticity: Disordered motor control* (pp. 17-24). Chicago: Year Book Medical Publishers.

Larson, C. R., Sutton, D., and Lindeman, R. C. (1974). Muscle spindles in non-human primate laryngeal muscles. *Folia Primatologia, 22,* 315-325.

Lashley, K. S. (1930). Basic neural mechanisms in behavior. *Psychological Review, 37,* 1-24.

Lindau, M., Jacobson, L., and Ladefoged, P. (1972). The feature advanced tongue root. *UCLA Working Papers in Phonetics, 22.*

Lindblom, B. (1982). The interdisciplinary challenge of speech motor control. In S. Grillner, B. Lindblom, J. Lubker, and A. Persson (Eds.), *Speech motor control* (pp. 3-18). London: Pergamon Press.

Love, R. J., Hagerman, E. L., and Taimi, E. G. (1980). Speech performance, dysphagia and oral reflexes in cerebral palsy. *Journal of Speech and Hearing Disorders, 45*, 59-75.

Lovell, M., Sutton, D., and Lindeman, R. (1977). Muscle spindles in non-human primate extrinsic auricular muscles. *Anatomical Record, 189*, 519-524.

Lucas Keene, M. F. (1961). Muscle spindles in human laryngeal muscles. *Journal of Anatomy, 95*, 25-29.

Lund, J. P., Richmond, F. J. R., Touloumis, C., Patry, Y., and Lamarre, Y. (1978). The distribution of ganglia tendon organs and muscle spindles in the masseter and temporalis muscles of the cat. *Neuroscience, 3*, 259-270.

Marsden, C. D. (1982). The mysterious motor function of the basal ganglia. *Neurology, 32*, 514-539.

McClean, M. D., Folkins, J. W., and Larson, C. R. (1979). The role of the perioral reflex in lip motor control for speech. *Brain and Language, 7*, 42-61.

Milhorn, H. T. (1966). *The application of control theory to physiological systems*. Philadephia: W. B. Saunders.

Milner-Brown, H. S., Stein, R. B., Lee, R. G., and Brown, W. F. (1980). Motor unit recruitment in patients with neuromuscular disorders. In J. E. Desmedt (Ed.), *Motor unit types, recruitment and plasticity in health and disease (Progress in clinical neurophysiology, Vol. 9)* (pp. 305-318). Basel: S. Karger.

Morasso, P. (1981). Spatial control of arm movements. *Experimental Brain Research, 42*, 223-227.

Muller, E. M., Abbs, J. H., and Kennedy, J. G. (1981). Some system physiology considerations for vocal control. In M. Hirano and K. Stevens (Eds.), *Proceedings of the conference on vocal fold physiology* (pp. 209-227). Tokyo: University of Tokyo Press.

Muller, E. M., and Brown, W. S. (1980). Variations in the supraglottal air pressure waveform and their articulatory interpretation. In N. J. Lass (Ed.), *Speech and language: Advances in basic research and practice* (pp. 317-389). New York: Academic Press.

Murphy, M. W. (1966). *Speech physiology problems in athetoid and spastic quadriplegic children*. Unpublished master's thesis, University of Iowa.

Nashner, L. M., and Grimm, R. J. (1978). Analysis of multiloop dyscontrols in standing cerebellar patients. In J. E. Desmedt (Ed.), *Cerebral motor control in man: Long loop mechanisms* (Vol. 4) (pp. 300-319). Basel: S. Karger.

Neilson, P. D., Andrews, G., Guitar, B. E., and Quinn, P. T. (1979). Tonic stretch reflexes in lip, tongue and jaw muscles. *Brain Research, 178*, 311-327.

Netsell, R. (1971-1976). Physiological studies of the dysarthrias. *Final Progress Report— NINCDS Research Grant*.

Netsell, R., and Abbs, J. H. (1975, October). *The modulation of perioral reflex sensitivity during speech movements*. Paper presented at the Acoustical Society of America, San Francisco.

Netsell, R., and Abbs, J. H. (1977). Some possible uses of neuromotor speech disturbances in understanding the normal mechanism. In M. Sawashima and F. S. Cooper (Eds.), *Dynamic aspects of speech production* (pp. 369-392). Tokyo: University of Tokyo Press.

Netsell, R., and Daniel, B. (1979). Dysarthria in adults: Physiological approach to rehabilitation. *Archives of Physical Medicine and Rehabilitation, 60*, 502-508.

Partridge, L. (1976). A proposal for study of a static description of the motor control system. In M. Shahani (Ed.), *The motor system: Neurophysiological and muscle mechanics* (pp. 363-370). New York: Elsevier.

Partridge, L. D., and Benton, L. A. (1981). Muscle, the motor. In V. B. Brooks (Ed.), *Handbook of physiology, Section 1 (Vol. II: Motor control, Part 1)* (pp. 43–106). Bethesda, MD: American Physiological Society.

Pedotti, A., Krishnan, V. V., and Stark, L. (1978). Optimization of muscle force sequencing in human locomotion. *Mathematical Biosciences, 38,* 57–76.

Penders, C. A., and Delwaide, P. J. (1973). Physiological approach to the human blink relflex. In J. E. Desmedt (Ed.), *New developments in electromyography and clinical neurophysiology* (pp. 649–657). Basel: S. Karger.

Petajan, J. H., Jarcho, L. W., and Thurman, D. J. (1969). Motor unit control in Huntington's disease: a possible presymptomatic test. In J. Chase (Ed.), *Advances in neurology* (pp. 163–176). New York: Raven Press.

Phillips, C. G., and Porter, R. (1977). *Corticospinal neurones. Their role in movement.* London: Academic Press.

Rack, P. M. H. (1981). Limitations of somatosensory feedback in control of posture and movement. In V. B. Brooks (Ed.), *Handbook of physiology, Section 1 (Vol. II: Motor control, Part 1)* (pp. 229–256). Bethesda, MD: American Physiological Society.

Robinson, D. A. (1981a). The use of control systems analysis in neurophysiology of eye movements. *Annual Review of Neuroscience, 4,* 463–503.

Robinson, D. A. (1981b). Control of eye movements. In V. B. Brooks (Ed.), *Handbook of physiology, Section 1 (Vol. II: Motor control, Part 2)* (pp. 1275–1320). Bethesda, MD: American Physiological Society.

Rosenbek, J. C., and LaPointe, L. (1978). The dysarthrias: Description, diagnosis, and treatment. In D. F. Johns (Ed.), *Clinical management of neurogenic communicative disorders* (pp. 251–310). Boston: Little, Brown.

Rubow, R. T. (1981). Biofeedback in the treatment of speech disorders. *Biofeedback Society of America Task Force Reports.*

Rubow, R. T., and Netsell, R. (1979). EMG biofeedback rehabilitation in facial paralysis: Ten year follow-up of a case study. *Proceedings of the Tenth Annual Meeting of the Biofeedback Society of America,* San Diego, California.

Sahrman, S. A., and Norton, B. J. (1977). The relationship of voluntary movement to spasticity in the upper motor neuron syndrome. *Annals of Neurology, 2,* 460–465.

Schonle, P. W. (1982). Personal communication.

Shahani, B. T., and Young, R. R. (1973). Blink reflexes in orbicularis oculi. In J. E. Desmedt (Ed.), *New developments in electromyography and clinical neurophysiology* (pp. 641–648). Basel: S. Karger.

Smit, A. (1969). *Relationship of select physiological variables to speech defectiveness of athetoid and spastic cerebral palsied children.* Unpublished master's thesis, University of Iowa.

Smith, L. L. (1964). *Restricted motility of the speech articulators, lung function, amount of air expired per unit of speech and speech defectiveness in adults with Parkinson's disease.* Unpublished master's thesis, University of Iowa.

Stalberg, E., and Young, R. R. (1981). *Clinical neurophysiology.* Boston: Butterworths International Medical Reviews.

Stevens, K. N., and House, A. S. (1955). Development of a quantitative description of vowel articulation. *Journal of the Acoustical Society of America, 27,* 484–493.

Stevens, K. N., and House, A. S. (1961). An acoustical theory of vowel production and some of its implications. *Journal of Speech and Hearing Research, 4,* 303–320.

Sussman, H. M., MacNeilage, P. F., and Hanson, R. J. (1973). Labial and mandibular dynamics during the production of bilabial stop consonants. *Journal of Speech and Hearing Research, 16,* 385–396.

Talbot, S. A., and Gessner, U. (1973). *Systems physiology.* New York: John Wiley and Sons.

Thumfart, W. (1981). Endoscopic electroneurography and neurography. In M. Sammii and P. Jannetta (Eds.), *The cranial nerves* (pp. 597–606). Berlin: Springer-Verlag.

Watson, C. (1973). Functional deficits and the patterns of degeneration following lesions of the face motor cortex in the *Macaca mulatta. Anatomical Review, 175,* 465.

Wyke, B. (Ed.) (1974). *Ventilatory and phonatory control systems.* London: Oxford University Press.

Walt Wolfram

The Phonologic System: Problems of Second Language Acquisition

Learning to speak a foreign language involves learning another phonologic system. While the acquisition of this second language system (L2) may be likened in some respects to learning the phonology of the first language (L1), there are obvious and important differences (Macken and Ferguson, 1981). In the acquisition of the native language phonologic system, certain natural and universal phonologic processes have to be overcome in learning the specific patterns of the adult language. In the acquisition of a foreign language as an adult, it is primarily the phonologic patterns of the first and native language that have to be overcome in learning the new system. Failure to overcome the L1 (i.e., native language) patterns of phonology in speaking the L2 (i.e., the target language) results in the classically defined "foreign accent." Technically, this is called language *interference* or *transfer*, referring to the fact that the patterns of the native language may be imposed on the target language.

The focus on language transfer in L2 phonologic acquisition is not intended to preclude other explanations. Certainly, some evidence suggests that other phenomena account for some adaptation of the L2 system as well (Tarone, 1976; Wode, 1977). For example, there may be a reactivation of the L1 developmental processes akin to those described in the recent emphasis on natural phonologic processes (Ingram, 1976; Stampe, 1973), or modifications that derive from particular L2 learning strategies (Wolfram, 1983). Nonetheless, the burden of explanation in adult L2 phonologic acquisition still rests on language transfer. This continued (and, in fact, renewed) emphasis on transfer in L2 phonology clearly contrasts with the trend in L2 syntax, where evidence over the past decade has emphasized the role of generalized learning strategies rather than language transfer (Burt and Kiparsky, 1972; Corder, 1981; Dulay and Burt, 1972).

In phonology, evidence (Oller, 1974; Sato, 1983) continues to point to the primary role of transfer for adult learners. Thus, a basic transfer model, with appropriate modifications, has weathered the challenge of empirically based L2 studies of the past decade. Given the state of the art, our goal is to present a coherent model that integrates current insights about variation and phonologic organization rather than simple recitation of recent research.

The range of transfer manifested by a given talker may vary, but in all cases we can expect the language codes to interact systematically. Speakers of a given native language background typically make similar kinds of "errors" when learning a foreign language, and this patterned behavior is the keynote to this discussion. We are dealing with systematic, patterned phonologic behavior that results from the normal interaction of two phonologic systems. While the resultant phonology may be quite different from the adult native speaker phonology, it can hardly be called a "disorder" in the traditional applications of this term. It is simply the normal result of imposing another phonologic system on one already established, and should be considered a kind of *interlanguage* norm. Nonetheless, this normal interlanguage behavior may lead to communication problems for talkers desiring to become more proficient in their phonology for various sociocultural reasons, so that it is a relevant topic for discussion here. In the following sections, we shall examine some aspects of phonologic organization in learning a second language, propose a model for understanding the acquisition of a second phonology, and finally discuss relevant pedagogic issues for language teachers, including diagnosis and remediation by speech-language pathologists.

The comparison of language systems related to foreign language learning has become a specialized field in its own right, often referred to as *contrastive linguistics*. Basic to this field is the comparison of structures in the native and target languages of the language learner in order to understand particular foreign language learner difficulties. While some aspects of contrastive linguistics have proved particularly troublesome on a theoretic and practical level (Wardhaugh, 1970), it is unarguable that the comparison of native and target language phonologies leads to considerable insight concerning the nature of learner problems. All levels of phonologic organization may be compared, including the underlying phonologic units, particular phonologic rules or processes, and surface phonemic contrasts. Traditionally, however, the emphasis has been on the interaction of systems on the more concrete levels of phonology—the surface phonemic contrasts. On the basis of a classic summary of inventories of phonemes and their allophones, Weinreich (1953) distinguished four different kinds of phonologic interaction and interference. These categories remain useful despite recent developments in redefining the basic units of a phonologic system.*

Underdifferentiation

This takes place when two or more contrastive sounds of the target language are treated as noncontrastive, because no phonologic contrast exists for these sounds in the native language. For example, Spanish does not contrast s and z; [z] is an allophone of [s]. English on the other hand, contrasts these sounds in items such as *sip* [sIp] and *zip* [sIp]. Thus, in learning English, a speaker of Spanish may not differentiate between the [s] and [z] contrast, possibly confusing items such as *sip* and *zip*, or *peace* and *peas*. Because underdifferentiation of this type can obviously lead to confusion among vocabulary items, it is considered one of the more serious types of phonologic interference. A similar problem of underdifferentiation might be faced by the English speaker learning an Asian language such as Hindi. In Hindi, the difference between aspirated and unaspirated stops is contrastive. English speakers who treat [p] and [p^h], or [k] and [k^h], as if they were part of the same contrastive unit (as they are in English) underdifferentiate the contrastive units of Hindi.

Overdifferentiation

In overdifferentiation, contrasts from the native language are applied to the sounds of the target language, even though they are not required by the target language phonologic system. For example, an English speaker learning Spanish might consider [s] and [z] to be contrastive items in Spanish because they are contrastive in English. But as we noted, [s] and [z] are not contrastive sounds in Spanish, so that their conceptual differentiation is not necessary. Similarly, a Hindi speaker learning English might treat [p] and [p^h] as if they were different contrastive units. Cases of overdifferentiation may not affect production in any significant way, but the learner's conception of contrastive units will differ from that of the native speaker. Understandably, overdifferentiation does not lead to the confusion among lexical items that underdifferentiation might. It is

---

*This section is adapted from Wolfram and Johnson (1982).

therefore not usually considered a problem in foreign language learning. Nonetheless, it must be recognized as one type of interaction between phonologic systems that affects the ways in which the units of the native language and the target language are conceptualized.

Reinterpretation of Distinctions

In the reinterpretation of distinctions, the contrast of units in the target language is maintained, but on a basis different from that found in the native language. Thus, phonetic features that are redundant in the target language may be used as the basis for maintaining contrast by the native language speaker. Consider how a speaker of German learning English may utilize vowel length contrastively in a context where an English speaker may utilize vowel length redundantly. In both instances, the end result is the differentiation of items, but on a different basis. German uses phonetic differences in vowel length to distinguish items. The difference between [štat] "city" and [šta:t] "state," and [kan] "can" and [ka:n] "boat," is indicated by the length of the vowel. In English, however, length is typically much more predictable on the basis of the following environment. Vowels are lengthened before voiced segments ([bI:d] "bid"), and unlengthened before voiceless segments ([bIt] "bit").

Another difference between German and English phonology relates to the voicing of obstruents (i.e., stops and fricatives) in word-final position. In German, only voiceless obstruents are produced in this position, whereas in English both voiced and voiceless obstruents are found. Using the German word-final devoicing pattern, German speakers will often devoice the final voiced obstruents on English items such as *bead, pig,* and *buzz.* Despite the devoicing of the final obstruents, however, contrast may be maintained for German speakers confronted with these English items. The German speaker who devoices final obstruents may use the length of the preceding vowel rather than the voicing contrast to distinguish items, producing *bead* [bi:t] and *beat* [bit], *pig* [pI:k] and *pick* [pIk], *buzz* [bʌ:s] and *bus* [bʌs]. In an informal experiment conducted by the author, it was clearly indicated that native German speakers were cueing on the vowel length rather than final voicing to distinguish these items. Thus, we see that English redundant features may take on distinctive status for speakers from a different language background.

Actual Phone Substitution

In phone substitution, the contrastive units of the native language and target language are comparable in terms of their contrastive status, but their phonetic production differs. For example, the German and French lateral *l* may be considered to be equivalent to English *l*, but the phonetic production may be different. German and French employ only the alveolar or "clear" [l], whereas English often produces an alveovelar lateral or "dark" [ł]. The difference in phonetic production may not lead to any particular confusion in terms of contrastive units, but the use of the English [ł] in speaking French or German will sound somewhat accented. Similarly, the exclusive use of [l] by French or German speakers using English will sound slightly accented in certain environments where English uses [ł].

Phonotactic Differences

We have just examined the interaction of the native and target languages only in terms of the basic inventory of units. But phonologic systems also are highly patterned in terms of the permissible sequences of sounds, referred to as *phonotactic patterning*. Thus, English has particular combinations of sounds in a linear string that may or may not be comparable to those found in other languages. Phonotactic differences are just as likely to lead to second language learning problems as are differences in the basic inventory of units.

There are several ways in which phonotactic differences may lead to problems for the second language learner. In some cases, the distribution patterns of segments within syllables may be different across language systems. Both English and Tagalog distinguish three nasals, [m], [n], and [ŋ], but English does not use [ŋ] in syllable-initial position, whereas Tagalog does. An English speaker confronted with items such as Tagalog [ŋaʔ] "really" and [ŋakŋa:k] "cry aloud" may therefore encounter difficulty producing the [ŋ] in these positions. This is a result not of a contrastive difference but of a difference in the distributional privileges within the syllable. Another difference in distribution between Tagalog and English is the occurrence of [h]. In Tagalog, [h] may occur in the syllable-final position, whereas in English it may not. Thus, Tagalog items such as [amah] "father" and [tu:boh] "tube" reveal a pattern not found in English. The native English speaker will tend to eliminate the final [h].

Major differences in phonotactics often concern sequences of segments of consonants or consonants and vowels. Syllable types and segment cluster types differ across phonologic systems, and these differences are often revealed in the kinds of problems found among second language learners. For example, Spanish does not permit syllable-initial sibilant + stop sequences, as in English *sp, st,* or *sk.* Thus, Spanish speakers impose the Spanish phonotactic system and produce these English clusters with a prothetic vowel ([ɛstʌdi] for *study* or [ɛskul] for *school*). In a parallel way, an English speaker learning German may be confronted with certain syllable-initial sequences not permissible in English. These include velar stops + nasals (German [knabə] "boy" and [gnadə] "mercy") and stops + fricatives ([psalm] "psalm" [pfʊnt] "pound"). Two possibilities exist here for imposing the English phonotactic structure. Speakers might use an epenthetic vowel to separate the nonpermissible English sequence ([kənabə]), or reduce the cluster by deleting one of the members ([nabə] or [fʊnt]). In both cases, the modification would result in a permissible English syllable type, but an unusual German pronunciation. Our examples might be expanded here, but the essential point remains the same: many second language learning problems may be attributable to differences in the sequencing of sounds rather than in the sound units themselves, and these differences must be taken into account along with differences in the inventory of units.

Phonologic Processes

Much recent work in phonology (e.g., Ingram, 1976; Wolfram and Johnson, 1982) has recognized that language differences are susceptible to a number of different phonologic processes that alter the shape of units. Because of the natural basis for various processes, it is not surprising to see similar processes in two different language systems. There is, for example, a class of nasal prefixes in Swahili that is conditioned by the place of articulation of the following segment (*m-bari* "clan," *n-devu* "beard," *ŋ-guzo* "post"). This *assimilation* is similar to the form changes found in English (*impossible, indefinite, inconclusive*). But while recognizing certain similarities in the types of phonologic processes found in different systems on the basis of some universal principles, we must also observe significant differences in detail as we compare phonologic systems.

Many language systems may employ *neutralization* of one type or another, but the particular details of neutralization will vary greatly. Thus, the English talker shows extensive neutralization of vowels in unstressed syllables, so most English vowels can reduce to [ə]. Spanish, on the other hand, reveals little vowel neutralization of this type, maintaining contrasts in unstressed syllables as well as stressed ones. By the same token, standard English does not have the broadly applied German rule of final obstruent devoicing. Neutralization of contrasts in unstressed syllables, or devoicing in word-final position, may qualify as natural processes, but the particular details of these processes and the extent of their operation show considerable variation between systems. Such diversity is an important aspect of comparing systems in a contrastive analysis.

Similarly, languages commonly have *deletion* processes, but they may differ in details. Thus, French has a rule in which many word-final consonants are deleted when the following word begins with a consonant (e.g., [pəti garsɔ] "little boy") but not when followed by a vowel (e.g., [pɔtit ami] "little friend"). The application of this rule to English by a native French speaker might result in the deletion of consonants in similar contexts in English, so that the talker might produce [bɛ gɛm] (bed game) but [bɛt ɔfər] (bet offer). In this instance, the primary difference is the transfer of a process or rule from the native language to the target language rather than a difference in the basic inventory or phonotactic structure of the language. Thus, the comparison of processes or rules across language systems is another dimension of phonologic organization that has to be taken into account in examining the interaction of two language systems. The application of native language processes to a second language will potentially create still another kind of phonologic interference.

The consideration of phonologic processes in L2 acquisition is a point at which the transfer model is in need of some qualification. Some phonologic processes appear to have a natural, universal basis rather than a language specific one, so that they may have an explanation that is independent of language. For example, Wolfram (1983) shows that certain final consonant deletion processes are operative in the L2 English of L1 Vietnamese speakers despite the fact that the particular final consonants are present in both the L1 and L2 languages. In a study of syllable structure processes by Tarone (1976), it was found that 10 per cent to 47 per cent of all L2 phonologic errors could not be attributed to a transfer source. Given such evidence, Mulford and Hecht (1980) suggest that there is an interaction between transfer and natural universal processes. They further suggest that the relative roles of universally based processes and transfer processes from L1 differ according to the class of sounds involved. They offer the following continuum of relative effect:

Vowels	Liquids	Stops	Fricatives/Affricates

←——→

Transfer   Developmental
processes   processes
predominate   predominate

Although such a continuum seems reasonable, it is still speculative, and in need of empirical justification. Furthermore, it seems much more applicable to children than adults. While adults certainly can reactivate L1 strategies to some extent in the L2 situation, current evidence (e.g., Oller, 1974; Sato, 1983) still points to the primary role of transfer.

Variation and Second Language Learning

At first glance, the phonology of a second language learner may appear to consist of a random set of language errors. While there is certainly fluctuation in the variants used as correspondences for the correct phonologic item in the target language where there are points of structural conflict between the native and target language, we can hardly conclude that they are unsystematic. Instead, we find a structured regularity that governs the fluctuation, and this regularity suggests a higher principle of language change. Language is a dynamic system, constantly undergoing change, and the way in which it changes follows a regular pattern, whether an entire system is changing its forms, a first language learner is acquiring the adult forms, or a second language learner is acquiring new forms. Ideally, the change moves from the categoric use of one form to another one, but the system passes through an orderly progression of variable stages as it goes from one extreme to the other. In second language learning, the stages are observed when a learner is required to learn a new unit in the second language. The orderly stages of progression in acquiring this unit can best be illustrated by taking the case of a typical "interference" variant and showing how it changes to the second language form. The model proposed here follows Wolfram (1978). For our illustrative purposes, we will take the case of the German speaker who is confronted with English [ə], in items such as *think, ether,* and *wreath.* German does not have the sound unit [ə], so the German speakers are confronted with acquiring this new phonologic form in the second language. Without a corresponding sound unit in German, speakers may use a unit from their native language in lieu of English [ə], and one of the common variants is [s], which is a unit in German.

In the first stage the use of [s] for [ə] may be categoric, so that [s] is always used in items such as *think* ([sɪŋk]), *ether* [isə] and *wreath* [ris]). In the next stage, we may begin to get [s] fluctuating with [ə] in a limited environment, perhaps only in word-initial position such as *think* [sɪŋk] and [əɪŋk]). Other environments, such as the intervocalic position of *ether* and the word-final position of *wreath,* would still evidence exclusive [s] use.

In the next stage, fluctuation between the correct English phone and the interference variant [s] may spread to a broader context, perhaps first to the intervocalic context of *ether* and then to the word-final position of *wreath.*

Following a stage of "maximal variability" (i.e., fluctuation in all environments), some environments will adopt the new variant categorically. Typically, this will taken place where the change to the new form was initiated originally. Thus, English [ə] may be adopted categorically in word-initial position, while continuing to fluctuate with [s] in intervocalic and final positions. Eventually, there is categorical adoption of the new variant in all the appropriate environments as the process of acquisition is completed. The logical stages of progression from the categorical use of the interference variant to the categorical acquisition of the new phone in the three environments is summarized in Table 3–1, where word-initial is E1, intervocalic E2, and word-final E3.

The model in this table provides an important starting point for seeing how new phonologic units in a second language are acquired. Naturally, this is an ideal; we know that many speakers' systems become "fossilized" so that they never complete the process of change. And, of course, the rate of passage from one stage to the next may vary greatly, so that no real-life time frame can be imposed on this progression. Nonetheless, we see that fluctuation occurs in a systematic way, constrained on the basis of different phonologic environments and moving in a regular progression from one stage to the next. Furthermore, different speakers go through the same stages in acquiring the new form.

An authentic model of second language phonologic acquisition will naturally have to represent additional dimensions of the interlanguage system. For instance, the notion of an "interference variant" needs some

Table 3–1. Stages in the Acquisition of a New Second Language Phonologic Unit

	E₁	E₂	E₃
Stage One (Categoric interference variant)	s	s	s
Stage Two (Limited variation)	s and ө	s	s
Stage Three (Expanded variation)	s and ө	s and ө	s
Stage Four (Maximal variation)	s and ө	s and ө	s and ө
Stage Five (Limited categorical adoption)	ө	s and ө	s and ө
Stage Six (Expanded categorical adoption)	ө	ө	s and ө
Stage Seven (Complete adoption)	ө	ө	ө

explanation. In the example in the table, it is suggested that the use of [s] for English [ө] was an interference form from the native language, based on our comparison of the two systems. Thus, equivalence between German [s] and English [ө] was assumed. But the notion of presumed equivalence between native and target language forms cannot always be predicted. In reality, some German speakers may use [t] instead of [s], or a given speaker may use both [t] and [s] for English [ө]. So, we cannot say that a single correspondence will always exist between the two language systems. For example, in one study of Japanese speakers producing the English consonant *r* (Dickerson and Dickerson, 1976), five different variants were observed, including the English target sound; and each of the ten subjects in the study showed the full range of variants indicated here:

Variants for English [r]
[ɾ] voiced nonretroflexed flap
[l] voiced lateral flap
[l] voiced lateral
[ɽ] voiced retroflexed flap
[r] voiced retroflexed semiconsonant

It is also necessary to clarify the nature of the relationship of phones in the native and target languages. We mentioned that the notion of equivalent structures in the native and target languages could not always be predicted, so that it is necessary to determine equivalence on an empirical basis. And, in the establishment of interference it is necessary to recognize productions that may be unique to the learner's system. In the study cited earlier, the range of phonetic variants reveals some productions that use phones in the native language, some that are phones in the target language, and some that may be unique to the learner's system. These unique sounds (which result as a product of interaction between systems) must be recognized as an authentic part of the interlanguage system.

In all of the preceding discussion, we have mentioned the important role of phonologic environment in determining variants. We may, for example, find a German speaker who uses [s] and [t] for English [θ] in initial position and [s] and [f] in final position. Or, the native Japanese speaker may use only [l] for English [r] preceding low vowels but [ɾ], [l], and [ɽ] before high vowels. The role of environment is important in determining the interlanguage variants that may occur and the range of fluctuation between variants. It should be noted that environment here must include all the dimensions found to be influential within any phonologic system, including the effect of neighboring sounds; the role of sounds in larger units such as syllables, words, and phrases; and prosodic features such as stress and intonation. Also, these different dimensions of environment may interact with each other, just as they may in a unitary phonologic system.

The model we propose here is one that accounts for the orderly progression from the units of one phonologic system to another. It takes into account the fluctuating nature of the interlanguage system while showing how the variability and change are highly systematic. Speakers of a new language do not suddenly awake with a new phonologic system. Instead, they go through an orderly progression of fluctuating variants, passing through inevitable stages as the process is carried to completion. In an important sense, the orderly acquisition of new forms in a second phonologic system recapitulates the process whereby all language systems undergo change.

Pedagogic Implications

The treatment of second language learning problems within the context of speech and language pathology has engendered considerable controversy during the past several years. The basic issue concerns the responsibility of speech pathologists to treat such problems. Some (Bjarkman and Buckingham, 1981; Gandour 1980) have argued that second language learning problems are not appropriately treated in a clinical context because they do not involve disorders in the traditional application of this designation. Furthermore, these problems are not best handled by those techniques characteristic of a clinical setting. From this perspective, these problems should be left in the hands of those specifically educated in the methods of teaching English as a second language (TESL).

Others within speech pathology (Dreher, 1981; Gillcrist, 1981) have maintained that speech pathologists can assume responsibility for treating problems of the second language learner because of their education regarding communication problems of all types. Furthermore, there is no evidence that the traditional therapy methods employed by speech and language pathologists are inappropriate or inferior to those used by TESL specialists. In some instances, there is also a practical argument because the speech and language pathologist may be the only individual available for referral within a particular real-life setting.

Unfortunately, the dispute has sometimes been reduced to a question of professional territorial rights and the consequences of treating second language problems in training speech pathologists. (For example, there have been extended arguments over the validity of clinical "clock hours" obtained in assisting persons learning English as a second language). With due respect to the vested interests of different service professions and the genuine need to clarify certifiable clock hours in student clinical education, the issue seems to be somewhat misdirected. Instead of arguing over who has the right and obligation to handle such cases, we are better served by delimiting the requisite knowledge and pedagogic base for the individual engaged in such activities. The professional affiliation seems not nearly as important as the requisite qualifications.

Before the requisite knowledge base is set forth, it is necessary to reiterate our philosophic perspective on interlanguage. Repeatedly, we have referred to this kind of behavior as the norm for those learning a second language, so that a clinical designation as a "disorder" is inappropriate. Consideration of these problems as if they were no different from traditionally designated functional and organic disorders can only have negative attitudinal consequences. We must always bear in mind that we are dealing with a pedagogic problem, not a clinical one, and any practical approach to teaching phonology to learners to English as a second language must start from that vantage point.

Several dimensions of a requisite knowledge base derive from our earlier discussion of phonologic acquisition in a second language. First, it is necessary for the instructor to understand the comparative phonologies involved in the language learning situation. Such structural knowledge serves as the basis for understanding the kinds of phenomena that emerge in the interlanguage. Even those sounds that may be unique to the language learning situation are best viewed in terms of adaptive strategies that derive from the interaction of two language systems. It must be remembered here that the talker is not simply attempting to learn an English phonology, but attempting to learn this phonology on the basis of competence in another system with similarities to, and differences from, the target language. Understanding the points of structural similarity and difference thus becomes the starting point for focusing on the nature of the interlanguage system. The structural knowledge involved should include those aspects of the system discussed earlier, including the inventory of phonologic units, the phonotactic structures, and the various phonologic processes that operate in the respective phonologies. The instructor who starts with such contrastive knowledge is at considerable advantage in focusing on points of conflict that will lead to problems in the acquisition of the second language phonology. Practically speaking, this means that an instructor teaching English to a speaker of Spanish, Japanese, or German should know something about the structure of the respective phonologies, because the learner will encounter different problems in accordance with the native language system.*

A second requisite for the instructor involves analytic ability in describing a phonologic system. The system of the language learner must be analyzed on the basis of the observed interlanguage forms. This analytic ability starts with a practical knowledge of phonetics that allows the instructor to transcribe all the sounds produced by the learner in adequate detail, and extends to ability to describe the inventory of phonologic contrasts, phonotactics, and processes that are utilized by a given talker. All talkers are not at the same stage in their interlanguage, and accurate diagnosis is dependent upon the ability to understand each person's phonologic behavior as a system. The instructor needs to know the details of the phonologic system as a basis for setting up relevant instructional focus. Effective diagnosis, which is the reasonable basis for subsequent instruction, presumes this essential analytic ability.

---

*We distinguish here between structural knowledge of a language, which involves familiarity with its organizational patterns, and speaking knowledge, which involves proficiency in using the language as a means of communication.

A third base of knowledge involves understanding the nature of the second language learning process. In a sense, this understanding parallels the need to understand the native language acquisition process if a speech-language pathologist is to work with children acquiring the native language system. Important practical corollaries follow from understanding a model of second language acquisition. For example, given the important role of phonologic environment in influencing interlanguage variants and the progressive utilization of new forms in terms of these environments, phonologic context must figure prominently in the development of instructional materials. Similarly, fluctuation between variants is to be expected, and differing levels of fluctuation (in addition to different variants) should be expected in the acquisition process. If instructional materials are to recapitulate the normal progression of acquisition in a second language, then a viable model of this process must provide a base.

Finally, those dealing with second language learners should be familiar with the instructional strategies utilized in teaching the second phonology. In this respect, the field of TESL has developed particular strategies for developing students' perceptual and productive capabilities in another phonology. However, it should be noted that the basic methods in TESL and speech pathology are probably not as different as they sometimes appear on the surface. Thus, both speech pathologists and TESL teachers may set up discrimination tasks as a means of focusing on target phonologic units. Similarly, both may concern themselves with accurate phonetic production of target phones, utilizing various linguistic and nonlinguistic tasks to enhance the accurate production of the target phone. Also, both focus on aspects of linguistic and nonlinguistic "generalization" or "transfer," so that use in an increasingly broad range of phonologic contexts, and facility along an increasingly spontaneous continuum of extralinguistic situations, constitute an essential pedagogic concern. The details of tasks may be structured somewhat differently in speech pathology and TESL, but the underlying pedagogic principles are quite similar. Thus, the adaptation of the pedagogic approach should not be too imposing a task for a resourceful speech-language pathologist. In the final analysis, we must be more concerned with the requisite knowledge and pedagogic base of the individuals who teach a second phonology than with their professional affiliation. Second language learners stand to profit most from those who can apply appropriate descriptive, analytic, and pedagogic strategies regardless of their professional affiliation.

Diagnosis and Remediation

For several reasons, issues of diagnosis and remediation are considerably more involved in an L2 than in an L1 system. Given the target norms of L2, it is essential to differentiate between a system differing from the target in accordance with the normal L2 phonologic acquisition process (i.e., *interlanguage norms*) and one which deviates from normal acquisition stages. The critical question is whether we can determine the difference between "normal" and "disordered" interlanguages, given that both will differ from the L2 target norms. The answer is complicated by several considerations related to the inherent nature of interlanguage. First, there is considerable fluctuation in how L2 target sounds may be modified. Thus, one speaker with a Vietnamese L1 background may use [t] for initial English [ɵ] and another may use [s], and both of these seem to be within normal limits. Furthermore, the same speaker may sometimes use [s] for [ɵ] and other times [t] for [ɵ] in the same item. This kind of fluctuation is a part of the normal developmental path, so that it is unrealistic to establish a unitary interlanguage norm.

Second, different persons may level or fossilize their interlanguage systems at varying stages. Thus, two persons with similar language backgrounds and similar exposure to the L2 may display quite different degrees of language transfer. While such differences indicate a range of proficiency levels in L2 acquisition, the situation seems relatively normal for interlanguage. Thus, we must recognize quite different individual proficiency levels within a broadly defined range of interlanguage normalcy.

Qualifications such as these certainly add complexity to an assessment task based on a developing L2 system. If the goal of the assessment is the identification of authentic phonologic disorders independent of language background, then assessment in the L1 certainly seems preferable. If this is not possible, then the assessment in L2 must proceed with the kinds of cautions discussed here. Realistic diversity in the interlanguage must be established as a baseline for assessment, just as normal dialectal variation must enter into the assessment of L1 clients with dialectally diverse backgrounds.

A speech-language pathologist called upon to serve a group for whom English is an L2 must usually accumulate data that can serve as a basis for establishing these kind of interlanguage norms. In many cases, the establishment of normal interlanguage for a particular group will have to be based on informal norms established by language-sensitive practitioners. For example, a speech pathologist asked to serve a Vietnamese refugee community will have to determine what the interlanguage norms are for that group. Thus, it may be determined that [t] and [s] for English initial [θ] are quite normal interlanguage norms based on an informal survey of talkers, but that an initial glottal stop [ʔ] for [θ] is not. From this perspective, the production of [sIn] or [tIn] for [θIn] would be considered normal, but [ʔIn] would not. Resourcefulness in such situations is obviously demanded, given the current scarcity of descriptions of L2 interlanguage systems, but the challenge seems appropriate for any speech pathologist serving such a population (Wolfram, 1979).

While the differentiation between normal interlanguage and disordered interlanguage looms important on a theoretical level, there is a practical point at which this issue may take a back seat to the practitioner's concern for basic intelligibility in the L2. When normal phonologic transfer imposes significant obstacles to intelligibility, then it seems appropriate for the speech pathologist to assist the development of the L2 phonology. The kinds of considerations that govern what aspects of the phonologic system are focused upon pedagogically, and the methods for modifying phonologic behavior, are not strikingly different in phonologic remediation and ESL training. For example, consider some of the factors that may enter into setting priorities for phonologic remediation:

1. The effect of pattern on intelligibility.
2. The generalization of the phonologic pattern.
3. The "functional load" of the phonologic opposition involved.
4. The fluctuation of the non-normative pattern.
5. The susceptibility to modification strategies.
6. The social obtrusiveness of the phonologic divergence.

These considerations may also serve the ESL teacher who adopts a systematic approach in setting priorities for developing phonologic materials in an L2.

The systematic organization of L2 pedagogy also parallels the classic considerations involved in the clinical approach to remediation in its concern for establishing the target behavior, generalizing the behavior linguistically and nonlinguistically, and stabilizing and retaining the behavior. A survey of remediation paradigms in speech pathology (e.g., Bernthal and Bankson, 1981; Winitz, 1975) and pedagogic approaches in ESL phonology (e.g., Goodman, 1980; Saville-Troike, 1976) finds many of the same kinds of drills, including techniques for phonetic establishment, discrimination, contrastive production, and generalization. If anything, the kinds of drills used in speech pathology are somewhat more exacting in pedagogic detail. Obviously, some adaptations will be made in ESL situations, given the dynamics of the systems involved. Thus, approaches to the treatment of underdifferentiation in L2 phonology may highlight discrimination training initially, whereas cases of phone substitution may focus on phonetic establishment. But even in these cases, similar strategies might derive from a comprehensive assessment of a phonologic disorder. In reality, then, the practical dimensions of L2 phonology seem quite susceptible to the traditional techniques utilized within the tradition of speech pathology. While the techniques designed to remediate phonologic disorders and to modify L2 interlanguage are common in many instances, there remains an important difference in perspective: divergence in L2 phonology is a normal part of the dynamics of adult second language learning, and any effort to increase proficiency in the L2 must highlight this normalcy rather than treat it as a basic disorder.

References

Bernthal, J. E., and Bankson, N. W. (1981). *Articulation disorders.* Englewood Cliffs, NJ: Prentice-Hall.

Bjarkman, P. C., and Buckingham, H. W. (1981). A response to Gandour (Letter to the editor). *Journal of Speech and Hearing Disorders, 46,* 220.

Burt, M. K., and Kiparsky, C. (1972). The Gooficon: *A repair manual for English.* Rowley: Newbury House.

Corder, S. P. (1981). *Error analysis and interlanguage.* Oxford: Oxford University Press.

Dickerson, L. J., and Dickerson, W. B. (1976). Interlanguage phonology: Current trends and future directions. In S. P. Corder and E. Roulet (Eds.), *Actes du ème colloque de linguistique appliquèe de Neuchâtel.* Geneva: Universite de Neuchâtel.

Dreher, B. B. (1981). Response to Gandour (Letter to the editor). *Journal of Speech and Hearing Disorders, 46,* 217-218.

Dulay, H., and Burt, M. K. (1972). Goofing: An indication of children's second language learning strategies. *Language Learning, 22,* 235-252.

Gandour, J. (1980). Speech therapy and teaching English to speakers of other languages (Letter to the editor). *Journal of Speech and Hearing Disorders, 45,* 133-135.

Gillcrist, M. M. (1981). A rationale for providing service to the limited English proficiency student. *Language, Speech, and Hearing Services in Schools, 12,* 145-152.

Goodman, B. (1980). Improving foreigners' pronunciation of American English. ERIC No. ED 192 608.

Ingram, D. (1976). *Phonological disability in children.* London: Edward Arnold.

Macken, M. A., and Ferguson, C. A. (1981). Phonological universals in language acquisition. In H. Winitz (Ed.), *Native language and foreign language acquisition.* New York: New York Academy of Sciences.

Mulford, R., and Hecht, B. F. (1980). Learning to speak without an accent: Acquisition of a second language phonology. *Papers Representing Child Language Development, 18,* 16–74.

Oller, D. K. (1974). *Toward a general theory of phonological processes in first and second language learning.* Paper presented at the meeting of the Western Conference on Linguistics, Seattle.

Sato, C. J. (1983). *Phonological processes in second language acquisition: Another look at interlanguage syllable structure.* Paper presented at the 17th Annual TESOL Convention, Toronto.

Saville-Troike, M. (1976). *Foundations for teaching English as a second language: Theory and method for multicultural education.* Englewood Cliffs, NJ: Prentice-Hall.

Stampe, D. (1973). *A dissertation on natural phonology.* Unpublished doctoral dissertation, University of Chicago.

Tarone, E. (1976). Some influences on interlanguage phonology. *Working Papers in Bilingualism, 8,* 87–111.

Wardhaugh, R. (1970). The contrastive analysis hypothesis. *TESOL Quarterly, 4,* 124–129.

Weinreich, U. (1953). *Languages in contact.* The Hague, Netherlands: Mouton.

Winitz, H. (1975). *From syllable to conversation.* Baltimore: University Park Press.

Wode, H. (1977). The L2 acquisition of /r/. *Phonetica, 34,* 200–217.

Wolfram, W. (1978). Contrastive linguistics and social dialectology. *Language learning, 28,* 1–28.

Wolfram, W. (1979). *Dialect differences and speech pathology.* Washington, DC: Center for Applied Linguistics.

Wolfram, W. (1983). *Vietnamese English pronunciation.* Unpublished manuscript, Center for Applied Linguistics, Washington, DC.

Wolfram, W., and Johnson, R. (1982). *Phonological analysis: Focus on American English.* Washington, DC: Center for Applied Linguistics.

Part Two

VOICE

William H. Perkins

Assessment and Treatment of Voice Disorders: State of the Art

In 1977, Paul Moore addressed the question of whether the major issues in voice disorders had been answered by research in speech science during the last 50 years. By way of softening his answer, which was "no," he reminded us that 300 years elapsed between the discovery of ether and its use as an anesthetic, 50 years between development of the laryngeal mirror and its use in diagnosis of laryngeal disease.

This is a review of what has been accomplished since 1976. (A "recent review" was operationally defined as work published during the last seven to eight years.) Although the answer for the voice clinician to Moore's question is still no, it is an answer that is changing rapidly in some areas. Of 170 articles reviewed, 132 were concerned with assessment and 38 with treatment, of which 27 described medical or surgical procedures for improving voice and only 11 dealt with voice therapy. As for assessment, of the 40 reports on acoustic methods, all but two involved detection of laryngeal pathology. Those two proposed an acoustic measure of vocal efficiency, the optimal target with which voice clinicians would presumably be primarily concerned, and both were written in German (Schultz-Coulon, Battmer, and Reichers, 1979).

By limiting this review to clinically relevant evidence (texts were included only if they reported data), what is presented is only the tip of the iceberg. With the growth of Japanese interest in voice science during the last decade, basic research in anatomy, physiology, and physics of voice has boomed, as has work in technology on measuring laryngeal function.

Two conferences on vocal fold physiology, one in 1980 at Kurume University, Japan, and the other in 1981 at the University of Wisconsin, provide a sense of the current frontiers. Topics ranged from the vascular network of the vocal fold, firing rate of motor units, neuromuscular control systems of phonation, and biorheology of vocal fold tissue to ultrasonic observation of vibratory action of inner layers of the vocal folds, computer simulations of cord vibration, interactions between glottal source and vocal tract, and relationships between glottal area time function and supraglottal pressure variation. Such topics as these, though not yet ready for clinical application, are all aspects of a common vocal mechanism that need basic understanding before a solid foundation for clinical application can be built (Stevens and Hirano, 1981). Unlike the 300 year delay for ether and the 50 years for the laryngeal mirror, clinical applications of voice research are already available for some aspects of assessment and are on the horizon for other problems of voice.

Assessment

Technology of Measurement

The development of instruments for measuring vocal function has attracted the largest body of scientific advances that are clinically useful. A conference organized by the Communicative Disorders Program of the National Institute of Neurological and Communicative Disorders and Stroke (NINCDS) in 1979 points up the priority of this area of advancement. The purpose of the conference was to identify objective, reliable, valid procedures for assessing voice disorders, which can permit communication of findings among clinics and clinical investigators. The voice scientists, speech pathologists, and laryngologists who participated concluded that fiberoptic, electromyographic, airflow, acoustic, and laryngographic techniques were highly relevant to the assessment of neurologic dysfunction, vocal cord lesions, morphologic changes of the cords, and abnormal phonatory function. They also concluded, however, that no technique could be singled out as the most effective (Ludlow and Hart, 1982).

Assessment of Laryngeal Pathology

Table 4-1 summarizes the assessment needs addressed by this conference. Judging from frequency of use in studies reported, acoustic

Table 4–1. Types of Measures Needed in the Management of Vocal Pathologies

Clinical Service	Measures Needed
Detection of changes in laryngeal tissues following completion of radiation treatment for laryngeal carcinoma.	Measures of changes in the stiffness and mass of the cords as may be reflected in phonatory functioning.
Assessment and reassessment of vocal nodules during voice therapy.	Objective, standardized, and reliable measures of the size and position of nodules from visual recordings. Measures of the effects of vocal nodules on phonatory function. Measures of differences in vocal cord positioning and vibratory patterns which may contribute to the development of the nodules.
Assessment and reassessment of recurrent laryngeal paresis/paralysis; abductor paresis/paralysis; superior laryngeal paresis/paralysis.	Objective, standardized, and reliable graphic measures of resting, inspiratory, and adducted positioning of the cords. Measures of vocal efficiency and range of phonatory functioning. Measures of muscle fiber activity in the vocalis, interarytenoid, posterior cricoarytenoid, and cricothyroid.
Diagnosis and assessment of "functional" phonatory disorders.	Measures of degree and type of deviation from normal in: Vocal cord positioning. Vibratory patterns. Patterns of intrinsic and extrinsic muscle fiber firing at rest and during phonation. Relative timing of adductor-abductor antagonistic muscle group contractions.
Assessment and reassessment of phonatory disorders associated with neuromuscular disorders.	Measures of degree and type of deviation from normal in: Muscle fiber firing at rest and during contraction. Synchronization of onset of firing in adductor and abductor muscle antagonists. Vibratory cycle. The rate of positioning of the vocal cords for phonation onset and offset during connected speech.
Detection of changes in esophageal speech which may be signs of carcinoma reoccurrence.	Measures of changes in: Rate of syllable production. Airflow during speech. Vocal efficiency for intensity. Median and range in fundamental frequency. Extraneous noise production during speech.

Ludlow, C. L. (1982). Research needs for the assessment of phonatory function. In C. L. Ludlow and M. O. Hart (Eds.), *Proceedings of the Conference on the Assessment of Vocal Pathology* (ASHA Reports 11) (p. 5). Rockville, MD: American Speech-Language-Hearing Association.

measures are the preferred technique for meeting as many of these needs as possible. This is not surprising, considering that these measures are nonintrusive, can be gathered and analyzed relatively easily, permit calibration and quantification, and provide inferences for a wide range of interpretations of normal and abnormal laryngeal conditions and patterns of vibration.

Acoustic Measures. Acoustic studies reported since 1976 have been concerned with two clinical topics: detection of pathologic laryngeal conditions and assessment of voice quality. In an excellent review, Davis (1979, 1982) analyzed various acoustic measures available and the clinical uses to which they can be put.

The underlying premise for detection of laryngeal pathology is that a deviant condition will result in an acoustic "signature" affecting fundamental frequency, intensity, or quality, singly or in combination. Pathology that affects vocal fold mass, elasticity, stiffness, or length will affect fundamental frequency. Paralysis of respiratory or laryngeal musculature will reduce sufficiency of subglottal pressure and, accordingly, of vocal intensity. The traditional early warning sign of laryngeal pathology, hoarseness, is heard as a deviant quality but can also involve fundamental frequency and intensity. A tumor or parlysis of one cord that produces asymmetric mass, stiffness, or elasticity will cause asymmetric cord vibration with consequent breathiness, reduced intensity, pitch perturbation (jitter), and amplitude perturbation (shimmer).

Much of the recent effort to detect pathology acoustically has used indirect rather than direct signals. The problem with direct signals is the resonance effect of the vocal tract, which, along with the glottal source component, constitutes the radiated sound. It is the glottal component, of course, which is affected by laryngeal pathology. Throat contact microphones, one type of direct signal that minimizes vocal tract resonances, also present problems: intervening neck tissue functions as a low pass filter, and the signal is sensitive to microphone placement. These difficulties have led to the use of a long metal reflectionless tube to separate the glottal source from resonance effects of the vocal tract. Although simple and inexpensive, it requires vocal tract adjustments that raise questions about the validity of the procedure (Monsen, 1982).

The more frequently used approach is *inverse filtering,* which requires computer analysis to filter out supraglottal resonance contributions to the signal. What remains is a more useful approximation of the glottal signal, which can be analyzed for effects of laryngeal pathology. Two methods of inverse filtering have been used. *Glottal inverse filtering* now uses digital computer techniques to estimate formant frequencies and band widths from which all but the glottal wave form is supposed to be removed. The resulting wave form, however, does not correspond satisfactorily with concepts of vocal cord closure (Davis, 1982; Hiki, Imazzumi, Hirano, Matsushita, and Kakita, 1976).

The other indirect method is *residue inverse filtering.* It is the inverse of the estimated lip radiation, vocal tract, and glottal spectral contributions to the speech signal. The signal that remains exhibits strong peaks at the start of each pitch period. The *residue* signal is obtained with a phase-insensitive autocorrelational method, which does not require the visual inspection of formants, marking of pitch periods, or controlled recording conditions necessary for glottal inverse filtering. Thus, the residual signal, although more of an abstraction than the glottal signal, is easier to obtain and has greater potential value for detecting laryngeal pathology (Davis, 1982; Markel and Gray, 1976). Although in some intermediate or advanced cases it does not seem to provide more information about the pathology than the unfiltered speech signal, in other early cases it has detected pathology that was not otherwise apparent (Davis, 1976).

Earlier work on acoustic effects of laryngeal pathology on periodicity of vocal cord vibration has continued (Kitajima and Gould, 1976; Murry and Doherty, 1980). Several approaches have been used. *Pitch period perturbation* is the time difference between durations of successive pitch periods in the vocal tone. Relative average perturbation, taking into account the slow smooth changes in pitch period that occur normally, provides a smoothed trend line against which rapid erratic perturbations can be measured. This measure has been refined into a frequency perturbation quotient (FPQ). Fundamental frequency perturbation, taking account of greater normal perturbation at higher frequencies, has provided a basis for distinguishing effects of laryngeal cancer between male and female voices. *Amplitude perturbation* is determined by correlograms of a series of amplitude values at each pitch period peak. This measure has been developed as an amplitude perturbation quotient (APQ). More recently, Davis (1976, 1982) used the residue signal, rather than the unfiltered speech signal, to devise an automated procedure for determining pitch and amplitude perturbation quotients (PPQ and APQ), which improve discrimination of pathologic from normal voice. Recognizing that the signal-to-noise ratio is higher between pitch peaks of the residue signal of pathologic than of normal voices, and that detection of fundamental frequency is made difficult by the "breathy" voice caused by pathology, Davis (1976) has also developed acoustic measures using these characteristics.

How to interpret pitch perturbation as evidence of pathology is confounded by its occurrence in normal voices (Horii, 1979). Exactly why it is greater in pathologic larynges is not entirely clear (Koike, Takahashi, and Calcaterra, 1977). For that matter, although earlier studies reported a relationship between perception of pathology and pitch perturbation, more recent work shows a negative relationship (Horii, 1979; Ludlow, 1982; Nichols, 1979).

Spectral analysis is another acoustic basis for detection of laryngeal pathology (Kitajima, 1981). Investigations over the last two decades have shown noise components in pathologic voices that mask formant and fundamental frequency characteristics. Observing that spectral flatness increases with spectral noise, Davis (1976) developed spectral measures for vocal assessment. Using features and signals obtained with residue inverse filtering, he developed a voice profile with which normal and pathologic voices can be differentiated. Although spectral flatness measures were useful in making the distinction, perturbation quotients were better, but still not infallible.

Spectrographic analysis has been used to study the breathiness of abductor spastic dysphonia and the strained voice arrests of adductor spastic dysphonia (Merson and Ginsberg, 1979; Wolfe and Bacon, 1976). Similarly, some correlations have been found between spectral characteristics and such voice qualities as overtight-breathy, hyper-hypokinetic, and nasality (Fritzell, Hammarberg, and Wedin, 1977; Gauffin and Sundberg, 1977; Lindblom, Lubker, and Pauli, 1977; Wirz, Subtelny and Whitehead, 1981).

Attractive as the potential of acoustic measures is for detecting laryngeal pathology, Ludlow (1982) points out that with the current state of knowledge, acoustic screening methods are not yet feasible. What these measures detect is hoarseness and roughness, qualities frequently found in voices not necessarily affected by pathology (Brindle and Morris, 1979; Emanuel and Austin, 1981; Emanuel and Scarzini, 1979, 1980; Hanson and Emanuel, 1979; Whitehead and Lieberth, 1979). Thus, until functional hoarseness can be reliably differentiated from pathologic hoarseness, acoustic methods will not become realistic tools of clinical assessment. Still, Hirano, Hiki, Imazzumi, Kakita, and Matsushita (1978) have demonstrated in a preliminary study of 217 patients with various pathologies that 84 per cent of them could be separated from 20 normal subjects. Similarly, 84 per cent of the cancer patients could be differentiated from those with other pathologies, and 70 per cent of patients with polyps, sulcis vocalis, and recurrent laryngeal paralysis could be differentiated. In a similar study of 30 patients, using long-term speech spectra, comparable results were obtained (Wendler, Doherty, Hollien, 1980). Whether their multivariate analysis of spectral harmonics, frequency perturbation, and amplitude perturbation will meet Ludlow's reservations remains to be determined.

Nonacoustic Measures. Various other measures have received recent attention as being clinically useful. What is searched for are quantitative measures of degree of laryngeal impairment that can provide a basis for comparison with the normal (Ludlow, 1982). Some have been in use for years; others seem to hold great potential but have barely been explored in laryngeal studies.

Ultrasound, the use of which has burgeoned in many areas of medicine, seems to have advantages for laryngeal inquiry. Using the principle of sonar, high frequency sound is reflected from internal structures that differ in acoustic reflective properties such as soft and hard tissues, fluids, and gases. Presumably, ultrasound could provide a nonintrusive method of visualizing the larynx, but extensive research will be needed before clinical merits can emerge (Hamlet, 1982).

Video nasopharyngoscopy has been used to visualize cord action in dysarthric speech (Ludlow and Bassich, 1981). A similar device, the laryngeal fiberscope with the lens positioned just below the velum, is routinely used in Japan for laryngeal diagnosis (Andrews, 1977; Fujimura, 1982; Parnes, Lavarato, and Myers, 1978; Sawashima, 1976). It has also been used with stroboscopic light (Gould, Kojima, and Lahiase, 1979; Saito, Fukuda, Kitahara, and Kokawa, 1978). The most recent advance is a stereofiberscope that permits three-dimensional visualization of the larynx (Fujimura, Baer, and Niimi, 1979). An alternative method of visualizing laryngeal pathology is computerized tomography. With reduced cost and radiation, the better information it provides makes it competitive with cinelaryngoscopy and laryngography (Ward, Hanafee, Mancuso, and Shallit, 1979). One of the costs in high speed cinematography, frame-by-frame analysis time, has been reduced with a video scanning technique for extracting glottal measurements (Childers, Paige, and Moore, 1976). On a much simpler and more practical level, a concave laryngeal mirror has been developed that magnifies and brightens the image (Janfaza, 1978).

Because air wastage tends to characterize laryngeal pathology and motor speech disorders, measures of *laryngeal management of the breath stream* are of clinical interest (Kelman, Gordon, Morton, and Simpson, 1981). Several noninvasive methods have been used. *Airflow wave form* at the vocal folds can be obtained from the oral air flow at the mouth with an inverse filter technique as well as with a refinement of the traditional pneumotachographic technique. A relatively simple clinical procedure for measuring *laryngeal airway resistance* has been developed (Merson and Ginsberg, 1979; Rothenberg, 1977, 1982; Smitheran and Hixon, 1981). Similarly, Forner and Hixon (1977) have simplified a kinematic method of measuring speech breathing that requires little training of clinician or client; is safe, precise, and rapid; and permits natural speech in real time. From an oscilloscopic display, changes of chest wall, and rib cage and abdomen contributions to lung volume, can be examined.

Whereas glottal air flow mainly reflects vocal fold movements when the glottis is open, *vocal fold contact area* yields information about the period of glottal closure. This information has been obtained with a laryngograph, a term preferred to glottograph. What is measured is current between electrodes on each side of the larynx. Current flow varies directly with the area of contact between the cords (Askenfelt, Gauffin, Sundberg, and Kitzing, 1980; Rothenberg, 1982; Teany, 1980).

Fourcin (1982) has presented evidence showing how laryngograph output can be analyzed to discriminate among pathologies and between normal and pathologic function. On the premise that different pathologies involve different vocal fold contacts, what the laryngograph presumably yields is a record of the performance of the vocal folds as they prepare to release acoustic pulses. Whether this record can overcome the difficulties of acoustic analysis and provide a basis for discriminating functional aperiodic vibration from pathologic aperiodicity remains to be determined. A difficulty that has often been encountered is the weakness of the signal obtained from some talkers (Rothenberg, 1982). Equally troubling in a comparison of laryngographic and stroboscopic measures of glottal openings and closings were wide variability and low correlations between the measures (Pederson, 1977).

Electromyography is another traditional tool that has been used in many studies of normal laryngeal function, but unlike its use with neuromuscular disorders, it has not been used for diagnosis of laryngeal muscle performance (Guidi, Bannister, Gibson, and Payne, 1981; Harris, 1982). Beyond its relevance for determining abnormalities of laryngeal motor firing, it may also prove essential to the determination of patterns of muscular contraction of functional dysphonia as they are distinguished from patterns of optimal vocal production.

Behavioral Measurement

For clinicians who have limited equipment, reliable behavioral procedures for assessing laryngeal functioning would be particularly useful. Only two studies of adults that address this need have been reported in the last five years. Gordon, Morton, and Simpson (1978) found that patients with additive laryngeal lesions had considerably reduced phonation times for some sustained vowels. These glottal margin tumors, such as nodules and polyps, presumably interfere with efficient cord closure. The consequences are decreased laryngeal airway resistance, increased air flow, and reduced phonation time.

As an indicator of adequacy of laryngeal function, an s/z ratio was devised and tested on 28 subjects with nodules or polyps, 36 dysphonic subjects with no laryngeal pathology, and 86 normally speaking subjects (Eckel and Boone, 1981). No differences were found among these groups in ability to sustain /s/. Similarly, normal speakers did not sustain /z/ much longer than did dysphonic speakers with no pathology, nor did their s/z ratios differ much from 1.0. The pathologic speakers differed significantly from both of these groups by ratios in excess of 1.4 95 per cent of the time, and by shorter durations of /z/. It should be noted, however, that some subjects from both nonpathologic groups showed shorter durations of /z/ and larger s/z ratios than did most of the pathologic subjects. Still, this behavioral screening measure is the most useful yet developed.

Voice Disorder Characteristics

With any disorder, assessment and treatment are dependent on the understanding of it. Most of the recent work on voice disorders has been concerned with the nature of the problems. Although it has not yet culminated in valid and reliable clinical methods, it is the forerunner of the development of such methods. Because it may soon result in the development of assessment procedures, it is reviewed in this section.

Spastic Dysphonia

In 1976, Dedo reported sectioning the recurrent laryngeal nerve as a treatment of spastic dysphonia. Whatever the ultimate merits of this procedure, its indisputable effect was that more recent inquiry has been devoted to this voice disorder than to any other. Whereas traditionally it was mainly considered to be a psychogenic disorder (Brodnitz, 1976), the tide of research abruptly swung to viewing it as a neuropathology. Because control of laryngeal muscle is related to that of middle ear muscles, acoustic reflexes as well as laryngeal nerves and muscles have been investigated (McCall, 1977). Although evidence of histopathology in the recurrent laryngeal nerve has been reported, other evidence has been negative (Aminoff, Dedo, and Izdebski, 1978; Bocchino and Tucker, 1978; Dedo, Izdebski, and Townsend, 1977; Dedo, Townsend, and Izdebski, 1978; Izdebski, 1977; Ravits, Aronson, DeSanto, and Dyck, 1979). Similarly, acoustic reflex differences have been found by some but not by others (Hall and Jerger, 1976; Sharbrough, Stockard, and Aronson, 1978). Still others have suspected focal dystonia of laryngeal musculature (Aminoff et al., 1978).

The meaning of this flurry of interest was the subject of a state-of-the-art conference in 1979 (Lawrence, 1979). The idea that spastic dysphonia is basically a neuropathology is attractive, but no one is certain whether the pathology, if it exists, is peripheral or central. Definitive answers are not yet available. A difficulty with accounting for a spastic condition with peripheral nerve pathology is that the symptom should be flaccidity rather than spasticity.

Perhaps the explanation, at least in part, lies in the evidence of two types of intermittent dysphonia, which in one case were both found in the same patient (Cannito and Johnson, 1981). Traditionally, spastic dysphonia is characterized by adductor spasms, resulting in intermittent strangulation of phonation that resembles essential voice tremor (Aronson and Hartman, 1981). By contrast, several patients have been reported with intermittent abductory spasms. Because the laryngeal behavior is different and the causes may be different, some have resisted the classification "spastic dysphonia—abductor type." Preferred alternatives are "intermittent abductory dysphonia" or "intermittent breathy dysphonia" (Bacon and Wolfe, 1980; Hartman and Aronson, 1981; Merson and Ginsberg, 1979; Parnes et al., 1978; Shipp, Mueller, and Zwitman, 1980; Zwitman, 1979). Whether the neuropathology of one is peripheral, and of the other is central, has not been established.

Motor Voice Disorders

Dysphonic effects of the various dysarthrias are often a consequence of difficulty in initiating and terminating phonation for onset and offset of voice during connected speech, especially in Parkinson's disease. Also affected in Shy-Drager syndrome, myasthenia gravis, Wilson's disease, amyotrophic lateral sclerosis, and tardive dyskinesia, as well as in Parkinson's disease, are abilities to control pitch, loudness, and quality (Dordain and Chevrie-Muller, 1977; Logemann, Fisher, Boshes, and Blonsky, 1978; Ludlow, 1982; Ludlow and Bassich, 1981; Portnoy, 1979; Williams, Hanson, and Calne, 1979). The involuntary grunting and throat-clearings of Gilles de la Tourette syndrome are among the less obtrusive symptoms of this bizarre disorder, which include coprolalia, echolalia, multiple tics, and involuntary jumping, squatting, and kicking. The cause of this dramatic disorder is uncertain, although recent evidence suggests a neurologic basis, a possibility supported by the tendency of affected children to have learning disabilities (Cohen, Shaywitz, Caparulo, Young, and Bowers, 1978; Golden, 1977).

Laryngeal Pathology

Some work has been done relating laryngeal function to voice disorders (Moore, 1976). Murry (1978) has shown that with the exception of a narrowed pitch range in laryngeal paralysis, fundamental frequency is not systematically different in laryngeal pathology from normal, perceptual impressions notwithstanding.

Paralysis. Frequently, a paralyzed vocal fold lies higher than the healthy one. Experimentation with simulated contraction of the lateral cricoarytenoid muscle suggests that this arytenoid displacement can be corrected (Baken and Isshiki, 1977). In somewhat surprising results of experimentation on the excised larynx, the effect of asymmetric tension in the vocal cords turned out opposite to expectation (Isshiki, Tanabe, Ishizaka, and Broad, 1977). Presumably, as cord tension increases, amplitude of vibration decreases. In computer simulation of this physiologic experiment, however, it was found that the tense cord (simulating the healthy cord) vibrated with somewhat greater amplitude than the "paralyzed" lax cord. Moreover, the lax cord dominated the tense one in determining pitch. Despite asymmetric tension (a simulation of unilateral paralysis), if the two cords started from a closed position, they vibrated at the same frequency, even though the tense cord opened faster and then had to wait for the lax cord to catch up. Thus, asymmetric tension alone did not result in hoarseness (Ishizaka and Isshiki, 1976; Isshiki, 1977a).

The implication of these experiments for clinical management of laryngeal paralysis is that if impaired cord resistance is not overpowered with excessive breath pressure, thereby permitting cord closure between vibratory cycles, a reasonably clear voice can be obtained. This brings into question the appropriateness of the widespread "effort" techniques intended to obtain reflexive closure of the cords by effortful lifting, pushing, coughing, or grunting. All of these procedures generate high levels of subglottal pressure, which would work against complete cord closure between cycles. Conversely, the clinical approach supported by this research is to strive for clear tone at a level of loudness as reduced as is necessary to obtain it. With clear tone, the clinician has evidence of symmetric cord vibration with each cycle, presumably beginning from a condition of closure.

Functional Pathology. Pivotal research has been concerned with the nature of vocal cord stress and its significance for vocal abuse in the development of functional pathology. In meticulous preliminary research, Hirano, Kurita, Matsuo, and Nagata (1980, 1981) have studied vocal fold reactions to stress that lead to acute inflammation, subepithelial bleeding, nodules, contact granulomas, polyps, and polypoid degeneration (Reinike's edema). They confirmed that all of these pathologies are largely a consequence of vocal abuse, with the exception of polypoid vocal fold.

Although polypoid hypertrophy is often thought to be basically similar to the polyp, it is not. Characterized by a chronic edematous lesion extending the length of the membranous vocal fold, usually bilaterally, polypoid hypertrophy appears to be caused primarily by smoking and age. Vocal abuse can aggravate the condition, but it is not likely to cause it. These conclusions are based on observations of 57 male and 40 female subjects. In 88 per cent, hoarseness did not begin until age 40, and then it progressed so slowly that most patients did not seek medical help for one to three years. Over three fourths of the patients smoked at least half a pack of cigarettes a day; otherwise, less than half showed any predisposing conditions such as excessive vocal abuse, air pollution, drinking, or the common cold.

Polyps and polypoid swelling both form in the superficial layer of the lamina propria. (The lamina propria of the mucosa, just beneath the thin epithelial surface of the cord, has three layers. The superficial layer is loose and pliable, with few fibers; the intermediate layer is composed chiefly of elastic fibers; and the deep layer consists mainly of collagenous thread-like fibers. The two deeper layers constitute the vocal ligament.) They differ, however, in form, location, and cause. Polyps develop as pedunculated tumors, ranging in size from small to large, attached to the middle of the membranous cord. Judging from data on 629 patients, polyps occur mainly in middle age, rarely in childhood, and somewhat more frequently in male than in female patients. They appear to be caused by a traumatic lesion of small vessels in the lamina propria during abusive phonation, often following a common cold. Neither smoking nor drinking appears to be much involved in causation. Apparently, mechanical stresses of deep layers of cord vibration rupture venules, which hemorrhage, giving the inital reddish appearance that changes to white as the hemorrhages in the polyp become old.

Nodules also develop in the superficial layer of the lamina propria, and at the same location on the cord as polyps. Mechanical vibratory stress in the nodule, however, appears confined to the cord edge, which is free of blood vessels, and activates proliferation of fibroblasts that produce collagenous fibers, which thicken the epithelium to form the whitish mass of the nodule. In 309 cases of nodule, no significant pathology of blood vessels was observed.

The relationship of age and sex to nodular development is somewhat puzzling. In children, far more boys than girls develop nodules, presumably because they yell more. In adults, nodules are rarely found in males, at least in Japan, but are as prevalent in middle aged women as in young boys. Polyps, on the other hand, are more frequently found in low pitch males than in high pitch females. This has led to the speculation that high pitches activate cord edge stress, leading to nodules, whereas low pitches activate deep layer stress, which ruptures blood vessels and causes polyps. How this explanation would account for polyps when they do occur in high-pitched women or nodules in adult low-pitch males has not been determined.

Hirano and colleagues (1980) differentiated acute from chronic reactions to vocal abuse, with nodules, polyps, and contact ulcers being chronic manifestations. Acute inflammation is a typical reaction to temporary excessive vocal abuse, such as yelling at a football game. The superficial layer of the lamina propria becomes edematous from leakage of serum and dilation of blood vessels. With increased stress, blood vessels rupture, resulting in subepithelial bleeding. Both of these acute conditions subside within a week or two of vocal rest and easy quiet phonation. Inflammation, the most frequent problem of professional speakers and singers, can also result from hormonal imbalance, such as that occurring during menstruation in some women, and upper respiratory infection (Schiff and Gould, 1978).

The effects of androgen on mutational voice change were studied in 35 cases of eunuchoidism. Treatment to lower the pitch to normal took 6 months to 2 years. Surprisingly, pitch changes often preceded structural development of the larynx. Apparently, mutational voice change may occur as a result of mode of laryngeal adjustments and changes in soft tissue (Hirose, Sawashima, Ushijima, and Kumamoto, 1977).

Respiration

Hixon, Mead, and Goldman (1976) and Forner and Hixon (1977) have pioneered in definitive studies of speech respiration. Among their recent contributions are investigations of the thorax, rib cage, diaphragm, and abdomen in normal and hearing impaired speech. In normal conversational speech, abdominal forces tune the diaphragm to facilitate minimal interruption of ongoing speech for needed inspiratory pauses. Respiration function in the hearing impaired differed from normal in several ways, including deviance in lung volume adjustments as well as in laryngeal and upper airway adjustments.

Comparisons have also been made of respiration in trained and untrained subjects (Baken, 1979; Baken and Cavallo, 1979, 1981; Proctor, 1979; Wilder, 1979). Although the rib cage and the diaphragm-abdomen, which are the two components of the chest wall, are linked within limits, they also can function independently. Thus, knowledge of the volume of air expired does not reveal relative activity of rib cage or abdomen. Presumably, an unlimited number of rib cage–abdominal patterns could be used to achieve the lung volumes and pressures needed for phonation. To the contrary, well defined prephonatory chest-wall adjustments were found in both trained and untrained talkers. They seem to represent an innate adjustment that has evolved to facilitate phonation. Trained subjects did differ in several ways, however, one of which was wider variations in patterns of chest wall adjustment.

Phonatory Control

Control of any phonatory episode involves the following sequence: prephonatory inspiration, which provides the necessary lung volume for the phrase of an intended length, loudness, pitch, and quality; prephonatory expiration and prephonatory tuning of the vocal folds for the intended utterance; phonatory expiration and modulation of laryngeal activity; and monitoring of the vocal output. Modulation of laryngeal activity is accomplished with three intrinsic reflexogenic systems, with receptors in the mucosa, joints, and muscles. The mucosal and muscle receptors are sensitive to the stretching force of expiratory pressure, whereas mechanoreceptors in the joints mediate cartilage adjustments during phonation (Gould, 1979; Wyke, 1979).

The role of feedback in voice control has also been studied in relation to nasality and laryngeal sensation (Garber and Moller, 1979; Horii and Weinberg, 1979; Leonard and Ringel, 1979; Sorenson, Horii, and Leonard, 1980; Stevens, Nickersen, Boothroyd, and Rollins, 1976). With normally hearing subjects, nasality has been shown to be under auditory feedback control. Lacking auditory feedback, visual feedback has been used to reduce nasality in the deaf. Presumably, phonatory control should be impaired by anesthetization of laryngeal mucosa. Although jitter increases as a result, especially at high frequencies, ability to match pitches was not affected in earlier experiments. Approaching the phonatory control system from a test of auditory and somesthetic feedback times, both sensory modalities were stimulated to determine minimal reaction times for phonatory initiation (Izdebski and Shipp, 1978). This novel tracking task placed greater dynamic demands on the mucosal feedback system, which, when anesthetized, resulted in impaired performance.

Talker Characteristics of Voice

A variety of vocal characteristics of talkers have been investigated, ranging from sex differences and effects on voice of smoking to perceptual systems of voice description. The area of greatest interest, however, has been the effects of age on voice.

Aging

Aside from voice disorders that are characteristic of various ages, such as mutational problems of adolescence and polyps of middle age, aging has effects on the voice that can be detected by observers. A fundamental difficulty in studying vocal aging is in how to define it. Should it be in terms of chronological age or in terms of decrement of vocal function? What should be the measures of perceptual, acoustic, physiologic, and anatomic characteristics? If aging effects are as variable as suspected, which populations should be studied? With these issues still unresolved, work in this area has been mostly exploratory and descriptive (Brodnitz, 1978, Weinberg, 1978; Wilder, 1978).

Beginning with preadolescence, the current description of voice at various ages is as follows. Because girls mature faster than boys, they approach adolescence with slightly lower speech-fundamental frequencies, (SFF), although a recent study suggests the opposite (Hasck, Singh, and Murry, 1980). During adolescence, their SFF becomes gradually lower until adulthood, at which time it remains essentially level until after menopause, when it lowers. In male subjects, who have been studied far more than female subjects, SFF drops about an octave in four to five years during puberty, then continues to lower gradually until about age 40, at which time it begins to rise slowly through the declining years. Pitch range increases during puberty, at least in males, and then declines in the aged. Some elderly voices exhibit tremor, breathiness, pitch variability, increased loudness, and increased noise at the expense of clear tone. Doubt has been cast, however, on jitter and shimmer as the reasons why aged voices are perceived as noisy and rough. Surprisingly, speed of speech is not reduced with age, but precision in achieving speech targets at fast rates is diminished (Hanley, Hanson, and Miller, 1978; Hartman, 1979; Hollien, 1978; Hollien and Tolhurst, 1978; Horii and Ryan, 1981; Horii and Weinberg, 1979; Stoicheff, 1981; Sweeting, 1979; Weinberg, 1978; Wilder, 1978).

This pattern must be recognized as being preliminary. Wide individual variations from it seem abundant, but little is known of these variations. For that matter, because of relatively few investigations, little is known of the female voice. What is known points to greater changes with age in the male than the female.

Recent histologic and laryngoscopic studies may account for some of these changes. Ossification and calcification of the larynx have been found to begin earlier and to be more extensive in male subjects than female subjects. In senility, men's vocal folds tend to atrophy, whereas those of women show mainly edema. That could explain why pitch becomes higher in the former and lower in the latter (Honjo and Isshiki, 1980; Kahane, 1980).

Perceptual Systems of Voice

Three approaches to the perceptual analysis of voice have been taken recently. Colton and Estill (1976, 1978) and Colton, Estill, and Gould (1977), in devising a system for categorizing voice quality, selected four qualities that could be perceptually distinguished: speech (as in everyday conversation), cry, twang, operatic ring. Their objective was to determine the acoustic and physiologic characteristics of these perceptual modes in order to fully describe the various qualities of the human voice.

In multidimensional analyses designed to differentiate between abnormal and normal voices, listeners used more dimensions to judge differences among pathologic voices than normal ones. Apparently, the perceptual strategy for judging normal voices of both sexes is to sort them according to sex and then make separate judgements for male and female subjects, possibly according to cultural stereotypes. Male subjects were judged for similarity on the basis of effort, pitch, and hoarseness; female subjects were characterized by effort, pitch, and nasality (Murry and Singh, 1980; Murry, Singh, and Sargent, 1977; Singh and Murry, 1978).

The third approach represents an attempt to delineate in measurable dimensions all of the independent perceptual elements by which vocal production is controlled. The purpose of this effort is to obtain the acoustic correlates of these perceptual dimensions that, by themselves, are impossible to verify and are very difficult, if not impossible, to measure reliably in a wide range of subjects (Ludlow, 1982). With acoustic correlates of these dimensions established, vocal production can be experimentally manipulated to determine patterns of vocal abuse and vocal efficiency (Perkins, 1978).

Sex Characteristics

Fundamental frequency, sound pressure level, and quality have been studied in male, female, and male transsexual subjects. The slight hoarseness that is reported in trained female singers during menstruation, presumably because of vocal fold edema, was not found in voices of normal untrained female subjects, possibly because they did not perform comparably strenuous vocal tasks (Schiff, 1977; Silverman and Zimmer, 1978). In another investigation, fundamental frequency-sound pressure level (f_0-SPL) profiles of young adult male and female subjects with normal voices were compared for maximum and minimum SPL with 10 per cent intervals of f_0. Male and female subjects were similar in f_0 range, SPL output throughout f_0 range, and SPL range. The profile has potential for graphing the range of frequencies at which the voice functions most efficiently.

In other experiments, fundamental frequency and vocal tract resonance were studied for their contribution to the perception of femaleness in the voice. In natural speech, f_0 was the major determinant in one study, but in another, vocal tract resonance played a major role. On the other hand, in the case of a male transsexual subject who had undergone hormone therapy and had raised her pitch, her voice was still discernibly different from a natural female voice. Interestingly, when trying to sound sexy, both males and females use lower pitches as well as slower rates (Bralley, Bull, and Gore, 1978; Brown and Feinstein, 1977; Coleman, 1976; Coleman, Mabis, and Hinson, 1977; Tuomi and Fisher, 1979).

Other Talker Characteristics

Isolated investigations of talker characteristics have ranged from vocal cues of schizophrenia to effects of a dental prosthesis on voice. In the latter study, use of an experimental dental appliance altered personal characteristics of voice to varying degrees for both listeners and speakers. In the former, schizophrenic talkers were differentiated from nonschizophrenic talkers, probably on the basis of vocal qualities, particularly flat inflection. Voice characteristics of depressive patients did not change significantly with treatment (Darby and Hollien, 1977; Hamlet, Geoffrey, and Bartlett, 1976; Todt and Howell, 1980; Tuomi and Fisher, 1979).

Two other studies were concerned with pitch and loudness. One tested the observation that talkers sound different to themselves than to listeners. Although this may be true for some aspects of voice, it is apparently not true in the perception of pitch. In the other, an investigation of intensity control, talkers appeared to regulate loudness in response to the sound of their voices in their own ears, rather than to maintain intelligible communication (Garber, Siegel, and Pick, 1980; Haskell and Baken, 1978).

Finally, the effect of voice disorders on judgments of a talker's personality and appearance were investigated. Hypernasality evoked more

negative evaluations than a harsh-breathy voice, but both were judged
negatively in comparison with normal voices (Blood, Mahan, and Hyman,
1979).

Treatment

The published literature on treatment of voice disorders has been
divided into three general topics. Under *voice therapy* are the articles dealing
with the nature of this treatment process, its application, and results.
Medical and surgical procedures deemed of interest to the speech
pathologist are included under *laryngeal pathology. Spastic dysphonia* is
discussed within a separate section for two reasons. First, it is the one
clinical entity that has attracted considerable attention, but more important,
the presumption of etiology that would be implied by inclusion under either
of the other headings was conveniently avoided.

To increase credibility of the recent advances reported, the articles
included in this chapter were subject to critical review, either by virtue of
being published in refereed journals, or as papers presented as proceedings
of scientific conferences. This criterion did not significantly exclude much
work on assessment, but the bulk of nonmedical voice treatment procedures
are not reported in journals. A major reason is that in recent years, criteria
for publication of any therapy includes evidence of effectiveness. Reed
(1980) has argued persuasively that as matters stand, the voice clinician
must rely on opinions expressed in textbooks of authors who use different
terms to describe different procedures based on different philosophies. He
concludes that there is little scientific evidence that therapy techniques
actually reduce vocal abuse.

Voice Therapy

Some considerations in approaching treatment of voice disorders have
been reported since 1976. One was an acoustic method of evaluating voice
improvement. Using a battery of acoustic measures, some (such as pitch
and amplitude perturbation) correlated well with a trained listener's
judgments of improvement in voice quality (Davis, 1982). Mysak (1977)
has proposed a systems approach to voice disorders that casts the clinical
problem in broad perspective of receptor, transmitter, facilitator, integrator,
effector, and sensor systems. Brodnitz (1981), drawing on his wealth of

experience, reminds the clinician that no amount of scientific progress will supplant the necessity of addressing the psychologic aspects of patients with voice disorders.

Two studies demonstrated that vocal performance can be changed with behavioral shaping procedures, and a footnote was added in another report warning of the hazards to health of using peanuts as reinforcers (Drudge and Philips, 1976; Lodge and Yarnall, 1981; Putnam, 1981).

Two cases, one treated with vocal rest, the other with a "pushing" technique, were reported. The traumatic effects on family, friends, and professional life of prolonged vocal rest following surgical removal of a nodule are described by the patient, a speech pathologist. As a consequence, she has sworn off complete vocal rest as routine therapy for patients recovering from laryngeal surgery (Fiedler, 1977). In the other case, a "hysterical" high pitch was lowered by obtaining low grunting sounds while the patient pulled herself down into her chair. Control and use of these pitched sounds were then extended (Aldes, 1981).

Therapy of vocal hyperfunction, the problem most frequently requiring intervention by voice clinicians, was the subject of only two investigations, both involving biofeedback. In one, EMG biofeedback from surface electrodes over the cricothyroid region was provided to six subjects with vocal hyperfunction. The three who had a normal larynx reduced EMG activity during speech and were judged to show improvement in quality. The other three, with spastic dysphonia or laryngeal lesions, did not improve (Prosek, Montgomery, Walden, and Schwartz, 1978). In the other study, five of seven improved (Stemple, Weiler, Whitehead, and Komray, 1980).

The full potential of biofeedback techniques will probably not be reached until far more is known about muscular activity during hyperfunction and optimal vocal function. Clearly, all laryngeal muscles do not relax during efficient phonation. With surface electrodes, biofeedback presently does not distinguish between those muscles that should relax and those that should contract.

Laryngeal Pathology

The primary purpose of phonosurgery is to improve voice. It takes five forms: extirpation of a lesion, laryngeal framework surgery to indirectly alter cord shape or mobility, direct cord surgery, neurosurgery to remobilize a paralyzed cord, and laryngeal reconstruction. The mechanisms of hoarseness, breathiness, roughness, and normal voice have been experimentally demonstrated to involve interactions among tightness of glottal closure, cord stiffness, and subglottal pressure. With closure too tight or pressure too high, roughness results. With incomplete cord closure, breathiness is heard (Isshiki, 1980).

Advances in phonosurgery since 1976 (other than for spastic dysphonia) have been mainly concerned with treatment of unilateral laryngeal paralysis. Isolated reports of management of other pathologies affecting voice range from procedures for papilloma to contact ulcers.

Laryngeal Paralysis

According to Tucker (1980), the most successful clinical strategy for unilateral laryngeal paralysis is patience. Out of 210 cases, 64 per cent recovered without therapy. Of the remainder, 26 per cent were helped with Teflon injections into the paralyzed cord to bring it into better approximation with the healthy cord. Similar success with Teflon has been reported by others (Reich and Lerman, 1978). Lewy (1976), who reviewed his results with 218 patients and reports on 1139 other cases, concluded that most persons recover voice. In a review of the literature, Montgomery (1979) indicated that when treatment is successful, the permanent level of improvement is reached in two to four weeks. A surgical correction for one of those causes of failure, excessive injection of Teflon, has also been devised (Horn and Dedo, 1980).

Two alternatives to vocal cord injection have been used to improve voice in cases of unilateral paralysis. (In bilateral paralysis, caused in over half of cases by thyroid surgery, restoration of the airway is the overriding concern. Preservation of whatever voice is possible is secondary; hence, the procedures are not classified as phonosurgery.) One is reinnervation of the paralyzed cord. Despite numerous earlier unsuccessful attempts, recent developments have provided some improvement in cases where the glottal chink was too great for vocal cord injection to be used (Isshiki, 1980; Sato and Ogura, 1978; Tucker, 1977, 1980). The other alternative that has produced dramatically improved voice in the few cases in which it has been used is to adduct the immobile arytenoid by applying tension to sutures, which simulates contraction of the paralyzed lateral cricoarytenoid muscle (Baken and Isshiki, 1977; Isshiki, 1977b; Isshiki, Tanabe, and Sawada, 1978).

Phonosurgery

Two procedures that have made phonosurgery possible are microlaryngeal techniques and laser surgery. With binocular microscope and stroboscopic illumination, the surgeon can make judgments on the basis of the vibratory pattern of the vocal cords. Preservation of mobility of the mucosa of the cords is especially important to prevention of hoarseness. Mucosal suppleness can be detected only when the cords vibrate, so the ability to observe them vibrating during surgery is a significant achievement in preservation of voice. The other procedure, laser surgery, often performed by use of the operating microscope, provides precision, safety, and prompt healing with minimal scarring when applied to small lesions such as nodules, polyps, papilloma, and cysts (Dedo and Izdebski, 1978; Isshiki, 1980).

The need to raise or lower pitch may arise from numerous conditions, not the least of which is transsexual operations. One condition that has been studied is the considerably higher fundamental frequency that follows treatment of asthma with prolonged administration of triamcinolone acetonide (Watkin and Ewanowski, 1979). Several experimental phonosurgical procedures have been used to change pitch. To raise it, cricothyroid approximation with sutures has been used to lengthen and thin the vocal folds. Also, injections of steroids to induce atrophy, and longitudinal incisions of the cords to weaken their resistance to elongation, have been attempted with limited success. To lower pitch, mass has been increased with vocal cord injections, neural supply to the cricothyroid muscle has been sectioned, and thyroplasty has been used in which portions of the thyroid cartilage were removed to shorten the cords. Although success is possible, these are procedures of last resort (Isshiki, 1980).

Other therapies of such lesions have also been reported. Skin grafts were used in 26 adults with papilloma; there was no recurrence in the transplant areas and voice was improved in 21 of the cases (Neumann and Ahmed, 1978). Medication was effective in relief of contact ulcers and granulomas caused by acid regurgitation secondary to hiatal hernia. For the mechanical causes of this functional pathology, which are usually habitual throat clearing and excessive glottal attacks, voice therapy was of value (Ward, Zwitman, Hanson, and Berci, 1980). To avoid the stiff mucosal scar, which impairs vibration, the traditional stripping of polypoid swelling was replaced with a sucking technique. Although this technique preserved the mucosal cord edge, voice improvement was not significantly better than with stripping (Hirano et al., 1981).

Spastic Dysphonia

Since the advent of surgical section of the recurrent laryngeal nerve as a treatment of spastic dysphonia, the procedure has been replicated with considerable success (Barton, 1979; Dedo, 1976, 1977; Levine, Wood, Batza, Rusnov, and Tucker, 1979). Similar improvement has been reported with modifications of the procedure, laryngeal nerve crush (a crushed nerve will regenerate, a sectioned nerve will not) being one example and selective section another. Selective section of the adductor, but not the abductor, branch of the recurrent nerve was attempted to preserve abduction during inspiration while retaining relief from hyperadduction during phonation (Biller, Som, and Lawson, 1979; Carpenter, Henley-Cohn, and Snyder, 1979; Lawrence, 1979).

At a symposium in 1979, these new surgical techniques and their results were discussed. All participants agreed that the cause of spastic dysphonia was unknown but that recurrent nerve section is the best treatment available. The typical result following surgery is relief from strain, but with an accompanying breathy, weak voice. Some reported that by the use of nerve crush, full voice returns when the nerve regenerates. Dedo attempted the same procedure, but spasticity returned along with nerve function. Iwamura described a technique in which selective section was done internally in the larynx instead of by the typical external procedure. Followup speech therapy was critical to his success. It apparently was also essential to Dedo's recurrent section procedure. DeSanto traced the results of sectioning in 27 patients whose voices were free of strain following surgery. Without further therapy, most improved for one month, then stayed the same. A few continued to improve, and 14 became worse (Lawrence, 1979).

The idea of intentionally inducing unilateral laryngeal paralysis, the consequence of recurrent nerve section, is troubling to many laryngologists. Although a case in which a sectioned recurrent nerve did regenerate has been reported, it is a rare exception (Wilson, Oldring, and Mueller, 1980). The predictable outcome is permanent paralysis with cord atrophy within a month. Although spasticity returns in 10 to 15 per cent of patients whose recurrent nerves are sectioned, it apparently results from development of compensatory attempts to achieve loudness (Dedo and Shipp, 1980). In one case, however, it resulted from reinnervation of the sectioned nerve.

The predictable outcome of recurrent nerve section is permanent paralysis. This traumatic outcome, coupled with the lurking suspicion that spastic dysphonia can result from many causes, including functional ones, impels a continuing search for less traumatic treatment (Isshiki, 1980; Lawrence, 1979). Still, it works well with some, and temporary chemical paralysis prior to surgery provides a reasonably accurate preview of the postsurgical voice (Izdebski, Shipp, and Dedo, 1979). Moreover, compensatory surgery is available to enlarge or thin the cord as necessary. Most important, voice therapy, designed along the lines of treatment of unilateral paralysis (which it is, indeed), is vital to optimize postsurgical vocal usage (Dedo and Shipp, 1980).

Summing Up

This review leaves no doubt that voice clinicians as well as voice scientists and laryngologists are searching for measures of laryngeal and vocal performance that are accurate and reliable. With them, communication among clinicians as well as scientists is enhanced. This objective is entirely commendable.

The picture that emerges is that virtually all of the recent advances have been in the detection and treatment of laryngeal pathology. Many of these advances have been accomplished by speech scientists and speech pathologists. They have played a dominant role in the development of noninvasive, acoustic, optic, behavioral, aerodynamic, and electro-myographic methods of assessing laryngeal pathology. The importance of this contribution cannot be diminished.

What is notable by its absence is any attention to the causes or treatment of functional dysphonia. What has been studied are the *consequences* of vocal abuse. Especially useful have been the investigations of vocal fold reactions to stress. However, neither laryngologists nor voice clinicians or scientists have shown any research interest in *causes* of vocal abuse. Neither have they shown much interest in its treatment, 2 case studies of biofeedback effects on hyperfunction out of 170 research reports being the sum total. Spastic dysphonia and laryngeal paralysis have dominated the literature on assessment as well as on treatment since 1976.

A question that arises is what role speech pathologists seek in the management of voice disorders. Judging from this review, the only activity in which their publications show interest is assessment of vocal function, especially in laryngeal pathology. This view is reflected in the most sophisticated scientific work and also in activities of the clinic as reflected in the following argument for the speech pathologists's use of fiberoptics in indirect laryngoscopy: "There is a growing recognition that the role of voice clinician goes beyond that of technician. . . . Such evaluations enable the speech pathologist to ask the laryngologist specific and relevant questions concerning each case, to note the surgeon's success in restoring normal tissue contour, and to interpret the laryngologist's findings. Thus, the speech pathologist becomes a more dynamic, vital, and integral member of the team" (Chapey and Salzberg, 1981, pp. 87–88).

Granting that skill in visualizing the larynx has merit for voice clinicians, it is puzzling how this skill, or other assessment techniques, moves speech pathologists beyond the role of technician and gives them more vital functions on the team of voice specialists. Presumably, each specialist can make a unique contribution to the remediation of a voice problem, but it is not clear how voice clinicians differentiate their contribution from that of the laryngologist. The first professional judgment to be made in managing a voice disorder is the diagnosis of the nature and cause of the laryngeal condition. Physicians can enlist whatever technical input is necessary from such procedures as laryngoscopy, radiography, histology, and acoustic analyses, but by virtue of their training and licensing, they are solely qualified to make a diagnosis. The only role in which the voice clinician can function in the diagnostic process is to provide technical support. This can be an important role, but it does not define a contribution that the speech pathologist is better qualified to make than anyone else.

As for treatment, surgical or medical intervention is, of course, the exclusive province of physicians. One of the most frequent problems they encounter, however, is functional dysphonia, for which neither surgical nor medical relief is appropriate. If the speech pathologist has a unique contribution, it appears to be as a specialist in the nature, causes, and treatment of vocal abuse. Yet, this is the area in which virtually no investigation could be found for this review.

Why have voice scientists and clinicians investigated what are essentially the laryngologist's problems rather than the speech pathologist's? Suspected reasons are dimly visible. One is that descriptions of vocal behavior, abusive as well as normal, have been so nebulous as to preclude definition and measurement. Feedback control of voice is by ear and by feel. Neither sensation lends itself to unambiguous description. The concept of hyperfunction is as close as clinicians have come to a causal explanation of functional dysphonia. It is only a description, however, of the general feeling of tightness and strain in the throat. Because vibratory characteristics, to say nothing of patterns of muscular contraction, of any type of vocal production are unknown (hyperfunctional, abusive, efficient, or whatever), acoustic and physiologic measures of clinical importance have not been developed. Only perceptual descriptions are available, and even when clinicians and scientists are trained in their use, they do not permit acceptably valid and reliable communication. Probably the fundamental deterrent to scientific investigation of causes of functional dysphonia is the lack of accurate measures of clinically relevant vocal behavior.

For this reason, and possibly others, voice therapy has been passed along from generation to generation as a clinical art, complete with idiosyncratic perceptual descriptions dispensed by authorities in their texts. Rarely have any of the multitude of techniques recommended been tested for effectiveness and subjected to the scrutiny of peer review in scientific journals. This does not mean they are useless, but that we have no knowledge of what they accomplish, if they accomplish anything. As matters stand, we have little evidence by which to select with confidence those methods that are appropriate for any particular voice disorder. Until such evidence becomes available, the answer to Paul Moore's question, "Have the major issues in voice disorders been answered by speech science?", will remain "no."

References

Aldes, M. (1981). Hysterical high pitch in an adult female: A case study. *Journal of Communication Disorders, 14,* 59-63.

Aminoff, M., Dedo, H., and Izdebski, K. (1978). Clinical aspects of spasmodic dysphonia. *Journal of Neurology, Neurosurgery, and Psychiatry, 41,* 361-365.

Andrews, A. *Gould-Andrews fiberoptic laryngoscope. (1977). In* V. Lawrence (Ed.), *Transcripts of the Sixth Symposium: Care of the professional voice.* New York: The Voice Foundation.

Aronson, A., and Hartman, D. (1981). Adductor spastic dysphonia as a sign of essential (voice) tremor. *Journal of Speech and Hearing Disorders, 46,* 52-58.

Askenfelt, A., Gauffin, J., Sundberg, J., and Kitzing, J. (1980). Vocal fundamental frequency, as measured from contact microphone and electroglottograph recordings. A comparison of contact microphone and electroglottograph for the measurement of vocal fundamental frequency. *Journal of Speech and Hearing Research, 23,* 258-274.

Bacon, M., and Wolfe, V. (1980). Response to Zwitman. *Journal of Speech and Hearing Disorders, 45,* 568.

Baken, R., (1979). Respiratory mechanisms: Introduction and overview. In V. Lawrence (Ed.), *Transcripts of the Eighth Symposium: Care of the professional voice. Part II. Respiratory and phonatory control mechanisms.* New York: The Voice Foundation

Baken, R., and Cavallo, S. (1979). Chest wall preparation for phonation in untrained speakers. In V. Lawrence (Ed.), *Transcripts of the Eighth Symposium: Care of the professional voice. Part II. Respiratory and Phonatory Control Mechanisms.* New York: The Voice Foundation.

Baken, R., and Cavallo, S. (1981). Prephonatory chest wall posturing. *Folia Phoniatrica, 33,* 193-203.

Baken, R., and Isshiki, N. (1977). Arytenoid displacement by simulated intrinsic muscle contraction. *Folia Phoniatrica, 29,* 206-216.

Barton, R. (1979). Treatment of spastic dysphonia by recurrent laryngeal nerve section. *Laryngoscope, 89,* 244-249.

Biller, H., Som, M., and Lawson, W. (1979). Laryngeal nerve crush for spasmodic dysphonia. *Annals of Otolaryngology, 88,* 531-532.

Blood, G., Mahan, G., and Hyman, M. (1979). Judging personality and appearance from voice disorders. *Journal of Communication Disorders, 12,* 63-67.

Bocchino, J., and Tucker, H. (1978). Recurrent laryngeal nerve pathology in spasmodic dysphonia. *Laryngoscope, 88,* 1274-1280.

Boone, D. (1983). Voice disorders in children and adults. *Seminars in Speech and Language, 4,* 189-286.

Bralley, R., Bull, J., Gore, C., and Edgerton, M. (1978). Evaluation of vocal pitch in male transsexuals. *Journal of Communication Disorders, 11,* 443-449.

Brindle, B., and Morris, H. (1979). Prevalence of voice quality deviations in the normal adult population. *Journal of Communication Disorders, 12,* 439-445.

Brodnitz, F. (1976). Spastic dysphonia. *Annals of Otology, Rhinology, and Laryngology, 85,* 210-214.

Brodnitz, F. (1978). Adolescent voice disorders. In B. Weinberg (Ed.), *Transcripts of the Seventh Symposium: Care of the professional voice. Part II: Life span changes in the human voice.* New York: The Voice Foundation.

Brodnitz, F. (1981). Psychological considerations in vocal rehabilitation. *Journal of Speech and Hearing Disorders, 46,* 21-16

Brown, W., and Feinstein, S. (1977). Speaker sex identification in Wilson's disease. *Folia Phoniatrica, 29,* 240-248.

Cannito, M., and Johnson, J. (1981). Spastic dysphonia: A continuum disorder. *Journal of Communication Disorders, 14,* 215-223.

Carpenter, R., Henley-Cohn, J., and Snyder, G. (1979). Spastic dysphonia: Treatment by selective section of the recurrent laryngeal nerve. *Laryngoscope, 89,* 2000-2003.

Chapey, R., and Salzberg, A. (1981). The speech clinician's use of fiberoptics in indirect laryngoscopy. *Journal of Communication Disorders, 14,* 87-90.

Childers, D., Paige, A., and Moore, G. (1976). Laryngeal vibration patterns: Machine-aided measurements from high-speed film. *Archives of Otolaryngology, 102,* 407-410.

Cohen, D., Shaywitz, B., Caparulo, B., Young, G., and Bowers, M. (1978). Chronic, multiple tics of Gilles de la Tourette's disease. *Archives of General Psychiatry, 35,* 245-250.

Coleman, R. (1976). A comparison of the contributions of two voice quality characteristics to the perception of maleness and femaleness in the voice. *Journal of Speech and Hearing Research, 19,* 168-180.

Coleman, R., Mabis, J., and Hinson, J. (1977). Fundamental frequency-sound pressure level profiles of adult male and female voices. *Journal of Speech and Hearing Research, 20,* 197-204.

Colton, R., and Estill, J. (1976). Perceptual differentiation of voice modes. In V. Lawrence (Ed.), *Transcripts of the Fifth Symposium: Care of the professional voice.* New York: The Voice Foundation.

Colton, R., and Estill, J. (1978). Mechanisms of voice quality variation: Voice modes. In V. Lawrence (Ed.), *Transcripts of the Seventh Symposium: Care of the professional voice. Part I: The scientific papers.* New York: The Voice Foundation.

Colton, R., Estill, J., and Gould, L. (1977). Physiology of voice modes: Vocal tract characteristics. In V. Lawrence (Ed.) *Transcripts of the Sixth Symposium: Care of the professional voice.* New York: The Voice Foundation.

Darby, J., and Hollien, H. (1977). Vocal and speech patterns of depressive patients. *Folia Phoniatrica, 29,* 279-241.

Davis, S. (1976). Computer evaluation of laryngeal pathology based on inverse filtering of speech. *SCRL Monograph, 13,* Santa Barbara, CA: Speech Communication Research Laboratory.

Davis, S. (1979). Acoustic characteristics of normal and pathological voices. In N. Lass (Ed.), *Speech and language: Research and theory.* New York: Academic Press.

Davis, S. (1982). Acoustic characteristics of normal and pathological voices. In Proceedings of the Conference on the Assessment of Vocal Pathology. *ASHA Reports, 11,* 97-115.

Dedo, H. (1976). Recurrent laryngeal nerve section for spastic dysphonia. *Annals of Otology, Rhinology, and Laryngology, 85,* 451-459.

Dedo, H. (1977). Surgical treatment of spastic dysphonia. In V. Lawrence (Ed.), *Transcripts of the Sixth Symposium: Care of the professional voice.* New York: The Voice Foundation.

Dedo, H., and Izdebski, K. (1978). The effects on voice upon removing certain vocal fold lesions. In V. Lawrence (Ed.), *Transcripts of the Seventh Symposium: Care of the professional voice. Part III: Medical/surgical therapy.* New York: The Voice Foundation.

Dedo, H., Izdebski, K., and Townsend, J. (1977). Recurrent laryngeal nerve histopathology in spastic dysphonia. *Annals of Otolaryngology, 86,* 806–812.

Dedo, H., and Shipp, T. (1980). *Spastic dysphonia: A surgical and voice therapy treatment program.* San Diego: College-Hill Press.

Dedo, H., Townsend, J., and Izdebski, K. (1978). Current evidence for the organic etiology of spastic dysphonia. *ORL, 86,* 875–880.

Dordain, M., and Chevrie-Muller, C. (1977). Voice and speech in Wilson's disease. *Folia Phoniatrica, 29,* 217–232.

Drudge, M., and Philips, B. (1976). Shaping behavior in voice therapy. *Journal of Speech and Hearing Disorders, 41,* 398–411.

Eckel, F., and Boone, D. (1981). The s/z ratio as an indicator of laryngeal pathology. *Journal of Speech and Hearing Disorders, 46,* 147–149.

Emanuel, F., and Austin, D. (1981). Identification of normal and abnormally rough vowels by spectral noise level measurements. *Journal of Communication Disorders, 14,* 75–85.

Emanuel, F., and Scarzini, A. (1979). Vocal register effects on vowel spectral noise and roughness: Findings for adult females. *Journal of Communication Disorders, 12,* 263–272.

Emanuel, F., and Scarzini, A. (1980). Vocal register effects on vowel spectral noise and roughness: Findings for adult males. *Journal of Communication Disorders, 13,* 121–131.

Fiedler, I. (1977). Vocal rest. *ASHA, 19,* 307–308.

Forner, L., and Hixon, T. (1977). Respiratory kinematics in profoundly hearing-impaired speakers. *Journal of Speech and Hearing Research, 20,* 373–408.

Fourcin, A. (1982). Laryngographic assessment of phonatory function. In Proceedings of the Conference on the Assessment of Vocal Pathology, *ASHA Reports, 11,* 116–127.

Fritzell, B., Hammarberg, B., and Wedin, L. (1977). Clinical applications of acoustic voice analysis, Part I. *Quarterly Progress and Status Report.* Stockholm: Speech Transmission Laboratory, Royal Institute of Technology.

Fujimura, O. (1982). Fiberoptic observation and measurement of vocal fold movement. In Proceedings of the Conference on the Assessment of Vocal Pathology. *ASHA Reports, 11,* 59–69.

Fujimura, O., Baer, T., and Niimi, S. (1979). A stereo-fiberscope with a magnetic interlens bridge for laryngeal observation. *Journal of the Acoustical Society of America, 65,* 478–480.

Garber, S., and Moller, K. (1979). The effects of feedback filtering on nasalization in normal and hypernasal speakers. *Journal of Speech and Hearing Research, 22,* 321–333.

Garber, S., Siegel, G., and Pick, H. (1980). The effects of feedback filtering on speaker intelligibility. *Journal of Communication Disorders, 13,* 289–294.

Gauffin, J., and Sundberg, J. (1977). Clinical applications of acoustic voice analysis, Part II. *Quarterly Progress and Status Report.* Stockholm: Speech Transmission Laboratory, Royal Institute of Technology.

Golden, G. (1977). Tourette syndrome. *American Journal of Diseases of Children, 131,* 531–534.

Gordon, M., Morton, F., and Simpson, I. (1978). Air flow measurements in diagnosis, assessment, and treatment of mechanical dysphonia. *Folia Phoniatrica, 30,* 166–174.

Gould, W. (1979). Interrelationship between voice and laryngeal mucosal reflexes. In V. Lawrence (Ed.), *Transcripts of the Eighth Symposium: Care of the professional voice. Part II. Respiratory and phonatory control mechanisms.* New York: The Voice Foundation.

Gould, W., Kojima, H., and Lambiase, A. (1979). A technique for stroboscopic examination of the vocal folds using fiberoptics. *Archives of Otolaryngology, 105,* 285.

Guidi, G., Bannister, R., Gibson, W., and Payne, J. (1981). Laryngeal electromyography in multiple system atrophy with autonomic failure. *Journal of Neurology, Neurosurgery and Psychiatry, 44,* 49–53.

Hall, J., and Jerger, J. (1976). Acoustic reflex characteristics in spastic dysphonia. *Archives of Otolaryngology, 102,* 411–415.

Hamlet, S. (1982). Ultra-sound assessment of phonatory function. In Proceedings of the *Conference on the Assessment of Vocal Pathology. ASHA Reports, 11,* 128–140.

Hamlet, S., Geoffrey, V., and Bartlett, D. (1976). Effect of a dental prosthesis on speaker-specific characteristics of voice. *Journal of Speech and Hearing Research, 19,* 639–650.

Hanley, T., Hanson, R., and Miller, A. (1978). Young adult and middle-aged voice. In B. Weinberg (Ed.), *Transcripts of the Seventh Symposium: Care of the professional voice, Part II: Life span changes in the human voice.* New York: The Voice Foundation.

Hanson, W., and Emanuel, F. (1979). Spectral noise and vocal roughness relationships in adults with laryngeal pathology. *Journal of Communication Disorders, 12,* 113–124.

Harris, K. (1982). Electromyography as a technique for laryngeal investigation. In Proceedings of the Conference on the Assessment of Vocal Pathology. *ASHA Reports, 11,* 70–87.

Hartman, D. (1979). The perceptual identity and characteristics of aging in normal male adult speakers. *Journal of Speech and Hearing Disorders, 12,* 53–61.

Hartman, D., and Aronson, A. (1981). Clinical investigations of intermittent breathy dysphonia. *Journal of Speech and Hearing Disorders, 46,* 428–432.

Hasek, C., Singh, S., and Murry, T. (1980). Acoustic attributes of pre-adolescent voices. *Journal of the Acoustical Society of America, 68,* 1262–1265.

Haskell, J., and Baken, R. (1978). Self perception of speaking pitch levels. *Journal of Speech and Hearing Disorders, 43,* 3–8.

Hiki, S., Imazzumi, S., Hirano, M., Matsushita, H., and Kakita, Y. (1976). Acoustical analysis for voice disorders. *Conference Record, 1976 IEEE International Conference on Acoustics, Speech, and Signal Processing.* Rome, NY: Canterbury Press.

Hirano, M., Hiki, S., Imazzumi, S., Kakita, Y., and Matsushita, H. (1978). Acoustical analysis of pathological voice. In V. Lawrence (Ed.), *Transcripts of the Seventh Symposium: Care of the professional voice. Part III: Medical/surgical therapy.* New York: The Voice Foundation.

Hirano, M., Kurita, S., Matsuo, K., and Nagata, K. (1980). Laryngeal tissue reaction to stress. In V. Lawrence and B. Weinberg (Eds.), *Transcripts of the Ninth Symposium: Care of the professional voice. Part I: Physical factors, vocal function and control.* New York: The Voice Foundation.

Hirano, M., Kurita, S., Matsuo, K., and Nagata, K. (1981). Vocal fold polyp and polypoid vocal fold (Reinike's edema). *Journal of Research in Singing, 4,* 33–44.

Hirose, H., Sawashima, M., Ushijima, T., and Kumamoto, Y. (1977). Eunuchoidism: Voice pitch abnormality as an autonomous syndrome. *Folia Phoniatrica, 29,* 261–269.

Hixon, T., Mead, J., and Goldman, M. (1976). Dynamics of the chest wall during speech production: Function of the thorax, rib cage, diaphragm, and abdomen. *Journal of Speech and Hearing Research, 19,* 297–356.

Hollien, H. (1978). Adolescence and voice change. In B. Weinberg (Ed.), *Transcripts of the Seventh Symposium: Care of the professional voice. Part II: Life span changes in the human voice.* New York: The Voice Foundation.

Hollien, H., and Tolhurst, G. (1978). The aging voice. In B. Weinberg (Ed.), *Transcripts of the Seventh Symposium: Care of the professional voice. Part II: Life span changes in the human voice.* New York: The Voice Foundation.

Honjo, I., and Isshiki, M. (1980). Laryngoscopic and voice characteristics of aged persons. *Archives of Otolaryngology, 106,* 149–150.

Horii, Y. (1979). Fundamental frequency perturbation observed in sustained phonation. *Journal of Speech and Hearing Research, 22,* 5–19.

Horii, Y., and Ryan, W. (1981). Fundamental frequency characteristics and perceived age of adult male speakers. *Folia Phoniatrica, 33,* 227–233.

Horii, Y., and Weinberg, B. (1979). Sensory contributions to the control of phonation. In V. Lawrence (Ed.), *Transcripts of the Eighth Symposium: Care of the professional voice. Part II. Respiratory and phonatory control mechanisms.* New York: The Voice Foundation.

Horn, K., and Dedo, H. (1980). Surgical correction of the convex vocal cord after teflon injection. *Laryngoscope, 90,* 281–286.

Ishizaka, K., and Isshiki, N. (1976). Computer simulation of pathological vocal-cord vibration. *Journal of the Acoustical Society of America, 60,* 1193–1198.

Isshiki, N. (1977a). Clinical implication of computer simulation of false voice. In V. Lawrence (Ed.), *Transcripts of the Sixth Symposium: Care of the professional voice.* New York: The Voice Foundation.

Isshiki, N. (1977b). Functional surgery of the larynx. In V. Lawrence (Ed.), *Transcripts of the Sixth Symposium: Care of the professional voice.* New York: The Voice Foundation.

Isshiki, N., (1980). Recent advances in phonosurgery. *Folia Phoniatrica, 32,* 119–154.

Isshiki, N., Tanabe, M., Ishizaka, K., and Broad, C. (1977). Clinical significance of asymmetrical tension of the vocal cords. *Annals of Otology, Rhinology, and Laryngology, 86,* 1–9.

Isshiki, N., Tanabe, M., and Sawada, M. (1978). Arytenoid adduction for unilateral vocal cord paralysis. *Archives of Otolaryngology, 104,* 555–558.

Izdebski, K. (1977). Some data on spastic dysphonia patients. In V. Lawrence (Ed.), *Transcripts of the Sixth Symposium: Care of the professional voice.* New York: The Voice Foundation.

Izdebski, K., and Shipp, T. (1978). Minimal reaction times for phonatory initiation. *Journal of Speech and Hearing Research, 21,* 638–651.

Izdebski, K., Shipp, T., and Dedo, H. (1979). Predicting postoperative voice characteristics of spastic dysphonia patients. *Otolaryngology Head and Neck Surgery, 87,* 428–434.

Janfaza, P. (1978). New magnifying laryngeal and nasalpharyngeal mirrors. *Archives of Otolaryngology, 104,* 740.

Kahane, J. (1980). Age related histological changes in the human male and female laryngeal cartilages: Biological and functional implications. In V. Lawrence and B. Weinberg (Eds.), *Transcripts of the Ninth Symposium: Care of the professional voice. Part I. Physical factors, vocal function and control.* New York: The Voice Foundation.

Kelman, A., Gordon, M., Morton, F., and Simpson, I. (1981). Comparison of methods for assessing vocal function. *Folia Phoniatrica, 33,* 51–65.

Kitajima, K. (1981). Quantitative evaluation of the noise level in the pathologic voice. *Folia Phoniatrica, 33,* 115–124.

Kitajima, K., and Gould, W. (1976). Vocal shimmer in sustained phonation of normal and pathologic voice. *Annals of Otology, Rhinology, and Laryngology, 85,* 377–381.

Koike, K., Takahashi, H., and Calcaterra, T. (1977). Acoustic measures for detecing laryngeal pathology. *Acta Otolaryngologica, 84,* 105–117.

Lawrence, V. (1979). *Spastic dysphonia: State of the art 1979.* New York: The Voice Foundation.

Leonard, R., and Ringel, R. (1979). Vocal shadowing under conditions of normal and altered laryngeal sensation. *Journal of Speech and Hearing Research, 22,* 794–817.

Levine, H., Wood, B., Batza, E., Rusnov, M., and Tucker, H. (1979). Recurrent laryngeal nerve section for spasmodic dysphonia. *Annals of Otology, Rhinology, and Laryngology, 88*, 527–530.

Lewy, R. (1976). Experience with vocal cord injection. *Annals of Otology, Rhinology, and Laryngology, 85*, 440–450.

Lindblom, B., Lubker, J., and Pauli, S. (1977). An acoustic-perceptual method for the quantitative evaluation of hypernasality. *Journal of Speech and Hearing Research, 20*, 485–496.

Lodge, J., and Yarnall, G. (1981). A case study of vocal volume reduction. Journal of Speech and Hearing Disorders, 46, 317–320.

Logemann, J., Fisher, H., Boshes, B., and Blonsky, E. (1978). Frequency and co-occurrence of vocal tract dysfunctions in the speech of a large sample of Parkinson patients. *Journal of Speech and Hearing Disorders, 43*, 47–57.

Ludlow, C. (1982). Research needs for the assessment of phonatory function. In Proceedings of the Conference on the Assessment of Vocal Pathology. *ASHA Reports, 11*, 3–8.

Ludlow, C., and Bassich, C. (1981). The differential diagnosis of syndromes of dysarthria using measures of speech production. In N. Lass (Ed.), *Speech and language: Advances in basic research and practice.* Academic Press.

Ludlow, C., and Hart, M. (1982). Preface. Proceedings of the Conference on the Assessment of Vocal Pathology. *ASHA Reports, 11*, v.

Markel, J., and Gray, A. (1976). *Linear prediction of speech.* New York: Springer-Verlag.

McCall, G. (1977). Studies in spastic dysphonia: Projected research concerned with central neurologic pathologies on laryngeal dysfunction. In V. Lawrence (Ed.), *Transcripts of the Sixth Symposium: Care of the professional voice.* New York: The Voice Foundation.

Merson, R., and Ginsberg, A. (1979). Spasmodic dysphonia: Abductor type. A clinical report of acoustic, aerodynamic, and perceptual characteristics. *Laryngoscope, 89*, 129–139.

Monsen, R. (1982). The use of the reflectionless tube to assess vocal function. In Proceedings of the Conference on the Assessment of Vocal Pathology. *ASHA Reports, 11*, 141–150.

Montgomery, W. (1979). Laryngeal paralysis: Teflon injection. *Annals of Otology, Rhinology, and Laryngology, 88*, 647–657.

Moore, G. (1976). Observations of laryngeal disease, laryngeal behavior and voice. *Annals of Otology, Rhinology, and Laryngology, 85*, 553–565.

Moore, P. (1977). Have the major issues in voice disorders been answered by research in speech science? A 50-year retrospective. *Journal of Speech and Hearing Disorders, 42*, 152–160.

Murry, T. (1978). Speaking fundamental frequency characteristics associated with voice pathologies. *Journal of Speech and Hearing Disorders, 43*, 374–379.

Murry, T., and Doherty, E. (1980). Selected acoustic characteristics of pathologic and normal speakers. *Journal of Speech and Hearing Research, 23*, 361–369.

Murry, T., and Singh, S. (1980). Multidimensional analysis of male and female voices. *Journal of the Acoustical Society of America, 68*, 1294–1300.

Murry, T., Singh, S., and Sargent, M. (1977). Multidimensional classification of abnormal voice qualities. *The Journal of the Acoustical Society of America, 61*, 1630–1635.

Mysak, E. (1977). Systems approach to voice disorders. In V. Lawrence (Ed.), *Transcripts of the Sixth Symposium: Care of the professional voice.* New York: The Voice Foundation.

Neumann, O., and Ahmed, M. (1978). A new approach to the treatment of laryngeal papilloma in adults. *Journal of Laryngology and Otology, 92*, 325–331.

Nichols, A. (1979). Jitter and shimmer related to vocal roughness. *Journal of Speech and Hearing Research, 22*, 670–671.

Parnes, S., Lavarato, A., and Myers, E. (1978). Study of spastic dysphonia using fiberoptic laryngoscopy. *Annals of Otology, Rhinology, and Laryngology, 87,* 322-326.

Pederson, M. (1977). Electroglottography compared with synchronized stroboscopy in normal persons. *Folia Phoniatrica, 29,* 191-199.

Perkins, W. (1978). Mechanisms of vocal abuse. In B. Weinberg (Ed.), *Transcripts of the Seventh Symposium: Care of the professional voice. Part II: Life span changes in the human voice.* New York: The Voice Foundation.

Portnoy, R. (1979). Hyperkinetic dysarthria as an early indicator of impending tardive dyskinesia. *Journal of Speech and Hearing Disorders, 44,* 214-219.

Proctor, D. (1979). Breath, the power source for the voice. In V. Lawrence (Ed.), *Transcripts of the Eighth Symposium: Care of the professional voice. Part II. Respiratory and phonatory control mechanisms.* New York: The Voice Foundation.

Prosek, R., Montgomery, A., Walden, B., and Schwartz, D. (1978). EMG biofeedback in the treatment of hyperfunctional voice disorders. *Journal of Speech and Hearing Disorders, 43,* 282-294.

Putnam, A. (1981). Caution. . .peanuts may be harmful to your clients' health. *Journal of Speech and Hearing Disorders, 46,* 220-221.

Ravits, J., Aronson, A., DeSanto, L., and Dyck, P. (1979). No morphometric abnormality of recurrent laryngeal nerve in spastic dysphonia. *Neurology, 29,* 1376-1382.

Reed, C. (1980). Voice therapy: A need for research. *Journal of Speech and Hearing Disorders, 45,* 157-169.

Reich, A., and Lerman, J. (1978). Teflon laryngoplasty: An acoustical and perceptual case study. *Journal of Speech and Hearing Research, 43,* 496-505.

Rothenberg, M. (1977). Measurement of air flow in speech. *Journal of Speech and Hearing Research, 20,* 155-176.

Rothenberg, M. (1982). Some relations between glottal air flow and vocal fold contact area. In Proceedings of the Conference on the Assessment of Vocal Pathology. *ASHA Reports, 11,* 88-96.

Saito, S., Fukuda, H., Kitahara, S., and Kokawa, N. (1978). Stroboscopic observation of vocal fold vibration with fiberoptics. *Folia Phoniatrica, 30,* 241-244.

Sato, F., and Ogura, J. (1978). Functional restoration for recurrent laryngeal nerve paralysis: an experimental study. *Laryngoscope, 88,* 855-871.

Sawashima, M. (1976). Fiberoptic observation of the larynx and other speech organs. In M. Sawashima and F. Cooper, (Eds.), *Dynamic aspects of speech production.* Tokyo: University of Tokyo Press.

Schiff, M. (1977). Medical management of acute laryngitis. In V. Lawrence (Ed.), *Transcripts of the Sixth Symposium: Care of the professional voice.* New York: The Voice Foundation.

Schiff, M., and Gould, W. (1978). Hormones and their influence on the performer's voice. In V. Lawrence (Ed.), *Transcripts of the Seventh Symposium: Care of the professional voice. Part III: Medical/surgical therapy.* New York: The Voice Foundation.

Schultz-Coulon, H., Battmer, R., and Reichers, H. (1979). The 3-kHz formant-a criterion for the evaluation of vocal efficiency? I. The untrained normal voice. II. The trained singing voice. *Folia Phoniatrica, 31,* 291-313.

Sharbrough, F., Stockard, J., and Aronson, A. (1978). Brainstem auditory evoked responses in spastic dysphonia. *Transactions of American Neurology, 103,* 198-201.

Shipp, T., Mueller, P., and Zwitman, D. (1980). Intermittent abductory dysphonia. *Journal of Speech and Hearing Disorders, 45,* 283.

Silverman, E., and Zimmer, C. (1978). Effect of the menstrual cycle on voice quality. *Archives of Otolaryngology, 104,* 7-10.

Singh, S., and Murry, T. (1978). Multidimensional classification of normal voice qualities. *Journal of the Acoustical Society of America, 64,* 81–87.

Smitheran, J., and Hixon, T. (1981). A clinical method for estimating laryngeal airway resistance during vowel production. *Journal of Speech and Hearing Disorders, 46,* 138–146.

Sorenson, D., Horii, Y., and Leonard, R. (1980). Effects of laryngeal topical anesthesia on voice fundamental frequency perturbation. *Journal of Speech and Hearing Research, 23,* 274–283.

Stemple, J., Weiler, E., Whitehead, W., and Komray, R. (1980). Electromyographic biofeedback training with patients exhibiting a hyperfunctional voice disorder. *Laryngoscope, 90,* 471–476.

Stevens, K., and Hirano, M. (Eds.) (1980). *Vocal fold physiology.* Tokyo: University of Tokyo Press.

Stevens, K., Nickersen, R., Boothroyd, A., and Rollins, A. (1976). Assessment of nasalization in the speech of deaf children. *Journal of Speech and Hearing Research, 19,* 393–416.

Stoicheff, M. (1981). Speaking fundamental frequency characteristics of nonsmoking female adults. *Journal of Speech and Hearing Research, 24,* 437–441.

Sweeting, P. (1979). Voice onset time and vowel duration in the normal aged population: Implications for phonatory control. In V. Lawrence (Ed.), *Transcripts of the Eighth Symposium: Care of the professional voice. Part II. Respiratory and phonatory control mechanisms.* New York: The Voice Foundation.

Teany, D. (1980). The electroglottograph as a clinical tool for the observation and analysis of vocal fold vibration. In V. Lawrence and B. Weinberg (Eds.), *Transcripts of the Ninth Symposium: Care of the professional voice. Part II: Vocal stress—Medical diagnosis/treatment.* New York: The Voice Foundation.

Todt, E., and Howell, R. (1980). Vocal cues as indices of schizophrenia. *Journal of Speech and Hearing Research, 23,* 517–526.

Tucker, H. (1977). Reinnervation of the unilaterally paralyzed larynx. *Annals of Otology, Rhinology, and Laryngology, 86,* 789–794.

Tucker, H. (1980). Vocal cord paralysis—etiology and management. *Laryngoscope, 90,* 585–590.

Tuomi, S., and Fisher, J. (1979). Characteristics of simulated sexy voice. *Folia Phoniatrica, 31,* 242–249.

Ward, P., Hanafee, W., Mancuso, A., Shallit, J., and Berci, G. (1979). Evaluation of computerized tomography, cinelaryngoscopy, and laryngography in determining the extent of laryngeal disease. *Annals of Otology, Rhinology, and Laryngology, 88,* 454–462.

Ward, P., Zwitman, D., Hanson, D., and Berci, G. (1980). Contact ulcers and granulomas of the larynx: New insights into their etiology as a basis for more rational treatment. *Otolaryngology and Head and Neck Surgery, 88,* 262–269.

Watkin, K., and Ewanowski, S. (1979). The effects of triamcinolone acetonide on the voice. *Journal of Speech and Hearing Research, 22,* 446–455.

Weinberg, G. (1978). Evolution/involution of the human voice summary with an introduction to age-associated voice disorders. In B. Weinberg (Ed.), *Transcripts of the Seventh Symposium: Care of the professional voice. Part II: Life span changes in the human voice.* New York: The Voice Foundation.

Wendler, J., Doherty, E., and Hollien, H. (1980). Voice classification by means of long-term speech spectra. *Folia Phoniatrica, 32,* 51–60.

Whitehead, R., and Lieberth, A. (1979). Spectrographic and perceptual features of vocal tension/harshness in hearing impaired adults. *Journal of Communication Disorders, 12,* 83–92.

Wilder, C. (1980). Vocal aging. In B. Weinberg (Ed.), *Transcripts of the Seventh Symposium: Care of the professional voice. Part II: Life span changes in the human voice.* New York: The Voice Foundation.

Wilder, C. (1979). Chest wall preparation for phonation in untrained speakers. In V. Lawrence (Ed.), *Transcripts of the Eighth Symposium: Care of the professional voice. Part II. Respiratory and phonatory control mechanisms.* New York: The Voice Foundation.

Williams A., Hanson, D., and Calne, D. (1979). Vocal cord paralysis in the Shy-Drager syndrome. *Journal of Neurosurgery and Psychiatry, 42,* 151–153.

Wilson, F., Oldring, D., and Mueller, K. (1980). Recurrent laryngeal nerve dissection: A case report involving return of spastic dysphonia after initial surgery. *Journal of Speech and Hearing Disorders, 45,* 112–118.

Wirz, S., Subtelny, J., and Whitehead, R. (1981). Perceptual and spectrographic study of tense voice in normal hearing and deaf subjects. *Folia Phoniatrica, 33,* 23–36.

Wolfe, V., and Bacon, M. (1976). Spectrographic comparison of two types of spastic dysphonia. *Journal of Speech and Hearing Disorders, 41,* 325–332.

Wyke, B. (1979). Neurological aspects of phonatory control systems in the larynx: A review of current concepts. In V. Lawrence (Ed.), *Transcripts of the Eighth Symposium: Care of the professional voice. Part II. Respiratory and phonatory control mechanisms.* New York: The Voice Foundation.

Zwitman, D. (1979). Bilateral cord dysfunctions: Abductor type spastic dysphonia. *Journal of Speech and Hearing Disorders, 44,* 373–378.

Bernd Weinberg

Speech Rehabilitation of the Laryngectomized Patient: Advances and Issues

An obvious and primary postsurgical rehabilitation objective for laryngectomized patients is the restoration of oral communication. Until recently, speech rehabilitation of laryngectomized patients has been accomplished chiefly with the time honored methods of esophageal speech or through the use of artificial larynges.

Unfortunately, major advances or improvements have not been made in the design of artificial larynges, and only slight improvements have been achieved in treatment for persons who use commercially available, artificial larynges. Although it is true that many laryngectomized patients are able to produce highly intelligible and functionally serviceable speech using these devices, studies dealing with important aspects of their use are scarce. The vocal output of users of artificial larynges is characterized by a non-normal, mechanical, or electronic quality with limited variation in f_o (pitch) or intensity (loudness). Given the state of technology, efforts should be made to design more efficient voicing sources to provide laryngectomized patients with more normal sounding vocal attributes.

The use of speech and vocal synthesis in the commercial sector has proliferated at an accelerating rate. For example, witness the extent to which people interact with large numbers of "voices" in a vast array of toys, business transactions, and so on. Undoubtedly, the quality of "voices" used in these commercial applications will improve to the extent that many people may not realize that they are interacting with nonhuman devices. It would be a sad commentary on our social system and values if, a decade from now, people interacted with a host of natural sounding, synthetic sources, while human talkers deprived of a normal voicing source, yet richly

This chapter was prepared, in part, through support from an NIH Grant (Linguistic Aspects of Speech After Laryngectomy).

endowed with normal linguistic performance and competence, continued to produce speech characterized by significant liability or absence of natural quality.

In recent years, a steady flow of information has resulted in improved understanding of esophageal speech production (see Weinberg, 1980, for a review). Although basic attributes of esophageal speech production are now more clearly understood, significant numbers of laryngectomized patients fail to develop functionally serviceable speech despite having been exposed to adequate therapy. Hence, advances in assessment and therapy for persons seeking to use esophageal speech produced on a conventional basis as a primary form of oral communication have been limited. The recent observations that some alaryngeal talkers are able to realize prosodic features and linguistic contrasts does represent an important advance in current understanding (Gandour and Weinberg, 1982, 1983; Gandour, Weinberg, and Garzione, 1983; Gandour, Weinberg, and Kosowski, 1983; McHenry, Reich, and Minifie, 1982; Scarpino and Weinberg, 1981). These recent observations have important clinical and basic scientific implications. For example, it now appears inappropriate to assume that talkers using some major forms of alaryngeal speech are unable to approximate normal linguistic-prosodic patterns (e.g., stress, intonation, juncture). The observation that some alaryngeal talkers are able to realize prosodic patterns suggests that such patients have the capacity to produce speech at proficiency levels exceeding those typically searched for by professional workers in the field.

Undoubtedly, the more striking advances in the field of speech rehabilitation for laryngectomized patients are those associated with techniques currently being advocated for surgical-prosthetic management. The major focus of this chapter will be to review the advances made and to examine some questions occasioned by these developments.

Surgical Prosthetic Approaches to Speech Rehabilitation

The more significant advances in the field of speech rehabilitation for laryngectomized patients are those related to surgical-prosthetic management. In the past decade, surgical-prosthetic approaches to speech restoration for laryngectomized patients have proliferated. Reviews of this recent proliferation are available in other sources (Shedd and Weinberg, 1980; Weinberg, 1980). The most significant contemporary advances in this field of endeavor relate to techniques and procedures advocated and used in conjunction with tracheoesophageal puncture (TEP) technique.

In 1980, Singer and Blom formally described an endoscopic technique for restoration after total laryngectomy. A comparable approach has been described by Panje (1981).

Technique Outcomes: Speech Results

The tracheoesophageal puncture approach to speech restoration for laryngectomized patients clearly represents a significant advance. At the time of this writing, carefully controlled studies have not been completed that enable us to specify the speech characteristics or levels of speech proficiency attained by patients undergoing this procedure. Informal descriptions of these attributes and levels have been published. For example, Singer and Blom (1980) initially described a two year, 60 patient experience with this method. Of the 60 patients, 54 (90 per cent) achieved what Singer and Blom refer to as "fluent voices and were satisfied with their communication ability" (p. 531). These patients achieved "satisfactory communication. . .regarded as intelligible and fluent to listeners" (p. 531). Conversely, the remaining six speakers (10 per cent) were classified as "nonfluent speakers or voice failures" (p. 531). In a more recent report, Singer, Blom, and Haymaker (1981) summarized their 40 month experience with 129 patients. Again using informal description, they indicated that "successful acquisition of voice occurred in 113 of the 129 patients (88%)" (p. 498).

The results of rehabilitation using the Singer-Blom method have also been described by others. For example, Wood, Rusnov, Tucker, and Levine (1981) recently summarized the results of experiences at the Cleveland Clinic with 30 total laryngectomy patients who underwent tracheoesophageal puncture. This group of clinicians categorized rehabilitation as successful "if the post-TEP [tracheoesophageal puncture] voice was judged better than the pre-TEP mode of communication by the patient, one or more family members, and the speech pathologist" (p. 493). On this basis 28 patients (93 per cent) were classified as successes, while two were regarded as failures.

Additional, independent descriptions of experiences with tracheoesophageal puncture have been offered by Wetmore, Johns, and Baker (1981). Their experiences reflect a multi-institutional (University of Virginia, University of Arkansas, University of Michigan) review of the Singer-Blom procedures completed on 63 patients. In this series, five patients (8 per cent) were regarded as "voice failures" (p. 675). These patients were unable to produce "fluent tracheoesophageal speech despite adequate clinical trial" (p. 675). Finally, Donegan, Gluckman, and Singh (1981) report a one year experience with 23 patients. From a speech perspective, these authors classified the rehabilitation outcome as successful "if the patient attained fluent and intelligible speech" (p. 495). Donegan and colleagues indicated that "only three of our failures were due to inability to produce fluent speech" (p. 496).

The Singer-Blom method is a *speech* restoration technique. Hence, a criterion by which the outcome of this method must be evaluated is efficiency and proficiency of speech production. Published accounts of outcome using speech criteria certainly indicate that the Singer-Blom approach represents an important advance. It appears that many patients undergoing this form of treatment develop speech that is characterized as "fluent and intelligible." Moreover, a significant number of them develop speech quickly, and many of them were previously unable to produce fluent or intelligible discourse using esophageal speech produced on a conventional basis, which suggests a significant advance in treatment regimens available to laryngectomized patients.

The problems associated with evaluation of treatment outcomes are numerous and are not unique to this field of endeavor. One major problem associated with the interpretation of published reviews of speech outcomes of this method relates to the failure to carefully specify speech and vocal outcomes. Methodologies are available that permit valid, reliable specification of speech and vocal attributes and proficiency levels. It is regrettable, therefore, that more specific, replicable forms of speech assessment were not undertaken on the patient series reviewed to date.

A second problem relates to an apparent failure to clearly distinguish the differences between the terms *voice* and *speech*. The Singer-Blom technique or similar techniques (e.g., Panje, 1981) represent *speech* restoration approaches. Virtually all the titles of papers dealing with these approaches (see References) identify the voice restoration aspects of the procedure. Although human voice production represents an essential part of the speech act, this multidimensional part of speech production is but one piece of an even larger, multidimensional communication process. Hence, future specification of outcomes for these methods might well define outcomes in terms of both vocal and speech communication efficiency, attributes, and proficiency.

In this context, there is the related issue of ascertaining and distinguishing influences of surgical-prosthetic intervention from those occasioned by associated behavioral or nonsurgical influences. To put it simply, the ultimate success or level of proficiency achieved by patients undergoing puncture-type methods of treatment is not solely dependent upon the surgical procedure or upon surgical-prosthetic interactions. Rather, outcomes are dictated by complex interactions among surgical, prosthetic, behavioral, and nonmedical therapeutic influences. The interactions among these influences merit more careful study and appreciation.

Finally, there is the important investigative advantage afforded by the development of puncture-type methods. These methods offer minimally invasive entry for monitoring key respiratory influences on speech and vocal production. The advent of puncture-type methods opens the door for the completion of important investigations aimed at enriching the current understanding of mechanisms underlying the regulation of essential aspects of alaryngeal voice (e.g., vocal fundamental frequency and intensity) and speech (e.g., prosody) production.

Nonspeech Outcomes

The tracheal puncture approach necessitates the creation of a connection between the trachea and the esophagus, the placement of a one-way valve into this connection, and the use of this surgical-prosthetic, pulmonary-digestive link to energize esophageal speech production. Successful culmination and continued use of this process of producing alaryngeal speech depends upon factors other than speech and voice limitation or failure.

Donegan and colleagues (1981) have addressed this issue succinctly. They state:

> A successful outcome was considered achieved if the patient attained fluent and intelligible speech *and* was willing and able to maintain the prosthesis unaided. Inability to achieve these goals was regarded as a failure. . . . We have included willingness and ability to maintain the prosthesis in the criteria for success. We feel this is necessary in that reporting results as fluency of speech only is not a true indication of how well these patients achieve vocal rehabilitation. Of the 23 patients in this series, 13 were deemed successful (56%), and there were 10 failures. Seven of the failures were due to the patients' inability to care for the prosthesis in a home setting despite having achieved fluent speech. The problems encountered included difficulty manipulating the prosthesis into position after cleaning and difficulty maintaining the prosthesis in position, and a few simply left the prosthesis out for prolonged periods allowing the fistula to close (pp. 495–496).

Donegan and colleagues (1981) acknowledge that the Singer-Blom technique "represents a dramatic advance in neoglottic surgery" (pp.

495–496), but they identified several nonspeech factors that may limit success or contribute to failure. In their series of 23 patients, 13 (56 per cent) were classified successful, whereas 10 were regarded as failures. Among the failure group, 7 failed because of factors unrelated to speech or vocal failure.

These patients were unable to care for the prosthesis despite having "fluent speech." Similar observations have been made by others. For example, Wetmore, Johns, and Baker (1981) noted that although 56 (89 per cent) of the 63 patients in their series developed speech, only 45 (71 per cent) have continued to use this modality. The main reasons for discontinuing use of this speech technique were inadvertent dislodgement of the prosthesis with subsequent closure of the TEP tract or patient noncompliance. Two patients in this series failed to use tracheoesophageal speech because of problems with aspiration. Wetmore, Johns, and Baker noted that "a minor degree of aspiration developed in five additional patients; thus aspiration was treated by cauterizing the TEP tract" (p. 674).

Wood and colleagues (1981) also commented about nonspeech factors that may limit the outcome of the tracheoesophageal puncture technique. In this series from the Cleveland Clinic, two patients required repeat punture for complete stenosis of the TEP tract following displacement of the prosthesis due to incorrect taping. One patient developed cervical cellulitis when the TEP was mistakenly placed too high in the trachea. One patient developed acute, symptomatic aspiration. This was resolved by use of "aggressive silver nitrate ($AGNO_3$) cautery of the fistula tract and reduction in the size of the stent" (p. 494).

Finally, there is the Singer, Blom, and Haymaker (1981) series of 129 patients. In this group, nine patients were unable to maintain the voice prosthesis in spite of speech acquisition. Singer and colleagues commented thus:

> Routine maintenance involves daily stoma hygiene, cleaning the prosthesis, and replacement with prescribed skin adhesives. Patients previously unable or unwilling to care for their tracheostomas were limited in their ability to handle the voice prosthesis. Visual problems, generalized infirmity, or disinterest precluded satisfactory adaptation to this method of vocal rehabilitation. Three patients with exceptionally low tracheostomas failed to use the prosthesis over time. In this group of failures, the prosthesis was removed and the puncture spontaneously closed in 12 to 24 hours. (p. 498)

These authors also commented

> Approximately 20% of the patients will experience occasional extrusion of the voice prosthesis, requiring replacement after dilatation of the tracheoesophageal puncture, and additional supervision of their stoma care regimen. Two of the patients accidently aspirated the voice prosthesis without consequence. The prostheses were retrieved with a flexible fiberoptic bronchoscope.

> Problems relating to the tracheoesophageal puncture procedure have remained minimal. One patient developed cervical subcutaneous emphysema after he inadvertently removed the stent. There have been four marked inflammatory reactions around the stoma in irradiated patients. This problem required the use of a silicone tracheal vent tube or laryngectomy tube until the reaction resolved.
>
> The most important group of problems is related to tracheal reflux. Although salivary contamination of the trachea can be a serious problem, no patients experienced aspiration pneumonia. Two patients had intractable leakage around the voice prosthesis and required a second procedure to close the puncture. Intermittent aspiration was reported by three patients three months to one year postoperatively. They were treated by repeated applications of electrocautery to the tracheoesophageal puncture to enhance stenosis. Nine others experienced minimal leakage which has been eliminated by a single application of electrocautery. (p. 498)

As indicated earlier, the problems associated with evaluation of the outcomes of surgical-prosthetic techniques are numerous and are not unique to this field of endeavor. It is apparent that, at a minimum, outcome must be evaluated in terms of both speech and nonspeech criteria. In recognition of this reality, Wood and colleagues (1981) offer patient criteria that they believe "largely determine the success or failure of this particular surgical procedure" (p. 492). Their criteria include adequate motivation and reasonable patient expectations; capacity of patients to learn; adequate manual dexterity and vision; adequate stomal size, maturity, and architecture; adequate physical health; and positive air insufflation test results.

Identification of these criteria highlights the fact that all patient series reviewed here embody sampling bias. Namely, patients considered for tracheoesophageal puncture are evaluated and are selected (or rejected) to undergo surgery and prosthetic management on some bases. This bias may exert a significant influence upon the outcome and makes comparative evaluation difficult to achieve.

Panje (1981) has addressed this problem. He indicated that "patient selection can significantly bias the end results to the point of misleading the observer to the effectiveness of the treatment or technique. Just as the attainment of esophageal speech is markedly influenced by patient anatomy, interest, intelligence and habits, so might these factors influence the success of prosthetic vocal rehabilitation" (pp. 118–119).

It is apparent that the tracheoesophageal puncture approach to speech restoration for laryngectomized patients represents a dramatic advance. Although this is true, the method is characterized by some relative liabilities. Thus, as is the case for esophageal speech and speech powered by artificial larynges, surgical-prosthetic assisted forms of speech are also not characterized by functional universality.

Esophageal Air Insufflation Testing

As part of the preoperative evaluation protocol used to assess a patient's candidacy for tracheoesophageal puncture, Singer and Blom (1980) have advocated routine, preoperative esophageal air insufflation testing. They stated

> The voice failures can be predicted preoperatively by the air insufflation test. The test is critical to successful patient selection. Limitation to airflow by this test correlated well with lack of initial voice fluency and the need for reeducation of the pharyngoesophageal muscles for voice production. To date there have been both false positives and negatives, but in limited numbers. We use the test as a relative guide to patient selection, and estimation of time involved for postsurgical rehabilitation. (p. 532)

Blom, Singer, and Haymaker (1982) commented that "in spite of a patent tracheoesophageal puncture and functional voice prosthesis, 16 patients failed to develop satisfactory speech. All were assessed by preoperative insufflation of the esophagus with voice failure correlating with complete cessation of airflow during speech or brisk esophageal distention. The 16 patients were predicted by insufflation" (p. 576). Thirteen additional patients exhibited limitation to airflow or lack of fluency, but they eventually acquired satisfactory tracheoesophageal speech.

These observations raise questions about the validity of the assertion that "voice failures can be predicted preoperatively by the air insufflation test (Singer and Blom, 1980)" (p. 552). Indeed, Donegan and colleagues (1981) have written that all patients in their series "were assessed preoperatively by the surgeon and the speech therapist. The air insufflation test was used in all patients in an attempt to predict the outcome of the procedure, but was found to be of limited value in predicting success or failure of the tracheoesophageal puncture" (p. 495).

Wood and colleagues (1981) relate that they "continue to use the air insufflation test for prognostic purposes despite a number of false-positive results" (p. 492). Panje (1981) has commented that "the air insufflation test has been advocated by some as a determinant of those patients who will do best with tracheoesophageal sound production. . . . However, both patients who failed to develop speech with Voice Button placement had had sound production on the administration of air into the esophagus via a small catheter, which seems to demonstrate the capricious nature of the test and the variability among patients" (p. 119).

It is clear that all "failures" may not be predicted preoperatively by air insufflation testing, although this form of testing does identify a subgroup of patients who cannot achieve airflow across the pharyngoesophagus during catheter-induced air insufflation and esophageal distention. Important questions are raised by the advocacy of esophageal air insufflation testing and the notation of variable responses to this form of assessment of pharyngoesophageal function. For example, what is the rate of prediction offered by preoperative air insufflation testing? Precisely what is predicted (e.g., ability to produce voice, sustain voice, use voice appropriately as part of the speech act)? In addition, specific details are needed on just how the air insufflation tests are conducted since there is a need to determine whether procedural variables used in the administration of this test influence outcome of test results.

Selective Myotomy for Voice Restoration

Speech and surgical specialists have often expressed the view that improvement in the rate and efficiency of voice reacquisition with esophageal phonation might occur if consideration was given to surgically altering the anatomy and physiology of the pharyngoesophageal (PE) segment. Singer and Blom (1981) have raised some provocative issues about the consequences of surgical alteration of the PE segment by proposing selective myotomy for voice restoration after total laryngectomy.

The observations of Singer and Blom (1981) have shown that some laryngectomized patients cannot achieve airflow across the pharyngoesophagus in association with insufflation of air into the esophagus, that parapharyngeal nerve block enabled these patients to temporarily achieve airflow across the pharyngoesophagus, and that selective, unilateral myotomy of the pharyngeal constrictors enabled these patients to achieve airflow across the pharyngoesophagus, produce voice, and achieve speech fluency. These observations emphasize the role played by altered function of the PE segment in influencing reacquisition of voice and speech following total laryngectomy, and they highlight the potential contribution surgical alteration of the PE segment may make to the voice and speech reacquisition process.

The observations made by Singer and Blom (1981) also raise some provocative questions. For example, they concluded that "airflow induced spasm of the cricopharyngeus and pharyngeal constrictor muscles seems to be an important factor in failures of more patients to acquire fluent speech" (p. 673). There appears to be little question about the fact that insufflation of air into the esophagus, coupled with esophageal distention, is associated with PE segment closure that is air tight in some laryngectomized patients. Although this is true, important issues related to this fact remain unclear.

For example, it is not known whether this form of air tight closure is induced by air flow. If flow cannot be passed across the pharyngoesophagus, such an explanation is doubtful. Other questions include determining the mechanisms underlying the production of air tight closure of the upper esophageal sphincter. Precisely how can or does the "air-filled and distended esophagus stimulate cricopharyngeal and pharyngeal constrictor muscle contraction?" (Singer and Blom, 1980 p. 673). How is this air tight response mediated? Is this response related to the method of surgical closure? Further consideration of the response of the normal PE sphincter to esophageal distention and air insufflation testing of this type is needed. Should this air tight response properly be regarded as spasm? If so, what triggers this spasmodic behavior? There are additional questions about whether this response is abnormal and why only a relatively small percentage of sampled laryngectomized patients exhibit this response. What is special about this group or subsample? Finally, there is a need to clarify the rationale for routinely performing selective, unilateral myotomy when only some patients exhibit this "problem" and when the mechanism underlying this response remains unclear.

Prothesis Design and Function

Puncture-type methods of speech restoration require the use of a one-way, tracheoesophageal puncture prosthesis. This prosthesis serves three primary functions: it maintains patency within the TEP; it permits air shunting between the trachea and the esophagus, and it functions as a one-way valve to prevent reflux of esophageal contents into the airway.

From a design perspective, tracheoesophageal puncture prostheses should be minimally resistive to airflow through them from the trachea to the esophagus, and maximally resistive to the flow of material entering the device from the esophagus. Minimal airway resistance of these prostheses to air flowing through them would be expected to enhance the efficiency of esophageal voice and speech production, while maximal resistance to flow reversal would attest to the competency of the device as a one-way valve.

At the time of this writing, two one-way valved prostheses have been developed for use in puncture-type approaches to speech rehabilitation. Singer and Blom (1980) have developed a duckbill prosthesis, while Panje (1981) has developed a four-flutter or flap, valved prosthesis. Both of these devices have apparently been developed on an empirical basis.

The opposition Singer-Blom prostheses offer to the flow of air through them has been calculated (Moon, Sullivan, and Weinberg, 1983; Weinberg, Horii, Blom, and Singer, 1982). The results of these works reveal that the overall airway resistance Singer-Blom prostheses offer to air flow is about 125 cm H_2O/LPS and that the overall resistance of these prostheses remains relatively constant as a function of increasing flow rate (0.05 to 0.2 LPS range). Average airway resistance for Singer-Blom prostheses is in excess of three times that offered by the normal human larynx during vowel production.

Weinberg (1982) has recently also calculated the resistance offered by prostheses developed by Panje (1981). The results of this work revealed that the opposition of Panje devices to airflow through them is more substantial. Resistance values for individual Voice Button prostheses ranged from 285 to 440 cm H_2O/LPS. These resistance values are higher than those calculated for opposition offered by esophageal voicing sources, suggesting that patients using Panje Voice Buttons may have to work more to overcome prosthetic opposition of air flow than they would to excite and sustain vibration of their voicing source. This situation would be expected to result in impoverished and inefficient production of voice and speech and it highlights the potential for modification in prosthesis design (Weinberg, 1982).

Further analysis of prosthesis function is expected to provide fundamental data critical to enlarging understanding of voice and speech production used by patients who speak with puncture methods, and to provide information essential to the future development of prosthesis modification. Tracheoesophageal puncture prostheses have apparently been developed on an empirical basis. Thus, basic studies aimed at defining the essential attributes of valve function are needed. These attributes can be studied using modeling approaches and computer-assisted design methods. It is expected that the results of such basic work will lead to enlightened understanding of prosthesis function and suggest potential modifications likely to enhance vocal and speech efficiency or valve competency. Basic studies of valve competency to combat flow reversal have apparently not yet been conducted.

As part of the general approach to developing a puncture-type method of speech restoration, Blom, Singer, and Haymaker (1982) have also developed a lightweight, two-way respiratory valve. This device permits two-way airflow at the stoma for vegetative breathing and converts to a one-way inspiratory valve with increased airflow. In the latter circumstance, air is diverted into the esophagus, eliminating the need for finger occlusion of the stoma. This device would be expected to represent a significant advance. The development of this device has also proceeded on an empirical basis, and basic research is needed before firm conclusions regarding its usefulness, function, or redesign can be made.

Speech Pathology: Roles and Contributions

The recent development of tracheoesophageal puncture-type approaches to speech restoration in no way diminishes the role of speech pathologists in the rehabilitation process offered to laryngectomized patients. Although these advances alter some of the functions speech pathologists play in this process, the contributions made by speech pathologists to rehabilitation continue to play a critical role.

As indicated earlier, puncture-type approaches to restoration represent speech reacquisition methods. The ultimate success of these methods depends primarily upon interactions, yet unspecified, among surgical, prosthetic, behavioral, and nonmedical therapeutic factors. The process of speech rehabilitation for patients using puncture-type methods involves far more than merely "restoring the voice or getting the voice back."

This writer is concerned about the apparently limited therapeutic management offered to patients undergoing tracheoesophageal puncture-type, surgical-prosthetic forms of treatment. The published reports reviewed in earlier sections of this chapter deal solely with the role of speech pathologists in patient selection, prosthesis fitting, and *voice* restoration. There is ample evidence to support this writer's view that the process of speech production is profoundly altered in patients who undergo these procedures. Restoration of speech involves much more than merely getting the voice back. Hence, speech pathologists must, at a minimum, routinely manage rate and temporal characteristics, enhance articulation and intelligibility attributes, eliminate extraneous behaviors and noises, and perfect realization of prosody and linguistic contrasts in patients who have undergone surgical-prosthetic treatment (see Weinberg, 1983, for details).

Speech pathologists who fail to address these facets of speech communication management may fail to fully comprehend speech restoration for laryngectomized patients and may seriously underestimate the contributions therapy can provide. This writer firmly believes that speech management dealing merely with prosthesis fitting and early voice return seriously undercuts the ultimate levels of speech proficiency that patients undergoing forms of surgical-prosthetic treatment might reasonably be expected to achieve. A comprehensive program of therapy must be offered and delivered to such patients (see Weinberg, 1983, for details). This program need not be long, however.

Clearly, therapy devoted solely to prosthesis fitting and voice return will lead to serious undercutting. On the other hand, efficient therapy devoted to patient selection, prosthesis fitting, voice return, *and* aspects of speech communication common to other forms of normal and alaryngeal speech would be expected to increase the prevalence of highly proficient alaryngeal speakers at the conclusion of speech rehabilitation. Further, speech pathologists can also contribute substantially to the improved development of sensitive and reliable outcome measures, so lacking in current reports. Failure to address speech rehabilitation in a comprehensive form seems likely to result in compromise and in diminished ultimate levels of speech attainment.

Conclusion

In this offering, some contemporary advances in the field of speech rehabilitation for laryngectomized patients have been reviewed. The more significant advances in this field are those related to surgical-prosthetic management. In addition to identifying advances in this field of endeavor, several important issues and questions raised by these advances have also been identified. It is clear that the field of speech rehabilitation for laryngectomized patients continues to be an exciting one. Advances have been made in both basic understanding and clinical application. It is hoped that in addition to providing information, the material discussed here will serve to interest others in the diverse problems associated with speech restoration following total laryngectomy, stimulate additional participation in this exciting arena of basic and applied research and rehabilitation, and highlight the need for continued interdisciplinary cooperation so essential to the improved quality of future rehabilitation of laryngectomized patients.

References

Blom, E. D., Singer, M. I., and Haymaker, R. C. (1982). Tracheostoma valve for postlaryngectomy voice rehabilitation. *Annals of Otology, Rhinology, and Laryngology, 91,* 576–578.

Donegan, J. O., Gluckman, J. L., and Singh, J. (1981). Limitations of the Blom-Singer technique for voice restoration. *Annals of Otology, Rhinology, and Laryngology, 90,* 495-497.

Gandour, J., and Weinberg, B. (1983). Perception of intonational contrasts in alaryngeal speech. *Journal of Speech and Hearing Research, 26,* 142-148.

Gandour, J., and Weinberg, B. (1982). Perception of contrastive stress in alaryngeal speech. *Journal of Phonetics, 10,* 347-350.

Gandour, J., Weinberg, B., and Garzione, B. (1983). Perception of lexical stresss in alaryngeal speech. *Journal of Speech and Hearing Research, 26,* 418-424.

Gandour, J., Weinberg, B., and Kosowsky, A. (1983). Perception of syntactic stress in alaryngeal speech. *Language and Speech, 25,* 299-304.

McHenry, M., Reich, A., and Minifie, F. (1982). Acoustical characteristics of intended syllabic stress in excellent esophageal speakers. *Journal of Speech and Hearing Research, 25,* 564-753.

Moon, J.B., Sullivan, J., and Weinberg, B. (1983). Evaluations of Blom-Singer tracheoesophageal puncture prostheses. *Journal of Speech and Hearing Research, 26,* 459-464.

Panje, W. R. (1981). Prosthetic vocal rehabilitation following laryngectomy. *Annals of Otology, Rhinology, and Larynogology, 90,* 116-120.

Scarpino, J., and Weinberg, B. (1981). Junctural contrasts in esophageal and normal speech. *Journal of Speech and Hearing Research, 46,* 120-126.

Shedd, D. P., and Weinberg, B. (1980). *Surgical-prosthetic approaches to speech rehabilitation.* Boston: G. K. Hall.

Singer, M. I., and Blom, E. D. (1980). An endoscopic technique for restoration of voice after laryngectomy. *Annals of Otology, Rhinology and Laryngology, 89,* 529-533.

Singer, M. I., and Blom, E. D. (1981). Selective myotomy for voice restoration after total laryngectomy. *Archives of Otolaryngology, 107,* 670-673.

Singer, M. I., Blom, E. D., and Haymaker, R. C. (1981). Further experience with voice restoration after total laryngectomy. *Annals of Otology, Rhinology, and Laryngology, 90,* 498-502.

Weinberg, B. (1980). *Readings in speech following total laryngectomy.* Baltimore: University Park Press.

Weinberg, B. (1982). Airway resistance of the Voice Button. *Archives of Otolaryngology, 108,* 498-500.

Weinberg, B. (1983). Speech and voice restoration following total laryngectomy. In W. H. Perkins (Ed.), *Current Therapy in Communication Disorders* (Vol. 4). New York: Thieme-Stratton.

Weinberg, B., Horii, Y., Blom, E., and Singer, M. (1982). Airway resistance during esophageal phonation. *Journal of Speech and Hearing Disorders, 47,* 194-199.

Wetmore, S. J., Johns, M. E., and Baker, S. H. (1981). The Singer-Blom voice restoration procedure. *Archives of Otolaryngology, 107,* 674-676.

Wood, B. G., Rusnov, M. G., Tucker, H. M., and Levine, H. L. (1981). Tracheoesophageal puncture for alaryngeal voice restoration. *Annals of Otology, Rhinology, and Laryngology, 90,* 492-494.

Thomas S. Johnson

Voice Disorders: The Measurement of Clinical Progress

Evaluation and treatment of voice disorders has had a long and curious development, with its roots primarily in vocal music and with some input from early medical science. Its strong connection with the musical and theatrical arts has greatly affected the contemporary practices of voice therapy (Brodnitz, 1971; Moore, 1977). Concurrent, sometimes controversial philosophies grew from those advocating a more symptomatic approach to vocal behavior and those who held that voice disturbance was reflective of personality disturbance. Hence, a wide variety of therapy approaches emerged, some of which have seemed foreign and strange to practicing speech-language pathologists. Symptomatic treatments were generally adapted from general speech, vocal music and theater, while psychiatric medicine contributed the personality theories. The belief held by a number of early writers that the voice is the "mirror of the emotions" and that it plays an important role in revealing information about the fears, anxieties, and emotional struggles of the individual (Brodnitz, 1971; Moses, 1954) has contributed significantly to the development of current evaluative and therapeutic processes for the management of voice problems.

Moore (1977), in his excellent and thought-provoking treatise on the major issues in voice disorders, reviewed 50 years of research and practice and made comparisons between then contemporary textbook writings in voice disorders and several classic publications of earlier years. His discussion indicated the following:

> Four features stand out in the recent publications: (1) voice disorders are described in greater detail and reflect an increased understanding of basic problems, but the problems are the same; (2) more attention is paid to specific vocal disorders such as laryngectomy; (3) there is a greater variety of therapeutic techniques; and (4) the major emphases in therapy remain as before: training in breath control (where indicated), relaxation and reduction of laryngeal

tension, training in listening, articulatory adjustments, and special techniques. These are applied to deviations in pitch, intensity, and quality (including the resonance disorders). Obviously, not much change in the basic clinical practices appears to have occurred over the years. (p. 156)

It is striking that the same conclusion could be drawn five years later from a review of more recent titles in the field. In completing such a review, the following conclusions were drawn: greater detail is available; still more attention is given special problems (especially spastic dysphonia); a somewhat increased variety of therapeutic techniques (though not greatly different) are described; and the major emphases remain essentially the same with the addition of some behavioral approaches and programmed formats. Current evaluation and therapeutic practices have been comprehensively described in recent years by Aronson (1980), Boone (1977), Cooper and Cooper (1977), Filter (1982b), Greene (1980), Murry (1982), and Wilson (1979). Contemporary voice therapy packaged kits have also been developed by Wilson and Rice (1977), Polow and Kaplan (1979), and Boone (1981). No attempt in this chapter will be made to review fundamental therapy approaches, as they are already available in these publications, and it is not the author's desire to add to the glut of restated, redescribed, widely known therapeutics.

The big disappointment with all of these publications is a significant lack of research data applied to validate the described clinical methodologies. Research on the clinical effectiveness of voice therapy procedures is regrettably sparse (Johnson, 1974; Michel and Wendahl, 1971; Moore, 1977; Reed, 1980). The overwhelming number of evaluative and treatment procedures described by the authors named have not been subjected to rigorous clinical research and contain few reports of precise data substantiating their effectiveness.

In recent years the field of communication disorders has experienced a demand for increased accountability. Such clinical accountability requires the development and use of objective measurement procedures (Reed, 1980). In the area of voice disorders, there has been a lack of such measurement techniques, and hence the therapeutic management of voice problems has had few accountability data available to it (Johnson, 1974; Lubker, 1979; Michel and Wendahl, 1971; Reed, 1980). Voice evaluation and measurement have long been practical problems for the voice clinician. Hence, the evaluative capability of clinicians has been limited chiefly to descriptive procedures, using subjective adjectives or adverbs, which have attempted to describe the acoustic perceptions of the voice. Such terms as hoarse, harsh, rough, sandy, breathy, and metallic, as well as many others (Laver, 1968; Perkins, 1971), have been used to describe the acoustic product of pathologic laryngeal physiology. Other descriptive systems have been proposed, but they suffer a lack of intra- and interexaminer reliability and are not sensitive to progressive change during voice management. Wilson's (1972) system offers descriptive information that is helpful in relating in a general way to the physiology of the laryngeal structures; however, agreement between judges is, in the author's experience, difficult to obtain, even using Wilson's prescribed training (Wilson and Rice, 1977). Additionally, other physiologic measures have simply not been precise enough or sensitive enough to the changes desired and those of most interest to the voice clinician. Further, a lack of standardization of evaluation procedures and a concurrent scarcity of normative data on vocal parameters also contribute to the imprecision of currently applied procedures to voice evaluation and measurement. An additional contributing force to this measurement dilemma faced by the voice clinician has been the historical reliance by the clinician on medical evaluation, chiefly that of indirect laryngoscopy. Even from a medical perspective, indirect laryngoscopy is at best an imprecise procedure, particularly for the purpose of reporting progress or improvement towards remediation of a laryngeal problem. The fleeting moment of visual observation interpreted through the subjective perception of the medical practitioner is not a very satisfactory procedure for monitoring laryngeal change over time. Recent advances in flexible fiberoptic systems hold promise in this regard; however, at present this technology is available only in larger medical facilities. The voice clinician then must look elsewhere to find a more satisfactory technique for achieving clinical accountability in voice therapy. The most exciting recent advances in the area of voice disorders, in the author's view, are investigations of the parameters of vocal functioning and of establishing ways and means of measuring them. For the first time, the profession is at the threshold of being able to validate years of clinical practice in voice disorders with efficient data collection techniques. These recent advances are the focus of the chapter to follow.

Voice as Behavior

The aforementioned notion that the voice is somehow the "mirror of the emotions" or the "barometer of the soul" seems to have created an aura about the voice that implies it is somehow different or in some ways mysterious and hence requires the use of mysterious procedures to correct it. One of the most important recent advances in the management of voice problems is the consideration that voice is behavior and is subject to what we know about the modification of, and change in, other types of behavior. In short, voice behaviors are classes of behaviors, which can be shaped and modified by use of principles of applied behavior analysis (Costello, 1977; Johnson, 1974; Miller, 1980; Mowrer, 1982).

In recent years, applied behavior analysis technology seems to have profoundly affected in all areas of educational intervention, including communicative disorders (Mowrer, 1982; Perkins, 1971). This movement has also had an impact on the management of voice disorders. Nell (1968) was the first writer who viewed the potential applicability of this evolving technology to voice problems. Hunsaker (1970) reported data on its applicability with a single subject, and other authors subsequently reported data indicating that vocal behaviors and behaviors associated with voice were manipulable response classes (Beck, 1976; Beste, 1971; Drudge and Phillips, 1976; Johnson, 1985; Parrish, 1972; Pierce, 1974; Rothwell, 1974; Smee, 1974). This finding allowed a rationale to develop, bringing the measurement of specific vocal behaviors into the context of "vocal hyperfunction" as originally proposed by Froeschels (1952) and augmented by Brodnitz (1971). In short, if vocal hyperfunction (i.e., vocal misuse and abuse) is responsible for a large majority of voice problems, as is argued by Brodnitz (1971), Perkins (1971), Boone (1977), Greene (1980), and others, then these abusive behaviors should be able to be accurately pinpointed, recorded, and subjected to experimental manipulation such as that advocated in the applied behavior analysis strategy.

Modification of Hyperfunctional Vocal Behavior

Most vocal problems in both children and adults have been primarily related to use, misuse, and abuse of the vocal mechanisms (hyperfunctional behaviors). The concept of vocal hyperfunction includes any behaviors that result in excessive muscular tension in the vocal tract. This excessive tension may come from any of the variety of vocal behaviors that induce tension into the vocal tract at any level. The laryngeal mechanism is largely a muscular system and functions in the same way as other muscular systems in the body in relation to hyperfunctional usage. To use the analogy of running and the muscular system of the legs, an individual could abuse or misuse the leg muscles in several ways: by running normally too long, or running too hard, or running in an abnormal fashion, putting too much stress on one leg or the other. Each of these activities could lead to a hyperfunctioning leg muscle system. The analogy holds true also for use of the vocal musculature. Additionally, prolonged hyperfunctioning of a muscle system fatigues the muscles to the degree that they finally become unable to produce a normal degree of muscle tone, and the condition of hypofunction sets in. As hypofunction increases, the muscular effort must also increase, adding more hyperfunctional usage to the system and fatiguing the muscles even more as the condition increases in severity in a vicious spiral. In laryngeal functioning, prolonged hyperfunctional use of the voice fatigues the vocal musculature to the degree that the muscles are unable to produce a normal degree of muscle tone, and a degree of hypofunction sets in. This hypofunction causes the vocal musculature to work even harder at producing appropriate phonation and in doing so adds more hyperfunction behavior, thus further fatiguing the musculature. More effort is added, and the condition worsens. This combined process of hyper- and hypofunctioning is an interesting phenomenon in the larynx, especially because the hyperfunctional behavior can also lead to the formation of organic-structural changes (such as nodules, thickened cords, and polyps) on the margins of the vocal folds. This further complicates the process and consequently affects the level of effort required for vocal fold functioning because of the increased mass of the folds generated by the presence of these vocal pathologies.

Several additional factors may interplay in this process of hyperfunction to produce a "hyperfunctional voice problem." These factors are susceptibility factors and relate to predisposing characteristics of the person with hyperfunctional vocal behavior. The combination of these susceptibility factors with hyperfunctional behavior (i.e., use, abuse, misuse) of the laryngeal mechanism can result in the formation of laryngeal pathologies and in the presence of vocal symptoms. Susceptibility factors include histologic differences in the basic cellular makeup of the individual laryngeal mechanisms, the presence of an invading bacterial or viral organism, the physical conditioning history of the individual's laryngeal mechanism, and other such factors that could increase an individual's susceptibility to the development of laryngeal problems. Figure 6–1 presents hypothetical examples of the combination of susceptibility factors and hyperfunctional behaviors in a general hyperfunctional equation relationship.

In Example 1, the individual has not conditioned his or her voice properly and then overuses the voice in singing, resulting in laryngeal inflammation and vocal disturbance. This example is representative of frequently seen cases in which voice majors who come to college with little vocal training or experience throw themselves completely into vocal

Susceptibility Factor		Hyperfunctional Behavioral Use, Abuse, Misuse	_yields_ →	Vocal Pathology Physiologic Change in Laryngeal Structure	_yields_ →	Vocal Symptoms
1. Lack of conditioning	+	Overuse of singing voice		Laryngeal inflammation and swelling		Vocal roughness and breathiness
2. Tissue susceptibility	+	Loud talking, yelling, screaming		Vocal nodules		Vocal roughness and breathiness
3. Presence of bacterial organism (developing upper respiratory infection)	+	Vocal usage at some level		Vocal polyp		Vocal roughness and breathiness
4. Irritated laryngeal mucosa due to tobacco or alcohol irritation	+	Hard attack phonation		Contact ulcer		Pain on voicing; Some roughness and glottal fry phonation

Figure 6–1. The hyperfunctional equation with four hypothetical examples of how it works.

performance and practice with little thought about the need to condition the vocal musculature. This situation is analogous to the nonrunner who decides to run in a marathon race with little though beforehand about a long and intensive program of physical conditioning.

Example 2 represents the frequently seen school child who seems not to yell or scream any more than his or her peers, but whose larynx has developed a set of vocal nodules. Histologic differences may be present in the individual larynx, and it is my (as yet unproved) hypothesis that such differences may ultimately account for one child developing nodules while another does not, when their levels of usage are strikingly similar.

Examples 3 and 4 provide additional hypothetical examples of how the hyperfunctional cycle can work to cause vocal problems.

The modification of hyperfunctional problems necessitates interrupting the hyperfunctional cycle and reducing the amount of potential hyperfunctional behavior, which, along with the susceptibility factors, has produced the vocal pathology. The clinician must remain aware and conscious of the susceptibility factors in planning and carrying out appropriate therapy procedures and, in some instances (e.g., lack of conditioning), build components into the total therapeutic plan to handle such factors.

The technology of applied behavior analysis suggests that behaviors be precisely defined so that they can be observed and counted readily. In attempting to interrupt the hyperfunctional cycle and reduce the amount of potential hyperfunctional behavior, the clinician needs to pinpoint carefully which of the client's behaviors is primarily responsible for the voice problem. Once the contributory behavior or behaviors are pinpointed precisely, and a baseline of those behaviors is obtained over a selected time, then the clinician must select a strategy to reduce the rate of occurrence of those behaviors. Respective pinpointed hyperfunction-producing behaviors associated with these problems include behaviors involved in phonation, respiration, and resonation. Specific examples include yelling, loud talking, coughing, throat clearing, strained phonation, hard attack phonation, pharyngeal tightness, inappropriate tongue carriage, restricted mouth opening, speaking on expiratory reserve air, and inadequate breath support.

In 1976, the author published a data-based program, the Vocal Abuse Reduction Program (VARP), based on seven years of supportive single-subject design research (Johnson, 1985). This program used a self-control management strategy from applied behavior analysis with a sensitive data collection procedure in the form of daily behavioral charting to produce a replicable, valid therapeutic procedure for affecting the reduction of hyperfunctional voice behaviors. The VARP also gave the clinician the opportunity to monitor progress continuously over the course of therapy by viewing the daily behavior records of vocally abusive behaviors. The VARP is a clinical management program that pinpoints vocal abuse and misuse behaviors for each client with such behaviors resulting in the formation of laryngeal pathologies (i.e., nodules, polyps, contact ulcers, and thickened cords), systematically and precisely reduces the pinpointed vocal abuse behaviors in specific high probability situations or time periods, and reduces or eliminates the abuse-generated laryngeal pathology and makes possible the establishment of normal voice quality. The VARP program is described in detail by Johnson (1984, 1985).

Figure 6–2 presents an example of the daily behavior chart obtained when the VARP program is used. The record indicates the rate of occurrence of abuse and misuse behaviors in selected time periods, which are gradually increased in length as control is obtained in each situation. The data themselves represent data collected by the client, who counts his or her own abuse and misuse behaviors with the assistance of a wrist counter.

This chart presents "yells" and "loud talk" behaviors occurring during specified situations over a 12 week management program with VARP. During the first 2 weeks, the behaviors were self monitored only during the morning recess period at school (20 minutes of monitored time). During weeks 3 and 4, the monitoring time was extended to include afternoon recess (totaling 35 minutes of monitored time). The magnitude of change during these first 4 weeks ranges from 1.7 behaviors per minute (or 34 yells–loud talks in 20 minutes) on the first data day to 0 yells–loud talk behaviors in 35 minutes on the final day of the fourth week. The rate of yelling and loud talking behavior may be seen to decelerate markedly during this period as a consequence of self-monitoring of those behaviors. In the fifth week, the monitored time is further extended to include a 35 minute lunch period (total monitored time, 70 minutes), with 3 days at the end of the week of no recorded yells or loud talk behaviors. In weeks 6 and 7, the time period is again extended to include after school until 6:00 PM, bringing the total monitored time to 220 minutes. Again, 3 days of no yells or loud talk behaviors appear at the end of week 7. The monitored time was then extended to include the entire day during weeks 8 through 12, with resulting low rates of yells and loud talk behaviors, including several full days of no self-observed loud talk and yell behaviors. On the third day of the eighth week, the client was seen by the laryngologist, who reported no remnant of the moderately large bilateral nodules. Rechecks by the examining laryngologist on the dates indicated at the top of the chart revealed no reoccurrence of the nodules. It is also interesting that good vocal quality did not return completely until the tenth week.

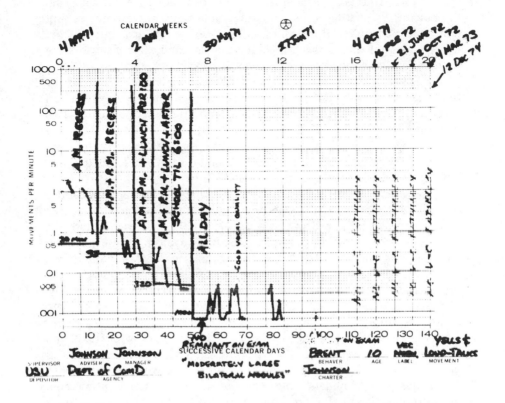

Figure 6-2. Example of daily behavioral chart of VARP intervention.

Intervention with VARP has been systematically studied in a series of similar single subject research projects at Utah State University. These successful systematic replications of VARP intervention have demonstrated the effectiveness and predictability of the VARP procedure.

Certainly, there are other methods for reducing hyperfunctional voice behaviors effectively; however, no reported procedures have the data base and predictive capability of the VARP procedure. For example, Wilson and Rice (1977) and Boone (1981) both describe abuse reduction programs but present no clinical data to support the procedures' effectiveness.

The recent interest in behavioral approaches to the study of the voice management process suggests some basic management principles.

1. Voice and voice disorders are not mysterious problems requiring unusual procedures to manage them effectively. Fundamental clinical processes are the same as those appropriate for communication disorders.

2. Voice and its associated features are behaviors. Hence, voice and the parameters relating to its physiology and pathology are not exempt from the principles of learning. Most voice problems spring from hyperfunctional action of the vocal mechanism, and these behaviors can be modified by applied behavior analysis procedures.

3. Some voice disorders have primarily an organic basis. Even so, the therapeutic and evaluative procedures used to facilitate a better voice can take advantage of what is known about the modification of behavior. This fact has been largely neglected in the voice therapy literature.

4. The utilization of careful stimulus programming, control, and precise consequence management is as facilitative in voice therapy as it is in other areas of speech-language pathology.

These principles suggest that there are many potential applications of applied behavior analysis technology to voice problems, whether hyperfunctional in nature or of an organic origin. At present, there is a great lack of material in the voice literature regarding these potential applications (Mowrer, 1982). In his review of instructional programs in the field, Mowrer laments the lack of such developed programs for the treatment of voice disorders. Additionally, Johnson (1974), Moore (1977), and Reed (1980) have all addressed the serious lack of research data addressing fundamental therapeutic management questions. The recent report by Drudge and Phillips (1976) is cited by both Mowrer (1982) and Reed (1980) as an example of the type of research that is seriously needed in voice therapeutics. Their 31 step program was designed to accomplish four major goals: elimination of vocal abuse, easy initiation of phonation, increased clear phonation time, and increased loudness without increase in laryngeal tension. Their program was criterion referenced, and they presented data on three subjects who successfully completed the program. Other behavioral programmed approaches to the management of voice problems have been studied by Smee (1974), Coachbuilder (1972), Greiner (1973), and Vance (1976). Briefly, these studies used the extended length and complexity of utterance therapy strategy (Ryan, 1974) to program for pitch disorders and quality problems. Data presented in these studies indicated the effectiveness of the programmed approach to the problems studied.

Clinical Assessment of Laryngeal Functioning

Reed (1980) indicated that the most fundamental need for voice research was to replace vague terms with measurable observations sensitive enough to allow the results to be interpreted by other investigators. Johnson (1974) echoed that concern and proposed a strategy and philosophy for what was termed a "functional voice evaluation format." Recently, Filter (1982b) reviewed much of the work completed in the voice evaluation area over the past several years. He described current case history procedures, screening procedures, perceptual description formats, associated behaviors, and additional data. Michel and Wendahl's (1971) landmark discussion concerning correlates of voice production suggested 12 parameters to be considered for investigation in the determination of pertinent measurable voice parameters. These 12 correlates form a basic set of measurable features of the voice, which, when investigated fully, could constitute a measurement battery to assess the adequacy of laryngeal or vocal functioning. Michel and Wendahl proposed "to present voice as a multidimensional series of measurable events, implying that a single phonation can be assessed in many different ways" (p. 267). The 12 correlates they proposed were vital capacity of the lungs, maximum duration of controlled sustained blowing, modal frequency level, maximum frequency ranges, maximum duration of sustained phonation, volume-velocity flow during phonation, glottal waveform, sound pressure level, jitter of the vocal signal, shimmer of the vocal signal, effort level (vocal), and transfer function of the vocal tract. Reed (1980), in discussing Michel and Wendahl's correlates, suggested six parameters that could serve as initial efforts to address the major concepts of voice quality: volume-velocity airflow, jitter, shimmer, effort level, electomyographic studies, and rise-fall time.

Since the 1960s, data from voice science laboratories have emerged signaling interest in the development of objective measurement parameters of the voice. An exhaustive review of this work is outside the scope of this chapter; however, much excellent laboratory work has yielded important information regarding the measurement of laryngeal function. Central to this work is that of Koike and colleagues (Hirano, Koike, and von Leden, 1968; Koike, 1968; Koike and Hirano, 1968; Koike, Hirano, and von Leden, 1967) Isshiki and associates (Isshiki, 1964, 1965; Isshiki, Okamura, and Morimoto, 1967; Isshiki, Okamura, Tanabe, and Morimoto, 1969; Isshiki and von Leden, 1964; Isshiki, Yanagihara, and Morimoto, 1966), Iwata and von Leden (1970), and Yanagihara and associates (Yanagihara and Koike, 1967; Yanagihara, Koike, and von Leden, 1966; Yanagihara and von Leden, 1967).

In another landmark article, Beckett (1971) suggested that several specific measures derived from the voice science laboratory could be clinically applied to patients with respirometric or voice disturbances. Additionally, he indicated that the respirometer was an effective, reliable means of obtaining those data clinically without the extensive instrumentation utilized in the voice science laboratory. Beckett proposed seven aerodynamic measures that could have diagnostic or clinical value. They included one-stage vital capacity (VC), phonation volume (PV), phonation time (PT), maximum predicted phonation time (MPT), mean flow rate (MFR), vocal velocity index (VVI), and phonation time–maximum predicted phonation time (PT/MPT).

Johnson and associates began in 1970 to apply such data gathering techniques on an experimental basis to clinical populations of voice disordered individuals, as well as to subjects without voice disorders. Initially, they conducted a series of studies that made use of precision measurement in combination with behavior modification techniques in persons with voice disorders (Beck, 1976; Hunsaker, 1970; Parrish, 1972; Pierce, 1974; Rothwell, 1974; Vance, 1976). These investigations culminated with the publishing of the Vocal Abuse Reduction Program as an effective data-based clinical voice management program (see earlier discussion). The cited thesis studies were single-subject design investigations of the effectiveness of the Vocal Abuse Reduction Program. With the establishment of this program as an effective, replicable, predictable clinical procedure, it became possible to utilize several experimental measurement procedures, as suggested by the work of Michel and Wendahl (1971) and that of Beckett (1971), for monitoring data as voice therapy progressed during VARP. Two investigators, Thompson (1976) and Smee (1974), demonstrated the feasibility of using experimental measurement procedures for monitoring client progress during voice management. This was done by tracking the measures over the course of treatment with several individual subjects, VARP being used as the intervention procedure.

Although the feasibility for the therapeutic tracking use of the procedure was demonstrated, the amount of information known about unimpaired performance on the individual measurements was minimal, and guideposts for interpreting the meaning of changes in those measurements were limited. Hence, a series of subsequent investigations was begun to study the use of these measures on the performance of varying age groups of children and adults without voice disorders (Child, 1979; Inglis, 1977; Lee, 1978; Taylor, 1980; Williams, 1977; Williams, 1979). The results of these investigations of subjects without voice disorders were summarized by Hammond (1981). The measurements included in the battery selected for study were vital capacity (VC), phonation volume (PV), phonation time (PT), phonation time ratio (PTR), maximum flow rate (MFR), phonation quotient (PQ), vocal velocity index (VVI), and phonation volume–vital capacity ratio (PV/VC). As indicated previously, these measures were originally derived from the voice science literature and were adapted for use as suggested by the work of Beckett (1971) and Michel and Wendahl (1971).

Table 6-1 provides a brief operational summary of the measurements and an abbreviation key used in the data tables that follow. The results of these investigations provide some preliminary data regarding the performance of children and adults with normal voices on the measurement battery.

Investigations with Children

Williams (1977) examined 60 elementary school children, 30 of whom were sixth graders, with a mean age of 11 years 9 months, a mean height of 58.3 inches, and a mean weight of 88 pounds. The remaining 30 children were third graders, with a mean age of 8 years 9 months, a mean height of 51.4 inches, and a mean weight of 63.5 pounds.

Respirometric and phonatory measures of vital capacity, phonation time, and phonation volume were obtained. From these three measurements, the other computational measures selected for the battery (Table 6-1) were obtained.

The children were sent singly to the testing room. On arrival, they were weighed and measured for height. They were then instructed to stand up straight and were given instructions on how to exhale into the respirometer to obtain vital capacity measurements, and then how to phonate /u/ into the respirometer for the measurement of phonation volume. Following vital capacity and phonation volume measurements, each child then sustained /a/ at conversational intensity for as long as possible, while being timed with a stopwatch for the phonation time measure. Three trails for each measure were obtained, and the maximum performance on each measure was used in the results.

Tables 6-2 and 6-3 summarize the results of the Williams study by age groups.

Child (1979) investigated 40 fourth grade children with a mean age of 10 years 2 months, a mean height of 55.0 inches, and a mean weight of 76.7 pounds. None of the subjects had had any discernible previous voice problems, nor did they have colds or any similar type of irritations that might have affected their vocal production ability. The same measurement battery used by Williams (1977) was also used in this study. In addition, Child was interested in the number of trials as a variable in the phonation time parameter.

Table 6-1. Descriptive Summary of the Measurements Used in the Investigations

Name	Definition	How Measured	Data Provide/Indicate
Vital capacity (VC)	Maximum volume of air that can be exhaled following maximum inhalation. Expressed in cubic centimeters.	Person exhales maximally into a respirometer after maximum inhalation.	Estimate of amount of air available for production of phonation
Phonation volume (PV)	Maximum volume of air that is used for maximally sustained phonation. Expressed in cubic centimeters.	Person phonates /a/ or /u/ into a respirometer after a maximum inhalation.	Actual phonated volume of air.
Phonation time (PT)	Maximum time an individual can sustain phonation after taking a minimum inhalation. Expressed in seconds.	Person is timed while phonating /a/ after maximal inhalation.	Durational performance measure for sustaining a vowel.
Phonation quotient (PQ)	Ratio of vital capacity and phonation time, providing an estimate of potential air flow. Expressed in cubic centimeters per second.	Computed measurement. Vital capacity/phonation time. $\frac{VC}{PT} = PQ$	Potential air flow; indirect air flow measurement.
Maximum predicted phonation time (MPPT)	Maximum phonation time of an individual as predicted by vital capacity. Expressed in seconds.	Computed measurement, vital capacity/110 $\times$ 0.67 male subjects; Vital capacity/110 $\times$ 0.59 female subjects (normal adults). (From Yanagihara and von Leden [1967])	Predicted phonation time as suggested by vital capacity.

Table 6-1 (continued).

Name	Definition	How Measured	Data Provide/Indicate
Phonation time ratio (PTR)	Ratio between phonation time and predicted phonation time. Expressed as a decimal value.	Computed measurement. Phonation time/maximum predicted phonation time. $\dfrac{PT}{MPPT}$	Indication of the relationship between predicted and actual phonation time.
Maximum flow rate (MFR)	Rate of air flow during phonation. Expressed in cubic centimeters of air per second.	Computed measurement. Phonation volume/phonation time. $\dfrac{PV}{PT}$	Indirect air flow measured using actual phonated air as measured by phonation volume and actual duration performance.
Vocal velocity index (VVI)	Ratio between maximum air flow and vital capacity during sustained phonation.	Computed measurement. Maximum flow rate/vital capacity. $\dfrac{MFR}{VC}$ (liters) (From Koike and Hirano [1968])	Hypotensive and hypertensive modes of phonation.
Phonation volume vital capacity ratio (PVVR)	Ratio between vital capacity and phonation time. Expressed as a decimal value.	Computed measurement. Phonation volume/vital capacity. $\dfrac{PV}{VC}$	Air consumption ratio between actual phonated air available for phonation and that actually used.

Table 6-2. Adjusted Means and Standard Deviations for the Third Grade and by Sex (Williams, 1977)

Measures	Total (n = 30)		Girls (n = 15)		Boys (n = 15)	
	Mean	SD	Mean	SD	Mean	SD
Height (in.)	51.4	2.8	52.4	3.0	50.3	2.1
Weight (lb.)	63.5	11.0	66.3	11.4	50.8	10.2
VC (cc)	1690.0	340.2	1620.4	329.4	1760.0	347.5
PV (cc)	1541.7	339.4	1480.0	322.8	1603.3	355.2
PT (s)	13.4	.4	13.6	5.2	13.3	2.5
PQ (cc/s)	132.3	41.8	133.3	46.5	131.2	38.2
MPT (s)	10.7	3.1	10.4	3.4	11.0	2.6
PTR (ratio)	1.3	.5	1.4	.6	1.3	.4
MFR (cc/s)	120.6	40.2	120.8	42.8	120.3	38.9
VVI (ratio)	72.6	23.8	76.5	29.3	68.7	16.7

Table 6-3. Adjusted Means and Standard Deviations for the Sixth Grade and by Sex (Williams, 1977)

Measures	Total (n = 30)		Girls (n = 15)		Boys (n = 15)	
	Mean	SD	Mean	SD	Mean	SD
Height (in.)	58.5	3.2	58.6	2.7	58.6	3.7
Weight (lb.)	88.0	17.4	85.3	15.1	90.5	19.4
VC (cc)	2289.6	352.1	2235.7	347.0	2340.0	361.6
PV (cc)	2096.5	356.5	2039.3	328.3	2150.0	384.5
PT (s)	16.9	4.5	15.8	4.1	17.8	4.7
PQ (cc/s)	145.1	.4	148.8	38.6	141.7	47.8
MPT (s)	14.0	2.8	13.3	2.0	14.8	3.2
PTR (ratio)	1.2	.3	1.2	.3	1.3	.4
MFR (cc/s)	134.2	44.1	137.0	41.1	131.5	48.0
VVI (ratio)	59.7	20.8	62.3	22.3	56.7	19.7

The mean and standard deviation for each of the vocal parameters, height and weight, were computed for the male population, the female population, and the total population. Table 6-4 presents the results.

Investigations with Adults

Inglis (1977) used 50 subjects, 25 female and 25 male, ranging in age from 18 to 25. The subjects had no previous history of laryngeal pathology respiratory disease or hearing loss.

The measurement battery previously described was administered. The mean and standard deviations were computed for each group: female, male, and total sample. The results of the study are listed in Table 6-5.

Taylor (1980) used the same battery to replicate the Inglis study. The study investigated the results from 60 young adults with ages ranging from 18 to 26 years (mean, 23 years).

The mean and standard deviation for the total population, female population, and male population were computed for each of the vocal parameters mentioned in the previous studies. The results of the study are shown in Table 6-6.

With these preliminary data available, clinicians may use the measurement battery to track change in their clients and to have a beginning reference from which to gauge client performance. It should be emphasized that these preliminary performance data should not be interpreted as representing what true normal performance should be, because of the small numbers of subjects and the developmental nature of the measurement battery.

Hammond (1981) reported the use of these measurements in successfully tracking the progress of a 9 year old client with vocal nodules who received VARP therapy. Phonation volume, phonation time, and the air flow measures (maximum flow rate and phonation quotient) appeared to be the most sensitive indicators of client progress in laryngeal function (i.e., reduction in size of the vocal nodules).

The following case report illustrates the potential use of these measures as clinical tracking data for the voice clinician.

A 28 year old woman was referred to the Utah State University Speech-Language and Hearing Center by a laryngologist who described the woman's voice pathology as "hypertrophic laryngitis and Reinke's edema." The client gave an extensive history that was consistent with a hyperfunctional genesis of the problem. She was the mother of seven

Table 6-4. Adjusted Means and Standard Deviations for the Total Population: Grade 4, Elementary Students, Ages 9; 3 to 10; 7 (Child, 1979)

Measures	Total (n = 40)		Girls (n = 20)		Boys (n = 20)	
	Mean	SD	Mean	SD	Mean	SD
Height (in.)	55.00	2.90	55.6	3.30	54.3	2.30
Weight (lb.)	76.70	15.50	80.7	17.40	72.7	12.50
VC (cc)	1997.60	335.20	1859.8	260.10	2135.5	350.60
PV (cc)	1761.30	348.80	1604.0	320.90	1918.5	307.80
PT (s)	17.60	5.10	15.1	4.30	20.2	4.70
PQ (cc/s)	125.80	38.00	133.7	44.60	109.8	25.80
MPT (s)	12.00	2.10	11.0	1.50	13.0	2.10
PTR (ratio)	1.50	.38	1.4	.42	1.6	.32
MFR (cc/s)	160.70	33.30	114.7	39.70	98.6	23.80
VVI (ratio)	54.50	17.70	61.8	19.40	47.1	12.40
PVR (ratio)	.88	.11	.86	.16	.90	.10

Table 6-5. Summary of Means and Standard Deviations for the Population, the Entire Female Population, and the Entire Male Population (Inglis, 1977)

Measures	Total Population		Female Subjects		Male Subjects	
	Mean	SD	Mean	SD	Mean	SD
Age (yr.)	21.7	2.3	20.6	2.0	22.8	2.0
Weight (lb.)	145.0	26.5	126.7	16.1	163.2	21.9
Height (in.)	68.6	3.8	65.7	2.4	71.5	2.4
VC (cc)	4196.0	921.0	3479.2	405.9	4930.0	666.5
PV (cc)	3732.0	832.7	3104.0	465.9	4360.0	588.6
PT (s)	23.8	6.6	22.8	4.1	24.8	8.4
PQ (cc/s)	187.6	61.6	157.2	35.6	217.8	67.7
MPT (s)	25.2	5.9	20.4	2.4	30.0	4.1
PTR (ratio)	1.0	.3	1.1	.3	.8	.3
MFR (cc/s)	166.6	52.3	140.9	34.4	192.3	55.0
VVI (ratio)	40.2	11.1	40.6	8.3	39.9	13.6
PVR (ratio)	.9	.2	.9	.1	.9	.1

Adult population age range: 18-25 years.

Table 6-6. Means and Standard Deviations for the Total Sample Population and by Sex (Taylor, 1980)

Measures	Total Population		Female Subjects		Male Subjects	
	Mean	SD	Mean	SD	Mean	SD
Height (in.)	67.9	3.6	65.1	2.5	70.8	2.1
VC (cc)	4174.8	932.5	3376.3	335.2	4973.3	580.9
PV (cc)	3821.3	940.9	3013.3	379.2	4229.2	554.1
PT (s)	25.5	2.89	22.9	5.8	28.0	8.9
PQ (cc/s)	176.00	56.50	157.0	43.70	195.00	61.40
MPT (s)	28.00	6.50	19.9	3.50	30.30	4.40
PTR (ratio)	1.03	.32	1.1	.34	.92	.29
MFR (cc/s)	161.00	52.70	140.0	40.50	181.00	55.40
VVI (ratio)	40.00	11.20	42.0	10.10	37.00	11.60

Adult population age range: 18–28 years.

children, ages 1 through 9, and observation and report information indicated that she used her voice extensively as the major control stimulus in the home. Yelling, screaming and "hollering" behavior were noted and were supported by reports from her family. Her 8 year old child remarked, "Mom yells at us a lot." The client presented a clinical picture of aphonic instances, occasional diplophonia, breathy production of voice, and observable laryngeal tension accompanied by observable general nervousness. The vocal measures were obtained from the client and were tracked on a monthly basis for the duration of her therapy. Table 6-7 presents her data, which reveal considerable change in the measures from the initial evaluation in April through the month of June. Her therapy program consisted of VARP programming adapted to her individual situation. Progress may be noted dramatically in her improvement during assessment periods, and in June the laryngologist indicated that there was only a small remnant of the pathology on one vocal fold. The reader should note particularly the improvements in phonation time and phonation volume, and the indirect air flow measures (PQ and MFR).

Other Measures

Eckel and Boone (1981) alluded to the clinical usefulness of objective measurements in monitoring client progress in their discussion of a 19 year

Table 6-7. Data from 28 year old Woman with Hypertrophic Laryngitis and Reinke's Edema: Measurements Over a Course of VARP Intervention

Measures	April	May	June
/s/ max	13 s	15 s	18 s
/z/ max	7 s	10 s	15 s
z/s ratio	.53	.67	.83
VC max	3800 cc	3800 cc	3925 cc
PV max	1850 cc	2200 cc	2650 cc
PV/VC ratio	.49	.58	.67
PT max	8 s	11 s	17 s
MPT max	22.4 s	22.4 s	23.1 s
PQ max	475 cc/s	345.5 cc/s	230.8 cc/s
MFR max	231.2 cc/s	200 cc/s	155.8 cc/s
VVI max	58	52.6	39.9

old university singer with bilateral nodules. Other investigators have similarly investigated various measurement procedures as possible correlates of laryngeal function. Gordon, Morton, and Simpson (1978) measured maximum phonation time for several vowels and reported greatly reduced times in persons with laryngeal pathologies. They also reported increased air flow rates during phonation of these patients. Boone (1977) discussed the use of the s/z ratio as an indicator of vocal fold pathology among voice clients. He reported that vocal folds with pathology appear to function less efficiently, resulting in a decrease in glottal resistance and increased airflow with shortened phonation times. Tait, Michel, and Carpenter (1980) studied children with normal voices, aged 5, 7, and 9, and found that they produced s/z ratios close to 1.0, with /z/ duration being typically slightly longer than the /s/. Eckel and Boone (1981) concluded that the s/z ratio used alone or in conjunction with other measures appeared to be an excellent indicator of poor laryngeal function resulting from glottal margin lesions. Inglis (1977) and Lee (1978) also studied the s/z ratio in their investigations and found them to be sensitive indicators of laryngeal function. Several investigators have reported data on the maximum duration of sustained phonation (phonation time) using sustained vowels (Child, 1979; Coombs, 1976; Kushner and Michel, 1978; Lewis, 1977; Mele, 1981;

Norwood, 1978; Ptacek and Sander, 1963; Wilson, 1979) and have suggested its clinical utility.

Smitheran and Hixon (1981) investigated a clinical method for estimating laryngeal airway resistance during vowel production and suggested that their procedure may be useful in discriminating between persons with normal laryngeal function and those with disordered laryngeal function. The procedure takes advantage of measuring oral pressure and airway opening flow by use of a specially designed utterance that alternates voiceless stop-plosives and voiced vowels. Oral pressure is obtained with an oral catheter, one end being placed in the oral cavity and the other coupled to a differential air pressure transducer. Airway opening flow is channelled through an anesthesia mask covering the mouth and nose. Flow from the mask is sensed by a pneumotachometer, also coupled to a separate air pressure transducer. The resultant conditioned data are recorded on a storage oscilloscope and a thermal recorder. The preliminary data gathered with the system supported the reliability and validity of the method as a way of estimating laryngeal airway resistance during vowel production. The authors cite exploratory clinical evidence to support the sensitivity of the method in detecting differences between persons with and without vocal pathology. This experimental procedure also appears to have great potential for use not only in discriminating between normal and disordered laryngeal functioning but also in the periodic tracking of clinical progress.

The results of these investigations suggest that a variety of noninvasive clinical measures are available to the clinician as potentially valuable sensors of clinical progress. Though many research data remain to be gathered in order to establish their scientific validity, initial investigations have demonstrated their usefulness and relative simplicity and convenience in clinical management.

In addition to these applied clinical techniques, the development of new high technology has created additional research capability to objectify elusive vocal parameters. Davis (1981) discussed techniques for obtaining acoustic measures of voices affected by laryngeal pathology. "These methods use digital computer techniques for voice analysis to extract from the speech signal acoustic measures of vocal function that could serve as clinical aids" (p. 77). Davis (1975, 1979, 1981) suggests that these techniques could produce a profile of acoustic characteristics that would be as useful to the laryngologist and speech-language pathologist as an audiogram is to the audiologist. His findings suggest that it is feasible to use quantifiable acoustic features to distinguish between subjects with and without pathologic voices and to use the analysis for assessing improvement during voice therapy. Davis's profile includes six features: pitch perturbation quotient (PPQ), amplitude perturbation quotient (APQ), pitch amplitude (PA), coefficient of excess (EX), spectral flatness of the inverse filter (SFI), and spectral flatness of the residue signal (SFR). His findings suggested that PPQ, APQ, and EX appeared to offer the most promise for monitoring improvement during voice therapy. Additionally, Gould (1975) and Kojima, Gould, Lambiase, and Isshiki (1980) have suggested additional types of laryngeal analysis procedures using acoustic and physiologic measurements. Perkins's chapter in this volume describes these advances in considerable detail.

Significant new voice analysis instrumentation is now available that undoubtedly will contribute significantly to research and development in the objective measurement of vocal function. Three instruments merit special mention. The Visi-Pitch* can accurately extract cycle to cycle fundamental frequency and can display each cycle in real time. The Voice Identification PM Series Pitch Analyzers[†] are microprocessor controlled and can extract precise acoustic information about both fundamental frequency and intensity. The third instrument meriting special mention is a group of new digital spectrographs*, which allow for detailed spectrum analysis with the newest in high speed components. These high technology instruments have the capability of greatly increasing our basic knowledge about the parameters of the human voice and will provide additional valuable clinical tracking capability to the voice therapy process. A thorough consideration of these potentially significant advances awaits data from ongoing investigations.

The implication of the advances in measurement capability discussed in this chapter is that clinicians can no longer justify a lack of precision on the implied or stated basis that measures of the voice are too difficult to obtain in the clinic. Measurement is a must in the clinical process with any communication disorder, and the area of voice disorders can no longer afford a nonmeasurement mode of operation in clinical management. Voice clinicians must take responsibility for finding and implementing reliable and sensitive clinical measures of vocal function within their clinical settings. The question regarding measurement is no longer "if," but rather "how." Such a consideration can only lead to further advances in the total management of voice problems.

FOOTNOTES

*Kay Elementrics Corporation, 12 Maple Ave., Pine Brook, NJ 07058.
[†]Voice Identification, Inc., P.O. Box 714, Somerville, NJ 08876.

Conclusion

In the author's view, the most significant advance in the voice disorders area is the research and development surrounding the measurement of clinical progress. Measurement as a process is basic to full understanding of a phenomenon. If a phenomenon cannot be measured, it cannot be studied, and further, if it cannot be studied precisely, it can never be understood fully. Such is the current status of vocal management. The excitement in participating in the emergence of these measurement procedures is the prospect that in a very short time the voice clinician will be able to validate voice therapy procedures advocated for many years but not validated, and to have an efficient resource available to precisely monitor progress during voice therapy. Moreover, with the development and refinement of these capabilities will come the continued gathering of data, the refining and sorting of effective and ineffective therapy techniques, and, perhaps, the burying forever of those which never did work.

References

Aronson, A. *Clinical voice disorders.* (1980). New York: Brian C. Decker.

Beck, M. A. (1976). *The remediation of vocal nodules in school children: A therapeutic program.* Unpublished master's thesis, Utah State University.

Beckett, R. L. (1971). The respirometer as a diagnostic and clinical tool in the speech clinic. *Journal of Speech and Hearing Disorders, 36,* 235, 241.

Beste, L. R. (1971). *Spastic dysphonia—a review of literature and case study.* Unpublished master's thesis, Utah State University.

Boone, D. R. (1977). *The voice and voice therapy* (2nd ed.). Englewood Cliffs, NJ: Prentice-Hall.

Boone, D. R. (1981). Boone Voice Therapy Kit. Gladstone, OR: C. C. Publications.

Brodnitz, F. S. (1971). *Vocal rehabilitation* Rochester, MN: Whiting Press.

Child, D. R. (1979). *Maximum phonation time: Optimum number of trials and normative performance on fourth grade children.* Unpublished master's thesis, Utah State University.

Coachbuilder, D. P. (1972). *Programming vocal exercises for the development of pitch.* Unpublished master's thesis, Utah State University.

Coombs, J. (1976). *The maximum duration of phonation of /a/ in normal and hoarse voiced children.* Unpublished master's thesis, Portland State University.

Cooper, M., and Cooper, M. H. (1977). *Approaches to vocal rehabilitation.* Springfield, IL: Charles C Thomas.

Costello, Janis M. (1977). Programmed instruction. *Journal of Speech and Hearing Disorders, 42,* 3–28.

Davis, S. B. (1975). Preliminary results using inverse filtering of speech for automatic evaluation of laryngeal pathology. *58,* s111 (abstract).

Davis, S. B. (1979). Acoustic characteristics of normal and pathological voices. In N. J. Lass (Ed.), *Speech and language: Advances in basic research and practice* (Vol. 1). New York: Academic Press.

Davis, S. B. (1981). Acoustic characteristics of laryngeal pathology. In J. K. Darby (Ed.), *Speech evaluation in medicine.* New York: Grune & Stratton.

Drudge, M. K. M., and Phillips, B. J. (1976). Shaping behavior in voice therapy. *Journal of Speech and Hearing Disorders, 41,* 398–411.

Eckel, F. C., and Boone, D. R. (1981). The s/z ratio as an indicator of laryngeal pathology. *Journal of Speech and Hearing Disorders, 46,* 147–149.

Filter, M. D. (Ed.) (1982a). *Phonatory voice disorders in children.* Springfield, IL: Charles C Thomas.

Filter, M. D. (1982b). Evaluation of children with phonatory voice disorders: Role of the speech-pathologist. In M. D. Filter (Ed.), *Phonatory voice disorders in children.* Springfield, IL: Charles C Thomas.

Froeschels, E. (1952). Chewing method as therapy: A discussion with some philosophical conclusions. *Archives of Otolaryngology, 56,* 427–434.

Gordon, M. T., Morton, F. M., and Simpson, I. C. (1978). Airflow measurements in diagnosis, assessment and treatment of mechanical dysphonia. *Folia Phoniatrica, 30,* 166–174.

Gould, W. J. (1975). Quantitative assessment of voice function in microlaryngology. *Folia Phoniatrica, 27,* 190, 204.

Greene, M. C. L. (1980). *The voice and its disorders* (4th ed.). Philadelphia: J. B. Lippincott.

Greiner, G. (1973). *A programmed therapy approach to pitch disturbances of the voice.* Unpublished master's thesis, Utah State University.

Hammond, J. (1981). *A precision approach to evaluation and therapy in voice.* Unpublished master's thesis, Utah State University.

Hirano, M., Koike, Y., and von Leden, H. (1968). Maximum phonation time and air usage during phonation. *Folia Phoniatrica, 20,* 185–201.

Hunsaker, J. C. (1974). *Behavior modification and functional voice disorders.* Unpublished master's thesis, Utah State University.

Inglis, J. M. (1977). *Obtaining normative data on vocal parameters in a group of adult speakers.* Unpublished master's thesis, Utah State University.

Isshiki, N. (1964). Regulatory mechanism of voice intensity variation. *Journal of Speech and Hearing Research, 7,* 17–29.

Isshiki, N. (1965). Vocal intensity and air flow rate. *Folia Phoniatrica, 17,* 92–104.

Isshiki, N., Okamura, H., and Morimoto, M. (1967). Maximum phonation time and air flow rate during phonation: Simple clinical tests for vocal function. *Annals of Otology, Rhinology, and Laryngology, 76,* 998–1007.

Isshiki, N., Okamura, H., Tanabe, M., and Morimoto, M. (1969). Differential diagnosis of hoarseness. *Folia Phoniatrica, 21,* 9–19.

Isshiki, N., and von Leden, H. (1964). Hoarseness: Aerodynamic studies. *Archives of Otolaryngology, 80,* 206–213.

Isshiki, N., Yanagihara, N., and Morimoto, M. (1966). Approach to the objective diagnosis of hoarseness. *Folia Phoniatrica, 18,* 393–400.

Iwata, S., and von Leden, H. (1970). Phonation quotient in patients with laryngeal diseases. *Folia Phoniatrica, 22,* 117–128.

Johnson, T. S. (1974). *A precision approach to hyperfunctional voice problems.* Logan, Utah: Utah State University.

Johnson, T. S. (1984). Treatment of vocal abuse in children. In W. H. Perkins (Ed.), *Current therapy of communicative disorders: Voice disorders.* New York: Thieme-Stratton.

Johnson, T. S. (1985). *Vocal abuse reduction program (VARP).* San Diego: College-Hill Press.

Koike, Y. (1968). Vowel amplitude modulations in patients with laryngeal diseases. *Journal of the Acoustical Society of America, 45,* 839-844.

Koike, Y., and Hirano, M. (1968). Significance of vocal velocity index. *Folia Phoniatrica, 20,* 285-296.

Koike, Y., Hirano, M., and von Leden, H. (1967). Vocal initiation: Acoustic and aerodynamic investigations of normal subjects. *Folia Phoniatrica, 19,* 173-182.

Kojima, H., Gould, W. J., Lambiase, A., and Isshiki, N. (1980). Computer analysis of hoarseness. *Acta Otolaryngology, 89,* 547-554.

Kushner, D., and Michel, J. (1978) *Maximum phonation times in 100 adults.* Paper presented to the Annual Convention of the American Speech and Hearing Association, San Francisco.

Laver, J. D. (1968). Voice quality and indexical information. *British Journal of Disordered Communication, 3,* 43-54.

Lee, R. L. (1978). *Phonation and respiratory production in cheerleaders.* Unpublished master's thesis, Utah State University.

Lewis, K. (1977). *The maximum duration of phonation of /a/ in children.* Unpublished master's thesis, Portland State University.

Lubker, J. F. (1979). Acoustic-perceptual methods for evaluation of defective speech. In N. H. Lass (Ed.), *Speech and language: Advances in basic research and practice* (Vol. 1). New York: Academic Press.

Mele, L. (1981). *Maximum phonation time in children four and five years of age.* Unpublished manuscript, James Madison University.

Michel, J. F., and Wendahl, R. (1971). Correlates of voice production. In L. E. Travis (Ed.), *Handbook of speech pathology and audiology.* New York: Appleton-Century-Crofts.

Miller, L. K. (1980). *Principles of everyday behavior analysis.* Monterey, CA: Brooks/Cole.

Moore, G. P. (1977). Have the major issues in voice disorders been answered by research in speech science? A 50 year retrospective. *Journal of Speech and Hearing Disorders, 42,* 152-160.

Moses, P. (1954). *The voice of neurosis.* New York: Grune & Stratton.

Mowrer, D. E. (1982). *Methods of modifying speech behaviors* (2nd ed.). Columbus, OH: Charles E. Merrill.

Murry, T. (1982) Phonation: Remediation. In N. J. Lass, L. V. McReynolds, and J. Northern (Eds.), *Speech, language and hearing: Pathologies of speech and language* (Vol 2). Philadelphia: W. B. Saunders.

Nell, G. W. (1968). An evaluation of behavior therapy in the handling of functional dysphonia in children. *Journal of the South African Logopedic Society, 15,* 14-18.

Norwood, E. D. (1978). *Variability in test-retest of maximum duration of sustained /a/ in children.* Unpublished master's thesis, Portland State University.

Parrish, M. L. (1972). *A therapeutic program for the remediation of vocal nodules in children.* Unpublished master's thesis, Utah State University.

Perkins, W. H. (1971). Vocal function: A behavioral analysis. In L. E. Travis (Ed.), *Handbook of speech pathology and audiology.* New York: Appleton-Century-Crofts

Pierce, G. L. (1974). *An analysis and reduction of breathiness with accompanying inspiratory speech.* Unpublished master's thesis, Utah State University.

Polow, N., and Kaplan, E. D. (1979). *Symptomatic voice therapy.* Tulsa: Modern Education Corporation.

Ptacek, P. H., and Sander, E. K. (1963). Maximum duration of phonation. *Journal of Speech and Hearing Disorders, 29,* 171-182.

Reed, C. G. (1980). Voice therapy: A need for research. *Journal of Speech and Hearing Disorders, 45,* 157-169.

Rothwell, R. (1974). *A therapeutic program for the remediation of hyperfunctional voice disorders in adults.* Unpublished master's thesis, Utah State University.

Ryan, B. P. (1974). *Programmed therapy for stuttering in children and adults.* Springfield, IL: Charles C Thomas.

Smee, J. S. (1974). *An analysis of contact ulcer reduction using the vocal abuse reduction program and vocal quality program.* Unpublished master's thesis, Utah State University.

Smitheran, J. R., and Hixon, T. J. (1981). A clinical method for estimating laryngeal airway resistance during vowel production. *Journal of Speech and Hearing Disorders, 46,* 138–146.

Tait, N. A., Michel, J. F., and Carpenter, M. A.(1980). Maximum duration of sustained /s/ and /z/ in children. *Journal of Speech and Hearing Disorders, 45,* 239–246.

Taylor, T. J. (1980). *Air flow parameters in college-age individuals.* Unpublished master's thesis, Utah State University.

Thompson, C. G. (1976). *The feasibility of using respirometer measurements as a monitoring agent of laryngeal functioning during vocal nodule rehabilitation.* Unpublished master's thesis, Utah State University.

Vance, S. E. (1976). *A therapeutic approach to an extended length of utterance program for extension and generalization of appropriate vocal quality production.* Unpublished master's thesis, Utah State University.

Williams, K. (1977). *Performances of elementary school aged children on respirometric and phonatory measures.* Unpublished master's thesis, Utah State University.

Williams, S. W. (1979). *A comparative analysis of the Collins P-900 9 liter respirometer and the dropper compact spirometer.* Unpublished master's thesis, Utah State University.

Wilson, D. K. (1979). *Voice problems of children.* Baltimore: Williams & Wilkins.

Wilson, F. B. (1972). The voice disordered child: A descriptive approach. *Language, Speech, and Hearing Services in the Schools, 4,* 14–22.

Wilson, F. B., and Rice, M. (1977). *A programmed approach to voice therapy.* Austin, TX: Learning Concepts.

Yanagihara, N., and Koike, Y. (1967). The regulation of sustained phonation. *Folia Phoniatrica, 19,* 1–18.

Yanagihara, N., Koike, Y., and von Leden, H. (1966). Phonation and respiration. *Folia Phoniatrica, 18,* 323–340.

Yanagihara, N., and von Leden, H. (1967). Respiration and phonation. *Folia Phoniatrica, 19,* 153–166.

Part Three

STUTTERING

STUTTERING

M. N. Hegde

Treatment of Fluency Disorders: State of the Art

Theories and Therapies

It is well known that stuttering is a "disorder of many theories" (Jonas, 1977, p. 7). As such, it is also a disorder of many therapies. It is generally thought that the treatment procedures of a disorder are derived from a theory of that disorder. It must be noted, however, that there are different kinds of theories and only a certain kind can tell the clinician how to treat the disorder. The philosophy of science recognizes two main types of theories: hypothetico-deductive and inductive. The hypothetico-deductive, the classic type, has had some remarkable success in the natural sciences. In order to develop this kind of theory, the researcher first defines some basic terms and then proposes a series of postulates that describe and explain the phenomenon under investigation. Often, these postulates themselves are not directly testable. Therefore, the researcher deduces some theorems from them. These theorems are experimentally tested, and when supported by the results, the theoretical postulates from which they were derived are said to be valid. In essence, deductive theories are predictive models based on logic and mathematics. If the predictions made by the theory are empirically supported, the theory is said to be validated. If not, the theory is appropriately modified or rejected.

The inductive theories, on the other hand, do not start out as predictive models. Instead, they stay close to experimental evidence. While the hypothetico-deductive theory emerges from a logical premise, the inductive theory emerges from data that are experimentally derived, are replicated to some extent, and are known to have a certain degree of generality. The scientist within the deductive framework first suggests a theory, albeit with some evidence, and then sets out a program of research to verify it. The scientist within the inductive framework first performs a series of experiments (and continues to do so) and then lets the results shape theoretic statements.

In the behavioral sciences, Hull's (1951) learning theory illustrates the hypothetico-deductive method, whereas Skinner's (1953, 1969, 1974) experimental analysis of behavior illustrates the inductive method. In the field of learning and conditioning, the Hullian type of deductive theories have not been very successful. Initially, Skinner's main concern was to isolate the controlling variables of behaviors and his theoretical analyses (1969, 1974) came after at least 30 years of experimental research. Skinner rejects theories that are devoid of *demonstrated* empirical relationships but not those based on controlled experimental evidence. Deductive theories have fared better in the natural sciences because of the relatively long tradition of experimental research and the ease with which certain physical and chemical phenomena can be controlled and manipulated. Validated deductive theories are just fine, but it takes a long time to validate them. Meanwhile, scientists and practitioners can get stuck with a theory that may eventually be rejected.

A theory, in its broadest sense, not only describes all aspects of a phenomenon, but also explains why it is taking place by specifying its controlling (independent) variables. By manipulation of the controlling variables, the event can be changed. As can be seen, the clinician needs access to controlling variables of a disorder in order to modify it. It is thus clear that in an applied discipline such as ours, only an inductive theory based on *already demonstrated* controlling variables of events can be of immediate practical significance. Hypothesized but not yet demonstrated cause-effect relationships are of no use to the clinician. Similarly, processes that are presumed to take place in the nervous system but are not manipulable, and fictional psychologic variables such as self-image, provide for neither theoretic rigor nor clinical strategy. As such, experimental research is not restricted to laboratory science. A clinical profession can make no progress without it.

It is both surprising and unfortunate that in the field of stuttering there are hardly any theories that are validated either deductively or inductively. It is surprising because stuttering has been one of the most researched of the speech-language disorders. It is unfortunate because a lack of agreement on the controlling variables of stuttering has led to fruitless theoretic controversies and inefficient therapeutic diversity. History supports the statement that stuttering is a disorder of many pseudo-theories and therapies. This may be largely due to an abundance of nonexperimental research.

From a historical perspective, it cannot be said that effective stuttering therapies have been derived from stuttering theories. Theories and therapies have often been on different courses, resulting in conceptual inconsistencies.

Therapies recommended by many have had very little logical or empirical connection with their own theoretical positions. For example, during the 1930s, when stuttering was explained at the University of Iowa on the basis of disturbed lateral dominance, recommended treatment was often psychologic. As noted by Bloodstein, "It is a curious feature of an essentially neurophysiological breakdown theory that it permits considerable emphasis in therapy on the stutterer's attitudes and adjustments" (1981, p. 345). In more recent years, West and Ansberry (1968) considered stuttering to be an organic disease due to subtle neurologic lesions and atavistic heredity; but when it came to stuttering therapy, they recommended, among other things, that the stutterer's self-confidence be developed (Hegde, 1970).

Many of the current research trends are based on neurophysiologic models of one kind or another. These models postulate that neurophysiologic, neuromotor, or central neural processes, or a combination thereof, are causally involved in stuttering. As yet, no clear cut treatment procedures have been derived from these theoretic positions, although this fact by itself does not necessarily cast doubt on the validity of those hypotheses.

A possible reason why neurophysiologic research has not suggested new or more effective treatments is that, for the most part, this kind of research has not been about the controlling variables of stuttering. It has been about stuttering itself. In other words, the dependent variable (stuttering), not its independent variable(s), has been studied at levels that were inaccessible before. Since by definition, treatment procedures are independent variables the manipulation of which will change the effect, research that focuses almost exclusively on the response properties may not lead to therapeutic tactics.

In the overall scheme of treatment development, neurophysiologic descriptions of stuttering can serve a more useful purpose than theories thereof. Such descriptions tell us about the neurophysiologic events that are a part of stuttering. A knowledge of these events can help us define the treatment targets better, although it does not determine the treatment variables. As long as we heed Perkins's (1981) caution that an integral part of an effect cannot be the cause of the total effect, we will not confuse cause-effect relations and hence will keep treatment targets and procedures separate.

The rest of this chapter concerns various aspects of stuttering treatment. First, we shall look at some treatment procedures whose application seems to have declined over the years. Second, we shall review a recent revival of a therapeutic philosophy concerning attitudinal therapy.

Third, we shall examine major contemporary approaches to stuttering therapy. Fourth, we shall identify elements that are common to several different treatment programs.

Noise, Rhythmic Stimulation, and Anxiety Reduction Procedures: Yet to be Proved

The scarcity of published reports suggests that the use of such techniques as masking noise, metronome-conditioned speech, and anxiety reduction procedures (involving biofeedback and systematic desensitization) has somewhat declined. The author realizes that statements such as this should be made with a good deal of caution, since stuttering treatment procedures are notorious for their rebirths, and, ipso facto, repeated deaths. Nonetheless, the effectiveness of some of these procedures has not been established, and sophisticated studies are simply lacking.

Noise as a Form of Treatment

Ever since it was found that different levels of auditory masking noise can reduce the frequency of stuttering, attempts have been made to develop treatment procedures based on this finding (Cherry, Sayers, and Marland, 1955; Shane, 1955). Unfortunately, the masking noise procedure always had technical problems. Since the initial masking units were bulky, the treatment was restricted to the clinical situation. Then came the portable electronic models, but they posed the problem of social acceptance. These units required the stutterer to wear double earphones, which tend to evoke undue social attention. The double earphones reduce some hearing acuity for the stutterer and suggest hearing loss to the listener. The most important reason for the decline of masking noise therapy may be its lack of long term effects, however.

There is a general agreement that masking noise of various intensities can reduce stuttering as soon as it is introduced, and perhaps over a short period of time. But the long term effects are a different story. A study by Garber and Martin (1974) has shown that when the masking noise is presented over four to six treatment sessions, there may be no consistent reduction in stuttering frequency across sessions as well as subjects.

The introduction of a voice activated noise unit called the Edinburgh Masker has rekindled some interest in the masking noise procedure (Dewar,

Dewar, and Barnes, 1976). The voice activated unit is technically more sophisticated in that it delivers noise only when the stutterer is talking. Unfortunately, the results of a study by Dewar and colleagues have established neither long term effects nor information on whether the stutterer can be eventually fluent without the masking noise. Further, Ingham, Southwood, and Horsburgh (1981) demonstrated experimentally the wide range of effects (and noneffects) the Edinburgh Masker can have on the stuttering of individual subjects during both oral reading and spontaneous monologue speech. Even if it becomes established that the effects of masking noise do not diminish over time for those subjects who show reliable reductions of stuttering, the procedure may not be acceptable to many stutterers if they have to wear the unit indefinitely.

Rhythmic Stimulation

As a form of stuttering therapy, rhythmic stimulation is both ancient and modern. The most researched signal is auditory, generated by a metronome of either the old desk variety or the modern behind-the-ear electronic model. When the stutterer times his or her syllables or words to the beats of a metronome, there is usually a reduction in stuttering and speech rate. The resulting "fluency" is somewhat deliberate and lacks the normal intonational patterns.

The most promising results with the rhythmic procedure were originally reported by Brady (1971). His Metronome Conditioned Speech retraining procedure was considered effective in 23 stutterers. A followup conducted at 6 to 44 months after therapy showed that 90 per cent of his stutterers had sustained significant improvement. Brady's (1971) promising report prompted a few additional studies, but unfortunately, the results have not been encouraging. Studies by Berman and Brady (1973), Adams and Hotchkiss (1973), Trotter and Silverman (1974), Ost, Gotestam, and Melin (1976), and Silverman (1976), while reporting some positive findings, have actually raised a number of questions about the metronome-conditioned speech. None of these studies have established generalized fluency sustained over a prolonged period of time without equipment. The personal experience of Silverman (1976) suggests that when the unit is used for a long period of time, it may cease to be effective in controlling stuttering.

Anxiety Reduction

In behavior therapy, anxiety reduction procedures such as systematic desensitization and biofeedback have not been very effective. When applied to stuttering, these procedures turn out to be indirect forms of treatment. In anxiety reduction procedures, the focus is on the psychophysiologic state of the speaker, not stuttered speech. In systematic desensitization (also known as reciprocal inhibition), the stutterer's anxiety and fear responses relative to the act of speaking and speaking situations are reduced. This is accomplished by teaching the client deep muscle relaxation and having the person imagine himself or herself speaking in difficult situations. Then, progressively more difficult situations are presented. When this is done repeatedly, the relaxation response is expected to reciprocally inhibit anxiety associated with speech tasks. The assumption has been that if a stutterer's anxiety is eliminated, stuttering will decrease. In biofeedback, various kinds of electronic instruments are used to display information concerning psychophysiologic functions such as muscle tension, blood pressure, and electromyographic activity. By and large, biofeedback as applied to stuttering is also designed to reduce the stutterer's anxiety and muscle tension with the assumption that a relaxed stutterer can speak without stuttering.

Both systematic desensitization and biofeedback seemingly make sense in view of the impression that anxiety and tension are often associated with stuttered speech. Unfortunately, the clinical application of these two procedures has been neither extensive nor very encouraging. Studies on reciprocal inhibition (Boudreau and Jeffrey, 1973; Burgraff, 1974; Moleski and Tosi, 1976; Tyre, Maisto, and Companik, 1973; Yonovitz, Shepherd, and Garrett, 1977), and biofeedback (Guitar, 1975; Hanna, Wilfling, and McNeil, 1975; Lanyon, Barrington, and Newman, 1976) have produced some positive findings, but data on the long term effects are lacking. The use of these two techniques does not appear to be on the increase. As we will see later, more successful techniques teach certain specific responses that lead to nonstuttered speech, and all of these responses are speech-related. Normally, a relaxed neuromuscular state may be a helpful background variable for fluency, but relaxation by itself does not teach the stutterer the skills necessary to produce nonstuttered speech.

A Philosophic Revival: Attitudinal Therapy

A therapeutic philosophy that has staged a sort of comeback relates to stutterers' attitudes and their therapeutic modifications. Historical research on stutterers' attitudes and feelings include two distinct perspectives. An empirical perspective has attempted to describe the kinds of attitudes and feelings the stutterer exhibits (see Bloodstein, 1981, for a review). As can be expected, a speech disorder such as stuttering is bound to have some effect on practically every aspect of the stutterer's life. The person who stutters may evoke unusual reactions from peers, parents, teachers, strangers, and prospective employers. Whether most listeners do indeed react negatively or not, the stutterer is likely to feel that they do. Stuttering can restrict social life and occupational choices. It may alter educational plans and create unpleasant family relationships. Ordinary speaking situations may be traumatic, and the stutterer may learn to avoid them.

Largely because of such personal experience, stutterers may come to entertain a set of beliefs about themselves in relation to their stuttering. The typical set of thoughts stutterers entertain about themselves, when verbalized, is often referred to as "self-image." Stutterers may also feel less confident about themselves because of repeated failures in speaking situations.

Although many clinicians and researchers may believe that for at least some persons stuttering produces personal, emotional, social, and cognitive effects, a controversy arises in regard to the role of these phenomena in the treatment of stuttering. Traditionally, it has been assumed that in order to achieve lasting fluency, attitudes must be changed; if the treatment is designed only to reduce stuttering and increase nonstuttered speech, maladaptive attitudes do not change, and these unchanged attitudes will soon wipe out the temporary and shaky fluency generated by a treatment procedure whose exclusive concern was to modify the stuttering/nonstuttering rates.

How are attitudes, feelings, and self-images changed? Generally, there is more written on the *need* for attitudinal therapy than on its procedures. Fortunately, Gregory (1979) has given some descriptions of procedures by which attitudes are thought to be changed. In essence, the modification of attitudes is attempted mostly at the verbal level. The clinician, assuming the role of a sympathetic listener, encourages stuttering clients to talk freely about feelings, attitudes, and thoughts concerning themselves and their stutterings. In addition, the clinician offers new information on stuttering, and interprets the stutterers' feelings and attitudes so they can understand them better. Finally, the stutterers' verbal expressions of appropriate attitudes and feelings are approved, while inappropriate statements may be disapproved or ignored.

Many treatment procedures that place an emphasis on directly modifying stuttering and/or nonstuttered response rates do not focus on the stutterer's feelings and attitudes. Specifically, procedures based on operant conditioning, and those that are designed to teach certain target behaviors aimed at altering the stutterer's manner of talking (e.g., slowed speech rate) typically do not attempt to manipulate feelings and attitudes (Costello, 1980; Ingham, 1975; Ryan, 1979; Webster, 1979). This has led to the criticism that behavioral treatment of stuttering can generate only limited fluency, which will not be sustained across time or situations (Sheehan, 1979).

Conceptually, attitudinal therapy would be needed only when certain attitudes cause stuttering or when attitudes and stutterings are independent of each other. Unfortunately, there exist virtually no empirical data showing that faulty attitudes exist before the onset of stuttering and hence cause the speech problem. Possibly as a consequence, most experts who advocate attitudinal therapy seem to do so on the assumption that attitudes and stutterings are independent of each other and hence need separate treatment (Erickson, 1969; Guitar, 1976).

The current interest in attitudinal therapy has been stimulated by the reports of Guitar and associates. Initially, Guitar (1976) reported that pretreatment attitudinal measures showed a moderate correlation with treatment outcome, as measured a year later. This report also indicated that pretreatment attitudes were independent of pretreatment stuttering frequency, suggesting that "attitude measures tap an entirely different dimension of stuttering than do counts of stutters and syllables" (Guitar, 1976, p. 598). The next report (Guitar and Bass, 1978) suggested that those stutterers who had "normalized" attitudes at the end of a behavioral (prolonged speech) treatment program were more likely to remain fluent after one year than those whose attitudes had not normalized. These two studies are thought to support the position that attitudes reflect something other than measures of stuttered speech, and that there is a need for attitudinal therapy.

Because of some methodologic and conceptual difficulties, it may be prudent not to conclude that the Guitar (1976) and Guitar and Bass (1978) studies support a need to modify the stutterer's attitudes. Ingham's (1979) critique of the Guitar and Bass paper has pointed out several of these problems and has prompted Guitar (1981) to reanalyze the original data with a more appropriate statistical procedure. On the basis of this reanalysis, Guitar later concluded that "there is not a significant difference in the stuttering frequency between the group that had normalized attitudes after treatment and the group that did not" (1981, p. 440).

A critical examination of research on attitudes and attitudinal therapy raises several questions, the most important being the following: What are attitudes? How are they measured? What are the effects of attitudinal and nonattitudinal therapy?

Traditionally, attitudes are considered to be certain mental states or predispositions to respond in some unspecified ways. In the context of stuttering, attitudes are often defined as either affective and cognitive responses to stimuli (Gregory, 1979) or as "strongly conditioned responses between the subject's stuttered speech and his environment" (Guitar, 1976, p. 598). However, when attitudes are defined as conditioned responses to stimuli, they then become behaviors, not mental states. Such a description negates the distinction between "attitudes" and "behaviors." In essence, the term attitude (as a mental state) may be a misnomer, and if the phenomenon can be described as behavior, then the term is also unnecessary.

If attitudes are certain kinds of behaviors, what kind are they? A potential answer to this question lies in the measurement procedure. Attitudes are typically measured through questionnaires, such as the Iowa Scale of Attitudes Toward Stuttering (Johnson, 1961) or the Erickson S-Scale (Erickson, 1969). In the latter scale, which has been used by several investigators, the stutterer is asked to respond (true or false) to such statements as these: "I would rather not introduce myself to strangers," and "I often feel nervous while talking." Such measures of "attitudes" constitute stutterers' verbal statements concerning their speech and how they feel about their speech performance. From a logical standpoint, such verbal statements and feelings are probably determined by the stutterer's stuttering in the particular situations being questioned.

A recent study by Ulliana and Ingham (1984) demonstrated that modified (S24, Andrews and Cutler, 1974) Erickson Scale responses were not independent of speech and stuttering behaviors. When stutterers were given an opportunity to suggest the basis of their responses to each of the scale items, it became evident that their own speech and stuttering behaviors largely determined the kinds of responses evoked by the questionnaire. Furthermore, actual measures of stuttering in certain scale-identified situations showed that situations associated with "negative attitudes" were also associated with a higher frequency of stutterings than situations associated with "positive attitudes." This led to the conclusion that measures of attitudes, at least on the popular S24 Erickson Scale, were not independent of stuttering.

It is thus evident that attitudinal therapy can hardly be justified on the assumption that stutterings and attitudes are two separate problems of a stutterer. In all likelihood, stutterers' verbal statements and feelings concerning their stuttering ("attitudes") are a direct result of the stuttering itself. In this case, what needs treatment is stuttering, and a successful treatment should eliminate whatever consequences the speech problem generated. Indeed, the results of attitudinal therapy and behavioral treatments that exclude it both support this contention.

Attitudinal therapy is nothing new, although controlled studies on its effects are not many. Broadly speaking, this therapy is not unlike psychotherapy and counseling, which have rarely been effective in reducing stuttering (Van Riper, 1973; Bloodstein, 1981). Long ago, Bryngelson found that a mere reduction of fear of stuttering and negative attitudes had no effect on stuttering frequency (Bloodstein, 1981). Van Riper reported that when he used psychotherapy and counseling aimed at stutterers' feelings and attitudes in the absence of direct procedures, he obtained "the poorest results of any program of therapy" ever employed (1973, p. 216).

An even more crucial question regarding the effectiveness of attitudinal therapy was raised by a study by Martin and Haroldson (1969). They treated one group of stutterers with "information-attitude" therapy and another group with "time-out from speaking." The subjects in both the groups responded to the Iowa Scale of Attitudes Toward Stuttering before and after the treatment. The results were that the time-out was effective in reducing stuttering, but the information-attitude therapy was not. But more importantly, the attitudinal therapy did not make a difference in the pre- and posttreatment scores on the attitudinal scale. In other words, attitudinal therapy may be ineffective not only in reducing stuttering, but also in eliminating negative attitudes.

The effects of behavioral treatments that do not include attitudinal therapy have shed some additional light on the relationship between attitudes and stutterings. The indications are that the degree to which the scores on an attitude scale would reflect "normal attitudes" after treatment is related to the extent of *generalized* fluency. For example, using the S24 Erickson Scale, Andrews and Cutler (1974) showed that a behavioral treatment program resulted in normalized attitudes, but only after stuttering was reduced in several everyday situations. As can be expected, stutterers continue to express negative verbal statements and feelings about situations in which they still stutter.

Additional data indicate that attitudes are effects of stuttering, and what needs treatment is just stuttering. The well known treatment programs of Webster (1979) and Ryan (1979) do not include direct procedures to change attitudes and feelings. Nevertheless, they have reported that as stutterers become more and more fluent, their unfavorable attitudes decrease.

The issue of attitudinal therapy, though an empirical one, has been argued for too long on logical grounds alone. As Webster (1979) has pointed out, "It is incumbent upon those who stress the importance of attitude change procedures to demonstrate the relationship of such procedures to the efficacy of therapeutic practice" (p. 221). It is surprising that the protracted debate on attitude change has not produced a single experimental study with appropriate methodology. Predictive and correlational studies do not produce definitive evidence. Also, it is best to avoid the questionable practice of arguing from negative evidence that might show that certain treatments do not produce lasting fluency. Shortcomings of direct treatment programs do not necessarily justify attitudinal therapy. What is needed is a series of controlled experiments in which attitudinal therapy is employed exclusively to demonstrate its effectiveness in reducing stuttering *and* negative attitudes.

Stuttering Therapies: An Overview

In this section, the major stuttering therapies being practiced today will be reviewed. It is recognized that classifying stuttering therapies into well known categories such as traditional versus current or operant versus nonoperant is not always satisfactory or justifiable (Sheehan, 1979). Organizing treatment procedures according to some general and noncontroversial principle can be useful, however. It appears that one such principle is the focus of therapeutic attention. Some techniques seek to modify the *form* of stuttering, not necessarily its frequency. On the other hand, several other techniques are designed to achieve a significant reduction in the frequency of stuttering behaviors. These techniques also seek to establish speech that is considered normal with regard to the parameters of fluency, although this secondary goal has remained somewhat elusive. As will be seen later, systematic studies on the nature of treated and untreated fluency are beginning to be reported.

Modification of the Form of Stuttering

The historical beginnings of the modern treatment of stuttering within the profession of speech-language pathology in the United States are associated with the names of Bryngelson, Johnson, and Van Riper. Bryngelson's initial treatment procedure, Johnson's extensive empirical research, and Van Riper's treatment regimen have created one of the most influential of stuttering therapies. Eventually, Van Riper, over several decades, refined a treatment program and thereby established a certain philosophy and strategy of stuttering therapy. Van Riper's approach is better known than many other approaches, and the sources are readily available (Van Riper, 1973, 1982).

The Van Riper therapy includes both indirect and direct procedures. The indirect procedures are counseling and psychotherapeutic discussions aimed at changing the stutterer's feelings, perceptions, and attitudes. The direct procedures, on the other hand, are concerned with stuttering itself, and their main goal is to modify the *form* of stuttering, not necessarily its frequency. In essence, Van Riper would teach the stutterer what to do when stuttering is expected (preparatory sets), when stuttering has actually begun (pull-outs), and when stuttering has occurred (cancellation). The stutterer's mastery of these skills results in less severe stuttering, or, as Van Riper has often put it, "fluent stuttering."

Two major philosophic assumptions characterize the Van Riperian approach to stuttering therapy. First, the approach, by seeking to modify only the form of stuttering, assumes that fluent speech may not be an appropriate therapeutic target for most stutterers. It is even suggested that the goal of fluent speech may be detrimental because any therapeutic shortcoming can only compound the considerable emotional and attitudinal problems the stutterer typically experiences.

Second, a significant goal of stuttering therapy is to help the stutterer live with the problem. A well adjusted stutterer who stutters with less abnormality is the final goal. Therefore, the stutterer's attitudes must be changed. The stutterer will have to stop avoiding speaking situations, speaking tasks, and stuttering. Instead, stuttering should be allowed to occur while its abnormality and associated negative emotions are controlled. In short, the stutterer should regain self-confidence and self-respect by accepting the realistic therapeutic goal of controlled stuttering.

Reduction in the Frequency of Stuttering

There are several therapy procedures that are non–Van Riperian in their basic assumptions. These procedures assume that fluent speech can and should be the target of stuttering therapy, mere modification of the form of stuttering is not sufficient, and the treatment target should be a significant reduction in stuttering frequency as well as severity. Some of these treatment procedures do not include attitudinal therapy. A few others do, but not necessarily for the purpose of having the stutterer "adjust" to his or her problems.

The argument in favor of the treatment approach seeking to reduce the frequency of stuttering can be summarized as follows. Whether fluency can be a treatment target or not should be treated as an empirical question, and should not be rejected out of hand. The assumption that fluency is unattainable is understandable in the light of disappointing results of historical therapies. It is true that ethical and scientific restraints prevent the clinician from holding out promises that cannot be kept. Nevertheless, scientific progress in the treatment of stuttering can be made only when presumed or demonstrated limits are repeatedly tested. The clinical scientist must operate on the basis that more effective treatment techniques can be developed.

If fluency is considered a possible treatment target for a majority of stutterers, then a mere modification of the form of stuttering is insufficient. A significant reduction in the frequency of stuttering, so that the parameters of fluency fall within normal limits, should be the treatment target. There is some evidence that with additional refinements in generalization procedures and the normalcy of treated fluency, this target is within the reach of many stutterers.

Several treatment programs seek to establish fluent speech in stutterers. A review of these procedures can hardly be exhaustive; only some of the major procedures that characterize the current state of the art can be reviewed here. Even then, only the salient features of selected techniques can be mentioned. Two criteria have guided the selection of procedures for review: some relation to recent advances, and empirical evidence concerning their effectiveness. Different research clinicians have described somewhat different treatment programs, but there seems to be a set of common procedures across several programs (Andrews, Guitar, and Howie, 1980; Andrews and Tanner, 1982; Azrin, Nunn, and Frantz, 1979; Bloodstein, 1975, 1981; Brutten, 1975; Costello, 1975, 1980; Howie, Tanner, and Andrews, 1981; Howie and Woods, 1982; Ingham, 1975; Ingham and Andrews, 1973; Ingham and Packman, 1977; Mowrer, 1975, 1979, 1982; Perkins, 1973a, 1973b; Ryan, 1974, 1979; Ryan and Van Kirk, 1974; Shames and Egolf, 1976; Shames and Florance, 1980; Sheehan, 1979; Webster, 1974; Williams, 1979, 1982, among others). In a later section we shall return to the issue of common elements across treatment programs.

For the most part, the strategy seeking a significant reduction in stuttering was developed within the behavioral framework. Later developments within this strategy were not necessarily restricted to the behavioral paradigm, however. Nevertheless, a non–Van Riperian approach to stuttering treatment owes its existence to the influence of the experimental and applied analyses of behavior.

Behavioral Treatment: Current Status

From the very beginning, behavioral research in stuttering was concerned with the effects of consequences made contingent on various speech behaviors of stutterers. In one strategy, punishing consequences were programmed for stuttering, or disfluencies, whereas in a second strategy, reinforcing consequences were programmed for nonstuttered speech. The first strategy seeks to directly decrease stuttering, while the second strategy seeks to directly increase fluency. These are only procedural differences, because both strategies have the same clinical goal of decreased rate of stuttering and increased rate of fluency (Hegde, 1978). Eventually a third strategy also emerged in which reinforcement and punishment procedures were combined in various proportions.

Punishment of Stuttering

The beginning of the behavioral treatment of stuttering is often associated with the 1958 study of Flanagan, Goldiamond, and Azrin. (For a comprehensive review of the experimental literature related to stuttering as operant behavior, see Costello and Ingham, 1984.) The study by Flanagan and colleagues demonstrated that stuttering can be punished (decreased) as well as reinforced (increased) by contingent consequences. Within the next few years, Goldiamond began to use an operant treatment procedure that used the delayed auditory feedback (Goldiamond, 1965).

Additional clinical procedures based on operant conditioning were somewhat slow to emerge, however. During the 1960s, the operant research on stuttering was firmly established, but it remained mostly experimental. A series of studies conducted by Martin and Siegel and their associates explored the effects of various stimuli delivered contingent on the stutterings and disfluencies of stutterers and normal speakers, respectively (see Siegel, 1970; Martin and Ingham, 1973, for reviews). The initial studies used electric shock as the contingent stimulus. In subsequent studies, the effects of verbal stimuli such as "wrong," time-out from speaking, response cost, and aversive noise were analyzed. The bulk of the evidence of these studies showed that stutterings and disfluencies of stutterers and nonstutterers can be reduced by a variety of consequences, which led to the conclusion that these behaviors were operant responses.

Beyond such a general conclusion, the studies of Martin and Siegel and their associates revealed several problems and complexities, however. Electric shock, which is known to be one of the most powerful of the punishing stimuli proved to be a weak punisher of stuttering. On the average, only 19 per cent of stutterings were reduced by contingent shock.

This was by no means an impressive punishment effect. The verbal stimulus "wrong," on the other hand, was more effective, reducing stuttering by an average of 38 per cent. With nonstuttering speakers, a much greater reduction (60 per cent) in disfluencies was observed when they were instructed not to repeat or interject *and* punished with "wrong."

Additional problems became evident when a later study by Martin, St. Louis, Haroldson, and Hasbrouck (1975) essentially contradicted the long series of earlier investigations. In this study, Martin and colleagues analyzed the effects of continuous shock, which was terminated every time the subject stuttered (negative reinforcement), and response contingent shock (punishment). In the former condition, two of the five adult stutterers stuttered more, just as expected. But the other three subjects did not show a clear cut, consistent increase in stuttering, a finding inconsistent with the negative reinforcement paradigm. In the second condition, only two of the five stutterers showed a decrease in stuttering. In two other subjects, stuttering decreased initially but increased subsequently. The remaining subject's stuttering did not change at all under the shock condition. Martin and colleagues therefore concluded that the results "yield only equivocal support to the notion that stuttering is an operant response class" (1975, p. 489).

Other studies have shown that stuttering, especially part-word repetitions and sound prolongations, either do not change or actually increase when response-contingent shock is presented (Hegde, 1971; Janssen and Brutten, 1973). On the basis of these and other kinds of evidence, Brutten and Shoemaker (1967) have suggested that part-word repetitions and sound prolongations are not operants. On the other hand, a recent study by Costello and Hurst (1981) has suggested that a different form of punishment (time-out) may be more effective in reducing a variety of stuttering topographies, including some considered to be nonoperants by Brutten and Shoemaker (1967).

Although a consistent reduction in stuttering in the laboratory under punishment contingencies may be sufficient ground to suggest that these behaviors are operant, it may not serve as an adequate basis to develop treatment procedures. Long term clinical effects of shock, verbal punishers, and noise have not been established. There is no evidence that this type of punishment leads to lasting fluency. As a result, there are no treatment procedures that exclusively depend on the presentation of aversive stimuli. Somewhat ironically, this is so not because some studies have shown stuttering to increase under shock conditions, but because the magnitude of the demonstrated effect of aversive stimulus presentation has not been of clinical significance in research with adult stutterers.

Another kind of punishment procedure has produced more consistent, and hence less controversial, results. The procedure considered so far involves the *presentation* of known aversive stimuli contingent on stuttering responses. In this other procedure, aversive stimuli are not presented. Instead, positive reinforcers are withdrawn, contingent on response. Time-out (from positive reinforcement) and response cost are the two specific forms of punishment involved in this procedure. In time-out, assumed positive reinforcers are withheld for a brief period, typically 10 seconds, immediately following every stuttering. The subject is not allowed to talk during this period of time-out. This procedure has not only produced more consistent effects on stuttering, but also effects of greater magnitude than the presentation of known aversive stimuli. Several studies indicate that it is possible to generate virtually stutter-free speech with time-out, especially in young stutterers.

Unlike aversive stimulus presentation, time-out has been used as a clinical treatment program. Costello (1975, 1980) has described this procedure in detail along with data on its effectiveness. A stable baseline of stuttering is first established while the client talks and receives the normal kinds of reinforcers from the clinician (attention, smiles, etc.). The treatment is then started. Every stuttering is followed by a 10 second silent period signaled by a "stop" from the clinician. The clinician also avoids eye contact during the time-out period. After the 10 second interval, the clinician re-presents eye contact, smiles, and asks the stutterer to continue. Costello (1975) has found this procedure to be effective in reducing stuttering in three adult stutterers. A notable aspect of the Costello program is that in the latter stages of therapy, the stutterer is asked to remain fluent without the time-out contingency, and the contingency itself is faded out. By the end of the treatment program the stutterers were able to maintain fluency without the treatment contingency. A seven year followup on one of the three clients indicated that the treatment gains were maintained (Costello, 1980). Effectiveness of time-out in obtaining significant reductions in stuttering with adult stutterers has been reported by other investigators as well (Adams and Popelka, 1971; Haroldson, Martin, and Starr, 1968; Martin and Berndt, 1970).

It is possible that the response cost procedure will also prove to be an effective treatment procedure. A study by Halvorson (1971) showed that when each stuttering resulted in the loss of a point on a counter, stuttering frequency decreased. When one of the three subjects could exchange the remaining points for money, there was even a greater reduction in stuttering during the response cost condition. Because of these positive findings, additional research with this procedure seems desirable.

By way of summary, it can be stated that punishment of stuttering with the presentation of aversive stimuli alone has not been a basis of successful treatment strategies. Researchers' interest in this type of punishment has mostly been theoretic (Hegde, 1979). On the other hand, stuttering-contingent withdrawal of positive reinforcers seems to provide a more effective treatment strategy. Evidence suggests that if stuttering is to be punished, time-out and response cost are better alternatives than the presentation of aversive verbal, faradic, and noise stimuli. It must be noted, however, that more research is still needed to establish the long term effects of time-out and response cost. We need more replications and followup data. Also to be noted is that the effects of any punishment procedure, including the presentation of aversive stimuli, can be enhanced by combining it with positive reinforcement for fluency. Indeed, verbal "no" and "wrong" are often presented contingent on stuttering when fluency is positively reinforced. In time-out, too, continuous reinforcement is provided as long as the subject does not stutter.

Reinforcement of Fluency

It is known that most stutterers speak most of their syllables and words without stuttering most of the time, and behavioral technology can decrease as well as increase behaviors. If punishment of stuttering is not very effective, socially undesirable, or tends to generate emotional side effects, then positive reinforcement of nonstuttered utterances can be an attractive alternative. In fact, one of the significant trends in recent years has been to manipulate the parameters of fluency. This has been done both within and outside the behavioral framework. We shall review some of the major procedures of this kind in this section, recognizing that not all of these procedures are explicitly behavioral. They all share one thing in common: the main focus is either the fluent utterance as a *terminal* response, or a series of responses that *result* in nonstuttered speech.

To begin with, attempts were made to positively reinforce fluent utterances as terminal responses. Most of these were case studies with children, which lacked adequate controls and measurement of dependent variables. A review of these studies can be found in Martin and Ingham (1973), and Hegde (1978).

Martin and Siegel (1966) demonstrated in a laboratory study that a combination of punishment of stuttering and reinforcement of fluency can be effective. The effects of the two procedures were confounded in that study, however. Another experimental study in which three adult stutterers were reinforced for speaking fluently was reported by Hegde and Brutten (1977). During the first two (baserate) and the last two (extinction) sessions of this experiment, disfluencies and fluent intervals were measured in the absence of reinforcement. During the middle two experimental sessions, every preselected interval of fluent oral reading was reinforced by the presentation of a dime. When compared to the baserate and the extinction sessions, all three subjects exhibited a greater number of fluent intervals when those intervals were reinforced.

Although it is evident that fluency can be technically reinforced, there are not many studies in which generalized fluency has been established exclusively through reinforcement procedures. It seems that when no attempt is made to alter the speech pattern of the stutterer, reinforcement of stutter-free utterances may not be powerful enough to generate clinically significant (and durable) fluency. This seems to be especially true with the adult stutterer.

Combined Reinforcement and Punishment and Procedures Requiring Altered Speech Patterns

It is thus clear that either the straightforward punishment of stuttering or an exclusive reinforcement of unaltered fluent utterances has not resulted in a comprehensive and successful treatment program for adult stutterers. Procedurally, the two distinct strategies can be combined, however. And this is exactly what is done in several clinical programs.

It is known that concurrent conditioning of reciprocal behaviors is more effective than the exclusive strategies of reinforcement or punishment. However, most of the treatment programs that use both reinforcement and punishment contingencies have also changed the response topography on which those contingencies are placed. Reinforcement is often made contingent not upon the typical stutter-free (fluent) utterance, but upon an *altered pattern* of speech (such as slow or prolonged speech). Treatment programs of this variety have been described by Ingham and Andrews (1973), Ingham (1975), Ingham and Packman (1977), Ryan (1974), Ryan and Van Kirk (1974), Mowrer (1975, 1979, 1982), Howie, Tanner, and Andrews (1981), Webster (1974, 1979) and others. Although there are significant differences across these treatment programs, all of them recognize the importance of the behavioral contingency involving reinforcing consequences programmed for target behaviors and punishing consequences provided for stuttered utterances.

Ingham and Andrews and their associates have conducted a significant series of experiments on stuttering therapy over the past several years. They have analyzed the effects of a variety of treatment procedures with one of the most rigorous measurement procedures ever used in the assessment of stuttering therapy. The treatment program administered by Ingham and Andrews and their associates in Australia is very intensive. In fact, the stutterers are hospitalized for three weeks, during which time they receive 12 hours of daily treatment. Because of their strong commitment to experimental methodology, the treatment program associated with the names of Ingham and Andrews has undergone considerable change over the years. It will not be possible to review all of those changes, although they are interesting from the clinical research viewpoint. (See Ingham, 1984, and Ingham and Lewis, 1978, for reviews, along with Howie, Tanner, and Andrews, 1981).

Initially, a form of rhythmic speech called syllable-timed speech was employed, but it was later abandoned. The authors then added a system of token economy to the prolonged speech method of Curlee and Perkins (1969). In this arrangement, hospitalized stutterers earned tokens by exhibiting nonstuttered speech in order to gain access to various activities, privileges, and necessities. Stuttering exhibited during the several daily assessment sessions resulted in the loss of tokens according to a predetermined schedule. Ingham and Andrews (Ingham, 1975; Ingham and Andrews, 1973) have also used delayed auditory feedback (DAF) to establish prolonged, nonstuttered speech which is eventually shaped back to normal rate. Systematic techniques designed to obtain generalization of treatment effects to the client's natural environment are included. Rate of speech and stuttering frequency are measured throughout the course of treatment and generalization phases.

A recent report describes the current program based on the Ingham and Andrews model as now used by Howie and colleagues (1981). The program is designed to teach Smooth Motion Speech, which is characterized by "slow onset of phonation, continuous airflow and movement of articulators throughout each utterance, and extension of vowels and consonant duration" (Howie et al., 1981, p. 104). The rate is initially slowed to about 50 syllables per minute (SPM). As a result, the speech is virtually stutter-free from the beginning. The normal rate is shaped while the client remains stutter-free in each of the successive stages of this shaping process. Instructions and modeling have replaced the delayed auditory feedback once used to initiate slow speech. Another significant change is that the token economy is no longer used. (See Howie and Woods, 1982, and Ingham, 1983, for an interesting exchange regarding this issue.) Informative feedback and small monetary rewards, which were found to be quite effective, are used to reinforce nonstuttered speech.

The report by Howie and colleagues (1981) offers data on 36 adult stutterers whose speech rate and percentage syllables stuttered were measured on the last day of treatment, after two months in the maintenance phase, and three to nine months after dismissal. Additional data were also offered on 43 stutterers who were followed up 12 to 18 months after treatment. The results showed that virtually all clients stuttered considerably less than before treatment. Varying degrees of relapse were evident in 30 to 60 per cent of the clients, however. Only 50 per cent of the treated clients were fully satisfied with their fluency. Howie and colleagues estimated that with their treatment procedure a stutterer "has a 70% chance of having substantially improved speech and increased speaking confidence 12 months after intensive treatment" (1981, p. 108).

Ryan's well known programmed approach to stuttering modification consists of two major strategies: delayed auditory feedback (DAF) and graduated increase in length and complexity of utterance (GILCU). The treatment of choice is DAF for older or more severely affected stutterers, and GILCU for younger or less severely affected stutterers (Ryan, 1979). Initially, DAF is used to establish slow, prolonged, nonstuttered speech. The amount of DAF is then faded in gradual steps, and the client approaches fluency with normal or near normal speech rate. Successful completion of graduated steps is verbally reinforced, and branching programs to counter failures are specified. An instance of stuttering requires the client to begin the treatment step anew. Both the GILCU and the DAF programs have establishment, transfer, and maintenance phases. Ryan and Van Kirk have offered data on a large number of clients, a majority of whom are reported to have sustained vastly improved fluency in their natural environments (Ryan, 1979).

Mowrer's (1975, 1979, 1982) stuttering treatment program contains several specific steps grouped into establishment, transfer, and maintenance phases. Reinforcing and punishing consequences are programmed for fluency and stuttering, respectively. The program establishes fluency in oral reading and conversational speech, starting with the oral reading of single words. The number of words read is increased gradually until a typical prose selection can be read at a rate of 100 or more words per minute. In most of the early steps, a 95 per cent fluency criterion is required, whereas in the final steps, 98 per cent fluency is expected. The next phase is designed to establish fluency in conversational speech. Transfer and maintenance phases follow. A notable feature of Mowrer's program is that during the initial steps of treatment, 1000 Hz tones are used as stimuli to evoke and time the fluent utterance. The tone stimuli are presented in such a way that the rate is reduced. Eventually, the tone is faded and the rate shaped back to normal. Mowrer (1975) has offered data on 20 stutterers who completed various stages of treatment. Those who were able to complete most of the steps of the program were able to achieve fluency at 99 per cent or better.

A program of research almost exclusively concerned with the direct treatment of stuttering is that of Webster (1974, 1979). Although Webster does not describe his current treatment procedure as being strictly operant, his methodologic and conceptual framework is almost identical to that of operant conditioning and radical behaviorism. Webster analyzes and treats stuttering and speech production strictly at the behavioral level, is highly skeptical of much of the current speculative theorizing, rejects indirect treatment of stuttering through reduction of anxiety or negative attitudes, and has repeatedly urged his colleagues to gather objective, empirical evidence so that we are not "doomed to live forever within the jungle of opinion" (Webster, 1979, p. 221).

Webster's Precision Fluency Shaping Program is another intensive treatment program. About 100 hours of direct treatment are given in a 19 day program. Earlier, Webster had used DAF to establish slow and nonstuttered speech, but later he abandoned it because it did not teach the stutterer those specific behaviors that resulted in fluency. Therefore, Webster began to search for those behaviors that seemed necessary for fluency. His current program consists of teaching stutterers the production of these assumed fluency prerequisites, which include the prolongation of speech sounds (which, ironically, was what he earlier used DAF to achieve), full breath, gentle initiation of phonation, and smooth syllable transitions. He uses an instrument known as the Voice Monitor for teaching appropriate voice onset responses.

Shames and his colleagues have developed and refined an operant therapy procedure aimed at stutter-free speech (Shames and Egolf, 1976; Shames and Florance, 1980). Like several other programs, the recent Shames and Florance program makes use of DAF in the initial phases to slow down the rate of speech and induce stutter-free speech. Continuous phonation throughout the utterance is also required. Establishment of the volitional control of speech is the major goal of the initial phase. In the second phase of treatment, stutterers learn procedures of self-monitoring and self-reinforcement of stutter-free speech. The third phase involves activities designed to promote generalization of treatment effects. In the fourth and the final phase, the stutterer is taught how to maintain stutter-free speech without constant monitoring. A five year followup is also a part of the treatment program. The followup data reported by Shames and Florance (1980) showed that 35 of 37 persons who were examined no longer stuttered, although no quantitative data have been offered. The authors were concerned about the fact that 38 per cent of those who started their treatment terminated it prematurely.

Therapeutic Packages

Another recent trend in stuttering therapy has been to combine several procedures into a therapeutic package. As our review so far suggests, exclusive use of a single technique is a less common practice. Most therapies are a combination of different procedures and targets. A therapeutic package developed by Perkins and his colleagues illustrates this. After obtaining some disappointing results with psychotherapy, Perkins began to analyze and treat stuttering at the behavioral level. He has found the objective behavioral approach to be more effective in reducing stuttering than the subjective and indirect psychotherapeutic approaches (Perkins, 1973a, 1973b, 1979). At the level of the dependent variable (responses), Perkins considers stuttering to be a discoordination of the basic processes involved in the production of speech (Perkins, Bell, Johnson, and Stock, 1979; Perkins, Rudas, Johnson, and Bell, 1976). From a conceptual standpoint, treatment is aimed at teaching the stutterer to use respiratory, phonatory, and articulatory processes in a coordinated manner to produce and maintain fluent speech. Perkins believes that treatment limited to a behavioral establishment of fluency is not complete, however. Psychotherapeutic discussions are also considered of value in coping with persistent use of avoidance tactics.

The initial goal of the Perkins program is to establish slow, nonstuttered oral reading with the help of 250 milliseconds of delayed auditory feedback. Prolongation of syllables is emphasized. In gradual steps, the duration of the delayed auditory feedback is reduced. The next goal is to teach a normal breathflow with easy vocal attacks. Speaking short phrases with sufficient air capacity and continuous airflow is the specific target. Normal prosody is then taught. Next, slow normal speech with DAF is established in conversational speech mode. Establishing a normal speech rate and fading the DAF are the next targets. A clear voice of sufficient loudness is also shaped. Finally, generalization procedures are implemented along with additional counseling (Perkins 1973a, 1973b).

Perkins, Rudas, Johnson, Michael, and Curlee (1974) have published data on the effectiveness of their treatment program. The effects of therapy are evaluated in terms of the number of syllables spoken and stuttered, along with judgments of normalcy of treated fluency, self evaluations, and personality measures. This evaluation has shown that in 17 stutterers, the percentage of syllables stuttered decreased from an average of 9.04 per cent before the treatment to 1.04 per cent at the end of the treatment. Six months later, the rate of stuttering was still only 1.73 per cent. The relapse of stuttering to varying degrees was a problem, however. Only 53 per cent of the treated clients maintained relatively permanent fluency.

Another therapeutic package whose predominant feature is regulated breathing has been described by Azrin and colleagues (1979). The regulated breathing component involves an extended duration of inhalation, an immediate exhalation of some air, and uninterrupted, smooth airflow throughout the utterance. The other components of the program include slightly prolonged vowels, general relaxation training, clear formulation of thoughts before speaking, deliberate pausing at natural junctures, and speaking only a few words at a time. Azrin and colleagues (1979) have reported that the method can eliminate stuttering rapidly. The authors have offered some evidence based upon the clients' own reports on the frequency of stuttering in natural environment. This certainly appears to be a desirable procedure, but its reliability is yet to be established.

There have been several attempts at replicating the results of Azrin and colleagues (1979), but unfortunately the results have not been consistent or supportive (Andrews and Tanner, 1982; Ladouceur, Boudreau, and Theberge, 1981; Poppen, Nunn, and Hook, 1977; Williamson, Epstein, and Coburn, 1981).

Some Critical Research Needs in Stuttering Therapy

A review of the current status of stuttering therapy suggests that although some significant progress has been made, there still are some critical research needs that the clinicians must be aware of. Issues that need to be researched include the effects of treatment components, both independent and interactive; "normalcy" of treated fluency; and generalization and maintenance of treatment effects.

Effects of Treatment Components

It is evident that regardless of theoretic differences, some components are common to several different treatment programs. To a certain extent, the appearance of therapeutic diversity may be due to differences in the language used to describe the same or similar target behaviors and procedures. It is probable that theoretic biases add certain components to a hypothetical treatment program while subtracting certain other components from it. How much of this addition and subtraction is only in the description of techniques and not in their practice is an interesting question, the answer to which might simultaneously delight and dismay clinicians practicing on the opposite sides of theoretic fences. In any case, the existence of common elements across treatment programs raises some important questions for the clinician. Essentially, we need to find out the relative effects of different treatment components along with their combined and interactive effects. It appears that the descriptions of several of the more successful treatment programs include some form of modified phonation, rate reduction, airflow management, and, to a lesser extent, relaxed movement of the articulators.

Modified phonation seems to have two components: gentle or soft vocal onset and prolongation of speech sounds. The prolonged speech technique has its historical roots (see Ingham, 1984), but the modern interest in it is due mostly to the work of Goldiamond (1965) involving delayed auditory feedback. Currently, prolonged speech is more often induced by clinician instructions and modeling. Much of the recent research on stuttering therapy with adult stutterers has been done with some form of prolonged speech. This has raised the possibility that several other techniques, such as "airflow therapy," "regulated breathing," or "rate control," among others, may be just variations of prolonged speech (Ingham, 1984). Furthermore, in their meta-analysis of stuttering treatment research, Andrews, Guitar, and Howie (1980) have concluded that "treatments based on training a stutterer in prolonged speech and gentle onset techniques are superior to other types of treatment" (p. 305).

A review of recent research on treatment of stuttering suggests that programs based on "pure paradigms" are relatively rare. Most treatment programs include different components, and unfortunately, the name of one of the components often becomes a label for the entire program. Azrin and Nunn's (1977) "regulated breathing" procedure is a case in point. Regulated breathing is but one component in the program, which includes relaxation, "deliberate pauses in speech, thinking out beforehand what you wish to say, adding stress sounds to words, and speaking a few words at a time" (p. 102). Thus, treatment labels (and even descriptions that are often vague) may not necessarily suggest the critical treatment factor in a program.

Equally significant is the possibility that a given treatment component may have effects on other components that are neither described nor measured by the clinical researcher. "Gentle phonatory onset," for example, may affect the rate of speech, which may then become an added and unidentified treatment component. Explicit management of breathstream can induce gentle onset and reduced rate. When the rate is slowed down, the breathing pattern may be changed. Mere simplification of response topography (single words, short phrases) may have an effect on speech rate, breathing patterns, and phonation. Until such possibilities are experimentally ruled out, it may be prudent not to identify the "most effective" treatment component nor to reduce different components to a single one, such as prolonged speech. As Ingham (1984) has pointed out, "it is far from clear which treatment component(s) is necessary either to establish improved speech or to transfer and maintain treatment effects" (p. 372).

What is urgently needed is an experimental analysis of the effects of specific treatment components on the frequency of stuttering. A recent report by Ingham, Montgomery, and Ulliana (1983) is noteworthy in this respect. Their study suggests that it is possible to gain experimental control over a narrowly defined behavior, such as specified durations of phonation. We can expect to understand the treatment process better with this kind of research, in which specific treatment targets are isolated and experimentally manipulated. Once the effects on stuttering of manipulation of different treatment targets are isolated, their interactive effects can be studied. Research on the interaction of different treatment targets and procedures can help combine the most effective treatment components into a single treatment package.

Normalcy of Treated Fluency

A majority of currently effective treatment techniques alter the normal prosodic features of speech. Whether the treatment component is regulated breathing, prolonged speech, gentle onset, or rate reduction, the resulting nonstuttered speech is often deliberate, slow, and devoid of typical intonational patterns. This result is not socially acceptable, and the therapeutic effects may not generalize or last, simply because of this problem. Therefore, concurrent with the establishment of nonstuttered speech, the clinician needs to shape the normal prosodic features.

It seems that before the clinician can shape the normal prosodic features of fluent speech, they must be identified. Research on this issue has barely begun. It is known that listeners can usually distinguish the speech of treated stutterers from that of nonstutterers (Ingham and Packman, 1978; Runyan and Adams, 1978, 1979). Some recent evidence suggests that a critical variable that sets the treated stutterer's speech apart from a nonstutterer's speech may be the rate (Prosek and Runyan, 1983).

It is evident that if the clinical objective is nonstuttered speech that is also not readily distinguished from the speech of normal speakers, shaping of the normal rate should be a part of treatment programs.

Some empirical issues are associated with the need to shape normal rate. Normal rate is a variable phenomenon across individuals. Even a given individual's rate may vary across situations. It is doubtful whether a "norm" can be used in the rate shaping process. It is probably necessary to find out, in replicated series, what speech rates minimize or eliminate discrimination between the speech samples of treated stutterers and normal speakers.

Another potential issue associated with rate control and shaping is whether treated stutterers can sustain both fluency and a rate that cannot be discriminated. Since it seems clear that a discriminated rate is not socially acceptable, clinicians will have to strive towards an indiscriminable ("normal") rate. Nevertheless, whether such an indiscriminable rate is also the one that can help maintain fluency in treated stutterers is yet to be researched.

Finally, the normalcy of treated fluency may not entirely be a function of a certain rate. Rate-related variables are in essence temporal, but there may be factors such as intonational patterns that may not be temporal but topographical. It is possible that in addition to shaping an indiscriminable rate, a certain intonational pattern may also have to be shaped. Clinical experience suggests that when clients begin to increase their rate, their intonational patterns also become indiscriminable. If this is experimentally verified, it would then mean that certain rate and intonational patterns belong to the same response class.

The process of establishing indiscriminable parameters of speech in stutterers may require both measurement procedures and descriptions of those parameters. Martin, Haroldson, and Triden (1984) have demonstrated that "speech naturalness" is a property that can be scaled. However, what temporal and topographical factors are necessary for a judgment of "naturalness" is not clear. As was suggested, rate and intonational patterns are among the most important of the variables. One can systematically manipulate (or shape) these variables independently to see how judgments of "naturalness" are affected.

Generalization and Maintenance of Treatment Effects

Recent advances in the treatment of stuttering suggest that it is possible to induce stutter-free speech patterns within the clinic setting in almost all stutterers, but the treatment effects do not always generalize; and if they do generalize, the effects may not be maintained over time. In the basic research on learning, generalization of conditioned behaviors was considered a natural consequence of stimulus and response similarity. In applied research, however, deficient behaviors that need extensive clinical treatment often do not generalize to the natural environment. This may be so because the treatment environment is unusual (highly discriminated), and the natural environment is still a discriminative stimulus for the deficient behaviors. In any case, only in recent years has the problem of generalization and maintenance been systematically addressed by applied researchers (e.g., Stokes and Baer, 1977).

Most of the researched stuttering treatment programs include a generalization or maintenance phase (Howie, Tanner, and Andrews, 1981; Ingham and Andrews, 1971; Ingham, 1984a; Mowrer, 1975; Perkins, 1973b; Ryan, 1974; Shames and Florance, 1980). There is some evidence, however, that a certain amount of generalization can be obtained in the absence of specific procedures. Most often, such unprogrammed generalization has been observed when child stutterers were treated with stuttering-contingent time out (see Ingham, 1984a, 1984b, for a review of studies on generalization tactics). Nevertheless, most stutterers, especially adults, need specific procedures to achieve generalized and maintained treatment effects.

There are several methodologic and conceptual issues relative to how generalization is programmed or measured (Ingham, 1984a, 1984b). Generalization typically refers to the occurrence of learned behaviors under various nontreatment conditions and response modes. However, when such generalization is not observed, specific procedures may be applied with the consequence that the resulting response rate may or may not be a product of pure generalization. For instance, the treatment variable may be introduced to the home situation, the parents of a stuttering child may be taught to manage the reinforcement contingencies, or an adult stutterer may be taught some self-management techniques. In situations such as these, it is difficult to determine when the treatment ends and the process of spontaneous generalization begins. Purely from a clinical standpoint, this may be a moot issue, however. If specific procedures are needed to obtain generalized and maintained fluency, they must then be implemented, regardless of whether the effects of such procedures would be considered (technically) to be generalization.

Various tactics for producing generalization have been identified in applied behavioral research (Stokes and Baer, 1977) and in the particular context of stuttering treatment (Ingham, 1984a, 1984b). In principle, generalization and maintenance procedures are designed to minimize discrimination between the stutterer's natural environment and the treatment setting, while simultaneously creating everyday discriminative stimuli for the treated fluency, and to teach self-monitoring skills so that certain treatment variables become ubiquitous.

The first set of techniques is based on the assumption that discrimination prevents generalization and that the client's everyday situations should contain stimuli associated with the target behaviors. Initially, the clinician and the treatment setting become the discriminative stimuli for stutter-free speech while those stimuli are absent in the stutterer's everyday situations. Techniques that minimize discrimination between the clinical setting and the natural environment can simultaneously create new discriminative stimuli for stutter-free speech in nonclinical settings. The latter phases of most treatment programs, for instance, are often loosely structured so that the highly discriminated treatment setting begins to approximate everyday situations. Informal treatment sessions may be held outside the typical clinical setting. The clinician may accompany the stutterer to a store or a restaurant, and manage the treatment contingencies in a subtle manner. Family members or even unfamiliar persons may be invited to the treatment sessions. Treatment may be shifted across response modes such as reading, monologue, and conversational speech. Parents, teachers, siblings, or spouses may be trained to reinforce stutter-free speech in home and school.

The second set of techniques is based on the assumption that if stutterers themselves can manipulate some treatment components, then technically the treatment can be applied in every situation. If the techniques used are effective at all, stutter-free speech should be durable across situations and over time. Those treatment models that teach the stutterer certain skills necessary for stutter-free speech are probably better able to exploit this strategy (Azrin and Nunn, 1977; Perkins, 1973a, 1973b; Webster, 1974). If skills such as reduced rate, gentle phonatory onset, or continuous airflow are part of the treatment program, the stutterer can be taught to maintain them in everyday situations as long as the resulting stutter-free speech is socially acceptable. Within the punishment strategy, there is some evidence that stuttering contingent time-out can be self-administered and thus can help sustain treatment gains (James, 1981; Martin and Haroldson, 1982).

It is evident that a variety of generalization and maintenance strategies have been a part of many treatment programs. Nevertheless, there are very few controlled studies showing that a given strategy was indeed effective. We do not know the relative effects of different strategies. It is possible that some of the generalization strategies are not effective at all. Once again, we need controlled research to document the independent, relative, and interactive effects of generalization and maintenance strategies.

Concluding Remarks

It is difficult to say that in the recent years some startlingly new or dramatically effective treatment procedures have been developed. Nonetheless, significant progress has been made in the treatment of stuttering. There is now a growing confidence within the profession that a more complete treatment of stuttering is within our reach.

In the judgment of this reviewer, it is better to focus research on stuttering therapy on the *response topography* that needs to be taught or modified, rather than on the procedure with which the targets are accomplished. A reasonably effective technology of behavior change is available, and has been for some time now. We know how to set occasions for responses and arrange consequences that produce desirable changes in those responses. Somewhat ironically, and as Webster (1979) has recognized, what we have been searching for is the target response itself. Much of the research efforts have been concerned with *what* to modify, not *how*. Note that gentle phonation or continuous airflow refer not to independent variables (treatment), but to dependent variables (responses). Additional research with this conceptual framework can be fruitful.

One would hope that in coming years, significant progress can be made in identifying critical treatment variables in relation to specific response properties. Most stuttering therapies are still a conglomeration of treatment variables and response topographies. There is no assurance that all of the described components of a treatment program are always used by the same clinician or replicated by others. We urgently need research that can identify independent, relative, and interactive effects of treatment components and the advantages of focusing on one or more specific response topographies.

Most researchers recognize that we need to develop more effective techniques of generalization and maintenance of treatment effects. Adequate long term followup and measurement of treatment effects through objective procedures are becoming a part of treatment programs. One can expect significant progress in all of these areas. Although there is plenty of room for improvement, research on stuttering therapy is more data based now than ever before, and this might be the most significant of the recent advances.

References

Adams, M. R., and Hotchkiss, J. (1973). Some reactions and responses of stutterers to a miniaturized metronome and metronome-conditioning therapy: Three case reports. *Behavior Therapy, 4,* 565–569.

Adams, M. R., and Popelka, G. (1971). The influence of "time-out" on stutterers and their disfluency. *Behavior Therapy, 2,* 334–449.

Andrews, G., and Cutler, J. (1974). Stuttering therapy: The relation between changes in symptom level and attitudes. *Journal of Speech and Hearing Disorders, 39,* 312–319.

Andrews, G., Guitar, B., and Howie, P. (1980). Meta-analysis of the effects of stuttering treatment. *Journal of Speech and Hearing Disorders, 45,* 287–308.

Andrews, G., and Tanner, S. (1982). Stuttering treatment: An attempt to replicate the regulated-breathing method. *Journal of Speech and Hearing Disorders, 42,* 138–140.

Azrin, N. H., and Nunn, R. G. (1977). *Habit control in a day.* New York: Simon and Schuster.

Azrin, N. H., Nunn, R. B., and Frantz, S. E. (1979). Comparison of regulated breathing versus abbreviated desensitization on reported stuttering episodes. *Journal of Speech and Hearing Disorders, 44,* 331–339.

Berman, P. A., and Brady, J. P. (1973). Miniaturized metronomes in the treatment of stuttering: A survey of clinicians' experiences. *Journal of Behavior Therapy and Experimental Psychiatry, 4,* 117–119.

Bloodstein, O. (1975). Stuttering as tension and fragmentation. In J. Eisenson (Ed.), *Stuttering: A second symposium.* New York: Harper and Row.

Bloodstein, O. (1981). *A handbook of stuttering* (3rd ed.). Chicago: National Easter Seal Society.

Boudreau, L. A., and Jeffrey, C. L. (1973). Stuttering treated by desensitization. *Journal of Behavior Therapy and Experimental Psychiatry, 4,* 209–212.

Brady, J. P. (1971). Metronome-conditioned speech retraining for stuttering. *Behavior Therapy, 2,* 129–150.

Brutten, G. J. (1975). Stuttering: Topography, assessment, and behavior change strategies. In J. Eisenson (Ed.), *Stuttering: A second symposium.* New York: Harper and Row.

Brutten, G. J., and Shoemaker, D. J. (1967). *The modification of stuttering.* Englewood Cliffs, NJ: Prentice-Hall.

Burgraff, R. I., (1974). The efficacy of systematic desensitization via imagery as a therapeutic technique with stutterers. *British Journal of Disorders of Communication, 9,* 134–139.

Cherry, C., Sayers, B., and Marland, P. M. (1955). Experiments on the complete supression of stammering. *Nature, 176,* 874–875.

Costello, J. M. (1975). The establishment of fluency with time-out procedures: Three case studies. *Journal of Speech and Hearing Disorders, 40,* 216–231.

Costello, J. M. (1980). Operant conditioning and the treatment of stuttering. In W. H. Perkins (Ed.), Strategies in stuttering therapy. *Seminars in Speech, Language and Hearing, 1,* 311–325. New York: Thieme-Stratton.

Costello, J. M., and Hurst, M. T. (1981). An analysis of the relationship among stuttering behaviors. *Journal of Speech and Hearing Research, 24,* 247–256.

Costello, J. M., and Ingham, R. J. (1984). Stuttering as an operant disorder. In R. Curlee and W. H. Perkins (Eds.), *Nature and treatment of stuttering: New directions.* San Diego: College-Hill Press.

Dewar, A., Dewar, A. D., and Barnes, H. E. (1976). Automatic triggering of auditory feedback masking in stammering and cluttering. *British Journal of Disorders of Communication, 11,* 19–26.

Erickson, R. L. (1969). Assessing communication attitudes among stutterers. *Journal of Speech and Hearing Research, 12,* 711–724.

Curlee, R. F., and Perkins, W. H. (1969). Conversational rate control therapy for stuttering. *Journal of Speech and Hearing Disorders, 34,* 245–250.

Flanagan, B., Goldiamond, I., and Azrin, N. H. (1958). Operant stuttering: The control of stuttering behavior through response-contingent consequences. *Journal of the Experimental Analysis of Behavior, 1,* 173–177.

Garber, S. F., and Martin, R. R. (1974). The effects of white noise on the frequency of stuttering. *Journal of Speech and Hearing Disorders, 17,* 73–79.

Goldiamond, I. (1965). Stuttering and fluency as manipulatable operant response classes. In L. Krasner and L. P. Ullman (Eds.), *Research in behavior modification.* New York: Holt, Rinehart and Winston.

Gregory, H. H. (1979). Controversial issues: Statement and review of literature. In H. H. Gregory (Ed.), *Controversies in stuttering therapy.* Baltimore: University Park Press.

Guitar, B. (1975). Reduction of stuttering frequency using analog electromyographic feedback. *Journal of Speech and Hearing Research, 18,* 672–685.

Guitar, B. (1976). Pretreatment factors associated with the outcome of stuttering therapy. *Journal of Speech and Hearing Research, 19,* 590–600.

Guitar, B. (1981). A correction to "A response to Ingham's critique." *Journal of Speech and Hearing Disorders, 46,* 440.

Guitar, B., and Bass, C. (1978). Stuttering therapy: The relation between attitude change and long-term outcome. *Journal of Speech and Hearing Disorders, 43,* 392–400.

Hanna, R., Wilfling, F., and McNeil, B. (1975). A biofeedback treatment for stuttering. *Journal of Speech and Hearing Disorders, 40,* 270–273.

Haroldson, S. K., Martin, R. R., and Starr, C. (1968). Time-out as a punishment for stuttering. *Journal of Speech and Hearing Research, 11,* 560–566.

Halvorson, J. (1971). The effect on stuttering frequency of pairing punishment (response cost) with reinforcement. *Journal of Speech and Hearing Research, 14,* 356–364.

Hegde, M. N. (1970). Stuttering: A case study in the scientific method. *Journal of the All India Institute of Speech and Hearing, 1,* 104–122.

Hegde, M. N. (1971). The effect of shock on stuttering. *Journal of the All India Institute of Speech and Hearing, 2,* 104–110.

Hegde, M. N. (1978). Fluency and fluency disorders: Their definition, measurement, and modification. *Journal of Fluency Disorders, 3,* 51–71.

Hegde, M. N. (1979). Stuttering as operant behavior. *Journal of Speech and Hearing Research, 22,* 657–671.

Hegde, M. N., and Brutten, G. J., (1977). Reinforcing fluency in stutterers. An experimental study. *Journal of Fluency Disorders, 2,* 21–28.

Howie, P. M., Tanner, S., and Andrews, G. (1981). Short- and long-term outcome in an intensive treatment program for adult stutterers. *Journal of Speech and Hearing Disorders, 46,* 104–109.

Howie, P. M., and Woods, C. L. (1982). Token reinforcement during the instatement and shaping of fluency in the treatment of stuttering. *Journal of Applied Behavior Analysis, 15,* 55–64.

Hull, C. L. (1951). *Essentials of behavior.* New Haven, CT: Yale University Press.

Ingham, R. J. (1975). Operant methodology in stuttering therapy. In J. Eisenson (Ed.), *Stuttering: A second symposium.* New York: Harper and Row.

Ingham, R. J. (1979). Comment on "Stuttering therapy: The relation between attitude change and long-term outcome." *Journal of Speech and Hearing Disorders, 44,* 397–400.

Ingham, R. J. (1983). On token reinforcement and stuttering therapy: Another view on the findings reported by Howie and Woods (1982). *Journal of Applied Behavior Analysis, 16,* 465–470.

Ingham, R. J. (1984a). *Stuttering and behavior therapy: Current status and experimental foundations*. San Diego: College-Hill Press.

Ingham, R. J. (1984b). Generalization and maintenance in the treatment of stuttering. In W. H. Perkins and R. Curlee (Eds.), *Nature and treatment of stuttering: New directions*. San Diego: College-Hill Press.

Ingham, R. J., and Andrews, G. (1971). Stuttering: The quality of fluency after treatment. *Journal of Communication Disorders., 4,* 279-288.

Ingham, R. J., and Andrews, G. (1973). An analysis of a token economy in stuttering therapy. *Journal of Applied Behavior Analysis, 6,* 219-229.

Ingham, R. J., and Lewis, J. I. (1978, Autumn). Behavior therapy and stuttering: And the story grows. *Human Communication,* pp. 125-152.

Ingham, R. J., Montgomery, J., and Ulliana, L. (1983). The effects of manipulating phonation duration on stuttering. *Journal of Speech and Hearing Research, 26,* 579-587.

Ingham, R. J., and Packman, A. (1977). Treatment and generalization effects in an experimental treatment for a stutterer using contingency management and rate control. *Journal of Speech and Hearing Disorders, 42,* 394-407.

Ingham, R. J., and Packman, A. (1978). Perceptual assessment of normalcy of speech following stuttering therapy. *Journal of Speech and Hearing Research, 21,* 63-73.

Ingham, R. J., Southwood, H., and Horsburgh, G. (1981). Some effects of the Edinburgh Masker on stuttering during oral reading and spontaneous speech. *Journal of Fluency Disorders, 6,* 135-154.

James, J. E. (1981). Behavioral self-control of stuttering using time-out from speaking. *Journal of Applied Behavior Analysis, 14,* 25-37.

Janssen, P., and Brutten, G. J., (1973). The differential effects of punishment of oral prolongations. In Y. Lebrun and R. Hoops (Eds.), *Neurolinguistic approaches to stuttering*. The Hague, Netherlands: Mouton.

Johnson, W. (1961). *Stuttering and what you can do about it*. Minneapolis: University of Minnesota Press.

Jonas, G. (1977). Stuttering: *The disorder of many theories*. New York: Farrar, Straus, & Giroux.

Ladouceur, R., Boudreau, L., and Theberge, S. (1981). Awareness training and regulated breathing method in modification of stuttering. *Perceptual and Motor Skills, 53,* 187-194.

Lanyon, R. I., Barrington, C. C., and Newman, A. C. (1976). Modification of stuttering through EMG biofeedback: A preliminary study. *Behavior Therapy, 7,* 96-103.

Martin, R. R., and Berndt, L. A. (1970). The effects of time-out on stuttering in a 12 year old boy. *Exceptional Children, 37,* 303-304.

Martin, R. R., and Haroldson, S. K. (1969). The effects of two treatment procedures on stuttering. *Journal of Communication Disorders, 2,* 115-125.

Martin, R. R., and Haroldson, S. K., (1982). Contingent self-stimulation for stuttering. *Journal of Speech and Hearing Disorders, 47,* 407-413.

Martin, R. R., Haroldson, S. K., and Triden, K. A. (1984). Stuttering and speech naturalness. *Journal of Speech and Hearing Disorders, 49,* 53-58.

Martin, R. R., and Ingham, R. J. (1973). Stuttering. In B. Lahey (Ed.), *The modification of language behavior*. Springfield, IL: Charles C Thomas.

Martin, R. R, and Siegel, G. M. (1966). The effects of simultaneously punishing stuttering and rewarding fluency. *Journal of Speech and Hearing Research, 9,* 466-475.

Martin, R. R., St. Louis, K., Haroldson, S. K., and Hasbrouck, J. (1975). Punishment and negative reinforcement of stuttering using electric shock. *Journal of Speech and Hearing Research, 18,* 478-490.

Moleski, R., and Tosi, D. J. (1976). Comparative psychotherapy: Rational emotive therapy versus systematic desensitization in the treatment of stuttering. *Journal of Consulting and Clinical Psychology, 44,* 309–311.

Mowrer, D. E. (1975). An instructional program to increase fluent speech of stutterers. *Journal of Fluency Disorders, 1,* 25–35.

Mowrer, D. E. (1979). *A program to establish fluent speech.* Columbus, OH: Charles E. Merrill.

Mowrer, D. E. (1982). Treatment procedures for stutterers. In D. E. Mowrer and J. L. Case, *Clinical management of speech disorders.* Rockville, MD: Aspen.

Ost, L. G., Gotestam, K. G., and Melin, L. A. (1976). A controlled study of two behavioral methods in the treatment of stuttering. *Behavior Therapy, 7,* 587–592.

Perkins, W. H. (1973a). Replacement of stuttering with normal speech: I. Rationale. *Journal of Speech and Hearing Disorders, 38,* 283–294.

Perkins, W. H. (1973b). Replacement of stuttering with normal speech: II. Clinical procedures. *Journal of Speech and Hearing Disorders, 38,* 295–303.

Perkins, W. H. (1979). From psychoanalysis to discoordination. In H. H. Gregory (Ed.), *Controversies about stuttering therapy.* Baltimore: University Park Press.

Perkins, W. H. (1981). Implications of scientific research for treatment of stuttering: A lecture. *Journal of Fluency Disorders, 6,* 155–162.

Perkins, W. H., Bell, J., Johnson, L., and Stocks, J. (1979). Phone rate and the effective planning time hypothesis of stuttering. *Journal of Speech and Hearing Research, 22,* 747–755.

Perkins, W. H., Rudas, J., Johnson, L., and Bell, J. (1976). Stuttering: Discoordination of phonation with articulation and respiration. *Journal of Speech and Hearing Research, 19,* 509–522.

Perkins, W. H., Rudas, J., Johnson, L., Michael, W. B., and Curlee, R. F. (1974). Replacement of stuttering with normal speech: III. Clinical effectiveness. *Journal of Speech and Hearing Disorders, 39,* 416–428.

Poppen, R., Nunn, R. G., and Hook, S. (1977). Effects of several therapies on stuttering in a single case. *Journal of Fluency Disorders, 2,* 35–44.

Prosek, R. A., and Runyan, C. M. (1983). Effects of segment and pause manipulations on the identification of treated stutterers. *Journal of Speech and Hearing Research, 26,* 510–516.

Runyan, C. M., and Adams, M. R. (1978). Perceptual study of the speech of "successfully therapeutized" stutterers. *Journal of Fluency Disorders, 3,* 25–39.

Runyan, C. M., and Adams, M. R. (1979). Unsophisticated judges' perceptual evaluation of the speech of "successfully treated" stutterers. *Journal of Fluency Disorders, 4,* 29–38.

Ryan, B. P. (1974). *Programmed therapy for stuttering in children and adults.* Springfield, IL: Charles C Thomas.

Ryan, B. P. (1979). Stuttering therapy in a framework of operant conditioning and programmed learning. In H. H. Gregory (Ed.), *Controversies about stuttering therapy.* Baltimore: University Park Press.

Ryan, B. P., and Van Kirk, B. (1974). The establishment, transfer, and maintenance of fluent speech in 50 stutterers using delayed auditory feedback and operant procedures. *Journal of Speech and Hearing Disorders, 39,* 3–10.

Shames, G. H., and Egolf, D. B. (1976). *Operant conditioning and the management of stuttering.* Englewood Cliffs, NJ: Prentice-Hall.

Shames, G. H., and Florance, C. L. (1980). *Stutter-free speech: A goal for therapy.* Columbus, OH: Charles E. Merrill.

Shane, M. L. S. (1955). Effects on stuttering of alteration in auditory feedback. In W. Johnson and R. R. Leutenegger (Eds.), *Stuttering in children and adults.* Minneapolis: University of Minnesota Press.

Sheehan, J. G. (1979). Current issues on stuttering and recovery. In H. H. Gregory (Ed.), *Controversies about stuttering therapy.* Baltimore: University Park Press.

Siegel, G. M. (1970). Punishment, stuttering, and disfluency. *Journal of Speech and Hearing Research, 13,* 677–714.

Silverman, F. H. (1976). Long-term impact of a miniaturized metronome on stuttering: An interim report. *Perceptual and Motor Skills, 42,* 13–22.

Skinner, B. F. (1953). *Science and human behavior.* New York: Macmillan.

Skinner, B. F. (1969). *Contingencies of reinforcement: A theoretical analysis.* New York. Appleton-Century-Crofts.

Skinner, B. F. (1974). *About behaviorism.* New York: Vintage Books.

Stokes, T. F., and Baer, D. M. (1977). An implicit technology of generalization. *Journal of Applied Behavior Analysis, 10,* 349–367.

Trotter, W. D., and Silverman, F. H. (1974). Does the effect of spacing speech with a miniaturized metronome on stuttering wear off? *Perceptual and Motor Skills, 39,* 429–430.

Tyre, T. E., Maisto, S. A., and Companik, P. J. (1973). The use of systematic desensitization in the treatment of chronic stuttering behavior. *Journal of Speech and Hearing Disorders, 38,* 514–519.

Ulliana, L., and Ingham, R. J. (1984). Behavioral and nonbehavioral variables in the measurement of stutterers' communication attitudes. *Journal of Speech and Hearing Disorders, 49,* 83–93.

Van Riper, C. (1973). *The treatment of stuttering.* Englewood Cliffs, NJ: Prentice-Hall.

Van Riper, C. (1982). *The nature of stuttering* (2nd ed.). Englewood Cliffs, NJ: Prentice-Hall.

Webster, R. L. (1974). A behavioral analysis of stuttering: Treatment and theory. In K. S. Calhoun, H. E. Adams, and K. M. Mitchell (Eds.), *Innovative treatment methods in psychotherapy.* New York: John Wiley & Sons.

Webster, R. L. (1979). Empirical considerations regarding stuttering therapy. In H. H. Gregory (Ed.), *Controversies about stuttering therapy.* Baltimore: University Park Press.

West, R., and Ansberry, M. (1968). *The rehabilitation of speech* (4th ed.). New York: Harper & Row.

Williams, D. E. (1979). A perspective on approaches to stuttering therapy. In H. H. Gregory (Ed.), *Controversies about stuttering therapy.* Baltimore: University Park Press.

Williams, D. E. (1982). Stuttering therapy: Where are we going—and why? *Journal of Fluency Disorders, 7,* 159–170.

Williamson, D. A., Epstein, L. H., and Coburn, C. (1981). Multiple baseline analysis of the regulated breathing procedure for the treatment of stuttering. *Journal of Fluency Disorders, 6,* 327–339.

Yonovitz, A., Shepherd, W. T., and Garrett, S. (1977). Hierarchical stimulation: Two case studies of stuttering modification using systematic desensitization. *Journal of Fluency Disorders, 2,* 21–28.

Language Disorders in Children

Recent Advances

Editor in chief, Speech, Language, and Hearing Disorders Series
William H. Perkins, PhD

Preface

I spend most of my professional energies in the study of adult language disorders, while maintaining an interest in child language disorders and their remediation. However, as knowledge in both areas has exploded, it has been increasingly impossible to keep in touch with changes and advances in the far larger, more often pacesetting area of child language. When I undertook to edit this volume, it was simultaneously a challenge and a wonderful opportunity to "catch up" on recent advances in child language. The trick, of course, was to choose the authors carefully and to learn from them as one occasionally reunited a split infinitive or knocked off an unintended redundancy. Because editing this book has been such a heady learning experience for me, and because it has allowed me to become relatively "caught up," I am very pleased to introduce *Language Disorders in Children* to its readers.

Laurence Leonard, who wrote his chapter while training for the Boston Marathon, initiates the volume with a thoughtful resume of the state of the art in the study of normal language acquisition. His chapter critically highlights recent developments, and carefully separates the significant from the merely trendy. He takes the important next step as well—relating advances in the general study of child language to their application to children with language disorders.

Following Leonard's chapter, Jacqueline Liebergott, Anthony Bashir, and Martin Schultz offer a new look at the knowns and unknowns about at-risk infants and their likelihood of developing speech and language disorders. Because the easy belief is that at-risk infants are at-risk for problems generally, the chapter may come as a surprise to a number of readers. The straightforwardness of its logic and clarity of its argument, however, cannot easily be dismissed. It is anticipated that this chapter will have great professional impact.

Three chapters next discuss children who have developmental disorders of language. An arbitrary editorial decision was made to split the population by age, into preschool children, school-age children, and adolescents. The preschool chapter by M. Jeanne Wilcox, and the school-age chapter by Lynn Snyder, relate meaningfully to each other and to Leonard's chapter, without sacrificing the important contrasts that necessarily differentiate diagnosis and treatment of language disorders in the two age groups. Wilcox' chapter not only sets the scholarly context for language remediation, but it provides a nuts-and-bolts application to treatment. Snyder's chapter offers an insightful analysis of the relationships between language and learning disorders, providing a model for subsequent study and clinical intervention as well.

Elizabeth Prather's chapter on language disorders in adolescents is a departure from the previous two, because the study of normal and disordered language lacks the interest and richness of data apparent in the study of preschoolers and school-age children. Prather's chapter is a crisp and pointed review of the little-studied area; but, its major focus must be seen as its plea for more information.

Children who acquire language disorders after a period of previously normal development are different in some substantial ways from children who have failed to develop language normally. However these differences are not well studied. In this volume's chapter on children with acquired seizure disorders, Jon Miller, Thomas Campbell, Robin Chapman, and Susan Weismer provide a germinal model for the study of children with acquired disorders of language. The work can serve as a model for other acquired language disorders in children, including such diverse problems as closed-head injury and sickle cell disease.

No matter how thoroughly trained the speech/language pathologist might be, if that training occurred 5 years or more ago, that training has failed to prepare for the present significant movement in nonvocal communication. Marie Capozzi and Beth Mineo provide readers with a thorough tutorial designed to acquaint them with the exploding and often confusing, field of augmentive communication and its accompanying technology. The comprehensive nature of their review should fill the void that exists for so many of us as a result of the recent rapid accumulation of techniques and instrumentation.

Rather than continue to preview the chapters in the book, it is important to let them talk for themselves. It has been very rewarding to work with these authors and to learn from them. I have no doubt that you will be similarly rewarded by what follows.

Audrey L. Holland
Editor

Laurence B. Leonard

Normal Language Acquisition: Some Recent Findings and Clinical Implications

For some time, speech-language clinicians have made considerable use of the available literature on normal language acquisition when devising assessment and treatment strategies for language-disordered children. This type of application is only as good as the source, however, and when new information is gained concerning the nature of language acquisition in normally developing children, aspects of adopted intervention strategies may need to be re-evaluated. It is appropriate, therefore, that a volume on recent advances in the study of language disorders also include a discussion of recent findings in the area of normal language acquisition.

The topics included in this chapter are those that seem to me to be both current and clinically applicable. In the interest of space, not all appropriate topics are represented. The final selection was based on the additional consideration that the chapter reflect findings covering a wide range of linguistic abilities acquired during childhood. These abilities are discussed more or less in developmental order.

As will be apparent in the chapters that follow, some of the findings reviewed here have served as the foundation for recent research with language-disordered children. In order to avoid duplication, this applied research will not be discussed. However, these studies are only just beginning to appear, and there are a number of clinical issues arising from the normal-language findings that have yet to be addressed. Some of these are noted at the end of each section of the chapter.

Normal Language Acquisition: Some Recent Findings

Early Comprehension and Production

Early comprehension

One trend seen in the literature on normal language development during the past several years is an increased interest in young children's comprehension skills. From Huttenlocher's (1974) classic report of early language comprehension, we had reason to believe that children as young as nine months of age may respond appropriately to words and short phrases. However, children at this young age are not the most co-operative of subjects, and, thus, assessment of comprehension has had to rely on informal techniques.

Chapman (1978) has described some of the limitations to interpretation that can arise from the use of such informal procedures. She identified several comprehension strategies used by young children that can give the impression they understand more than they actually do. Some of these strategies are based on nonlinguistic cues and require no language comprehension. One such strategy is acting on objects that are noticed. Such a strategy might be seen in cases where an adult places an object in front of the child and says, "Pick up the X." Another nonlinguistic strategy is the imitation of the actions of others. For instance, the child may hold his arms up if, along with asking "Up?" the adult begins to reach for the child.

Other strategies may require lexical comprehension on the part of the child, but an uncritical assessment of the child's response may lead to the interpretation that he or she understands sentences. The strategy of doing what is usually done in the situation serves as a good example. For instance, when faced with an array consisting of a toy truck, brush, doll, and block, a child might respond correctly to the request, "Brush the dolly's hair," by comprehending the word "hair" and performing the usual action done with hair.

More recently, Oviatt (1980) has developed a method for assessing lexical comprehension in young children that allows one to draw more definitive conclusions concerning a child's comprehension ability than seems possible with most informal measures. This method is basically a training procedure. The child is provided with exposures to previously unknown object and action names. Following this exposure period, the child's comprehension of each word is tested. One important feature of this approach is that it allows one to compute the consistency of the child's response to the word relative to his or her response to a control word and his or her response when no word is provided.

Oviatt's (1980) procedure for assessing comprehension of an object name can serve as an illustration. A highly salient referent (a live rabbit or hamster housed in a transparent travel case) was placed to the side of the child. For three minutes the child was permitted to observe the animal, while the experimenter and the child's parent named it a total of 24 times. The child was then distracted with novel toys for the following three minutes. The experimenter then gained the child's attention and asked the child to locate the target referent ("Where's the rabbit?"), a nonexistent referent ("Where's the kawlow?"), and, in some cases, a familiar referent ("Where's the book?") in alternating order. Instances where the child gazed back at the target referent constituted the measure of interest. Along with determining the rate of responding to the target and control questions, the frequency with which the child gazed back at the target referent when no question was asked was also considered, for purposes of determining a base rate. A child was credited with recognitory comprehension of the word if he or she showed no gazing responses to control questions and responded to the target questions at a rate that exceeded base rate. Oviatt found that on such tasks, recognitory comprehension seemed to show an abrupt emergence at approximately 10 to 11 months of age, and appeared very consistent by ages 12 to 14 months. Similar findings were seen for object and action names.

The clinical implications of the work of Chapman (1978) and Oviatt (1980) are substantial. With regard to the former, it seems that there are several factors unrelated to lexical comprehension per se that might allow a child to respond as if he or she understands the word being tested. Proper assessment of understanding of the word, then, would require elimination of these factors during testing. Requests for an action (e.g., "Wave bye-bye"), for example, should not be accompanied by behaviors the child can imitate, nor should they be made only when situational clues are available (e.g., "Go peek-a-boo," as the child is handed a blanket). Likewise, assessment of the child's comprehension of object names should include requests for objects when other objects are also present, and in situations in which the requested objects are not usually present (e.g., "Where's the ball?" requested at the snack table) as well as in situations in which they are.

It appears that the Oviatt (1980) procedure holds much promise for clinical application. The tasks currently available for assessing early lexical comprehension in language-disordered children require the child to perform acts such as retrieving or pointing to the correct referent from an array of objects, or performing, or making a doll perform, a requested action. Yet, young children just beginning to attach meanings to words exhibit only a recognitory comprehension of such words. Thus, if the clinical goal is to determine a language-disordered child's readiness for comprehension training, Oviatt's procedure would seem to be most appropriate. Once the child has shown evidence of comprehending words and the clinical focus shifts to an assessment of the number of words comprehended, existing tasks might then be employed.

Word Production

Along with gaining a greater understanding of children's early lexical comprehension, we have been able to form a clearer picture of their early production of words. Much of the work devoted to word production has focused on factors that influence a young child's tendency to use a particular word. One such factor is the phonological composition of the word. For a number of years, diary and naturalistic studies of young children have included the observation that many seem to avoid use of certain forms of adult words (Ferguson, Peizer, & Weeks, 1973; Macken, 1976; Menn, 1976; Vihman, 1976). According to these accounts, a few lexical types are selected that serve as the basis of the child's production system and attempts at other kinds of lexical items are avoided. Interestingly, children seem to vary in the particular adult forms selected and avoided. Some children have primarily selected words with labial or apical consonants in the initial position (Leopold, 1947), others have selected words with word-initial velars (Menn, 1971), and others have attempted words with word-initial fricatives (Ferguson & Farwell, 1975). The initial consonant seems to serve as a primary determiner in these cases (Shibamoto & Olmsted, 1978). However, in some instances, children's selection and avoidance tendencies may involve an interaction between the initial consonant and the syllable shape of words (Macken, 1976).

One of the difficulties in interpreting reports of phonological selection and avoidance tendencies in young children has been that there was no way to rule out the possibility that they were not simply a reflection of the differential frequencies of consonants and syllable shapes in the speech heard in the child's environment. However, more recently, investigations controlling for this frequency of exposure factor have appeared in the literature. Schwartz and Leonard (1982) found that children with expressive lexicons of approximately five words were more likely to acquire the use of new words that contained consonants they had previously produced accurately than words containing consonants they had shown no prior evidence of attempting, even when both types of words had been exposed with equal frequency. Leonard, Schwartz, Morris, and

Chapman (1981) reported identical findings for children with expressive lexicons of approximately 50 words.

Another factor that may influence children's use of new words is unsolicited imitation. Although young children vary considerably in the degree to which they engage in such behavior, imitation seems to play a role in lexical acquisition for those children who do imitate. Two hypotheses concerning the influence of imitation on lexical acquisition have been explored. The first is that imitated words are acquired more readily in production as a result of the imitation process. This hypothesis is at the heart of studies conducted by Bloom, Hood, and Lightbown (1974) and Ramer (1976). These investigators examined the lexical items used by young children and determined whether such usage was imitative or spontaneous. They found it was proper to speak of two populations of words in a child's speech—words used spontaneously and words used imitatively. Further, they observed a progression across time as imitation of a particular lexical item decreased while the spontaneous use of the lexical item increased. Such findings led to the interpretation that imitation could serve as a vehicle through which words might be introduced more readily into the lexicon. As imitation was not viewed as necessary for the normal acquisition of all of the child's words, the facilitative effects of imitation were assumed to apply only to those words the child chose to imitate.

More recently, a second hypothesis has been investigated. Leonard, Schwartz, Folger, Newhoff, and Wilcox (1979) attempted to determine whether imitated words were acquired more readily in production than words that were not imitated. These investigators presented novel words and their referents to children in sessions designed to simulate informal play. During these sessions, the children's imitative and spontaneous use of the words was noted. Leonard et al. observed that the first spontaneous use of nonimitated words required no more stimulus exposures than the first spontaneous use of previously imitated words. However, in a follow up study, Leonard, Chapman, Rowan, and Weiss (1983) observed that spontaneous usage was more frequent for words that had been both imitated and used spontaneously (regardless of whether imitation preceded spontaneous use or vice versa) than for words that had been used spontaneously without having been imitated. In addition, words that were produced correctly on a post test were usually those that had been previously imitated. These findings led Leonard et al. to propose that imitation may facilitate lexical acquisition.

Until the mid-1970s, studies of children's early word usage centered principally on the types of words produced (e.g., Nelson, 1973) and the semantic boundaries reflected in such usage (Clark, 1973). In recent years, increasing attention has been placed on the communicative functions served by the child's early word usage (Coggins & Carpenter, 1981; Dale, 1980; Halliday, 1975). One of the most detailed studies on this topic is that of McShane (1980), in which the communicative functions expressed by six children—presented in Table 1-1— were studied longitudinally from approximately age 12 to 24 months. Communicative attempts by the child were assigned to one of the communicative function categories along with a designation of whether the attempt was expressed lexically.

Not surprisingly, the percentage of communicative attempts taking lexical form increased with age. The communicative functions expressed most frequently in lexical form were requests, naming, and answers. However, each of the six children also used lexical items to serve attention, description, information, giving, doing, imitation, follow-on, and question functions. Five of the six children used words to express a determination function. These findings suggest that young children used their relatively limited lexicons to convey a variety of communicative intentions.

The recent findings concerning young children's word productions and the factors influencing them seem to offer some new considerations for clinical management. If language-disordered children are found to show the same phonological selection and avoidance tendencies seen in young normally developing children, it would appear that an additional factor could be considered when selecting the words to include in lexical training. That is, along with selecting words according to their communicative significance for the child (Holland, 1975) and their semantic properties (Lahey & Bloom, 1977), the phonological composition of the words relative to the child's own phonological characteristics might be considered. For example, it could prove useful to select for training those words that conform to the child's phonological characteristics, particularly if a priority is being placed on increasing lexicon size as efficiently as possible.

A finding that unsolicited imitation facilitates the acquisition of words in language-disordered children might also have implications for clinical management. Such a finding could suggest a possible modification in current lexical-training procedures. Specifically, it might prove useful to provide a number of exposures of a word to which the child need not respond (but may choose to imitate) in addition to the formal stimuli (e.g., imitative prompts, questions) to which the child is required to respond.

At present, relatively little is known about the communicative functions served by the early lexical usage of language-disordered children. However, judging from the available data for young normally developing children, there are a variety of communicative uses to which a relatively limited expressive lexicon can be put. It might be important, therefore, to insure that our lexical-training procedures include provisions for associating a new word with more than one communicative function where applicable. Before a child is assumed to have acquired the use of a word, he or she might be required to use it in more than one way (e.g., requesting and naming; doing and description). If a child has acquired the use of a number of words, yet fails to use any to serve a particular communicative function typically seen in young normally developing children, specific attempts to increase awareness of this function might be instituted.

Language Learning Styles

In recent years, one of the most important lessons we have learned about young children's language development is that children may follow different routes, yet still acquire language in a normal manner and at a normal rate. The study that first opened our eyes to this fact was performed by Nelson (1973). In an examination of the first 50 words used by young normally developing children, Nelson observed some clear differences in the distribution of words across lexical categories. The most striking differences between the children was in the number of general nominals used, such as names of objects, animals, and substances. Over half of the lexical items used by some of the children took the form of general nominals. These children were termed "referential speakers" since they seemed to display an object-oriented language. The other children—termed "expressive speakers"—made less use of general nominals and appeared to display a social-interaction language. Compared to the referential speakers, the expressive speakers showed greater use of personal-social words, such as *pat-a-cake* and *whoops*. These differences in lexical orientation were related to later differences between the children. For example, at 24 months of age, the referential speakers displayed larger vocabularies than the expressive speakers (see, also, Nelson, 1975). On the other hand, the expressive speakers used a larger number of phrases early in the language-acquisition period than did the referential speakers. The latter group appeared, instead, to follow a gradual progression from the single- to the two-word-utterance stage.

It now seems that the styles identified by Nelson (1973) may apply as well to young children who have been studied by other investigators. For example, Dore (1974) observed the linguistic development of two children and noted that one child used many object names and progressed from the single- to the two-word stage in a discrete fashion, while the other child, from the outset, used a number of phrases identifiable more from their intonation than from their phonetic accuracy. Peters (1977) also described a young child with limited intelligibility who used phrases identifiable from their intonation contours, as well as a number of personal-social words. Other investigators have observed differences in lexical usage

Table 1-1
McShane's (1980) Communicative function categories.

CATEGORY	DEFINITION	EXAMPLE
Regulation		
Attention	An utterance that attempts to direct the attention of another person to an object or event.	*look,* as the child points to an object and looks up at the listener.
Request	An utterance that requests that another person do something for the child, or requests permission to do something.	*juice,* as the child holds out a glass to the mother.
Vocative	An utterance that calls another person to locate him or her or to request his or her presence.	*Mommy* (spoken loudly) as the child goes from room to room in search of mother.
Statement		
Naming	An utterance that makes reference to an object or person by name only.	*car*, as the child points to a car.
Description	An utterance that makes some statement, other than naming, about an object, action, or event.	*gone*, as the child arrives at the location where a desired object is usually found, but is unable to find it.

Table 1-1
McShane's (1980) Communicative function categories.

CATEGORY	DEFINITION	EXAMPLE
Information	An utterance that makes a statement about an event beyond the "here-and-now," excluding acts the child is about to perform.	*chick*, as the child looks at the visitor. The mother then comments "We saw some chicks at the farm yesterday, didn't we?"
Exchange		
Giving	An utterance spoken while giving or attempting to give an object to another person.	*here*, as the child hands a doll to the father.
Receiving	An utterance spoken while receiving an object from another person.	*thank you*, as the child takes the offered cookie.
Personal		
Doing	An utterance describing an act the child is performing or has just performed.	*down*, after the child has just put a box of blocks on the floor.
Determination	An utterance specifying the child's intention to carry out some act immediately.	*out*, spoken immediately before standing up and walking toward the door.

Table 1-1
McShane's (1980) Communicative function categories.

CATEGORY	DEFINITION	EXAMPLE
Refusal	An utterance used to refuse an object or request to do something.	*no*, as the mother hands the child a hat to put on the doll.
Protest	A "high-pitched" utterance expressing the child's displeasure with an action by another person.	*don't!*, as the child's brother starts to take the play phone away from the child.
Conversation *Imitation*	An utterance that imitates all or part of a preceding adult utterance with no intervening utterance on the child's part.	*fish*, in response to the father's utterance "What a big fish."
Answer	An utterance spoken in response to a question (excluding imitations).	*shoe*, in response to the mother's question "What's this called?"
Follow-on	An utterance serving as a conversational response that is neither an imitation nor an answer.	*yeah*, in response to the visitor's comment "Let's see what's in the box."
Question	An utterance that requests information from another person.	*what's that?*, as the child looks first at a microphone, then at the visitor.

(Snyder, Bates, & Bretherton, 1979), the types of multi-word utterances acquired (Lieven, 1980) and patterns of play behavior (Rosenblatt, 1975; Wolf & Gardner, 1979) that may parallel the style differences reported by Nelson. Some caution should be taken in interpreting the literature on language-learning style, however. Nelson (1981) has raised the possibility that the two styles may represent two extremes on a continuum, and that some children may fall at neither extreme. Further, Peters has noted that the speaking situation at hand may dictate the degree to which a child exhibits behaviors associated with one or another style.

Assuming that style distinctions can be made with language-disordered children, determination of a child's style may have important implications for the selection of additional words to include in lexical training. A study of young normally developing children by Leonard et al. (1981) offers an illustration. These investigators presented novel object and action words and referents to referential and expressive speakers for 10 sessions. The referential speakers acquired a greater number of the object words than the expressive speakers. However, the two groups did not differ in their acquisition of the action words. Such a finding suggests that for language-disordered children exhibiting a referential style, introduction of new general nominals might lead to more rapid lexical learning than would be the case if other types of words had been selected for training. At some point, of course, such a concentration on words of a particular type should give way to a more balanced distribution of lexical types. However, this approach of selecting words in keeping with a child's language-learning style may have some benefits in cases where the child's lexical growth is proceeding rather slowly.

Early Combinatorial Speech

Early Comprehension of Word Combinations

Prior to their production of true word combinations, young children show evidence of comprehending two-word utterances to a limited degree. In some cases this comprehension may be more apparent than real, as when a child responds correctly to the request "Throw ball," not because he or she understood the relational aspects of the utterance, but because he or she understood the word "ball" and performed the action typically associated with the ball (Chapman, 1978). However, there is evidence that children at this stage in linguistic development can make inferences about the relationship between two words. Sachs and Truswell (1978) presented young children with a comprehension task involving familiar words in novel combinations arranged in sets of four-way minimal contrasts (e.g., "Pat teddy, " "Kiss book, " "Pat book, " "Kiss teddy"). Ten of the 12 children studied performed well on this task and the remaining children responded correctly to some of the instructions. It should be noted that this did not constitute evidence of syntactic comprehension, for the children's responses to requests such as "Teddy kiss" were not tested. It is possible that under such circumstances children might adopt the strategy of acting as agent themselves (Chapman, 1978). However, their successful performance on the Sachs and Truswell task indicates that late in the single-word utterance stage, children can process more than one word in the utterances directed toward them.

The Sachs and Truswell (1978) task seems to have considerable potential for use in clinical settings. Through use of minimal contrasts, nonlinguistic and single-lexical-item response strategies are obviated, enabling the clinician to determine whether the child can comprehend both components of certain two-word utterances. Successful performance on this task might serve as a criterion for the child's entry into two-word-utterance production training.

Two Word Utterance Usage

For more than a decade, the study of children's two-word utterances has included a consideration of the types of meanings they convey. This work has led to the impression that, regardless of the language being acquired, young children seem to express the same relatively small set of meanings. These include noting identification, disappearance, recurrence, location, or properties of things, as well as the actions of those things, and the agents performing these actions.

In the past few years, however, the analysis of the relational meanings reflected in children's early word combinations has seemed much less straightforward than previously presumed. During this period, several papers have pointed out a number of difficulties involved in placing two-word utterances into semantic-relation categories (Duchan & Lund, 1979; Howe, 1976; 1981; Rodgon, 1977). The most serious problem is that the semantic relations often ascribed to children may not reflect the relational meanings that are actually operative in their speech. This concern has been tempered somewhat by recent arguments that the analysis of children's utterances in their situational context does not constitute imposing adult semantic categories upon the data, but rather deriving categories from the data (Bloom, Capatides, & Tackeff, 1981). Nonetheless, all investigators now seem to agree on the importance of securing firm evidence from the child's speech before assuming that a particular semantic relation is operative in his or her linguistic system.

A method of analysis that seems capable of providing such evidence was developed by Braine (1976), and has since been expanded by Ingram (1979). One of the major features of this approach is that the child's word combinations are assumed to be unanalyzed wholes unless the data can show otherwise. This applies not only to highly routinized forms such as "Thank you" and "What's that?"—but also to forms such as "That ball" and "More juice," which, on first impression, might be assumed to have been generated by means of a rule for combining words. Particular attention is paid to whether or not a word that appears in one combination is also seen in combination with other words (e.g., "Throw ball," "Throw block"). The type of meaning that seems to be reflected in these combinations is then examined. Finally, the child's utterances are examined for word combinations that are unlikely to have been heard in the speech of others (e.g., "That feet").

Application of this analysis procedure to young children's word combinations led Braine (1976) to conclude that semantic relation categories such as action + object, possession, and the like may often be inappropriate for these children. For example, some children exhibit word-combination patterns that seem to be lexically based (e.g., "Open box," "Open door," "Open window"). It seems that such patterns represent cases where the child has focused on a particular word in a particular word position, and has observed the words it combines with in the speech of others. Thus, the utterances produced by the child may not have been generated by a rule for combining words. In other cases, the word combinations seem to reflect a productive rule, as evidenced by the use of clearly novel word combinations (e.g., "Open orange" [=Peel the orange], in addition to "Open box," "Open door"). However, the rule still applies only to specific lexical items (e.g., *Open* + X). When the child's word-combination rules transcend specific lexical items, they often embody meanings that are too narrow for the traditional semantic-relation categories. For example, Braine has reported evidence for a word-combining rule that might be characterized as Act-of-Oral-Consumption + Object-Consumed (e.g., "Eat banana," "Bite banana," "Eat cookie," "Bite cookie". This is to say that positional consistency obtained only in word combinations related to the acts of eating and drinking.

Thus, these findings indicate that young children's two-word utterances may represent (1) memorization of a number of combinations into which particular words may enter, (2) productive rules applied only to specific words, (3) productive rules conveying meanings that cross lexical boundaries, but are narrower than traditional semantic relation categories, as well as (4) semantic relation rules of the traditional type. Such findings suggest that the assessment of the meanings reflected in the two-word utterances of language-disordered children should be performed with greater care than previously presumed. There seem to be two ways of accomplishing this. One way is to collect speech samples from the child that are larger than the 50- or 100-utterance samples ordinarily obtained in clinical settings. A second approach is to follow up a standard (smaller) speech sample with probes aimed at discovering the bases and nature of the two-word utterances noted in the sample. For example, if the utterance "Little baby" was noted in a child's sample, the clinician might select object and/or pictorial stimuli designed to determine whether the child can use "Little " in combination with other words, whether his or her use of "Little " is part of a relatively narrow word-combining rule (e.g., Size + X, as in "Little baby, " "Little ball, " "Big ball, " "Big dog") or, instead reflects a broader rule that corresponds to a semantic relation such as attribution.

Longer Word Combinations

Shortly after productive two-word utterances are heard in young children's speech, their sentences seem to lengthen almost daily. By the time many children reach two years of age, three-word utterances are almost as common as two-word utterances, and four- and five-word utterances are not out of the ordinary. However, the rapidity of this progression from two-word utterances to those of longer length should not be taken to mean that the process is unpatterned. For example, Bloom, Miller, and Hood (1975) have noted several conditions that seem to increase or decrease the likelihood that an utterance will contain three versus two constituents. While use of verb inflections, prepositions, noun inflections, and determiners seem equally likely in two- or three-constituent utterances, the expression of negation, recurrence, possession, and attribution seem less likely in three-constituent utterances. Similarly, verbs previously used by the child appear as likely to occur in three- as in two-constituent utterances, but newly acquired verbs are usually restricted to two-constituent utterances. Finally, differences can be seen in the distribution of two- and three-constituent utterances in discourse. While two-constituent utterances often serve as the first utterance in a sequence, utterances containing three constituents often serve as expansions of a prior utterance.

The findings of Bloom et al. (1975) seem to have a great deal of potential for clinical application. For example, for language-intervention procedures in which several linguistic features serve as simultaneous goals, the clinician might be able to model certain combinations of features (e.g., Agent + Action + Location utterances which also contain a preposition such as "Mommy sit on bed") that, when attempted by the child, have a reasonable likelihood of being produced accurately. If children prove more able to produce three-constituent utterances when such utterances serve as expansions, the clinician employing a modeling approach might alter the procedure to accommodate such expansions. For example, rather than describing three pictures using an Agent + Action + Object construction and then presenting the child with a fourth picture to which he or she is asked to respond, the clinician might describe each of the three pictures with a two-part response, composed of a two-constituent description followed by a three-constituent expansion (e.g., "Ride bike." "Daddy ride bike."). The clinician might then provide a two-constituent description of a fourth picture and ask the child to provide the follow-up utterance. Finally, the Bloom et al. findings regarding the relative use of new and old lexical items in three-constituent utterances suggest that training activities designed to facilitate the child's production of longer utterances should make use of lexical items, particularly action words, which the child has been using for some time (Bloom & Lahey, 1978).

Grammatical Inflections

As children's utterances increase in length, function words and grammatical inflections begin to appear. Fourteen of these words and inflections comprise the grammatical morphemes examined in Brown's (1973) well-known longitudinal study. He noted that these morphemes are acquired in an approximately consistent order across children, a finding generally supported by the cross-sectional findings of deVilliers and deVilliers (1973). While Brown found evidence that the syntactic and/or semantic complexity of the morphemes may be partly responsible for their order of acquisition, he found no evidence that acquisition order was related to the frequency with which the morphemes were used in parental speech. More recently, a lively debate has surfaced in which it has been claimed, after further analysis of Brown's data, that parental input frequency is a factor in acquisition order (Moerk, 1980) and that syntactic and semantic complexity are not (Block & Kessel, 1980). Pinker (1981) has re-examined each of these newer claims in detail and has concluded that they are based on faulty interpretations of the statistical analysis used. Pinker's arguments appear reasonable and, thus, for the time being, Brown's original conclusions still stand.

Investigations of children's use of grammatical inflections have not been limited to those concerned with the sequence in which inflections appear, or the factors responsible for this sequence. One of the most informative studies pertaining to grammatical inflections, in fact, dealt with the types of verbs with which the verb inflections -*ing*, -*s* and -*ed* (the latter considered along with irregular past forms) typically co-occur in young children's speech (Bloom, Lifter, & Hafitz, 1980). Action verbs that occurred with -*ing* were found to name events extending over time (durative) in which there was no immediate and clear result (noncompletive). Examples include *play, ride,* and *write*. The action verbs associated with -*s* were typically completive and durative, in that the completed action leaves a relatively permanent state of affairs, as seen in "This goes here" or "It fits." Action verbs associated with -*ed* and irregular usage usually named nondurative, completive events (e.g., *jump, bite*). The tendency for an action verb to be associated primarily with one type of inflection was seen principally when the verb was newly acquired. Unlike most action verbs, those that seemed to serve as "all-purpose" verbs with rather general meanings (e.g., *do, make, get*) often occurred with more than one inflection.

Bloom et al. (1980) also noted a difference between types of state verbs. Those that named internal, nonshared events, such as *want* and *like*, were rarely inflected. However, those that referred to observable processes (e.g., *look, lay, sleep*) were more likely to be inflected.

The finding that young children seemed to make use of different inflections according to whether a verb is durative or nondurative, or completive or noncompletive, led Bloom et al. (1980) to propose that aspect rather than tense may motivate children's early inflectional usage. That is, the use of verb inflections did not seem closely tied to the relationship between the time that the action or state occurred and the time when the utterance referring to the action or state was produced. This usage did seem related to the temporal contour of particular events, however, such as whether an action was momentary in time or extended over a considerable period of time.

The Bloom et al. (1980) findings make it clear that when teaching language-disordered children the use of verb inflections, considerable attention should be paid to the semantics of the verbs used. It seems more likely that the durative, noncompletive nature of verbs such as *play* may be particularly conducive to -*ing* training, while the nondurative, completive character of verbs such as *jump* may facilitate the acquisition of -*ed*. The use of -*s* might be fostered by the introduction of completive, but durative, verbs such as *fit*. At some point, of course, the child will need to demonstrate evidence of the ability to use more than one inflection with the same verb. Training activities with this as their goal might include in the early stages "all-purpose" verbs (e.g., *do, make*) whose meanings are sufficiently broad to accommodate a number of aspectual contours.

Conversational Skills

Contingent and Adjacent Speech

The child-language literature since the mid-1970s has reflected a growing interest in the nature of the development of children's conversational skills. One area of investigation has been the relationship between the child's utterances and preceding adult utterances, and how this relationship changes across time. The available evidence suggests that from at least the age of 21 months, children's utterances more often than not temporally follow an adult utterance (Bloom, Rocissano, & Hood, 1976). However, approximately one-third of these adjacent utterances do not share the same topic as the prior adult utterance. Another 10% to 25% represent imitations of the adult utterance. Contingent utterances—those that share the same topic and add new information—represent approximately 25% of the child's adjacent utterances. Bloom et al. noted that by the time the child has reached three years of age, the percentage of adjacent utterances falling into the first two categories is much lower, while contingent speech may represent as much as 50% of the child's adjacent speech.

The fact that children's unsolicited imitations are quite frequent at a point in their development when their contingent speech is low has led a number of investigators to propose that one function of imitation may be to enable children to participate in conversation at a time when their limited linguistic ability restricts the amount of original and relevant information they can provide (Keenan, 1974; Mayer & Valian, 1977; McTear, 1978). Only Boskey and Nelson (1980) have studied this issue in systematic fashion, by asking children predesigned questions that they could and could not answer during the course of a play activity. Boskey and Nelson found unanswerable questions were likely to result in imitation, while relevant verbal responses were more frequent for answerable questions. Thus, some support can be found for the hypothesis that young children may imitate when they have nothing else to say. Along with facilitating the child's acquisition of specific linguistic material (as discussed above), then, imitation may assist the child during conversational participation.

It appears that children's developing use of contingent speech represents more than a simple increase in the proportion of adjacent utterances that add new information to the topic. Bloom et al. (1976) noted that the proportion of contingent utterances that followed from the situation or action pertaining to the adult's utterance (contextually contingent speech) decreased across time, while the proportion of contingent utterances showing structural continuities with the clause structure of the adult utterance (linguistically contingent speech) increased. Two main types of linguistically contingent speech were identified. The first type involved intraclausal relations, in which the child's utterance changed or added information to the same clause structure seen in the adult utterance. Interclausal relations represented the second type. In this case, the child's utterance added information with another clause that was grammatically subordinate to the clause of the adult utterance. Both types of linguistically contingent speech increased across time relative to the use of contextually contingent speech. However, utterances involving interclausal relations emerged several months after those involving intraclausal relations.

One form of contingent speech that has received considerable investigative attention is the contingent query, a device seemingly used by the child to regulate the verbal interaction. Research conducted by Garvey (1977; 1979) indicates that the various forms of the contingent query are well learned by three years of age. Contingent queries seem to serve several different functions. They can serve as requests for repetition, confirmation, specification, or elaboration. Examples of each of these functions appear in Table 1-2.

An inspection of the types of utterances young children use following an utterance by their co-conversationalist offers a number of insights regarding possible intervention strategies with language-disordered children. First, it appears that the child's use of imitation during conversation might be regarded as an acceptable response to a preceding utterance by another. As there is no evidence to date that imitation facilitates the child's acquisition of new conversational devices, it should probably not represent a target for training. However, the information contained in the child's imitation could be acknowledged and the imitation itself accepted as an appropriate conversational turn, unless the clinician has reason to believe the child can respond with an information-bearing comment of his or her own.

Active attempts to teach the child the use of contingent speech might commence with intraclausal relations between the adult utterance and the child's response. For example, within a modeling framework, the clinician might present a picture to the model and child, saying "The truck is pulling a car." The model might respond with "A broken car" or "Train can pull car. " Providing the child with a number of such examples might enable him or her to discover some ways to add information to a preceding utterance produced by another. Once a child shows use of contingent speech involving intraclausal relations, modeling might focus on interclausal relations. Contingent utterances of this type seem to require greater grammatical sophistication on the child's part. Therefore, it would be necessary to precede such training with a careful consideration of the child's grammatical skills. Examples of interclausal relations might include the clinician's description of a picture, "The girl is carrying some popcorn," followed by the model's comment "She's gonna eat it."

Table 1-2
Illustration of the functions of contingent queries proposed by Garvey (1979).

FUNCTION	PRECEDING UTTERANCE	CONTINGENT QUERY*
Request for Repetition	"Let's take the truck."	"The what ╱"
Request for Confirmation	"The bike is too small for Daddy."	"The black one ╱"
Request for Specification	"Hold onto the box. You don't want to break it."	"What ╲"
Request for Elaboration	"Hurry up. We're gonna go now."	"Where ╲"

*╱ indicates phrase-final rise in intonation, ╲ indicates phrase-final fall in intonation.

The specific functions served by contingent queries make them good candidates for inclusion in a language-treatment program. Contingent queries serve as signals to the co-conversationalist that the message was not fully understood. The specific form of the query indicates to the co-conversationalist which aspect of the message needs to be repeated, specified, etc. Given that a number of language-disordered children experience comprehension difficulties, a means to indicate that a message was not fully understood as spoken would be highly useful. Again, a modeling framework might be appropriate. For example, the clinician might tell a brief story about two girls who are bored and who decide they are going to go outside "to look for it" (deliberately not being clear as to the referent). The model might then respond, "What ╲," a query for specification. Following a number of queries by the model, the child could be given the charge of providing feedback to the clinician.

Turn-Taking

Another area of active research in recent years is that of children's conversational turn-taking. Much of this work has focused on child-child interactions. Although children seem to be provided with a framework for turn-taking when they are still infants (Ninio & Bruner, 1978), it appears that the proper timing and monitoring of turns are not well established until the early elementary school years. For example, while children six to eight years of age show only minimal overlap in their conversational turns, overlap is much higher in children under four-and-one-half years of age. These younger children are also less able to time their interruptions so they occur at a syntactic or prosodic boundary in the other speaker's utterance. Not surprisingly, younger children show greater difficulty in timing during triadic versus dyadic interaction than older children (Ervin-Tripp, 1979). Along with impressions of the nature and frequency of interruptions, we have impressions of children's reactions to interruptions. Common remedies, regardless of age, seem to be immediate repetition or an increase in volume. Children above the age of four-and-one-half years, however, seem less likely to ignore interruptions than younger children. Frequently, these children stop speaking when such interruptions occur (Ervin-Tripp, 1979).

Of course, not all turn exchanges are mistimed. Garvey and Berninger (1981) have attempted to determine the duration of the pause between one child's utterance and the follow-up utterance of a second child. Such switching pauses are shorter for children approximately five years of age than for children approximately three years of age. For both age groups, pauses are relatively short when the first utterance follows a conventional pattern, has a predictable response, and the response can be selected from a limited set of alternatives or involves only repetition or confirmation:

Child A: "I know where this goes."
Child B: "Where \ "

However, pauses are longer for cases where the response is both less predictable and requires the formulation of linguistic elements new to the discourse:

Child A: "What do you call this?"
Child B: "I'm not sure. Maybe an igloo."

Garvey and Berninger (1981) have also studied the behavior of children when they receive no response to an utterance for which one was expected. In these cases, younger as well as older children seem to follow up their original utterance with another. Repetition appears to be most frequent followed by a change of force (e.g., "I'm going to put this near the window. . .All right?") and paraphrase. Older children seem more likely than younger children to follow up with a change of force if the original utterance was a declarative. Finally, older children seem to wait longer for a response than younger children if the original utterance was an interrogative. Garvey and Berninger suggest that older children may have more confidence in the turn-transfer effects of interrogatives.

The available evidence regarding children's developing turn-taking skills has implications for intervention. For example, children for whom conversational turn-taking is a clinical goal might first be encouraged to participate in dyads. If a child must interact with more than one other child at a time, as is often the case in some preschool language-stimulation programs, the child's conversations may amount to frequent and ill-timed interruptions—or the opposite extreme, a reluctance to actively participate. Triadic communication, then, might be reserved as a later goal of intervention. A child's ability to take conversational turns might be promoted by insuring that a number of the utterances initially directed his or her way have predictable responses whose formulation can be based on a small set of response alternatives, and where, in some cases, simple repetition or confirmation is appropriate.

Wh-Questions

It seems safe to say that one of the reasons why clinicians pay close attention to the literature on normal children's language acquisition is to collect information concerning the sequence in which particular linguistic features might be taught to language-disordered children. In no area is this more true than in the area of *wh*-question acquisition. Previous research with normally developing children has suggested that *wh*-questions emerge in a particular sequence. *What* and *where* questions emerge relatively early, for example, while *why* and *when* questions appear later. These findings have provided clinicians with an approximate order in which *wh*-questions might be trained.

In the past five years, however, we have learned a great deal more about factors that may contribute to the observed sequence of acquisition, and the specific conditions that must be present in order for the sequence to hold. For example, Tyack and Ingram (1977) found that the transitivity of the verb and the sentence constituent represented by the *wh*-word influenced the *wh*-question comprehension of children aged four to five-and-one-half years. While *where* questions containing intransitive verbs were relatively easy for the children, *where* questions with transitive verbs were more difficult. Questions in which *who* served as the object of the sentence ("Who is the girl touching?") were more likely to be comprehended than questions in which *who* served as the subject of the sentence ("Who is touching the girl?").

An investigation by Wootten, Merkin, Hood, and Bloom (1979) has provided considerable insight into the factors involved in the sequence of acquisition seen in children's production of *wh*-questions. The children, studied from approximately 22 to 36 months of age, showed the same general order of acquisition reported in earlier studies, with *what* and *where* questions emerging early, followed by *how, who,* and *why* questions. This sequence seemed attributable in part to the syntactic function served by the *wh*-words. With the exception of *who*, those that serve as *wh*-pronominals asking for the particular constituent they replace, such as *what* or *where*, tended to appear earlier in the children's speech. Those that are *wh*-sententials asking for information pertaining to semantic relations among all the constituents of a sentence (*how* and *why*), appeared later. The somewhat late appearance of *who* questions seemed due to the fact that, unlike the other *wh*-pronominals, *who* was not used by the children in identifying questions (such as "Who's that?") during the early phases of the study. This may have been due to the fact that, at younger ages, children's contact with persons whose identity they might question is relatively limited.

Another factor that Wootten et al. (1979) identified as having a possible bearing on the observed order of emergence was the distribution of verb types with *wh*-words. *What, where,* and *who* questions usually occurred with the copula or the pro-verbs *do* and *go. How* questions were used with verbs that named specific actions and states (*eat, sleep*), as well as with pro-verbs and the copula. *Why* questions, on the other hand, were primarily used with verbs that referred to specific actions and states. This finding suggested the presence of a developmental interaction between the syntactic function of a *wh*-word and the semantic complexity of the verbs used with it.

Finally, Wootten et al. (1979) examined the children's use of *wh*-questions containing no verbs. Those that represented agrammatical constructions ("Where dog?") decreased in frequency over time. On the other hand, an increase across time was seen in the frequency of questions that were elliptical ("What book?" "Why?"), serving as responses to an utterance produced by another.

These recent findings provide additional details that should probably be considered when teaching *wh*-questions to language-disordered children. Although the order of emergence of *wh*-questions reflected in the literature can serve as a general guide for training, it seems essential that the clinician insure that the particular features of *wh*-questions responsible for this order be incorporated into training. For example, *what* questions may be taught first, but only those that serve as identifying questions. Other types of *what* questions might be introduced later. *Where* questions containing intransitive verbs should probably be introduced before those that contain transitive verbs. The acquisition of the later-emerging questions, such as *how* and particularly *why,* seem to be predicated on an ability to use a variety of verbs referring to specific states and actions. Therefore, it would seem important to conduct a detailed assessment of a child's ability with specific verbs before such *wh*-questions are introduced in training.

Complex Sentences

Structure and Meaning

Not long after their second birthday, young children begin to show use of complex sentences that are built up of combinations of simpler sentences. This building-up process can be accomplished through use of one of three different types of syntactic structures. In one type, the simpler sentences are joined by a co-ordinating conjunction such that neither component is subordinate to the other. The second type involves complementation, in which a subordinate sentence fills an empty syntactic slot (e.g., direct object) of the sentence into which it is embedded ("I like eating ice cream"). The third type involves relativization. In this case, a subordinate sentence modifies a constituent of the sentence into which it is embedded (e.g., "There's the man who talks to chairs").

Children's acquisition of complex sentences does not vary only according to the type of syntactic structure involved. Additionally, it varies according to (1) whether or not a sentence connective is used (e.g., *and, because, what, that*), (2) the semantic relations expressed in the complex sentence, and (3) the presence of certain syntactic and/or cognitive processing constraints associated with the complex sentence. For example, when complex sentences containing connectives are considered, it appears that conjunction structures generally emerge in children's speech before structures involving complementation, while complementation structures emerge before structures with relativization (Bloom, Lahey, Hood, Lifter, & Fiess, 1980). However, the first complex sentences in children's speech involve object complementation where no connective is required, as in "I want see Ernie" (Limber, 1973). Sentences of this type often emerge shortly after the same verbs have been used with direct objects, as in "I want car" (Bowerman, 1979). Even conjunction structures first appear as juxtaposed sentences with no connective, such as "(There) my paper, pencil" (Clancey, Jacobsen, & Silva, 1976; Limber, 1973).

An examination of the order of emergence of sentence connectives reveals only a rough order of acquisition, for certain connectives seem quite variable in their point of emergence. The connective *and* typically appears before all others. The connectives *and then* and *because* are usually among the first several to emerge, *that* and *how* among the last (Bloom et al., 1980; Bowerman, 1979). As noted above, this general order may be due in part to the type of syntactic structure in which each connective is involved. For example, *and, and then,* and *because* are often used in conjunction structures, *how* in complementation structures and *that* in complementation and relativization structures.

The sequence of emergence of connectives also seems related to the semantic relations into which they may enter. Bloom et al. (1980) identified a number of such relations in their data. Additive relations were observed quite early. These involved the simple joining of elements whose combination did not create a meaning different from the meaning of each element separately ("Maybe you can carry that and I can carry this"). Other early emerging relations were temporal in character, in which one element of the sentence typically described an event that preceded or followed in time the event noted in the other element, as in "I going this way to get the groceries, then come back." Causal relations, too, emerged relatively early. In sentences of this type, one element of the sentence usually referred to an intended or ongoing action, and the other provided a reason for, or result of, the action ("Get them 'cause I want it"). Among the later emerging relations were adversative and notice relations. The former represented cases in which the information in one element contrasted with that of the other, as in " 'Cause I was tired. But now I'm not tired." Notice relations were seen when the first element of the sentence called attention to a state or action mentioned in the second ("Watch what I'm doing"). Bloom et al. noted that the connective *and* was often used with additive, temporal, and causal relations (among others), *and then* with temporal relations, *because* with causal relations. Later emerging connectives, on the other hand, were more often used with later emerging semantic relations, or were not used frequently with any other semantic relations.

An investigation focusing specifically on causal relations was performed by Hood and Bloom (1979). They noted that children's early expressions of causality make reference to the nonoccurrence of an event or the nonexistence of a state of affairs ("It can't go, 'cause it's too little"), requests for action by the listener ("Move over. Because the train hurt you"), and intended actions ("I want some milk 'cause I have a cold). Bloom and Hood observed differences among their subjects in terms of whether the cause element of the utterance typically preceded or followed the effect element. Interestingly, these order differences seemed to be established before the children began to use connectives. Further, for most of the children, it appears that the dominant order could have dictated which connective was acquired first. Those children who showed a dominant cause/effect order acquired *so* before *because*. Those who exhibited an effect/cause tendency acquired *because* before *so*. The children who showed no preferred order began to use *so* and *because* at approximately the same point in time.

Several studies have reported constraints on the use of certain complex sentences that may relate to processing difficulties and/or the extent to which certain syntactic operations can apply in particular sentence positions. For example, subject complementation and relativization ("The woman who fell went to the hospital") emerge later in children's speech than (nonparticipial) object complementation and relativization, respectively (Limber, 1973). Recently, several studies have focused on the constraints involved in the use of co-ordination with *and*. Lust (1977) presented data from elicited imitation experiments suggesting that young children have difficulty with sentences in which redundant elements have been deleted (phrasal co-ordination, as in, "Mary cooked the meal and ate the bread"), and perform at higher levels with sentences in which redundant elements are included (sentential co-ordination, as in, "Mary cooked the meal and Mary ate the bread"). In addition, when children delete redundant elements, they are more likely to do so when the element to be deleted follows the one to be retained (forward deletion, as in, "Kittens hop and φ run") than when it precedes the element to be retained (backward deletion, as in "Kittens φ and dogs hide").

Unfortunately, the elicited imitation data collected by deVilliers, Tager Flusberg, and Hakuta (1977) were not in accord with those of Lust (1977). These investigators found no evidence that sentential co-ordination was easier than phrasal co-ordination or that forward deletion was more likely than backward deletion. In order to gain greater insight into this issue, deVilliers et al. examined longitudinally collected spontaneous speech samples for instances of co-ordination with *and*. The children were observed to use phrasal co-ordination prior to sentential co-ordination. In addition, cases of forward deletion were more prevalent than those of backward deletion. More recently, Lust and Mervis (1980) performed a cross-sectional examination of young children's spontaneous speech, and reported that cases of forward deletion emerged earlier, and were more frequent, than instances of backward deletion. They also interpreted their data as supporting the view that sentential co-ordination was more frequent in the children's speech than phrasal co-ordination. An examination of their data, however, suggests that this is true only for children at the third highest level of mean-utterance-length studied (mean=4.15 morphemes). Although the evidence reported thus far concerning sentential versus phrasal co-ordination is not sufficiently clear to permit conclusions to be drawn, it does appear that forward deletions are more likely in young children's speech than backward deletions. As noted by deVilliers et al., this may possibly be due to the difficulty of planning for compound sentence subjects, given the right-branching structure of English.

The available evidence regarding children's acquisition of complex sentences offers a number of possibilities for clinical application. It may be important to insure that the child juxtaposes sentences in his or her speech before requiring production of sentences joined by a connective. In the case of causal relations, it might be useful to consider the order in which cause and effect elements are used by the child when selecting the causal connective to introduce in training.

It is clear that the teaching of connectives should involve more than the systematic introduction of connectives in the order seen in normal children's acquisition, with *and* presented before *and then* and *because*, etc. It seems important to insure that an early emerging connective (e.g., *and*) is first trained in utterances that express appropriate early emerging semantic relations (e.g., additive, temporal relations). Whether prior to or after the appearance of sentential conjunction, if it seems helpful to teach a child the use of phrasal conjunction, utterances with forward deletion appear to be the most appropriate to introduce—at least, at the outset.

Finally, the literature suggests that complementation and relativization might be better introduced in object position before subject position during training. It may also prove important to insure that the child can already use complement-taking verbs with direct objects prior to the commencement of complementation training.

Communication Usage

The growing complexity of utterances within the productive capabilities of children approaching age three allows them to use speech in the service of many communicative functions. Dore (1977) has described a number of these functions in a study of the speech used by seven children, ages 34 to 39 months when interacting with their peers and their nursery-school teacher. Thirty-two different functions, or illocutionary acts, were noted in the children's speech. The most common (each constituting from 7% to 10% of the utterances observed) included requests for action, requests for information about the identity, location, or property of an object, labeling of an object or event, descriptions of an event, and reports of the child's internal state. Protests, claims, the expression of rules, compliances with the action requests of others, and requests for permission to perform acts are examples of other functions seen with some regularity. Quite clearly, by the time children reach three years of age their communicative as well as structural capabilities are considerable.

Findings such as Dore's can be valuable to clinicians as guides in selecting communicative situations that might be employed in the clinical setting. It seems reasonable to assume that children who have had practice in using utterances serving a variety of functions may be better able to communicate at home, in the school room, and on the playground. Knowledge of the communicative functions expressed by young children can also provide clinicians with information concerning the lexical and syntactic forms that might be taught to the child. For example, permission requests ("May I go outside?") require the ability to use modals and to transpose elements. The expression of rules ("We should't put our feet on the table") requires use of conditionals and/or modals. Unless the child has acquired these forms, his or her expression of these communicative functions may be quite inadequate.

Texts

Cohesion

Thus far, discussion of children's linguistic development has centered on the comprehension and production of words and sentences. Yet, effective communication often requires the speaker to produce a series of sentences that are logically and structurally connected, as when a story is being told, instructions for the performance of some task are being given, and so on. The process of relating elements of the discourse (or text) together is termed "cohesion." To date, Halliday and Hasan (1976) may have provided the most complete description of the cohesive devices used by competent speakers of the language. These include, among others, anaphoric reference, cataphoric reference, ellipsis, and lexical cohesion. In anaphoric reference, features such as pronouns or definite articles are used to refer back to a previously established referent ("Gina is sick today. She has the flu"). In cataphoric reference, pronouns or demonstratives direct the listener to coming elements of the text ("After he warms up, Edwin is going to be unstoppable"). Ellipsis refers to the deletion of information available in an immediately preceding portion of the text ("Do you like to dance? I do"). In the case of lexical cohesion, a synonym or superordinate is used to refer back to a previously noted referent ("Suddenly, a lion appeared. The beast let out a terrifying roar.").

Relatively little is known about children's use of some of these cohesive devices. It appears that they follow up their own utterances with ellipsis less frequently than those of an interactant, and the percentages of ellipsis of the former type only increase from approximately 10% to 25% during the span from age five through nine years. In addition, for children in this age range, lexical cohesion usually represents no more than repeating the name of a referent in a subsequent utterance, perhaps to signal a continuity of meaning ("Erika wanted to take a walk. But it was raining outside. So Erika watched television instead") (Fine, 1978).

There has been considerable research on both anaphora and cataphora. Much of this work has been concerned with within-sentence anaphoric ("John said that he was going") and cataphoric reference ("Although he was in pain, the runner kept going") (Lust, 1981; Maratsos, 1973; Solan, 1981). However, a few studies focusing on between-sentence anaphora have appeared. These have dealt with use of the definite article. For example, Warden (1976) presented adults and children, ages three, five, seven, and nine years, with three drawings representing sequential events that formed a story. The stories were constructed so that as the subject told a story conforming to the picture sequence, at least two of the referents would each be mentioned twice. Of particular interest to Warden, of course, was whether the children would describe the referent the first time with the indefinite article *a* and, subsequently, with the definite article *the* ("A dog is chasing a hen" [picture 1]. "A cow stops the dog and the hen hides" [picture 2]. "The hen lays an egg" [picture 3]). Warden found that all of the subjects typically used the definite article when describing a referent that had already been mentioned (reaching 100% by age 7). However, the tendency to use the indefinite article when describing a referent introduced for the first time appeared to develop later. Only about one-half of the 3-year-olds' descriptions of newly introduced referents made use of the indefinite article. This percentage was approximately 80% for the 9-year-olds. Using a task similar to that of Warden, Emslie and Stevenson (1981) found evidence that when children are provided with aids to help them remember which referents had and had not appeared before, 3-year-olds' performances more closely approximate that of older children and adults.

Although a great deal more needs to be learned about cohesion in the speech of children, a few features appear in the literature that warrant consideration for possible clinical application. For instance, it seems that ellipsis might be modeled for a child through a two-person interaction in which one speaker's utterance can serve as an elliptical response to an utterance of the other speaker. Given the finding that ellipsis is more likely to follow an utterance of another than an utterance produced by the child, such a tack might be more successful than modeling a monologue in which a speaker responds elliptically to his or her own previous utterance. It also appears that the task used by Warden (1976), and refined by Emslie and Stevenson (1981), serves as an effective means of tapping young children's use of article anaphora, and may therefore prove quite useful as an assessment and/or training procedure with language disordered children.

Story Schemata

A number of psychologists have recently directed their efforts toward a characterization of the structure of stories and other types of prose. This work has indicated that stories, for example, have suprasentential structure, and that persons listening to stories use this structure as an aid to comprehension and recall. The structure of stories has often been described in terms of a grammar consisting of rewrite rules capable of generating well-formed stories, or of breaking them down into constituent units. The constituent units proposed have varied somewhat from investigator to investigator. The story-grammar structure proposed by Mandler and Johnson (1977) involves a setting followed by one or more episodes. Each episode has a beginning, a reaction of a character to the event in the beginning, an attempt to deal with the problem created in the beginning, an outcome of the attempt, and an ending.

When people listen to stories, they use pre-existing schemata acquired through previous experience with the structure of stories, as well as experience with various types of event sequences in the world. These two sources of experience have constituted two interrelated areas of investigation into children's comprehension and recall of stories. Representative of the first area is a study by Mandler (1978). The goal of this study was to determine whether two-episode stories whose structure conformed to the story grammar of Mandler and Johnson (1977) would be better recalled than two-episode stories with a structure characterized by an interleaving of the events of the two episodes. The elementary school-age children serving as subjects recalled more information and showed fewer distortions with the properly structured stories. Interestingly, interleaved stories were often recalled in a properly structured, rather than interleaved, form. Similar findings have been reported by Brown and Murphy (1975) and Stein and Glenn (1979).

As noted above, story schemata that serve as a guide to comprehension and recall are based not only on prior experience with the structure of stories, but also on world knowledge. The latter refers to expectations built up from knowledge of sequences of actions called for in familiar situations. These have been termed "scripts" (Schank & Abelson, 1977). Recently,

McCartney and Nelson (1981) presented evidence that script-based knowledge can play an important role in the story recall of kindergarten and second-grade children. Stories were devised that dealt with activities common to young children, such as eating dinner and preparing for bed. The particular events included in the stories were based, in part, on responses from preschoolers to questions concerning "what happened" during these activities. Along with the events that were hypothesized to conform to the children's scripts, "filler" events were added to the stories. These events enriched the story, but were not central to the activities. McCartney and Nelson found that central events were better recalled than filler events. For example, in a story about dinner time, the children usually recalled the main character being called to dinner, the commencement of eating, and the character's request to be excused, but often failed to recall the announced dinner menu or the topic of conversation during the meal. The older children out-performed the younger children, but primarily in recall of filler events. The two age groups were similar in recalling central events.

It seems that our developing knowledge of the structure of stories might be put to good clinical use. For example, the basic constituents of stories (setting, beginning, reaction, etc.) might be made explicit for language-disordered children, not only to aid comprehension but to serve as a means of ordering their comments when telling a story. The available evidence concerning children's scripts might be used by clinicians as a guide to the kind of information in a story that children may, and may not, be expected to retain. In addition, poor recall of central story events by children who seem to possess sufficient language-comprehension ability for the task might raise the possibility that the child's previous world experience with these events is limited, or is different from that of most children.

Figurative Language

In recent years, a number of studies dealing with children's comprehension and use of nonliteral, or figurative, language have appeared. These investigations have been concerned with riddles, proverbs, idioms, and metaphors. The majority of these studies have focused on metaphors. A metaphor represents the use of words in which one element, the topic, is compared to another, the vehicle, on the basis of shared attributes, the ground (Gardner, Winner, Bechhofer, & Wolf, 1978). For example, in "A shadow is a piece of night, " the topic, "a shadow" is compared to the vehicle, "a piece of night" on the basis of the shared quality of darkness, the ground.

Early work on children's understanding of metaphors suggested that this ability does not appear until children reach approximately nine years of age. However, an abundance of more recent studies suggests that this is not the case. For example, Gardner (1974) found that children as young as 3 years of age could attribute terms such as *happy* and *sad* to colors and auditory tones. Gentner (1977) observed that 4- and 5-year- olds were able to assign body parts (e.g., *knee, mouth*) to pictures of objects such as trees and mountains. These findings suggest that when metaphoric ability is assessed using simple directions, a nonverbal response mode, and familiar words and materials, evidence for metaphoric ability is seen at much younger ages. (In fact, when metaphoric ability is assessed completely independent of language, it is possible that even infants show a limited skill in this area [Wagner, Winner, Cicchetti, & Gardner, 1981]).

Although a basic ability to comprehend metaphoric language emerges early, it is clear that metaphoric ability continues to develop across time. Younger children seem to perform better on metaphors for which they can select the topic that goes with a vehicle provided them (therefore allowing more flexibility in the shared attributes that are criterial) than on metaphors for which all three elements are already provided (Winner, Engel, & Gardner, 1980). They perform better when they can choose from among several possible meanings of a metaphor than when they must explain its meaning (Winner, Rosenthiel, & Gardner, 1976). Not surprisingly, such children understand "frozen" forms, which, due to their frequent use, may have lost their metaphoric quality (e.g., "I ate up a storm") better than novel forms (Pollio & Pollio, 1979). Cross-sensory metaphors ("Her perfume was bright sunshine") are also better understood than psychological-physical metaphors ("The prison guard was a hard rock") (Winner et al., 1976). In addition, similarity metaphors, where objects are compared on the basis of shared features ("The stars are a thousand eyes") seem to be comprehended better by young children than proportional metaphors, where three objects are mentioned and a fourth must be inferred to complete a proportion ("My head is an apple without any core") (Billow, 1975). Performance on each of these more difficult types of metaphors increases with age. Finally, a word should be said about the production of metaphors. Although very young children show evidence of using words that serve as comments of analogy (e.g., Winner, 1979), it is nonetheless the case that the production of novel, appropriate metaphors is infrequent through adolescence, and does not seem to show a developmental increase until after seven years of age (Gardner, Kircher, Winner, & Perkins, 1975).

For many clinicians, a language-disordered child's understanding of metaphoric language would be an achievement beyond expectations.

Indeed, the severity of the linguistic difficulties experienced by many language-disordered children make the acquisition of some of the basic, literal aspects of language enough of a challenge. Nonetheless, figurative language appears not only in conversational speech, but in school activities and upper-elementary-grade textbooks (Ortony, Reynolds, & Arter, 1978). Thus, for the language-disordered child who functions linguistically at or above the four-year level, comprehension of metaphoric ability might constitute a reasonable clinical goal. Much more research needs to be done in this area, but the available work suggests a few directions for possible clinical application. For example, the child might be initially presented with words only, rather than sentences that must be treated in a nonliteral manner. Applying the qualities of the word's referent to referents pertaining to another modality (cross-sensory application) may prove most successful in the early phases of training. Initially, the child might be required only to point to his or her choice. When sentence metaphors are eventually introduced, they might first take the form of similarity metaphors, presented in a multiple-choice-task format.

Summary

In this chapter, a number of findings pertaining to normal language acquisition have been reviewed, with an eye toward how they may have relevance to clinical management. The abilities discussed have ranged from comprehension of the child's first word to appreciation of the relations expressed in a metaphor. The developmental relevance of this literature to clinical activities, then, is difficult to deny. Less certain is the degree to which the reviewed findings should serve as the basis for altering current assessment and training procedures. This question can be answered only if clinicians attempt to incorporate this information in their clinical work, or, better, put some of the possible applications to the test in controlled clinical research.

References

Billow, R. A cognitive developmental study of metaphor comprehension. *Developmental Psychology*, 1975, *11*, 415-423.

Block, E., & Kessel, F. Determinants of the acquisition order of grammatical morphemes: A re-analysis and re-interpretation. *Journal of Child Language*, 1980, *7*, 181-188.

Bloom, L., Capatides, J., & Tackeff, J. Further remarks on interpretive analysis: In response to Christine Howe. *Journal of Child Language*, 1981, *8*, 403-412.

Bloom, L., Hood, L., & Lightbown, P. Imitation in language development: If, when, and why. *Cognitive Psychology*, 1974, *6*, 380-420.

Bloom, L., & Lahey, M. *Language development and language disorders.* New York: Wiley, 1978.

Bloom, L., Lahey, M., Hood, L., Lifter, K., & Fiess, K. Complex sentences: Acquisition of syntactic connectives and the semantic relations they encode. *Journal of Child Language*, 1980, *7*, 235-262.

Bloom, L., Lifter, K., & Hafitz, J. Semantics of verbs and the development of verb inflection in child language. *Language*, 1980, *56*, 386-412.

Bloom, L., Miller, P., & Hood, L. Variation and reduction as aspects of competence in language development. In A. Picke (Ed.), *Minnesota symposia on child psychology* (Vol. 9). Minneapolis: University of Minnesota Press, 1975.

Bloom, L., Rocissano, L., & Hood, L. Adult-child discourse: Developmental interaction between information processing and linguistic knowledge. *Cognitive Psychology*, 1976, *8*, 521-552.

Boskey, M., & Nelson, K. Answering unanswerable questions: The role of imitation. Paper presented to the Boston University Conference on Language Development, Boston, MA., 1980.

Bowerman, M. The acquisition of complex sentences. In P. Fletcher & M. Garman (Eds.), *Language acquisition*. Cambridge, Eng.: Cambridge University Press, 1979.

Braine, M. Children's first word combinations. *Monographs of the Society for Research in Child Development*, 1976, *41* (Serial No. 164).

Brown, A., & Murphy, M. Reconstruction of arbitrary versus logical sequences by preschool children. *Journal of Experimental Child Psychology*, 1975, *20*, 307-326.

Brown, R. *A first language: The early stages.* Cambridge, MA: Harvard University Press, 1973.

Chapman, R. Comprehension strategies in children. In J. Kavanaugh & W. Strange (Eds.), *Speech and language in the laboratory, school, and clinic*. Cambridge, MA: MIT Press, 1978.

Clancey, P., Jacobsen, T., & Silva, M. The acquisition of conjunction: A cross-linguistic study. *Papers and Reports on Child Language Development*, 1976, *12*, 71-80.

Clark, E. What's in a word? On the child's acquisition of semantics in his first language. In T. Moore (Ed.), *Cognitive development and the acquisition of language*. New York: Academic Press, 1973.

Coggins, T., & Carpenter, R. The communicative intention inventory: A system for observing and coding children's early intentional communication. *Applied Psycholinguistics*, 1981, *2*, 235-252.

Dale, P. Is early pragmatic development measurable? *Journal of Child Language*, 1980, *7*, 1-12.

deVilliers, J., & deVilliers, P. A cross-sectional study of the acquisition of grammatical morphemes. *Journal of Psycholinguistic Research*, 1973, *2*, 267-278.

deVilliers, J., Tager Flusberg, H., & Hakuta, K. Deciding among theories of the development of coordination in child speech. *Papers and Reports on Child Language Development*, 1977, *13*, 118-125.

Dore, J. A pragmatic description of early language development. *Journal of Psycholinguistic Research*, 1974, *3*, 343-350.

Dore, J. Children's illocutionary acts. In R. Freedle (Ed.), *Discourse production and comprehension*. Norwood, NJ: Ablex, 1977.

Duchan, J., & Lund, N. Why not semantic relations? *Journal of Child Language*, 1979, *6*, 243-251.

Emslie, H., & Stevenson, R. Pre-school children's use of the articles in definite and indefinite referring expressions. *Journal of Child Language*, 1981, *8*, 313-328.

Ervin-Tripp, S. Children's verbal turn-taking. In E. Ochs & B. Schieffelin (Eds.), *Developmental pragmatics*. New York: Academic Press, 1979.

Ferguson, C., & Farwell, C. Words and sounds in early language acquisition: English initial consonants in the first 50 words. *Language*, 1975, *51*, 419-439.

Ferguson, C., Peizer, D., & Weeks, T. Model and replica phonological grammar of a child's first words. *Lingua*, 1973, *31*, 35-65.

Fine, J. Conversation, cohesive and thematic patterning in children's dialogues. *Discourse Processes*, 1978, *1*, 247-266.

Gardner, H. Metaphors and modalities: How children project polar adjectives onto diverse domains. *Child Development*, 1974, *45*, 84-91.

Gardner, H., Kircher, M., Winner, E., & Perkins, D. Children's metaphoric productions and preferences. *Journal of Child Language*, 1975, *2*, 125-141.

Gardner, H., Winner, E., Bechhofer, R., & Wolf, D. The development of figurative language. In K. Nelson (Ed.), *Children's language* (Vol. 1). New York: Gardner Press, 1978.

Garvey, C. The contingent query: A dependent act in conversation. In M. Lewis & L. Rosenblum (Eds.), *Interaction, conversation, and the development of language*. New York: Wiley, 1977.

Garvey, C. Contingent queries and their relations in discourse. In E. Ochs & B. Schieffelin (Eds.), *Developmental pragmatics*. New York: Academic Press, 1979.

Garvey, C., & Berninger, G. Timing and turn taking in children's conversations. *Discourse Processes*, 1981, *4*, 27-58.

Gentner, D. Children's performance on a spatial analogies task. *Child Development*, 1977, *48*, 1034-1039.

Halliday, M. *Learning how to mean*. London: Edward Arnold, 1975.

Halliday, M., & Hasan, R. *Cohesion in English*. London: Longman, 1976.

Holland, A. Language therapy for children: Some thoughts on context and content. *Journal of Speech and Hearing Disorders*, 1975, *40*, 514-523.

Hood, L., & Bloom, L. What, when, and how about why: A longitudinal study of early expressions of causality. *Monographs of the Society for Research in Child Development*, 1979, *44* (Serial No. 181).

Howe, C. The meanings of two-word utterances in the speech of young children. *Journal of Child Language*, 1976, *3*, 29-47.

Howe, C. Interpretive analysis and role semantics: A ten-year mésalliance? *Journal of Child Language*, 1981, *8*, 439-456.

Huttenlocher, J. The origins of language comprehension. In R. Solso (Ed.), *Theories in cognitive psychology*. Hillsdale, NJ: Lawrence Erlbaum, 1974.

Ingram, D. Early patterns of grammatical development. Paper presented at the Conference on Language Behavior in Infancy and Early Childhood, Santa Barbara, CA, 1979.

Keenan, E. Conversational competence in children. *Journal of Child Language*, 1974, *1*, 163-184.

Lahey, M., & Bloom, L. Planning a first lexicon: Which words to teach first. *Journal of Speech and Hearing Disorders*, 1977, *42*, 340-350.

Leonard, L. Chapman, K., Rowan, L., & Weiss, A. Three hypotheses concerning young children's imitation of lexical items. *Developmental Psychology*, 1983, *19*, 591-601.

Leonard, L., Schwartz, R., Folger, M., Newhoff, M., & Wilcox, M. Children's imitations of lexical items. *Child Development*, 1979, *50*, 19-27.

Leonard, L., Schwartz, R., Morris, B., & Chapman, K. Factors influencing early lexical acquisition: Lexical orientation and phonological composition. *Child Development*, 1981, *52*, 882-887.

Leopold, W. *Speech development of a bilingual child. Volume II. Sound learning in the first two years*. Evanston, IL: Northwestern University Press, 1947.

Lieven, E. Different routes to multiple word combinations? Paper presented at the Stanford Child Language Research Forum, Stanford, 1980.

Limber, J. The genesis of complex sentences. In T. Moore (Ed.), *Cognitive development and the acquisition of language*. New York: Academic Press, 1973.

Lust, B. Conjunction reduction in child language. *Journal of Child Language*, 1977, *4*, 257-288.

Lust, B. Constraints on anaphora in child language: A prediction for a universal. In S. Tavakolian (Ed.), *Language acquisition and linguistic theory*. Cambridge, MA: MIT Press, 1981.

Lust, B., & Mervis, C.A. Development of coordination in the natural speech of young children. *Journal of Child Language*, 1980, *7*, 279-304.

Macken, M. Permitted complexity in phonological development: One child's acquisition of Spanish consonants. *Papers and Reports on Child Language Development*, 1976, *11*, 28-60.

Mandler, J. A code in the node: The use of a story schema in retrieval. *Discourse Processes*, 1978, *1*, 14-35.

Mandler, J., & Johnson, N. Rememberance of things parsed: Story structure and recall. *Cognitive Psychology*, 1977, *9*, 111-151.

Maratsos, M. The effects of stress on the understanding of pronominal coreference in children. *Journal of Psycholinguistic Research*, 1973, *2*, 1-8.

Mayer, J., & Valian, V. When do children imitate? When imitate? When necessary. Paper presented at the Boston University Conference on Language Development, Boston, MA, 1977.

McCartney, K., & Nelson, K. Children's use of scripts in story recall. *Discourse Processes*, 1981, *4*, 59-70.

McShane, J. *Learning to talk*. Cambridge, Eng.: Cambridge University Press, 1980.

McTear, M. Repetition in child language: Imitation or creation? In R. Campbell & P. Smith (Eds.), *Recent advances in the psychology of language: Language development and mother-child interaction*. New York: Plenum Press, 1978.

Menn, L. Phonotactic rules in beginning speech. *Lingua*, 1971, *26*, 225-251.

Menn, L. *Pattern, control, and contrast in beginning speech: A case study in the development of word form and word function*. Unpublished doctoral dissertation, University of Illinois, Champaign, 1976.

Moerk, E. Relationships between parental input frequencies and children's language acquisition: A reanalysis of Brown's data. *Journal of Child Language*, 1980, *7*, 105-118.

Nelson, K. Structure and strategy in learning to talk. *Monographs of the Society for Research in Child Development*, 1973, *38*, Serial No. 1-2.

Nelson, K. The nominal shift in semantic-syntactic development. *Cognitive Psychology*, 1975, *7*, 461-479.

Nelson, K. Individual differences in language development: Implications for development and language. *Developmental Psychology*, 1981, *17*, 170-187.

Ninio, A., & Bruner, J. The achievement and antecedents of labelling. *Journal of Child Language*, 1978, *5*, 1-16.

Ortony, A., Reynolds, R., & Arter, J. Metaphor: Theoretical and empirical research. *Psychological Bulletin*, 1978, *85*, 919-943.

Oviatt, S. The emerging ability to comprehend language: An experimental approach. *Child Development*, 1980, *51* 97-106.

Peters, A. Language learning strategies: Does the whole equal the sum of the parts? *Language*, 1977, *53*, 560-573.

Pinker, S. On the acquisition of grammatical morphemes. *Journal of Child Language*, 1981, *8*, 477-484.

Pollio, M., & Pollio, H. A test of metaphoric comprehension and some preliminary data. *Journal of Child Language*, 1979, *6*, 111-120.

Ramer, A. The function of imitation in child language. *Journal of Speech and Hearing Research*, 1976, *19*, 700-717.

Rodgon, M. Situation and meaning in one- and two-word utterances: Observations on Howe's "The meanings of two word utterances in the speech of young children." *Journal of Child Language*, 1977, *4*, 111-114.

Rosenblatt, D. Learning how to mean: The development of representation in play and language. Paper presented at the Conference on the Biology of Play, Farnham, Eng., 1975.

Sachs, J., & Truswell, L. Comprehension of two-word instructions by children in the one-word stage. *Journal of Child Language*, 1978, *5*, 17-24.

Schank, R., & Abelson, R. *Scripts, plans, goals and understanding*. Hillsdale, NJ: Lawrence Erlbaum, 1977.

Schwartz, R., & Leonard, L. Do children pick and choose? Phonological selection and avoidance in early lexical acquisition. *Journal of Child Language*, 1982, *9*, 319-336.

Shibamoto, J., & Olmsted, D. Lexical and syllabic patterns in phonological acquisition. *Journal of Child Language*, 1978, *5*, 417-456.

Snyder, L., Bates, L., & Bretherton, I. The transition from first words into syntax: Continuities from 13 to 20 months. Paper presented at the Boston University Conference on Language Development, Boston, 1979.

Solan, L. The acquisition of structural restrictions on anaphora. In S. Tavakolian (Ed.), *Language acquisition and linguistic theory*. Cambridge, MA: MIT Press, 1981.

Stein, N., & Glenn, C. An analysis of story comprehension in elementary school children. In R. Freedle (Ed.), *New directions in discourse processing*. Norwood, NJ: Ablex, 1979.

Tyack, D., & Ingram, D. Children's production and comprehension of questions. *Journal of Child Language*, 1977, *4*, 211-224.

Vihman, M. From pre-speech to speech: On early phonology. *Papers and Reports on Child Language Development*, 1976, *12*, 230-244.

Wagner, S., Winner, E., Cicchetti, D., & Gardner, H. "Metaphorical" mapping in human infants. *Child Development*, 1981, *52*, 728-731.

Warden, D. The influence of context on children's use of identifying expressions and references. *British Journal of Psychology*, 1976, *67*, 101-112.

Winner, E. New names for old things: The emergence of metaphoric language. *Journal of Child Language*, 1979, *6*, 469-491.

Winner, E., Engel, M., & Gardner, H. Misunderstanding metaphor: What's the problem? *Journal of Experimental Child Psychology*, 1980, *30*, 22-32.

Winner, E., Rosenthiel, A., & Gardner, H. The development of metaphoric understanding. *Developmental Psychology*, 1976, *12*, 289-297.

Wolf, D., & Gardner, H. Style and sequence in early symbolic play. In N. Smith & M. Franklin (Eds.), *Symbolic functioning in children*. Hillsdale, NJ: Lawrence Erlbaum, 1979.

Wootten, J., Merkin, S., Hood, L., & Bloom, L. *Wh*-questions: Linguistic evidence to explain the sequence of acquisition. Paper presented to the Society for Research in Child Development, San Francisco, 1979.

Jacqueline Weis Liebergott
Anthony S. Bashir
Martin C. Schultz

Dancing Around and Making Strange Noises: Children at Risk

One of the more familiar vaudeville routines goes something like this: "Daddy, why are you out in the backyard dancing around and making strange noises?" "I'm performing an incantation to ward off white elephants," answers the father. Delighted to be able to outwit her father, the child says, "But, Daddy, I don't see any white elephants." And the ever-wise father retorts, "Exactly."

In an attempt to modify, if not ward off, the effects of handicapping conditions, speech-language clinicians are joining with other developmental specialists in early intervention programs for young handicapped and at-risk children. Our involvement in these programs suggests that we share with our colleagues the belief, or hope, that early intervention will enhance the child's developmental status. We also believe that as language clinicians we have a major role in achieving this improved outcome. Inherent in our belief is the idea that we can identify and assess infants and young children who may be at risk for language disorders. Similarly, we believe that we can use our findings to design effective models of intervention, as well as to determine therapeutic goals.

This chapter addresses some of the issues involved in the identification and assessment of children at risk for language impairments. It is apparent that the potential for future developments in these areas will be more exciting than the present state of the art.

At-Risk Children: Problems in Determination

A series of problems and questions arise when the label "at risk" is used to designate the developmental status of a child. The clinician might ask: "What is the child at risk for? What event or criteria did you use in making your determination? What were the key elements in the child's history or the family history that made you concerned for the possibility of later developmental or communicative problems? What clinical assessment scales or measurements were used to determine the child's status?" In answering these questions, different aspects and perspectives concerning the problem emerge. As speech-language clinicians, our primary concern is the identification of those children who are specifically at risk for language problems. As yet, however, we are not able to specify what types of differences in communicative behaviors place the very young child at risk. Consequently, we have relied on approaches that use the presence of a variety of antecedent conditions to say that a child is at risk for future language problems.

Such an approach is seen in the works of Tjossem (1976) and Ramey, Trohanis, and Hostler (1982). They distinguish three kinds of risk factors. These factors are established risk, environmental risk, and biological risk. The groupings are not mutually exclusive.

1. *Established Risk.* "This term refers to the infant whose early appearing and aberrant development is related to diagnosed medical disorders of known etiology and which have relatively well known expectancies for developmental outcome within specified ranges of developmental delay" (Ramey, Trohanis, & Hostler, 1982, p. 8). Children with Down's syndrome, deafness, or hearing impairment are in this category.

2. *Environmental Risk.* "When the life experiences of a biologically sound infant are limited to the extent that, without corrective intervention, they impart a high probability for delayed development, the infant is at environmental risk" (Ramey et al., 1982, p. 8). Notice the tautology implicit in this definition, since the judgment concerning the need for intervention has become part of the definition. Abused and/or neglected children and failure-to-thrive children are suspected by some to be at-risk for a language impairment.

3. *Biological Risk.* "This term specifies the infant who presents a history of prenatal, perinatal, neonatal and early development events suggestive of biological insult to the developing central nervous system and which, either sing-

ly or collectively, increase the probability of later appearing aberrant development" (Ramey et al., 1982, p. 8). Among these conditions are anoxia, very low birth weight, prematurity at birth, respiratory-distress syndrome, metabolic disturbances, and central-nervous-system disorders.

The approach that uses antecedent conditions to identify children at high risk has several inherent problems. First, as pointed out by Cairns and Butterfield (1981), two types of inappropriate expectancies occur. Some of the children with a history of certain antecedent conditions do not develop poorly, while some children with no early indications of problems do not do well. Further, the various categories defining risk represent a not well-understood continuum, and there is uncertainty concerning the eventual communicative status of children in many of these categories. For example, we have more informatioin about the consequences of deafness and Down's syndrome on communicative status than we have about the effects of such conditions as failure to thrive, prematurity of birth, or metabolic disease. Finally, given the variability in outcomes associated with histories of different antecedent conditions, little is to be gained from a *strict* reliance on established, environmental, and biological risk factors for identifying children with potential problems.

To elaborate some of the issues and limitations related to the use of antecedent conditions for determining whether a child is at risk for later language disorders, we have chosen to focus on biological risk factors, specifically infants born prematurely. We first discuss what is known about the existence of handicapping conditions in general in this population, and then describe what is known about their speech and language status.

Prematurity

Field (1979) makes a distinction between "healthy" and "sick" premature infants. "Sick" premature infants are those suffering from complications in addition to prematurity. These complications include asphyxia, respiratory-distress syndrome, metabolic disorders, and such central-nervous-system complications as subependymal-intraventricular hemorrhage. The outcome for infants with one or more of these complications is less favorable than for those who are free of complications.

Approximately 7% of all pregnancies end before term (Pilliteri, 1981). According to Fitzhardinge (1980), in the absence of asphyxia, the prognosis for infants weighing between 1,500 and 2,500 grams is very good. The introduction of the neonatal intensive-care unit and advances in the medical management of these infants have reduced neonatal mortality and morbidity (Field, 1979; Thompson & Reynolds, 1977). For infants weighing between 1,000 and 1,500 grams, survival rates from 1947 to 1968 were 40% to 50%, whereas data collected in the late 1970s showed survival rates approaching 75% to 95% for low-birth-weight infants managed within intensive-care units (ICUs) (Thompson & Reynolds, 1977). Iatrogenic problems of the ICUs of the late 1960s and early 1970s have also decreased, as neonatologists have learned more about appropriate management of respiratory complications, temperature control, and metabolic, biochemical, and nutritional needs (Koops & Harmon, 1980). The outlook for babies born weighing less than 1,000 grams, whose weight is appropriate for their gestational age, is also improving, but Thompson and Reynolds (1977) report that the number of survivors remains below 30%. Similarly, the incidence of severely handicapping conditions in this group remains high. In data reported by Kitchen, Ryan, Rickards, et at., (1980), there was a survival rate of 47.7% for those weighing under 1,000 grams in 1978, as compared to 6.4% in the early 1970s. Changes in numbers of children with serious handicaps have also occurred. For example, Lubchenco (1976), describing children born in the 1950s and early 1960s, reported an incidence of cerebral palsy in low-birth-weight infants of 32%; more recent studies report incidences of cerebral palsy as ranging from 2.4% (Kitchen et al., 1980) to 4% (Fitzhardinge & Ramsay 1973; Stewart & Reynolds, 1974).

Although the presence of severe handicapping conditions has decreased, the numbers of children who have mild and moderate disabilities that may relate to problematic educational outcomes or disruption in social interaction patterns persist. Thompson and Reynolds (1977) state that additional information on the subtle educational, speech, hearing, and behavioral disabilities of low-birth-weight infants is necessary if we are to appreciate the problems encountered by those who survive. Fitzhardinge (1980) suggested that the identification of later language and learning problems evidenced by surviving infants was complicated by the lack of sensitive assessment measures of the less severe conditions.

Studies of speech and language acquisition involving direct assessment of young children's communicative behavior are few. The children evaluated in these studies are sometimes not clearly described and, because evaluation procedures and ages of assessment differ markedly, it is difficult to make comparisons across studies. Furthermore, it is all too obvious that there are insufficient valid and reliable instruments for measuring the language of very young children. This issue is discussed at length in a later section of this chapter.

Kastein and Fowler (1959) reported data on the speech and language abilities of 66 premature infants evaluated at two years of age. No descriptions of what characterized the children's prematurity or their neonatal course were provided. Of these 66 children born at a time when 50% was the survival rate for premature infants, 58% were considered to have "retardations of language and speech development." DeHirsch, Jansky, and Langford (1964) also studied the language abilities of premature children born in the 1950s. They evaluated 51 prematurely born children and 66 maturely born children. The two groups were evaluated at 5.8 years on the average. The premature children had birth weights ranging from 1,000 to 2,239 grams. Both groups had normal intellectual achievement on the Stanford-Binet Intelligence Scale, Form L. Fifteen different measures of speech and language were used. Significant differences were found between the two groups on 7 of the measures: handtapping patterns, language comprehension, word finding, number of words used, mean length of the five longest utterances, sentence elaboration, and definitions. DeHirsch et al. suggested that these differences resulted from the premature children's "lingering neurophysiological immaturity," directing the argument to the issue of delay-versus-deficient language. Unfortunately, the important question—"will the noted language difference affect the child's achievement of educational and social success?—was left unanswered, and remains so to this day.

The results of the Collaborative Perinatal Project of the National Institute of Neurological and Communication Disorders and Stroke (Lassman, Fisch, Vetter, & LaBenz, 1980) provide us with data collected on the largest published sample of premature children evaluated for speech and language abilities. Their sample of approximately 20,000 children included 917 premature children ($\leq$ 36 weeks and $\leq$ 2,500 grams) and 100 low-birth-weight children ($\leq$ 1,500 grams) born in the early 1960s. The speech and language abilities of these children were assessed at 3 and 8 years of age. When the 917 premature children were compared to the entire 8-year-old sample, the premature children performed more poorly in articulation, language comprehension and production, word identification, and concept development. Further, the 100 low-birth-weight children performed even more poorly than the children with birth-weights between 1,500 and 2,500 grams. No tests of statistical significance were performed on these data, since the study designers believed that statistical significance did not necessarily indicate clinical significance. The authors interpreted their findings much like DeHirsch et al., suggesting that eventually the majority of premature children would reach normal developmental levels. Like many others, this study did not address the question of whether or how early reductions in speech and language abilities of these children might be related to later educational status and social development.

Ehrlich, Shapiro, Kimball, and Huttner (1973) evaluated the language and speech abilities of 181 high-risk children at five years of age. Twenty-nine measures were used to assess these children, including the Peabody Picture Vocabulary Test, Templin-Darley Articulation Screening Test, the Illinois Test of Psycholinguistic Abilities, the Wechsler Pre-School and Primary Scale of Intelligence, and the Leiter. Although children having evident neurological abnormalities (reported in their intensive care unit records) were excluded from the study, at the time of the assessment six of the children demonstrated neurologic and sensory problems, three evidenced mild retardation, two had cerebral palsy, two had visual impairments, and two had sensorineural hearing loss. Significant correlations were found between language ability and each of these antecedent conditions: respiratory-distress syndrome, birth weights of less than 2,500 grams, and shortened gestational age. Only 16% of the total sample was functioning normally, 30% was reported as needing "close watching," and 54% was recommended for follow-up.

It is important to remember that the children included in the above reported studies were born in the 1950s and 1960s, a time when catastrophic outcomes were common. What of the children of the 1970s? Fitzhardinge (1980) in a study of full-term, small-for-gestational-age children, reported that 13 of 39 boys and 15 of 67 girls had significant speech problems. Twenty-two children had problems that persisted into school age. She concluded that although improved nutrition during the neonatal period may have reduced the incidence of speech and language delay and disorders below that seen in the survivors of the 1960s, specific learning disabilities and language disorders will most likely be evident in the apparently normal 1970s survivors as they grow older.

Blackstone (1980) reported on the language status of three groups of at-risk children studied at 24 months of age. These groups consisted of low-birth-weight infants, full-term infants who manifested seizure disorders, and children of low birth weight who manifested seizure disorders. Children were evaluated using the *Denver Developmental Screening Test* (DDST) and a protocol to assess communication development. The results indicated a higher incidence of problems in the risk groups, when their performances were compared to available norm-referenced data. Nearly one-half of the infants with seizure disorders were severely handicapped. Most of the low-birth-weight children had normal DDST scores and normal neurological exams at 24 months, but their language status was judged by the speech-language clinician to be "questionable." The results from the group of children with low birth weights and seizures fell between the other two groups.

Blackstone argues that the questionable status of language abilities in these children, who otherwise have normal DDST exams, may reflect the kinds of language behaviors assessed at 2 years. The nature of the children's problems may be subtle. To assess children's language behavior, the *Sequenced Inventory of Communication Development* (SICD) and the *Receptive Expressive Emergent Language Scale* (REEL) were used. Correlation coefficients between a subject's performance at 2, 4, 6, 9, 12, and 18 months were compared to performance at 24 months. Neither the SICD nor the REEL test was useful in predicting performance in other than severely impaired children before 1 year of age; both tests were most predictive of 24-month scores at 18 months of age. Blackstone suggested a need to develop more sensitive developmental indices.

Hubatch, Johnson, Kistler, and Rutherford (1981) conducted a study of 10 low-birth-weight infants (780 to 1,730 grams) all of whom experienced respiratory-distress syndrome and required mechanical ventilation. These infants were compared to a group of 10 normal children matched for MLU. The premature children averaged 23 months of age and the normal children were 19 months old. All children were in the one-word stage. The premature children performed within normal limits on the Bayley Mental Development Index; the normal children did likewise on the DDST. Results indicated that the groups differed on measures of receptive and expressive language as well as in their developmental histories. The children with low birth weights and respiratory distress performed significantly more poorly in receptive vocabulary, and made fewer utterances. They also imitated less and said their first words later. Hubatch et al. state that the reason for differences was not known. They concluded that the group of children with low birth weight and respiratory-distress syndrome were "at risk" for later communication disorders.

Findings of these studies of children born prematurely highlight some of the issues and limitations involved in attempting to predict language outcomes on the basis of antecedent conditions. Some of the issues are the following:

1. While advances in the medical care of children born prematurely have resulted in a reduction of catastrophic outcomes, there is variability in the developmental status of the children who survive. This makes it difficult to use the presence of an antecedent condition to identify children, since there exist problems of prediction secondary to the extended range of outcome possibilities.

2. Children born prematurely and who have had additional complications, such as asphyxia, respiratory-disease syndrome, or subependymal-intraventricular hemorrhage, may be at greater risk for language disorders. However, only longitudinal studies of the children and the individual varia-

tions in language acquisition and development will allow us to identify those genuinely at risk for later linguistic disorders.

3. Studies of children whose birth weights are less than 1,500 grams suggest that, for some, problems during the preschool years persist as disorders of reading and written language. However, the presence of later educational disorders in children with early language disorders is not restricted to children with low birth weight. The findings of later academic problems are similar to those reported on other groups of children, and these later studies have implicated early disruptions in speech and language development as precursors of later learning disabilities (Aram & Nation, 1980; Snyder, this volume; Strominger & Bashir, 1977).

4. The lack of appropriate measurements of early language behavior that can be useful as predictors of later language abilities makes the identification of children at risk for communication disorders difficult.

5. The historical presence of an antecedent condition alerts the clinician that the child may be at greater risk for later language disorder. However, because of variability in developmental outcomes, assessments of the child's cognitive and linguistic behavior is necessary to determine accurately the scope of the disabilities, and, therefore, the need for intervention. Miller (1982), in a consideration of etiology and language disorders, states that: "identifying the primary etiologic agent can predict an increased potential for language deficits, serving as an "at risk" register for language disorders [and as such can only] serve as a first level screen in early identification. . .(p. 64).

Review of these studies indicates the need for more precise information relating later speech and language outcomes to earlier perinatal and medical problems. Such documentation requires longitudinal studies ensuring an adequate understanding of neonatal complications and their impact on developmental language disorders. Further insights can be expected from the routine and periodic measures that would be taken of emerging speech and language during such longitudinal investigations. Additionally, comparable longitudinal data must be forthcoming on normal children developing language, so as to describe normal variability in the emergence of communication. We must move from a determination of at-risk-by-reference-to-antecedent conditions to a determination of at-risk-by-reference-to-indices-of-linguistic-and-communicative behaviors that have *predictive validity* for the later language status of the child.

Indices of Language Development: The Need

Clinicians' abilities to identify and to provide high quality service to children at risk are restricted by the lack of evaluation instruments that directly assess children's prelinguistic and early linguistic behaviors. We believe that the optimum way to develop indices for identification and assessment is through the study of the cognitive, affective, and linguistic status of the child, as well as the specific patterns of parent-child interaction that may affect the child's linguistic development.

Identification and assessment must incorporate a probabilistic perspective, since there presently are no clear clinical indices available that allow us to distinguish between children who demonstrate slow language development from those children who demonstrate "genuinely" altered language development. Leonard (1972) made the following comments concerning the probabilistic nature of early identification:

> The future linguistic behavior of children who use restricted utterances made up of early developing structures. . .proves difficult to predict. If such a child is three or older, it is not worth the risk of waiting to see whether his language develops further, for the social and educational developments in his near future will demand a more sophisticated linguistic system. And if the child is not yet three years of age? Many of us may not treat such a child because he may be a "late developer. " A few of us may recommend some sort of language intervention, but all of us are just guessing (p. 441).

The development of better assessment indices will increase the probability of identifying those children who are not at risk, those who are at risk for language disorder, and those who will require services. The need for what we call indices of language development results from seven considerations.

First, the measures designed for assessment of children whose language abilities are below the three-year level usually consist of a limited number of restricted tasks intended to do little more than assess major language milestones. For example, the *Receptive-Expressive Emergent Language Scale* (REEL) designed by Bzoch and League (1971) consists of a total of 66 items assessing receptive language and 66 items assessing expressive language. The test has three expressive items and three receptive items at each age interval, and extends across the range 3 months to 36 months. Age levels are divided into 2, 3, and 4-month intervals, so that six behaviors are assessed in each 3-month period. The *Preschool Language Scale* (revised form), another frequently used test, designed by Zimmerman, Steiner, and Evatt (1979), assesses children at 6-month intervals from 12 months to 7 years of age. This test contains only eight items at each age level, four measuring auditory comprehension and four measuring verbal abilities. The clinician has only eight different behaviors by which to reach a clinically competent decision, and to design a therapy plan. The *Reynell Developmental Language Scales* (Reynell, 1969) is probably one of the more sophisticated procedures and yet it too contains only a limited number of tasks for the assessment of any one stage of development. In addition, as Menyuk (1979) points out, many of the behaviors on standardized tests are difficult to quantify, e.g., how does one objectify "enjoys making sounds" or "combines sounds?" An analysis of the items of the *Denver Developmental Screening Test* allows the same conclusions (Miller, 1982).

Second, most assessment procedures are designed to obtain preliminary information about a child's language status; they cannot be used directly to prescribe the goals of intervention (Siegel, 1979). The clinician presently must rely on his or her own abilities to make a prescriptive determination. While clinicians engage in prescriptive determination, it is unclear that the results of their assessment allow them to direct intervention toward those aspects of language deficit that may best respond to environmental intervention (Menyuk & Wilbur, 1981). This is true because we are uncertain about which aspects of language behavior are influenced specifically by environmental factors. However, there are data that indicate a general compensatory or ameliorative influence of "good" home environments (see Siegel, 1982), and several studies that document the success of early intervention programs (Heber & Garber, 1975; Kysela, Hillyard, McDonald & Ahlsten-Taylor, 1981).

Third, the tasks included on currently available instruments assess discrete abilities not necessarily related to later linguistic accomplishments. Currently, we do not have the knowledge necessary to construct assessment instruments allowing for the specific assessments of earlier behaviors that serve as important precursors or predictors of the child's later linguistic development. For example, while we know that children produce increasingly diversified phonological units before the development of first words, we do not know how this phonological experimentation influences the emergence of first words or determines the course of later phonological development. Similarly, we do not know what earlier behaviors support the emergence of first words and what the influence of early acquisition of first words has on subsequent development of other linguistic and cognitive strategies.

Fourth, most assessment procedures do not measure language in terms of the interactive functions it serves for children and their communicative partners (McLean, 1979). Rees (1978) noted that current tests fail to explore the pragmatics of language. Moreover, such intervention efforts based on test results usually address only those abilities assessed, such as acquisition of vocabulary, development of syntax, and/or acquisition of speech sounds.

Fifth, since the currently available assessment instruments consist of a small number of items at each level, the clinician is limited in his or her ability to monitor effects of intervention. This issue can be addressed only by having an appraisal system that is sensitive to the changes occurring in the process of acquiring language. For example, the monitoring of the child's acquisition of a first lexicon should include some way of assessing both number and kind of words that the child knows as well as ways in which the child can use these words to communicate information, needs, and intent. Current assessment instruments do not provide this, since their principal goal is to determine if the child comprehends or produces a few commonly used object labels or actions.

Sixth, since a significant discrepancy from expectation must be present for the diagnosis of a language disorder to be made, intervention must wait until that significant difference has occurred. This is so because the determination of who is language impaired and who is not is based almost exclusively on the age at which the child accomplishes developmental milestones. Most often, clinicians use as a "rule of thumb" that the child must be a year behind in some or all aspects of language behavior. For a young child below the age of 3, this may mean that the child is not only a year behind before receiving assistance, but that the child has not mastered a significant proportion of language mastered by comparable peers. Therefore, a system of appraisal needs to be constructed examining component process as well as rate of emergence.

Seventh, while the role of the environment in the children's acquisition of language is receiving increasing attention in the literature on acquisition (Chapman, 1981; Furrow, Nelson, & Benedict, 1979; Snow & Ferguson, 1977), it is seldom considered in assessment. An exception to this can be seen in the work of those involved in the predictions of at-risk children. Sameroff and Chandler (1975) note that failures in the prediction of developmental disorders result from a lack of adequate knowledge regarding the complex and mutual influences between the child and the environment. These interactional influences serve to ameliorate or exacerbate the effects of earlier insults or trauma. Sameroff and Chandler conclude that developmental problems require developmental approaches for analysis. Cornell and Gottfried (1976) review some relevant studies of the ability of "stimulating" environments to compensate for developmental delay and for inadequate environments to increase delay.

Siegel (1982), in a recent study of 80 low-birth-weight children (birth weights less than 1,501 grams) and 68 full-term infants, attempted to increase the predictability of infant tests for assessing language and cognitive abilities using the Caldwell Inventory of Home Stimulation (HOME) (Elardo, Bradley, & Caldwell, 1975), along with the Uzgiris and Hunt Scale (1975) and the Bayley Infant Development Scales (1969). Children were assessed with the Bayley and Uzgiris-Hunt Scales at 4, 8, 12, and 18 months. The Caldwell Inventory was administered at 12 months of age. Outcome status was determined at two years of age by re-administering the Bayley Scales, the Hunt-Uzgiris Scales, and the Reynell Developmental Language Scales. Siegel found significant correlations between early measures and developmental outcomes particularly on certain subscales. She reported that children classified as being at risk in infancy, but who showed normal language and cognitive development at two years of age, came from families who scored higher on the HOME Scale. In contrast, children who were not classified as being at-risk in infancy, but who demonstrated later language or cognitive difficulty came from families who scored lower on the HOME Scale.

This type of data reinforces the need to include in assessment indices measures of the child's linguistic environment. Since at present we are unsure about the role of the environment in acquisition and its relation to developmental outcomes, here, too, we must be cautious. For example, Murphy (1982) studied phonetic development and mother responsiveness in a group of twelve children who differed in their rate of lexical acquisition. She found that the mothers' responsiveness to structured vocalizations (defined as vocalizations that contained at least one syllabic segment) did not influence strongly the rate of lexical acquisition. Mothers' responsiveness scores were higher for children whose lexical acquisition was more rapid than were mother's responsiveness scores for children whose lexicons developed more slowly. However, differences were minimized when the number of structured vocalizations were equated. Menyuk (1979), reviewing some of the results of mother-infant interaction studies, stated that perhaps only extreme variations in the amount and kind of speech provided by the caretaker will have an effect on the rate or quality of linguistic behaviors during the *early* years.

In reviewing studies of mothers' speech to children during the second year of life, Chapman (1981) suggested this stage as one in which the mother's verbal interaction with the child may play a differential role in development. She concluded that linguistically responsive—rather than linguistically stimulating—environments may accelerate acquisition. Longitudinal studies using appropriate assessment measures, and including outcome measures, should begin to yield *clinically* relevant answers to issues of environmental influence. We need to answer questions concerning matters like, "What is the mother responsive to?" and "What kinds of behavior in the child does her responsiveness affect?"—so that we may design more effective intervention programs.

What to Assess and How

This chapter began by describing an adult incantation for warding off white elephants. When we get down to the issue of what behaviors to assess and how, the white elephant problem becomes clearer. If the literature provided us with descriptions of linguistic differences between normally developing and impaired children, then the question of what, how, and when to measure would be simplified. This, however, is not the case. Johnston (1982) reviewed studies that attempted to find differences in syntax, grammatical morphology, relational semantics, lexical semantics, and pragmatics. She drew similar conclusions. Johnston stated that "research to date revealed virtually no consequence of learning language out of phase. Language disordered children may learn to speak slowly and late, but little else about their language has proved remarkable" (p. 789). The implication for assessment, and therefore prediction, appears to be that either we stop looking for differences or that we alter the way in which we attempt to isolate differences.

Johnston suggests that differences can be described perhaps by the simultaneous investigation of different aspects of linguistic behavior. As an example, she suggests that the appearance of inflectional morphemes such as progressive -ing and plural -s may accompany the production of complex rather than simple sentences in language-impaired children. It is interesting to note that as support for the above hypothesis, she cites four case studies which followed children longitudinally, rather than cross-sectional experimental investigations (Bax & Stevenson, 1977; Kerschensteiner & Huber, 1975; Trantham & Pederson, 1976; Weiner, 1974). Her own longitudinal work with Schery (Johnston & Schery, 1976) on the development of grammatical morphemes in language-impaired children, seems to support her hypothesis as well. She concluded that differences may appear once different aspects of the linguistic system are studied. To her suggestion, we would add that this research *should* be longitudinal, and that if prediction is a goal, follow-up analysis is necessary to determine the relations between earlier and later language behaviors.

The results of studying relations among different aspects of the grammar should advance our ability to define what constitutes a language disorder. Additionally, these studies should include the study of patterns of coherence and dissociation in linguistic, cognitive, and affective domains.

This approach may be critical for the objectification of the clinician's belief that many children who are language-impaired are different, not just delayed. The principal reason for this belief may derive from the fact that the clinician uses information from multiple domains. In general, during the course of assessment, clinicians focus simultaneously on the data from formal measurement of language abilities, on other data derived from their interactions with the child, and the family, historical information, and on data from other assessments. All of these sources allow the clinician to form hypotheses used directly in the diagnostic decision that a child is language-impaired. Indeed, the clinical diagnosis is based on information about the status of the child, and these data are derived by direct or observational information from at least three domains of behavior; for example, linguistic, cognitive, and affective.

Cross-domain research and studies of different aspects of the linguistic system appear to be a productive means for determining parameters of language impairment. We would like to offer an additional suggestion on how we might objectify clinical intuitions of difference. It would seem that time spent by a child within a stage must be included when matching children for linguistic development. Investigators (Leonard, 1979; Morehead & Ingram, 1973) have found that differences resulting from the analyses of children's production disappear when children are matched for MLU or Brown's stages of development, or both. Miller and Chapman (1981) investigated the relation between age and MLU in 123 normal-developing children between 17 and 59 months of age. Their children spent an average of 3.3 months in each of Brown's stages (ranges 3.1 to 3.9). We know it takes longer for language-impaired children to learn to speak, and that they may remain at a particular stage for a much longer time. It is possible, then, that when we match impaired children with children who move rapidly from stage to stage, we may be obscuring "time-in-stage differences" in results.

One potential design for investigating differences may be to match language impaired children with normal children when the language-impaired child has been in one of Brown's stages for a similar period of time. This means that both groups of children would need to be followed longitudinally until they have been in a stage for an equivalent amount of time. They would then be assessed at this point, (e.g., 2 months after their MLU had reached 2.0, but remained less than 2.5, if we use a change in MLU of 0.5 to indicate a change in stage). It would then be interesting to continue to follow these children using this same assessment procedure to describe the differences in the emerging patterns.

Another major issue facing those interested in assessment and prediction is the evaluation of age norms for the acquisition of certain language behaviors. Studies of different aspects of language acquisition show large variability, even among the normal population. Some examples may prove interesting. Menyuk (1978) describes the variability found in Brown's study of normally developing children (1973). Brown found that the age for achieving an MLS 2.5 was 25 to 30 months, for an MLU of 3.5 was 24 to 35 months, and for an MLU of 4.5 was 32 to 48 months. Menyuk found even wider discrepancies when she evaluated Morehead and Ingram's (1973) data on normal developing and developmentally dysphasic children. Whereas the normal children reached an MLU of 2-plus at 20 months of age, the dysphasic children did not reach this MLU until 60 months. This represents a difference of 40 months in age for attainment. The age discrepancy between the groups increased for attainment of an MLU of 5.5, the groups now differing by 71 months of age.

Nelson (1973) and Benedict (1979) report similar amounts of variability when studying normal children's acquisition of a first lexicon. For example, Nelson (1973) studied eighteen children and found that they reached a productive vocabulary of 50 words at an average age of 19.6 months, with a standard deviation of 2.89—but the range was 14 to 24 months. Benedict (1979) using a similar procedure with eight children, found a mean of 18.8 months and a range of 13 to 22 months. Reporting on the comprehension of 50 words, however, she found still smaller variability; that is, a mean age of 13.5 months, and a range of 10.2 to 16.5 months. If one were to presume that this small amount of data reflected the range seen in the normal population, one might conclude that it is reasonable to attempt to separate normal/at-risk children by acquisition rate. However, it would be necessary to determine the relation between lexical acquisition and other measures of language before one could determine accurately a ceiling score that could be used to determine the presence of a language disorder.

Hubbell (1981) expressed similar concern over age ranges provided by many standardized tests. He cited as one example the item in the *Denver Developmental Screening Test* that assesses comprehension of three prepositions. This item was passed by 25% of the children at 2.7 years, 50% at 3.1 years, 75% at 3.4 years, and 90% at 4.5 years. He concluded that these age ranges "encompass virtually half the children's total life span at the time the testing was done." The problem is to differentiate between children who are developing language normally, albeit at a slower rate, from those children who evidence altered acquisitional patterns that persist into the school years. It is likely that the relation between various aspects of language, or the *patterns* formed by different variables between groups at different developmental stages, may be more important than differences in rate.

A final issue that must be considered in the assessment and prediction of children with language impairments is how to evaluate the cognitive behaviors that have been identified as relating to language development (Bloom, 1970, 1973; Bowerman, 1974; Brown, 1973; Morehead & Ingram, 1973). Menyuk (1979) argued that some cognitive measures, for example, the *Bayley Scales of Infant Development,* are simply measuring limited aspects of linguistic development, rather than measuring cognitive development per se. Similarly, standardized performance tests that yield results showing language-impaired children operating within the "normal range" may not be measuring appropriate nonlinguistic behaviors. Many researchers have investigated cognitive functioning in language-impaired children and found that some of them appear to evidence nonlinguistic deficits (Brown, Redmond, Bass, Liebergott, & Swope, 1975; Folger & Leonard, 1978; Johnston & Ramstad, 1978; Lovell, Hoyle, & Siddall, 1968; Snyder, 1975). However, the developmental consequences of these nonlinguistic deficits remain speculative. Assessment and description of children's cognitive behavior may yield useful information for the content of therapy, but we have yet to determine the contribution made by nonlinguistic behavior to specific aspects of language acquisition.

There is a multitude of linguistic behaviors that can be used for constructing indices of language development (Miller, 1981; 1982). These behaviors have been discussed in the normal-language-acquisition literature, and a few have been investigated in children with language impairments. The usefulness of these measures (i.e., behaviors across linguistic domains) for predicting later language development cannot be discussed at this time because outcome studies have yet to be done.

In summary, to construct indices of language development for the identification and assessment of children at risk for language disorders, we will need to engage in:

1. Longitudinal study of larger groups of normal children, as well as subgroups of language-impaired children.

2. Measurement of children's linguistic behavior that allows for simultaneous investigation of different aspects of linguistic behavior.

3. Studies of patterns of coherence and dissociation in linguistic, cognitive, and affective domains.

4. Studies of the relation between earlier and later language ability as they relate to linguistic and school outcomes.

Those interested in pursuing the construction of clinically useful assessment procedures must be prepared for the constraints of such research. They will need to face the reliability and validity issues described above.

They will need to find methods for dealing with the variability in language acquisition they will inevitably find. While group trends may be a sufficient first approximation, the final question relates to the single child and the determination of his or her needs. The issues are important.

Acknowledgements

This work was supported in part by grant number G008006727 from the Office of Special Education and Rehabilitative Services, U.S. Department of Education, to M.C. Schultz. The authors gratefully acknowledge the additional support of the Esther S. and Joseph M. Shapiro Center for Research in Communicative Disorders and the Hazel Moore Graves Memorial Fund.

References

Aram, D.M., & Nation, J.E. Preschool language disorders and subsequent language and academic difficulties. *Journal of Communication Disorders,* 1980, *13,* 159-170.

Bax, M., & Stevenson, P. Analysis of a developmental language delay. *Proceedings of the Royal Society of Medicine,* 1977, *70,* 727-728.

Bayley, N. *Bayley Scales of Infant Development.* New York: Psychological Corporation, 1969.

Benedict, H. Early lexical development: Comprehension and production. *Journal of Child Language,* 1979, *6,* 183-200.

Blackstone, S.W. *Communication assessment of high risk infants.* Unpublished doctoral dissertation, University of Pittsburgh, 1980.

Bloom, L. *Language development: Form and function in emerging grammars.* Cambridge, MA: MIT Press, 1970.

Bloom, L. *One word at a time.* The Hague: Mouton, 1973.

Bowerman, M. Discussion summary—development of concepts underlying language. In R.L. Schiefelbusch & L.L. Lloyd (Eds.), *Language perspectives—Acquisition, retardation, and Intervention.* Baltimore: University Park Press, 1974.

Brown, J., Redmond, A., Bass, K., Liebergott, J.W., & Swope, S., *Symbolic play in normal and language-impaired children.* Paper presented at the Annual Convention of the American Speech and Hearing Association, Washington, D.C., November, 1975.

Brown, R. *A first language: The early stages.* Cambridge, MA: Harvard University Press, 1973.

Bzoch, R., & League, R. *Assessing language skills in infancy.* Gainsville, FL: Tree of Life Press, 1971.

Cairns, G.F., & Butterfield, E.C. Assessing language-related skills of prelinguistic children. *Allied Health and Behavioral Sciences,* 1981, *1,* 81-130.

Chapman, R.S. Mother-child interaction in the second year of life. In R. Schiefelbusch & D.D. Bricker (Eds.), *Early language: Acquisition and intervention.* Baltimore: University Park Press, 1982.

Cornell, E.H., & Gottfried, A.W. Intervention with premature infants. *Child Development,* 1976, *47,* 32-39.

DeHirsch, K., Jansky, J., & Langford, W.S. The oral language performance of premature children and controls. *Journal of Speech and Hearing Disorders,* 1964, *29,* 60-69.

Ehrlich, C.H., Shapiro, E., Kimball, B., & Huttner, M. Communication skills in five-year-old children with high risk neonatal histories. *Journal of Speech and Hearing Research,* 1973, *16,* 522-529.

Elardo, R., Bradley, R.H., & Caldwell, B.M. The relation of infants' home environments to mental tests performance from six to thirty-six months: A longitudinal analysis. *Child Development,* 1975, *46,* 71-76.

Field, T. Interaction patterns of preterm and term infants. In T. Field, A.M. Sostek, S. Goldberg, & H. Shuman (Eds.), *Infants born at risk: Behavior and development.* New York: Spectrum Publications, 1979.

Fitzhardinge, P. Current outcome: ICU populations. In A.W. Brann & J.J. Volpe (Eds.), *Neonatal neurological assessment and outcome.* Columbus, OH: Ross Laboratories, 1980.

Fitzhardinge, P.M. & Ramsay, M. The improving outlook for the small prematurely born infant. *Developmental Medicine and Child Neurology,* 1973, *15,* 447-459.

Folger, M., & Leonard, L.B. Language and sensorimotor development during the early period of referential speech. *Journal of Speech and Hearing Research,* 1978, *21,* 519-527.

Furrow, D., Nelson, K., & Benedict, H. Mothers' speech to children and synthetic development: Some simple relationships. *Journal of Child Language,* 1979, *6,* 423-442.

Heber, R., & Garber, H. The Milwaukee project: A study of the use of family intervention to prevent cultural-familial retardation. In B. Friedlander, G. Steritt, & S. Kirk (Eds.) *Exceptional infant,* (Vol. 1). New York: Brunner/Mazel, 1975.

Hubatch, L.M., Johnson, C.J., Kistler, D.J., & Rutherford, D.R. *Language development of high risk infants.* Paper presented at the Annual Convention of the American Speech-Language-Hearing Association, Los Angeles, November, 1981.

Hubbel, R. *Children's language disorders: An integrated approach.* Englewood Cliffs, NJ: Prentice-Hall, 1981.

Johnston, J. The language disordered child. In N.A. Lass, L.V. McReynolds, J.L. Northern, & D.E. Yoder (Eds.), *Speech, language and hearing, Vol. II. Pathologies of Speech and Language.* Philadelphia: W.B. Saunders, 1982.

Johnston, J., & Ramstad, V. Cognitive development in preadolescent language-impaired children. In M. Burns & J. Andrews (Eds.), *Selected papers in language and phonology.* Evanston, IL: Institute for continuing Professional Education, 1978.

Johnston, J., & Schery, T. The use of grammatical morphemes by children with communication disorders. In D. Morehead & A. Morehead (Eds.), *Normal and deficient child language.* Baltimore: University Park Press, 1976.

Kastein, S., & Fowler, E.P. Language development among survivors of premature birth. *Archives of Otolaryngology,* 1959, *69,* 131-135.

Kerschensteiner, M., & Huber, W. Grammatical impairment in developmental aphasia. *Cortex,* 1975, *11,* 264-282.

Kitchen, W.H., Ryan, M.M., Rickards, A., McDougall, A.B., Billson, F.A., Keir, E.H., & Naylor, F.D. A longitudinal study of very low birthweight infants. IV: An overview of performance at eight years of age. *Developmental Medicine and Child Neurology,* 1980, *22,* 172-188.

Koops, B.L. & Harmon, R.J. Studies on long-term outcome in newborns with birthweights under 1,500 grams. *Advances in behavioral pediatrics* (Vol. 1). New York: JAI press, 1980.

Kysela, G., Hillyard, A., McDonald, L., & Ahlsten-Taylor, J. Early intervention: Design and evaluation. In R. Schiefelbusch & D. Bricker (Eds.), *Early language intervention.* Baltimore: University Park Press, 1981.

Lassman, F.M., Fisch, R.O., Vetter, D.K., & LaBenz, E.S. *Early correlates of speech, language and hearing: The collaborative perinatal project of the national institute of neurological and communicative disorders and stroke.* Littleton, MA: PSG Publishing, 1980.

Leonard, L.B. What is language deviant? *Journal of Speech and Hearing Disorders,* 1972, *37,* 427-446.

Leonard, L.B. Language impairment in children. *Merrill-Palmer Quarterly,* 1979, *25,* 205-232.

Lovell, K., Hoyle, H., & Siddall, M. A study of some aspects of the play and language of young children with delayed speech. *Journal of Child Psychology and Psychiatry,* 1968, *9,* 41-50.

Lubchenco, L.O. *The high risk infant.* Philadelphia: W.B. Saunders, 1976.

McLean, J.E. Sequenced inventory of communication development. In F.L. Darley (Ed.), *Evaluation of appraisal techniques in speech and language pathology.* Reading, MA: Addison-Wesley Publishing, 1979.

Menyuk, P. Linguistic problems in children with developmental dysphasia. In M. Wyke (Ed.), *Developmental dysphasia.* London: Academic Press, 1978.

Menyuk, P. Methods used to measure linguistic competence during the first five years of life. In R.B. Kearsley & I.E. Sigel (Eds.), *Infants at risk: Assessment of cognitive functioning.* Hillsdale, NJ: Lawrence Erlbaum Associates, 1979.

Menyuk, P., & Wilbur, R. Preface to special issue on language disorders. *Journal of Autism and Developmental Disorders,* 1981, 11.

Miller, J. *Assessing language production in children.* Baltimore: University Park Press, 1981.

Miller, J.F. Identifying children with language disorders and describing their language performance. In J. Miller, D.E. Yoder, & R. Schiefelbusch (Eds.), *Contemporary issues in language intervention.* Rockville, MD: The American Speech-Language-Hearing Association, 1982.

Miller, J.F., & Chapman, R.S. The relation between age and mean length of utterance in morphemes. *Journal of Speech and Hearing Research,* 1981, *24,* 154-161.

Morehead, D.M., & Ingram, D. The development of base syntax in normal and linguistically deviant children. *Journal of Speech and Hearing Research.* 1973, *16,* 330-352.

Murphy, R.L. *Predicting lexical acquisition.* Unpublished master's thesis, Emerson College, 1982.

Nelson, K. Structure and strategy in learning to talk. *Monographs of the society for research in child development,* No. 149, 1973.

Pillitteri, A. *Maternal-newborn nursing.* Boston: Little, Brown & Co., 1981.

Ramey, C.T., Trohanis, P.L., & Hostler, S.L. An introduction. In C.T. Ramey & P.L. Trohanis (Eds.), *Finding and educating high-risk and handicapped infants.* Baltimore: University Park Press, 1982.

Rees, N.S. Pragmatics of language: Applications to normal and disordered language development. In R. Schiefelbusch (Ed.), *Bases of language intervention.* Baltimore: University Park Press, 1978.

Reynell, J. *Reynell Developmental Language Scales.* Windsor, Eng.: NFER Publishing, 1969.

Sameroff, A.J., & Chandler, M.J. Reproductive risk and the continuum of caretaking causality. In J. D. Horowitz (Ed.), *Review of child development research* (Vol. 4). Chicago: University of Chicago Press, 1975.

Siegel, G.M. Appraisal of language development. In F.L. Darley (Ed.), *Evaluation of appraisal techniques in speech and language pathology.* Reading, MA.: Addison-Wesley Publishing, 1979.

Siegel, L.S. Reproductive, perinatal and environmental factors as predictors of the cognitive and language development of preterm and full-term infants. *Child Development,* 1982, *53,* 963-973.

Snow, C.E., & Ferguson, C.A. *Talking to children: Language input and acquisition.* Cambridge, Eng.: Cambridge University Press, 1977.

Snyder, L. *Pragmatics in language disabled children: Their prelinguistic and early verbal performances and presuppositions.* Unpublished doctoral dissertation, University of Colorado, 1975.

Stewart, A.L., & Reynolds, E.O. Improved prognosis for infants of very low birth weight. *Pediatrics,* 1974, *34,* 724-735.

Strominger, A., & Bashir, A. *A nine-year follow-up of language disordered children.* Paper presented at the Annual Convention of the American Speech-Language-Hearing Association, Chicago, November, 1977.

Thompson, T., & Reynolds, J. Neonatal intensive care. *Journal of Perinatal Medicine,* 1977, *5,* 59-75.

Tjossem, T.D. Early intervention: Issues and approaches. In T.D. Tjossem (Ed.), *Intervention strategies for high risk infants and young children.* Baltimore: University Park Press, 1976.

Trantham, C.R., & Pederson, J. *Normal language development.* Baltimore: Williams & Wilkins, 1976.

Uzgiris, I.C., & Hunt, J.M. *Assessment in infancy: Ordinal scales of psychological development.* Urbana, IL: University of Illinois Press, 1975.

Weiner, P. A language delayed child at adolescence. *Journal of Speech and Hearing Disorders,* 1974, *34,* 302-312.

Zimmerman, I., Steiner, V., & Evatt, R. *Preschool language scale.* Columbus, OH: Charles E. Merrill, 1979.

Jon F. Miller
Thomas F. Campbell
Robin S. Chapman
Susan E. Weismer

Language Behavior in Acquired Childhood Aphasia

Most children learn to talk easily and rapidly despite variation in environment and endowment. Among the exceptions are children with mental deficiency, hearing impairment, central-nervous-system impairment affecting the speech production mechanism, emotional disturbance, or extreme environmental deprivation. For these children, the cause of the language deficit is evident. Another group of children, for no identified reason, begins the language-acquisition process late and progresses more slowly and with more difficulty than their peers. These children have been variously labeled developmentally aphasic, dysphasic, language-impaired, language-disabled, and language-disordered (Johnston, 1982; Leonard, 1979). The children in this latter group are considered to have developmental disorders specific to language learning that result in significant rate differences for at least some aspects of the language system.

Acquired Childhood Aphasia

This chapter is about yet another group of children, who differ from all the preceding groups in that they start out learning language normally, achieving developmental milestones at the appropriate rate. Their progress is disturbed as a direct result of neurological impairment. A variety of etiologies are associated with this group, including cerebral trauma, head tumors, cerebrovascular abnormalities, and seizure disorders. These children have acquired language disorders and are generally refered to as *acquired aphasics*.

Within this group of acquired childhood aphasics is a group whose language disturbance is accompanied by a seizure disorder and/or abnormal electroencephalographic (EEG) findings (Landau & Kleffner, 1957). These children have increasingly been the subject of investigation, particularly case reports (e.g., Campbell, 1982; Cromer, 1981; Deonna, Fletcher, & Voumard, in press). The cases available in the literature are quite diverse in presenting symptoms, degree of pathology, course, resolution, and outcome of the neurological and language deficit. The onset of the disorder may be gradual or acute, with deficits lasting from a few days to years. Some children have been reported to recover completely, some remain the same, and others display progressive disorders (Mantovani & Landau, 1980).

These cases provide a unique opportunity for studies that improve our understanding of deficits associated with a particular diagnosed neurological impairment in the developmental period. A detailed review of this literature will provide insight into the complexity of this disorder, and the theoretical and clinical issues raised in determining prognosis and constructing behavioral and medical intervention programs. Of special interest in this chapter will be the linguistic outcomes of the various onset, severity, and descriptive characteristics associated with acquired aphasia accompanied by seizure disorders.

Acquired Childhood Aphasia Secondary to a Convulsive Disorder

Landau and Kleffner (1957) originally reported examples of acquired aphasia associated with a convulsive disorder and paroxysmal EEG abnormalities. They described five children, ages five to nine years, who displayed both receptive and expressive language deficits following a normal period of speech and language development. The regression in these children's language abilities was either accompanied, preceded, or followed by seizures and other neurological manifestations. In some, the onset of the syndrome was noted to be gradual, while in others it was sudden. Improvement of speech and language skills in one child occurred with no intervention whatsoever; however, in four cases, improvement was aided by medication for seizures and language intervention. Their case reports included little information regarding specific speech and language behaviors displayed before, during, or following the disorder.

In the twenty-five years since Landau and Kleffner's first report, case studies have followed that have added fragmentary information to this puzzling clinical disorder. Twenty-six published articles describing the disorder have verified many of Landau and Kleffner's original observations. Still, virtually no data have been presented in recent years to provide new insight into the mechanisms underlying the neurological and language dysfunctions. Description of this population of children as reported in the literature follows.

Sex

Tables 3-1 through 3-3 present a review of the 94 cases of this syndrome reported in the literature. Examination of Table 3-1 reveals that in the 75 cases which present gender data, males were affected 65% of the time. The overall ratio of approximately two males to every female has also been reported in an earlier review by Cooper and Ferry (1978).

Time and Rate of Onset

Time of onset ranges from 1-1/2 to 13 years. Deonna, Beaumanoir, Gaillard, and Assal (1977) note that most of these children experience initial language loss between the ages of 3 and 7 years. In 25% of the cases reviewed (Table 3-1), the onset of the language regression was gradual, occurring over a period of longer than six months. In the remainder, language loss was more abrupt. In some cases, it occurred within a matter of hours or days. Language use during the early phases of this disorder has frequently been characterized as fluctuating, with performance varying widely across days or within a day.

Neurological Characteristics

Aside from the seizure (EEG abnormalities were the basis for case selection), the clinical neurological examination for these children was essentially normal. One case of flattening of the lower face, facial apraxia, and incoordination and clumsiness was reported (Gascon, Victor, Lombroso, & Goodglass, 1973; Landau & Kleffner, 1957). As indicated in Table 3-2, all cases that reported EEG results (84) revealed abnormal electrical discharges from one or both temporal lobes.

Of the 68 children who displayed some type of seizure (general, psychomotor, myoclonic, minor motor, petit mal, or complex partial), 43% experienced seizures before the dysphasia, 16% displayed co-occurrence of seizures and language regression, and 41% reported the language disorder to have occurred before onset of the seizures. Language regression in this final group of children has been noted to have occurred from six months (Shoumaker, Bennett, Bray, & Curless, 1974) to two years (Gascon et al., 1973) before onset of seizures.

Table 3-1

Sex, time, and rate of onset characteristics reported in 26 studies of acquired childhood aphasia secondary to a convulsive disorder. (NR = no report)

Author	N	Sex		Time of Onset		
		Male	Female	Age, yrs.	6 mos.	6 mos.
Landau & Kleffner (1957)	5	2	3	3.5-9	2	3
Barlow (1968)	1	1	0	8.5	NR	NR
Stein & Curry (1968)	1	0	1	2.6	0	1
Worster-Drought (1971)	14	5	9	3-7	0	14
Gascon, Victor, Lombroso, & Goodglass (1973)	3	3	0	3.5-6	2	1
Harel, Walsh, & Menkes (1973)	1	1	0	3	NR	NR
Deuel & Lenn (1974)	3	NR	NR	NR	NR	NR
Huskisson (1974)	1	1	1	4.10	0	1
McKinney & McGreal (1974)	9	6	3	3-13	NR	NR
Shoumaker, Bennett, Bray, & Curless (1974)	3	3	0	5-6	1	2
Lou, Brandt, & Bruhn (1977)	4	2	2	3.4	3	1
Deonna, Beaumanoir, Gaillard, & Assal (1977)	6	5	1	3.5-9	1	5

Deuel & Lenn (1977)	1	0	1	4	1	0
Rapin, Mattis, Rowan, & Golden (1977)	3	3	0	1.5-3	0	3
Campbell & Heaton (1978)	1	1	0	5	1	0
Cooper & Ferry (1978)	3	3	0	2.5-10	0	3
Koepp & Lagenstein (1978)	1	1	0	4.5	0	1
Kracke (1978)	7	NR	NR	3-5	NR	NR
van Harskamp, van Dongen, & Loonen (1978)	1	1	1	4	0	1
Jordan (1980)	1	1	0	5	NR	NR
Mantovani & Landau (1980)	3	1	2	3-6	2	1
de Negri (1980)	8	NR	NR	3-6	NR	NR
Deonna, Fletcher, & Voumard (in press)	1	1	0	2.5	0	1
Waisman Study (1981)	6	5	1	2.5-7	4	2
Holmes & McKeever (1981)	2	NR	NR	NR	NR	NR
Campbell (1982)	5	4	1	2.5-8	0	5
Totals	**94**	**49**	**26**	**1.5-13**	**17**	**45**

Table 3-2
Seizure status in 26 studies of acquired childhood aphasia secondary to a conculsive disorder. (NR = no report)

Author	Abnormal		Seizures Precede Aphasia	Co-occur	Aphasia Precedes Seizures
	N	EEG Seizures			
Landau & Kleffner (1957)	5	5	5	4	0	1
Barlow (1968)	1	1	1	1	0	0
Stein & Curry (1968)	1	1	1	NR	NR	NR
Worster-Drought (1971)	14	14	14	NR	NR	NR
Gascon et al. (1973)	3	3	3	1	1	1
Harel et al. (1973)	1	1	1	0	0	1
Deuel & Lenn (1974)	3	NR	NR	NR	NR	NR
Huskisson (1974)	1	1	NR	NR	NR	NR
McKinney & McGreal (1974)	9	9	7	4	0	3
Shoumaker et al. (1974)	3	3	2	0	0	2
Lou et al. (1977)	4	4	3	2	1	0
Deonna et al. (1974)	6	6	5	2	1	2
Deuel & Lenn (1977)	1	1	1	1	0	0
Rapin et al. (1977)	3	3	2	0	0	2

Study						
Campbell & Heaton (1978)	1	1	1	0	0	1
Cooper & Ferry (1978)	3	3	3	0	2	1
van Harskamp et al. (1978)	1	1	1	0	0	1
Jordan (1980)	1	1	1	NR	NR	NR
Kracke (1978)	7	NR	NR	NR	NR	NR
Koepp & Lagenstein (1978)	1	1	1	0	0	0
Mantovani & Landau (1980)	3	3	3	0	0	0
de Negri (1980)	8	8	8	NR	NR	NR
Deonna, et al. (in press)	1	1	1	1	NR	NR
Waisman Study (1981)	6	6	6	3	1	2
Holmes & McKeever (1981)	2	2	2	NR	NR	NR
Campbell (1982)	5	5	5	1	1	1
Totals	**94**	**84**	**68**	**19**	**7**	**18**

Audiological Characteristics

Because the language disorder typically includes disturbance of comprehension as well as production skills, the children often give the impression of having become deaf. Those studies that do include audiological information, however, typically indicate normal hearing sensitivity for pure tones throughout the entire frequency range. Normal early components of auditory-evoked potentials have also revealed normal hearing sensitivity in several cases (Gascon et al., 1973). Speech audiometric tests are often not attempted in light of the severe receptive and expressive language deficit. Waters (1974) cautions that interpretation of any behavioral audiological test may present problems.

Behavioral Characteristics

Behavioral abnormalities have been frequently noted in this population of children (Campbell & Heaton, 1978; Deonna et al., 1977; Deuel & Lenn, 1977; Gascon et al., 1973; Shoumaker et al., 1974; Stein & Curry, 1968). Behaviors such as inattention, withdrawal, aggressiveness, temper outbursts, refusing to respond, and, in some cases, hyperactivity, have been observed. Mantovani and Landau (1980) speculated that behavioral problems in this group of children "may reflect a primary disinhibition at limbic or diencephalic levels" (p. 528). It is equally likely, however, that such behaviors may be secondary reactions to the sudden loss in communication abilities. This interpretation is supported by the fact that many of these behaviors disappear once the child is provided with an alternative communication system (Campbell & Heaton, 1979). Deonna et al. (1977) note that "a bizarre, sudden, or insidious onset or language regression in a previously normal child, with no other evidence of organic illness, can easily be mistaken for a psychiatric reaction" (p. 272).

Cognitive Characteristics

Of the 72 cases that provide results of cognitive testing, over 85% show normal intellectual functioning, as indicated by a nonverbal performance IQ score of 90 or above, assessed with a variety of nonverbal measures. Comparable measures prior to seizures or language loss, however, have not been available. The difference between verbal and nonverbal cognitive abilities can vary considerably. In their discussion of nine adult cases who were followed up 10 or more years after onset of the disorder, Mantovani and Landau (1980) found a discrepancy of 12 to 15 points between verbal and performance scores on the Wechsler Adult Intelligence Scale (WAIS).

Language Characteristics

All 94 review cases displayed both receptive and expressive language deficits. Waters (1974), Campbell and Heaton (1978) and Jordan (1980), among others, report that difficulties in auditory comprehension appear first, followed by expressive speech and language difficulties. Communication problems recur or persist beyond six months in 94% of the cases (see Table 3-3). Reports from parents reveal that these children do not carry out verbal commands which they could perform previously, and, in certain respects, give the appearance of being deaf. For one 9-year-old male reported by Campbell and Heaton (1978), spoken commands were responded to by puzzled expressions and a shoulder shrug, or the commands were ignored completely. Worster-Drought (1971), in a review of 14 children, found that some were capable of understanding simple commands, while others appeared to be almost oblivious to verbal stimuli. The child reported by Stein and Curry (1968) comprehended better when visual cues were used to enhance spoken language; however, even when lip-reading cues were made available, comprehension remained poor. Campbell and Heaton (1979) reported that reading comprehension abilities displayed by their children were often far in advance of their ability to comprehend speech. Spontaneous speech, in particular, poses major comprehension problems for many of these individuals. For example, a 15-year-old boy, whose speech and language eventually returned to normal, stated that connected speech sounded like "blah, blah, blah" to him (Landau & Kleffner, 1957).

In addition to deficits in comprehension of speech, auditory receptive problems have also been observed in discriminating and recognizing nonspeech sounds (Stein & Curry, 1968; Campbell & Heaton, 1978).

Expressively, some children became totally mute. Some use jargon-like speech characterized by isolated production of consonants or vowels. And, in many cases, they resort to gestures and grunts. Others display a variety of misarticulations, inappropriate substitutions of words, and word-retrieval problems. One child, who subsequently improved, said that he understood what was said to him, but could not recall the words he wanted to say (Landau & Kleffner, 1957).

Voice quality is affected in some children. Worster-Drought (1971) and Cooper and Ferry (1978) report that some children retain normal quality and suprasegmental characteristics, while others shift to a high fundamental frequency lacking normal inflection. Their speech is similar to that of deaf children. Results of instrumental assessments of voice quality and suprasegmental characteristics have not been reported. Nor does the literature contain precise descriptions of these children's articulatory, phonological, syntactic, or semantic systems.

Table 3-3
Duration of language disorder reported in 26 studies of acquired aphasia secondary to a convulsive disorder.

		Duration of Language Deficit		
	N	*< 6 mo.*	*> 6 mo.*	*Recur*
Landau & Kleffner (1957)	5	0	3	2
Barlow (1968)	1	0	1	0
Stein & Curry (1968)	1	0	1	0
Worster-Drought (1971)	14	0	14	0
Gascon et al. (1973)	3	0	2	1
Harel et al. (1973)	1	0	1	0
Deuel & Lenn (1974)	3	0	3	0
Huskisson (1974)	1	0	1	0
McKinney & McGreal (1974)	9	3	6	0
Shoumaker et al. (1974)	3	0	2	1
Lou et. al. (1977)	4	1	3	0
Deonna et al. (1977)	6	0	5	1
Deuel & Lenn (1977)	1	0	0	1
Rapin et al. (1977)	3	0	3	0
Campbell & Heaton (1978)	1	0	0	1
Cooper & Ferry (1978)	3	0	3	0
Kracke (1978)	7	0	7	0
Koepp & Lagenstein (1978)	1	0	1	0
van Harskamp et al. (1978)	1	0	1	0
Jordan (1980)	1	0	0	1
Mantovani & Landau (1980)	3	0	3	0
de Negri (1980)	8	NR	NR	NR
Deonna et al. (1981)	1	1	0	0
Waisman Study (1981)	6	0	6	0
Holmes & McKeever (1981)	2	0	2	0
Campbell (1982)	5	0	3	2
Totals	**94**	**5**	**71**	**10**

(NR = no report)

Relationship Among EEG, Seizures, and Language Deficit

The relationships among the EEG disturbance, seizures, and the language disorder have not been clearly demonstrated. However, Mantovani and Landau (1980) stated that

> our data do not indicate that the absence of seizures is a decisive factor for therapeutic response or ultimate outcome. Until more is known about pathogenesis, we prefer to continue the original designation, because we believe that paroxysmal EEG is the pathophysiologic definition of convulsive disorder (p. 528).

Landau and Kleffner (1957) originally adopted a similar point of view when they stated: "The seizure manifestations have been readily controlled medically and are not closely correlated with the aphasic symtoms. In all cases a severe paroxysmal electroencephalographic abnormality, usually diffuse, is observed" (p. 530).

The nature of the relationship of the EEG disturbance to the language disorder, however, remains ambiguous. Landau and Kleffner (1957) noted that "electroencephalographic improvement tended to parallel improvement in speech re-education" (p. 530). Shoumaker et al., (1974) also reported that improvement in speech correlated with a decrease in the abnormalities on the EEG. In all three of the patients observed by Shoumaker and colleagues, the greatest spike-wave discharges were noted when the language disorder was at its peak; and language improvement was not observed until the abnormal electrical activity had disappeared. They further stated that improvement in speech/language functioning was not sudden once the discharges decreased, and, in one case, it lagged for 2 to 3 months. Rose (1969), in fact, noted that recovery of speech/language skills (not further specified) may lag behind EEG improvement up to 6 months.

Conversely, Worster-Drought (1971) and Rapin, Mattis, Rowan, and Golden, (1977) have reported persistent speech and language problems despite subsequent normal EEGs. In addition, Campbell and Heaton (1978) describe a boy who suddenly acquired a severe speech and language deficit after 5 years of normal language development. Medical reports revealed that the child presented normal EEG tracings 2 months after the onset of the disorder, but language skills never returned to normal. As can be surmised from these few studies, the relationship between the EEG disturbance and the language disorder remains unclear, and is likely to remain so until more is known about the cause of the disorder.

Pathogenesis

Deonna, Beaumanoir, Gaillard, and Assal (1977) suggest that the variability in these children's recovery of speech and language abilities may relate to differing pathogeneses. Although data to support such a notion are not available, several hypotheses have been proposed. Landau and Kleffner (1957) discuss the possibility that regression in speech and language skills may result from the functional ablation of the primary cortical language areas by persistent electrical discharges in these regions. This hypothesis is supported by Sato and Dreifuss (1972), who posit that the language regression in one child was due to continuous bilateral synchronous temporal spike activity, which caused a dysfunction of both hemispheres.

Gascon et al. (1973, p. 162) state that "EEG discharges are a cortical manifestation of a lower level subcortical de-afferenting process." This hypothesis implies that the electrical discharges displayed by these children are a secondary factor, and are not directly responsible for the aphasia. These authors suggest that there is some subcortical involvement of the auditory pathways. However, case reports reveal normal hearing- and auditory-evoked response profiles in some of these children (Campbell, 1982; Waisman Study, 1981), indicating integrity of the auditory pathways. Such cases argue against the hypothesis.

Gascon et al. (1973) further speculate that the cause of the disorder might be some pathogenetic mechanism that is related in an unknown way to the convulsive disorder. Deonna et al. (1977) suggest that these children may have an "unusual genetic or acquired pattern of cerebral organization which renders them particularly sensitive to brain damage or seizure activity as far as language is concerned" (p. 271).

Pathoanatomical studies to support these hypotheses are limited. McKinney and McGreal (1974) examined brain tissue taken from one child. No abnormalities were noted. However, they believe that the fluctuating course in many of these patients indicates an inflammatory mechanism. This follows Worster-Drought's (1971) hyphothesis that there is an active low-grade selective encephalitis which affects the temporal lobes. Results from a cortical biopsy reported by Lou, Brandt, and Bruhn (1977) clearly showed inflammation of the meninges with leukocyte infiltration and thickening. The results also revealed gliosis and loss of neurons, suggesting a meningoencephalities of the "slow virus" type. Rasmussen and McCann (1968) report similar findings in adults with prolonged temporal lobe seizures.

If an inflammatory process were localized in the region of the temporal lobe, it certainly could result in both language dysfunction and seizures. However, additional pathoanatomical investigations suggest other possible causes. Rapin et al. (1977) found a small vascular anomaly in the left angular gyrus of one of these children. In a second child, they found diminished vascularization in the area of the left middle cerebral artery.

Interpretation of these findings is limited because there have been no occasions for pathoanatomic studies close in time to symptom onset. Until noninvasive means of assessing cortical structure and function are better developed, the true cause and nature of the syndrome will remain a matter of speculation.

Prognosis

The long-term course of the disorder remains unclear. Several researchers (most notably Gascon et al., 1973; Landau & Kleffner, 1957; Mantovani & Landau, 1980; Rapin et al., 1977; Worster-Drought, 1971) have reported a number of children who regained normal receptive and expressive language skills following their sudden loss. A review of the reported cases, however, indicates that more than 80% of the children display both receptive and expressive language deficits that persist longer than 6 months. According to Gascon et al. (1973), the degree of residual language loss ranges from verbal-auditory agnosia with no verbal communication, to mild deficits in academic areas such as spelling and reading. In a survey of 45 case studies, Cooper and Ferry (1978) reported that 42% of the children were left with a severe auditory-comprehension deficit, 24% had moderate-to-mild deficits, and 33% made a complete recovery. The explanation for this variability in recovery remains one of the most puzzling features of the disorder.

Grouping according to the limited descriptive data available does not appear to simplify prognosis. Based on general clinical features (onset characteristics, number of seizures, and the course of the language disorder), Deonna et al. (1977) propose three different clinical varieties of the syndrome.

One group consists of those children in whom language development is abruptly interrupted in association with seizures. The language deficit persists for variable amounts of time (anywhere from a few days to several years) and Deonna et al. (1977) suggest that the recovery is "too rapid to be explained by a shift in speech dominance" (p. 270). They further suggest that the language disorder may represent "a functional disconnection of language mechanisms without any newly acquired lesion" (p. 270).

The second group includes children who show little or no improvement in verbal communication skills after a major seizure, or following repeated episodes of language fluctuation. Recovery for these children, when it occurs, has been reported to take place in the course of months or years. Deonna et al. speculate that if recovery does take place, one might assume that the other hemisphere has "taken over speech." Limited empirical data are available to support this speculation.

The third group concerns those children who gradually develop a moderate-to-severe deficit in auditory comprehension. Children in this group may experience few or no seizures, and, often, appear to be deaf. Variable degrees of recovery have been reported in this group of children. In many cases, little improvement has been reported after several years.

These three groups, constructed on the basis of differing types of onset (sudden, fluctuating, or gradual) and presence or absence of seizures, each display varying rates and degrees of recovery. It remains unclear whether the language abilities of the children within each group were homogeneous in nature. Thus, grouping by onset characteristics does not appear to create groups more homogeneous in prognosis.

Illustrations of New Directions for Research

As the preceding summary makes clear, children with acquired aphasia associated with convulsive disorders show a variety of patterns of onset and recovery. The language disorder may itself be the earliest symptom of central-nervous-system disease, and the last to recover, if recovery takes place at all. How is the clinician to predict the course of recovery and make recommendations for treatment in the face of this variability in patterns of onset and recovery? One promising direction for new research, we believe, comes from a far more detailed description of the children's speech and language skills than previous studies have provided—a study began early after onset and continued longitudinally. Particularly, we advocate the detailed comparison of language skills to other intellectual skills measured nonverbally; of comprehension skills to production skills; and of each to the normal developmental progression. In a later section of this paper, children participating in the pilot study of acquired aphasia carried out at the Waisman Center (1981) will be used to illustrate this approach. Groups homogeneous with respect to the pattern, type, and degree of delay or disorder are far more likely to show similarities in cause, recovery, and effective treatment approaches.

When detailed descriptions of children's cognitive and communication skills are available, a second promising line of new research can then be followed: that of comparing different subsets to discover which share similar problems. We illustrate this second direction for research by comparing three acquired-aphasic and three language-disordered learning-disabled children in a final section of this paper.

Describing Language Skills
of Children with Acquired Aphasia

Over a 24-month period, children suspected of acquired aphasia associated with seizures or abnormal EEGs were seen at an experimental neurogenics clinic at the Waisman Center. The number of visits for each child varied depending upon when during this 24-month period he or she was initially seen. Generally, children were seen for re-evaluation at approximately three-month intervals. The protocol for evaluating language and cognitive functioning in these children was constructed to span a broad developmental range, to include comprehension measures of both vocabulary and syntax, to include production measures of both vocabulary and syntax based on free-speech samples, and to use cognitive measures that were nonverbal in their requirements for both understanding the directions and answering. If children showed very little comprehension on the standard tests, then written testing, or spoken testing with the addition of lip-reading cues, was attempted. Specific procedures included the following:

Standard Assessment Protocol for Pilot Subjects

Comprehension
1. Lexical Comprehension Items
   (Miller, Chapman, Branston, & Reichle, 1980).
2. Peabody Picture Vocabulary Test (Dunn & Dunn, 1981).
3. Simple Sentence Test Procedure (Chapman & Miller, 1980).
4. Miller-Yoder Test of Grammatical Comprehension (Miller & Yoder, 1972).
5. Revised Token Test (McNeil & Prescott, 1978).
6. Comprehension in Routine Contexts (Miller & Chapman, 1980).

Production Data
1. Conversation with the clinician about current activities and events.
2. Narration—Story-telling about an event, movie, TV show of interest to the child.

Production Analysis
1. Assigning Structural Stage (ASS) (Miller, 1981).
2. MLU/Age Predictions (Miller & Chapman, 1981).
3. Lexical Analysis (Miller & Chapman, 1982).
4. Productivity Analysis (Miller & Chapman, 1982).

Cognitive Assessment

Nonverbal cognitive testing was carried out for each subject whose cognitive abilities had not been previously assessed, using one or more of the following procedures as appropriate:

1. 2—24 months—Piagetian procedures for the sensorimotor period (Miller, Chapman, Branston, & Reichle, 1980).
2. 25—42 months—Leiter International Performance Scale (Leiter, 1969).
3. 42 months—10 years—Columbia Mental Maturity Scale (Burgemeister, Blum & Lorge, 1972).
4. 10 years and up—WISC Performance Scale (Wechsler, 1974).

Procedures appropriate to the child's developmental level were given over one to two continuous days, interspersed with neurological and other behavioral clinical evaluation procedures, including hearing and speech motor control assessment.

Pilot Data

An initial goal of this pilot project was to evaluate similarities and differences in child performance, relative to developmental history and neurological status. After careful examination of cognitive and linguistic data, eight of the sixteen children evaluated fell outside even the most general definition of acquired aphasia in children. Significant cognitive or emotional deficits were uncovered—or a developmental language delay was evident—throughout the developmental period, but no seizure activity was noted.

The remaining eight children could be classed as follows: (1) those whose history of language development could not be clearly established as normal, but who evidenced seizure activity and language deficits affecting both comprehension and production—these were not further classified; (2) children meeting the definition of acquired aphasia who showed no oral language comprehension skills and little productive language, possibly an auditory agnosia group; and (3) children meeting the definition of acquired aphasia whose language comprehension was moderately affected with more severe deficits in language production. It will be helpful to review each group in more detail at this point before moving on to specific comparisons of selected subjects.

Children with Seizures But No History
of Normal Language Development

Three children in the group of eight did not meet the definition of acquired aphasia because no history of normal speech and language development was reported; all, however, displayed a seizure disorder and abnormal EEGs. A brief discussion of each of these children's cognitive, language, and speech performance will help illustrate the point that language disorders—developmental or acquired—can be heterogeneous.

The disorder for one male who was 5 years, 3 months of age was characterized by fluctuation in language and cognitive skills accompanied by repeated episodes of seizures. History indicated that the development of language was generally slow, but he was producing 2- and 3-word utterances by 4 years. During his fourth year, a notable regression in cognitive and language skills was noted in association with seizures. At the time of assessment, cognitive abilities were estimated to be at the 6-month level of functioning (Piagetian sensorimotor stage III). These findings indicate approximately a 57-month difference between his chronological age (63 months) and estimated mental age (6 months). In relation to his cognitive skills, which were estimated to be at the 40-45-month level prior to the seizure disorder, this 57-month difference represents a significant regression in cognitive functioning. Comprehension testing revealed no response to either verbal or nonverbal auditory stimuli. His ability to comprehend language was estimated to be well below the 12-month level of functioning. Expressive speech and language skills were characterized by "grunts" and the production of a few vowel sounds (/a/ and / ə /). No evidence was given that he was attaching meaning to these productions. As was the case with both cognitive and receptive language skills, expressive speech and language abilities were well below the one-year level.

A second child, who was 10 years, 5 months of age, also displayed a language deficit associated with a seizure disorder and abnormal EEG results. For this child, previous reports revealed a long history of language and cognitive delay. However, in contrast to the first child, there was virtually no regression observed in communication and cognitive abilities, even after episodes of seizure activity. Assessment results showed a mild delay in cognitive functioning (based on nonverbal measures). Both lexical and syntactic comprehension were at approximately the 7-year level (CA=10;5). Expressive language was characterized by developmental articulation and syntax errors, and mean length of utterance in morphemes (Brown, 1973) was beyond Stage V. In addition, difficulty in recalling appropriate lexical items was noted during conversational speech.

A third child, 8 years, 4 months of age, also presented a history of general language delay similar to child 1 and child 2. Once again, seizure activity and abnormal EEGs were reported. However, unlike the two previous children, assessment results indicated that nonverbal cognitive abilities were within normal limits. Lexical as well as syntactic comprehension were at the seven-year level of functioning. Expressive language was characterized by both developmental and nondevelopmental syntactic errors. As was the case for child 2, word-finding problems were observed in conversational speech.

Children with Acquired Aphasia, No Comprehension, and Little Production: Auditory Verbal Agnosia?

Two of the children in the pilot study, ages 6 years, 10 months, and 11 years, 8 months, displayed both receptive and expressive language deficits following a normal period of language development. The disturbance in language abilities was associated with seizures and abnormal EEG results. For these children, the language disturbance was characterized by complete loss of auditory comprehension and expressive language abilities, despite retention of age-appropriate cognitive functioning, as measured by nonverbal tasks.

Comprehension data for both children indicated that they were able to discriminate between nonspeech sounds with a high degree of accuracy. As these sounds (environmental sounds and musical instruments) became less familiar, accuracy decreased. Their ability to discriminate between various types of linguistic stimuli was at chance levels. Baseline scores on the Peabody Picture Vocabulary Test could not be obtained when administered with only auditory cues (auditory only = hearing only the spoken lexical item), nor when given using both auditory and visual cues (auditory + visual = hearing the spoken lexical item and seeing the clinician's facial/oral structures). Each child's ability to comprehend language was aided by gestures, signs, and comprehension strategies. Their ability to comprehend spoken language was below the 12-month level of functioning, as indicated by informal comprehension testing. Finally, for the 11-year-old, it is interesting to note that, despite his deficit in auditory comprehension of spoken language, he was capable of correctly matching several orthographically presented words to an appropriate picture. When the PPVT and the Miller-Yoder Test of Grammatical Comprehension were presented orthographically, scores on these measures improved considerably. Due to the 6-year-old's low reading level, comprehension of language could not be tested by orthographic presentation. For both children, auditory comprehension (on the basis of acoustic cues alone) was stable and nonexistent across the 18 to 24 months that they were followed.

On initial evaluation, expressive speech and language for the 11-year-old was characterized by the spontaneous production of several CV, VC, and CVC combinations. Although these productions were mostly unintelligible, he appeared to be attaching meaning to these sound combinations. Production of consonant-vowel combinations, as well as monosyllable words, was enhanced, somewhat, when a model was presented which he could imitate. Based on diagnostic data from this child, it appears that when certain combinations of cues were presented by the clinician (auditory, visual, and orthographic), correct production was enhanced. In addition, during production of isolated phonemes and consonant-vowel combinations, movements of the articulators were apraxic-like. Furthermore, pitch, loudness, and voice quality were not within normal limits. For example, fundamental frequency was extremely high in conversational speech (440 to 460 cycles per second) and there were difficulties in regulating intensity. Voice quality was similar to that of a deaf child. Over the 24-month period this child was followed, little change in expressive speech and language skills were observed.

The 6-year-old, on the other hand, presented virtually no expressive speech and language during the intial assessment. However, for this child, gains in productive speech were documented across the 18 months she was followed. At first, imitation of sounds and words, or spontaneous production of vowels were observed. During later evaluations, expressive speech and language consisted of several 1- and 2-word utterances with good intelligibility.

Three distinguishing characteristics of these two children include (1) a disturbance in normal language development, (2) presence of seizures and abnormal EEG findings, and (3) the retention of normal nonverbal cognitive functions. A fourth, and possibly the most interesting aspect, of the disorder in these children is related to their unique comprehension abilities. That is, regardless of their ability to discriminate between certain nonlinguistic auditory stimuli, they, in essence, display verbal auditory agnosia (pure word deafness). As noted by Rapin et al. (1977) and Campbell and Heaton (1979), among others, sight-word-reading vocabulary is typically in advance of such children's auditory receptive language skills. In some, visual communication functions are remarkably preserved, and many can be taught to read and write quite well. Higher levels of comprehension abilities assessed through other channels in these children are striking, especially when they are compared to congenitally hearing-impaired children learning oral and written language. Comprehension skills in this latter group for written language are greatly delayed. Assuming that the two children described above might have begun learning language over again through lip reading, sign, and written programming after the onset of the convulsive disorder, they came much further in comprehension than one could reasonably expect under the circumstances.

Thus, these two children, along with similar cases described in the literature, indicate that the language loss at the time of the seizure episodes was not irrevocable. Rather, these case descriptions suggest that the links between acoustic input and meaning, and between meaning and expression, were severed—double dissociation, in the aphasiologist's terms. If this hypothesis is so, one should be able to demonstrate extraordinarily rapid acquisition of language through an augmentative system (e.g., signing and writing) that maps directly into previously acquired linguistic knowledge. Furthermore, one could predict that expression in such an augmentative system would be representative of language organization prior to the disorder. Neither of these hypotheses is true for congenitally hearing-impaired children, nor should they prove true if the seizure disorder, in fact, "erased" prior language learning. At present, the disturbance in linguistic competence (as opposed to language performance measured through verbal language comprehension and production) in these children is poorly understood and, thus, is a good candidate for further inquiry. The study of these childrens' language learning and knowledge, through augmentative procedures, may provide important pieces of information to this puzzling question.

Children with Acquired Aphasia, Variable Comprehension, and Delayed Production with Word Finding Problems

The last three children in the pilot study showed auditory comprehension and expressive speech and language abilities which appear to be both quantitatively and qualitatively different from those previously described. These three children (ages 9, 10, and 11 years) also experienced a normal period of speech and language development. Between ages 4 and 7 years, disturbances in receptive and expressive language skills were observed, accompanied by a seizure disorder. The disturbances in communication abilities proved to be less severe than the loss displayed by the children presented previously. When improvement in speech and language took place, it was sudden. Psychological and school reports indicated that nonverbal cognitive abilities were not affected and the major educational deficits occurred in academic areas, such as spelling and reading. Our clinical observations of these three children indicate that, although they are capable of functioning in a normal educational setting, they continue to display specific receptive and expressive language deficits which interfere with the normal learning process. Expressive speech and language is characterized by developmental and nondevelopmental syntactic errors, word finding problems, and other communication breakdowns. Aside from developmental articulation errors, speech is relatively intelligible. In terms of receptive language, variable auditory comprehension of the same word or strings of words has been observed from moment to moment. In addition, all three of these children claim that they have increased difficulty processing spontaneous speech when it is produced at rates they perceive as being faster than normal.

The description of the abilities of these three children is continued in the following section, where we compare their productive language to learning-disabled language-disordered children with no history of seizures or sudden disturbance of language functioning.

Comparing the Expressive Language of Aphasic and Learning Disabled Children

Do children with acquired aphasia associated with a seizure disorder show productive language similar to children with language deficits accompanied by learning disabilities? Descriptive and causal models attempting to explain the performance of language-delayed learning-disabled children have been primarily unidimensional, and presented as hypotheses about the impaired processes. These hypotheses include deficits in:

1. Short-term memory
2. Rate of auditory processing
3. Auditory sequencing
4. Linguistic processing
5. Phonological processing
6. Attention
7. Production-span capacity
8. Rhythmic ability
9. Hierarchical planning
10. General representation

It can be argued that all of these conditions simply co-occur with delayed onset and slow rates of language acquisition. Or, one could argue they are the result, rather than the cause, of the language disorder. At present there are no direct prognostic links from deficits in any specific process or physiological condition to the course, sequence, rate, and extent of language and communication development; but, children have not been grouped by detailed patterns of language deficit prior to the investigation of these factors, and comprehension status, in particular, has seldom been documented.

Each of the hypotheses proposed above predicts certain outcomes for language comprehension and language production independently; and each hypothesis could be extended, if warranted by similarities in functioning, to children with acquired aphasia. Short-term memory deficits, slow rate of auditory processing, deficits in linguistic and phonological processing, and attentional deficits would result in a disturbance in language comprehension. Reduced production-span capacity would directly affect language production at a variety of levels. Sequencing deficits, defective rhythmic abilities, hierarchical planning deficits, and general representational deficits would impair both language comprehension and production. When detailed language-performance data become available on children within each of the two groups, it may be possible to predict processing deficits with sufficient specificity to test them experimentally. Here, we illustrate one fragment of the comparison in language skills necessary to warrant the hypothesis that similar processing problems may be at work for the two different groups.

In order to examine the question of whether acquired aphasic and language disordered children showed similar deficits in talking, analyses of productive language were carried out using a computer program entitled Systematic Analysis of Language Transcripts (SALT) (Miller & Chapman, 1982). This program permits transcripts to be typed in, stored, and analyzed for both adults and children for the following measures: mean length of utterance in words and morphemes; distribution of utterances by word and morpheme length; distribution of number of utterances per speaking turn; total number of words; total number of different words; type-token ratio; frequency of occurrence of each word in the sample; bound morpheme frequency table; question, negation, conjunction, modal verb, semi-auxiliary frequency tables; and a search routine to recall utterances containing specific words, word sets, or word strings. The latter can be used to analyze subjects' use of vocabulary containing various semantic fields, such as time words, mental verbs, and words making indefinite reference.

Aphasic Children

The aphasic children selected for comparison were three boys, ages 9;10, 10;0, and 11;6, who fell into the third group described previously. These children had experienced a normal period of speech and language development. Between the ages of 4 and 7 years, a disturbance in auditory comprehension and expressive language skills was noted, accompanied by a seizure disorder and abnormal EEGs, which were characterized by a left temporal lobe focus. At the time of testing, all children displayed normal nonverbal cognitive abilities, and were attending a normal educational classroom. Descriptive data consisting of age, sex, developmental history, time of onset, seizure history, EEG findings, educational history, and cognitive, comprehension, and productions levels are summarized in Table 3-4.

Learning-Disabled Children

The language-delayed learning-disabled children selected for comparison with the aphasic children were two boys and one girl, ages 11;2, 11;3, and 10;11, who had been identified as learning-disabled by the public schools. Medical history revealed that none of these children had displayed seizures or other neurological abnormalities. At the time of testing, all showed a 28 to 36 point gap between verbal and performance scale IQ scores on the Wechsler Intelligence Scale for Children (Revised), with performance scale scores being the higher of the two. All were attending a class for children with specific learning disabilities. Descriptive data for these children are summarized in Table 3-5.

Language Samples

Spontaneous language samples were obtained under two conditions: (1) a conversational condition in which the child engaged in dialogue concerning past, present, and future events, and (2) a narrative condition in which the child described a television show from memory. Conversational and narrative language samples from acquired aphasic and LD (learning-disabled) children were analyzed for a variety of lexical and productive characteristics.

Mean Length of Utterance

Tables 3-6 and 3-7 present word and morpheme summaries for conversation and narration conditions for both aphasic and LD children. With regard to utterance length for complete and intelligible utterances, mean length of utterance (MLU) in morphemes (Brown, 1973) for the conversational condition ranged from 4.22 to 5.86 for the aphasic children, and from 4.73 to 5.47 for the LD children. During the narrative condition, MLU ranged from 4.67 to 8.10 for the aphasic group, and from 5.43 to 8.69 for the LD children. As these data indicate, similar ranges for MLU were obtained for aphasic and LD groups, for both conditions. However, with the exception of LD6, each aphasic and LD child presented a greater MLU for narration than conversation.

Table 3-4.
Descriptive characteristics of the aphasic children.

Category	*Children*		
	AP1	*AP2*	*AP3*
Age	9;10	11;6	10;0
Sex	Male	Male	Male
Developmental History	Normal until age 4;0 when seizures began.	Normal until age 5;6 when seizures began.	Mild early expressive language delay; first word at 18 months; 2-word utterances at 42 months.
Time of Onset of Language Disturbance	4;0	5;0-7;0	5;0
Seizure History	Several petite mal and motor seizures - Abnormal EEG— Predominately left temporal region.	Several motor seizures at night— Abnormal EEG— left temporal region.	Several motor seizures at night— Abnormal EEG— left temporal region

Educational History	Attended a special school for aphasic children from 4;0 to 7;0—Currently in a normal 4th grade class.	Has always been in a normal educational classroom setting.	Has always been in a normal classroom setting.
Cognition	80%-ile—Ravens Matrices	60%-ile—Ravens Matrices	WISC-R V 90 P 118 FS 104
Comprehension	PPVT—6;2 Miller-Yoder—100%.	PPVT—9;2 Miller-Yoder—100%.	PPVT—6;5 Miller-Yoder—100%.
Production	MLU 5.10 Word retrieval problems.	MLU 5.86 Word retrieval problems.	MLU 4.22 Word retrieval problems.

Table 3-5
Descriptive characteristics of the learning-disabled children. (NA = not available)

Category	Children		
	LD1	*LD2*	*LD3*
Age	11;2	11;3	10;11
Sex	Male	Male	Female
Developmental History	Normal	Normal	Normal
Time of Onset of Language Disturbance.	N/A	N/A	N/A
Seizure History	N/A	N/A	N/A
Educational History	Has been in both normal and LD classroom—currently in a LD classroom.	Has been in normal and LD classrooms—currently in LD classroom.	Has been in both normal and LD classrooms—currently in LD classroom.
Cognition	WISC-R V 98 P 121 FS 104	WISC-R V 95 P 123 FS 108	WISC-R V 81 P 117 FS 97
Comprehension	PPVT—11;0 Miller-Yoder—100%.	PPVT 10;5 Miller-Yoder—100%.	PPVT 9;10 Miller-Yoder—100%.
Production	MLU 5.77 Word retrieval problems.	MLU 5.31 Word retrieval problems.	MLU 6.05 Word retrieval problems.

Utterance Types

Tables 3-8 and 3-9 summarize frequency and percentage of utterance types for both groups of children. As can be seen in these two tables, percentage of complete and intelligible utterances in the conversational condition was high, ranging from 88.89% to 96.61% for the aphasic group, and from 96.26% to 100.00% for the LD group. In the narrative condition, percentage of complete and intelligible utterances ranged from 83.75% to 96.67% for the three aphasic children, and from 78.16% to 98.88% for the three LD children. As shown, the percentage of complete and intelligible utterances is similar for each group, for both conversational and narrative conditions. However, for the majority of children, the percentage of complete and intelligible utterances decreases slightly in the narrative condition.

Communication Breakdowns

Conversational and narrative samples were also analyzed in terms of communication breakdowns, defined as including:

1. Garbles, which involve:
   a. filled pauses
   b. part-word repetitions
   c. whole-word repetitions
   d. phrase repetitions
   e. word/phrase replacements
   f. word/phrase revisions;
2. Incomplete utterances (abandoned utterance attempts); and
3. Unintelligible or partially unintelligible utterances;

Table 3-10 provides a summary of the overall percentage of communication breakdowns for each child per-language-sample-condition (i.e., conversation vs. narration). Based on this summary information, several points can be made. First, it is evident that for both groups, the percentage of communication breakdowns was higher for the narrative sample than for the conversational sample. It is possible to speculate that the higher percentage of communication breakdowns in the narrative condition was due to increased processing demands involved in reconstructing and reorganizing information from memory. Alternately, it could be reasoned that communication breakdowns occurred more frequently during the narrative sample as a result of attempts to produce longer and more syntactically complex utterances. The data in Table 3-11 seem to support the latter interpretation. As previously noted, MLU for complete and intelligible utterances in the narrative sample (for all subjects except LD6) was higher

Table 3-6
Aphasic children word and morpheme summaries.

	Conversation					
	Child AP1 Con		Child AP2 Con		Child AP3 Con	
	Total Utterances	Complete and Intelligible	Total Utterances	Complete and Intelligible	Total Utterances	Complete and Intelligible
No. Different Words	183	174	135	129	153	142
Total No. Words	534	490	341	307	360	305
TTR (First 50 utterances)	---	0.50	---	0.45	---	0.54
MLU in Words	4.64	4.58	5.33	5.39	3.75	3.81
MLU in Morphemes	5.15	5.10	5.83	5.86	4.12	4.22
Brown's Stage	Post V	Post V	Post V	Post V	Late V	Late V

Narration

	Child AP1 Nar		Child AP2 Nar		Child AP3 Nar	
	Total Utterances	*Complete and Intelligible*	*Total Utterances*	*Complete and Intelligible*	*Total Utterances*	*Complete and Intelligible*
No. Different Words	143	126	178	160	126	116
Total No. Words	375	302	619	479	274	237
TTR (First 50 utterances)	---	0.42	---	0.40	---	0.50
MLU in Words	6.15	6.29	6.96	7.15	4.09	4.09
MLU in Morphemes	6.84	6.98	7.85	8.10	4.63	4.67
Brown's Stage	Post V	Post V	Post V	Post V	Post V	Post V

Table 3-7.
Learning-Disabled children word and morpheme summaries.

	Conversation					
	Child LD1 Con		Child LD2 Con		Child LD3 Con	
	Total Utterances	Complete and Intelligible	Total Utterances	Complete and Intelligible	Total Utterances	Complete and Intelligible
No. Different Words	221	221	165	164	329	320
Total No. Words	662	657	456	454	1060	985
TTR (First 50 utterances)	---	0.53	---	0.49	---	0.51
MLU in Words	4.98	5.05	4.65	4.73	5.52	5.47
MLU in Morphemes	5.68	5.77	5.22	5.31	6.09	6.05
Brown's Stage	Post V	Post V	Post V	Post V	Post V	Post V

Narration

	Child LD1 Nar		Child LD2 Nar		Child LD3 Nar	
	Total Utterances	Complete and Intelligible	Total Utterances	Complete and Intelligible	Total Utterances	Complete and Intelligible
No. Different Words	205	202	136	133	196	170
Total No. Words	706	693	371	349	472	335
TTR (First 50 utterances)	---	0.40	---	0.38	---	0.55
MLU in Words	7.84	7.87	6.87	7.12	5.36	4.93
MLU in Morphemes	8.66	8.69	7.44	7.71	5.85	5.43
Brown's Stage	Post V	Post V	Post V	Post V	Post V	Post V

Table 3-8
Aphasic children frequency and percentage of utterance types.

	Conversation					
	Child AP1 Con		Child AP2 Con		Child AP3 Con	
	Number	*%*	*Number*	*%*	*Number*	*%*
Total Utterances (Speaker Attempts)	115	---	64	---	97	---
(Utterances with Garbles)	36	31.30	12	18.75	27	27.84
Complete Utterances	**112**	**97.39**	**59**	**92.19**	**90**	**92.78**
Unintelligible	0	---	0	---	4	4.44
Partly intelligible	5	4.46	2	3.39	6	6.67
Complete and intelligible	107	95.54	57	96.61	80	88.89
Incomplete Utterances	**3**	**2.61**	**5**	**7.81**	**6**	**6.19**
Unintelligible	0	---	0	---	0	---
Partly intelligible	0	---	1	20.00	0	---
Incomplete and intelligible	3	100.00	4	80.00	6	100.00

Narration

	Child AP1 Nar		Child AP2 Nar		Child AP3 Nar	
	Number	%	Number	%	Number	%
Total Utterances (Speaker Attempts)	61	---	89	---	67	---
(Utterances with Garbles)	26	42.62	31	34.83	26	38.81
Complete Utterances	54	88.52	80	89.89	60	89.55
Unintelligible	0	---	0	---	0	---
Partly intelligible	6	11.11	13	16.25	2	3.33
Complete and intelligible	48	88.89	67	83.75	58	96.67
Incomplete Utterances	7	11.48	9	10.11	7	10.45
Unintelligible	0	---	1	11.11	0	---
Partly intelligible	0	---	0	---	1	14.29
Incomplete and intelligible	7	100.00	8	88.89	6	85.71

Table 3-9
Learning-disabled children frequency and percentage of utterance types.

	Conversation					
	Child LD1 Con		Child LD2 Con		Child LD3 Con	
	Number	%	Number	%	Number	%
Total Utterances (Speaker Attempts)	133	---	98	---	192	---
(Utterances with Garbles)	25	18.88	27	27.55	42	21.87
Complete Utterances	**130**	**97.74**	**96**	**97.96**	**187**	**97.40**
Unintelligible	0	---	0	---	1	0.53
Partly intelligible	0	---	0	---	6	3.21
Complete and intelligible	130	100.00	96	100.00	180	96.26
Incomplete Utterances	**3**	**2.26**	**2**	**2.04**	**5**	**2.60**
Unintelligible	0	---	0	---	0	---
Partly intelligible	0	---	0	---	0	---
Incomplete and intelligible	3	100.00	2	100.00	5	100.00

Narration

	Child LD1 Nar		Child LD2 Nar		Child LD3 Nar	
	Number	*%*	*Number*	*%*	*Number*	*%*
Total Utterances (Speaker Attempts)	91	---	55	---	90	---
(Utterances with Garbles)	26	28.57	25	45.45	44	48.89
Complete Utterances	89	97.80	50	90.91	87	96.67
Unintelligible	0	---	0	---	4	4.60
Partly intelligible	1	1.12	1	2.00	15	17.24
Complete and intelligible	88	98.88	49	98.00	68	78.16
Incomplete Utterances	1	1.10	4	7.27	1	1.11
Unintelligible	0	---	0	---	0	---
Partly intelligible	0	---	0	---	0	---
Incomplete and intelligible	1	100.00	4	100.00	1	100.00
Communication						
Gesture	1	1.10	1	1.82	2	2.22

Table 3-10
Percentage of utterances containing communication breakdowns by sample condition.

Children	Conversation	Narrative
AP1	32	54
AP2	30	56
AP3	34	46
LD1	21	28
LD2	26	47
LD3	25	56

than MLU for complete and intelligible utterances in the conversational sample. Furthermore, within each language sample condition, the MLU for the utterances containing garbles is higher in every case than the MLU for the entire sample. That is, utterances in which filled pauses, part-word repetitions, etc., occurred were generally longer than those without these types of commmunication breakdowns. Words and phrases within garbles were, of course, excluded from the MLU count—only the remainder of the utterance was counted.

Also evident in Table 3-10 is the fact that the acquired aphasic group had somewhat higher percentages of communication breakdowns for the conversational condition (ranging from 30-34%) than the LD group (ranging from 21-26%). However, two of the three LD children (LD3 and LD6) evidenced percentages of breakdowns in the narrative conditions which were nearly identical to those of the aphasic children. The third LD child (LD2) demonstrated relatively low percentages of communication breakdowns across both sample conditions.

Data on the various categories of communication breakdowns for the acquired aphasic children and the LD children are presented in Tables 3-12 and 3-13, respectively. In Table 3-14, these data are summarized in terms of mean percentages exhibited by both groups for each breakdown category in the conversational condition and the narrative condition. The results of these analyses point to several similarities between the two groups. It is evident that the finding regarding higher percentages of communication breakdowns on the narrative samples than the conversational samples also generally hold true for the individual categories of breakdowns. More importantly, the pattern of types of communication breakdowns that occur most frequently were very similar across groups. Regardless of language-sample condition (conversational vs. narrative), the breakdown types most common in aphasic and LD children were filled pauses and word/phrase revisions. Filled pauses in the transcripts of the aphasic children consisted exclusively of fillers "um" or "uh", as in "well (um) when (um um) we play tag," while interjections such as "and my sister is (oh boy is tw) twelve" were used by the LD children in addition to fillers. Word revisions, such as in the utterance "go to my (cousin) cousin's house," usually involved the addition of a grammatical marker to the unmarked form. Phrase revisions, for example "in fourth grade (um I was like, I came, I came like) I was asleep" entailed syntactic reformations at the phrase level.

Communication breakdowns exhibited by the acquired aphasic children and the LD children appear to be related, at least in some instances, to word-retrieval difficulties. There were varying degrees of evidence in the transcripts indicative of word-finding problems. Some of the most obvious, but infrequent, cases involved repairs, or instances in which the child eventually recalled the appropriate word, as illustrated by the following example: "It's only hard to because they always put these (uh, a lot of, uh, hum) *things* on it, (uh) *words*. A lotta *words* on it." There were 10 instances of these types of repairs in the aphasic transcripts (based on a total of 509 utterances) and 6 instances (in 659 total utterances) in the LD transcripts. Direct remarks such as "oh, what is it called" or "starts with a Y" also provided clear indications of word-finding problems. Such comments, however, were rare. Other evidence of difficulties in word retrieval included the use of semantically or phonologically related words for the intended word, such as the use of "remind" for "remember," or "where" for "when". There were 10 instances of semantically similar word replacement in the transcripts of the aphasic children and only 1 instance in the transcripts of the LD children. Phonological replacements occurred 3 times in the aphasic samples and once in the LD samples. A less direct form of evidence for word-retrieval problems involved the use of indefinite reference terms where definite reference was called for, including deictic terms with no clear referent, and nonspecific terms such as "stuff" and "things." In the aphasic transcripts, indefinite reference terms appeared 46 times as compared to 31 times in the LD transcripts (which is a difference of 9% compared to 5% of the total utterances).

Whether word-finding problems can eventually be shown to be the root of the other communication breakdowns observed, or not, the overall comparison of language use in the two groups reveals striking similarities. Naive listeners could not distinguish among brief segments of narration from

Table 3-11
Mean utterance length in morphemes of total samples and the utterances containing garbles by child.

	Conversational Sample		Narrative Sample	
Child	Total Sample	Utterances with Garbles	Total Sample	Utterances with Garbles
AP1	5.10	6.90	6.98	10.15
AP2	5.86	9.42	8.10	10.92
AP3	4.22	6.05	4.67	5.70
LD1	5.77	7.20	8.69	13.52
LD2	5.31	8.67	7.71	10.2
LD3	6.05	8.70	5.43	7.79

Table 3-12
Percentage of aphasic children's total utterances containing each type of communication breakdown.

Child/Sample	Filled Pauses	Part-word Repetition	Whole-word Repetition	Phrase Repetition	Word/Phrase Replacement	Word/Phrase Revision	Incomplete Utterance	Unintelligible Utterance
AP1 CON	11	1	7	7	4	10	3	4
AP1 NAR	21	0	12	10	7	18	12	10
AP2 CON	6	2	9	2	2	9	8	5
AP2 NAR	23	1	15	5	6	9	10	16
AP3 CON	12	3	4	4	0	12	5	9
AP3 NAR	15	3	6	12	0	15	10	5

Table 3-13
Percentage of learning-disordered children's total utterances containing each type of communication breakdown.

Child/Sample	Filled Pauses	Part-word Repetition	Whole-word Repetition	Phrase Repetition	Word/Phrase Replacement	Word/Phrase Revision	Incomplete Utterance	Unintelligible Utterance
LD1 CON	8	2	2	3	2	5	2	0
LD1 NAR	13	2	2	2	4	8	1	1
LD2 CON	7	2	7	5	2	10	2	0
LD2 NAR	24	2	7	5	5	24	7	2
LD3 CON	10	3	4	2	2	6	3	4
LD3 NAR	23	2	10	3	7	10	1	21

Table 3-14
Mean percentage of total utterances containing each type of communication breakdown by sample condition for acquired aphasic and learning-disabled children.

Children and Sample	Filled Pauses	Part-word Repetition	Whole-word Repetition	Phrase Repetition	Word/Phrase Replacement	Word/Phrase Revision	Incomplete Utterance	Unintelligible Utterance
Aphasic Conversation	10	2	7	4	2	10	5	6
Aphasic Narration	20	1	11	9	4	14	11	10
LD Conversation	8	2	4	3	2	7	2	1
LD Narration	20	2	10	3	5	14	3	8

children in each of the groups. This comparison suggests that similar processes may be at work for the two groups studied: the acquired aphasic children, with only moderate delays in comprehension and production skills, and the learning-disabled children with specific language deficits.

Summary

We have reviewed the work on children with acquired aphasia associated with a seizure disorder, and concluded that detailed descriptions of communication functioning may improve our ability to predict the course of the disorder, monitor the child's improvement, or select appropriate intervention techniques for the child's current status. New directions for research were illustrated through detailed descriptions of communicative functioning in eight children, documenting the potential divergence in linguistic comprehension skills among children, and—through a comparison of a subgroup of acquired aphasic children with language-delayed learning-disabled children of a similar age and linguistic level— documenting the similarities in production characteristics of the two groups. We believe that the research strategy of creating homogeneous groups through detailed description, and comparing homogeneous subsets of language-disordered children will improve the clinician's ability to predict the course of recovery and make recommendations for treatment.

Acknowledgments

Support for this project came in part from research grants to the first author from the Graduate School Research Committee, University of Wisconsin-Madison, MRRC core support to the first and third authors through the Waisman Center on Mental Retardation and Human Development, University of Wisconsin-Madison, NICHD, NIH, Grant No. 2-P30-HD-03352-14, and support from University Affiliated Facility Project No. MCT-000915-13 to the Waisman Center. Portions of this work were conducted as part of a clinical research project coordinated by Dr. Kurt Hecox.

References

Barlow, C.F. Acquired disorders of communication in childhood. In A. Dorfman, (Ed.), *Child care in health and disease.* Chicago: Year Book Medical, 1968.
Brown, R. *A first language.* Cambridge, MA: Harvard University Press, 1973.

Burgemeister, B., Blum, L., & Lorge, I. *Columbia Mental Maturity Scale* (3rd Ed.). N.Y.: Harcourt, Brace & Jovanovich, 1972.

Campbell, T.F. *Effects of presentation rate and divided attention on auditory comprehension in acquired childhood aphasia.* Unpublished doctoral dissertation, University of Wisconsin, 1982.

Campbell, T.F. & Heaton, E.M. An expressive speech program for a child with acquired aphasia: A case study. *Canadian Journal of Human Communication,* 1978, Summer, 89-102.

Campbell, T.F., & Heaton, E.M. An expressive language program for a child with acquired aphasia. Paper presented at the Annual Convention of the American Speech-Language-Hearing Association, Atlanta, 1979.

Chapman, R., & Miller, J. *The simple sentence comprehension procedure.* Unpublished paper, University of Wisconsin-Madison, 1980.

Cooper, J.A., & Ferry, P.C. Acquired auditory verbal aphasia and seizures in childhood. *Journal of Speech and Hearing Disorders,* 1978, *43,* 176-184.

Cromer, R. Hierarchical ordering disability and aphasic children. In P. Dale & D. Ingram (Eds.), *Child language—An international perspective.* Baltimore: University Park Press, 1981, pp. 319-330.

de Negri, M. Some critical notes about "the epilepsy-aphasia syndrome" in children. *Brain Development,* 1980, *2,* 81-85.

Deonna, T.H. Beaumanoir, F., Gaillard, F., & Assal, G. Acquired aphasia in childhood with seizure disorder: A heterogeneous syndrome. *Neuropadiatrie,* 1977, *8,* 3, 263-273.

Deonna, T., Fletcher, P., & Voumard, C. Temporary regression during language acquisition: A linguistic analysis of a 2½ year old child with epileptic aphasia. *Developmental Medicine and Child Neurology,* in press.

Deuel, R.K., & Lenn, N.J. Acquired epileptic aphasia. Paper presented at the Child Neurology Society Meeting, Madison, WI, 1974.

Deuel, R.K., & Lenn, N.J. Treatment of acquired epileptic aphasia. *Journal of Pediatrics,* 1977, *90,* 959-961.

Dunn, L.M., & Dunn, L.M. *Peabody Picture Vocabulary Test-Revised.* Circle Pines, MI: American Guidance Service, 1981.

Gascon, G., Victor, O. Lombroso, C.T., & Goodglass, H. Language disorder, convulsive disorder and electroencephalographic abnormalities. *Archives of Neurology,* 1973, *28,* 156-162.

Harel, S.H., Walsh, G.O., & Menkes, J.H. Syndrome of acquired aphasia with epileptic electroencephalographic discharges. Paper presented at the Child Neurology Society Meeting, Nashville, Tenn., 1973.

Holmes, G.L., & McKeever, M. Aphasia with EEG abnormalities: Evaluation using EEG telemetry and videotape recording. *Neurology,* 1981, *31,* 102.

Huskisson, J.A. Acquired receptive language difficulties in childhood: A case study. *British Journal of Disorders of Communication,* 1974, *8,* 54-63.

Johnston, J. The language disordered child. In N. Lass, L. McReynolds, J. Northern, & D. Yoder (Eds.), *Speech, language and hearing: Vol. II. Pathologies of speech and language.* Philadelphia: W.B. Sanders, 1982, 780-801.

Jordan, L.S. Receptive and expressive language problems occurring in combination with a seizure disorder: A case report. *Journal of Communication Disorders,* 1980, *13,* 295-303.

Koepp, P., & Lagenstein I. Acquired epileptic aphasia: Letter to the editor. *The Journal of Pediatrics,* 1978, *99,* 164.

Kracke, I. Perception of rhythmic sequences by receptive aphasic and deaf children. *British Journal of Disorders of Communication,* 1978, *13,* 43-51.

Landau, W.M., & Kleffner, F.R. Syndrome of acquired aphasia with convulsive disorder in children. *Neurology,* 1957, *10,* 915-921.

Leiter, R.G. *Leiter International Performance Scale.* Los Angeles: Western Psychological Services, 1969.

Leonard, L. Language impairment in children. *Merrill-Palmer Quarterly,* 1979, *25,* 205-232.

Lou, H.C., Brandt, S., & Bruhn, P. Progressive aphasia and epilepsy with a self-limited course. In J.K. Penry (Ed.), *Epilepsy: The eighth international symposium.* New York: Raven Press (1977).

Mantovani, J.F., & Landau, W.M. Acquired aphasics with convulsive disorder: Course and prognosis. *Neurology,* 1980, *30,* 524-529.

McKinney, W., & McGreal, D.A. An asphasic syndrome in children. *Canadian Medical Association Journal,* 1974, *110,* 637-639.

McNeil, M.R., & Prescott, T.E. *Revised Token Test.* Baltimore: University Park Press, 1978.

Miller, J. *Assessing language production in children.* Baltimore: University Park Press, 1981.

Miller, J., & Chapman, R. Comprehension in routine contexts, Unpublished paper, University of Wisconsin-Madison, 1980.

Miller, J., & Chapman, R. The relationship between age and mean length of utterance in morphemes. *Journal of Speech and Hearing Research,* 1981, *24,* 154-161.

Miller, J., & Chapman, R. Users Manual: (SALT) Systematic Analysis of Language Transcripts. Unpublished document, University of Wisconsin-Madison, 1982.

Miller, J.F., Chapman, R., Branston, MB. & Reichle, J. Language comprehension in sensorimotor stages V and VI. *Journal of Speech and Hearing Research,* 1980, *23,* 284-311.

Miller, J.F., & Yoder, D.E. *The Miller-Yoder Test of Grammatical Comprehension.* Madison, WS: The University Book Store, 1972.

Rapin, I., Mattis, S., Rowan, A.J., & Golden, G.G. Verbal auditory agnosia in children. *Developmental Medicine and Child Neurology,* 1977, *19,* 192-207.

Rasmussen, T., & McCann, W. Clinical studies of patients with focal epilepsy due to chronic encephalitis. *Transactions of the American Neurological Association,* 1968, *93,* 89-94.

Rose, F.C. Receptive aphasia in childhood. Proceedings of the Society of British Neurological Surgeons. *Journal of Neurology, Neurosurgery and Psychiatry,* 1969, *32,* 65. (Abstract)

Sato, S., & Dreifuss, F.E. Electroencephalographic findings in a patient with developmental expressive aphasia. *Neurology.* 1972, *23,* 181-185.

Shoumaker, R.D., Bennett, D.R., Bray, P.F. & Curless, R.G. Clinical and EEG manifestations of an unusual aphasic syndrome in children. *Neurology,* 1974, *24,* 10-16.

Stein, L.K., & Curry, E.K.W. Childhood auditory agnosia. *Journal of Speech and Hearing Disorders,* 1968, *28,* 361-370.

Van Harskamp, F., Van Dongen, H.R., & Loonen, M.C.B. Acquired aphasia with convulsive disorders in children: Case study with seven years follow-up. *Brain and Language,* 1978, *6,* 141-148.

Waisman Study. Experimental neurosensory language disorders clinic. Waisman Center of Mental Retardation, University of Wisconsin-Madison, 1981.

Waters, G.V. The syndrome of acquired aphasia and convulsive disorder in children. *Journal of the Canadian Medical Association,* 1974, *110,* 611-612.

Wechsler, D. *Wechsler Intelligence Scale for Children (WISC).* New York: Psychological Corporation, 1974.

Worster-Drought, C. An unusual form of acquired aphasia in children. *Developmental Medicine and Child Neurology,* 1971, *13,* 563-571.

M. Jeanne Wilcox

Developmental Language Disorders: Preschoolers

The current emphasis on pragmatic aspects of communication has resulted in an investigative trend that has important implications for the structure and content of early language intervention. Specifically, studies of child language acquisition have been broadened to include an examination of communicative, rather than purely linguistic, competence. Many early investigations of child language, being largely influenced by Chomsky's works (1957, 1965) focused primarily on the acquisition of linguistic competence (Braine, 1963; Brown, Cazden, & Bellugi, 1973; Brown & Hanlon, 1970; McNeill, 1970). The influence of such investigations has been manifested in a variety of syntactically based early language intervention protocols (e.g., Miller & Yoder, 1972; Stremel & Waryas, 1974). More recently, as a pragmatic view of communication has taken hold, specialists concerned with normal, as well as disordered, child language have realized that linguistic competence is only one portion of the process of language acquisition (Bates, 1976; Hymes, 1971; Lakoff, 1972; Rees, 1978). The focus in studies of child language has therefore shifted from linguistic to communicative competence. As a result of this shift, it has become generally accepted that linguistic structures cannot be studied in normal populations, or treated in disordered populations, without reference to the context in which communication naturally occurs.

The general purpose of this chapter is threefold. First, a brief review of clinically applicable findings pertaining to the acquisition of communicative competence will be conducted. Second, the integration of these findings into current research focusing on language-disordered preschoolers will be considered. Finally, a treatment model for preschool language intervention will be presented in detail. The model, which is based upon current findings in the normal literature, serves as an example of the application of normal developmental literature to the treatment of language-disordered children.

The Acquisition of Communicative Competence: Implications for Language-Disordered Children

Communicative competence can generally be regarded as the ability to convey effectively and efficiently an intended message to a receiver. As such, this ability requires not only knowledge of the conventional communicative code, but also knowledge pertaining to socially appropriate communicative behaviors. As researchers have attempted to describe the acquisition of communicative competence, several areas have received attention. These include communication prior to speech, analyses of the contexts and functions of communication, the role of environmental communicative input, and children's observance of socially appropriate communicative conventions. Investigation in each of these areas has yielded a wealth of information that merits consideration in the management of young language-disordered children.

Prespeech Communication

Whereas language development was once viewed as beginning with the first word, it has become increasingly clearer that, prior to actual word production, children have developed rich communicative systems. Various researchers have examined children's prespeech communicative abilities (Barten, 1979; Bates, Camaioni, & Volterra, 1979; Bruner, 1975; Carter, 1978; Clark, 1978). It appears that there is a phase of development in which children intentionally communicate without actually using words. Generally, these communications seem to occur by means of gestures which may or may not be accompanied by vocalizations. Several investigators have systematically observed and described such gestural systems (Bates et al., 1979; Carter, 1978; Halliday, 1975).

Results of investigations, such as those cited above, have implied that there is a continuous flow of development from early gestural systems to speech. However, the specific transition from gestural communication to speech has not been specified. Nor is it clear the degree to which early gestures, per se , are required for later speech development. Most children communicate with gestures prior to words. However, when early words emerge, they do not simply replace gestures (Wilcox & Howse, 1982). On the contrary, early words are most often expressed as accompaniments to gestures (Snow, 1981). Further, as verbal development progresses, many gestures increase in frequency (Wilkinson & Rembold, 1981). Thus, prespeech gestural systems do not seem to serve as mere symbols to be later replaced by verbal behavior. Such gestures would seem to play a broader role in the acquisition of communicative competence.

The issue thus becomes one of identifying the role of prespeech communication in overall communicative development. This issue has been addressed by various researchers (Bruner, 1979; Dore, 1974; Halliday, 1975). The bulk of the research suggests that while children are engaging in prespeech communication, they are acquiring important sociocommunicative information. In this way, children who are not yet capable of verbal representation are using gestures as devices for extracting and putting into use knowledge about the communicative process.

The specification of knowledge gained during prespeech communication is particularly important for professionals concerned with programming for the nonverbal language-disordered child. It would seem that prior to the commencement of a verbal intervention plan, it is necessary to ascertain a child's understanding of the communicative concepts that are normally established during prespeech communciation.

For the clinician, the issue becomes one of being able to define operationally the type of communicative knowledge gained during prespeech communication. More specifically, what must a child understand about communication before she or he can engage in effective verbal interactions? The answer to this question seems to lie in the studies of children's language that have focused on early communicative functions.

Social Communicative Functions

Analyses of children's prespeech as well as early verbal communications have indicated that young children are capable of expressing a variety of social language functions, Halliday (1975) has described in detail the emergence of a social language system. Although many other investigators have observed and described prespeech and early verbal communications (e.g., Bates et al., 1979; Carter, 1978; Dore, 1974), Halliday's account relates most directly to the exemplary treatment model to be discussed later in this chapter and will, therefore, be the only description considered here. Further, Halliday's description accounts for the transition from preverbal to verbal development and does not attempt to describe child communication within the boundaries of adult meaning. Essentially, Halliday directly observed a child's emerging communication and formulated hypotheses conerning the social language functions. He described a total of seven language functions, which are, in order of emergence, as follows:

1. INSTRUMENTAL, in which language is used to satisfy material needs.
2. REGULATORY, in which language is used to control actions of other persons.
3. INTERACTIONAL, in which language is used to establish and maintain contact with other persons.
4. PERSONAL, in which language is used to inform others of one's own behavior.
5. HEURISTIC, in which language is used to explore and obtain explanations about the environment.
6. IMAGINATIVE, in which language is used to create a pretend environment.
7. INFORMATIVE, in which language is used to give information to someone who it is believed did not possess the information.

The first three functions, termed pragmatic, are interpersonal in nature, and generally relate to using communication to act upon the environment. These functions, as such, require some sort of response from the environment. The remaining functions, termed mathetic, are ideational in nature and represent the use of communication to code experiences. The informative function, which emerges significantly later than the others, is the one that indicates that the child is using language in the adult sense, or engaging in true language. The mastery of the other six functions is regarded as necessary for true language production.

Overall, Halliday has suggested that children learn, and with prespeech communicative forms, convey these meanings (excepting the informative) well before they have a conventional verbal means of expression. These social meanings then provide the foundation for the later expression of conventional language forms.

Initially, children learn the interpersonal nature of communication. After they have begun to express various interpersonal functions, they then differentiate the interpersonal from the ideational, and express functions in one mode (interpersonal or ideational) or the other. At this point there is no longer a one-to-one correspondence between a communication and a function. Rather, a communication may be used to express more than one function.

Halliday's description of prespeech and early verbal communication has important clinical applications. For the professional working with a nonverbal or low-verbal disordered child, it provides a means of assessing the current status of communication. Specifically, the clinician can ascertain whether a child understands the interpersonal nature of communication by noting nonverbal use of the instrumental, regulatory, and interactional functions. Such an assessment is particularly important for treatment programming. If a child does not understand that communication can be used to act upon the environment, then the establishment of such would be prerequisite to verbal intervention.

Environmental Communicative Input

As investigators have examined the role of input language, it has become clear that there are a number of ways in which input may influence, either positively or negatively, the language acquisition process (Cross, 1978; Gleason & Weintraub, 1978; Nelson, 1973). Although there are still many gray areas with respect to the influences of input, some general statements can be made.

It has been well documented that adults modify speech addressed to young children (Cross, 1977; Gleason & Weintraub, 1978; Lieven, 1978; Newhoff, Silverman & Millet, 1980; Newport, Gleitman, & Gleitman, 1977; Snow, 1972, 1977). However, the reason why such modifications might occur is not entirely clear. Some researchers have suggested that input is modified so as to teach children language. Others have suggested that teaching is not the primary goal, rather, the input is modified to achieve communication with children on their level. Still others have suggested that the input is modified so as to maintain a flow of conversation with children, therefore providing an appropriate model of conversational exchanges. Gleason and Weintraub (1978) have suggested that input plays different roles according to the age of the child. They described input to children under 12 months of age as serving primarily to establish an affectional bond. Input to children learning language (12 to 48 months) was viewed as facilitatory with respect to abstraction of linguistic knowledge. Finally, input to children over four years of age was characterized as providing information about the world.

There appears to be no clear agreement as to why children receive a specialized form of input. From the input literature, however, it is possible to extract those types of input that seem to exert a positive influence on the language-acquisition process. These are summarized in Table 4-1. As can be seen in the table, the first type of input described relates to expansions. It appears that expansions preserving a child's semantic intent exert a positive influence on language acquisition (Cross, 1977, 1978). Such expansions can occur in the form of noun phrase, pronoun, or verb phrase expansions. Examples of each of these forms of expansions can be seen in the table.

Table 4-1
Adult interactive strategies exerting positive influences on child language behavior.

1. **Comments in the form of expansions preserving a child's semantic intent.**

   a. Noun phrase expansions: An utterance incorporating the noun phrase topic.

   >Child: *kitty jump*
   >Adult: *the kitty is on the chair*

   b. Pronoun expansions: An utterance that incorporates the child's topic by using pronominalization.

   >Child: *kitty jump*
   >Adult: *she is jumping*

   c. Verb phrase expansions: An utterance preserving the topic expressed by the child in the verb phrase, but using a lexical item not found in the child's noun phrase.

   >Child: *kitty jump*
   >Adult: *the dog is jumping, too*

2. **Allowing the child to select the topic of joint (i.e., adult-child) attention.**

3. **Feedback responding to the truth value of a child's utterance, rather than linguistic accuracy.**

   >Child: *kitty jump*
   >Adult: *yes, the kitty is jumping*

A second factor in adult-child interaction that can influence language acquisition pertains to synchrony of the adult with the child's level. Specifically, children gain the most verbally when the adult is in cognitive as well as verbal synchrony with the child. Behaviorally, such synchrony can be facilitated by allowing the child to take the lead and, therefore, direct the activity or interaction.

This particular input variable becomes especially important when we consider the nature of most current treatment procedures. In many treatment programs, a child is presented with stimuli previously selected by the clinician. These stimuli may be objects or pictures that the clinician perceives as being within the child's conceptual abilities; but, in fact, there is the risk of a mismatch with respect to adult-child synchrony. The risk is particularly high in early language intervention, as it is apparent from the normal literature that an adult meaning system cannot be imposed on child language. It may be that in a situation in which the clinician has selected the stimuli, and the child is making minimal progress in treatment, the stimuli selected by the clinician are simply beyond the child's conceptual level. By allowing the child to select the topic of joint attention, it cannot be guaranteed that a mismatch in synchrony will not occur. Rather, the assumption is made that if the child is allowed to take the lead, it further reduces the possiblility of a mismatch that may impede treatment progress.

Nelson (1977) has examined the influences of these first two input variables in the language of normal children. In this study, an experimenter engaged in play with the children. During the play sessions, semantically related expansions of the children's preceding utterances were provided. The utterance types modeled by the experimenter (in the form of expansions) represented syntactic structures not used by the children at the initiation of the study. Following termination of experimental procedures, the children were observed to use the modeled syntactic forms. It was concluded that the procedures resulted in the acquisition of new syntactic forms by the children.

The final input variable to be discussed relates to the way adults respond to children's utterances. Children seem to derive maximum benefit from input that responds to the truth value, rather than the linguistic accuracy, of their utterances. This point has been discussed by various investigators (Bowerman, 1976; Bruner, 1975; Nelson, 1973). Nelson noted that there are some mothers who function in a directive mode and seemingly attempt to teach their children correct words. In doing such, they were observed to correct their children's inaccurate productions. Nelson concluded that this style of interaction slowed the children's language learning. Bruner, in his studies of mother-child interaction, supported Nelson's view of negative feedback. He suggested that maternal corrections have an undesirable effect on the communicative interaction. Bowerman provided a detailed discussion on the role of negative feedback in language acquisition. Following a review of various studies, she suggested that "feedback about inadequate performance is neither required for language learning nor does it particularly accelerate its pace" (1976, p. 170).

This rather ominous view of negative feedback has important implications for treatment procedures currently practiced with language-disordered children. Clearly, many treatment procedures rely on correction of inaccurate responses. In view of current information relative to negative feedback, this mode of treatment should probably be modified. However, as Bowerman has pointed out, most information relative to the role of negative feedback has been derived from normal populations. It may be that with disordered children, who have obviously not acquired language in a normal manner, negative, as well as positive, feedback is necessary for the accurate formulation of linguistic hypotheses.

Conversational Conventions

Another aspect of communicative competence relates to the ability to engage appropriately in a communicative interaction. Such appropriateness goes beyond the individual utterance level and focuses more on conversatioinal behaviors. Generally, three basic skills are required in order to engage in a socially appropriate conversational interaction. As described by Wilcox and Webster (1980), they are (1) the initiation and maintenance of a communicative interaction, (2) consideration of the listener's perspective when encoding messages, and (3) appropriate responses to listener feedback. Initiation and maintenance of an interaction relies heavily on nonverbal behavior, such as gaze regulation, use of silences, timing of speech, and turn-taking. Consideration of the listener's perspective requires awareness of shared, as well as unshared, information between speaker and listener. Appropriate responses to listener feedback require answering questions and appropriately repeating or recoding utterances as indicated by the listener feedback.

Numerous investigators have examined the development of communicative conventions in normal children (Gallagher, 1977; Garvey, 1977; Wellman & Lempers, 1977; Wilcox & Webster, 1980). In general, evidence indicates that children have a basic understanding of these skills by age four. Further, it has been suggested that these skills may function independently of the level of linguistic development. Clinically, this means that an evaluation of linguistic skills is not sufficient to ascertain functioning in terms of communicative competence. Assessment procedures should also include provisions to evaluate children's awareness of socially appropriate communicative conventions.

The need for evaluating both aspects (i.e., linguistic as well as socially appropriate interpersonal skills) of a child's communication is further substantiated in a recent study by Blank, Gessner, and Esposito (1979). The investigation consisted of the analysis of the communicative behavior of a child (age 3;3) while interacting with his parents over a 10-week period. The child was initially referred for an evaluation because of his refusal to interact with anyone other than his parents. Analysis of the linguistic aspects of the child's speech (e.g., semantic relations and syntax) revealed age-appropriate behavior. However, analysis of the child's interpersonal communicative functioning revealed numerous difficulties. Most noticable was his inability to use or comprehend gestures (e.g., pointing) or to appropriately respond to utterances. His responses, when made, were usually irrelevant to the preceding comment.

Communicative Competence: Studies with Language-Disordered Children

Communicative Functions

One of the first investigations of language-disordered children's use of communicative functions was conducted by Snyder (1975). Her participants included 15 language-disordered and 15 normal children, all functioning at the one-word stage of language production. The children were presented with tasks designed to elicit imperative and declarative functions. Responses were scored on a five-point scale ranging from nonverbal to verbal behavior. On both function measures, the language-disordered children produced fewer verbal functions, and were observed to engage in more nontask responses than the normal children.

In a more recent investigation, Leonard, Camarata, Rowan, and Chapman (1982) also examined the communicative functions of young language-disordered children. The participants in the study included 14 normal and 14 language-impaired children. Both groups of children were functioning at the single-word stage of language production. Spontaneous language samples were obtained from all children and were then analyzed using McShane's (1980) classification of communicative functions. The classification system included the following major functions:

1. **Regulation**—attempts to control other persons' behaviors
2. **Statement**—utterances that name, describe, or provide information about a situation not in the here and now
3. **Exchange**—utterances made when a child is giving or receiving objects from another person
4. **Personal**—utterances about what the child is doing, or about to be doing, as well as refusals and protests
5. **Conversation**—utterances in response to preceding utterances produced by other people.

Results indicated that the groups of children were highly similar in their use of the functions with two exceptions. The normal children produced more statement functions in the form of naming, while the language-disordered children produced more conversation functions in the form of answering. Since statement functions are child-initiated, while the conversation functions are not, it could be said that the language-disordered children were less likely to spontaneously initiate verbal communications.

In another recent investigation, communicative functions served by echolalic behavior in autistic children was examined (Prizant & Duchan, 1981). Four children diagnosed as autistic, and ranging in age from 4;8 to 9;3, were videotaped in a variety of natural settings. Of particular interest were the children's echolalic utterances. By viewing such utterances in their natural contexts, the authors posited seven different functions the echoic utterances seemed to be serving. The majority of the children's echoic utterances fell into four categories that appeared to be communicative in nature. These included turn-taking, declaration, affirmation, and request.

These preceding studies of communicative functions produced by language-disordered children contain a wealth of information applicable to the treatment process. First, they provide guidelines for assessment and treatment by specifically identifying various communicative functions. Second, they alert one to the possibility that there may be differences in language-disordered children's use of functions as compared to normals. Finally, the study by Prizant and Duchan importantly emphasizes the need to evaluate the communicative use of behaviors that are frequently regarded by clinicians as undesirable and noncommunicative in nature.

Conversational Skills

Another important aspect of language-disordered children's communicative competence pertains to their conversational functioning beyond the level of expressing functions. These aspects of communication are frequently referred to as discourse abilities and include behaviors mentioned in the first section of this chapter. These are (1) initiating and sustaining a communicative interaction, (2) considering a listener's perspective when encoding messages, and (3) responding to listener feedback.

Initiation of a communicative interaction involves obtaining attention and then asserting the desired message. Typically, initiation comprises nonverbal behaviors, such as eye contact and body position, as its first steps. For example, to initiate an interaction, a potential speaker will usually look at, then lean or walk toward, a potential listener. If necessary, these nonverbal behaviors may be supplemented, especially in young children, by verbal attention-getters, such as "Hey, " "Look, " or by producing the name of the person whose attention is desired.

Investigators who have examined initiation abilities of language-disordered children have suggested that appropriate initiation skills may represent a problem area (Dukes, 1981; Lucas, 1980). It appears that some language-disordered children not only have difficulty appropriately obtaining attention for purposes of initiation, but they also attempt to initiate communication at inappropriate times. Further, it has been suggested that once attention has been obtained, some children with language disorders may have difficulty asserting their desired message for reasons unrelated to their linguistic deficits. Hence, potential problems with initiation may be at the verbal (asserting a message) or nonverbal (eye contact, body posture) level.

The ability to sustain a communicative interaction involves a variety of behaviors. These include turn-taking conventions, the production of utterances appropriate and relevant to preceding utterances, acknowledgement and/or answers to questions, and requests for clarification of ambiguous messages. Various studies have found deficits in language-disordered children with respect to these abilities (Donahue, Pearl, & Bryan, 1980; Dukes, 1981; Lucas, 1980; Miller, 1978). Language-disordered children have been observed to violate turn-taking conventions, produce irrelevant utterances, ignore questions, and, infrequently, request clarification of ambiguous or nonunderstood messages. In general it can be said that some language-disordered children may have problems maintaining control of a communicative interaction for a sufficient length of time to express a desired message.

Another aspect of conversational proficiency relates to the consideration of a listener's perspective when encoding utterances. Basically, this means that a speaker must be able to integrate verbal and contextual information in such a way that the utterance produced is as informative as the situation requires. The degree of speaker informativeness required will depend on different factors. One factor pertains to a speaker's awareness of information already available to, or shared by, a listener. Such information can be apparent from linguistic or nonlinguistic context. A second factor pertains to a speaker's awareness of listener limitations that may require modifications of his or her normal communicative behavior.

Although little research has focused on young language-disordered children's abilities to consider a listener's perspective, there are two recent studies relating to aspects of this skill. Shatz, Bernstein, and Shulman (1980) examined language-disordered children's responses to indirect directives (e.g., "Can you put the dolly in the bed?"). Utterances such as these are frequently referred to as indirect requests. For example, "Can you put the dolly in the bed?" is literally a question about one's ability to perform the stated action. If a listener had both arms in casts, then a literal interpretation of this utterance would be appropriate. However, in a context in which there are no apparent limitations on a listener's mobility—which is to say that listener's mobility is shared information—then the utterance would be regarded as a request to perform the stated action. Thus, appropriate interpretations of utterances coded in an indirect format rely on the listener's ability to compare the utterance with the context in which it is produced.

Shatz et al. examined aspects of language-disordered children's abilities to encode context by noting their responses to indirect, as well as direct, sentence forms. In the study, five language-disordered children ranging in age from 5 to 6 years served as participants. In an initial experiment, the children were seen in a familiar therapy room equipped with toys, and presented with direct ("Put the ball in the truck. ") and indirect ("Can you put the ball in the truck?") requests. Results indicated that the children performed the requested action the majority of the time.

A second experiment was conducted that more specifically examined the children's abilities to consider contextual cues. In this experiment, the children were presented with test utterances only in the *can + you* format. However, this time the utterances were preceded by verbal information designed to foster either (1) literal interpretation of the utterance as a question ("Can you run fast?") or (2) interpretation of the utterance as a request ("Can you give me the toy?"). Results indicated the the children had difficulty using the information given in the prior linguistic context, particularly when the context indicated that the appropriate interpretation would be as a question.

Fey, Leonard, and Wilcox (1981) examined language-disordered children's abilities to modify their speech as a function of listener age. Six language-disordered children, ranging in age from 4;3 to 6;5 served as participants. The participants were observed in a free-play setting with (1) a language-normal child of the same age and (2) a language-normal child who was younger, but exhibited linguistic abilities similar to the disordered child. The results indicated that the participants simplified their speech somewhat when communicating with the younger children. Specifically, they exhibited a shorter mean preverb length, while also using more sentence forms designed to engage the younger children in an interaction.

At this time, general conclusions cannot be drawn with respect to language-disordered children's abilities to consider a listener's perspective. It would be most prudent to say that perspective-taking, as described previously, is an important skill for effective communication. It may constitute a problem area for some children, especially when they are required to evaluate prior linguistic context.

The final aspect of conversational proficiency to be discussed concerns responses to listener feedback indicating a lack of understanding. More specifically, a speaker must be able to provide clarification of utterances that a listener has indicated are ambiguous. Some research has focused on this ability in language-disordered children. Gallagher and Darnton (1978) examined these children's attempts to clarify their utterances in response to the question "What?" Results indicated that the majority of the time, the children recoded their original utterances.

Pearl, Donahue, and Bryan (1979) also examined language-disordered children's responses to clarification requests. The children were provided with three types of feedback, (1) explicit ("Tell me more") (2) implicit ("I don't understand"), and (3) facial feedback which consisted of a puzzled look. Results indicated that the children attempted to clarify utterances in response to all types of feedback.

From research conducted thus far, it would appear that language-disordered children recognize the need to clarify ambiguous messages. However, the degree to which their clarifications are successful has yet to be determined. Hence, the ability to clarify an ambiguous utterance successfully also merits consideration for potential treatment content.

The Integration of Communicative Competence into Early Language Intervention: An Exemplary Treatment Model

As a professional concerned with the management of language-disordered children, my primary interest in studies of the nature of children's communication is their application to the treatment process for disordered populations. Throughout the first two sections of this chapter, as well as in the chapter by Leonard (this volume), brief suggestions were made in this regard. As is all too often the case with disordered populations, specific studies of the treatment process are relatively few in number. Further, as the idea of communicative competence is relatively new, the number of available references is even further reduced (Leonard, 1981). Hence, a specialist who recognizes the need to improve a child's communicative, rather than purely linguistic, competence must frequently review the literature and then develop his or her own procedures.

It is my intent to devote the remainder of this chapter to a discussion of the ways in which the literature I have previously reviewed can be applied to the treatment process. To accomplish this, I will present, in detail, an exemplary treatment model for preschool language intervention. The model is not intended to be all-inclusive. Rather, it illustrates one way in which aspects of linguistic, as well as communicative, competence can be treated.

In the more recent literature, there are other treatment procedures reflecting current trends in the study of child language. Taenzer, Cermak, and Hanlon (1981), as well as Culotta and Horn (1982), describe procedures that incorporate important pragmatic variables or modify spontaneous communicative behavior. Dukes (1981) outlines an approach based on group activities that focuses on several aspects of communicative competence, including nonverbal as well as verbal skills. Finally, Lucas (1980) describes procedures oriented toward the appropriate use of linguistic forms in social settings.

The treatment model to be discussed here incorporates several of the parameters of communicative competence addressed in previous sections of this chapter. First, the importance of prespeech communication is recognized by including procedures designed to establish social language functions expressed during prespeech communication. Second, input behaviors found to have a positive influence on language acquisition are utilized in the intervention procedures. Specifically, these include (a) semantically related expansions of child utterances, (b) child-directed interactions, and (c) clinician feedback responding to the truth value of child utterances. Third, to enable modification of spontaneous communicative behavior, treatment takes place in a free-play setting in which few restrictions are placed on the child's verbal or nonverbal behavior. By staging the treatment setting in this manner, children's utterances are not treated in isolation. Rather, the focus of treatment is on conversational competence. This setting also allows the clinician to model socially appropriate communicative conventions (i.e., initiating and sustaining a communicative interaction, consideration of a listener's perspective, and appropriate responses to listener feedback).

The treatment protocol is divided into three phases. The first phase is referred to as nonverbal intervention. This phase is designed to establish intentional communication in the form of gestures and/or vocalizations. The second phase establishes initial verbal skills in the form of a core lexicon. The final phase focuses on expansion of verbal skills beyond the single-word level. Each of these phases will be considered separately.

Nonverbal Intervention

This first part of the protocol is designed for children who do not understand the interpersonal nature of communication. Typically, such children exhibit no identifiable forms of intentional communication. The assumption is made that the ability to manipulate the environment intentionally is necessary for language development. Hence, the goal at this phase of intervention, which is based upon Halliday's (1975) model of language acquisition, is to establish the following social meanings: interactional, instrumental, and regulatory. These meanings will then serve as the basis for later conventional expressions.

The procedures and goals for this initial intervention are summarized in Table 4-2. Upon completion of this phase of the protocol, a child will (1) understand that communication can be used to obtain attention and (2) understand that communication can be used to obtain assistance in achieving desired ends. Operationally, this translates into the goals listed in Table 4-2. Although the interactional function appears first in the outline, it is not necessarily trained first. In reality all three functions (interactional, instrumental, and regulatory) can be the focus of training at the same time.

The first step in establishing the interactional function requires the clinician to attend to the child's behavior and comment about the child's activity or focus of attention. At this point, the basic idea is for the child to begin to understand that his or her activities are of interest to the clinician. Over time, this adult interest will take on the properties of a reinforcer for the child. The child will in turn start engaging in behaviors to obtain attention from the clinician.

At this step of intervention, it is critical that the clinician follow the child's lead. This means that no attempts should be made to direct the play activities, other than imposing limits on potentially harmful behaviors. The clinician, by behaving in this essentially nondirective fashion, is facilitating adult-child synchrony. In this way, the clinician's comments, which can be regarded as verbal expansions of the child's nonverbal interactions, are more likely to be within the child's conceptual sphere. Clinician comments about the child's activities should be of a simple linguistic form, generally at the single- or two-word utterance level.

Eventually, the clinician will begin to place contingencies on the child that concern his or her attending behavior. However, at least three unconditional sessions are initially required. The actual number of such sessions will vary depending on how frequently the child is seen for treatment. For example, if a child is seen for treatment on an infrequent basis (i.e., once a week) a larger number of unconditional sessions will probably be required.

After the initial unconditional sessions, the clinician can begin placing contingencies on attending. Attention is therefore withheld in an attempt to elicit some form of appropriate attention-getting behavior from the child. The actual behaviors to be evoked will vary from child to child, and should be predetermined by the clinician. Generally, appropriate attention-getting behavior will take the form of eye contact or gestures which may or may not be accompanied by a vocalization.

As the clinician begins to place contingencies on attending, the child may initially make no attempt to get attention from the clinician. If this

Table 4-2
Nonverbal intervention.

---

1. **Interactional Function**
    Goal: Establish appropriate attention-getting behavior
    a. Attend to child's behavior and comment
    b. Place contingencies on giving attention

2. **Instrumental/Regulatory Function**
    Goal: Establish a clear signal indicating assistance is required
    a. Anticipate need for assistance, and comply
    b. Place contingencies on providing assistance

---

occurs, the clinician should return to the first step for a session and continue to probe by periodically witholding attention. As the child initially begins to make attempts to obtain attention, she or he may exhibit very slight moving-toward behaviors. Such behaviors should be noted, reinforced with attention, and then incorporated into a procedure of successive approximation to achieve the desired end goal.

The establishment of the instrumental and regulatory functions also relies on the clinician following the child's lead and then verbally expanding the child's nonverbal interactions. In the case of these functions, the procedures initially require the clinician to anticipate a child's need for assistance, and comply. For example, the child may be looking at a toy on a high shelf. The clinician would then get the toy and give it to the child, while making a comment such as "here."

As with the interactional function, at least three sessions should be unconditional. It is initially necessary to establish the pattern that the clinician can, and is willing to, assist the child. After the initial unconditional sessions, the clinician can begin to place contingencies on providing his or her assistance. Specifically, the clinician does not provide assistance until the child makes some attempt to engage it. Again, the process of successive approximation should be employed to establish the desired target response.

Once these interpersonal functions have been established a child is ready to begin initial verbal intervention. To determine such readiness, a productivity criterion is used. That is, a child is required to demonstrate productive use of the interpersonal communicative functions (interactional and instrumental and/or regulatory). A function is regarded as being productive if it is expressed in at least five different contexts during a given treatment session. To ensure a degree of stability, two consecutive probes meeting this criterion are required.

Productivity, rather than percentage of use was selected as a criterion as percentages can often be misleading. A child may be producing a function 90% of the time. However, if that function is always in the same context it may be that a child has not actually acquired the communicative behavior in a manner that is useful for communication. That is to say that the child may not have acquired a generalizable communicative behavior. Thus, in keeping treatment data, percentages are still recorded but productive use of a behavior is used for purposes of determining acquisition.

Table 4-3 displays data on a child who was exposed to this initial phase of intervention. The female child was 3;10 at the time of intervention. The initial diagnostic evaluation revealed no verbal communication and little-to-no nonverbal communication. Parental reports confirmed the diagnostic impressions. Initial baseline observations were conducted to assess percentage of time spent engaging in the interpersonal communicative functions as well as the number of different contexts in which the functions were expressed. Interpersonal communications were identified as those instances in which the child sought the attention or assistance of the clinician. Three baseline observations were made via videotape. During this time the clinician and the child were in a large room equipped with various age-appropriate toys. The clinician was instructed to "engage in play with the child." Each baseline session was thirty minutes in duration.

The videotapes were reviewed and the duration of each interpersonal communicative act was timed. The percentage of time spent engaging in interpersonal communication as well as the number of different contexts was then computed for the child. Once the baseline data were obtained, treatment began. The child was seen four times weekly in individual treatment that was thirty minutes in duration.

The child was initially exposed to three unconditional treatment sessions. Contingencies were then placed on the clinician's attention and compliance during the fourth session. The data displayed in Table 4-3, therefore, represent the baseline information, the first three unconditional treatment sessions, and weekly probes. As can be seen from the Table, the child reached criterion during the fourth week of treatment. Treatment was extended for an additional week to ensure stability.

Initial Verbal Intervention

This phase of the treatment protocol is designed for children who exhibit intentional communication, but do not code it in conventional terms. The general idea is to establish a core lexicon. Various investigators (e.g.,

Table 4-3
Data: Nonverbal intervention.

Session Type	% Time Engaged Interpersonal Communication Functions	Number of Different Contexts	
		Interactional	Regulatory/ Instrumental
Baseline	08	1	1
Baseline	06	1	1
Baseline	09	1	1
Treatment No. 1 (no contingencies)	12	1	2
Treatment No. 2 (no contingencies)	10	1	2
Treatment No. 3 (no contingencies)	11	1	2
Weekly Probe No. 1 (contingencies)	20	2	3
Weekly Probe No. 2 (contingencies)	24	2	2
Weekly Probe No. 3 (contingencies)	39	4	3
Weekly Probe No. 4 (contingencies)	51	5	5
Weekly Probe No. 5 (contingencies)	56	6	5

Bowerman, 1976; Holland, 1975) have provided guidelines for selection of such a core, and the reader is referred to them for purposes of devising an appropriate initial lexicon. The primary focus of this section will be on procedures for establishing whatever core lexicon has been selected. The procedures for this phase of intervention are summarized in Table 4-4.

The initial lexicon is trained in the context of the interactional, instrumental, and regulatory functions. As with the first phase of the protocol, there is no order to the establishment of the functions. Rather, the context dictates what particular function will be verbally coded.

The general procedures for establishing the initial words are very similar to the procedures outlined for establishing the interpersonal functions in phase 1 of the protocol. The actual steps to be followed are listed in Table 4-4. As can be seen, the clinician's attention and assistance are serving as the means for establishing the target words. A child either beginning, or moving into, this second phase of the protocol already understands the interpersonal communicative functions, and, as such, can be regarded as motivated to communicate. Essentially, in this second phase of treatment, the child will begin mapping conventional verbal signs upon interpersonal functions that are already in use.

As with phase 1 of the protocol, the initial treatment sessions should be conducted with no contingencies. Thus, for at least three sessions, the clinician will follow the child's lead and expand the nonverbal communicative acts in the form of words from the core lexicon. Hence, all clinician comments will initially be in the form of a single-word utterance. Following these unconditional sessions, the clinician may then begin to introduce contingencies in the forms of steps 2 and 3 (appearing in Table 4-4). The intermediate step, in which any vocalization is accepted, is necessary only for those children who do not accompany their nonverbal communications with vocalizations. Since many children will spontaneously do this while expressing social functions (Halliday, 1975), this step will not be necessary for all children.

In terms of size of the core lexicon, it is recommended that 10 to 15 words be initially selected. As with phase 1 of the protocol a productivity criteria is employed. Specifically, when a child is using a given lexical item in at least five different contexts, he or she is regarded as ready to incorporate that item in more complex linguistic structures.

Table 4-5 displays data obtained from a child who was exposed to this second phase of the treatment protocol. The data is in percentage form so as to display an overall picture of the types of communicative behaviors. The male child was aged 2;10 at the initiation of treatment. The diagnostic evaluation revealed intentional communication expressed primarily with gestural symbols. The only conventional linguistic sign was 'mama.' This

Table 4-4
Initial Verbal Intervention

1. **Interactional Function**
   a. Child demonstrates attention-getting behavior, clinician attends and provides word for joint focus of attention.
   b. Contingencies placed on attending: Clinician withholds attention until child pairs nonverbal signal with a vocalization. Clinician then attends and provides word for joint focus of attention.
   c. Contingencies placed on attending: Clinician withholds attention until child utilizes word (or acceptable approximation). Clinician then attends and expands with two-word utterance.

2. **Instrumental/Regulatory Function**
   a. Child produces signal for assistance, clinician provides assistance and produces word.
   b. Contingencies placed on providing assistance: Clinician doesn't assist until child pairs nonverbal signal with a vocalization. Clinician then complies and produces desired word.
   c. Contingencies placed on providing assistance: Clinician doesn't assist until child uses word (or acceptable approximation). Clinician then complies and expands with a two-word utterance.

sign was regarded as productive. Parental reports confirmed the findings in the diagnostic evaluation.

The child was seen for individual treatment four times weekly. Each session was thirty minutes long. Baseline information was obtained for the first three sessions via videotape. During baseline collection, the clinician was simply instructed to "engage in play with the child." The tapes were reviewed and the communicative acts were coded with respect to (1) the social language function and (2) the means used to express the function. The interactional, instrumental, and regulatory functions were consistently used. The means of expression were coded as gestural, gesture and vocalization, single-word utterances, and two-word utterances. Percentages in each of these categories were computed. The baseline information appearing in the table represents the mean of these sessions. Additionally, contexts of each word production were noted (e.g., "truck" while pushing the truck; "truck" while pointing to a truck out of reach). These notations then served as the basis for determining word productivity.

Following baseline, treatment procedures began. The goal was to establish a core lexicon of at least 15 words. Weekly probes were obtained by video recording during the last treatment session in each week. During the fourth week, the established criterion was met for seven of the target words. At this point, the clinician began modeling two word utterances incorporating these words while she continued to model single word responses for those words that were not yet productive. The effects of this can be seen with the resulting increases in two-word responses. These expanded child responses incorporated the productive lexical items.

Expansion of Verbal Skills

This phase of the protocol is designed for children who are ready to expand verbal skills beyond the single-word level. The procedures in this phase can be used to establish use of semantic relations, grammatical morphemes, kernel-sentence structures, or transformational structures. The specific target selected simply varies according to a child's needs. To determine the appropriate target structure, it is recommended that a spontaneous language sample be obtained and analyzed. Miller (1981) has several suggestions and recommendations for the specifics of such an analysis. Once the analyses of the language sample have been done, it is recommended that the clinician consult developmental norms for purposes of determining appropriate target responses for the child.

In terms of specific procedures, as with phases 1 and 2 of the protocol, it is important for the clinician to follow the child's lead. To facilitate this, the clinician should engage in imitative play. This means that the clinician watches the child and then plays in exactly the same way as she or he does. For example, if a child begins stacking blocks, the clinician will also stack blocks. With many children, this imitative play will not be necessary, as the children themselves will specify what they want the clinician to do. For example, a child may be engaging in a pretend cooking activity in which he will give the clinician instructions such as, "Put the plate there" or "Pour the milk now," and so on. So the general rule is for the clinician to engage in imitative play unless otherwise specified by the child.

The other two input facilitators appearing in Table 4-1 of this chapter are also used by the clinician. Specifically, the clinician expands child utterances in the form of the selected target response and, when a child uses the target response, responds to the truth value. Table 4-6 summarizes the steps and procedures for this phase of the protocol. As can be seen upon examining the table, when the child makes a comment, the clinician expands with the target response. If the child is quiet, the clinician will code the

Table 4-5
Data: Initial verbal intervention.

Session	Gesture %	Gesture and Vocalization %	Single-Word %	Two-Word %
Baseline	91	05	04	00
Week 1[1]	90	03	07	00
Week 2[2]	51	19	30	00
Week 3	52	15	33	00
Week 4	25	18	56	00
Week 5[3]	16	14	70	00
Week 6	11	19	65	05
Week 7	07	10	65	18

[1]No contingencies placed on clinician attention and assistance

[2]Contingencies placed on clinician attention and assistance

[3]Clinician began modeling two-word utterances for productive lexical items

nonverbal behavior in the form of the target response. If the child produces the target response, the clincian will confirm the truth value and expand one level beyond the target response. Essentially, unless the child actually produces the target response, all clinician verbal behavior will be in the form of the desired target response.

The criterion for acquisition of a given structure varies as a function of the selected target response. If a target behavior is a grammatical morpheme, the criterion for termination of treatment is 50% usage in obligatory contexts for two consecutive treatment sessions. A relatively liberal criterion is employed because experience with the protocol has indicated that at a time in which children are using a grammatical morpheme during 50% of the required contexts, they have, in effect, acquired the structure and are able to stablize use on their own. However, once criterion has been reached, the clinician should monitor the structure for a few sessions. If there appears to be a pattern of decreased use, then that structure should again be the focus of treatment.

If the target behavior is a semantic relation, kernel structure, or transformation, the same criterion used in phases 1 and 2 is employed. However,

Table 4-6
Expansion of verbal skills.

---

1. Identify verbal target (e.g., agent + action)
2. Child initiates activity and clinician imitates play unless otherwise specified by the child.
3. Clinician verbal behavior:
   a. If child makes a comment, the clinician expands in the form of the verbal target.

      Child: *doggie* (as making dog jump)
      Clinician: *doggie jump* (while also making dog jump)

   b. If child is quiet, the clinician does the nonverbal behavior in the form of the target structure.

      Child: making dog jump
      Clinician: doggie jump (while also making dog jump)

   c. If child produces target structure, the clinician responds to the truth value, then expands the utterance.

      Child: *doggie jump*
      Clinician: *yes, doggie jumping*

---

productivity is defined in terms of word combinations rather than non-linguistic contexts. Specifically, a given structure is regarded as productive if it occurs at least five times in combination with different words for two consecutive treatment sessions.

Since all treatment sessions take place in a free play, spontaneous context, it is not necessary to gather additional samples for purposes of determining whether criterion has been reached. The clinician is, in fact, treating spontaneous speech. Hence, an analysis of the child's language used during a treatment session will yield the desired information. To chart a given child's progress, it is recommended that weekly analyses be conducted.

Table 4-7 displays data from a child exposed to this phase of the treatment protocol. The male child was age 3;8 at the initiation of treatment. His mean length of response in morphemes was 2.29. The initial treatment goal was to establish productive use of the subject + verb + object (SVO) sentence structure. Once productivity of this structure was acquired, the goal was to establish use of the present progressive within the same kernel structure. Hence, data on both structures was recorded from the outset of treatment. Although the table displays percentage of use, productivity as previously defined was the criterion employed.

Table 4-7
Results of expansion of subject + verb + object (SVO) skills.

Session	SVO %	SVing0 %
Baseline	01	00
Week 1	02	00
Week 3	20	00
Week4[1]	24	00
Week 5	28	14
Week 6	30	20
Week 7[2]	35	34

[1]SVO was productive during this weekly probe

[2]SVing0 was productive during this weekly probe

The child was seen twice weekly for treatment. Each treatment session was one and one-half hours in duration and consisted of individual and group treatment. For the first four weeks of treatment the clinician modeled only the SVO sentence structure. Analysis of the sample obtained during the fourth week indicated that the structure was productive. The clinician then began modeling the SVO sentence structure with the present progressive form. This structure was productive during the seventh week of treatment.

Orazi (1981) also conducted a study analyzing the effectiveness of phase three of the treatment protocol. The subjects consisted of seven language-disordered children. The children ranged in age from 3;5 to 4;7 at the initiation of treatment. They ranged in mean length of utterance in morphemes from 2.52 to 4.70. All children demonstrated absence of use of the yes/no question transformation upon analyses of spontaneous language samples. For purposes of evaluating treatment effectiveness, children were assigned to either an experimental or control group. Thus, four children received treatment and three received no treatment. Those assigned to the experimental group were exposed to treatment, designed to establish use of the yes/no question transformation, until productivity of the structure was obtained. Once they met criterion, experimental-control comparisons were made. The experimental group demonstrated significant gains in the target structure as compared to the control group.

Summary and Conclusions

Several recent trends in the child language literature that have important implications for preschool language disorders have been considered. These include the relationship of prespeech communication to later verbal communication, the role of environmental communicative input in children's language acquisition, and young children's knowledge with respect to socially appropriate communicative conventions.

A developmentally based treatment protocol has been discussed. The protocol is designed for preschool language-disordered children. The procedures incorporate adult behaviors found to have a positive influence on child language behavior. The protocol further includes provisions to establish, if necessary, socio-communicative knowledge regarded as necessary for verbal development. The remaining phases of the protocol include procedures for establishing an initial lexicon and, then, expansion of the lexicon in terms of semantic relations, kernel sentences, grammatical morphemes, and transformations.

Through presentation of data at each phase of the protocol, it can be seen that the procedures are effective in establishing the desired behaviors. However, there are aspects of the procedures that require further evaluation. First, the clinician is, in effect, treating spontaneous speech. Therefore, the assumption is made that generalization is, in fact, occurring outside the treatment setting. However, this assumption has not yet been verified. Second, it would be useful to determine whether the protocol can be utilized to establish social language functions other than the interactional, instrumental, and regulatory. It also seems possible that the protocol could serve as a basis for parent training. In instances where a clinician has a particularly large potential case load, explorations with adaptations of the model for parents might be a viable alternative to lengthy waiting lists. Finally, I want to again emphasize that this model serves only as one example of a treatment procedure focusing on the development of linguistic and communicative competence. In many cases, the clinician may be faced with a case in which she or he will rely on a mixture of approaches in order to achieve treatment goals.

Acknowledgments

I wish to thank Ann Grant-Harbin and Kay Halfhill for their assistance in gathering data on the treatment protocol. A special thanks is extended to Marilyn Newhoff for her input in development of the treatment protocol.

References

Barten, S. Development of gesture. In N. Smith & M. Franklin (Eds.), *Symbolic functioning in childhood*. Hillsdale, NJ: Lawrence Erlbaum, 1979.

Bates, E. *Language and context: The acquisition of pragmatics*. New York: Academic Press, 1976.

Bates, E., Camaioni, L., & Volterra, V. The acquisition of performatives prior to speech. In E. Ochs & B. Achieffelin (Eds.), *Developmental pragmatics*. New York: Academic Press, 1979.

Blank, M., Gessner, M., & Esposito, A. Language without communication: A case study. *Journal of Child Language*, 1979, *6*, 329-352.

Bowerman, M. Semantic factors in the acquisition of rules for word use and sentence construction. In D. Morehead & A. Morehead (Eds.), *Normal and deficient child language*. Baltimore: University Park Press, 1976.

Braine, M. The ontogeny of English phrase structures: The first phase. *Language*, 1963, *30*, 1-14.

Brown, R., Cazden, C., & Bellugi, U. The child's grammar from I to III. In C. Ferguson & D. Slobin (Eds.), *Studies in child language development*. New York: Holt, Rinehart & Winston, 1973.

Brown, R., & Hanlon, C. Derivational complexity and order of acquisition in child speech. In J. Hayes (Ed.) *Cognition and the development of language*. New York: Wiley, 1970.

Bruner, J. The ontogenesis of speech acts. *Journal of Child Language*, 1975, *2*, 1-19.

Bruner, J. Learning how to do things with words. In D. Aaronson & R. Reiber (Eds.), *Psycholinguistic research: Implications and applications*. Hillsdale, NJ: Lawrence Erlbaum, 1979.

Carter, A. From sensori-motor vocalizations to words: A case study in the evolution of attention-directing communication in the second year. In A. Lock (Ed.), *Action, gesture, and symbol*. New York: Academic Press, 1978.

Chomsky, N. *Syntactic structures*. Cambridge, MA: MIT Press, 1957.

Chomsky, N. *Aspects of a theory of syntax*. Cambridge, MA: MIT Press, 1965.

Clark, R. The transition from action to gesture. In A. Lock (Ed.), *Action, gesture, and symbol*. New York: Academic Press, 1978.

Cross, R. Mothers' speech adjustments: The control of selected child listener variables. In C. Snow & C. Ferguson (Eds.), *Talking to children: Language input and acquisition*. Cambridge, Eng: Cambridge University Press, 1977.

Cross, T. Mothers' speech and its association with rate of linguistic development in young children. In N. Waterson & C Snow (Eds.), *The development of communication*. New York: Wiley, 1978.

Culatta, B., & Horn, D. A program for generalization of grammatical rules to spontaneous discourse. *Journal of Speech and Hearing Disorders*, 1982, *47*, 174-180.

Dore, J. A pragmatic description of early development. *Journal of Psycholinguistic Research*, 1974, *3*, 343-350.

Donahue, M., Pearl, R., & Bryan, R. Conversational competence in learning disabled children: Responses to uninformative messsages, *Applied Psycholinguistics*, 1980, *1*, 387-403.

Dukes, P. Developing social prerequisites to oral communication. *Topics in Learning and Learning Disabilities*, 1981, *1*, 47-58.

Fey, M., Leonard, L., & Wilcox, K. Speech style modifications of language-impaired children. *Journal of Speech and Hearing Disorders*, 1981, *46*, 91-96.

Gallagher, T. Revision Behaviors in the speech of normal children developing language. *Journal of Speech and Hearing Research*, 1977, *20*, 303-318.

Gallagher, T., & Darnton, B. Conversational aspects of the speech of language-disordered children: Revision behaviors. *Journal of Speech and Hearing Research*, 1978, *21*,118-135.

Garvey, C. The contingent query: A dependent act in conversation. In M. Lewis & L. Rosenblum (Eds.), *Origins of behavior, Vol. 5: Communication and the development of language*. New York: Wiley, 1977.

Gleason, J. & Weintraub, S. Input language and the acquisition of communicative competence. In K. Nelson (Ed.), *Children's language: Vol. I.,* New York: Gardner Press, 1978.

Halliday, M. *Learning how to mean: Explorations in the development of language*. New York: Elsevier, 1975.

Holland, A. Language therapy for children: Some thoughts on context and content. *Journal of Speech and Hearing Disorders*, 1975, *40*, 514-523.

Hymes, D. Competence and performance in linguistic theory. In R. Huxley & E. Ingram (Eds.), *Language acquisition: Models and methods*. New York: Academic Press, 1971.

Lakoff, R. Language in context. *Language*, 1972, *48*, 907-927.

Leonard, L., Facilitating linguistic skills in children with specific language impairment. *Applied Psycholinguistics*, 1981, *2*, 89-118.

Leonard, L., Camarata, S., Rowan, L., & Chapman, D. The communicative functions of lexical usage by language-impaired children, *Applied Psycholinguistics*, 1982, *3*, 109-126

Lieven, E. Conversations between mothers and young children: Individual differences and their possible implication for the study of language learning. In N. Waterson & C. Snow (Eds.), *The development of communication*. New York: Wiley, 1978.

Lucas, E. *Semantic and pragmatic language disorders: Assessment and remediation*. Rockville, MD: Aspen, 1980.

McNeill, D. *The acquisition of language: The study of developmental psycholinguistics*. New York: Harper & Row, 1970.

McShane, J. *Learning to talk*. Cambridge, Eng.: Cambridge University Press, 1980.

Miller, L. Pragmatics: An assessment/intervention model used with an autistic child. Paper presented at the Annual Convention of the American Speech Language Hearing Association, San Francisco, 1978.

Miller, J. *Assessing language production in children*. Baltimore: University Park Press, 1981.

Miller, J., & Yoder, D., A syntax teaching program. In J. McLean, D. Yoder, & R. Schiefelbusch (Eds.), *Language intervention with the retarded*. Baltimore: University Park Press, 1972.

Nelson, K. Structure and strategy in learning to talk. *Monographs of the Society for Research in Child Development*, 1973, *38*, (1-2, Serial No. 149).

Nelson, K.E. Facilitating children's syntax acquisition. *Developmental Psychology*, 1977, *13*, 101-107.

Newhoff, M., Silverman, L., & Millet, A., Linguistic differences in parents' speech to normal and language-disordered children. *Proceedings from the Symposium on Research in Child Language Disorders*. Madison: University of Wisconsin, 1980.

Newport, E., Gleitman, L., & Gleitman, H. I'd rather do it myself. In C. Snow & C. Ferguson, (Eds.), *Talking to children: Language input and acquisition*. Cambridge, Eng.: Cambridge University Press, 1977.

Orazi, D. *A play-oriented approach to early language intervention*. Unpublished master's thesis, Kent State University, 1981.

Pearl, R., Donahue, M., & Bryan, T. Learning-disabled and normal children's responses to requests for clarification which vary in explicitness. Paper presented at the Boston University Conference on Language Development, 1979.

Prizant, B., & Duchan, J. The functions of immediate echolalia in autistic children. *Journal of Speech and Hearing Disorders*, 1981, *46*, 241-249.

Rees, N. Pragmatics of language: Applications to normal and disordered language development. In R. Sehiefelbusch (Ed.), *Bases of language intervention.* Baltimore: University Park Press, 1978.

Shatz, M., Bernstein, D., & Shulman, M. The responses of language-disordered children to indirect directives in varying contexts, *Applied Psycholinguistics,* 1980, *1,* 295-306.

Snow, C. Mothers' speech to children learning language. *Child Development,* 1972, *43,* 549-565.

Snow, C. The development of conversation between mothers and babies. *Journal of Child Language,* 1977, *4,* 1-22.

Snow, C. Social interaction and language acquisition. In P. Dale & D. Ingram (Eds.), *Child language: An international perspective.* Baltimore: University Park Press, 1981.

Snyder, L. *Pragmatics in language-deficient children: Prelinguistic and early verbal performatives and presuppositions.* Unpublished doctoral dissertation, University of Colorado, 1975.

Stremel, K., & Waryas, C. A behavioral psycholinguistic approach to language training. In L. McReynolds (Ed.), *Developing systematic procedures for training children's language.* American Speech and Hearing Association Monographs, 1974, *18.*

Taenzer, S., Cermak, C., & Hanlon, R. Outside the therapy room: A naturalistic approach to language intervention. *Topics in Learning and Learning Disabilities,* 1981, *1,* 41-46.

Wellman, H., & Lempers, J. The naturalistic communicative abilities of two-year olds. *Child Development,* 1977, *48,* 1052-1057.

Wilcox, M., & Howse, P. Children's use of gestural and verbal behavior in communicative misunderstandings. *Journal of Applied Psycholinguistics,* 1982, *3,* 15-28.

Wilcox, M., & Webster, E. Early discourse behavior: An analysis of children's responses to listener feedback. *Child Development,* 1980, *51,* 1120-1125.

Wilkinson, L., & Rembold, K. The form and function of children's gestures accompanying verbal directives. In P. Dale & D. Ingram (Eds.), *Child language: An international perspective.* Baltimore: University Park Press, 1981.

Lynn S. Snyder, Ph.D.

Developmental Language Disorders: Elementary School Age

When language-disordered children enter elementary school, they seem to disappear. The prevalence of language disorders in preschool children is just above 3% (Leske, 1981). This figure abruptly declines to a figure somewhat closer to 1% in the school-aged population. It would be rewarding to surmise that our programs for the early identification and intervention of language disorders have been so successful that they account for this decline. Unfortunately, as our colleagues working in the schools will tell us, this is not the case.

What, then, is the nature of the great disappearing act that language-disordered children perform when they enter school? To answer this question, we need only look at one other prevalence figure: the prevalence of learning disabilities. It emerges at the elementary school level and ranges between 2% and 8% in the various states (Sheppard, 1981). Careful study of these figures reveals that over time, they changed from 3% to 5% in states like Colorado, where the term "perceptual and communicative disorder" is used in lieu of the term "learning disability." It tends to be lower in states that separate language from learning disabilities.

This great disappearing act is also evident in research. In contrast to the numerous studies of language disorders in preschool children, relatively few studies have been conducted on school-aged children. There are, however, many studies of the language deficits of learning-disabled children.

When language-disordered children enter elementary school, they often come to be associated with different labels: learning-disabled, language- and learning-disabled, reading-disabled, or even dyslexic. It is not that language-disordered children radically change when they reach 6 or 7 years of age. Rather, their problems in processing and producing oral language make it difficult for them to acquire written language: the ability to read, spell, and write composition. In addition, other youngsters are added to their ranks: children who find it difficult to learn written language. Systematic assessment reveals that these children also sustain underlying oral language deficits (Lerner, 1977). It is not surprising that the United States Office of Education defines learning-disabled children as those with intact sensory functioning, normal psychosocial development, general cognitive abilities in the normal range, who demonstrate "a disorder in one or more of the basic psychological processes involved in understanding or using language, spoken or written" (USOE, 1977, p. 65083). This disorder is reflected in a significant discrepancy between age or general abilities and academic achievement. This population, then, seems to constitute the greater proportion of school-aged children with language disorders.

This chapter will examine the semantic, syntactic, morphological, and pragmatic processing and production deficits of these language-disordered youngsters. Since many school-aged children with language disorders have been identified as "learning disabled," or with some similar label, much of the discussion will reference studies of learning-disabled, language- and learning-disabled, reading-disabled, and dyslexic children.

Lexical Processing and Production

The semantic component of language refers to the meaning carried by words. Often our concern with meaning directs our attention to the *lexicon*, or internal dictionary, that one carries in one's head. Although the communicator's internal dictionary is not organized alphabetically like Webster's, it does contain many similar types of information. As Fillmore (1971) pointed out, one's knowledge of a word includes several components. Much like Webster's, it includes information about the phonetic shape of the word, or how it should be pronounced. Like Webster's, it also includes information about the syntactic class to which the word belongs—noun, verb, etc., its primary referential meaning, and any alternate multiple meanings it may carry. The literature suggests that school-aged language-disordered children seem to encounter difficulty processing and producing lexical items.

Word Comprehension

The problems that school-aged language-disordered children encounter with lexical comprehension are not apparent if we look at their ability to comprehend the primary meaning of single words on vocabulary tests such as the *Peabody Picture Vocabulary Test* (PPVT) (Dunn, 1965; Dunn & Dunn, 1981). In fact, studies comparing normal and language/learning-disabled children's comprehension of items on experimental measures (Wiig & Semel, 1973; Wiig, Semel, & Crouse, 1973) indicate that the normal and language/learning-disabled subjects performed similarly on the PPVT. Likewise, Semel and Wiig (1975) found no significant difference between matched normal and language/learning-disabled children's comprehension of vocabulary items on the *Assessment of Children's Language Comprehension* (ACLC) (Foster, Giddan, & Stark, 1973). Rather, school-aged language-disordered children seem to differ from their normal counterparts in their comprehension of specific word categories.

School-aged language/learning-disabled youngsters appear to have particular difficulty comprehending words that express spatial, temporal, and kinship relations. Wiig and Semel (1973) compared the ability of matched normal and language/learning-disabled children to comprehend sentences that employed spatial, temporal, and kinship words, as well as passive constructions and comparative form markers. They found that the language/learning-disabled children performed significantly lower than the normal children on each of these word and form categories. Despite the fact that the youngsters had comparable PPVT scores, they experienced difficulty comprehending the words in these specific categories. If we examine these categories more closely, we find that they are composed of relational words. They do not refer to events, actions, or objects. Rather, these words refer to relationships between objects and/or persons. For example, spatial relationships are often marked by spatial prepositions. Temporal relationships are expressed by the prepositions "before" and "after. " Kinship terms such as "aunt, " "uncle, " and the like relational nouns expressing a familial relationship between two or more persons. These relational words, then, require that the child keep more than one referent in mind. This may be an aspect of lexical processing that is more difficult for language-disordered children.

Word Retrieval

Clinical descriptions of school-aged language/learning-disabled children (DeHirsch, Jansky, & Langford, 1966; Johnson & Myklebust, 1967; Wiig

& Semel, 1976, 1980) have reported that some of these youngsters have difficulty retrieving or accessing words from their lexicon. Typically, these observations have been made while the children were engaged in conversational exchanges. Consequently, it is not always clear whether formulation deficits were also implicated.

In recent years, however, empirical support for these reports has appeared in the literature. Mattis, French, and Rapin's (1975) neuropsy-chological study compared the performance of reading-disabled or dyslexic children, brain-damaged dyslexics, and brain-damaged children with no reading deficits on a variety of cognitive and linguistic measures. They identified three subtypes of disorders that accounted for most of their subjects. The largest subtype demonstrated language deficits. These were characterized by language comprehension problems, syntactic production deficits, poor speech sound discrimination problems, and "anomia," or naming problems. Similarly, Denckla's (1978) retrospective study of dyslexic children seen by her clinic identified three subgroups or subtypes of reading-disabled children. Anomia, or naming problems, was a characteristic attributed to two of the three subgroups that she identified. These studies support the idea that some language/learning-disabled youngsters have word retrieval problems.

More direct tests of these observations can be found in confrontation naming studies which bypass the confounding effects of formulation factors. Denckla (1972) studied the ability of dyslexic, or reading-disabled, boys to name colors and pictured objects. She found that they only experienced color-naming difficulty under rapid and repetitive naming conditions, where they had been instructed to name the colors as quickly as possible. Subsequently, Denckla and Rudel (1976b) examined the rapid automatized naming (RAN) of matched dyslexic, normal, and nondyslexic "low achieving" children between 7 and 12 years of age. Studying the response latencies during the tasks, they found that the dyslexic children were the slowest to respond and name the depicted items, while the normal controls were the fastest. In a similar study, Denckla and Rudel (1976a) compared the performance of dyslexic children, adequate readers with other types of learning problems, and matched normal children between 8 and 11 years of age. All subjects were asked to rapidly name pictured objects. The dyslexic children made more errors than the other groups of children, particularly on low freqeuency words. Error analysis revealed that the majority of the dyslexic children's errors were circumlocutions phonetically similar to the target word. By contrast, the majority of the errors made by the other learning-disabled groups were wrong names that seemed to be visually perceptually based, e.g., a pair of dice was named "Swiss Cheese."

More recently, Wolf (1979) conducted an in-depth study of the word-finding abilities of matched good and poor readers between 6 and 11 years of age. She administered the *Peabody Picture Vocabulary Test;* the *Boston Naming Test;* a picture-naming task in which the stimuli were visually distorted; a rapid automatized naming test for colors, numbers, and letters; phonological (e.g., name as many things as you can that begin with "f") and semantic (e.g., name as many animals as you can) verbal fluency measures; as well as reading tests. She found that the good readers performed significantly better than the poor readers on all naming tests, except the RAN numbers and the visually distorted pictures. The poor readers were particularly deficient in their performance on both measures of verbal fluency. These findings suggest that school-aged learning-disabled children, specifically those with reading deficits, also seem to sustain word-finding problems.

In the same year, German (1979) compared the ability of matched normal and language/learning-disabled children (8 to 11 years of age) on vocabulary comprehension and naming tasks. The groups demonstrated comparable age, general intelligence scores, *Peabody Picture Vocabulary Test* scores, and socioeconomic status. Asking these subjects to name items in pictures, to complete open-ended sentences, and to name objects described, German found that the language/learning-disabled children made significantly more word-finding errors than their matched controls. They found low frequency words in the cloze condition and the naming-to-description condition particularly difficult. Subsequent group analyses revealed that 43% of the learning-disabled children were classified as poor retrievers, performing more than one standard deviation above the mean error rate of the normal children.

Recently, Wiig, Semel, and Nystrom (1982) compared the rapid-naming skills of a group of language/learning-disabled 8- and 9-year-olds with a group of academically achieving 8- and 9-year-olds with normal language development. They assessed the children's ability to rapidly name pictured objects, colors, geometric forms, and colored geometric forms. Their data revealed that the language/learning-disabled children performed significantly worse than their age peers for both time and accuracy when naming pictured objects and colored forms. The total naming time of the language/learning subjects increased as their accuracy decreased. Those language/learning-disabled children who had demonstrated word-finding problems in their spontaneous speech, performed above +1 SD of the mean naming time of the normal group on the object naming measure. These data offer further confirmation of the word-retrieval problems found among school-aged language/learning-disabled children.

Summary

The research of the last decade suggests that many school-aged language-disordered children have lexical processing and production deficits. Although they often demonstrate comparable understanding of single vocabulary words on vocabulary measures, they often have difficulty understanding relational words. Likewise, a number of school-aged language-disordered children have difficulty retrieving words, making more errors in producing names than their normal peers. Thus, selected aspects of the lexicon and the ability to access the words it contains prove difficult for some school-aged language-disordered children.

Syntactic Processing and Production

Some school-aged language-disordered children sustain lexical deficits. In addition, some of these youngsters also seem to have difficulty comprehending and using the syntax and associated morphology of language.

The earlier clinical accounts of DeHirsch et al. (1966) and Johnson and Myklebust (1967) reported that language/learning-disabled children experienced difficulty comprehending and producing syntactic structures. Johnson and Myklebust's anecdotal information suggested a considerable range of severity, with some children sustaining severe deficits. By contrast, the DeHirsch et al. accounts did not reflect this degree of severity. Jansky's later descriptions (1975) characterized the syntactic formulation deficits of language/learning-disabled children as more "subtle." She observed that their spoken language often appears adequate, although it is not really articulate. Sentence formulation is often awkward, characterized by many sentential fragments, simple sentence forms, and the repeated use of stereotypic phrases. Delayed morphological development, particularly in the use of irregular past-tense markers and an over-extended use of pronouns, is also observed. Jansky suggested that these types of problems seem to call less attention to themselves, merely giving one the impression that the child has a less verbal cognitive style. Consequently, these language problems often go unidentified until the children enter school and begin to have problems learning to read and spell. These early observations clearly suggest that language/learning-disabled children may sustain syntactic deficits. Confirmation of these clinical observations came somewhat later with the research of the 70s.

Comprehension of Syntactic and Morphological Forms

One of the earliest tests of the notion that language/learning-disabled children had problems understanding syntactic forms and morphological markers is found in the Wiig and Semel (1973) study discussed earlier. In addition to their comparison of normal and language/learning-disabled children's comprehension of relational terms, they also studied their ability to comprehend passive sentence forms and comparative morphological markers. The language/learning-disabled children also performed significantly worse than their age mates on these items.

More recently, Dixon (1982) compared the ability of 8- and 9-year-old reading-disabled children, age-matched controls, and reading-level controls on several measures of oral language. Despite a number of significant differences between the two groups, she found that the groups were comparable in their comprehension of spoken syntactic and morphological forms. She had assessed their comprehension with the Grammatic Understanding subtest of the *Test of Language Development* (TOLD) (Newcomer & Hammill, 1977). However, this subtest of the TOLD does not seem to adequately sample the syntactic processing that develops during the school years.

Byrne (1981) addressed this question by comparing good and poor second-grade readers' comprehension of late-maturing structures. These included the *John is easy / eager to please* type of constructions identified by Chomsky (1969), and reversible center-embedded, improbable center-embedded, and control relative clause constructions. The *easy / eager to please* constructions were adapted from Cromer (1970), and systematically varied subject, object, and ambiguous adjectives. The following are examples taken from each *easy / eager to please* construction type (Bryne, 1981, p. 206):

Subject-Adjective: *The bird is happy to bite.*

Object-Adjective: *The bird is tasty to bite.*

Ambiguous-Adjective: *The bird is nice to bite.*

Each child was requested to act out the test sentences using hand puppets. Byrne found that while all of the children understood subject-adjective sentence forms equally well, the poor readers tended to assign the logical subjects to the surface structure subject in the object-adjective sentences more frequently than the good readers. Comprehension of the relative clause constructions was assessed by asking the children to point to the one of two pictures that correctly depicted the test sentence. The following are items taken from each of the relative clause construction types as assessed by Byrne (1981, p. 207):

Control sentence: *The fish is biting a yellow frog.*

Reversible sentence: *The cow that the monkey is scaring is yellow.*

Improbable sentence: *The horse that the girl is kicking is brown.*

Again, the poor readers tended to use less mature syntactic processing strategies on these relative clause comprehension tasks. Although both good and poor readers were comparable in their ability to process the reversible clause constructions, the poor readers tended to make more errors on the improbable relative clause sentences. Again, they were more easily seduced into using a less mature syntactic processing strategy. In this case, they used a "probable event" strategy (deVilliers & deVilliers, 1973), in which they ignored the underlying syntactic form and chose the picture depicting the event most likely to occur in the real world. Byrne's data, then, provide nice evidence for the syntactic comprehension deficits sustained by school-aged language/learning-disabled children.

Production of Syntactic and Morphological Forms

Given this evidence for syntactic and morphological processing deficits in language/learning-disabled children, it is not unreasonable to expect that they will also sustain production deficits.

In an early effort to compare the productive language of matched 7 year-old good and poor readers, Fry (1967) and Schulte (1967) subsequently summarized in a paper by Fry, Johnson, and Muehl (1970) exhaustively analyzed oral language samples collected from subjects. They found that the language of the poor readers was characterized by a lower type-token ratio, less frequent use of subject-verb-object frames, and clauses as direct objects, indirect objects, and complements than their normal peers. Transformational analyses revealed that the poor reader's sentences contained fewer transformations than their age mates. Lastly, the poor readers made significantly more errors in subject-verb agreement. Thus, these studies of the syntactic maturity of children with reading problems demonstrate that they often have deficient syntactic formulation.

Recently, Donohue, Pearl, and Bryan (in press) compared the length and syntactic complexity of the sentences produced by matched normal and learning-disabled children. Language samples were collected from the subjects during a classical referential communication task, in which they described figures to an examiner who could not see them. The description of each item would then allow the examiner to select the correct referent from an array set before her. Using the T-unit analysis technique (Golub

& Kidder, 1974; Hunt, 1965), they found that the language/learning-disabled children produced significantly fewer words per T-unit and fewer words per main clause than their normal peers. However, there was no difference in the productivity measures for the two groups. They produced similar numbers of words and T-units. Thus, while the language/ learning-disabled children said as much as their age mates, the syntax of their utterances was not as complex.

A number of studies have examined the ability of language/learning-disabled children to produce appropriate morphological markers. Wiig, Semel, and Crouse's (1973) study of normal, high-risk, and language/learning-disabled children examined their performance on Berko-Gleason's (1958) measure and the Auditory Association subtest of the *Illinois Test of Psycholinguistic Abilities* (ITPA) (Kirk & McCarthy, 1961). The language/learning-disabled youngsters performed significantly worse than their age mates on both measures of inflectional morphology. Again, the data point to linguistic production deficits in school-aged language/learning-disabled children.

In a somewhat different study, Vogel (1975, 1977) compared the ability of matched normal and dyslexic second graders on a variety of linguistic and suprasegmental measures. These included a standardized version of Berko-Gleason's (1958) tasks, the *Berry-Talbott Test* (1966), and the Grammatic Closure subtest of the ITPA. She found that the dyslexic children performed significantly worse than their age mates in their ability to morphologically mark real and nonsense words embedded in sentence contexts, as seen in their performance on the ITPA subtest and the Berry-Talbott measures, respectively. These data also corroborate other findings and reports of deficits in the productive morphology of learning-disabled children.

Hook's (1976) study explored the inflectional morphology of matched normal and learning-disabled fourth-grade children. Using the same measures as Vogel, she replicated Vogel's findings in this older age group.

Subsequently, Moran and Byrne (1977) explored one aspect of inflectional morphology—verb-tense markers—in greater depth. Noting Leonard's (1972) observation that the inappropriate use of verb forms has often characterized deviant language skills, they systematically compared the ability of matched groups of normal and language/learning-disabled children to produce appropriate verb-tense markers. They sampled their subjects' ability to produce three regular past-tense verbs formed by adding /-d/, /-t/, and /-əd/. In addition, they also examined the formation of seven irregular verb categories based upon Greenbaum, Quirk, Leach, and Svartnik's (1972) classification system. Analysis of their data revealed that the language/learning-disabled children made significantly more errors across all ten categories. In addition, it appeared that they used qualitatively different strategies for marking past tense. For example, they often avoided using past-tense markers by frequent use of the form "did" with an uninflected form of the verb—"she did climb." In addition, the language/learning-disabled children were three times more likely than their normal age mates to produce an uninflected root verb than a past-tense marker. They were also more likely to use redundant markers than their normal peers, e.g., "jumpted." Thus, their inflectional morphology was not only significantly different from that of normal children, it also appeared to be somewhat deviant.

Dixon's (1982) comparison of age-matched, reading-level matched, and reading-disabled 8- and 9-year-olds also included a measure of productive inflectional morphology. She found that the reading-disabled group performed significantly worse than both their age-matched and reading-level matched controls. Clearly, the early clinical observations of Johnson and Myklebust (1967) and DeHirsch et al. (1966) that noted the language/learning-disabled child's difficulty marking word inflections have been well supported by empirical studies.

If these youngsters are deficient in their productive syntax and morphology, it might be interesting to know whether they can recognize and/or correct ungrammatical productions. Liles, Schulman, and Bartlett (1977) compared the ability of normal and language-disabled 5- to 7-year-olds to make judgments of grammaticality, and to correct ungrammatical sentences. They found that the language-disabled youngsters attempted to correct only 78% of the agrammatical sentences in contrast to 97% attempted by their controls. Further, approximately 90% of the corrections made by the controls in each error category—syntactic agreement, lexical violation, and word order—were correct. By contrast, the language-disordered children were able to correctly revise only 21% of the sentences assessing syntactic agreement, 42% of the lexical violations, and 41% of the word-order errors. These data suggest that school-aged language-disordered children have difficulty recognizing syntactic errors when they occur and knowing how to revise them acceptably. In light of earlier evidence for syntactic production deficits in school-aged language-disordered children, these results are not unreasonable.

Summary

School-aged language/learning-disabled children seem to have difficulty processing and producing syntactic and morphological forms, and they seem to be late at learning those underlying syntactic structures that develop during the elementary school years. Similarly, the transformational complexity of their productive output is also reduced. They also seem to have difficulty producing appropriate irregular morphological forms and handling syntactic agreement. Thus, even during the elementary school years, language/learning-disabled children have difficulty with the syntactic component of language.

Pragmatic Processing and Production

With the publication of Bates' *Language and Context,* (1976), basic and applied psycholinguistic research took a new direction. Our post-Chomskian fascination with children's developing comprehension and production of syntactic forms gave way to a concern with how these forms were mobilized to achieve communicative goals. Observers of normal and disordered child language studied the functions of the child's utterances or the uses to which they were put, in addition to the syntactic forms they assumed. Thus, they looked at the types of speech acts children performed with their utterances. These included direct and indirect requests or directives (Ervin-Tripp, 1977), acknowledgments, solicitations, responses, and threats (Dore, 1978). It became apparent that by the time children entered elementary school, they comprehended and had productive control over many direct and indirect ways of requesting things, acknowledging and answering others, and achieving a variety of social goals (Ervin-Tripp, 1977).

It also became obvious that children not only could accomplish these pragmatic or functional goals on the utterance level, but could amortize their requesting strategies across conversational turns (Ervin-Tripp, 1977). Thus, they gradually "set up" their listener during the course of the conversation. In addition, they learned to initiate, develop, and maintain conversational topics, structure their discourse narrative, and revise their utterances (Gallagher, 1977). Similarly, they were increasingly able to process larger units of narrative discourse and acquired the ability to draw inferences between utterances in discourse (Johnson & Smith, 1981; Stein & Glenn, 1979).

Just as language/learning-disabled children experience difficulty with the structural aspects of language, they often find it difficult to handle the functional or pragmatic aspects of the system.

Processing Pragmatic Structures

The psycholinguistic study of the pragmatic aspects of language has suggested some underlying functional organization to language in addition to its structural organization (Bates, 1976; Clark & Haviland, 1977; Greenfield & Smith, 1976; Kintsch, 1974, 1977). Individuals are able to go beyond identification of the syntactic frame to understand the speaker's underlying intention. Children learn to do this as well. They come to realize that one communicative intention can be expressed with many different syntactic forms. Conversely, they also learn that one syntactic form can express many different communicative intentions.

Sentences also seem to have a specific functional organization. The topic of a conversational point is systematically identified by a variety of syntactic and lexical devices. In English, it is usually expressed by the subject of a sentence. Once the topic has been identified or named, the conversational partners consider it "given" information. They then make comments or share "new" information about it (Haviland & Clark, 1974). This topic/comment organization of language occurs at both the sentence and the discourse, or conversational, level. At the sentence level, speakers identify their topic and comment about it. In discourse, they identify main topics and subtopics, often nesting subtopics within the main topics. They make comments that are related to those topics or subtopics (Bates & MacWhinney, in press). Using syntactic devices to mark new topics, they direct the flow of conversation from one topic to another.

Individuals seem to expect speakers to adhere to this functional organization of topic ("given" information) and comment ("new" information). Clark and Haviland (1977) suggest that, in a sense, conversational partners have a given-new contract. The speaker assumes that the listener knows a particular piece, or pieces, of information. This "given" information forms the topic for the comment, or " new, " information the speaker wishes to share. His listener locates the given information in the utterance and searches his memory for this piece of world knowledge. He then attaches the new information to it. Thus, conversational speakers must consider or estimate the "given" information—the prior knowledge, beliefs, assumptions, and experiences—they share with their listeners. In this way, they keep the given-new contract and insure effective communication.

Speakers and listeners seem to adhere to the given-new contract on both the sentence and discourse level. At the sentence level, speakers use syntactic and lexical devices to signal given and new information. Their listeners use their own linguistic knowledge of these devices to isolate given and new pieces of information.

On the discourse level, the "given" part of the contract can take on interesting charcteristics. A speaker may assume that a listener has some knowledge of events, such as going to a movie or a bank. He assumes that the listener has organized the basic information contained in those events in a way similar to his own. Consequently, they share the same "script"

(Schank & Abelson, 1977) for the event. For example, they both know that one purchases a ticket for the movie, gives it to the usher, is admitted, enters the theater area, seats oneself, views the film, and leaves. While each may have some different specific scripts, e.g., for drive-in movies or for a subscription series at the art museum, they share a generic script that organizes the component events and identifies the roles assumed by the participants. Scriptal information seems to facilitate comprehension of longer units of discourse, particularly narrative discourse or stories (Rumelhardt, 1980). The listener activates his script for the event that has been given. He then attaches the pieces of new information contained in the narrative to the component events and roles of the script that he has activated (Anderson, Spiro, & Anderson, 1978). The listener and reader have scripts for stories, as well as for events. These are often referred to as story schemata (Kintsch, 1974) or story grammars (Mandler & Johnson, 1978; Stein & Glenn, 1979). These types of structures seem to organize and facilitate the comprehension of discourse narratives (Kintsch & Kintsch, 1979).

Lastly, when speakers fail to indentify a "given" referent clearly or consistently, listeners use their scripts to draw inferences. They use their scripts to construct information the speaker has not explicitly stated (Haviland & Clark, 1974; Kintsch, 1974, 1977). For example, referring to Mary as "she" in a sentence during a new subtopic forces the listener to draw an inference that "she" refers to the woman, Mary, who was discussed several sentences earlier. Or, take the following sentences used by Clark and Haviland (1974): *Horace got some picnic supplies out of the trunk. The beer was warm.* It was never explicitly stated that Horace had packed beer. However, listeners seem to activate their "picnic" scripts, which suggest that picnic supplies often include beer. Thus, they infer that Horace had included beer in his picnic supplies (Haviland & Clark, 1974).

Listeners seem to engage in many types of functional or pragmatically based operations as they process sentence and discourse level information.

Sentence Level Processes

At face value, it seems that it must be difficult to figure out a speaker's underlying intention even when it differs from the syntactic form of the sentence. Children, however, seem to master this skill during their preschool years (Shatz, 1978). In an early effort to determine whether 5- to 7-year-old language-disordered children can comprehend indirect speech acts, Prinz (1977; in press) compared their ability to comprehend direct and indirect requests with younger normal children at comparable language levels.

He found that the language-disordered children did not differ significantly from the normal children with whom they had been matched.

Other pragmatic structures processed at the sentence level included identification of given and new information. This has been explored recently in learning-disabled youngsters. Donohue (1981a), using Hornby's (1971) experimental paradigm, compared the ability of matched normal and learning-disabled children to comprehend and use syntactic devices that indicated given vs. new information. At this point, the discussion will be confined to the comprehension phase of the experiment. Specifically, she asked each child to listen to sentences, and indicate which of two pictures was described. The sentences took one of five syntactic forms, and described an actor-action-object relationship. However, since the test sentences did not accurately describe either of the pictures, the child's answer indicated the sentential component that he regarded as the given information. Although Donohue observed the expected developmental and sentence-type effects, she found no significant differences between the performance of the normal and learning-disabled children.

At this point, the available literature suggests that school-aged language-disordered children seem to process sentence-level pragmatic structures as well as their peers. They can comprehend a variety of indirect requests. In addition, they seem to be able to understand the various syntactic devices used to signal given vs. new information.

Discourse Level Processes: Conversation

Although school-aged language-disordered children seem to have mastered pragmatic processing at the sentence level, this does not seem to hold true at the level of discourse. This can be seen in a study of their ability to understand conversational rules, as well as in a number of studies of their narrative discourse processing.

Comparing the conversational skills of matched normal and learning-disabled school children, Donohue, Pearl, and Bryan (1980) studied their ability to request clarification of messages based on the informational adequacy of the message. Using the classic referential paradigm of screened interlocutors, Donohue et al. asked each child to identify a drawing from a plate containing four choices. The child was instructed by one examiner that his "partner" behind the screen could give him clues which would help him choose the correct picture. If he was not sure which drawing was the correct choice, he could ask her questions. This examiner also ran trial items with the child to insure that he understood the task, as well as the opportunity to query the speaker. His "partner," a second examiner, entered, sat behind the screen, and described each item to the child. The messages differed in the amount of information the child needed to correctly identify the picture, being either fully informative, partially informative, or uninformative. The first examiner was present on the child's side of the screen, recording the child's responses. Subsequently, the child was asked to judge messages given by other people. The child had to indicate whether the message would allow a listener to choose the correct drawing.

Analysis of the subjects' responses to the communication task revealed several significant differences. First, there were clear developmental effects in children's ability to realize when they were given inadequate clues. Older children were more likely to recognize less-adequate messages, request clarification, and, thus, choose the correct drawing. The learning-disabled children did not differ from the normal children in their ability to use the informative messages to select a correct picture. However, they were less likely to request clarification of the less-informative messages. Consequently, they had greater difficulty than their age mates in making the correct choices from the less-informative clues. Analysis of the children's performance on the appraisal task revealed that most of the learning-disabled children were able to *recognize* less-adequate messages. Analyses of request forms they produced indicated that they had the necessary linguistic skill to request clarification of messages. Despite these abilities, they made fewer requests for clarification. Donohue et al. suggest that they failed to understand their role as a conversational listener. The learning-disabled subjects did not seem to realize that, as listeners, they were obligated to let the speaker know when a message was unclear. These findings, then, suggest that some aspects of processing conversational discourse pose problems for the school-aged language/learning-disabled child.

Discourse Level Processes: Narratives

In addition to processing conversation, individuals also process discourse narratives or stories they hear. Professionals, using an educational model, have traditionally referred to this as listening comprehension (Durrell, 1965). Others, (e.g., Graybeal, 1981) refer to it as memory. Cognitive and experimental psychologists (Freedle, 1977; Just & Carpenter, 1977; Kintsch, 1974, 1977; Rumelhardt, 1980) have typically considered it discourse comprehension. Using a variety of recognition, verification, and recall experiments, the cognitive psychologists cited above and their colleagues have observed that individuals seem to understand discourse in terms of their schemata or knowledge of scripts, narratives, and other aspects of the world (Rumelhardt, 1980).

Individuals make such strong use of this strategy that when a narrative contains information that does not match the listener's, they understand the story only in terms of their own schemata—thus, "misunderstanding" the story. For example, in his now-classic experiment, Bartlett (1932) asked subjects to listen to an American Indian story. The narrative schema, or story structure, of the Indian myth was quite different from the structure of Western European narratives. When his subjects retold it, their versions did not resemble the original story. What they had done was to interpret the Indian tale in terms of the Western European tale "script" they knew so well. They changed the Indian tale to conform to their own story scripts! These results were recently replicated in a study by Kintsch and Green (1978), where subjects were presented with schema-conforming stories and Alaskan Indian myths. Anderson, Spiro, and Anderson (1978) suggest that these scripts or schemata are "ideational scaffolding." The listener takes in information, activates the schema or generic script that matches it, and anchors to it the information in the narrative. Thus, the listener understands the new information presented to him in relation to his existing knowledge.

The ability to process units as large as narrative discourse or stories develops during middle childhood. The amount of information children can understand and recall from stories increases as a function of age (Christie & Schumacher, 1975; Mandler & Johnson, 1977; Stein & Glenn, 1979). This developmental trend continues throughout the elementary school years (Stein & Glenn, 1979). School-aged children seem to remember story settings, beginnings, and outcomes best (Mandler & Johnson, 1977; Stein & Glenn, 1979). As they mature, they seem to acquire improved recall for the main characters' internal reactions and outcomes.

Many language/learning-disabled children seem to have difficulty with this type of processing. Have you ever tried to get them to tell you about a recent movie or television show they have seen?

A study of the discourse-processing of normal and reading-disabled children conducted by Weaver and Dickenson (1979) also included reading Stein and Glenn's (1979) stories to the children and asking the dyslexic subjects to recall the narratives. They compared their performance to that of Stein and Glenn's sample. Examining the number of ideas recalled, they found no significant differences between the two groups. However, their reading-disabled children included those with both high and low verbal abilities. When Weaver and Dickenson conducted a within-group analysis of the performance of their reading-disabled subjects, they found that the poor readers with high verbal ability recalled significantly more ideas than those with low verbal ability. These data lend further support for the presence of discourse-processing deficits in *some* reading-disabled youngsters.

In a similar study, Graybeal (1981) compared the ability of matched school-aged normal and language-impaired children to recall stories read to them. She tested each language-impaired child to determine that she or he possessed the vocabulary and syntactic comprehension skills needed to process the stories. Each child listened to and was asked to recall two stories, structured after Mandler and Johnson's (1977) story grammar. She found that the normal children recalled significantly more information than the language-impaired children. Again, the available evidence suggests that language-disordered children sustain discourse-processing deficits.

One might argue, however, that the language/learning-disabled children described here performed poorly because they may have had productive-language deficits. All of these studies asked subjects to retell the stories. If—as we know—language/learning-disabled children also have productive-language deficits, then these deficits might limit the amount of information they produce during recall. Snyder, Haas, and Becker (1982) investigated this question, asking normal and language/learning-disabled children probe-recall questions after they had retold a story. Once again, the normal children recalled significantly more information than the learning-disabled. And, they continued to recall more information during probe-recall questions that required little productive language. Thus, school-aged language/learning-disabled children seem to sustain true deficits in discourse-processing which do not seem to be related to the confounding effect of productive language deficits.

Discourse Level Processes: Inferences

The work of Clark and Haviland (1977), Keenan and Kintsch (1974), Trabasso and Nicholas (1977), and others have clearly demonstrated that listeners go beyond the information that is explicitly contained in the message. Using their schemata, or scripted knowledge, and the assumptions they share with the speakers, they interpret messages and construct meanings that were never explicitly stated. They draw inferences such as the types described earlier as well as a variety of others (Trabasso & Nicholas, 1977).

Young children acquire the ability to draw inferences. They develop the ability to answer questions about implied information (Kail, Chi, Ingram, & Danner, 1977; Paris & Upton, 1976), to make transitive inferences when they have encoded the premises (Riley & Trabasso, 1974; Trabasso, 1975), and to infer antecedent states and causes and predict outcomes in situations with familiar scripts (Gelman, Bullock, & Meck, 1980). In addition to these "local" inferences, they also acquire the ability to make "global" inferences, which draw upon information that has occurred in previous episodes or scenes in the story (Johnson & Smith, 1981).

Just as learning-disabled youngsters have difficulty mobilizing their schemata for story comprehension, they also have difficulty mobilizing them to draw inferences. In the previously cited study by Weaver and Dickenson (1979), they found that the reading-disabled children made significantly fewer minor inferences than normally developing children.

Ellis-Weismer (1981) compared the inferential skills of school-aged language-disordered children to one group of normal children with comparable nonverbal cognitive abilities, and another group of normal children at a similar level of language comprehension. Specifically, she examined their ability to draw spatial and causal inferences from short narratives presented in two ways: verbally and pictorially. She found that under both conditions, the language-disordered children performed like the normal children with similar comprehension skills. The normal children with similar nonverbal cognitive abilities performed significantly better than these two groups in the verbal condition for both explicitly stated information and information that had to be inferred. On the pictorial condition, they performed better only on the inferential items. These findings seem to offer support for the notion that language-disordered children sustain deficits in their inferential abilities.

Lastly, the Snyder et al. (1982) study cited earlier also investigated the ability of language/learning-disabled sixth-grade children to draw inferences. Using a probe-question paradigm, they assessed their subjects' ability to draw a variety of inferences: spatial, causal, world knowledge, and social motivational. Overall, they found that the language/learning-disabled were less proficient at drawing inferences than their age mates.

These studies provide some baseline indices that language/learning-disabled children may sustain a variety of discourse processing deficits.

Producing Pragmatic Structures

Pragmatic competence typically includes the ability to produce—as well as process—the various pragmatic structures. This includes the production of a wide variety of speech acts, particularly formulation of indirect forms. It also includes the ability to revise one's utterances in response to the needs of the listener. And, it goes beyond the sentence level to the production of effective conversations. Recent research has begun to focus on the ability of school-aged language-disordered children to produce pragmatic structures.

Producing Pragmatic Structures: Sentence level

Young children can produce a wide variety of speech acts by the time they enter elementary school. This is not necessarily true, however, of language-disordered children. Prinz (1977) compared the performance of young normal children matched with language-impaired children for linguistic level. In a free-play situation, he found that the language-disordered children used fewer declarative hints and more interrogatives to request actions and objects than the younger normal children. In an experimental situation in which its subjects requested things from a hand puppet, Prinz found that the language disordered children used fewer formal linguistic devices, e.g., contrastive stress, conditional mood, and so forth, to signal polite requests.

In a subsequent study, Prinz (in press) studied the requesting strategies of language-disordered children from 3½ to 8 years of age. During the free-play condition in this study, he made a "doctor" kit available to the children. Prinz found that, in this situation, the proportion of indirect requests produced by the language-disordered children decreased as a function of age. This observation is at variance with the literature on the normal development of request forms (Ervin-Tripp, 1977; Garvey, 1975). His findings, however, may be related to the use of the "doctor" kit. Research on requests produced during role-playing in this situation (Andersen, 1977, 1978) has revealed that high proportions of direct requests are associated with these types of roles. Thus, the increased proportion of direct requests produced by the older language-disordered children may have reflected their growing awareness of the sociolinguistic aspects of role-playing.

Prinz's findings are somewhat difficult to judge. His initial study observed distinct deficits in the requesting behavior of language-disordered children. His subsequent study revealed developmental trends similar to those observed in normal children. Since the latter study was a single-group investigation, it is difficult to know whether the requests produced by his language-disordered subjects were deficient, despite the developmental effects observed.

More recently, Donohue (1981b) compared the requesting strategies of matched normal and learning disabled children. Asking the children to request a newspaper from imaginary listeners with rather different power and familiarity characteristics, she analyzed the politeness of their requests and the nature of their appeals. She found that the two groups did not differ in the variety of request forms produced. Interestingly, the learning-disabled girls were more polite to all listeners. When the children's responses to the power vs. intimacy dimensions of their listeners were examined, Donohue found that the normal boys were more polite to nonintimate listeners, while the learning-disabled boys were more polite to low-power or low-dominance listeners. Thus, the learning disabled boys did differ in the politeness of their request, but they did not understand the conversational implications of the intimacy and power of the listener. In that these learning-disabled boys were able to vary their request forms, Donohue has interpreted this as evidence for a deficit in social cognition.

Producing Pragmatic Structures: Conversation

An important aspect of conversational competence is the ability to communicate new information to a listener effectively. In an early effort to study this skill, Meline (1978) compared school-aged language-disordered children with younger normal children who had similar levels of productive language development. Using the screened-listener paradigm, he asked each child to direct an adult listener in placing blocks into a pattern that matched the child's pattern. When one judged communicative effectiveness in terms of whether the listener chose the correct referent, the language-disordered children performed more successfully than their language-matched controls. However, when one compared the children in terms of the proportion of communicatively effective responses to the quantity of verbal output, the group differences disappeared. Preliminary data on a group of normal age peers revealed that they performed better than the language-disordered children. Thus, the language-disordered children in his study were not as communicatively effective as their more linguistically advanced age mates. Yet, they performed better than younger, linguistically similar children. They seemed to achieve this communicative success by saying more to their listener.

Perhaps one of the more challenging pragmatic tasks for an individual is engaging a listener in conversation, particularly a noncompliant, or socially powerful, listener, and achieving one's social goals with that person. This task might not be so tricky if listeners did not behave so unpredictably. Despite its difficulty, normal children seem to acquire the skill gradually, becoming remarkably proficient by adolescence. This is not so true of language/learning-disabled children.

In a rather interesting study of normal and learning-disabled children, Bryan, Donohue, and Pearl (1981) examined their conversational persuasion skills. Each child and two of his classmates were asked to rank-order gift choices for their class. Each subject was then taken aside. Half of the subjects in each group were given a "pep talk," and told that they had made good choices and should convince the others to make the same choices. The other half of the subjects were simply told "okay" and directed to the testing location. Analysis of the findings revealed that the learning-disabled children were less conversationally persuasive than their normal peers. The "pep talk" did not have any effect on their efforts. The learning-disabled children appeared to be more conversationally compliant than their peers. In addition, they did less to regulate or direct the flow of the conversation, making fewer attempts to monitor the conversation and fewer bids to hold the conversational floor. Thus, the learning-disabled children appeared to be less dominant, less assertive, and more compliant conversational partners.

In another attempt to examine learning-disabled children's ability to regulate and direct a conversation, Bryan, Donohue, Pearl, and Sturm (1981) studied their conversational skills when they were placed in a dominant role. They compared the conversational skills of matched normal and learning-disabled second- and fourth-grade children. Each child was placed into a pretend "TV Talk Show" situation where she or he was cast as the show's host. An academically achieving classmate was cast as the "talk show guest." Analysis of the children's conversations revealed that the learning-disabled children and their normal controls participated with the same frequency in the conversation, taking a similar number of conversational turns. In general, the learning-disabled children asked fewer questions. Specifically, they asked fewer open-ended questions than the normal children. Consequently, their "guests" were less likely to provide elaborated answers to questions, and in fact, they tended to ask their learning-disabled "hosts" more single-response questions. Not surprisingly, more role switching occurred when the learning-disabled children were "hosts" than when the nondisabled children assumed that dominant role. Despite the fact that this situational context clearly placed learning-disabled children in the socially dominant role, they were less able to benefit from this conversational advantage than their peers. Even when the "deck is loaded" in their favor, learning-disabled children continue to be more deferential and less assertive conversational partners.

In general, language/learning-disabled children seem to be less assertive conversational partners and to have difficulty understanding their role and all that it entails.

Summary

Although elementary school-age language/learning-disabled children seem to comprehend a wide variety of indirect and direct speech acts, they appear to have problems producing indirect forms. They also seem to have difficulty processing and producing the pragmatic aspects of discourse. They find aspects of both conversational and narrative discourse problematic and their comprehension of narrative discourse does not seem as complete or as organized as their age mates. As conversational partners, language/learning-disabled children seem to be more passive and agreeable partners, who cannot control the flow of conversation even when its direction is their responsibility. Thus, school-aged language-disordered children appear to have significant problems handling the pragmatic aspects of language.

Specific Cognitive Deficits

Both language-disordered children and learning-disabled children are characterized by their intact general cognitive abilities. Their language deficits, therefore, are not related to some form of mental retardation. In fact, the disorder is defined in terms of the discrepancy between the child's linguistic skills—oral and/or written—and general cognitive abilities. A few recent studies, however, have suggested that such a child may sustain impairment or delayed maturation of one specific cognitive skill—anticipatory imagery. *Anticipatory imagery* refers to the ability to look at an object or form, represent it mentally, and be able to rotate the mental visual symbol so that its position in space after several successive rotations can be anticipated (Piaget & Inhelder, 1971). This skill is typically assessed with spatial rotation tasks such as the higher level items of the *Ayres Space Test* and the *Minnesota Paper Form Board*. On the *Ayres Space Test*, for example, in the higher level items a puzzle form and two puzzle pieces are placed before the child, with the pieces partially rotated. Only one piece actually fits the puzzle. The child must determine—without touching or manipulating the stimuli—the piece that will actually complete the puzzle. In contrast to the static imagery of visual discrimination and visual-closure tasks, anticipatory imagery is considered dynamic and highly representational.

Recent interest in this ability of school-aged language-disordered youngsters was sparked by Johnston and Ramstad's (1977) study. Motivated by aspects of the relationship between language and cognition, they administered a series of classical Piagetian tasks to language-impaired preadolescents between 10 and 12 years of age. Their initial analyses revealed that all but one of their subjects had not reached the concrete operational stage level of performance on more than half of the tasks in their battery. In a subsequent task analysis, they separated their tasks into those that had required the processing of more complex verbal stimuli vs. those that had required the ablity to anticipate transformed physical states. Johnston and Ramstad found that all of their subjects experienced greatest difficulty on those tasks requiring anticipatory imagery. By contrast, they had the least difficulty on those tasks using complex verbal stimuli. This was a rather startling result for *language*-disordered children! They concluded that their language-disordered subjects' concomitant delays in anticipatory imagery might be related to a more basic deficit in the ability to mobilize symbols.

Subsequently, Murphy (1978) and Murphy and Stephens (in preparation) sought to compare the anticipatory imagery of normal and language-disordered children between 5 and 8½ years of age. Their subjects were matched for chronological age and performance on the *Raven's Coloured Progressive Matrices*. The language-disordered youngsters, however, did not seem to demonstrate particularly significant impairment. Ten of their eleven subjects scored *at* or just below the *28th* percentile, with one scoring at the 60th percentile on the Developmental Sentence Scoring (DSS). Such scores seem to represent the low end of the normal range. On a language-screening measure, only eight subjects failed the syntactic screening. Murphy and Stephens administered a series of Piagetian anticipatory imagery tasks and psychometric spatial tasks requiring anticipatory imagery. They found no significant differences between the two groups. These results are not surprising. First, they matched their groups on performance on the Ravens Matrices, a task which requires some anticipatory imagery at some levels. Second, a number of their "language-disordered" subjects did not appear to demonstrate a *significant* discrepancy between productive language abilities and general cognitive abilities. For the *most part*, they seem to have been comparing high verbal and low verbal *normal* children.

Another test of these notions was in a study by Savich (1980). She compared the ability of age-matched normal and language-disordered children between 7½ and 9½ years of age. The language-disordered children demonstrated language performance beyond one standard deviation below the mean on a standardized measure. They also demonstrated general cognitive abilities within the normal range. Savich assessed her subjects' visual analytic and visual gestaltist abilities, as well as their anticipatory imagery, using Piagetian and psychometric measures. Her findings indicated that the language-disordered children were far less accurate on all tasks requiring anticipation of the transformation of visual state or mental rotation, as well as on the visual analytic task. By contrast, they performed as well as their peers on one of the two gestaltist measures. Savich felt that these findings supported the specific cognitive deficit hypothesis: the ability to represent or symbolize information, and transform the symbolic representation a number of times, regardless of sensory channel—auditory/vocal or visual—is deficient in school-aged language-disordered children.

These studies provide some recent support for the link between specific cognitive abilities and language development. The results of the Johnston and Ramstad (1977) and Savich (1980) studies suggest that anticipatory imagery—that cognitive ability which makes its greatest developmental strides from 7 to 11 years of age—is deficient in school-aged language-disordered youngsters. Interestingly, Khami's (1981) comparative study of normal and language-disordered preschoolers demonstrated no significant group differences for one traditional test of anticipatory imagery, mental displacement, and differences for another test—haptic recognition. Although Khami interpreted the language-disordered children's deficient haptic recognition as evidence of deficits in anticipatory imagery, it is interesting to note they were similar to their normal counterparts on the more traditional measure of anticipatory imagery. Examining the distribution of his scores, it appears that all of his subjects were still at the early levels of skill development for that task. This skill is not expected to make its greatest gains for another 2 to 3 years. Consequently, one would not expect differences to emerge until that time.

Regardless of the differences between Khami's (1981) interpretation of his results and the interpretation put forward here, the critical point is the observed deficit in mental rotation or anticipatory imagery skills of language-disordered children. Since Strauss and Lehtinen (1947), we have alluded to the concomitant visual perceptual deficits of language-disordered and learning-disabled children. These findings suggest that they may not sustain deficits at the level of visual feature analysis. Rather, the "visual perceptual" deficits that we observe may be symptomatic of underlying representational, or even sequential, analytic deficits.

Recent Advances and an Age-Old Dilemma: Identification and Assessment of School-Aged Language-Disordered Children

Significant Discrepancy

The growing interest of our consumers, and our corresponding need for accountability, as well as the increased rigor demanded by our own research, have mandated that clinicians demonstrate that language-disordered youngsters' communicative skills are significantly discrepant from their general cognitive abilities. Translated operationally, this means that they should perform beyond -1 standard deviation below the mean, plus the test's standard error of measurement. The mean, however, is the mean projected given the child's general cognitive abilities. In some instances the term "general cognitive abilities" is interpreted as the child's nonverbal IQ. In other instances it is interpreted as his full scale IQ.

While this appears to be a rather straightforward standard, it is difficult to implement, particularly with school-aged children. First, a number of our existing diagnostic tools fail to report the standard error of measurement, or figures from which it might be derived. Second, we lack a sufficient number of standardized measures that extend beyond 8 years of age.

Only recently, have a few measures emerged that can be used with youngsters older than 8 years. These include Wiig and Semel's (1981) *Clinical Evaluation of Language Function* (CELF); *The Word Test* (Jorgensen, Barrett, Huisingh, and Zachman, 1981); and Gardner's *One Word Expressive Vocabulary Test* (1980). Third, none of the syntactic and pragmatic processing and production abilities thought to emerge during the elementary school years are sampled by our existing diagnostic measures of language development. Understandably, we need not apologize for our failure to do this in the pragmatic domain. Sufficient basic information has yet to be developed for normal children. However, we can hardly make this claim relative to the syntactic domain. Carol Chomsky's work emerged in 1969, followed closely by Kessel's (1970). More than a decade has passed since this research was conducted. Fourth, the problem is compounded by our lack of consensus regarding what constitutes a significant discrepancy in language development. Do we agree with Stark and Tallal's (1981) criteria, which suggest that the child must demonstrate both a receptive *and* expressive deficit? Or, can we include the group of youngsters whom they had observed exhibiting deficits in expressive skills alone? Similarly, how shall we regard the language/learning-disabled child? Is this a "mixed disorder" (Stark & Tallal, 1981)?

Thus, despite our new knowledge, it remains difficult to adequately identify and assess school-aged children with significant discrepancies in their oral language development.

The Territorial Imperative

The great disappearing act performed by elementary-school language-disordered children raises an uncomfortable issue: territorial rights. If we consider the logistics and administrative demands to report the number of children who receive special services, it becomes important to identify those children needing language intervention. Our ability to identify the underlying oral-language deficits of "learning-disabled" youngsters has been limited by the paucity of appropriate measures of syntactic development. Consequently, many of these youngsters are seen by special educators who focus their efforts on the children's visual-perceptual, visual-motor, and written-language skills. Current research, however, suggests that the majority of these youngsters sustain underlying oral-language deficits. If more viable measures of the syntactic development of school-aged children were available, some of them might be identified for language-intervention programming. Surely, a combined approach might prove more effective for these children.

One wonders, however, if we are afraid to assert our territorial rights.

Or, are we afraid to infringe upon the territorial claims of other professions—despite the mounting evidence for underlying oral language deficits in "learning" disabled children?

Conclusion

Current research suggests that language-disordered children of elementary school age sustain significant deficits in the processing and production of oral language. Unfortunately, our ability to identify and document these deficits beyond the experimental setting has been limited. Consequently, our charge seems clear. We need to translate our empirically derived knowledge of the normal and disordered language development of elementary-school children into tools for clinical assessment. Admittedly, this is not an easy task, but we would hope that some of our colleagues will rise to the challenge.

References

Andersen, E. Young children's knowledge of role-related speech differences: A mommy is not a daddy is not a baby. *Papers and Reports in Child Language Development,* 1977, *13,* 91-98.

Andersen, E. Will you don't snore please? Directives in young children's role-play speech. *Papers and Reports in Child Language Development,* 1978, *15,* 140-160.

Anderson, R. C., Spiro, R. J., & Anderson, M.C. Schemata as scaffolding for the representation of information in connected discourse. *American Educational Research Journal,* 1978, *15,* 433-440.

Bartlett, F.C. *Remembering.* Cambridge, Eng: Cambridge University Press, 1932.

Bates, E. *Language and context: Studies in the acquisition of pragmatics.* New York: Academic Press, 1976.

Bates, E., & MacWhinney, B. Functionalist approaches to grammar. In L. Gleitman & E. Wanner (Eds.), *Language acquisition: The state of the art.* New York: Cambridge University Press, in press.

Berko, J. The child's learning of English morphology. *Word,* 1958, *14,* 75-96.

Berry, M., & Talbott, S. *Berry-Talbott Language Tests, 1: Comprehension of Grammar.* Rockford, IL. 1966.

Bryan, T., Donohue, M., & Pearl, R. Learning disabled children's peer interactions during a small group problem solving task. *Learning Disability Quarterly,* 1981, *4,* 13-22.

Bryan, T., Donohue, M., Pearl, R., & Sturm, C. Learning disabled children's conversational skills: The "TV Talk Show." *Learning Disability Quarterly,* 1981, *4,* 250-259.

Byrne, B. Deficient syntactic control in poor readers: Is a weak phonetic memory code responsible? *Applied Psycholinguistics,* 1981, *2,* 201-212.

Chomsky, C.S. *The acquisition of syntax in children from 5 to 10.* Cambridge, Mass: MIT Press, 1969.

Christie, D.J., & Schumacher, G.M. Developmental trends in the abstraction and recall of relevant versus irrelevant thematic information from connected verbal materials. *Child Development*, 1975, *46*, 598-602.

Clark, H.H., & Haviland, S.E. Comprehension and the given-new contract. In R.O. Freedle (Ed.), *Discourse production and comprehension* (Vol. 1) Norwood, NJ: Ablex, 1977.

Cromer, R.F. "Children are nice to understand": Surface structure clues for the recovery of a deep structure. *British Journal of Psychology*, 1970, *61*, 397-408.

De Hirsch, K., Jansky, J., & Langford, W.S. *Predicting reading failures.* New York: Harper & Row, 1966.

Denckla, M.B. Color-naming defects in dyslexic boys. *Cortex*, 1972, *8*, 164-176.

Denckla, M.B. Retrospective study and dyslexic children (1975). Reported in A.L. Benton & D. Pearl (Eds.), *Dyslexia: An appraisal of current knowledge.* New York: Oxford University Press, 1978.

Denckla, M.B., & Rudel, R. Naming of object drawings by dyslexic and other learning disabled children. *Brain and Language*, 1976, *3*, 1-16. (a)

Denckla, M.B., & Rudel, R. Rapid "automatized" naming (R.A.N.): Dyslexia differentiated from other learning disabilities. *Neuropsychologia*, 1976, *14*, 471-479. (b)

deVilliers, J. & deVilliers, P. Delopment of the use of word order in comprehension. *Journal of Psycholinguistic Research*, 1973, *2*, 331-341.

Dixon, N.D. *Reading disability, language impairment and reading strategies: Implications for differential diagnosis.* Unpublished doctoral dissertation, University of Colorado, 1982.

Donohue, M. Learning disabled children's comprehension and production of syntactic devices for making given versus new information. In Chicago Institute for the Study of Learning Disabilities, Abstracts of Research Reports, 1981. (a)

Donohue, M. Requesting strategies of learning disabled children. *Applied Psycholinguistics*, 1981, *2*, 213-234. (b)

Donohue, M., Pearl, R., & Bryan, T. Learning disabled children's conversational competence: Responses to inadequate messages. *Applied Psycholinguistics*, 1980, *1*, 387-404.

Donohue, M., Pearl, R., & Bryan, T. Learning disabled children's syntactic proficiency on a communicative task. *Journal of Speech and Hearing Disorders*, in press.

Dore, J. Conversation and preschool language development. In P. Fletcher & M. Garman (Eds.), *Language acquisition.* Cambridge, Eng.: Cambridge University Press, 1978.

Dunn, L. *Peabody Picture Vocabulary Test.* Circle Pines, MI: American Guidance Services, 1965.

Dunn, L., & Dunn, L. *Peabody Picture Vocabulary Test—Revised.* Circle Pines, MI: American Guidance Services, 1981.

Durrell, J. *The Durrell analysis of reading difficulty* New York: Harcourt, Brace & Jovanovich, 1965.

Ellis-Weismer, S. *Constructive comprehension processes exhibited by language impaired children.* Unpublished doctoral dissertation, Indiana University, 1981.

Ervin-Tripp, S. Wait for me, roller skate! In S. Ervin-Tripp & C. Mitchell-Kernan (Eds.), *Child discourse*, New York: Academic Press, 1977.

Fillmore, C.J. Types of lexical information. In D.D. Steinberg & L.A. Jakobovits (Eds.), *Semantics: An interdisciplinary reader in philosophy, linguistics and psychology.* Cambridge, Eng: Cambridge University Press, 1971.

Foster, C., Giddan, J., & Stark, J. *Assessment of children's language comprehension.* Palo Alto, CA: Counseling Psychologists Press, 1973.

Freedle, R.O.(Ed.), *Discourse production and comprehension.* Norwood, NJ: Ablex, 1977.

Fry, M.A. *A transformational analysis of the oral language structure used by two reading groups at the second grade level.* Unpublished doctoral dissertation, University of Iowa, 1967.

Fry, M.A., Johnson, C.S., & Muehl, S. Oral language production in relation to reading achievement among select second graders. In D.J. Bakker & P. Satz (Eds.), *Specific reading disability: Advances in theory and method.* Rotterdam: Rotterdam University Press, 1970.

Gallagher, T.M. Revision behaviors in the speech of normal children developing language. *Journal of Speech and Hearing Research,* 1977, *20,* 303-318.

Gardner, R. *One-Word Expressive Vocabulary Test.* Novato, CA: Academic Therapy Publications, 1980.

Garvey, C. Requests andd responses in children's speech. *Journal of Child Language* 1975, *2,* 41-60.

Gelman, R., Bullock, M., & Meck, E. Preschooler's understanding of simple object transformations. *Child Development,* 1980, *51.* 691-699.

German, D.J. Word finding skills in children with learning disabilities. *Journal of Learning Disabilities,* 1979, *12,* 43-48.

Golub, L., & Kidder, C. Syntactic density and the computer, *Elementary English,* 1974, *51,* 1128-1131.

Graybeal, C.M. Memory for stories in language-impaired children. *Applied Psycholinguistics,* 1981, *2,* 269-283.

Greenbaum, S., Quirk, R., Leach, G., & Svartnik, J. *A grammar of contemporary English.* New York: Seminar Press, 1972.

Greenfield, P., & Smith, J. *The structure of communication in early development.* New York: Academic Press, 1976.

Haviland, S.E., & Clark, H.H. What's new? Acquiring new information as a process in comprehension. *Journal of Verbal Learning and Verbal Behavior,* 1974, *13,* 515-521.

Hook, P.E. *A study of metalinguistic awareness and reading strategies in proficient and learning disabled readers.* Unpublished doctoral dissertation, Northwestern University, 1976.

Hornby, P. Surface structure and the topic-comment distinction: A developmental study. *Child Development,* 1971, *42,* 1975-1978.

Hunt, K.W. Grammatical structures written at three grade levels. *National Council of Teachers of English,* No. 3, 1965.

Jansky, J. The marginally reading child. *Bulletin of Orton Society,* 1975, *25,* 69-85.

Johnson, D.J., & Myklebust, H.R. *Learning disabilities: Educational principles and practices.* New York: Grune and Straton, 1967.

Johnson, H., & Smith, L.B. Children's inferential abilities in the context of reading to understand. *Child Development,* 1981, *52,* 1216-1223.

Johnston, J., & Ramstad, V. Cognitive development in preadolescent language-impaired children. Paper presented at the Annual Convention of the American Speech and Hearing Association, Chicago, 1977.

Jorgensen, C., Barrett, M., Huisingh, R., & Zachman, Z. *The Word Test.* Moline, IL.: Lingui Systems, Inc., 1981.

Just, M.N., & Carpenter, P. (Eds.), *Cognitive processes in comprehension.* Hillsdale, NJ: Lawrence Erlbaum Associates, 1977.

Kail, R., Chi, M., Ingram, A., & Danner, F. Constructive aspects of children's reading comprehension. *Child Development,* 1977, *48,* 684-688.

Keenan, J.M., & Kintsch, W. The identification of explicity and implicity presented information. In W. Kintsch, *The representation of meaning in memory.* Hillsdale, NJ: Lawrence Erlbaum Associates, 1974.

Kessel, F.S. The role of syntax in children's comprehension from ages 6 to 12. *Society for Research in Child Development Monograph,* 1970, (Serial No. 139).

Khami, A.G. Nonlinguistic symbolic and conceptual abilities of language-impaired and normally developing children. *Journal of Speech and Hearing Research,* 1981, *24,* 446-453.

Kintsch, E., & Kintsch, W. The comprehension of texts. In R. McLean (Ed.), *Reading.* Belmont, Victoria: Deakin University Press, 1979.

Kintsch, W. *The representation of meaning in memory.* Hillsdale, NJ: Lawrence Erlbaum, 1974.

Kintsch, W. On comprehending stories. In M.A. Just & P. Carpenter (Eds.), *Cognitive processes in comprehension.* Hillsdale, NJ: Lawrence Erlbaum, 1977.

Kintsch, W., & Green, E. The role of culture-specific schemata in the comprehension and recall of stories. *Discourse Processes,* 1979, *1,* 1-13.

Kirk, S., & McCarthy, J. *The Illinois Test of Psycholinguistic Abilities.* Champaign-Urbana: University of Illinois Press, 1961.

Leonard, L.B. What is deviant language? *Journal of Speech and Hearing Disorders,* 1972, *37,* 427-446.

Lerner, J.W. *Children with learning disabilities* Second ed. Boston: Houghton Mifflin, 1977.

Leske, M.C. Speech prevalence estimates of communicative disorders in the U.S. *Asha,* 1981, *23,* 229-237.

Liles, B., Schulman, M., & Bartlett, S. Judgements of grammaticality by normal and language-disordered children. *Journal of Speech and Hearing Disorders,* 1977, *42,* 199-209.

Mandler, J.M., & Johnson, N.S. Remembrance of things parsed: Story structure and recall. *Cognitive Psychology,* 1977, *9,* 111-151.

Mattis, S., French, J., & Rapin, I. Dyslexia in children and young adults: Three independent neurological syndromes. *Developmental Medicine and Child Neurology,* 1975, *17,* 150-163.

Moran, M.R., & Byrne, M.C. Mastery of verb tense markers by normal and learning disabled children. *Journal of Speech and Hearing Research,* 1977, *20,* 529-542.

Meline, T. Referential communication by normal and language deficient children. Paper presented at the annual convention of the American Speech and Hearing Association, San Francisco, 1978.

Murphy, V.H. *A comparison of four measures of visual imagery in normal and language disorderd children.* Unpublished master's thesis, Northern Illinois University, 1978.

Murphy, V.H., & Stephens, M.I. A comparison of four measures of visual imagery in normal and language disordered children. In preparation.

Newcomer, P., & Hammill, D. *Test of Language Development.* Austin, TX: Empiric Press, 1977.

Paris, S., & Upton, L. Children's memory for inferential relationships in prose. *Child Development,* 1976, *47,* 660-668.

Piaget, J., & Inhelder, B. *Mental imagery in the child.* New York: Basic Books, 1971.

Prinz, P. The comprehension and production of requests in language disordered children. Paper presented at the Second Annual Boston University Conference on Language Development, Boston, October 1977.

Prinz, P. Requesting in normal and language disordered children. In K. Nelson (Ed.), *Children's language* (Vol. 3). New York: Gardner Press, in press.

Riley, C., & Trabasso, T. Comparatives, logical structures, and encoding in a transitive inference task. *Journal of Experimental Child Psychology,* 1974, *17,* 187-203.

Rumelhardt, D.E. Schemata: The building blocks of cognition. In R.J. Spiro, B.C. Bruce, & W.F. Brewer (Eds.), *Theoretical issues in reading comprehension.* Hillsdale, NJ: Lawrence Erlbaum, 1980.

Savich, P.A. *A comparison of the anticipatory imagery and spatial representation ability of normal and language disordered children.* Unpublished doctoral dissertation, University of Colorado, 1980.

Schulte, C. *A study of the relationship between oral language and reading achiement in second graders.* Unpublished doctoral dissertation, University of Iowa, 1967.

Schank, R.C., & Abelson, R.P. *Scripts, plans, goals and understanding.* Hillsdale, NJ: Lawrence Erlbaum, 1977.

Semel, E., & Wiig, E. Comprehension of syntactic structures and critical verbal elements by children with learning disabilities. *Journal of Learning Disabilities,* 1975, *8,* 53-58.

Shatz, M. On the development of communicative understanding: An early strategy for interpreting and responding to messages. *Cognitive Psychology,* 1978, *10,* 217-301.

Sheppard, L. Evolution of the identification of perceptual-cognitive disorders in Colorado. Final Report. Boulder: Laboratory of Educational Research, University of Colorado, 1981.

Snyder, L.S., Haas, C., & Becker, L.B. Discourse processing in normal and language and learning disabled children. Unpublished manuscript, 1982.

Stark, R., & Tallal, P. Selection of children with specific language deficits. *Journal of Speech and Hearing Disorders,* 1981, *46,* 114-122.

Stein, N., & Glenn, C. An analysis of story comprehension in elementary school children. In R. Freedle (Ed.), *New directions in discourse processing.* Hillsdale, NJ: Ablex, 1979.

Strauss, A., & Lehtinen, L. *Psychopathology and education of the brain-injured child.* New York: Grune & Stratton, 1946.

Trabasso, T. Representation, memory and reasoning: How do we make transitive inferences? In A. Pick (Ed.), *Minnesota Symposium on Child Psychology* (Vol. 9). Minneapolis: University of Minnesota Press, 1975.

Trabasso, T., & Nicholas, D. Memory and inferences in the comprehension of narratives. Paper presented at the Conference on Study of Children's Judgements, Kassel, Germany, June 1977.

U.S. Office of Education. Assistance to states for handicapped children. Procedure for evaluating specific learning disabilities. *Federal Register,* 1977, *42,* 65082-65085.

Vogel, S.A. *Syntactic abilities in normal and dyslexic children.* Baltimore: University Park Press, 1975.

Vogel, S. Syntactic abilities in normal and dyslexic children. *Journal of Learning Disabilities,* 1977, *7,* 47-53.

Weaver, P., & Dickenson, D. Story comprehension and recall in dyslexic students. *Bulletin of Orton Society,* 1979, *29,* 157-171.

Wiig, E.H., & Semel, E.M. Comprehension of linguistic concepts requiring logical operations by learning disabled children. *Journal of Speech and Hearing Research,* 1973, *16,* 627-636.

Wiig, E.H., & Semel, E.M. *Language disabilities in children and adolescents.* Columbus, OH: Charles C. Merrill, 1976.

Wiig, E.H., & Semel, E.M. *Language assessment and intervention for the learning disabled.* Columbus, OH.: Charles E. Merrill, 1980.

Wiig, E.H., & Semel, E.M. *Clinical evaluation of language function.* Columbus, OH.: Charles E. Merrill, 1981.

Wiig, E.H., Semel, E.M., & Crouse, M.B. The use of English morphology by high-risk and learning disabled children. *Journal of Learning Disabilities,* 1973, *6,* 457-465.

Wiig, E.H., Semel, E.M., & Nystrom, L.A. Comparison of rapid naming abilities in language learning disabled and academically achieving eight-year-olds. *Language, Speech and Hearing Services in the Schools,* 1982, *13,* 11-23.

Wolf, M. The relationship of word-finding and reading in children and aphasics. Unpublished doctoral dissertation, Harvard University, 1979.

Elizabeth M. Prather

Developmental Language Disorders: Adolescents

When asked to write this chapter on adolescent language disorders, I could think only of the many unknowns. For the past five years, I have gathered considerable information on the language of the adolescent, including normative data, differential diagnoses, and clinical treatment. Yet, we clinicians still seem like "babes in the woods," perhaps similar to our state 20 years ago regarding childhood language development and disorders. I have accepted the challenge of writing this chapter, not so much from the standpoint of what we know but from that of what we don't know, and in the belief that it may stimulate much needed research.

Normative Data—A Description of Language in Older Children and Adolescents

The discussion in this chapter is limited to students from fifth and sixth grades to the twelfth grade. The normative data have all been derived from standardized tests, and some are much more complete than others. We will see that from ages 11 to 18 years, some characteristics of language commonly show no improvement or change in development. Others demonstrate marked change, while yet others have not been investigated at the adolescent level.

Language Similarities from
Upper Elementary to High School

There is little evidence to suggest that students in high school perform appreciably better on language tests (from the view of speech-language pathology) than students in fifth and sixth grades. Two explanations probably account for this lack of change in test scores. First, current tests may be insensitive to the progress students make in language facility from fifth grade to high school. In other words, we may be testing the wrong factors. Second, there is the possibility that little changes in the student's ability to manipulate some aspects of language meaningfully beyond at least the fifth grade level. This latter possibility may reflect either a plateau or the upper end of certain language rule learning. We would, of course, expect increases in vocabulary as a result of content teaching in classroom curricula, and in the social use of language because of the growing importance of the peer group, but, perhaps, skills like repeating sentences verbatim, understanding subtle syntactic changes, and explaining the meaning of a known concept do not substantially increase during adolescence.

A review of current clinical language tests, all published in 1980, indicates little progress in students' abilities from the upper elementary to the high-school level, as exemplified in the following two screening tests and two more complete diagnostic batteries.

On the *Clinical Evaluation of Language Function Advanced Level Screening Test* (Semel & Wiig, 1980b), the mean number of items passed by fifth-grade students was 35.2, while the mean number passed by twelfth-grade students was only 39.6 from a total of 52 items. Tenth-grade students earned a mean score of only 35.1, slightly lower than fifth-grade. This total increase of approximately four items in seven years should be considered minimal.

Prather, Breecher, Stafford, and Wallace (1980) showed, on the *Screening Test of Adolescent Language* (STAL), that fifth-grade students earned a mean of 14.81 items, while ninth-grade students earned a mean score of 17.86. Most of the improvement resulted from the vocabulary subtest. The increase of essentially 3 items (from a total of 23 items) spans a four-year period, and indicates only slightly better sensitivity to change.

Semel and Wiig (1980b) devised their screening test from a more comprehensive diagnostic battery, *Clinical Evaluation of Language Function* (CELF) (1980a). As of this writing, the CELF does not include means and standard deviations for each grade level, but does show a "criterion score" for each grade level on each of the 13 subtests. The criterion scores are used to determine whether further "extension testing" is needed, reflecting perhaps a lower limit of normal performance for students at each grade level. On 6 of the 13 subtests, *no change* is reflected in the criterion scores from the sixth through the twelfth grades. On the other 7 subtests, the change varies from 2 items (2 subtests) to 4 items (2 subtests) to 8 items (3 subtests). The 3 subtests reflecting the greatest change, approximately one point per year, are as follows:

1. Processing relationships and ambiguities. Examples resemble:
   a. Mary followed Joe, and Joe followed Ann.
      Did Ann follow Mary?
   b. Better late than never. Does it mean: Don't
      be late?
2. Producing word associations. This task requires the student to name as many words as possible within two categories, and is timed.
3. Producing model sentences. The student repeats both meaningful and nonmeaningful "sentences" verbatim.

"Producing formulated sentences" is one of the subtests on which there is no change from sixth through twelfth grades. In this subtest, the student is given 12 words and asked to make a meaningful sentence with each. She or he can receive up to 8 points per sentence, depending on grammatic/syntactic complexity. A score of 3 is given to a simple sentence with phrase(s). The criterion score for this subtest is 35 for all seven grade levels, just under an average of 3 points per sentence. This lack of change over the 7 years is interesting in light of the ways speech-language pathologists program language-delayed students to use complex, compound, and embedded sentences. Perhaps if we knew more about "normal language" in adolescents, we would alter many of our current treatment goals.

The *Test of Adolescent Language* (TOAL) (Hammill, Brown, Larsen, & Wiederholt, 1980) includes normative data from ages 11 to 18½ years, also a span of 7 years. This more complete diagnostic test includes eight subtests of vocabulary and grammar across the four dimensions of listening, speaking, reading, and writing. It is not surprising that students show relatively less growth on the 4 grammar subtests than on the 4 vocabulary subtests, reaffirming the premise that syntactic/grammatic skills are well established by the eleventh birthday in normally developing students. The total change in group means between 11 and 18½ years in the speaking/grammar subtest (repeating sentences verbatim) was 2.3 more items correct in the 7-year span. Among the four dimensions, listening and speaking scores increased less than reading and, especially, writing scores. This result would also be expected if one assumes that the hierarchy of language development proceeds from listening to speaking to reading to writing. The normal developmental period for the reading and writing dimensions of language seems to extend at least into the teen years.

In summary, the clinical tests we are using lack sensitivity to change in the reception and expression of oral language from ages 11 to 18 years. We apparently cannot use existing tests to detect changes in many of the syntactic, grammatic, and memory aspects of language that are tested so heavily at earlier age levels.

Language Differences from Upper Elementary to High School

Evidence is available from other standardized tests that language facility indeed increases among students from fifth through twelfth grades. One very obvious example is that of vocabulary. On the *Peabody Picture Vocabulary Test—Revised Form L* (Dunn & Dunn, 1981), a raw score of 114 converts to an age-equivalent score of 11 years. In contrast, a raw score of 150 converts to an age-equivalent score of 18 years, 1 month. In other words, the high-school senior is expected to identify approximately 36 more items than the fifth-grader, a substantial increase. The more difficult items include terms from the study of geography, mathematics, anatomy, and physics, as well as less common adjectives and verbs.

Performance on the verbal scale of the *Wechsler Intelligence Scale for Children* (WISC) (1949) also shows considerable change from age 11 years to the ceiling age (15 years, 11 months) on 4 of the 6 subtests. The greatest increase is on the vocabulary subtest, which requires the student to define words orally. Many of the high-level, less common words would be known through academic coursework, readings, or exposure to specific experiences, i.e., *hara-kiri, ballast, mantis,* and *chattel.* The information subtest also increases in expectation from ages 11 to 16. The increase reflects greater knowledge, primarily in the areas of geography, history, and the sciences.

Two additional subtests of the WISC, general comprehension and similarities, show some change, but less than vocabulary and information. The general comprehension subtest, except for the 4 lowest-level items, requires the student to answer "why" questions (cause-effect relationships) of increasing difficulty. The similarities subtest (identifying key components of likeness) increases in difficulty for the older student by the inclusion of more abstract concepts, for example, *liberty-justice, first-last,* and *49-121.*

The two subtests of the WISC which show essentially no increase across the five years are arithmetic and digit span. The arithmetic items, beyond the low-level, block manipulations, are all short "story problems," which the subject hears (10 items) or reads (3 items). All require only basic arithmetic concepts of addition, subtraction, multiplication, and division of whole numbers or fractions. The digit-span task for auditory memory is scored by adding the number of digits correctly recalled on the two tasks of forward and backward repetition. The average 11-year-old student earns a score of ten digits (perhaps six forward and four backward) while the 15- to 16-year-old student earns a score of eleven digits. This failure to see an increase in memory span resembles the sentence-repetition performances described earlier in other language tests.

Other evidence in language growth through the teen years can be found in the various school achievement tests used throughout the country (*Peabody Individualized Achievement Test*, Dunn & Markwardt, 1970; *California Achievement Tests*, CTB/McGraw-Hill, 1977; *Wide Range Achievement Test*, Jastak, 1946; and *Metropolitan Achievement Tests*, Prescott, Balow, Hogan, & Farr, 1978). All of these tests measure various aspects of reading and vocabulary, and are dependent on academic achievement.

In summary, tests of vocabulary, abstract-concept explanations, and general knowledge of academic content areas show marked improvement in scores from the fifth to the twelfth grades, and reflect the expected semantic growth resulting from increased reading and exposure to many learning experiences. Curricular materials from classrooms at various grade levels reflect this semantic development.

Language Processes Not Yet Described

To my knowledge, no standardized tests for adolescents are available that tap pragmatic aspects of language, including topic maintenance, sensitivity to misunderstandings, and group problem-solving strategies. We certainly can predict that changes are expected in these areas as well as other areas related to the social use of language as the peer group gains importance. Much research is needed to identify and quantify some of the key components of language usage among adolescents.

Assessing Expected Competencies Among Adolescents

Clinicians would like to find discreet types of language disorders among adolescents. In theory, such findings would simplify remedial programming. Just as there are many dimensions of language, we can assume that there are also many possible dimensions to language disorders evidenced singly and in combination. We can also assume that there are as many etiological variables affecting language performance in adolescents as there are in younger children and adults.

No one questions the evidence that students who are mentally retarded, severely and multiply handicapped, autistic, hearing-impaired, and/or brain-damaged from trauma are likely to have difficulty manipulating the code system of language. We do, however, assume that the specific configuration of difficulties will differ both within and across etiological categories. Likewise, to expect that we can find a few distinct "types" of language problems in adolescents has to be totally unrealistic.

A group of special interest is the "learning disabled." I call it a "group" because, by educational placement, these students are apparently assumed to share at least some common characteristics. McGrady (1980, pp. 509-562) presents an excellent discussion on the diverse ways in which the term "learning disability" has been used and defined. He points out that, through use of behavioral testing, we now see school districts claiming 5% to 20% or more of their students as learning disabled. This incidence is in sharp contrast to the 1 to 2 % of students expected to have neurologically significant specific learning disabilities. The difference, according to McGrady, is that many students who are simply "underachievers and slow learners" have been labeled as "learning disabled." Many of these students are merely victims of poor teaching, or have come from families that do not value academic achievement. To expect that large segments of these students will have a specific "type" of language disability (e.g., poor auditory memory, language-processing problems, auditory figure-ground confusions, morphological/syntactical problems, word retrieval problems) is unrealistic, even if we could isolate and define the parameters of such specific deficits.

Assessment among adolescents includes at least two discrete tasks. The first is screening to determine which students need a more complete diagnostic evaluation. The second is the evaluation used to (1) determine whether a communication problem exists; (2) document the language disorder; and (3) program remedial or compensatory training.

Language Screening

Screening students for all types of communication disorders is an important task in school settings. In some districts, routine screening occurs at certain grade levels, while in other districts more reliance is placed on teacher and parent referrals.

Screening protocols for language among older students have posed real problems for us. Because of the lack of normative data, clinicians have relied heavily on short "informal" dialogues and monologues. Asking students such questions as "How many brothers and sisters do you have? What are their names and ages? How long have you lived in Phoenix?" is useless if used with this older age group to identify possible language problems. These questions are typically answered well by students in the primary grades. Simple monologues also may be equally ineffective. In an early draft of the STAL (Prather et al., 1980), we had included a subtest that required the student to relate a story from sequenced picture cues. We had to eliminate the subtest because of our inability to attain scoring reliability among various examiners. Some examiners gave maximum credit to a story told with correct grammar, paying little attention to content elaboration, complexity of sentence structure, or the sequencing of ideas. Some of these informal approaches for language screening, then, are no doubt ineffective, and result in highly variable judgments within and between school districts. To my knowledge, no researchers have extended the work of O'Donnell, Griffin, and Norris (1967) on T-Unit norms from the elementary to the high-school level, nor have the six production indices used by Ludlow (1977, pp. 97-134) with adult asphasics been normed on adolescents. Such approaches might be worthwhile.

One mini-screening test (Prather, Brenner, & Hughes, 1981), requiring approximately 90 seconds per student, has been devised for the mass screening of older students. It includes five items: two in vocabulary, one in sentence repetition, one in explanation of cause effect, and one in sentence explanation. The normative data indicate that the test passes approximately 75% of students from regular classrooms (sixth to twelfth grades). Additional screening time can then be spent with the 25% who fail.

Two more complete language-screening tests are available for use with adolescents. Both provide a standardized protocol for screening, and both tap several aspects of language. The STAL (Prather et al., 1980) requires approximately 7 minutes per student, while the Advanced Level CELF Screening Test (Semel & Wiig, 1980b) requires approximately 15 minutes. A student may "fail" either screening test because of poor performance on any one subtest, or because of a low total score. Both tests seem useful in identifying students whose language skills differ markedly from their peers and who may profit from more complete assessment.

Speech-Language Evaluations

Two excellent sources on expected language competencies are available (Bassett, Wittington, & Staton-Spicer, 1978; Simon, 1979). Both force the clinician to focus on specific features of speaking and listening that require assessment. Bassett et al. suggest guidelines for minimal speaking and listening competencies for high-school graduates, and urge that we assess not memorized facts, but the students' ability to use speaking and listening skills for tasks encountered in adult living. They divide 19 competencies among four areas. The first area is the use of the verbal and nonverbal codes to understand and express meaning. It includes such skills as understanding directions, using language appropriate to given situations, speaking clearly and loudly enough to be heard and understood, and using nonverbal signs (gestures and facial expressions) that are appropriate to the situation. The second assesses understanding of oral messages and includes skills such as identification of the main idea in messages; distinguishing fact from opinion, and information from persuasion; and recognizing when another has not understood your message. The third area measures elements selected and arranged to produce spoken messages. It includes skills such as expressing ideas clearly and concisely, defending a point of view, sequencing information so that others can understand, asking questions to obtain information, giving accurate and concise directions, and summarizing messages. Their last area looks at resolving conflicts in human relationships, and includes skills that can be assessed as describing another's point of view and differences of opinion, expressing feelings to others, and performing social rituals.

To assess all of these functional communication skills suggested by Bassett et al. (1978) requires that we approach assessment from a pragmatic level. They do not, however, include any suggestions for formal assessment. Simon (1979) not only presents a model for expressive communicative competence, but also suggests ways to obtain evidence of competence and incompetence. The reader is strongly urged to refer directly to Simon's Appendix 4, pages 69-76. It is filled with suggested activities for observing a student's use of language, including the seven functions of language as described by Halliday. These are: instrumental, regulatory, interactional, personal, heuristic, imaginative, and informational. In addition, Simon's battery includes phonology, morphology, syntax, semantics, and a few suggestions for observing receptive language. Her suggested approaches to the evaluation and treatment of language problems are not limited to the adolescent level; she includes much information on younger children as well. She has, however, incorporated many suggestions specific to the intermediate and junior high-school level.

In addition to specifying which aspects of language need to be tested, and how each might be observed, Simon (1979) also provides a system to organize accumulated data on each student, so that the strengths and weaknesses in speech and language become evident. She uses some standardized test scores to include with the documentation of the need for speech-language services. She agrees, however, with Leonard, Prutting, Perozzi and Berkley (1978), who advocate use of informal, descriptive evaluation procedures for communicative competence, and she states that our knowledge of the nature of effective communication exceeds our development of formal evaluation instruments. Thus, her format for organizing assessment information and writing comprehensive treatment objectives is a strong contribution to the working clinician.

Two recent diagnostic measures previously mentioned in this chapter— CELF and TOAL— are now available for use with adolescents. However, neither provides the types of functional assessment advocated by Simon (1979) and Bassett et al. (1978). Both the CELF and the TOAL are designed to reflect various patterns of strengths and weaknesses. The CELF includes 13 subtests across many aspects of receptive and expressive language. Normative data are severely limited in this first edition, and the test protocol does not provide for basal and ceiling scores. With some students, the need to administer all items in each subtest seems unnecessarily redundant.

The TOAL does provide basal and ceiling scores for its 8 subtests; administration time, however, ranges from one to three hours per student. The test is especially helpful to those clinicians who want language measures related to reading and writing (4 of the 8 subtests). Many of the listening and speaking test items are constructed to reduce guessing by requiring the two most appropriate choices from a set of four or five foils.

No assessment tools of interactive communication have been standardized on adolescents at this time. We can hope that research is under way which will help the clinician identify and assess those competencies that are expected in adolescent students. It may be possible to start a standardized functional communication procedure for adolescents with the *Communication Abilities in Daily Living* (Holland, 1980), capitalizing on her previous research with adult aphasics.

In addition to the observations and tests used to assess language competence, other school personnel and records are helpful. Besides the classroom teacher, the psychologist and counselor are especially important. Psychometric data and achievement test scores may be particularly helpful in understanding the nature of a possible language problem.

Treatment with Older Language-Impaired Students

Can language problems be remediated at these older age levels, or should we attempt to teach compensatory and coping strategies? In a possibly parallel situation, Darley (1972) wrote a treatise on the efficacy of language rehabilitation with aphasic adults. He concluded at that time that no generalizations to the population of aphasic patients was possible, and urged that future investigations specify the nature of the language problem treated, the objective measurement of relevant behavioral changes, and the nature, intensity, and quality of therapy provided. Darley's article, though over 10 years old, and directed to the effectiveness of treatment with aphasic patients, is applicable today to the treatment of language disorders in adolescents. Essentially no data for the latter population, beyond case studies, are available, however. The nature of the language problems has not been identified, the measurements for change have been gross, and the definitions of treatment inadequate.

The nature of treatment varies greatly across our field. The need for an individualized educational plan for each student suggests that it varies depending on the needs, strengths, and weaknesses of each individual. Yet, variability in approaches far exceeds student differences. It is not possible to include a thorough discussion of treatment in the context of this chapter, but a few of the major issues should be mentioned.

1. **Teaching to the student's weakness vs teaching to the student's strengths.** Teaching to the weaknesses suggests that (a) it is possible to determine the underlying nature of the language problem through diagnostic tests, and (b) remediation techniques are, or can be, effective in eliminating or greatly reducing the underlying problem. One is reminded here of programs designed to increase auditory memory or auditory processing based on the hypothesis that weaknesses in these areas have caused the problem. Two sources (Hammill & Larsen, 1974; Rees, 1981) are especially enlightening on the limited payoff of such approaches.

Teaching to the strengths suggests that (a) it is possible to determine the aspects of language the student handles well; and (b) remediation techniques that capitalize on these strengths will help the student compensate for the weaknesses. Such approaches always start with what the student "can do" and build to higher levels of achievement through progressive *successes*.

2. **Listening and speaking vs listening, speaking, reading, and writing.** The role of the clinician in treatment of reading and writing disorders is not clear. Whether we believe we should, or should not, be involved in the teaching of reading and written language depends heavily on personal philosophies, education, and experiences. For the most part, however, our training institutions are failing to ensure background in the areas of reading and written language.

3. **Syntactic-grammatic emphasis vs conceptual-semantic emphasis.** The ease with which syntax and grammar can be tested and programmed, and the changes documented, has probably resulted in a heavy grammatic emphasis in treatment programs. We know far less about which

concepts precede others in normal development (especially at the older age levels), or how to teach "concepts."

4. Language "brain twisters" vs functional communication. Many language "exercises" have been developed, even though the student rarely has an opportunity to use the new skill. I am reminded of a mother who recently brought her 14-year-old daughter to our clinic for service. This mother desired functional language skills, like answering the phone and taking accurate messages, rather than the learning of what "raining cats and dogs" means, an unusable skill, in her opinion, which the previous clinician had emphasized.

5. Motivation problems. It is a common complaint among clinicians that older students neither want their services nor are motivated for improvement. Furthermore, some say that services at the high-school level are not crucial, because students, once scheduled, do not show up for treatment sessions. All of us have failed at times to relate to and motivate the older student, usually one who has had several years of previous experience in speech-language therapy.

It seems obvious that students who are discouraged because of lack of progress would like to stop what has become a defeating and punishing experience. I have heard students state openly that "Speech therapy has not helped before, why would it help now?" Some have been forced to drill in areas of weakness, which has amplified their feelings of failure. We recently worked with a young college student who had many years of treatment, along with placement in a self-contained learning-disability classroom. For the past six years, he had struggled unsuccessfully to increase his auditory and visual memory span. At the time he entered our clinic, he presented a severe communication problem, including: lack of eye contact even on an occasional basis; a slow monotonous rate of speech, with frequent sentence revisions and interjections; very poor intelligibility, resulting from reduced mouth opening and limited articulatory movements; and no seeming desire to attempt changes. Any confidence he once had as a speaker had apparently been obliterated by inappropriate prior treatment, and the severity of his communication problem had increased rather than decreased.

Most students who truly have a communication disorder *and* hold the belief that speech-language therapy will be beneficial do not have motivation or attendance problems. An approach that I have used with considerable success might be termed the "three-week bargain." It involves a student-clinician agreement to commit themselves to three weeks of effort prior to rejecting the service. The clinician then must target and program for a high level of success on a change that is important to the student, not one that seemingly has no application to his or her life. Students often will discuss changes that *they* would like to make and the clinician might wisely heed their words.

Not all clinicians relate well with older students, just as some fail with preschoolers, and others with adults. Those who work well with adolescents seem to relate in straightforward, honest ways, avoiding false enthusiasm and condensension. Students are treated like adults and the responsibility for change is placed directly with them, not the parents.

It is not possible at this time to document the effectiveness of any of the above treatment approaches from controlled research. Logic, however, suggests that some approaches make more sense than others. If treatment is effective, then those approaches that help an individual student communicate in daily life seem preferable. If treatment is ineffective, why work to perfect skills in verbal exercises like repeating word strings, rearranging words from cut-up written sentences, or defining obscure and rarely used idioms?

Logic also suggests that we capitalize on each student's strengths and use those strengths to compensate as much as possible for weaknesses. For example, students can be encouraged to use short simple sentences effectively, rather than be forced to produce complex and embedded sentences which, for them, are meaningless.

Some clinicians organize the content of their treatment programs almost entirely from classroom curricula. From a logical standpoint, this simple approach seems excellent. It is very easy for them to obtain desk copies of the texts used at various grade levels. Many topics are covered at several intervals throughout the curriculum; for example, state history may be introduced in the fourth grade, and continued in the seventh and tenth grades. Using materials from the lower grade levels may be appropriate with students who do not have the basic concepts on which the new material is based. Content for all language targets (vocabulary, grammar, discourse, verbal explanations, cause-effect relationships, etc.) can be taken from the topics currently being studied in the student's classroom. From my discussions with many school clinicians, it almost seems as if this basic approach to treatment is so obvious that it is often overlooked. We state that language problems interfere with academic success. If so, then it seems advisable to program treatment using content on which academic success will be measured. The lack of normative data on expected competencies also supports use of school curricular materials. Moreover, such materials contain the vocabulary and concepts expected at the various grade levels.

Finally, the issue of teaching various subskills versus teaching directly to the problem needs comment. Perhaps you have heard about the reading teacher who started remediation with the sixth-grader by doing arm muscle exercises to increase his ability to hold a book. I hope we are less ridiculous.

Until we have evidence to the contrary, the shortest, most direct approach to a functional target is preferred.

Summary

From the foregoing discussion, we have seen that research data on adolescent language disorders are limited. Standardized test results from speech-language pathology, psychology, and education were used to describe language skills in older students and adolescents. In the areas of syntax, grammar, and auditory memory, test results indicate little improvement among normally developing students beyond the fifth-grade level. The semantic aspects of language, on the other hand, increase markedly between the fifth and twelfth grades. This increase in vocabulary, abstract concept development, and general knowledge is expected from academic curricula, extended reading, and exposure to many learning experiences. In other areas of language, specifically pragmatics and the social use of language, no normative research data are available to document expected competencies across the adolescent years.

The assessment and treatment of expected competencies with the older, language-impaired student were also discussed. The lack of research greatly hinders our ability to recommend specific procedures or protocols. I have attempted, however, to suggest that we emphasize *functional* communication skills both in assessment and treatment. Such an approach says that if our intervention makes a difference, it will be in those aspects of language the student encounters in daily living. By using content material from classroom curricula, for example, students are exposed to the vocabulary and concepts needed for school achievement—those with which they are likely to be more familiar.

References

Bassett, R.E., Whittington, N. & Staton-Spicer, A. The basics in speaking and listening for high-school graduates: What should be assessed? *Communication Education,* 1978, *27,* 293-303.

The California Achievement Tests. Monterey, CA: CTB/McGraw-Hill, 1977.

Darley, F.L. The efficacy of language rehabilitation in aphasia. *Journal of Speech and Hearing Disorders,* 1972, *37,* 3-21.

Dunn, Lloyd M., & Dunn, Leota M. *Peabody Picture Vocabulary Test—Revised* (Form L). Circle Pines, MN: American Guidance Service, 1981.

Dunn, L.M., & Markwardt, F.C. *Peabody Individualized Achievement Test.* Circle Pines, MN: American Guidance Service, 1970.

Hammill, D.D., Brown, V.L., Larsen, S.C., & Wiederholt, J.L. *Test of Adolescent Language: A Multidimensional Approach to Assessment.* Austin, TX: Services for Professional Educators, 1980.

Hammill, D.D., & Larsen, S.C. The effectiveness of psycholinguistic training. *Exceptional Children,* 1974, *40,* 5-14.

Holland, A. *Communicative abilities in daily living.* Baltimore: University Park Press, 1980.

Jastak, J. *Wide Range Achievement Test.* Wilmington, DE: Charles L. Story, 1946.

Leonard, L.B., Prutting, C., Perozzi, J.A., & Berkley, R.K. Nonstandardized approaches to the assessment of language behaviors. *Asha,* 1978, *20,* 371-397.

Ludlow, C. Recovery from aphasia: A foundation for treatment. In M. Sullivan & M.S. Kommers (Eds.), *Rationale for adult aphasia therapy.* Omaha: University of Nebraska Medical Center, 1977.

McGrady, H.J. Communication disorders in specific learning disabilities. In R.J. Van Hattam (Ed.), *Communication disorders: An introduction.* New York: Macmillan, 1980.

O'Donnell, P.D., Griffin, W.J., & Norris, R.C. Syntax of kindergarten and elementary school children: A transformational analysis. Research Report No. 8. NCTE Committee on Research, 508 S. 6th Street, Champaign, IL, 1967.

Prather, E.M., Breecher, S.V., Stafford, M.L., & Wallace, E.M. *Screening Test of Adolescent Language* (STAL). Seattle: University of Washington Press, 1980.

Prather, E.M., Brenner, A.C., & Hughes, K.S. A mini-screening language test for adolescents. *Language, Speech, and Hearing Services in Schools,* 1981, *12,* 67-73.

Prescott, G.A., Balow, I.H., Hogan, T.P., & Farr, R.C. *Metropolitan Achievement Tests: Survey Battery.* New York: Psychological Corp., 1978.

Rees, N. Saying more than we know: Is auditory processing disorder a meaningful concept? In R. Keith, *Central auditory and language disorders in children.* San Diego: College-Hill Press, 1981.

Semel, E., & Wiig, E. *Clinical Evaluation of Language Function* (CELF). Columbus, OH: Charles E. Merrill, 1980. (a)

Semel, E., & Wiig, E. *Clinial Evaluation of Language Function Advanced Level Screening Test.* Columbus, OH: Charles E. Merrill, 1980. (b)

Simon, C.S. *Communicative competence: A functional-pragmatic approach to language therapy.* Tucson, AZ: Communication Skills Builders, 1979.

Wechsler, D. *Wechsler Intelligence Scale for Children* (WISC). New York: Psychological Corporation, 1949.

Marie Capozzi
Beth Mineo

Nonspeech Language and Communication Systems

The emergence of nonspeech communication as a unique discipline is a recent phenomenon. Although estimates concerning the birth of this discipline vary, it is safe to say that most of the influential developments have occurred in the last decade. The complex and varied needs of the nonspeaking population—those who cannot manage a productive system of spoken language (Schiefelbusch & Hollis, 1980) —require that speech and language clinicians be "renaissance people," knowledgeable not only in all aspects of speech and language development, but also in psychology, child development, physical therapy, occupational therapy, and, to some degree, in engineering, computer science, and design.

This relatively new discipline, once regarded as peddling "gadgetry," is finally gaining the respect and recognition it deserves. The goal of the nonspeech-language interventionist is to facilitate independent communication for nonspeakers of all ages, physical abilities, and cognitive levels. This does not mean that every person will be handed a microprocessor-based system and be expected to say something movingly profound. It does mean that we have at our disposal a wide range of devices—some extremely simple and others employing quite sophisticated technology— and a wealth of information gained from recent research which allows us to provide services that have a lasting impact on our clients.

Professional organizations and a limited number of universities have begun to acknowledge the discipline and its accomplishments. We stress the importance of this chapter's information for all speech and language clinicians—for nonspeakers are found in schools, hospitals, and private clinics. In many instances, the clinician must not only fulfill the typical role, but is often required to serve as the co-ordinator of a transdisciplinary habilitation/rehabilitation team. Although this chapter has application for clinicians working with the entire range of communicatively handicapped persons, its primary focus is the assessment of and subsequent intervention with school-aged children who have not acquired vocal speech due to cognitive delay, and those who cannot functionally communicate via the vocal channel due to neuromuscular involvement, i.e., cerebral palsy, head trauma, or degenerative disease.

We tend to take speech for granted until we are forced to deal with its absence, as in the case of aphasia or debilitating and/or progressive dysarthria. Consider, on the other hand, the child born with so severe a physical disability that he or she is not only precluded from developing speech, but also from motorically manipulating the world. From infancy, the establishment of bonding relationships through feeding, sucking, and vocalizing are disrupted. The physical impairment interferes with the child's ability to "make something happen in his world" (Morris, 1981) by exploration and manipulation of toys and objects through mouthing, kicking, pushing, hitting, etc. Further, severely handicapped children have difficulty evoking vocal and physical feedback from parents and others. Parent interactions which are

> normally warm and rewarding may become situations of frustration and tension for caregivers who are uncomfortable in dealing with the physically handicapped child's erratic, involuntary, and spastic or athetoid reflexive movements. Motor-related handicaps can thus result in social/emotional, interactional, motivational, and communicative handicaps (Harris-Vanderheiden, 1976, p. 235).

As a result of this "experiental deprivation" (Goodenough-Trepagnier & Prather, 1981, p. 323), it is our belief that the conceptual formulations of these children differ from those of normal children, although comprehensive and early intervention to facilitate prelinguistic and linguistic achievement may alter these differences.

Many factors contribute to the decision to augment a child's communication. Primary among these is the inability to speak; other factors, such as physical and cognitive abilities, are vital in determining the type of augmentative system to be prescribed. Decisions about candidate selection and the intervention techniques used in designing and developing a communication system are generally contingent on analyzing the child's linguistic, cognitive, and physical status. Abilities in these areas cover a wide range, and each child presents unique combinations of strengths and weaknesses. For example, at Pioneer Center (a Pittsburgh public school for multiply handicapped children), there is Jennifer, a bright and very social 13-year-old, who has severe cerebral palsy along with cognitive and educational levels that are generally age-appropriate. Diana, another cerebral-palsied nonspeaker, is not only severely motorically and visually impaired, but also is cognitively handicapped. In contrast to these two severely physically handicapped students, Janice has full control over her hands and oral structures, yet fails to be an effective functional communicator due to profound mental retardation.

The purpose of this chapter is to: (1) describe the assessment procedures vital for determining a nonspeaking child's present level of functioning in both physical and communication realms, (2) review methods of intervention towards the goal of independent communication, and (3) acquaint the reader with trends in the development of communication devices.

Assessment Aspects

Physical Status

The physical assessment evaluates the child's ability to control and coordinate movement patterns. The precision with which these patterns are executed is inversely related to severity of impairment. Children who display minimal motor dysfunction have increased options in selecting and using efficient communication systems. Examples include children whose oral structures may be moderately involved, and whose oral speaking can be characterized as functional in a variety of settings. Other children may not be functional oral speakers, but can maintain efficient-to-adequate control of the upper extremities (hands, fingers), allowing for the development of "signing" systems. The children addressed in this section have physical conditions that result in severe motoric disabilities of the oral channel, thereby precluding the development of independent functional speech. These severely handicapped children are unable to inhibit abnormal reflexes and involuntary muscle action, and to coordinate and control muscle movement patterns necessary for normal communication acquisition.

A transdisciplinary team usually is responsible for assessing the motor functioning of physically handicapped children. Speech pathologists, along with physical and occupational therapists, assess the physical status of the child, and determine muscle function capabilities for using communication and environmental control devices. In addition, physical and occupational therapists are responsible for the child's correct positioning in different situations, i.e., in standing tables, on a prone board, on a mat, in a travel chair, in a wheelchair insert or corner seat. Therapeutic positioning and comfortable seating are essential for purposes of evaluation and training, as they facilitate concentration for learning and reduce fatigue.

The purpose of the physical assessment is to determine an anatomic site at which a controlled behavior can become both functionally reliable and voluntary. This purposeful movement activates an interface (the means by which a user communicates with his device), which in turn acts upon the device (see section on interfaces).

A number of variables must be considered when evaluating the adequacy of a particular anatomic site (hand, head, foot, etc.). These factors are delineated in Table 7-1.

Because they are the most natural sites for interfacing with a device, the hands and fingers are generally assessed first in a physical evaluation. Children with neuromuscular disabilities who exhibit limited range of motion, inability to cross midline, or abnormal reflex patterns are often precluded from exercising certain manual movements.

Although the head is often considered as an interface site before other body parts, a thorough evaluation of hand, finger, and foot control is warranted. If a reliable control site can be discovered from among these body parts, then the head and eyes can remain unencumbered. In turn, this freedom from unnatural attachments, such as head and chin pointers, allows for more natural communication via eye gaze and facial expression, vital elements in human nonverbal communication.

The foot is often overlooked or underrated as an interface site. Not only can the foot often be reliably controlled, but it may also be trained to activate as many as 225 different switch positions by slight alterations of its orientation in space (Eulenberg, 1982). A seemingly unrefined foot movement may become quite purposeful by virtue of a simple modification in the foot's elevation or attitude.

When evaluation of the extremities fails to reveal reliable voluntary control, the head and neck must then be considered as possible interface sites. Assessment of these anatomic sites involves, as did the others, an evaluation of movement range, resolution and control, force and endurance.

Speech and Language
Cognitive Prerequisites to Language

Cognition is defined as the mediation and organization of thought, perceptions, and experiences, and the product of these processes. Our cognitive "stockpiles" increase as we experience meaningful interactions

Table 7-1
Factors to consider when evaluating accuracy of motion.

1.	*Range of Motion*	Maximal distance of body motion sweeping across the vertical and horizontal plane. Data are generally obtained from a zero reference point, the position at rest (Coleman, Cook, & Meyers, 1980).
2.	*Resolution of Motion*	Minimal movement that can be reliably and accurately executed (Coleman et al., 1980).
3.	*Force*	Amount of pressure exerted by a given body part.
		Measurement can be obtained by using a calibrated strain-gauge bridge (Coleman et al., 1980) or by using commercial switches that are pregauged and have a narrow range of adjustment capability.
4.	*Control*	Consistency and reliability of voluntary motion for a given body site.
		Data on speed, accuracy, and reliability of purposeful movement can be obtained by using a stop watch or establishing criteria trials.
		The presence of abnormal reflexes, spasticity, and tremors may compromise speed and accuracy, and require adjustment in switch location.
5.	*Endurance*	Duration of optimum level of functioning for a given body site, i.e., the length of time a child can execute a particular movement before fatigue occurs.

with our environment. These interactions occur through observation, and both mental and motoric manipulation of events, objects, and ideas. Normally developing children independently and frequently conduct these manipulations; handicapped children, due to physical and/or intellectual impairment, often cannot proceed beyond rudimentary cognitive levels without outside intervention.

The responsibility of the "interventionists"—parents, teachers, speech pathologists, and others—is to see that the child receives the greatest possible exposure to various environments, and, if necessary, to help him or her to see relationships and develop concepts. Many researchers believe that linguistic achievement depends on the acquisition of certain cognitive prerequisites, although their acquisition in and of itself is not the only determining factor (Bloom, 1970; Bowerman, 1974; Chapman & Miller, 1980; Cromer, 1974). Among the necessary prelinguistic processes are visual tracking and visual search, object permanence, means-end relationships, objective causality, imitation, functional classification of objects, functional object grouping, and seriation (Bricker & Bricker, 1974).

Although their conceptual development may be qualitatively different from normal acquisition, physically and/or mentally handicapped children are required to communicate with normal speakers using conventional language structure and strategies. Therefore, the child's level of proficiency in understanding and using "normal" language must be evaluated.

Prelinguistic abilities are actually cognitive abilities achieved as children interact with and, thereby, learn to understand their environment. These abilities may be evaluated by observing children in interaction with their surroundings, noting their expectancies and intentions, and monitoring the purposiveness of their actions. Their physical handicaps may require that the environment be modified to allow them to act upon it. For example, only after children begin to understand the causal relationships between themselves and their surroundings are they prepared to apply the concept of causality to language. They observe relationships between words and actions, and come to realize that actions or vocalizations effect an environmental change.

True linguistic operations include: "yes/no" responding; representation of objects, ideas, and feelings via vocalization, pictures, or more abstract symbols; and combinations of these representations into acceptable structures. Nonspeakers' abilities in these areas are evaluated by both conventional and nonconventional means.

A major consideration in naturalistic assessment is the child's preferred mode of response. By definition, the nonspeaker does not or cannot functionally utilize the oral musculature for verbal communication; therefore, responses must be channelled through other modalities. Evaluation of affirmation/negation ability may reveal a "yes" response to be a traditional head nod, or no more than a brief upward eye gaze. Regardless of the method used to communicate, the most important considerations are the consistency and appropriateness of the response.

The child's ability to identify objects and indicate choices can be evaluated by presenting him or her with an array of objects or pictures, and instructing the child to choose among them. Having determined the child's physical capabilities as well as limitations, the array may be modified to correspond to his or her response mode. This may necessitate transferring the display to an augmentative device.

In terms of production, the child functions at a holophrastic (one-word) level when he or she can consistently choose one item from an array. Expansion and diversification of the array's vocabulary permit word combinations, allowing the user to communicate with more grammatically advanced structures. Evaluation of the progression from one-word to multiword utterances involves manipulation of the number of selections presented, the various word classes, and the degree of complexity and abstractness of the representations.

These prelinguistic and linguistic categories are broad parameters of the speech/language assessment. More detailed information regarding specific areas may be gained through use of commercially available language-evaluation materials, again modfied to suit the child's response mode. Of equal importance is identification of those sensory channels most efficient and effective for each individual. With the accumulated information regarding the child's speech and language, physical and cognitive capabilities, the process of identifying appropriate augmentative systems continues.

Communication Systems

Augmentative communication refers to any system employed to enhance the communicative effectiveness of a message-sender. The system used may reflect the user's language or may introduce a new way of expressing ideas. The range of systems available for communication enhancement falls into three major categories: gestural systems, language boards, and electronic devices. These categories, as will be shown, are not mutually exclusive.

Providing the appropriate augmentative system involves much more than the introduction of a device. It also requires:

1.   Determination of the appropriate semantic-transfer system;
2.   Thorough instruction in the capabilities and limitations of the system;

3. Continued training and practice with the system; and
4. On-going re-evaluation of the system's effectiveness.

Gestural Systems

Gestural systems include manual sign languages, pantomine, yes/no indications, eye blink encoding, gestural Morse code, pointing, and other formalized and informal gesture systems (Silverman, 1980). Manual sign language systems, among which are Signed English, Standard, American Indian, American Sign Language, and Rochester systems, have continued to be applied as augmentative modes. The various systems differ in their iconicity and their similarity to the syntax of spoken English. To detail these variations would exceed the scope of this chapter; excellent references in this area include texts by Wilbur (1979) and Klima and Bellugi (1979). Silverman (1980) describes both the sign language systems and other gestural modes.

Manual sign language as an augmentative system is limited by the degree of physical coordination necessary for its use. Signs may be modified to require use of only one hand and to necessitate fewer discrete movements. These concessions notwithstanding, a major difficulty remains—gestures are effective as an expressive mode only as long as they are decoded correctly. The person relying solely on a gestural system will suffer from the effects of a pervasive language barrier in a real-world situation, not unlike the tourist in a foreign country whose knowledge of the native tongue is limited to words for "bathroom" and "How much is it?"

Language Boards

The second type of system involves use of language boards, which assume many forms and employ a wide variety of semantic-transfer systems. Language boards are usually two-dimensional arrangements of visually represented objects and ideas from which the user selects his choice. Language boards may be mounted on wheelchair trays or folders, attached to ambulation equipment or furniture, or worn on the user's body. On nonelectronic language boards, lexical choices are indicated primarily by direct selection; this, and other methods of selection will be discussed later in the chapter.

Language boards may employ a variety of semantic-transfer systems. "Semantic-transfer system" means a system for communicating meaning from a sender to a receiver. An all-encompassing term such as this is necessary for describing all levels of units found in a communication system.

A symbol, according to Silverman (1980), is a sensory (visual, auditory, or tactile) image, or sign, that suggests, or stands for, something else by reason of relationship (association) or convention. The most common symbols are our alphabet and number systems; despite their frequent use, they are among the most complex symbolic possibilities for use on a language board. More basic systems involve use of drawings at various levels of cognitive complexity. To clarify this issue, try the following exercise:

Read each statement and imagine the object or symbol described.
See if you can visualize the progression from concrete to abstract.

A life-size red rose

A minature red rose

A full-size color photograph of a red rose

A scaled-down color photograph of a red rose

A colored line drawing of a red rose

A black and white drawing of a red rose

A stylized rendition of a red rose

What you just encountered was a hierarchical arrangement based on level of abstraction. Silverman (1980) states, "The *level of abstraction* of a picture is a function of the amount of detail (or information) present in the object or event depicted that is included in the picture. The more detail (or information) omitted, the higher the level of abstraction (p. 9)."

Level of abstraction is an important consideration when designing a board for a cognitively impaired person. The cognitive prerequisites to language discussed earlier are necessary for symbolization (allowing one unit to represent another). If this cognitive/linguistic milestone has not been reached, the child will not be able to conceptualize the derivation of the symbol from its referent. These same symbols may still be taught, yet in a remedial manner (Guess, Sailor, & Baer, 1974). In addition to the level of abstraction, it is necessary to consider other dimensions in the creation of a language board, including degree of complexity, degree of ambiguity, size, and the number of messages that can be encoded (Silverman, 1980).

By degree of complexity we mean the "busy-ness" of the symbol. For instance, a representation of "Mom" would be better expressed by a simple picture of the child's mother against a plain background than a picture of Mother, dressed in her Easter finery, posed with the family in front of a blossoming cherry tree.

The latter image is also useful in our illustration of degree of ambiguity; the photograph described could be used to represent Mom, family, springtime, Easter, standing, tree, and so on; in other words, it is ambiguous.

One aim in determining units for a language board is to reduce the degree of complexity. We concur with Silverman (1980) that "reducing complexity is one way of reducing ambiguity" (p. 90).

Picture size is a major consideration in designing a language board. Not only is size related to level of abstraction, but it is a crucial factor in regard to the user's visual abilities. Many small pictures grouped closely together necessitate not only finer visual discriminations, but also adequate figure-ground manipulation (i.e., singling out the desired picture from the background of the entire display).

It is also necessary to consider the number of messages that can be encoded with the chosen "vocabulary." Central to this determination are the child's level of functioning, and his environmental and educational needs. For the cognitively impaired, functional communication might best be facilitated by a language board picturing immediate environmental needs (cup, dish, toilet, etc). The more linguistically advanced will need to communicate basic needs as well as more complex ideas. One educational goal might be to foster correct sentence structure by the use of a language board. In this case, verbs and functor words would be included in the display.

Decisions regarding symbol inclusion are often difficult. Silverman (1980) suggests the following guideline: "The smallest set of pictures should be selected by which necessary messages can be encoded" (p. 90). McDonald and Schultz (1973) propose a complementary solution: The child should have different boards for different situations (home, classrooms, etc.).

The "rose" exercise presented earlier illustrated the levels of abstraction found in symbolic representation. Recall the most abstract version of the rose—of all the possibilities, this depiction has the least resemblance to the actual rose. It is this type of graphic representation that we shall next discuss.

Pictures are a very basic form of representation. Even more basic would be actual objects representing other objects (doll shoe for child's shoe). More complex than either of these options would be symbols that bear less, little, or no resemblance to their referents. This more complex type of symbol will first be generally addressed, and a review of some semantic-transfer systems currently in use for augmentative purposes will follow.

Symbols function at three levels of complexity, which have been described by Shane and Blau (1981). The first, in which the idea or object is clearly depicted at a concrete level, is known as the *pictographic*, or iconic level. Pictures and picture-like drawings fit into this category. A more complex level is the *ideographic*, or relational, symbol; in this case, the user must decipher the meaning from the symbol or combination of symbols presented to him. At this level, the symbol does not directly resemble its referent; however, prior explanation of the symbol's relation to the referent, or familiarity with the symbol's components, allows the user to derive meaning from it (see the Blissymbol examples that follow). The third level is the *arbitrary* level, at which the symbol has no discernible relationship to its referent. The written word is an example of this third level of complexity. These symbolic levels will become more clearly delineated as examples of each are encountered in the following discussion of symbol systems.

Blissymbolics is a symbol system originally devised for international, translinguistic communication by Charles Bliss (1965). Based on Chinese-type ideographic symbols, it is semantically based and relates to no specific language. Although Blissymbolics has not been widely accepted for its original purpose, it has found application as a semantic-transfer system for handicapped children (Archer, 1977; Carlson, 1976; Harris-Vanderheiden, 1976; Silverman, McNaughton & Kates, 1978), for it serves as a bridge between pictures and the written word.

The Blissymbol system contains approximately 100 basic symbols which, alone or in combination, can represent a surprisingly large number of ideas. In addition to representing objects and ideas, the symbols encode tense, inflection, and other grammatical indicators. Manipulation of the basic symbols along the dimensions of size, combination, and relative placement allow for almost limitless expression. All three levels of complexity (pictographic, ideographic, and arbitrary) are represented in this system.

○ represents "eye"

⌒ represents "car"

⌁ represents "electricity"

□ represents "thing"

Thus, combining them, □○⌒⌁ represents television, i.e., a thing run on electricity which we can see and hear.

Such symbols, when paired with various grammatical class indicators, take on different, yet related, meanings.

□ denotes a noun

∧ denotes a verb

∨ denotes an adjective

⌒ represents "ear"

⌒ represents "to hear"

⌒ represents "auditory"

These isolated examples are not intended to provide a lesson in Blissymbolics, but rather to illustrate its fascinating workings. A summary of the system is provided by Silverman (1980), and the Blissymbolics Communication Institute (Toronto) publishes many materials, including the *Handbook of Blissymbolics for Instructors, Users, Parents and Administrators* (Silverman et al. 1978).

While Blissymbolics are international in nature, the Rebus system employs English vocabulary and phonology. Rebus symbols are primarily pictographic, but the pictures themselves are often combined with English phonemes or morphemes represented orthographically.

Rebuses are used to teach reading (Woodcock, 1958, 1965, 1968; Woodcock, Clark, & Davies, 1968, 1969) and facilitate language acquisition (Clark, Moores, & Woodcock, 1973), as well as serve as a semantic-transfer system on an augmentative device.

Another symbol system emerged from the Premacks' investigation of a chimpanzee's ability to learn human language (Premack, 1970, 1971; Premack & Premack, 1972, 1974). As the semantic-transfer system in these experiments, pieces of plastic, arbitrary in their design, were used. This system was applied to individuals who were unable to manipulate other types of linguistic units (Carrier & Peak, 1975). They developed the *Non-Speech Language Initiation Program (Non-SLIP)* to provide a "very carefully structured, finely graded, set of procedures for starting children through the process of learning communication skills" (Carrier & Peak, 1975, p. 10). Its primary use has been in teaching the basics of symbolic representation (Silverman, 1980).

As noted previously, alphabet and numbers are the semantic-transfer systems most apparent in our daily encounters. These systems may be represented in various configurations on a language board, such as:

1.   an ordered alphanumeric line (A,B,C. . .and 1, 2, 3. . .);

2.   placement based on frequency of occurrence; or

3.   placement based on correspondence to the typewriter keyboard (referred to as "qwerty" in reference to the first six keys on the conventional keyboard's top alphabet row).

Morse code takes symbolization one step beyond the alphabet by requiring further symbolization of an already arbitrary system. Although Morse code can be represented visually (- . . , - . -), it is primarily an auditory system in which alphabet letters are encoded by sequences of long and short bursts of sound. Application of technology to augmentative systems has allowed Morse code to become a viable semantic-transfer system for handicapped users.

The symbol systems described previously are by no means the only ones in use on language boards. Items for inclusion on a board are often chosen from the child's personal lexicon. For example, pictures or drawings of the child's toys can be represented on the board in place of a generic representation of "toy." These familiar items are not only the most

FIGURE 7-1
Rebus symbols.

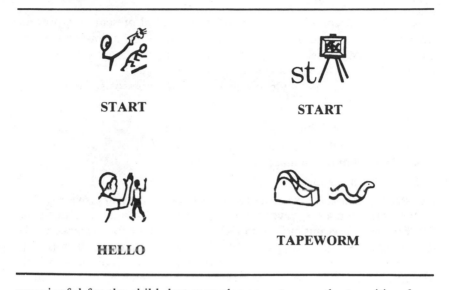

START	START
HELLO	TAPEWORM

meaningful for the child, but may also serve to ease the transition from one communication system to another.

Selection Modes

The use of electronic communication devices requires speech and language therapists to learn a few new terms and concepts if they are judiciously to choose the appropriate device for a given child. In this section, we will discuss these concepts, beginning with selection mode. "Selection mode" refers to the general means by which a user gets to (or "accesses") his semantic-transfer system. Thus, selection modes represent the various ways a child can access his vocabulary. The two types of selection modes are direct selection and scanning. The choice of one mode over the other depends on the child's physical and cognitive abilities; the primary difference between them is speed of communication.

The first of these modes, direct selection, is precisely that: the user directly indicates his chosen item on a display. Shane and Blau (1981) state that direct selection can be achieved by the use of:

1. an extremity (fist, elbow, finger, toe, etc.);
2. an extremity plus __ (splinted hand, hand-held pointer);
3. the eyes (directed gaze);

4. a rod (head or chin pointer, etc.); and

5. a light beam (mounted on body or held in hand or mouth).

Scanning is accomplished by halting a sequential presentation process when the desired choice is reached. Scanning is generally a slower and more complex mode of selection because the user must contend with the undesired choices as well as the desired ones.

Shane and Blau (1981) identified the various types of scanning as:

1. assisted scanning;

2. stepped scanning;

3. linear scanning;

4. row-column scanning; and

5. directed scanning.

Assisted scanning occurs when the user is required only to provide replies of the "affirmative/negative" type to a series of choices. A student at Pioneer Center uses this method to spell messages in the following way: (1) the child's communication partner determines if the message begins with a consonant or a vowel; (2) if it is a consonant, the child indicates in which half of the alphabet it occurs; and (3) letters are presented until the child indicates that his chosen letter has been reached with an upward eye movement indicating "yes."

The other four types of scanning are typically encountered when using electronic devices. At the risk of jumping ahead too quickly, Figure 7-2 shows a grid typical of those found on scanning devices to illustrate these other variations.

Stepped scanning requires the user to proceed one-at-a-time through the various selections. To reach the number 10 by stepped scanning, the user moves the indicator light (in the upper left corner of each cell) from 1 to 2, 2 to 3, and so on until he reaches 10. This requires 9 activations of the scanner.

Linear scanning also proceeds through all the selections before the desired one is reached, the difference being that it does not require an activation for each step. To access the number 10 requires 2 activations—one to begin the scan and one to stop it when it reaches the number 10. Although this method requires fewer activations, both the stepped and linear scanning methods share the drawback of the relatively long period of time required to scan every cell.

Row-column scanning somewhat alleviates this problem by scanning rows (on the horizontal axis) and columns (on the vertical axis), rather than individual cells. In this mode, all the lights in Row 1 glow first. The desired

FIGURE 7-2
Scanning device grid.

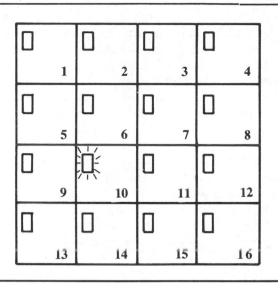

selection being in Row 3, the device continues scanning, next lighting up Row 2 and then Row 3, at which point the user indicates the row of choice by an activation of some kind. The device then begins scanning columns, proceeding from left to right. The scan stops at the second column, at which an activation lights up the number 10. This process requires three more activations than does linear scanning, yet is more efficient in terms of time.

Directed scanning occurs when the user communicates to the device the direction and amplitude of the scan. To access the number 10 in this mode, the user directs the device, using a joystick (the control stick similar to those found on many arcade games) to go over one column and down three rows. This requires more controlled movements on the part of the user, but markedly increases efficiency of communication. To further improve the rate of communication, these various scanning methods may be combined and modified in accordance with the user's needs.

Some approaches to nonspeech communication mention a third selection mode known as encoding. This technique employs coded information, selected either directly or by scanning, to access a larger lexicon. For instance, a student's language board may have expanded to include 500 items, yet the child lacks the range of motion necessary for direct selection over such a large area. As a solution, the rows may be labelled with alphabet letters and the columns with numbers, allowing the child to "encode" his choice by indicating the letter and number corresponding to his selection. Rather than consider encoding to be a third type of selection mode, we believe that it is more aptly termed a cognitive strategy (Shane & Blau, 1981), for it involves cognitive manipulation of predetermined codes, which are subsequently selected either directly or by scanning.

These selection modes—direct selection, scanning, and their related cognitive strategies—are the means by which the user accesses his semantic-transfer system. We will now turn our attention to the communication between the user and the device, and a new concept.

Interfaces

Knowledge of the child's physical, cognitive, and speech and language abilities is the prerequisite for making an informed choice regarding an augmentative communication device. The results of the physical assessment are particularly relevant, because they determine the type and placement of the chosen interface. An interface is the means by which the user communicates with his device, that is, how he makes his system work. Physically able persons use interfaces, too—consider remote-controlled televisions, light switches, and automatic garage-door openers. A requirement of all effective interfaces is that they be responsive to the capabilities of their user (Coleman et al., 1980). Figure 7-3 illustrates a variety of interfaces currently in use.

When choosing an interface, it is helpful to evaluate several switches at more than one anatomic site. The initial physical assessment serves as a good starting point, for it provides information as to the sites with most reliable control. Ongoing assessment of this type is also vital, because control may be trained and refined through practice. Evaluation of interfaces should entail quantification, as this allows for objective decision-making regarding final site/interface selection. Barker and Hastings (1981) suggest as the two major factors in this assessment, *tracking / select time* and *accuracy.* The first of these refers to the amount of time required for the user to move from a resting position to activation of the interface (tracking time), or from one aspect of the interface to another (select time). A temporal measurement in and of itself carries little meaning, unless it is accompanied by some indication of the appropriateness of the response; thus, an accuracy measure, when paired with a time measure, provides a more complete indication of the functionality of the site/interface match. It may be the case that one of these factors takes precedence over the other; for instance, when given the choice between a fast, yet inaccurate, interface site and a slower, more accurate one, the decision usually favors the latter option.

FIGURE 7-3
Zygo interfaces for "single switch" users.

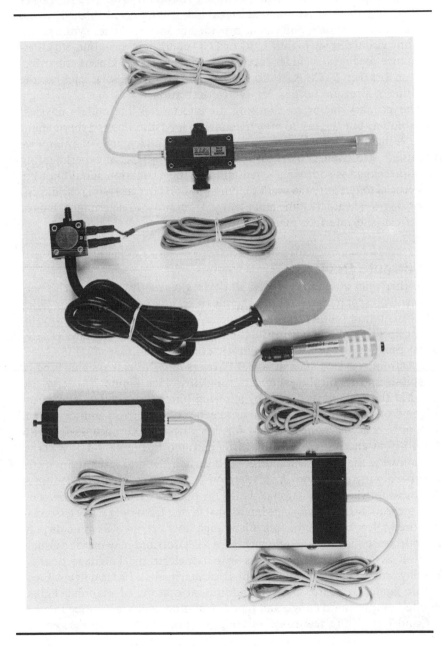

If one is to select an adequate interface, it is also important to consider the amount and type of feedback the child requires. Interfaces provide both environmental and performance feedback (Barker & Cook, 1981; Barker & Hastings, 1981). Environmental feedback is conducted through visual and auditory channels, and can be provided by buzzers, voice synthesizers, and any visual display (lights, LED or LCD characters, printout, etc.). Performance feedback includes tactile, proprioceptive, or kinesthetic information (Barker & Cook, 1981; Barker & Hastings, 1981), such as the amount of pressure needed for switch activation.

The primary factor in choosing an interface is the child's physical capabilities, but the key to effective interface positioning is experimentation. A slight variation in the switch's height or attitude (angle) may improve the user's effectiveness markedly. Although the process of experimenting with placement is somewhat serendipitous, the evaluation should not be; it is crucial to quantify the user's abilities (and preferences) along the dimensions discussed earlier—time and accuracy— in order to determine the most beneficial site/interface match.

Electronic Devices

Rather than attempt to review all devices currently available, this section will present a representative sample of commercial devices. The order of presentation follows the developmental hierarchy discussed previously in the speech and language evaluation section; the following devices augment prelinguistic as well as linguistic communication.

Electronic devices, such as signal boxes (similar to call-systems used in hospitals and on airplanes) and adapted toys (See Figure 7-4) serve the child at the prelinguisitc stage by allowing him to manipulate and effect his environment. "Yes/no" responses may be coded with an auditory signal box or by a device made expressly for this purpose. One such device, with both visual and auditory feedback, is pictured in Figure 7-5.

Following the progression introduced earlier, the next level of linguistic complexity involves choosing a selection from an array; this procedure is the basis for the introduction of language boards. Electronic devices may also serve as a sort of language board, displaying from only a few to several hundred selections. Converting a language board to an electronic display may decrease the motor requirements for selection and may provide visual, as well as auditory feedback. As with nonelectronic language boards, displays are primarily two-dimensional arrangements of lexical items. Electronic language boards have the additional options of scanning lights, printed output (hard copy), and taped or synthesized speech (See Figures 7-6 and 7-7). With a few exceptions (e.g., Prentke Romich Express systems

FIGURE 7-4
Toys.

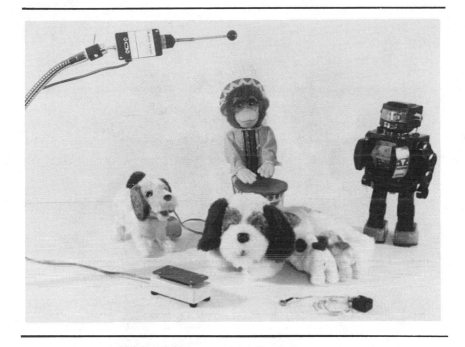

and Phonic Ear Vois 140), electronic language boards are designed to respond to only one selection mode, be it scanning or direct selection. These boards may employ any complexity level of semantic-transfer units, from photographs to words to the alphanumeric components of our language.

Keyboard instruments, on the other hand, rely strictly on alphanumeric characters for message coding. Modifications have been designed to accommodate the user's sensory and physical limitations. Keyboards are expanded (i.e., the keys are distributed over a larger area) to aid the person with poorly defined fine-motor movements; for those with limited range of motion, such as the inability to cross midline, keyboards may be reduced in size. Keyguards (see Figure 7-8) are designed for securing placement of the key selector (e.g., hand, chin, or head pointer). Figure 7-9 illustrates keyboards with liquid crystal (LCD) and light-emitting diode (LED) displays for providing visual feedback.

Microcomputers are another kind of keyboard instrument, but, unlike conventional keyboard devices, microprocessor-based systems have memory, storage, and programming capabilities. They may serve as aids for oral and

FIGURE 7-5
Zygo model 20 2-light choice indicator.

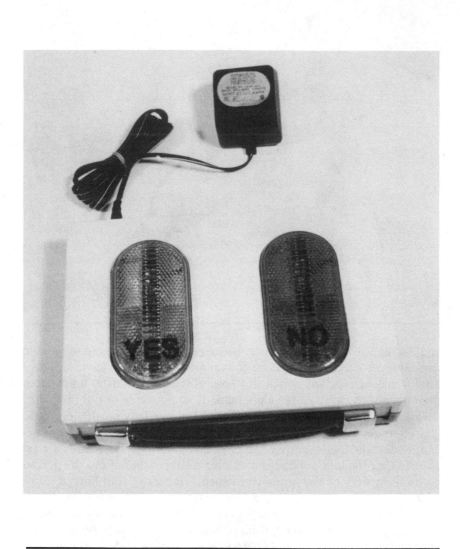

written communication, education, entertainment, and vocations. As with other systems, one of the primary problems our students encounter is that of access (interface) to the device. Resolution of access problems will

FIGURE 7-6
Zygo model 16 electronic communication system.

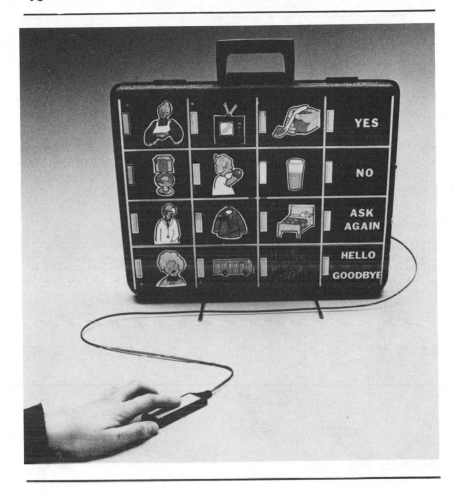

convert potential application of microprocessor-based systems into realities (Nelson et al., 1980).

The basic components of microcomputer devices are the hardware and software elements. "Hardware" refers to the actual machinery, i.e., the mechanical and electrical parts of the system. The significant part of the hardware is the silicon chip, smaller than a fingernail, which controls the "software" by completing the instruction of the software specifies. Thus, the software component refers simply to a set of instructions to make the machinery respond to the user's directives. The following paragraphs will

FIGURE 7-7
Zygo model 100 with model 2016 — display/printer.

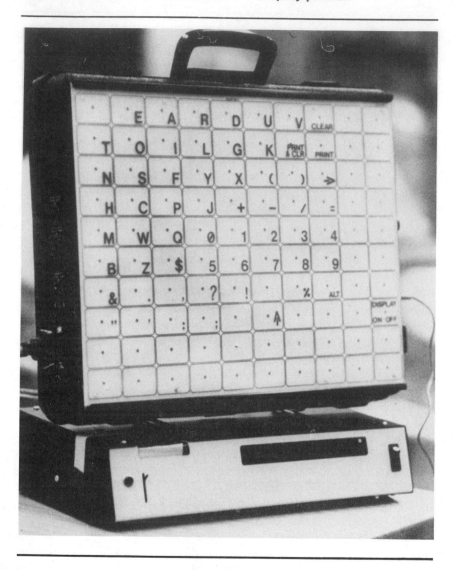

address two types of microcomputer devices as these systems apply to nonspeaking physically handicapped children.

Figure 7-10 illustrates the type of microprocessor-based devices which have preprogrammed lexicons of phrases, letters and phonemes. These

FIGURE 7-8
Canon Communicator with keyguard.

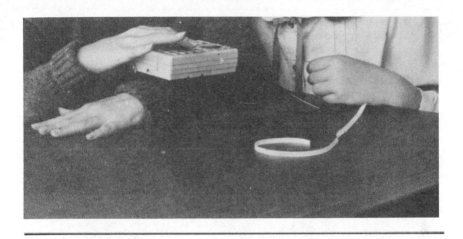

portable systems have memory capability, visual display (LED and LCD), and offer vocal and/or hard copy (printed) output. The devices shown in Figures 7-10 through 7-12 illustrate instruments that have preprogrammed lexicons, as well as capability to allow the user to program a personalized vocabulary, to control environmental operations of powered wheelchairs, appliances, lights, radios, tape recorders, etc., to select printed versus visual versus vocal output, and to interconnect to a general purpose computer. The Semantically Accessible Language Board (SAL) displayed in Figure 7-12 utilizes the basic elements of other systems previously mentioned, with additional software components such as "text-to-speech" capability. This allows for a synthetic speech production of a printed input; for example, selection of the keys C-H-R-I-S results in the synthesized articulation of "Chris."

Some students are able to use ready-made over-the-counter general purpose microcomputers rather than customized instruments. These popular systems, such as the Apple and TRS-80, are flexible, "portable," and moderately prices in a highly competitive market, and offer increased availability of educational and recreational software. Several manufacturers have so miniaturized the entire microcomputer system that "pocket" computers are now readily available and affordable. These small versions permit increased portability, while retaining the majority of the features of their larger counterparts.

FIGURE 7-9
Sharp Memowriter and VIP Communicator.

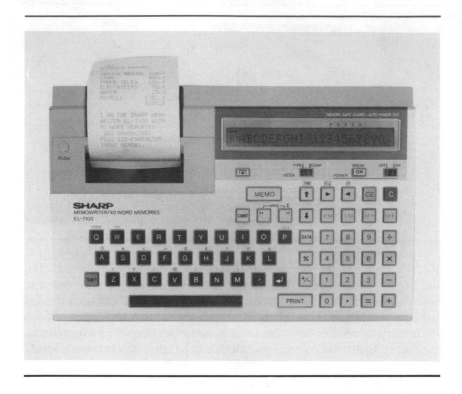

Some general examples of microcomputer applications are:

1. storage and retrieval of information;
2. text editing of oral annd written communication;
3. composition of oral and written communication;
4. operation of common environmental appliances; and
5. provision of computer-assisted instruction for educational, vocational, and personal purposes (Rogers, Fine, Kuhlemeir, & Bowen, 1980).

Although microcomputers are traditionally direct-selection devices, minimal hardware and/or software modifications render these devices responsive to scanning techniques and encoded input (Morse code, etc.). A microcomputer's inherent flexibility enables the device to be modified as the user's physical and cognitive skills develop beyond the scope of his current system (Heckathorne, Doubler, & Childress, 1980).

FIGURE 7-10
Phonic Ear Vois 130 and Phonic Ear Vois 140.

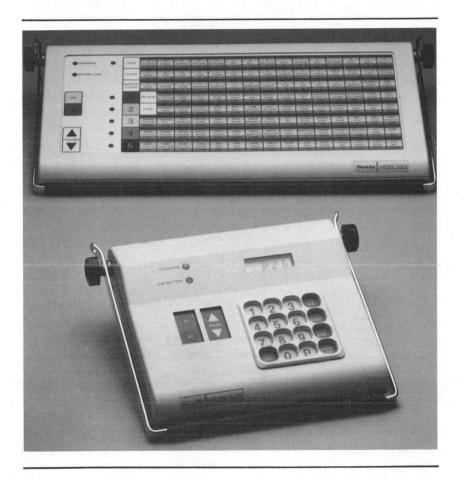

Case Histories

We have previously charted the course to follow when matching an augmentative device to a nonspeaker's needs. The procedure entails first assessing the child's abilities, the device's or system's capability, and then employing this information to interface the child to the device. To better illustrate this process, case histories of three children are pertinent. All of the students attend Pioneer Center and have been mentioned earlier in this chapter.

FIGURE 7-11
Prentke Romich Express 3.

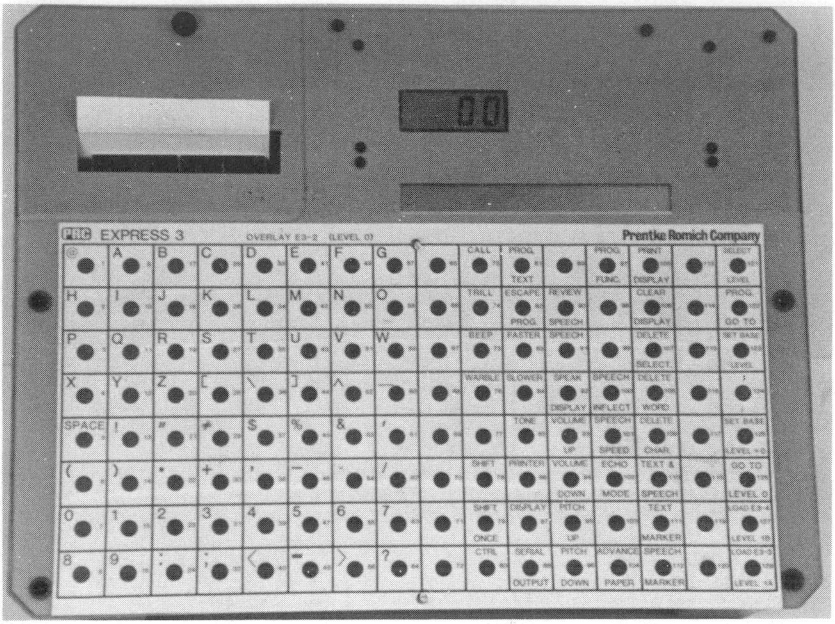

Diana (10 years old) is severely cerebral-palsied, visually impaired and mentally retarded. Her extreme physical disability prohibits not only functional oral communication, but also fine motor coordination. Gross motor movements are characterized by extension and spasticity. Results obtained from structured observations and informal assessment suggest that Diana is functioning at a prelinguistic level. She does not visually track, and is only now achieving the concept of causality. Although she sometimes indicates affirmation by an "eyes up" motion, this response is not consistent.

Physical assessment suggests that getting Diana interfaced to a simple switch is a difficult task, as she exhibits little reliable voluntary movement. Various anatomic sites and switches have been considered, and, at the present time, she is using a tread switch with performance and environmental feedback at her hand to access a tape recorder and toys. Seating modifications designed to minimize the effects of her spasticity include securing her in a corner seat to maintain midline arm postures and shoulder

FIGURE 7-12
Semantically Accessible Language (SAL) board.

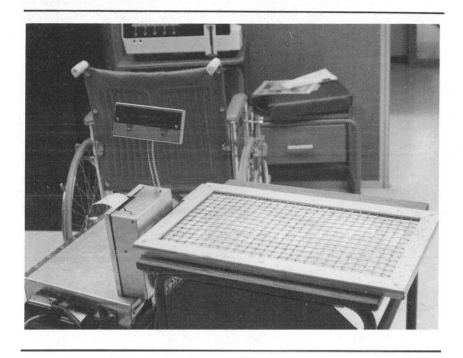

alignments, supporting her trunk with a vest, and stabilizing her free arm. Afforded opportunities to explore the function of the switch, Diana observed that its activation resulted in a pleasurable event (hearing music or voices on tape). Through repeated practice, she has begun to establish a cause-and-effect relationship between these two events. Establishment of this relationship is a vital step on the language acquisition hierarchy.

Janice (age 14), on the other hand, has progressed beyond prelinguistic behaviors to meaningful use of a limited number of language units. She has many physical problems (repaired cleft palate, Down's syndrome, arthrogryposis); until recently, her physical problems precluded walking. However, her hands and oral structures are physically capable of the activity necessary for communication. The hindrance to language development is Janice's low cognitive ability, but her increasing age makes the need for a functional method of communication all the more urgent.

Janice lacks the motivation to learn language because she seems to be unaware of the power that language wields. Therapeutic goals focus on providing Janice with a taste of communication's potency in the belief that once she experiences it, language will become naturally reinforcing.

To this end, Janice was first introduced to different augmentative devices in the hope that their novelty would spark interest and experimentation. A language board "notebook" was provided as well as a language board on her walker; a simple scanner and an eye-gaze system were also introduced. Janice's interest in these systems was short-lived, possibly because she failed to comprehend the communicative potential of her new "toys."

Attention was redirected to Janice's own communicators—her hands and mouth. Her language at this point was primarily nonfunctional, comprised of unrefined gestures, babbling, and some sterotypical phrases. Efforts were concentrated on helping Janice to see that her behaviors could exert control over her world. To this end, manual signs representing functional concepts such as "open, " "put in, " and "sleep" were modeled, shaped, prompted, and reinforced. This approach has proven successful and continues to be implemented in Janice's communication program.

Jennifer (13 years old) is extremely motivated and independently "explores" strategies to augment her communication. She is severely physically impaired due to cerebral palsy and requires total assistance for basic living functions. Although spelling and comprehension of spoken language are appropriate for her age and grade level, her academic performance in reading and arithmetic is not.

Physical assessment revealed the absence of any natural voluntary hand or foot movement for executing purposeful control. Seated and posture-stabilized, Jennifer directly accessed language boards and keyboard devices. Her experiences with these systems—Micon, HandiVoice 120 and typewriter keyboard—were at best frustrating compromises. Speed and accuracy, necessary in interaction, were virtually nonexistent.

Preferring to have her eyes and head free to explore her world, Jennifer refused to use obtrusive head or chin pointers, as well as electronic scanning instruments. However, her positive experiences with an unobtrusive small headlight pointer modified these attitudes. Available on her wheelchair tray is a 7 × 6 language board matrix displaying the alphabet, key words, phrases, and syllables. Her transmission of information is presently limited by her receiver's abilities to read and synthesize the selections at her rate of output, and the absence of voice and paper printout.

Currently these problems are tentatively resolved. Using a microcomputer with a customized interface which accepts the headlight input, Jennifer generates and transmits information. The continued availability of the relatively inexpensive microcomputer instruments will provide Jennifer educational, recreational, and vocational opportunities.

Recent Trends

Hardware

The gap between nonspeakers and their vocal counterparts has narrowed in the past decade, due to the application of technology in the area of augmentative communication. Unfortunately, most nonspeech communication continues to lack the speed and flexibility of normal interactions. Clinical applications have indicated that the most efficient and effective means of alleviating this problem is not through introduction of individual customized devices, but through modifications to readily available general purpose computers (GPCs), such as those made by Radio Shack, Atari, Apple, and Texas Instruments.

One GPC may now, by virtue of software and interface options, subsume the role of myriad customized devices. The same unit may serve as a keyboard device, an environmental control system, a scanner, a call system, a printer, and a voice synthesizer. The trend indicates that pocket computers will offer the full capabilities of a microcomputer.

The approach to interfacing is moving toward utilizing more natural movements in the control of devices, and away from requiring the user to adapt to contrived environments. For example, harnessing the voluntary control of Jennifer's head to direct a lightbeam is much less intrusive than subjecting her to an unnatural arm posture for the purpose of accessing a keyboard.

Tapping the intact abilities of nonspeakers is the most natural interfacing strategy. Such vital bodily activities as eye gaze, blood flow, muscular contraction, and even brain waves can be trained through biofeedback techniques to become reliable means by which to control a device (Beal, 1982). Even nonspeech vocal productions may be shaped and employed as a control mode.

Although there are many techniques for monitoring eye gaze, all are based on the observation that eye movement capabilities are generally intact in cerebral-palsied persons (Anderson, 1977; Fincke & O'Leary, 1980). One method used to determine eye position picks up electrical signals from the eye muscles that are amplified, filtered, interpreted and then mediated through a microcomputer for the purpose of controlling various devices (Laefsky & Roemer, 1978).

Other systems monitor eye gaze by detecting the corneal reflection of an infrared light source (Fincke & O'Leary, 1980; Rinard & Rugg, 1978; Rosen & Durkee, 1978). These systems contain computers that determine where the user is looking, relative to a display, by employing data from eye direction and, in some cases, from orientation of the head as determined by ultrasonography.

Other systems employ eye gaze as a sort of joystick control, requiring the user to gaze in one of several specific directions. Combinations of these signals designate various alphanumeric, punctuation, and control symbols via a coded input (Rosen & Durkee, 1978).

Speech recognition is the process by which a microprocessor is controlled through spoken input. Only ten years ago scientists predicted that this century would not see sophisticated applications of the speech-recognition technique (Doddington & Schalk, 1981); 1980s' technology has already proven them wrong. Not only can our machines talk to us via synthetic speech, but we can control them via verbal requests. Voice data entry becomes necessary when: (1) other body parts are occupied or otherwise unable to input data; and (2) the task requires mobility, thereby precluding stationary communication with the computer.

To commend speech recognition as an interface method for nonspeakers seems paradoxical, yet one must bear in mind that a nonspeaker is one for whom speech is a nonfunctional communication mode. This is not to say that a nonspeaker has no vocal output; rather, that his or her vocal productions are generally unintelligible and therefore not useful in reciprocal speech systems.

Speech recognition systems for the functional nonspeaker are programmed to be responsive to whatever consistent vocalizations the user produces. These may range from unintelligible renditions of words to single vowel productions; however, regardless of the level of complexity of production, the vocalization must be consistent to enable the computer to recognize the features by which intentions are classified. As Doddington and Schalk (1981) commented, "Consistency is an elusive goal," and not a problem limited solely to the speaker. Changes in the environment (affecting noise and reverberation) and in microphone placement can contribute to inconsistency (Doddington & Schalk, 1981). These problems are at present being addressed by research (Eulenberg, 1982).

As we attempt to utilize more natural movement in interfacing, the trend is toward maximizing the information that can be gained by a single input, thus minimizing the energy required. Whereas a single switch traditionally permits an all-or-nothing, on/off choice, proportional control allows for gradations of switch inputs. Although proportionally controlled interface systems are primarily used for the operation of wheelchairs, these same principles are being applied to communication devices as well.

Software

Employing innovative interfacing techniques is not the only means by which to make a general purpose computer (GPC) compatible with a user's needs; software design can further simplify and systematize communication via computer. A GPC's greatest attribute is its ability to store and retrieve tremendous amounts of information. When this capacity is fully exploited, the system demands some sort of organizational network to make information retrieval more efficient. This is especially relevant for the physically handicapped user who cannot afford to expend energy in numerous key selections.

Innovative software design is the solution to this problem. One general approach involves revising programs designed to be accessed directly, by making them responsive to selection by scanning. In this way, the user need only input signals to direct the scanning, rather than expend several keystrokes in typing a message. Other software changes may rearrange and/or systematize the information to make selection more efficient. Three examples of these specific modifications to software—chunking, predictive scanning, and layered hierarchies—are detailed below.

The chunking system, developed by Goodenough-Trepagnier and Prather (1979), and based on traditional orthography, employs phoneme sequences, as well as individual alphabet letters, in its semantic transfer system. The sequences were chosen in terms of frequency of occurrence in English, and require the user to activate fewer selections than would be necessary in a purely single-character system. Chunking has application not only to microcomputers (Goodenough-Trepagnier, Goldenburg, & Fried-Oken, 1981) but to nonelectronic language boards as well. Including more phoneme sequences on the display reduces the selection gestures, thus increasing communication rate (Goodenough-Trepagnier & Prather, 1981).

Another time- and effort-saving software design involves prediction of subsequent units from those previously entered. Prediction of this sort works at all linguistic levels—phonetic, morphological, syntactic, and semantic. It is in essence a "most likely to succeed" guessing game, in that the computer decides what letter is most likely to succeed the input "T R E" (Lee, 1982) or what word is most likely to complete the phrases, "The squirrel ran up the __ ." Some programs are designed to expand telegraphic sentences; for instance, the user would input "I go home", and the computer would produce "I am going home" (Hillinger, Fox, & Wilson, 1981).

Predictive scanning was introduced as a solution to the often tedious nature of row-column scanning. In this latter method, the user must wait until his selection is approached by the scanner and has no means by which to "skip over" the undesired selections. Predictive scanning's "dynamic matrix" changes the actual configuration of the letters so that the ones "most likely to succeed" are the easiest and fastest to access (Jones, 1981).

The use of predictive scanning has increased communication speed from 200% to 400% (Jones, 1981).

The final software design method to be discussed is that of hierarchical arrangements of information. These layered hierarchies, or menus, are arranged so that the information contained becomes increasingly specific as the progression through them continues. For instance:

> Selecting VERBS from the main menu yields a menu of verbs in the infinitive form; selection of one of these infinitives yields a sub-menu—a list of conjugations of that verb. When one of these is selected, it is appended to a message. Theoretically, a word list could contain menus to an arbitary degree; however, in practial use, there has never been a need for more than 3 layers of menu (Buus, 1981, p. 132).

Menus may also be based on alphabetization, word frequency, or situational constraints (Campbell and Nieves, 1981).

Permutations and Combinations

Systematic Evaluation

Computers, previously discussed as instructional and communication devices, may also assist in the systematic assessment of a child's abilities. Not only has software been designed to evaluate cognitive and perceptual abilities, but microprocessor-based systems have been devised to evaluate the child's capacity for device control.

Barker and colleagues developed a control evaluator and trainer kit to assess anatomic sites systematically (Barker & Cook, 1981; Barker & Hastings, 1981). The Barker system, a portable self-contained micro-processor-based evaluation-and-training device, uses performance and environmental feedback to facilitate quantitative measurements of control. Anatomic sites are ranked in terms of the user's ability to exercise purposeful movement or the range over which voluntary control can be effectively exercised (Barker & Cook, 1981; Barker & Hastings, 1981).

Firmware

The need for hardware and/or software modifications decreases the number of commercial computer programs available to physically disabled individuals. Further, adaptations can be exorbitantly expensive simply because these programs are not easily changed. At the University of Washington and at the Trace Center-University of Wisconsin a technique that uses an adaptive-firmware card has been developed for the Apple II.

The firmware card allows the disabled client to use standard commercial software without the expense of hardware and/or software modifications. Thus, a vast library of commercial programs becomes readily available to the user.

The adaptive-firmware card makes the computer think that the keyboard is actually providing the input. The insertion of the card into the microcomputer provides a variety of "transparent" inputs, including scanning, Morse code, and direct selection (Schwejda & Vanderheiden, 1982). These inputs are referred to as "transparent' because they work in conjunction with other programs, without requiring that these programs be altered in any way. The keyboard input can come from a variety of interfaces, such as single-switch, dual switches, joysticks, or paddle controls.

Another technique currently being investigated at the Trace Center-University of Wisconsin is the design of universal keyboard emulators to work with a variety of personal computers and terminals. The keyboard emulators not only mimic the actual keyboard of the computer, but are also invisible to the system. The microcomputer is deceived into thinking the message originated from direct keyboard input, rather than through an emulator. With the emulator installed, normal use of the computer keyboard can continue. The application of this technique will allow handicapped clients to use nonstandard input devices such as communication aids or other micro and hand-held computers.

Hybrid Lightbeam/Sensor Technique

The combination of two types of head/light-pointing techniques has resulted in the improved "hybrid light" developed at the Trace Center-University of Wisconsin (Vanderheiden, 1982a, 1982b, 1982c). This new selection device has as its ancestor the humble headstick, a simple wand attached to the head by means of a hat-like contraption. It allows the user to directly select elements from a language board. The headstick, like all other devices, has both benefits and drawbacks. The benefit is that the head can be one of the body parts with the most precise voluntary movement. A very obvious drawback is the unnatural appearance and cumbersome handling of the large apparatus.

A selection mechanism using lights need not be large and cumbersome, yet it should allow the user to take advantage of good voluntary head control. These considerations prompted development of two types of electronic headsticks in use today.

The first is simply a lightbeam-emitting device akin to a tiny flashlight mounted on a band around the user's head. This allows the user to direct the light beam onto whatever he intends to indicate, which may be not only selections on a language board, but also choices among foods in a meal, people in a room, or various toys. The benefit of this system is the constant visual feedback provided by the lightbeams regarding head position. The drawback, at the present time, is the unavailability of a commercial system responsive to this type of light input.

The other type of device employs a photoreceptive sensor, rather than an actual light in the head-mounted apparatus. This is then used in conjunction with a discrete LED device, such as the Express III (see Figure 7-11). Behind each selection block on the face of the device is a small LED. When the user centers the light-sensitive receptor worn on the head over this spot, the message is relayed to the device, and that unit is thus selected. The drawback of this system is that the "sweet spot" for selection is very small, and only when the user can center the sensor over the spot for the designated time is the selection accomplished. The device gives no visual feedback as to location of the sensor, simply an all-or-nothing activation of the individual LEDs.

The Trace Center's "hybrid light" is a combination of devices; it contains both the photoreceptive sensor and the lightbeam device. The photoreceptor works as before, allowing communication with a device for printing, display, and storage of the message; the addition of the lightbeam allows the user to constantly monitor his or her head positions, correcting minor excursions from the "sweet spot" with relative ease. In addition, the lightbeam may be used for selection in the absence of the user's electronic communication system.

Summary

The handicapped population benefits from our society's technological advances. Granted, not every nonspeaker can take advantage of highly sophisticated computers, nor can applications of technology solve every problem and overcome every limitation. In the hands of knowledgeable professionals, however, these new devices and systems can change lives.

In this discipline the human factor, rather than the machine, is the critical component. Employing information from assessments of both physical and cognitive functioning, professionals determine the status and needs of the nonspeaker. Knowledge of available systems and interfacing techniques allows the professional to match the user with appropriate devices.

Even if this "matchmaking" is successful, it should never be the end of the line. Communication enhancement is not an event; it is a process. We revise our prescriptions as our clients change and grow, as we learn more, and—last, but not least—as technology continues to advance.

References

Anderson, K.E. An eye-position controlled typewriter. *Proceedings of the Workshop on Communication Aids for the Non-Verbal Physically Handicapped,* June 1977, 137-141.

Archer, L. Blissymobolics—A non-verbal communication system. *Journal of Speech and Hearing Disorders,* 1977, *42,* 568-579.

Barker, M.R., & Cook, A.M. A systematic approach to evaluating physical ability for control of assistive devices. *Proceedings of the Fourth Annual Conference on Rehabilitation Engineering,* 1981, 287-289.

Barker, M.R., & Hastings, W.R. Control evaluator and trainer kit. *Proceedings of the Johns Hopkins First National Search for Applications of Personal Computing to Aid the Handicapped,* 1981, 175-177.

Beal, J. Mind to mind communication. In Communications and the future, panel presented at Meeting of the World Future Society's Fourth General Assembly, Washington, D.C., 1982.

Bliss, C.K. *Semantography (Blissymbolics)* (2nd ed.). Sydney, Aus.: Semantography (Blissymbolics) Publications, 1965.

Bloom, L. *Language development: Structure and function in emerging grammars.* Cambridge, Mass. MIT Press, 1970.

Bowerman, M. Discussion summary—development of concepts underlying language. In R.L. Schiefelbusch & L.L. Lloyd (Eds.), *Language perspectives—Acquisition, retardation and intervention.* Baltimore: University Park Press, 1974.

Bricker, W.A., & Bricker, D.D. An early language training strategy. In R.L. Schiefelbusch & L.L. Lloyd, (Eds.), *Language perspectives—Acquisition, retardation and intervention.* Baltimore: University Park Press, 1974.

Buus, R. A computer communication aid for the nonverbal handicapped. *Proceedings of the Johns Hopkins First National Search for Applications of Personal Computing to Aid the Handicapped,* 1981, 131-135.

Campbell, R.S., & Nieves, L.A. Communication and environmental control system. *Proceedings of the Johns Hopkins First National Search for Application of Personal Computing to Aid the Handicapped,* 1981, 114-115.

Carlson, F.L. *An adapted communication project for a nonspeaking child.* Paper presented at the 51st Annual Convention of the American Speech and Hearing Association, Houston, November 1976.

Carrier, J.K., Jr., & Peak, T. *Program Manual for Non-SLIP (Non-Speech Language Initiation Program).* Lawrence, KS: H & H Enterprises, Inc., 1975.

Chapman, R.S., & Miller, J.F. Analyzing language and communication in the child. In R.L. Schiefelbusch (Ed.), *Nonspeech language and communication: Analysis and intervention.* Baltimore: University Park Press, 1980.

Clark, C.R., Moores, D.F., & Woodcock, R.W. *Minnesota Early Language Development Sequence.* Minneapolis: Research, Development & Demonstration Center in Education of Handicapped Children, University of Minnesota, 1973.

Coleman, C.L., Cook, A.M. & Meyers, L.S. Assessing non-oral clients for assistive communication devices. *Journal of Speech and Hearing Disorders,* 1980, *45,* 515-526.

Cromer, R.F. The development of language and cognition: The cognition hypothesis. In D. Foss (Ed.), *New perspectives in child development.* Baltimore: Penguin, 1974.

Cromer, R.F. The cognitive hypothesis of language acquisition and its implications for child language deficiency. In D. Morehead & A. Morehead (Eds.), *Normal and deficient child language.* Baltimore: University Park Press, 1976.

Doddington, G.R., & Schalk, T.B. Speech recognition: Turning theory to practice. *IEEE Spectrum,* September 1981, *18,* 26-32.

Eulenberg, J. Personal communication, February 18, 1982.

Eulenberg, J. Personal communication, July 19, 1982.

Fincke, R. & O'Leary, J.P., Jr. The design of a line of gaze interface for communication and environment manipulation. *Proceedings of the International Conference on Rehabilitation Engineering,* 1980, 96-97.

Goodenough-Trepagnier, C., Goldenburg, E.P., & Fried-Oken, M. Nonvocal communication system with unlimited vocabulary using Apple and SPEEC Syllables. *Proceedings of the Fourth Annual Conference on Rehabilitation Engineering,* 1981, 173-175.

Goodenough-Trepagnier, C., & Prather, P. *Manual for teachers of SPEEC.* Boston: Tufts-New England Medical Center, 1979.

Goodenough-Trepagnier, C., & Prather, P. Communication systems for the nonvocal based on frequent phoneme sequences. *Journal of Speech and Hearing Research,* 1981, *24,* (3), 322-329.

Guess, D., Sailor, W., & Baer, D.M. To teach language to retarded children. In R.L. Schiefelbusch & L.L. Lloyd (Eds.), *Language perspectives—Acquisition, retardation and intervention.* Baltimore: University Park Press, 1974.

Harris, D., & Vanderheiden, G. Enhancing the development of communicative interaction. In R.L. Schiefelbusch (Ed.), *Nonspeech language and communication: Analysis and intervention.* Baltimore: University Park Press, 1980.

Harris-Vanderheiden, D. Blissymbolics and the mentally retarded. In G.C. Vanderheiden & K. Grilley (Eds.), *Non-vocal communication techniques and aids for the severely physically handicapped.* Baltimore: University Park Press, 1976.

Heckathorne, C.W., Doubler, J.A., & Childress, D.S. Experiences with microprocessor-based aids for disabled people. *Proceedings of the Johns Hopkins First National Search for Applications of Personal Computing to Aid the Handicapped,* 1981, 53-56.

Hillinger, M., Fox, B., & Wilson, M. Computer-enhanced communication systems for the Apple II. *Proceedings of the Johns Hopkins First National Search for Applications of Personal Computing to Aid the Handicapped,* 1981, 16-18.

Jones, Randal L. Row/column scanning with a dynamic matrix. *Proceedings of the Johns Hopkins First National Search for Applications of Personal Computing to Aid the Handicapped,* 1981, 6-8.

Klima, E., & Bellugi, U. *The signs of language.* Cambridge, MA: Harvard University Press, 1979.

Laefsky, I.M., & Roemer, R.A. A real-time control system for CAI and prothesis. *Behavioral Research Methods and Instrumentation,* 1978, *10,* (2), 182-185.

Lee, S.A. A microcomputer-based VOCA for the non-vocal. *Proceedings of the Fifth Annual Conference on Rehabilitation Engineering,* 1982, 141-143.

McDonald, E.T., & Schultz, A.R. Communication boards for cerebral palsied children. *Journal of Speech and Hearing Disorders,* 1973, *38,* 73-88.

Morris, S.E. Communication/interaction development at mealtimes for the multiply handicapped child: Implication for the use of augmentative communication systems. *Language Speech and Hearing Services in Schools,* 1981, *12* (4), 216-232.

Nelson, D.J., Park, G.C., Farley, R.L., & Cote-Baldwin, C. Providing access to computers for physically handicapped persons: Two approaches. *Proceedings of the Fourth Annual Conference on Rehabilitation Engineering,* 1981, 140-142.

Non-speech communication: A position paper. *Asha,* 1980, *22* (4), 267-272.

Premack, A.J., & Premack, D. Teaching language to an ape. *Scientific American,* 1972, *277,* 92-99.

Premack, D. A functional analysis of language. *Journal of Experimental Analysis of Behavior,* 1970, *14,* 107-125.

Premack, D. Language in chimpanzee? *Science,* 1971, *172,* 808-822.

Premack, D., & Premack, A.J. Teaching visual language to apes and language deficient persons. In R.L. Schiefelbusch & L.L. Lloyd (Eds.), *Language perspectives—Acquisition, retardation and intervention.* Baltimore: University Park Press, 1974.

Rinard, G., & Rugg, D. Application of the ocular transducer to the ETRAN communicator. Conference on Systems and Devices for the Disabled, Houston, 1978.

Rinard, G., & Rugg, D. Communication/control application of the ocular transducer (Technical note 78-001), Denver Research Institute, University of Denver.

Rogers, J.T., Fine, P.R., Kuhlemeir, K.V., & Bowen, R.L. C2E2: A micro-computer system to aid the severely physically disabled in activities of daily living. *Proceedings of the International Conference on Rehabilitation Engineering,* 1980, 36-38.

Rosen, M.J., & Durkee, W.K. Preliminary report on EYECOM. Conference on Systems and Devices for the Disabled, Houston, 1978.

Schiefelbusch, R.L., & Hollis, J.H. A general system for nonspeech language. In R.L. Schiefelbusch (Ed.), *Nonspeech language and communication: Analysis and intervention.* Baltimore: University Park Press, 1980.

Schwejda, P., & Vanderheiden, G.C. Adaptive-firmware card for the Apple II. *Byte,* September 1982, *7* (9), 276-314.

Shane, H., & Blau, A. Paper presented at the Northeast Regional Conference of the American Speech and Hearing Association, July 1981.

Silverman, F.H. *Communication for the speechless.* Englewood Cliffs, NJ: Prentice-Hall, 1980.

Silverman, H., McNaughton, S., & Kates, B. *Handbook of Blissymbolics for instructors, users, parents and administrators.* Toronto: Blissymbolics Communication Institute, 1978.

Vanderheiden, G.C. Hybrid optical headpointing technique. *Proceedings of the Fifth Annual Conference on Rehabilitation Engineering,* 1982, 24. (a)

Vanderheiden, G.C. Lightbeam headpointer research. *Communication Outlook,* 1982, *4,* 11. (b)

Vanderheiden, G.C. Trace-hybrid lightbeam/sensor techniques. *Communication Outlook,* 1982, *3,* 6-7. (c)

Weiss, L. Personal communication, February 5, 1982.

Wilbur, R.B. *American sign language and sign systems.* Baltimore: University Park Press, 1979.

Woodcock, R.W. An experimental test for remedial readers. *Journal of Educational Psychology,* 1958, *49,* 23-27.

Woodcock, R.W. (Ed.) *The rebus reading series.* Nashville, TN: Institute on Mental Retardation & Intellectual Development, George Peabody College, 1965.

Woodcock, R.W. Rebuses as a medium in beginning reading instruction. *IMRID Papers and Reports,* 1968, *5* (4).

Woodcock, R.W., Clark, C.R., & Davis, C.O. *The Peabody rebus reading program.* Circle Pines, MN: American Guidance Service, 1968.

Woodcock, R.W., Clark, C.R., & Davies, C.O. *The Peabody Rebus Reading Program-Teacher's Guide.* Circle Pines, MN: American Guidance Service, 1969.

Language Disorders in Adults

Recent Advances

Editor in chief, Speech, Language, and Hearing Disorders Series

William H. Perkins, PhD

Preface

It has been a pleasure to edit this book. Part of the pleasure has come from having had the opportunity to share ideas and to interact with this enthusiastic and knowledgeable group of contributors. The major reason, however, is that it has been a significant learning experience for me. I regard this volume as a "state of the art" book about some major problems and issues concerning adult language disorders, and what can (or cannot) be done about a fair sampling of them. I have learned mightily in the process of working with these authors, and by virtue of it, catching up on new material, new research, new trends, and developing concepts about language and its disorders in adults.

The profession of Speech-Language Pathology and Audiology celebrated its 50th birthday a few years ago, and 1981 marked the occasion of 50 years of systematic treatment for aphasia by American speech-language pathologists. Nevertheless, most professions surely mature more slowly than do the people who practice them, and this one is no exception. In recent years, our still only dawning maturity has resulted in restructuring some of the methods that constitute clinical practice, some redefinition of the people and the problems we treat, some refocusing of clinical perspective generally, and even some returns to a few early beliefs that were discarded in the profession's brash adolescence. The content of this book reflects the profession's growth.

In this volume, some old problems such as aphasia are presented in a variety of new ways. Other problems, notably language disorders in dementia, closed head injury, and in patients with right-hemisphere damage, are singled out and emphasized as different from, and justifiably separated from, the aphasias that result from focal damage, usually to the left hemisphere. The coverage of non-speech language and communication in adults reflects a broadening of perspective in a field that used to be held in thrall by the spoken and written word and their respective forms of comprehension. Although the profession has long recognized the importance of understanding disordered language in children in the context of normal acquisition of language, this volume puts adult language disorders into their appropriate lifespan developmental context as well. Finally, throughout the book, concern for the patient-as-a-person is manifested.

Ideally, an introduction should simply set the stage, whet the readers' appetites, properly raise their levels of anticipation for the heady content to follow. So I will be brief in describing the topics and the authors, preferring to let them speak for themselves. Nonetheless, it is irresistible not to add my own perspective to what is covered in this volume, chapter-by-chapter.

Robert T. Wertz opens the book with a comprehensive overview of language disorders of adulthood, stressing recent trends in their study, diagnosis, and treatment. A crucial feature of Wertz' review is its breadth, and its inclusion of some new concerns, such as the language of schizophrenia, usually ignored by speech/language pathologists. My belief is that this chapter may well influence the direction of adult language pathology for some years to come.

G. Albyn Davis' chapter on normal adult language has the very difficult goal of summarizing a broad literature on language and normal aging, most of it coming from other disciplines, including geriatric psychology and sociology. His conclusion that surprisingly little of real substance is known about how language might change across the adult lifespan is a sobering one. Nevertheless, Davis has carefully described the crucial issues and has suggested many areas for future research, in addition to suggesting strategies for such study.

Three chapters are devoted specifically to the topic of aphasia. Aphasia has been split into mild, moderate, and severe forms of the disorder for consideration here. This split is a result of my belief that different treatment principles and goals for treatment derive from a consideration of the severity of the problem, as well as from the specific aphasic syndrome a patient is manifesting.

It is largely through the work of Nancy Helm-Estabrooks that aphasiologists are reconsidering the idea that severe aphasia, particularly global aphasia, is hopeless. She has been responsible for the development of techniques specifically directed to such patients and has been careful to quantify their effectiveness. In her chapter on severe aphasia in this book, she shares not only her approaches to such patients, but also her unique way of thinking about them.

Jennifer Horner has taken the territory about which aphasiologists appear to have known the most for the longest, the problems of the moderately impaired patient. She has fitted these problems with a new suit of clothes, partly fashioned by her own clinical experience, but also influenced by her understanding of neuropsychology and its potential for contributing to aphasia rehabilitation in very direct ways.

Craig Linebaugh has filled a very tough assignment, describing the treatment of aphasic patients whose impairments are mild. The importance of developing keener insight into the mildly impaired aphasic patient is great, for not only are they virtually ignored in clinical texts, but they are the patients with the highest likelihood of returning to their pre-aphasia lifestyles and vocations.

Before leaving the subject of aphasia, it is pertinent to add that medical advances themselves have led us to consider more explicitly those patients whose aphasias are at the poles of severity. Better medical management of stroke has resulted in more survivors who might previously have died, and possibly thereby has forced the more severely impaired upon our consciousness. Better medical management has also lessened the likelihood of severe stroke, and similarly left the aphasiologist with a significantly larger number of mildly impaired patients. The example aptly illustrates that not only self-contemplation but medical, social, and philosophic concerns interact to bring about advances in the profession.

In a related field, Penelope Meyers has broken new ground with her comprehensive chapter on the problems of patients who have incurred right-hemisphere deficits. Few students of aphasia rehabilitation have been required to study right-hemisphere problems, yet speech-language pathologists are increasingly being called on to work with the visuospatial, language, and cognitive deficits that occur as a result of damage to the formerly "minor hemisphere. " Meyers' chapter breaches this void.

Kathryn Bayles has filled a similar need with her broad overview of dementia. Dementia is another problem that has recently begun to attract the attention of speech-language pathologists who work with adults. As aging generally has become the focus of national concern, professional interest in one of its major disorders has also increased. Yet, few speech-language pathology curricula are prepared to teach the clinician about dementia, and few clinicians are prepared to develop a principled stance about their role in working with dementia, either as it occurs in pure form, or as it might accompany aphasias and other disorders of aging. At the same time, speech-language pathologists increasingly find employment in chronic care facilities, nursing homes, and institutions for the aging and infirm. Bayles' chapter provides the background against which the speech-language pathologist can develop his or her own principled beliefs.

As the nation's largest killer of people under the age of 35, closed-head injury is increasingly recognized as a major American problem. And those who survive head injury have rapidly swelled the clinical caseloads of aphasiologists, who, in working with these patients, are beginning to recognize the limitations of the well-known treatments for aphasia. Chris Hagen, whose work with the head-injured has considerably influenced most of the systematic treatment programs for the problem, has provided for this volume a meticulously detailed, comprehensive approach.

No volume purporting to discuss recent advances in language disorders could avoid having a chapter on nonspeech language and communication if it chose to be worthy of the title. And this book's final chapter by Kathryn Yorkston and Patricia Dowden serves simultaneously to educate the speech-language pathologist about the importance of understanding nonspeech language advances and to give a very current overview of this, probably the profession's most rapidly advancing topic.

It is past time to stop my own enthusiasm and let readers get down to the business of stirring up their own. In closing, allow me to share a final rumination and speculation. As this volume was planned and as it has developed over the past year, I became fascinated with trying to imagine what I would have expected of it, had I been planning it 20, or even 10, years ago. I do not think I would have come close to what every reader will recognize as the new directions, new problems, and new solutions presented here. And it is also fascinating to think what might be encountered in a *Recent Advances* 10 or 20 years in the future. I expect that it will be at least as unpredictable. The great satisfaction of this profession is the surprises it holds and the constancy of its change.

Audrey L. Holland
Editor

Robert T. Wertz

Language Disorders in Adults: State of the Clinical Art

On February 26, 1885, William Osler began his "State of the Art" Gulstonian Lectures on malignant endocarditis. He summarized the past, defined his present purposes, and predicted the future.

> Mr. President and gentlemen—It is of use, from time to time, to take stock, so to speak, of our knowledge of a particular disease, to see exactly where we stand in regard to it, to inquire to what conclusions the accumulated facts seem to point, and to ascertain in what direction we may look for fruitful investigations in the future. (Osler, 1885, p.1)

Fair enough! But, Osler's task was, for him, an easy one. First, he knew what he was talking about. Much of what was known about malignant endocarditis had resulted from his labors. Second, the etiological, clinical, and anatomical characteristics of the disease had been fairly well ascertained. And, third, he was ready with a review of over two hundred cases he had seen in the General Hospital in Montreal.

A similar attempt to present the clinical state of the art on language disorders in adults can agree with the utility of Osler's purpose. It is of use to take stock—to determine where we are, what we know, and where we might go. However, the task is exceedingly more difficult. First, even though all language disorders in adults are frequently collapsed into one, aphasia, there are others. Second, no single individual is sufficiently knowledgeable to complete the task. Third, each chapter in this volume represents a "state of the art" on a specific language disorder, or a portion of a specific language disorder, and, therefore, may render what follows superficial and redundant. And, fourth, any attempt to state "the state of the art" is historical before it reaches print.

Even though one may not succeed, one can try. So, what follows is one person's "state of the art" filtered through his information, his misinformation, and his biases. My purpose is to examine what I think we know today about managing language disorders in adults that I am not certain we knew ten or more years ago. Specifically, I will discuss six conditions in which adult language may go awry—normal, older individuals who may find themselves in an abnormal environment; confusion; schizophrenia; right hemisphere involvement; dementia; and aphasia. Because this is an attempt to state the "state of the *clinical* art," each condition will be considered under what I believe are the four steps in clinical management— appraisal, diagnosis, prognosis, and treatment. I will attempt to determine whether our science has influenced our service, if research has reached reality, whether our data are reflected in our deeds.

The Disorders

Any attempt to list, lacks. One person's pathologies include another's "no problems." One person's exclusions contain another's emphasis. Conversely, while some societies have no name for "it," others have several. So, while my list of potential language disorders in adults may be limited, I will attempt to describe each in order for others to identify that which they label differently. These are the language disorders that find their way to our clinical door.

Environmental Influence on the Normal Aged

Getting old affects more than the bladder. Davis, in this volume and elsewhere (Beasley & Davis, 1981), tells us what can go wrong with communication as one migrates through life's later decades. Certain performances decline as the organism ages, and older folk venture into the period when the nervous system is attacked more frequently by disease. For example, the incidence of cerebral vascular accident is greater after 65 than before 45. Some carry their communication problems with them as they travel further into life. All of these conditions exist, and they coexist. The individual whose stuttering began at 6 and accompanied him or her through life can be battered by a stroke in his 60s, a time when he or she is beleaguered by presbycusis and the physiologic decline that comes with years lived. Attempts to study aging make the strongest scientists weep.

Another complication in any attempt to bring order to aging is the variability in performance among older individuals. Forty-year-old nervous systems seem to reside in some who are 80, and 90-year-old nervous systems are housed in some who are 60. Set out to collect "normative" data on the elderly and you are certain to return with a sack full of extremely large standard deviations.

But, some do survive the rigors of living with their faculties in fine fettle. They function until they find themselves in an environment that erodes their intact skills. Holland (1978) and Lubinski (1981) have documented the disastrous effects an abnormal environment can have on a normal older person's communicative ability. We see these individuals in our clinics. They may have entered our medical centers with down-stream problems—an ornery prostate or arthritis, but after a few weeks, a consult is sent by the ward physician to please evaluate Mr. Boomis' confusion, or "this 80-year-old male's dementia. " Similarly, social circumstances that dictate the elderly leave the stimulating environment of their familiar neighborhood and take up residence in a nursing home, or other extended care facility may lead, eventually, to language deficit. Holland (1980) reports that normal older individuals in institutionalized settings achieve lower scores on her measure, *Communicative Abilities in Daily Living* (CADL), than normal older individuals who reside in noninstitutionalized environments.

Thus, custody appears to confound cortex, at least the cortex utilized for communication. I list this condition as a potential language disorder in adults, and label it as language deficit in a normal older person residing in an abnormal environment. Lubinski (1981) uses the phrase "a communication-impaired environment" to describe a setting where there is reduced opportunity for successful, meaningful communication. This typifies some, not all, of our acute and chronic care facilities, where at least one in five of our nation's elderly will spend time prior to demise.

A specific set of symptoms to identify the normal older person whose language has eroded as a result of residing in a communication-impairing environment is difficult to list. Obler and Albert (1981) have provided some clues for identification. They indicate that the expected ravages of age affect naming skills and auditory comprehension in the healthy elderly. To cope, the healthy oldster utilizes strategies—syntax to cue naming ability and context to improve comprehension. Dropped into an unfavorable environment where few listen or speak, the healthy elderly find their strategies no longer result in solutions, and they abandon them. They cease attempting to convey and seek information when faced with misinformation or no information. Because communication is a "use it or lose it" phenomenon, the lack of use results in loss.

So, impaired language in the normal aged exists and it confronts the speech pathologist. It needs to be identified, to be differentiated from disorders—confusion, aphasia, dementia—it may masquerade as, and it needs to be managed appropriately.

Language of Confusion

Observe a group of medical residents being quizzed for a diagnosis by a senior physician and you hear an interesting dialogue. "What is your diagnosis young doctors?" asks the senior staff member. "Pneumonoultramicroscopicsilicovolcanoconiosis," replies the first-year resident. "Yes," responds the mentor, "there is one case reported in the entire history of medicine. Do you believe we have another?" We ignore the most probable and remember the odd, the bizarre, the interesting.

Similarly, the language of confusion is rare, but, if we have seen it, we remember it by its bizarre characteristics. And, like the young doctors, our memory may tempt application when the term is inappropriate. Darley, in a paper presented to the American Speech and Hearing Association (1969), has defined the language of confusion as:

> Impairment of language accompanying neurologic conditions; often traumatically induced; characterized by reduced recognition and understanding of and responsiveness to the environment, faulty memory, unclear thinking, and disorientation in time and space. Structured language events are usually normal and responses utilize correct syntax; open-ended language situations elicit irrelevance, confabulation.

Neurologists (Mayo Clinic, 1976) identify this condition as "confused state" or "confusion." Speech Pathologists (Halpern, Darley, & Brown, 1973) use Darley's term, the "language of confusion." Though rare, usually less than five percent of the language disorders we see in our clinic, it exists and requires our attention. These patients are not aphasic, and they are not demented. They need to be identified and to be managed appropriately.

Schizophrenia

Jaffe (1981) asked if a schizophrenic patient suffered a left hemisphere CVA with subsequent Wernicke's aphasia, would anyone notice? A partial answer to Jaffe's question is, probably, the speech pathologist would not. We know language deficit in aphasia, but I am not certain we know language deficit in schizophrenia. We see few patients who demonstrate the language of confusion because it is rare. We see few schizophrenic patients. Less than 1% of the referrals sent to our clinic are from the psychiatric wards. Consult a list of references in schizophrenia or, more specifically, references on the language of schizophrenic patients, and you will find few contributions by speech pathologists. Yet, language is disrupted in schizophrenic patients, and should it come to our attention, we need to identify it and differentiate it from other language disorders.

DiSimoni, Darley, and Aronson (1977) have reviewed language involvement in schizophrenia. They tell us schizophrenic patients may not use language for informational purposes, their prosody may be abnormal, they may dwell on certain themes and perseverate in their ideas, their performance may vary with the mode of stimulus presentation, they may display disrupted syntax, they may be disoriented, they may confabulate, and their verbal and written responses may be paraphasic.

As is true with most language disorders, language disturbance in schizophrenia varies with severity, and, specifically in schizophrenia, severity is linked with time postonset. Darley (1982) reports that as duration of the illness increases, performance declines. Deterioration of language in schizophrenic patients may migrate through the language performance displayed by a confused patient to, eventually, the language performance displayed by a demented patient.

Some (Chapman, 1966) suggest that an aphasia exists in schizophrenia. Others (Benson, 1973) do not. Some (Elmore & Gorham, 1957) do not differentiate the language of schizophrenic patients from the language of chronic brain syndrome patients, who are usually classified as demented. Whether the same as or different from, most agree language is not normal in schizophrenia. Therefore, it qualifies as a language disorder one may see in adults.

Right Hemisphere Involvement

Myers (1978, 1979), as she does in this volume, directs our attention to a communication deficit that may be present following right hemisphere damage. For years, we have suspected that the right hemisphere did something, that it was more than a spare if the left was damaged. Joynt and Goldstein (1975) have listed what may go wrong when the right hemisphere is damaged. The problems include: spatial perception and body image disorders, visual perception disorders, constructional disabilities, auditory perception disorders, somatosensory disorders, speech disorders, and motor impersistence. These have been studied by neurologists and psychologists. One wonders, what is left for the speech pathologist in the right hemisphere patient? A lot, Myers and West (1978) tell us.

Patients who suffer damage to the right hemisphere may have few overt language deficits, but they have difficulty communicating. Myers (1978) suggests that to communicate means more than just to impart. It also means to take part. While the right hemisphere patient's ability to impart may approach normality, his or her ability to participate is abnormal.

Historically, damage to the right hemisphere is reported to result in a variety of language deficits. Eisenson (1962) believes the right hemisphere patient has difficulty with high level language functions. Critchley (1962) reports difficulty in auditory and visual identification of language. Swisher and Sarno (1969) note difficulty in comprehending lengthy auditory stimuli. Weinstein (1964) observed naming errors. Archibald and Wepman (1968) reported aphasic-like responses on the *Language Modalities Test for Aphasia* (LMTA) (Wepman & Jones, 1961). And, several (Denny-Brown, Meyers, & Horenstein, 1952; Hecaen & Marcie, 1974; Metzler & Jelinek, 1977) have observed writing disturbance.

So, right hemisphere involvement appears to result in both nonverbal and verbal deficits. To these, Myers (1978, 1979) adds a disruption in cognitive style. The symptoms are inability to use visual imagery, inability to understand figurative language, altered affect, and an abnormal sense of humor. Together, they influence the way patients look at the world, the way they integrate what they see and hear, and the way they respond. Abnormal cognitive style has been described by Gardner (1975):

> The right hemisphere patient appears unconcerned about his message, insensitive to his situation or to the environment. He resembles a language machine, a talking computer that decodes literally, gives the most immediate response, insensitive to the ideas behind the question or the implications of the questioner. (p. 296)

Myers (1978) adds that the right hemisphere patient misses nuances and subtleties. His or her sense of humor, if present, is caustic. These patients are verbally dependent. They ignore context. They cannot, or do not, do what normals and aphasic patients do—fill in what is not present in the words.

Until recently, right hemisphere patients were not referred to the speech pathologist, or were referred "for our interest." More and more, they are being referred for evaluation and for treatment. Their problems and what we may be able to do about them classify them for inclusion in a list of language disorders in adults.

Dementia

"Mind! Mind!" one of my aphasic friends used to say when his brain and tongue failed to connect. His "mind" was fine. He was aphasic. Not so, for many who suffer dementia, more accurately, the dementias. Literally, the term means "deprived of mind. " Estimates indicate 5% of our fellow citizens over 65 are severly demented. Another 10% are reported to be mildly to moderately demented.

The dementias result from brain diseases that erode mental abilities. Memory slips as does attention, judgment, and ability to learn. A few dementias are treatable. Most are not. Bayles, in this volume and elsewhere (Bayles, 1982b), tells us dementia is the chronic, progressive deterioration of intellect due to changes in the central nervous system. The culprits include Alzheimer's disease, now considered the same as senile dementia or senile brain disease; multiple infarcts; ideopathic Parkinson's disease; Huntington's disease; Creutzfeldt-Jakob disease; Pick's disease, and Korsakoff's disease. Causes of dementia with a brighter future, in that they may respond to treatment, are intoxication, poor nutrition, subdural hematoma, depression, tumor, metabolic disorders, and occult hydrocephalus (Foley, 1972).

Speech pathologists are attracted to dementia by its language symptoms. The intellectual loss is measured and documented by psychologists. The language deficits are measured and documented in the speech clinic. Darley (1969, 1982) has classified these as the language of generalized intellectual impairment. His definition is:

> Deterioration of performance on more difficult language tasks; reduced efficiency in all modes; greater impairment evident in language tasks requiring better retention, closer attention, and powers of abstraction and generalization; degree of impairment roughly proportionate to deterioration of other mental functions. (in a paper presented to the American Speech & Hearing Assn., 1969)

We see these patients, and our task is to separate them from patients with other language disorders. Our contribution transcends deciding that this patient is less intelligent than he sounds, hence, demented, and that patient is more intelligent than he sounds, hence, aphasic. We can step beyond diagnosis and document change over time, and we can manage demented patients as well as our tools and talents permit.

Aphasia

If neurologists, neuropsychologists, neurolinguists, and speech pathologists know anything, they know aphasia. In fact, they know enough to disagree on its definition and the words to be used in talking about it. Most agree that aphasic patients have difficulty in auditory comprehension, reading, oral-expressive use of language, and writing. However, confusion can arise, as Rosenbek (1983) points out, when books are titled *Aphasia, Alexia, and Agraphia* (Benson, 1979a). This might imply that aphasia involves listening and speaking, but not reading and writing. One must read the text to discover that all four are impaired in aphasia. Further, some have narrowed aphasia's boundaries to relate exclusively to "a disturbance in verbal language as opposed to other forms of language, for example, the language of gestures or of facial expression " (Damasio, 1981, p. 52).

The tendency to limit aphasia or to subdivide it into the aphasias can be contrasted with Darley's (1982) general definition of it as:

> Impairment, as a result of brain damage, of the capacity for interpretation and formulation of language symbols; multimodality loss or reduction in efficiency of the ability to decode and encode conventional meaningful linguistic elements (morphemes and larger syntactic units); disproportionate to impairment of other intellective functions; not attributable to dementia, confusion, sensory loss, or motor dysfunction; and manifested in reduced availability of vocabulary, reduced efficiency in application of syntactic rules, reduced auditory retention span, and impaired efficiency in input and output channel selection. (p. 42)

Darley prefers his aphasia lean, without adjectives. He draws support for his point of view from the Schuell, Jenkins, and Carroll (1962) factor analysis of results obtained on the *Minnesota Test for Differential Diagnosis of Aphasia* (Schuell, 1965a). The failure to find several dimensions led Schuell et al. to conclude that aphasia is a general language deficit that is not modality specific. This lack of evidence for a taxonomy or a dichotomy—sensory-motor, receptive-expressive, input-output—is amplified by Darley. Differences among aphasic patients, he believes, may not indicate different types of aphasia, but the presence of two disorders, for example, aphasia and apraxia of speech. Further, severity of aphasia confounds taxonomy and does not justify the conclusion that there are different aphasic types. Finally, Darley points out that time postonset erodes severity and differences. There is a migration among aphasic types as time postonset increases and severity decreases (Kertesz & McCabe, 1977; Wertz, Kitselman, & Deal, 1981). Thus, unlike a rose, a Wernicke's not always is a Wernicke's is a Wernicke's.

This "aphasia is one" point of view coexists in the literature and the clinic with the position that stresses classification. Classification of the aphasias is a core course in the curriculum of most neurologists, neuropsychologists, neurolinguists, and some speech pathologists. The systems popularized by Benson (1979a), Kertesz (1979), and Goodglass and Kaplan (1972) are used, and when clinicians with differing points of view meet to discuss a patient, confusion can result. And, the terminological debate is bound to become more complex. As we learn more about the contribution of subcortical structures to speech and language (Ojemann, 1975), subcortical aphasic syndromes find their way into the literature (Benson, 1979a; Alexander & Lo Verme, 1980).

While one may not agree, one can become bilingual. Rosenbek (1983) suggests settling on the best available definition of aphasia and the most clinically useful classification of people with it, because our failure to do so may affect our clinical practice. So, while we may not agree on what to call it, we seem to recognize it when we see it. This is fortunate, because we see a lot of it.

The State of the Art

These are the disorders that fill our literature and find their way to our clinic. The list is not exclusive, and little attention has been given to the possibility of coexisting disorders. Further, the literature contains debate on whether the language deficits in one disorder really represent another disorder.

Recently, we reviewed the percentages of different neurogenic speech and language disorders referred to our clinic during a one-year period. The figures were: aphasia, 28%; language of confusion, 6%; language of generalized intellectual impairment, 8%; dysarthria, 38%; apraxia of speech, 9%; and undetermined, 11%. The exercise told us more than we wanted to know, but it did not tell us enough about what we need to know. For example, disorders coexist. All of the apraxia of speech patients demonstrated coexisting aphasia. Apraxia of speech was just the most salient symptom. What was represented under the undetermined label? Here we put the right hemisphere patient, the rare schizophrenic patient, the patient with bilateral head trauma, and the ones we just could not label.

So, our list lacks. If it matters what you call it, and I believe it does, we need to find some names and apply them appropriately. For example, referrals from psychiatry, though few, are not all schizophrenic. Some have affective disorders, and not all schizophrenic patients demonstrate a thought disorder. Further, where do we put the bilateral head trauma patient with brain stem involvement? If the latter affects speech, dysarthria is an appropriate label, but what about the patient's language deficits? Are they aphasic? Holland (1982a) argues they are not, really. Or, at least, they differ from aphasia subsequent to a left hemisphere cerebral vascular accident. But what if both hemispheres are injured? Do these patients behave the way right hemisphere patients do? Somewhat, but not totally. Damage both sides of the brain and behavior differs from that seen following lateralized damage. Porch (1973) presents percentiles on his test, the *Porch Index of Communicative Ability* (PICA), for patients who have bilateral damage. The percentiles differ from those he presents for patients with left hemisphere damage. Is it useful to label the bilateral patients aphasic? I am not certain it is. But, is the language of generalized intellectual impairment more appropriate? Yes and no. And, what about the language disorder in dementia? Is it aphasic? Appell, Kertesz, and Fishman (1981) argue that it is. I (Wertz, 1982) have rebutted this—it is not.

Not long ago, I ran across a review of a book that was titled *Progress in Anatomy* (Harrison & Holmes, 1981). I wondered, how can there be progress in anatomy? Anatomy is. One studies it; not about it. Yet, some are studying about it. Similarly, we can make my error when we think language disorders in adults *are*; that we have compiled and completed the list. The state of the art in the labels we use is not etched. It is evolving. Two disorders appear in this chapter—environmental influence on the normal aged and schizophrenia—that did not appear in a survey I did five years ago (Wertz, 1978).

Appraisal

One way to test the validity of a list of language disorders is to pass it through a sieve of clinical scrutiny. Do patients find a place to abide on the list? Are there leftovers? Clinical scrutiny is another way of saying appraisal.

Appraisal, I believe, is a process of collecting data—biographical, medical, and behavioral. The purpose of appraisal is to find out what a patient has to tell you about his or her problem. Its ends are to make a diagnosis, formulate a prognosis, and either focus treatment or justify a decision not to treat.

There have been several influences on appraisal of language disorders in adults in recent years. First, available tests, at least for aphasia, abound. Second, neurospychology has come out of the laboratory into life. Third, speech pathologists are beginning to realize that tests for aphasia are not the only—or best—tools for appraising other language disorders. Fourth, neurology has evolved from safety pin and mallet to some highly sophisticated neuroradiological techniques.

In 1979, 14 tests for appraising acquired language dysfunction were reviewed (Darley, 1979a). These included: the *Aphasia Language Performance Scales* (ALPS) (Keenan & Brassell, 1975); the *Appraisal of*

Language Disturbance (ALD) (Emerick, 1971); *Boston Diagnostic Aphasia Examination* (BDAE) (Goodglass & Kaplan, 1972); *Examining for Aphasia* (Eisenson, 1954); *Functional Communication Profile* (FCP) (Sarno, 1969); *Halstead Aphasia Test, Form M* (Halstead, Wepman, Reitan, & Heimburger 1949); *The Language Modalities Test for Aphasia* (LMTA) (Wepman & Jones, 1961); *The Minnesota Test for Differential Diagnosis of Aphasia* (MTDDA) (Schuell, 1965a); the *Neurosensory Center Comprehensive Examination for Aphasia* (NCCEA) (Spreen & Benton, 1969); the *Orzeck Aphasia Evaluation* (AE) (Orzeck, 1964); the *Porch Index of Communicative Ability* (PICA) (Porch, 1973); the *Sklar Aphasia Scale* (SAS) (Sklar, 1966); the *Token Test* (TT) (DeRenzi & Vignolo, 1962); and the *Word Fluency Measure* (WF) (Borkowski, Benton & Spreen, 1967). Additional measures that have appeared subsequently are: the *Communicative Abilities in Daily Living* (CADL) (Holland, 1980); the *Revised Token Test* (RTT) (McNeil & Prescott, 1978); and the *Western Aphasia Battery* (WAB) (Kertesz, 1982). While most of these tests were designed to appraise aphasia, they have been applied with other langauge disorders.

More and more, neuropsychologists are involved in the clinical management of language-disordered adults, and their primary involvement has been in appraisal. Certainly, the contribution of neuropsychology to clinical management is not new in some settings. For example, there is a rich history in the Boston Veterans Administration Medical Center on the clinical contributions of neuropsychology, and the *Boston Diagnostic Aphasia Examination* (Goodglass & Kaplan, 1972) is a significant part of the testimony. Other medical settings have been slower to add clinical neuropsychologists, but, today, most psychology services contain both psychologists and neuropsychologists.

One product of the clinical growth in neuropsychology has been the development of tests. And, a significant representative in this development was the standardization of Luria's (1970) clinical tools into the *Luria-Nebraska Neuropsychological Battery* (Golden, Hammeke, & Purisch, 1980). Like any new test, the Luria-Nebraska has attracted converts and controversy. Criticism has ranged from the general to the specific. Crosson and Warren (1982) suggest the test may not be valid for patients with language disturbance. Their use of it failed to distinguish between patients with language disturbance and patients with other deficits, and they were unable to differentiate among types of language disturbance. Spiers (1981) believes the test is not capable of providing a comprehensive assessment of neuropsychological functioning in its present form. Delis and Kaplan (1982) reported an aphasic patient whose performance on the Luria-Nebraska was not consistent with his language behavior, or with the localization of his lesion. Holland (1982b) suggests that the problem with the language sections in the Luria-Nebraska is the language. Her analysis of the 269 items in the test revealed that 139 required speech as a response. She recommends not using the test in its present form with language problems if one hopes to measure anything other than language contamination. She concludes that the battery may also penalize, inappropriately, the demented patient and the less well educated, and that it does not indicate where, or how, to focus treatment. Parsons (1982) has pointed out that part of the problem, and the reactions to the Luria-Nebraska, may be cultural. He suggests that Luria's techniques were qualitative and flexible. Conversely, the Luria-Nebraska is quantitative and standardized. This clash of two cultures, Parsons concludes, results in what happens whenever two cultures clash—conflict. Whatever the state or the fate of the Luria-Nebraska, it represents the clinical activity (perhaps storm) and active involvement neuropsychology has with language disorders in adults.

Speech pathologists have had the tendency to use old tools to appraise problems that are new to them. We have taken our trusted tests for aphasia and attempted to measure language deficits in dementia, confusion, and the right hemisphere patient. Some—for example, Halpern, Darley, and Brown's (1973) use of an adaptation of Schuell's (1957) short examination for aphasia to differentiate among four different disorders—have been more successful than others. Our use (Deal, Deal, Wertz, Kitselmann, & Dwyer, 1979) of the PICA to evaluate language deficits in right hemisphere patients led to the conclusion that there must be a more appropriate measure for that population. Fortunately, there is a growing trend to leave aphasia tests to the evaluation of aphasic patients and select or develop other measures for the other language disorders. Myers (1979) is refining a battery to appraise the right hemisphere patient, and Bayles (1982b) has developed a battery for appraising language deficits in dementia.

Finally, advances in neuroradiologic techniques have changed our previous practice, where neurologists localized lesions by observing language behaviors and compared their results with neuropsychology's localization, which was also based on observing language behavior. This circular approach has been shattered by transmission computerized tomography (CT) to localize the site of structutral lesions and positron emission tomography (PET) to reveal the functional locus of lesions.

Environmental Influence
on the Normal Aged

If the normal aged person's communication is influenced by his or her environment, adequate appraisal requires a look at both the individual and the individual's environment. The task is to determine whether the environment is the culprit, or whether the real villain is some other cause that may erode communication.

Lubinski (1981) discusses what to look for in order to detect a communication impairing environment. One problem is that there may be no one looking. Surveys by Mueller (1978) and Mueller and Peters (1981) indicate that many institutionalized environments do not provide speech and language services. Therefore, in the absence of a communication specialist, the influence of the environment on communication is not appraised.

But, if one does look, what does one look for? Lubinski (1981) recommends appraising opportunities for successful, meaningful communication; places within the setting to have a private conversation; administration and staff attitudes about the value of communication and their communicative behavior with patients; patients' values and attitudes about communication; rules that govern communication in the setting; and the influence of the physical design of the setting on communication. Her suggestions come from observation of institutional environments and interviews (Lubinski, Morrison, & Rigrodsky, 1981) with residents living in institutions.

If 15% of our nation's elderly are demented, 85% are aphasic, confused, schizophrenic, or normal. The task of appraisal is to find out who is who. Unfortunately, as Lubinski (1981) points out, none of the popular tests is designed to sort the normal aged suffering communication deficit arising out of environmental influences from those with other language deficits. None focuses on the communication needs of the institutionalized person—ability to communicate health care and personal needs, interaction with the staff or fellow residents or family. The measure that comes the closest is the CADL (Holland, 1980), and its use tells us older persons perform worse than younger persons, and institutionalized persons perform worse than noninstitutionalized persons (Holland, 1978). So, age itself, as well as being old in an institutionalized environment, can have an effect on useful communication.

Appraisal of the aged, like all appraisal, requires collecting biographic, medical, and behavioral data. One seeks explanations. For example, sensory deficits may erode mental abilities. Snyder, Pyrek, and Smith (1976) found a relationship between vision and mental status in their elderly subjects. Performance on the *Mental Status Questionnaire* (Kahn, Goldfarb, Pollack, & Peck, 1960) dropped as visual acuity became worse. A similar case can be made for hearing (Beasley & Davis, 1981). Further, one wants to rule out drug effects. Although the elderly make up only 10% of the population, they use 25% of all prescription drugs sold. Finlayson and Martin (1982) suggest age-related changes alter drug absorption. A therapeutic dose for an older person may be 50% less than that for a younger person.

The appraisal tools we have are many, but appropriate ones for the aged may be few. The use of the CADL to tap environmental influences was documented above. Duffy and Keith (1980) provide data about normal performance on the PICA (Porch, 1973). Their results indicate PICA test scores drop and test time increases as age increases. However, they were able to differentiate 92% of their normal sample from aphasic patients.

Others have devised measures to meet their needs. Keenan (1979) uses conversation with elderly patients in a custodial facility to rate: hearing, comprehension, and alertness; voice and articulation; rate, prosody, and fluency; vocabulary and grammar; talkativeness; and content and relevance. He begins with how the patient talks and whether the patient believes he has a problem. Keenan combines his observations of behavior with an assessment of physical, psychological, and environmental influences. To this he adds the patient's willingness to work on the problem, if one is present. Brandt, Rose, and Lucas (in press) have devised a similar approach for use in nursing homes.

Another appraisal technique we have used with other disorders is diagnostic treatment. We let the patient tell us what he or she has by the response to what we do with him or her. While environmental influence on communication may not be distinguishable from other disorders when appraised, it should change if its causes are removed or manipulated. Folsom (1968) has used reality orientation to change a diagnosis from dementia to normal aging. Diagnostic therapy might employ similar methods to make a diagnosis in patients whose communication is influenced by where they reside.

Language of Confusion

Appraisal of confusion seeks answers to four questions posed by Darley (1964). First, is the patient oriented in place and time? The confused patient is not. Second, does the patient stay in contact with the examiner? The confused patient does not if given the opportunity to wander. Third, how aware is the patient of the inappropriateness of his or her responses? The confused patient is not aware he or she is inappropriate. Fourth, how well structured are the patient's responses? The confused patient has normal sentence structure and decent vocabulary.

Answers to the above questions come from behavioral measures. Also, there are some useful signs in the patient's biographical and medical data. For example, an accurate biography is needed to determine if the patient confabulates when queried about himself or herself and his or her past.

Medical signs have been provided by Halpern, Darley, and Brown (1973). Eighty percent of their patients had a rapid onset, less than 10 days. All of their patients were less than 3 months postonset when evaluated. All patients displayed either diffuse or disseminated lesions. Half of the sample suffered trauma, and 30% suffered hemorrhage of hematoma.

Behavioral appraisal requires presenting tasks that flush the confused language. Chedru and Geschwind (1972) studied patients in an acute confusional state and compared their performance with control subjects. Tests that differentiated the confused from the nonconfused were temporal-spatial orientation tasks, digit span, writing, word fluency, and imitation of movements. Tests that did not differentiate were comprehension tasks, oral spelling, praxis tasks, visual recognition tasks, proverb interpretation, and spontaneous speech. Geschwind (1974a) has elaborated on the use of writing tasks, particularly copying, writing words from dictation, and writing sentences on a specific topic. He reports confused patients' writing is not very legible, letters and words are spaced poorly, and it contains syntactic and spelling errors.

Halpern, Darley, and Brown's (1973) results run contrary to those of Chedru and Geschwind (1972). Both observed disturbance in writing from dictation, but that is where the similarity ends. Halpern et al. found confused patients were deficient in arithmetic, reading comprehension, relevance, adequacy, and auditory comprehension. Syntax; naming; auditory retention, measured partially by digit span; and fluency were less impaired. The primary measure that differentiated confused patients from those with aphasia, dementia, and apraxia of speech was relevance, tapped primarily by proverb interpretation and spontaneous speech. Mills and Drummond (1980) have contested the naming results of Halpern et al. by suggesting the need for more detailed analysis. Comparing naming errors on high uncertainty and low uncertainty stimuli, response time, and semantic analysis of errors, Mills and Drummond differentiated confused patients from aphasic patients.

While the reports on language behavior in confusion do not agree, they do suggest appraisal tasks. Apparently, confused patients will identify themselves when asked to write and when asked to speak with few constraints imposed by the examiner. In confusion, we look for irrelevance and confabulation.

Schizophrenia

Most agree that the schizophrenic patient has a problem, but few agree on what constitutes the problem. Darby (1981) describes schizophrenia as a group of diseases with a symptom complex that produces massive disruption in thinking, mood, and behavior. Not all symptoms are present in every patient, and symptoms vary with time—from time to time, and as time postonset increases.

Debate rages on whether the schizophrenic patient has a language disorder. Benson (1975) holds that schizophrenia is characterized by abnormality in thinking, and this is mirrored in the patient's speech. He suggests it is unusual for the patient to have a breakdown in language. The schizophrenic patients he sees demonstrate intact speech and language, a sizable vocabulary, and corrrect use of grammar and syntax. It is the bizarre content of the patient's language that characterizes what is called "schizophrenic language." Brown (1972) agrees. Schizophrenic patients do not reveal a breakdown in language; they reveal a breakdown in thought. So, he suggests, there is not schizophrenic speech or language, there is schizophrenic thought that may be reflected in the patient's speech and language. Chaika (1974) disagrees and lists six features that characterize schizophrenic speech: disrupted phonological rules, disruption in matching semantic features, preoccupation with too many semantic features, influence by previously uttered words rather than the topic, disrupted syntax, and failure to self-monitor. But, Fromkin (1975) disagrees with Chaika. Except for problems in sequencing ideas, Fromkin points out that Chaika's features are prevalent in normal speech.

Whether the problem is one of thought or one of language, or both, language is used to identify schizophrenia. Chapman (1966) observed three features in schizophrenic verbal behavior: intermittent episodes of word-finding difficulty, inability to "screen out" unwanted words, and involuntary echoing of what is heard. Ostwold (1963) found prosodic abnormality in the speech of a sample of schizophrenic patients. Similarly, Todt and Howell (1980) found schizophrenic patients could be differentiated from normals on the basis of vocal qualities—less inflection, poorer enunciation, more repetitions and substitutions, and a significantly slower oral reading rate. Using a type-token ratio analysis to measure vocabulary diversity, Fairbanks (1944) found schizophrenic patients used fewer different words in speaking and writing than normals. A replication of Fairbank's effort by Feldstein and Jaffe (1962), however, showed no significant differences between schizophrenic patients and normals. Rochester, Martin, and Thurston (1977) observed that their schizophrenic patients were adequate communicators; however, the schizophrenic speech samples could be distinguished from nonschizophrenic samples with 75% accuracy. They relate that the schizophrenic speaker makes the listener's task difficult by requiring him to search for information which is never clearly given and by providing few conjunctive links between clauses.

Several investigations have compared schizophrenic patients with aphasic patients or used aphasia tests to seek language disturbance in schizophrenia. Taylor, Greenspan, and Abrams, (1979) administered an aphasia screening test to schizophrenic patients, patients with affective disorders, and normals. Their schizophrenic group made significantly more total errors and demonstrated temporoparietal signs including anomia, neologisms, and letter and number agnosias. Farber and Reichstein (1981) compared schizophrenic patients with "formal thought disorders," manic and depressed patients, and normals on the BDAE (Goodglass & Kaplan, 1972) and the Token Test (DeRenzi & Vignolo, 1962). The schizophrenic patients displayed significantly more errors on the Token Test and on the repetition of phrases BDAE subtest. The authors suggest that there is a subgroup of schizophrenic patients that could be labelled schizophasic schizophrenia. Conversely, Strohner, Cohen, Kelter, and Woll (1978) found no significant differences between schizophrenic patients, aphasic patients, and normals on a task of matching familiar environmental sounds with pictures. Horsfall (1972), using the PICA (Porch, 1973), observed his sample of schizophrenic patients were less severe than a sample of aphasic patients and a sample of bilateral brain-injured patients; however, the test profiles did not reveal useful differences among groups. Rausch, Prescott, and De Wolfe (1980) compared schizophrenic patients, aphasic patients, and normals on a word-ordering task. The aphasic group made significantly more errors and took longer to complete the task than the other two groups, and schizophrenic patients did not differ from normals except on items that required rearranging words to make sentences containing direct and indirect objects. Finally, Gerson, Benson, and Frazier (1977) found six differentiating characteristics when they compared schizophrenic patients with aphasic patients who had posterior lesions. First, the schizophrenic patients' responses were longer. Second, the aphasic patients were aware of their language deficit and disturbed by it, but the schizophrenic patients were not. Third, the aphasic patients used nonverbal substitutes or pauses to enlist the aid of the examiner. The schizophrenic patients did not. Fourth, the aphasic patients substituted letters, words, or neologisms. The schizophrenic patients did not. Fifth, vagueness in the aphasic patients' responses resulted from shifts in subject matter. And, sixth, aphasic patients displayed no persisting themes in their responses, but the schizophrenic patients produced bizarre themes and repeated them throughout their responses.

Benson (1973) suggests using six tasks to differentiate schizophrenic patients from aphasic patients: conversation, comprehension of spoken language, repetition, confrontation naming, reading, and writing. Di Simoni, Darley, and Aronson (1977) report that schizophrenic patients can be differentiated from aphasic patients on the measure used by Halpern, Darley and Brown (1973). In addition, they used Part V of the Token Test (DeRenzi & Vignolo, 1962); the Word Fluency Measure (Borkowski, Benton, & Spreen, 1967); a general information test; and a Temporal Orientation Test (Benton, Van Allen, & Fogel, 1964) to obtain a comprehensive sample of schizophrenic language. They observed that their sample had the most difficulty with relevance, arithmetic, and reading comprehension. Best performance was in syntax, adequacy, and naming. Only two of 27 patients displayed any articulatory deficits. Seventy percent of the sample performed within normal limits on Part V of the Token Test. Conversely, 75% fell below 80% correct on the general information test. The authors conclude that language disturbance in their sample was mild. The patients had no difficulty in making their wishes known. Performance on open-ended questions was much worse than on short-answer, specific questions. On the former, the patients displayed a wealth of extraneous conversation and irrelevant responses.

So, what does one use to appraise language in schizophrenic patients? If the tasks are to determine the presence or absence of deficits and to differentiate schizophrenia from other language disorders, the methods suggested by Benson (1973) and those employed by Di Simoni, Darley, and Aronson (1977) seem appropriate. One needs to include tasks that permit the schizophrenic patient to reveal his primary disorder—irrelevance. Conversation and open-ended questions should suffice. Appraisal may not answer the question of whether the patient's communication disorder results from disrupted thought or disrupted language. But, appraisal must determine whether a deficit is present and whether it differs from other language disorders.

Right Hemisphere Involvement

Appraisal of patients who have suffered a right hemisphere lesion presents similar problems to those encountered in appraising the schizophrenic patient. First, the problem is not clear. Is it disrupted language, or is it disrupted communication in patients with fairly intact language? Second, no ready-made tests or test batteries are available, so the appraiser must roll his own. Third, speech pathologists do not have a lengthy history of contact with the right hemisphere patient and are just beginning to learn what to look for.

Earlier, I suggested that the right hemisphere patient may have one or more of three problems—disrupted speech and language, disrupted nonverbal communication, or disrupted cognitive style. The speech has been described as "copious and inappropriate; as confabulatory, irrelevant, literal, and occasionally bizarre" (Myers, 1979, p. 38). Appraisal's task is to find out which, why and whether anything can be done about it.

We (Deal et al., 1979) followed tradition and used a measure—the PICA (Porch, 1973), traditionally used with aphasic patients—to look at behavior in right hemisphere patients. Using a discriminant function analysis (Porch, Friden, & Porec, 1976), 62% of our sample could not be distinguished from aphasia, 31% could, and 7% fell in a grey area—not aphasia, but not not aphasia. The PICA subtests that differentiated right hemisphere patients from aphasic patients were VIII, matching pictures with objects; XI, matching identical objects; A, writing the function of objects; and F, copying geometric shapes. Right hemisphere patients displayed relative difficulty on subtests VIII, XI, and F. Aphasic patients displayed relative success on these tasks. Right hemisphere patients did fairly well on subtest A. Aphasic patients found this task the most difficult one in the battery. We presented percentiles for right hemisphere performance to provide a measure of severity, but we concluded that there are probably more appropriate measures for detecting communication deficit in right hemisphere patients.

Myers (1979) reported her initial results with a battery she is developing to appraise right hemisphere patients. It includes the BDAE (Goodglass & Kaplan, 1972); the Hooper Test of Visual Organization (Hooper, 1958); a retelling a story task that presents the same information in three contexts—one emphasizing spatial context, one emotional context, and one noncanonical context—and an intensive interview with the patient and a family member. Initial results indicate that performance on the BDAE was within normal limits. However, verbal performance on the Cookie Theft picture, when filtered through the Yorkston and Beukelman (1977) analysis, contained mostly itemized responses and very few inferences. Right hemisphere performance on the Hooper was significantly lower than normal performance. Myers concluded that the right hemisphere patient has difficulty integrating information on a formal and a perceptual level. The deficit is represented in verbal expression. If the patient is irrelevant, Myers suggests investigating the reasons for it. Is it truly confabulatory and bizarre, or does it consist of related but unintegrated bits of information? The reason for irrelevance may surface when one compares responses on highly structured questions to responses on open-ended questions.

Myers and Linebaugh (1981) have appraised one aspect of cognitive style in right hemisphere patients, the ability to comprehend figurative language. Their right hemisphere patients gave literal responses indicating a lack of comprehension. Even though they demonstrated decent language skills, they were unable to use context to gain meaning, the way many aphasic patients and normals do.

Adamovich and Brooks (1981), recognizing that language batteries appropriate for left hemisphere patients do not provide a sufficient evaluation of communication deficits in right hemisphere patients, combined several measures to compare right hemisphere patients with normals. Their measures included: the BDAE (Goodglass & Kaplan, 1972); the Revised Token Test (McNeil & Prescott, 1978); the Hooper Test of Visual Organization (Hooper, 1958); the Detroit Test of Learning Aptitude (Baker & Leland, 1967); the Word Fluency Measure (Borkowski, Benton, & Spreen, 1967); and the Boston Naming Test (Kaplan, Goodglass, & Weintraub, 1976). They observed that right hemisphere patients had significant deficits in auditory comprehension, verbal expression, and reading, when performance was compared with their normal sample. They concluded that the deficits appeared to result from cognitive and linguistic lack rather than problems in visual perception, organization, or memory.

Given our present knowledge and our present ability to appraise the right hemisphere patient, Myers' (1979) suggestion to look at three areas appears wise. We need to tap speech and language ability to determine the presence or absence of specific or general problems, evaluate nonverbal communication, and appraise cognitive style. Some of our existing measures are appropriate for the first. Tools for the latter two are being developed and await refinement.

Dementia

Appraisal of the demented patient requires a look at biographical, medical, and behavioral data. Knowing a patient's biography may indicate how far the dementia has progressed, how far the patient has fallen. Knowing the medical history may assist in determining whether one is dealing with a true dementia or, perhaps, a pseudodementia resulting from depression. And, even if the dementia is real, the medical record may indicate whether it is one that may respond to treatment. Further, information about rapidity of onset, hemispheric localization, and whether the lesion is focal, diffuse, or disseminated may assist in differentiating dementia from aphasia.

Behavioral data on language abilities in demented patients come from two sources: the use of tests developed to appraise other disorders and the use of tests specifically designed to appraise dementia. Halpern, Darley, and Brown (1973) studied demented patients with their adaptation of

Schuell's (1957) short examination for aphasia. They found demented patients made more errors on tasks of adequacy, reading comprehension, arithmetic, and auditory comprehension, and fewer errors on tasks of fluency, writing to dictation, relevance, and syntax. Our replication (Deal, Wertz, & Spring, 1981) of their effort resulted in only somewhat similar results. While we agreed on the difficulty of tasks of adequacy and arithmetic and the ease of tasks of fluency, relevance, and syntax for demented subjects, we disagreed on writing to dictation and auditory retention tasks. Both were among the most difficult for our patients, but both were among the easiest for Halpern and colleagues' patients.

Appell, Kertesz, and Fishman (1981) used the WAB (Kertesz, 1982) to evaluate a group of patients with Alzheimer's disease. They report the patients' performance was aphasic. Patients were classified as global, Wernicke's, transcortical sensory, or anomic types. In addition, the sample showed severe deficits on other subtests—reading, writing, praxis, and construction—not used to measure aphasia on the WAB.

Watson and Records (1978) gave the PICA (Porch, 1973) to a sample of demented patients and a sample of aphasic patients. While the aphasic group was more severe, the demented group showed marked language deficit (60th percentile overall) on the PICA. Watson and Records suggest performance on specific subtests discriminated between aphasic and demented patients. The demented group had relatively more difficulty with primarily visual subtests—VIII, XI, E, and F—and relatively less difficulty with auditory subtests—VI, X, B, and C. The aphasic sample showed opposite performance, more difficulty with auditory than visual subtests.

Schwartz, Marin, and Saffran (1979) and Bayles and Boone (1982) report that semantic knowledge deteriorates in dementia, but there is relative preservation of syntactic and phonologic abilities. Horner and Heyman (1982) agree, but they suggest that as severity increases, demented patients begin to show syntax and phonologic errors, as well as semantic errors.

Some have attempted to develop measures for appraising language deficit in dementia. For example, Nelson and O'Connell (1978) developed the New Adult Reading Test (NART), a measure that assesses familiarity with words rather than the ability to decode unfamiliar words phonetically. Demented patients had no significant difficulty reading NART words; therefore, Nelson and O'Connell suggest performance will provide an estimate of premorbid intelligence.

Hughes, Berg, Danziger, Coben, and Martin (1982) have developed a clinical scale to determine the severity of dementia. Their Clinical Dementia Rating (CDR) uses a patient interview and tasks from a variety of tests to rate performance in six areas: memory, orientation, judgment + problem solving, community affairs, home + hobbies, and personal care. Ratings range from CDR 0, healthy; through CDR 0.5, questionable dementia; CDR 1, mild dementia; CDR 2, moderate dementia; to CDR 3, severe dementia.

Bayles (1982b) has developed a battery of measures to detect the presence and to rate the severity of dementia. Discriminant function analyses (Bayles, 1982a; Bayles & Boone, 1982) indicate that language tests are extremely sensitive in detecting dementia. Patients are classified as mild, moderate, or advanced on the following measures: receptive pragmatics, vocabulary, sentence error correction, visual/spatial, verbal reasoning, mental status, story retelling, sentence disambiguation, verbal description, and picture naming.

While we no longer rely exclusively on tests for aphasia to detect the presence and severity of dementia, our tools to evaluate the language of generalized intellectual deficit are few. Bayles (1982b) has demonstrated that language measures are as good as, if not better than, other psychometric measures for evaluating demented patients. Thus, the utility of appraising language deficits in demented patients has been established and justifies additional effort.

Aphasia

Each of the 17 tests listed at the beginning of this section were, primarily, designed to appraise aphasia. So, the problem in appraising aphasic patients is not a paucity of tools, but a problem in selecting among existing tools. Each of the existing measures has its strengths and its weaknesses. None constitute an adequate appraisal by itself. Typically, clinicians combine several measures into a battery and supplement the battery with additional measures if the patient's behavior dictates. This has been the approach with individual patients and with large, controlled studies of aphasia (Ludlow, 1983; Wertz et al., 1981). Unfortunately, the controlled studies are that, controlled, and do not have the flexibility of day-to-day patient management. Nevertheless, what is used to appraise a patient in a large, controlled study probably represents the state of the art, or at least one version of it, at the time the study is being conducted.

Table 1-1 shows the measures we are using in the current Veterans Administration Cooperative Study, "A Comparison of Clinic, Home, and Deferred Treatment for Aphasia." It differs from the battery we used in the first VA Cooperative Study (Wertz et al., 1981), and it differs from the battery employed in the Viet Nam Head Injury Study (Ludlow, 1983). It is more extensive than most clinicians employ with individual patients,

TABLE 1-1
Measures used to appraise aphasic patients in the Veterans Administration Cooperative Study, "A Comparison of Clinic, Home, and Deferred Treatment for Aphasia."

MEASURE	PURPOSE
Porch Index of Communicative Ability (Porch, 1973)	Quantified measure of communicative ability
Boston Diagnostic Aphasia Examination (Goodglass & Kaplan, 1972)	Provides type of aphasia and extends language sampled on the PICA
Communicative Abilities in Daily Living (Holland, 1980)	Measures "functional" communicative ability
Token Test (Spreen & Benton adaptation, 1969)	Extends measures of auditory comprehension
Reading Comprehension Battery for Aphasia (LaPointe Horner, 1979)	Extends measures of reading comprehension
Motor Speech Evaluation (Wertz & Rosenbek, 1971)	Determines the presence and severity of apraxia of speech and/or dysarthria
Coloured Progressive Matrices (Raven, 1962)	Estimate of nonverbal intelligence

but certain patients, in some clinics, may receive all of the measures listed at some time during the course of their management. The measures listed in Table 1-1 are not prescriptive. They are descriptive. They represent the "best" available tools, our biases; the most comprehensive, our needs; and economy, our limitations.

Probably, the most identifiable activity in appraising aphasia during the past 10 years has been the emphasis placed on "functional" communicative ability. The previous 10 years, 1965 through 1975, had seen the development of several standardized tests. The past ten years have seen a move to determine whether behavior on these standardized tests reflects what a patient does or does not do in nontest environments. Holland's CADL (1980) represents an organized means of evaluating functional language skills. Other measures include speech samples; for example, conversation on the BDAE (Goodglass & Kaplan, 1972) and WAB (Kertesz, 1982), or the length and complexity analysis suggested by Keenan and Brassell (1974).

Holland (1982c) cautions that the best measure of functional ability is to observe a patient communicating without prompts in the right environment.

So, the state of the art in appraising aphasic patients is characterized not by poverty but by preference. There are sufficient measures to select among, and the selection is influenced by the clinician's bias. Those who modify aphasia with adjectives select the BDAE or the WAB. Those who do not, pick a PICA or the MTDDA. Usually, patient performance, not clinician perference, dictates the measures used to supplement the primary measure or measures. This is as things should be.

The State of the Art

We have a wealth of measures for some disorders and few measures for other disorders. This prompts borrowing from the rich to appraise the poor. Recent experience indicates it may be better to develop appropriate measures for disorders that lack them, rather than apply tests designed for other disorders. When we use an aphasia test to appraise disorders other than aphasia, there is a good chance of finding aphasia in confusion, aphasia following a right hemisphere lesion, aphasia in dementia, etc. Not only do we need to develop appropriate measures for the environmental influences on the normal aged, for the language of confusion, and for schizophrenia, we also need to refine the batteries being developed by Myers (1979) for the right hemisphere patient and by Bayles (1982b) for the demented patient.

The purposes of appraisal, I believe, are to collect sufficient data to make a diagnosis, state a prognosis, and, if appropriate, focus therapy. I am not certain we are very efficient or reliable on any of these, especially on differentiating among disorders. Darley (1979b) seemed to agree. He suggested constructing tests trimmed down to those components that allow precise differentiation among disorders. An example of this type of appraisal measure might resemble Buschke's (1975) proposed method for evaluating language competence that is shown in Table 1-2. While Buschke intended his measure for aphasic patients, it may be useful in differentiating among language disorders. For example, if the required response eliminates the need for elaborate verbal, gestural, or written output, the aphasic patient may have the opportunity to display linguistic competence. Similarly, the demented patient may be identified by a lack of cognitive competence, the confused patient by irrelevance, etc. Thus, not only do we need measures to tell us that a disorder is present, we need measures to tell us that a disorder differs from other disorders.

TABLE 1-2
Method for evaluating language competence. (Adapted from Buschke, 1975)

PURPOSE	TASK	STIMULI	RESPONSE
Lexical Competence	Distinguishing real English words from paralogs	Hotel Vumac	Yes = real No = not real
Semantic Competence	Distinguishing meaningful sentences from nonsensical but grammatical strings of words	"Black clouds mean sudden storms. " "Rich clouds have important persons. "	Yes = makes sense No = does not make sense
Syntactic Competence	Distinguishing grammatical strings from random word strings	"Wild gentlemen mean clear battles. " "Animal skies famous sudden buy. "	Yes = right order No = wrong order
Cognitive Competence	Distinguishing true from false sentences	"Some dogs have short tails. " "Snow is soft and warm. "	Yes = true No = false

Finally, we need to become better at playing the game of appraisal. The appraisal room is an abode of boredom, confusion, and fear; fear of being found out, fear of failure. Our appraisal story is uneven. We are better at the middle, the testing, than we are at the beginning, preparing the patient for testing, and at the end, explaining to the patient how he or she did. Wheelchairs can become tumbrels as they roll to the place of appraisal. We can execute a patient with abundance. We have added new measures, but we have discarded few of the old measures. Our tests may corrode what a patient can do. There is a need for ecological evaluation, one that avoids erosion of what the patient brings with him to the appraisal session.

Diagnosis

Diagnosis involves putting a label on what one observes. We match the appraisal data—biographical, medical, behavioral—with our definitions and look for a best fit. Some signs have diagnostic significance and indicate the presence of one disorder, but not others. For example, Geschwind (1974b) suggests mutism is uncommon even in the most severe aphasia. Certain psychotic syndromes, however, may present with mutism. In dementia, mutism indicates the dementing process has progressed to the point where the patient has nothing more to say. Diagnosis, therefore, is the use of appraisal data to determine who is who.

Environmental Influence on the Normal Aged

The label "environmental influence" is applied when the person's environment is the culprit and there is no evidence of an organic or psychiatric cause of the communication deficit. Therefore, we must rule out the language of confusion, schizophrenia, a right hemisphere lesion, dementia, and aphasia. And, we must provide evidence that the person's environment has eroded communication skills that were intact until the environment worked its influence.

Biographical data should certify that the normal aged person was, indeed, normal. We look for evidence that indicates communication skills were appropriate for the person's age until entering his or her present environment. We seek intellectual and educational information from the person's past to estimate "premorbid"—in this case, prior to entering the present environment—abilities. We seek to avoid false accusation of the environment when potential causes may be lifelong low intelligence or illiteracy. And, we seek information on how communicative the person was prior to being institutionalized. A taciturn nontalker probably will not become verbose after entry into a nursing home.

Medical data are essential. We look for a clean bill of neurologic health. If we do not have a neurologic evaluation that concludes there is no evidence of CVA, trauma, degeneration, etc., we request that an evaluation be conducted. Confusion, aphasia, and right hemisphere signs erupt. Dementia and schizophrenia may creep. So, we look at performance and change in performance over time. Similarly, we look for sensory deficits— hearing, visual—that may interfere with communication and explain some of the patient's deficit. And, finally, the patient's medication—types, dosage—need to be explored to determine their possible influence on communication. The medical data, therefore, tell us that the normal aged person's communicative deficits cannot be explained by an organic cause, a psychiatric problem, sensory deficit, or medications. The lack of these prompt us to probe the environment for an explanation.

If we confuse environmental influences on communication with one of the other disorders being discussed here, we are likely to confuse it with dementia. The lack of an abrupt onset usually rules out confusion, aphasia, and right hemisphere involvement. Schizophrenia often can be ruled out because it leaves a trail. Seldom does it occur abruptly simply because the person's living environment has been changed. Schizophrenia, typically, has its onset in adolescence or early adulthood. Its onset in an elderly person would be considered a psychiatric curiosity.

Differentiating environmental influence on communication from dementia is more difficult. Bayles' (1982b) mildly demented patients differed from her normal age-matched controls, but not markedly. Holland's (1980) CADL data on institutionalized older persons show deficits, but they are not marked. Could they represent the early stages of dementia? Possibly. Our behavioral data may show deficits, but these data must be expanded to show not only what the patient can do, but also what he or she could do if environmental conditions were more favorable. Thus, we may need to manipulate our measures and probe areas of deficit by indicating that we are really interested in what the patient has to say and whether he or she understands what is said to him or her. We may need to suggest that a patient use coping strategies; for example, the use of context to improve comprehension and word finding, to determine whether skills are just rusty and not eroded. Sometimes, a final decision must await observation of change in the patient's communication after the environment is manipulated.

Some of the normal aged person's communication deficit may result from depression. Blazer and Williams (1980) report that 5 to 44% of the elderly are depressed. If severe, depression may masquerade as dementia. Finlayson and Martin (1982) label this condition pseudodementia. It shares similar signs with dementia, including lack of self care, restlessness, irritability, loss of creativity, somatic complaints, disorientation, and memory and concentration difficulties. Table 1-3 contrasts pseudodementia resulting from depression with true dementia. There are significant differences betweeen the two, and correct diagnosis requires that we look for these differences.

Finally, even after organic and psychiatric causes have been ruled out, diagnosis of environmental influence on communication requires documenting the presence of detrimental environmental influences. We look for the conditions listed earlier—a lack of opportunity for successful communication; no place to have a private conversation; low priority on communication by administration, staff, and patients; rules that restrict communication; and physical barriers that prevent communication.

TABLE 1-3
Comparison of pseudodementia and dementia. (After Finlayson &
Martin, 1982)

PSEUDODEMENTIA	*DEMENTIA*
Onset quite abrupt	Onset insidious
Progression usually rapid	Progression usually slow
Patient aware of deficits	Patient not as aware
Complaint of memory loss	Patient tries to hide loss (confabulates)
Global responses ("I don't know.")	Near-miss answers
Patient gives evidence of deficits	Patient emphasizes accomplishments
Impairment not usually worse at night	Usually worse at night
Mood depressed	Patient is typically "happy"
History of psychiatric disturbance common	Psychiatric history not common
Suicide risk considerable	Suicide risk much lower

Language of Confusion

Confused language fascinates. It must be differentiated from the bizarre responses and preoccupation with specific themes seen in the schizophrenic patient, the sometimes irrelevant responses made by the patient with a right hemisphere lesion, and the irrelevant respones that may flow from the aphasic patient with a severe auditory comprehension deficit that prevents him from understanding what was requested. Similarly, the normal aged in an impoverished communication environment, or the demented patient may appear confused, because he or she is not oriented to date, to place, or to his or her condition. But, unlike the patient with the language of confusion, neither confabulate.

Biographical information provides data to identify the confused patient's confabulation. Knowing that a patient parked cars for a living assists in identifying a tale of being a fish farmer as confabulation. Biographical information provides an accurate data base.

Medical data confirm the presence of bilateral brain injury, often traumatically induced, as a cause of confused language. The absence of brain damage or the presence of unilateral damage lead us to look elsewhere for a diagnosis, perhaps schizophrenia or environmental influence, when there is no evidence of brain damage, and, perhaps, right hemisphere deficits or aphasia, when there is a unilateral lesion.

The behavioral data, however, pull the confused patient's covers. The absence of word-finding deficits and the good syntax, coupled with irrelevance and confabulation, signify confusion. Halpern, Darley, and Brown (1973) report that the confused patient may show the specific deficits seen in aphasia and dementia—reading and writing deficits and a lack of adequacy—but the patient's lack of relevance differentiates confusion from those with aphasia or dementia.

Schizophrenia

Schizophrenic patients may masquerade as demonstrating another disorder. Sometimes, their bizarre responses are difficult to differentiate from the irrelevance and confabulation seen in the language of confusion. Their "word-salad" composed of real words, phonemic substitutions, verbal substitutions, and neologisms may make their speech unintelligible and similar to that seen in some aphasic patients. What Kleist (1960) has called "ethical flattening" and "affective blunting" in schizophrenia may be difficult to differentiate from similar behavior in a patient with a right hemisphere lesion. Again, one turns to the appraisal data to determine who is who.

Biographical information should indicate that a schizophrenic patient's history was influenced by the onset of psychiatric disturbance some time in late adolescence or early adulthood. His or her educational and work history may reveal how schizophrenia has influenced his or her life. Medical data should indicate the history of psychiatric disturbance and the lack of focal or diffuse cerebral pathology as an explanation for past and present behavior. Kitselman (1981) suggests that when an adequate history is available, differentiating schizophrenia from aphasia is not difficult. Similarly, the history coupled with behavioral data should permit differentiating schizophrenia from other disorders.

Di Simoni, Darley, and Aronson (1977) report that both relevance and reading comprehension are impaired in schizophrenia. Halpern, Darley, and Brown (1973) report similar results for confused patients. However, examination of both sets of data indicates relevance is more impaired than reading comprehension in schizophrenia, and the reverse is seen in confusion. Further, schizophrenic patients make more fluency errors, relative

to their performance on other tasks, and fluency errors were the least frequently occurring problem—relative to their performance on other tasks—
in confused patients. Finally, a comparison of the two reports indicates
schizophrenic patients make about 50% fewer total errors than are made
by confused patients. Nevertheless, Di Simoni et al. found schizophrenic
patients deteriorate as time postonset increases. At some point in time,
the schizophrenic patient may be difficult to differentiate from the confused patient. One must look at the medical data. The presence or absence
of demonstrable brain injury will tip the diagnostic decision.

Differentiating schizophrenia from aphasia, according to Benson (1975),
should not be difficult. He suggests schizophrenic "word-salad" is seen
only in chronic, severe schizophrenia and, therefore, if present, usually
represents a true aphasia when there is no history of mental problems.
When in doubt, Benson recommends using a test of auditory comprehension to differentiate aphasia from schizophrenia. Horsfall's (1972) PICA
data indicate that his sample of schizophrenic patients showed they were
less severe than a sample of aphasic patients and a sample of bilaterally
damaged patients. These results are shown in Figure 1-1. His schizophrenic
sample performed at approximately the 85th percentile overall on left
hemisphere norms and at the 95th percentile overall on bilateral norms.
Because a difference in severity may imply differences in the pattern of
performance that do not exist, I have equated performance among the
three samples by using 85th percentile left hemisphere and 95th percentile
bilateral norms from the PICA manual. This manipulation is shown in
Figure 1-2. When performance is equated for severity with aphasia and
bilateral brain injury, there is little in the test profiles that differentiates
schizophrenic patients from the other two groups.

Di Simoni et al. (1977) report that impaired relevance and relatively intact writing, reading, and listening abilities differentiate the schizophrenic
patient from the aphasic patient. Even the older, long-time postonset
schizophrenic patient in their sample was more likely to resemble dementia than aphasia. Thus, diagnosis of schizophrenia can be made by noting
the presence of a high degree of irrelevance, an absence of signs that indicate central-language impairment, and an absence of brain injury.

Right Hemisphere
Involvement

To diagnose right hemisphere involvement, one looks for information
in the biographical data indicating that the patient was a normal communicator prior to suffering a right hemisphere lesion. We check education to rule out illiteracy. The medical data should show the presence of

FIGURE 1-1
PICA Ranked Response Summary comparing performance by schizophrenic, aphasic, and bilateral brain-injured patients. (After Horsfall, 1972).

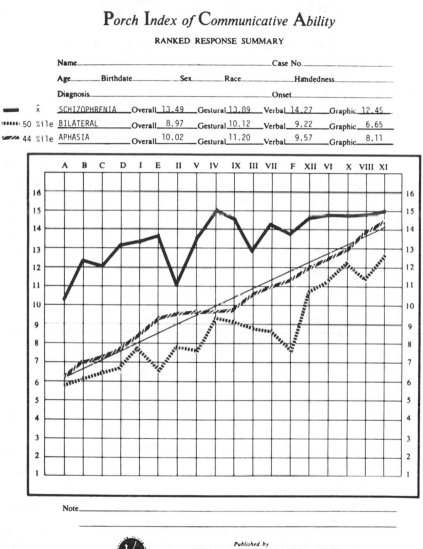

Porch Index of Communicative Ability

RANKED RESPONSE SUMMARY

Name_____Case No._____

Age_____Birthdate_____Sex_____Race_____Handedness_____

Diagnosis_____Onset_____

x̄   SCHIZOPHRENIA   Overall 13.49   Gestural 13.89   Verbal 14.27   Graphic 12.45

50 %ile BILATERAL   Overall 8.97   Gestural 10.12   Verbal 9.22   Graphic 6.65

44 %ile APHASIA   Overall 10.02   Gestural 11.20   Verbal 9.57   Graphic 8.11

Note_____

Published by
CONSULTING PSYCHOLOGISTS PRESS
577 College Avenue   Palo Alto, California

FIGURE 1-2
PICA Ranked Response Summary comparing performance by schizophrenic patients with aphasic and bilateral brain-injured patients who have been equated for severity. (After Horsfall, 1972)

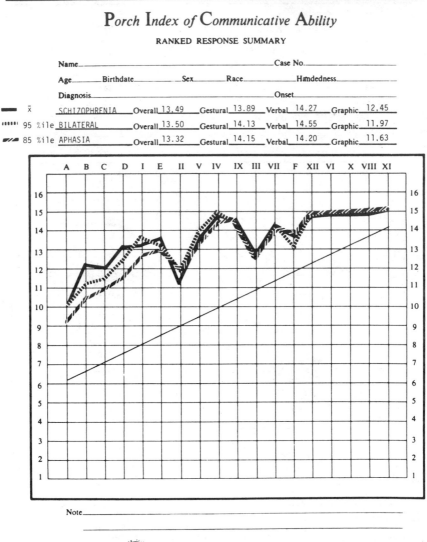

Porch Index of Communicative Ability

RANKED RESPONSE SUMMARY

Name		Case No.		
Age___Birthdate___ Sex___ Race___			Handedness	
Diagnosis		Onset		

		Overall	Gestural	Verbal	Graphic
x̄	SCHIZOPHRENIA	13.49	13.89	14.27	12.45
95 %ile	BILATERAL	13.50	14.13	14.55	11.97
85 %ile	APHASIA	13.32	14.15	14.20	11.63

Note_____

Published by
CONSULTING PSYCHOLOGISTS PRESS
577 College Avenue   Palo Alto, California

a right hemisphere lesion and its suspected cause. In the behavioral data provided by other disciplines, we look for the presence of other disorders—spatial perception and body image disorders, visual perception disorders, constructional disabilities, auditory perception disorders, somatosensory disorders, motor impersistence—which suggest right hemisphere involvement. In our language data, we look for behavior that differentiates the patient from those who are aphasic, demented, and schizophrenic.

Though rare, some individuals demonstrate "crossed aphasia." This condition, today, refers to aphasia in a right-handed person following damage to the right hemisphere (Hecaen & Albert, 1978). Estimates of incidence range from 0.4% (Hecaen, Magurs, Remier, et al., 1971) to 10% (Branch, Milner, & Rasmussen, 1964). These patients appear to be aphasic and should be diagnosed as such. They are not the patients being discussed here who demonstrate communicative deficits subsequent to a right hemisphere lesion. Nevertheless, the latter group have been described as displaying "aphasia-like" behavior (Archibald & Wepman, 1968), and 62% of our right hemisphere sample resembled aphasia on the PICA (Deal et al., 1979). So, they may create a diagnostic dilemma.

The general sign that differentiates the patient with right hemisphere communication impairment from the left hemisphere aphasic patient is the former's relatively good language, which contrasts sharply with his impaired communication. Myers' (1979) specific signs—failure to integrate information on a perceptual level, tendency to itemize rather than interpret information, irrelevance, better performance on structured tasks than on open-ended tasks, lack of affect, caustic sense of humor—tend to help separate right hemisphere communication deficit from aphasia.

Medical data differentiate the right hemisphere patient from the demented patient. The former has a unilateral, usually focal, lesion, and the latter has bilateral, diffuse, disseminated, or multifocal lesions. Similarly, the presence of a unilateral, right hemisphere lesion differentiates the right hemisphere patient from the schizophrenic patient who has no evidence of brain injury.

Dementia

Wells (1982) discusses two types of errors that can be made in diagnosing dementia. The first is a failure to recognize dementia, thus labeling the patient's problem as functional. The second is the reverse of the first; diagnosing dementia when the problem is functional, and not organic. Usually, either error occurs when dementia and depression coexist, as they frequently do. The main source of error, Wells believes, is to assume that cognitive loss automatically indicates organicity. While cognitive deficit is a primary sign of an organic syndrome, Wells does not believe it is diagnostic of it. He does not think any neuropsychological measure of cognition can be devised to differentiate dementia from functional disorders that resemble it. He suggests a diagnosis of dementia is appropriate only when there is approximately the same amount of impairment in cognition, behavior, and affect. Diagnosing dementia, therefore, may be more difficult than one might expect.

Certainly, environmental influence on the communication of the normal aged can be considered functional. It is necessary to differentiate them from demented patients. The influence of depression on behavior in older persons was discussed earlier, and differential diagnostic signs provided by Finlayson and Martin (1982) were listed. Nevertheless, Bayles (1982b) relates that misdiagnosis occurs in approximately 15% of demented patients. Her cluster analyses (Bayles, 1982a) identified 83% of her demented sample and 77% of her normal sample correctly. Bollinger (1970) reported little difficulty in differentiating normals from demented patients on the PICA. His normal sample performed significantly faster than his demented patients, and the latter identified themselves by writing performance that was significantly worse than their gestural and verbal performance. Thus, utilization of data in the three areas requested by Wells (1982)—cognition, behavior (for our purposes, language behavior), and affect—plus medical evidence of bilateral brain injury, should be sufficient to differentiate the normal aged in a communication-impairing environment from the demented person.

The patient with the language of confusion may masquerade as a demented patient. Halpern et al. (1973) have demonstrated that the key diagnostic sign to differentiate between the two disorders is relevance. In their samples, the confused group made 40% relevance errors and the demented group made only 10% relevance errors. Reading was similar in the two groups, but writing to dictation differed. Confused patients made 44% writing errors and demented patients only 10%. The presence of bilateral brain injury does not tell who is who. Both of Halpern and associates' groups tended to be bilateral. However, rapidity of onset and duration of symptoms differed. Eighty percent of the confused patients had a rapid onset—less than 10 days—and 90% of the demented group had a slow onset. Similarly, 100% of the confused patients had a duration of symptoms of less than 3 months. Conversely, 90% of the demented patients had a duration of symptoms of over 3 months. Combined medical and language data, therefore, assist in differentiating dementia from confusion.

A similar approach can be used to differentiate dementia from schizophrenia. Di Simoni et al. (1977) have shown relevance errors abound in schizophrenic patients, 45%, and Halpern et al. (1973) have demonstrated they are rare in dementia, 10%. Fluency errors were the fourth most frequent type in the Di Simoni et al. schizophrenic sample. Fluency errors were the least frequent type in the Halpern et al. demented sample. Di Simoni et al. do note that the older, long-time postonset schizophrenic patient may, eventually, resemble the demented patient. However, for most, comparing the language behavior of the two groups and the presence of bilateral injury in dementia, and its absence in schizophrenia, should sort out dementia from schizophrenia. If one is still puzzled, a look at the age of onset may make the decision. Dementia is a problem that occurs in later life, and schizophrenia, typically, has its onset in late adolescence or early adulthood.

Demented, or aphasic, or both? This question plagues clinicians, and, gradually, they are beginning to line up behind one of the three possibilities. I stand in the queue that differentiates the language deficit in dementia from that seen in aphasia. While some of the language behavior in the demented patient resembles that seen in aphasia, I see no useful purpose served by talking about aphasia in dementia. Yet, some do.

Ernst, Dalby, and Dalby (1970) reported "aphasic symptoms" in dementia. Watson and Heilman (1974) believe aphasia may be seen in degenerative diseases, such as Alzheimer's and Pick's. Hecaen and Albert (1978) report that aphasia may suddenly appear in a previously demented patient. Appell et al. (1981) administered the WAB (Kertesz, 1982) to a sample of Alzheimer's patients and concluded that all were aphasic. And, Horner and Heyman (1982) differentiate between focal aphasia and dementia, but they label the language deficits in the latter, Alzheimer's aphasia.

Conversely, Rochford (1971) has demonstrated that the naming deficit in dementia results from visual misrecognition of the stimulus and not the linguistic anomic deficit seen in aphasia. Halpern et al. (1973) observed that reading comprehension was the second most frequent error in their demented patients, and it was the third least frequent error in their aphasic sample. In addition, their aphasic patients had severe auditory retention deficits, but their demented patients had only moderate difficulty on auditory retention tasks. Finally, fluency errors were frequent in the aphasic patients, 33%, but they were rare, 9%, in their demented sample. They concluded that the language of intellectual impairment seen in their demented patients could be differentiated from aphasia by comparison of each group's profile of deficits on a battery of language tests. Our replication (Deal, Wertz, & Spring, 1981) of their effort, including the use of Q-correlations to provide an index of similarity between profiles, tended to pick out the aphasic patients, 17 of 21, but was less than adequate for classifying the demented patients, only 8 of 15. Nevertheless, when we used all data—biographical, medical, and behavioral—all patients, aphasic and demented, were diagnosed correctly. Thus, Well's (1982) requirement for more data than that provided by a neuropsychologic measure, appears sage. When combined data are used, typically, one can differentiate dementia from aphasia and from other disorders.

Aphasia

Because diagnosis of aphasia is being discussed last, there appears to be little left to say about differentiating it from other disorders. But, for a patient to be labeled aphasic, he or she must meet one's definition of aphasia. And, as was true with the other disorders, we scan the biographical, medical, and behavioral data for evidence.

Information about premorbid literacy and intelligence should be obtained. Diagnosis of aphasia may be complicated in patients who lacked education or had diminished intelligence at onset. Sensory deficits—vision, hearing—if present must be identified and weighed in the diagnostic decision. We must have evidence of unilateral, typically left hemisphere, brain damage. And, we must see a general language deficit that crosses all communicative modalities—auditory comprehension, reading, oral expressive language, and writing. Deficits in all areas need not be, and usually are not, equal, but to be aphasic, one must show deficits in all areas.

The latter requirement creates an interesting difference in the identification of aphasia between those who do and those who do not use adjectives to modify it. The former group, generally, utilize the BDAE or WAB to detect the presence, severity, and type of aphasia. Neither instrument requires the examiner to use reading and writing performance to diagnose aphasia. Both utilize conversation, picture description, verbal repetition, naming, and auditory comprehension to make the diagnosis, estimate severity, and determine type. The latter group, those who do not type, typically include reading and writing performance along with auditory comprehension and oral expressive performance to make a diagnosis and determine severity. I do not imply that those who type aphasia would do so if the patient displayed no deficits in reading or writing. But, it is interesting to note that even though the BDAE and the WAB contain excellent means for appraising reading and writing, performance in these areas is not required to make a diagnosis of aphasia.

As with several other disorders, Halpern et al. (1973) provide a profile for aphasia. The most salient subtests in their battery were tasks of auditory retention, auditory comprehension, and fluency. Deficits in these areas tended to differentiate their aphasic patients from their demented and confused groups. In addition, their aphasic sample displayed more total language deficit than the other groups studied. Our use (Deal et al., 1981) of the Halpern et al. profile for aphasia successfully classified 17 of 21 aphasic patients. When we combined language performance with medical data—all aphasic patients had a rapid onset, less than 10 days; all had a left hemisphere lesion; and all had a focal lesion—we had no difficulty in differentiating aphasia from dementia.

A persisting problem in the diagnosis of aphasia is not necessarily its identification but whether it is present in the other disorders being discussed here. For example, is aphasia the communicative deficit in the normal aged person, the schizophrenic patient, the confused patient, the patient with a right hemisphere lesion, and the demented patient? I believe it is not very useful to say it is. While we seem to know more about aphasia than we do about the other disorders, calling the language deficit in the other disorders aphasia does not add to our knowledge; it complicates it.

However, disorders can, and do, coexist. We talk about apraxia of speech coexisting with aphasia (Darley, 1982; Wertz, 1978). Why not aphasia coexisting with dementia? If we can tease out evidence for the presence of two disorders in coexisting aphasia and apraxia of speech, for example, articulatory errors indicating apraxia of speech and semantic and syntax errors indicating aphasia, we might be able to identify aphasia coexisting with dementia. Some (Appell et al., 1981) argue that the language deficit in dementia is aphasia. Others (Hecaen and Albert, 1978) suggest that the two coexist. I believe neither position is correct or, at least, very useful. Unlike coexisting aphasia and apraxia of speech, where the former is a language disorder and the latter is a motor speech disorder, both aphasia and the demented patient's language of generalized intellectual impairment are language disorders. Calling one the other or indicating the coexistence of two language disorders in the same patient does not assist in patient management.

I (1982) have utilized Watson and Records' (1978) PICA data to demonstrate that the langauge deficits in aphasia and dementia differ. Figure 1-3 shows PICA performance by their aphasic and demented samples. Performance in the aphasic sample has been equated for severity with the demented sample. The demented patients do better on more difficult writing tasks—Subtest A, B, and C; worse on most verbal tasks—Subtests IV, IX, and XII; worse on auditory tasks—Subtests VI and X; and worse on visual tasks—Subtests VIII and XI. If one compares PICA Subtest percentiles, as shown in Figure 1-4., the profiles of the two groups differ even more markedly. Finally, use of the Porch et al. (1976) discriminate function analysis, which requires multiplying selected subtest

FIGURE 1-3
PICA Ranked Response Summary comparing performance by aphasic patients with performance by demented patients. The samples have been equated for severity. (After Watson & Records, 1978)

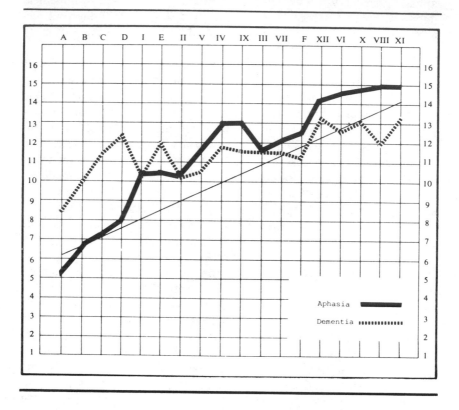

percentiles by an appropriate weight to obtain a discriminate score, indicates that the demented sample is not aphasic. Scores larger than $-.211$ represent aphasia, and scores less than $-.279$ are considered nonaphasic. My calculations for Watson and Records' demented sample yield a score of $-.612$, clearly nonaphasic.

A final problem in the diagnosis of aphasia is determining when a patient is no longer aphasic. Some suffer a mild aphasia, others improve to a point where they no longer are aphasic on the measures we use. Duffy (1981) has discussed this "grey area" between mild aphasia and normal language ability. His PICA data (Duffy & Keith, 1980) show that scores achieved by left brain-injured patients above the 90th percentile overlap with scores achieved by normal subjects. Other tests for aphasia—Token

FIGURE 1-4
Comparison of PICA subtest percentile performance by demented and aphasic patients. (After Watson & Records, 1978)

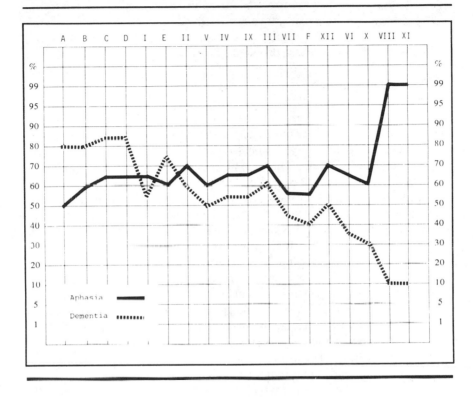

Test, Word Fluency Measure, BDAE—contain similar problems in differentiating mild aphasia from no aphasia. Presently, one of the best solutions to the dilemma is to ask the patient, "Is your language as good as it was before your stroke?" The sanity of this approach is well documented in Moss's (1972) account of his own aphasia.

State of the Art

As we mature, we become more and more adroit at differentiating among language disorders and less and less prone to abet mislabeling. However, problems persist. Only recently have we discovered some disorders, for example, communication deficit in the normal aged brought on by environmental influence; and only recently have we probed problems we have known exist, for example, communication deficits in schizophrenia and following a right hemisphere lesion. We lack measures to explore the new, and we tend to apply measures for the new that may be appropriate only for the old. For example, appraising right hemisphere deficit with a measure appropriate for aphasia may result in identifying the former as the latter. We have not resolved the dilemma of coexisting disorders. Does a patient display more than one type of language disorder, or does the way we appraise problems dictate a "two for" when only one exists? Finally, time postonset confounds. What begins as one disorder may gradually assume the characteristics of another.

Progress in differentiating one disorder from another has been steady but not rapid. Efforts akin to those of Halpern et al. (1973) and Di Simoni et al. (1977), that compare one disorder with another on the same measure, are marked by their rarity. Table 1-4 shows data adapted from reports by Halpern et al., and Di Simoni et al. that differentiate among aphasia, dementia, the language of confusion, and schizophrenia. Absent are similar data for environmental influence on the normal aged and right hemisphere involvement. When the state of the art is written on diagnosis in 5 years, one would hope that the missing data will have been provided, or, perhaps, a new measure that tells who is who will have replaced our current tools.

I believe what you call it is important; that determining who is who is useful. Certainly, the words are not important, but what the words imply should make a difference. Diagnosis is more than arranging phonemes to create labels that differ one from the other. Diagnosis carries implications that transcend the labels. It implies prognosis, and it dictates appropriate management. Sometimes, we suffer the same fate as our patients whose ideas, like most of their ideas, pass through their minds without words, and any attempt to form the ideas into words fails, indeed may chase the ideas from their minds. Clinicians, like their patients, continue to seek the right words to label what they observe.

Prognosis

Attempts to prognose are exercises in augury. We utilize what the patient brings with him or her—a biography, medical data—and combine these with what he or she has to tell us about his or her problems—behavioral data—and the diagnosis to predict his or her future. Nothing is more important to the patient, and unfortunately, this is what we do less well than anything else.

Usually our prognostic statements are a best guess, and the precision we are capable of is restricted to predicting change on a specific language measure. What we can do may have little to say about what the patient will

TABLE 1-4
Salient speech and language behaviors for four language disorders.

	APHASIA	DEMENTIA	CONFUSION	SCHIZOPHRENIA
M O S T	Adequacy	Adequacy	Reading Comprehension	Relevance
	Auditory Retention	Reading Comprehension	Writing to Dictation	Reading Comprehension
I M P A I R E D	Fluency	Auditory Retention	Relevance	Fluency
			Adequacy	
L E A S T	Reading Comprehension	Relevance	Auditory Retention	Auditory Retention
	Writing to Dictation	Writing to Dictation	Fluency	Writing to Dictation
I M P A I R E D	Relevance	Fluency		Adequacy

Generally, "most impaired" indicates percent of error is above the mean percent of total errors for each disorder, and "least impaired" indicates percent of error is below the mean percent of total errors for each group. (Adapted from Di Simoni, Darley, & Aronson, 1977)

be able to do. We are not very good at stating prognosis for "What." Dresser, Meirowsky, Weiss, McNeel, Simon, and Caveness (1973) indicated that 75% of their sample of Korean War veterans with head trauma were involved in some kind of employment 15 years after onset. Such reports are very rare.

Frequently, prognosis must be filtered through whether the patient will or will not receive treatment. Jellinek and Harvey (1982) report 73% of their brain-injured sample were considered appropriate for vocational and/or educational rehabilitation, but only 51% of these received a rehabilitation program. None of the patients who did not receive rehabilitation returned to work or school, whereas 78% of those who were treated did. Thus, treatment appears to influence prognosis.

Finally, our ability to state a patient's future is better for some language disorders than it is for others. For example, we are better at prognosticating for the aphasic patient than we are for the normal aged in a communication-impairing environment. The following is what I think we know, but mostly, what I think we do not know about prognosis for the different language disorders being discussed here.

Environmental Influence on the Normal Aged

I find no empirical evidence to indicate that the normal aged person in a communication-impairing environment has a bright or a bleak future. By definition, we might assume that the patient's future depends upon modification of the environment. If it can be changed to promote a favorable climate for communication, the patient's future should be promising. If it cannot, lack of change or additional erosion should be the result. But, we do not know. Only a few treatment studies, to be discussed later, imply that patients in a custodial setting improve if given appropriate stimulation. However, it is not clear whether these patients are those whose communication deficits result from environmental influence, or whether they should be placed in another diagnostic group.

Thus, we can say little about the normal aged person's potential for regaining environmentally eroded communication skills. Can what has been lost be regained? Are there variables which may predict who is most resistant to environmental influences? Will improvement result if the environment becomes more favorable? We do not know. Of course, we could find out. Comparison of language behavior pre- and post-environmental manipulation appears to be a first step.

Language of Confusion

One might expect the patient with the language of confusion to have a favorable prognosis. Chedru and Geschwind (1972) used the adjective "acute" to modify confusional state. So, change is expected. But, in what direction? Brosin (1967) suggests confusion is a disorder caused by reversible, temporary, diffuse disturbance in brain function. He believes it is usually brief, but he cautions it may persist up to 1 month or longer and may end in health and cure, death, or chronic disease. Pick a prognosis from this description. Reversible, temporary, brief, health and cure imply a favorable future for the confused patient. Death or chronic disease forecast something else. Again, I have found no empirical evidence to predict who can expect what.

My clinical experience indicates that patients who are correctly diagnosed as demonstrating the language of confusion can expect to improve rapidly and markedly. One returned to his previous position as a high school mathematics teacher within a year postonset. Another went back to parking cars. My clinical experience also indicates that the confused patient who does not make marked and rapid improvement may receive a change in his or her diagnosis. Lack of positive change may shift the confused patient's diagnosis to dementia or language disturbance undetermined. Because the language of confusion is rare, few clinicians see enough of it to build a data base for prediction.

Perhaps what causes the confusion may hold an answer. For example, the acute cases studied by Chedru and Geschwind (1972) included patients with acute alcoholic intoxication, barbituate intoxication, those undergoing electro-convulsive therapy, and those undergoing general anesthesia. All of these conditions could be expected to improve, and Chedru and Geschwind report they did. However, we know little about the future for the tumor, trauma, infection, and hematoma cases studied by Halpern et al. (1973).

Schizophrenia

A few pieces of information are beginning to emerge to assist in predicting the schizophrenic patient's future. However, none are specifically applicable for predicting change in the schizophrenic patient's language behavior.

Negative prognostic signs include age, duration, and intelligence. Di Simoni et al. (1977) report older schizophrenic patients and those who are a long time postonset have more severe language deficits, often resembling the language of confusion or dementia. Rioch and Lubin (1959) have observed that schizophrenic patients with IQs below 90 do not respond favorably to long-term intensive psychotherapy. However, their patients with IQs at, or above, 110 varied in their response to treatment and did not permit prediction. Pollack, Levenstein, and Klein (1968) suggest that patients with higher IQs do better in treatment than those with lower IQs.

A positive prognostic sign appears to be the patient's social milieu. Klonoff, Fibiger, and Hutton (1970) observed that ambulatory outpatients performed better than nonambulatory inpatients on the Halstead-Reitan battery. Caton (1982) found that the quality of a patient's living environment and the relationship with significant others are critical in determining whether he or she will require hospitalization. Interestingly, Caton also observed that the patient's length of hospitalization bore no relationship with subsequent hospitalization, treatment compliance, or social functioning in the community.

Thus, older, long-time postonset, low intelligence schizophrenic patients with unfavorable living environments and poor relationships with significant others appear to have a poor prognosis for improvement. Conversely, younger, close-to-onset schizophrenic patients, with favorable living environments, and good relationships with significant others have a brighter future. That is not much on which to hang a prognosis. But, it is a beginning.

Right Hemisphere Involvement

What we know about prognosis for the right hemisphere patient is sparse, but what we do know indicates the prognosis is not very good. Prognostic information comes from two sources, examination of variables that may predict whether the patient will return to work, and comparison of improvement in patients with right hemisphere lesions to improvement made by patients with left hemisphere lesions.

Weisbroth, Esibill, and Zuger (1971) examined the influence of seven variables on the probability of the right hemisphere patient returning to work. They found no predictive information in age and education. Gender; ambulation; use of the affected upper extremity; and cognition, measured by performance on a block design task, all had prognostic significance. More females in their right hemisphere sample returned to work than males. More patients who could walk, and who had some use of their affected upper extremity, returned to work than those who were nonambulatory, and/or had minimal use of their affected upper extremity. Those with better cognition were more likely to return to work. In the Weisbroth et al. sample of 28 patients, only 11 returned to work. The average time postonset when they re-entered the world of work was 19 months. All who returned to work had received an average of 10 months of vocational rehabilitation.

Right hemisphere patients make less gain in developing self-care activities than left hemisphere patients, even though they receive longer inpatient rehabilitation (Gordon, Drenth, Jarvis, Johnson, & Wright 1978). Even after discharge, Forer and Miller (1980) and Lorenze and Canero (1962) report that the right hemisphere patient demonstrates greater impairment in activities of daily living than the left hemisphere patient. Golper (1980) compared right and left hemisphere patients on a verbal picture description task at 1 week and 1 month postonset. The left hemisphere patients improved the efficiency of their verbal communication. The right hemisphere patients continued to give redundant statements and irrelevant remarks, indicating that their recovery of language was characterized by less efficiency than the left hemisphere patients.

Based on the minimal information available, the patient with a right hemisphere lesion, therefore, has a guarded prognosis. Less than half return to work. Their ability to walk, their use of their involved upper extremity, and their cognitive ability appear to predict whether they will become employed. Even though they have less language deficit than the left hemisphere patient, their communication skills continue to be impaired.

Dementia

Causes of dementia can be divided into those that are treatable and those for which there is no treatment. Prognosis is, of course, better for patients with a treatable cause than for those with an untreatable cause. Prognosis is best for those who have been misdiagnosed—for example, pseudodementia resulting from depression.

The most frequent cause of dementia is Alzheimer's disease. It strikes, typically, in the 4th or 5th decade of life, and the downhill course may continue for up to 10 years before death intervenes. Older Alzheimer's patients may survive only a few years. Thus, dementia resulting from Alzheimer's disease has a poor prognosis for improvement. Prognosis, like diagnosis, is complicated in Alzheimer's disease, because its presence is usually verifiable only at autopsy (Friedland, 1982). Thus the patient is typically labeled as demonstrating Alzheimer's "type" dementia. Nevertheless, these patients constitute the overwhelming majority of demented patients, and their future is bleak.

Treatable dementias are few. Freeman and Rudd (1982) found only 16 patients with a potentially reversible cause in a sample of 110 who had progressive intellectual deterioration. Twelve of the 16 responded favorably to medical, surgical, and psychiatric treatment. Their underlying illnesses included normal-pressure hydrocephalus, subdural hematoma, depression, hempatic encephalopathy, and chronic drug overdose. The intellectual deterioration in this group was of short duration, and all patients showed less cortical atrophy on their computed tomographic scans than patients with idiopathic dementia. The average age of the treatable patients did not differ significantly from the average age of the patients with idiopathic dementia.

Therefore, prognosis in dementia is poor, except for patients with a potentially treatable cause. The latter group can be identified by a shorter duration of symptoms and less cortical atrophy on CT scans.

Aphasia

We have used three methods to predict the aphasic patient's future: prognostic variables, behavioral profiles on language measures, and statistical prediction. The first approach utilizes biographical, medical, and behavioral characteristics to predict change or the lack of it. The second involves evaluating a patient, constructing a profile of performance, and comparing this with change made by previous patients with a similar profile. The third employs multiple regression techniques to predict performance on a measure of aphasia at different points in time postonset. Use of prognostic variables and the behavioral profile are limited to forecasting with an adjective—good, fair, guarded, poor. Unfortunately, prognostic variables coexist, and a patient may have both favorable and unfavorable signs. We do not know how positive and negative signs interact to influence change. The behavioral profile approach is hampered by inability to classify some patients into a specific prognostic group. Finally, statistical prediction has promise, but it is not sufficiently developed for use with individual patients.

Over the years, we have observed the influence of specific variables on change in aphasia. Some have withstood the test of time. Others have not. Table 1-5 shows the conclusions I reached in a recent review (Wertz, 1983a) regarding the influence of selected variables on improvement in aphasia. Age, formerly believed to have prognostic importance, has not held up as a significant sign in recent reports. Education, premorbid intelligence, and occupational status have always been debatable as prognostic indicants, and they remain so today. Etiology has an influence on the patient's future. Aphasia resulting from closed head trauma improves more than aphasia resulting from CVA (Alajouanine, Castaigne, L'Hermitte, Escourolle, & De Ribancourt, 1957; Eisenson, 1964; Kertesz & McCabe, 1977; Luria, 1963). The size of the lesion and its localization influence recovery. Yarnell, Monroe, and Sobel (1976) and Rubens (1975) are consistent in their observations that patients with small lesions, a single lesion, and lesions that avoid the temporal-parietal region have a better prognosis than those with large lesions, multiple or bilateral lesions, and damage in the temporal-parietal cortex. Health, severity, and time postonset have held up as useful prognostic signs. Patients in good health postonset improve more than those in poor health (Anderson, Bourestom,

TABLE 1-5
Selected variables suggested to have an influence on improvement in aphasia. + = agreement, ? = conflicting reports.

VARIABLE	STATUS
Age	?
Education	?
Premorbid Intelligence	?
Occupational Status	?
Etiology	+
Size of Lesion	+
Localization	+
Health	+
Severity	+
Time Post onset	+
Type of Aphasia	?

& Greenberg, 1970; Eisenson, 1949, 1964). Almost everyone who has looked suggests that less severe patients at onset have a better future than those with more severe aphasia (Basso, Capitani, & Vignolo, 1979; Hartman, 1981; Kertesz & McCabe, 1977; Sarno & Levita, 1979; Schuell, Jenkins, & Jimenez-Pabon, 1964). The closer to onset, the more improvement a patient can expect (Basso et al., 1979; Deal & Deal, 1978; Kertesz & McCabe, 1977; Vignolo, 1964; Wertz et al, 1981). Finally, the influence of type of aphasia is debatable. Kertesz and McCabe (1977) and Lomas and Kertesz (1978) report anomic and conduction types have the best prognosis. Prins, Snow, and Wagenaar (1978) found no influence of type of aphasia on improvement.

Therefore, the prognostic variable approach for stating an aphasic patient's prognosis indicates that a patient who suffered closed head trauma resulting in one small lesion that does not involve temporal-parietal cortex, who is in good health, mildly aphasic, and less than a month postonset has an excellent prognosis for improvement. Unfortunately, most of our patients do not display this kind of syzygy. Positive and negative signs coexist, and coexistence complicates prediction.

Schuell (1965b) and Keenan and Brassell (1974) have popularized the behavioral profile approach. Language data are used to construct the profile, and the profile is compared with previous patients' profiles. Schuell developed five major prognostic groups and two minor syndromes based on her retrospective look at initial MTDDA performance by patients whose improvement or lack of it was documented. Initial profiles for patients who showed marked improvement were used to forecast a positive prognosis, and initial profiles for patients who displayed limited recovery were used to predict a poor prognosis. This approach permits making an early, data-based prediction. Problems arise when a patient's performance cannot be classified in one of Schuell's prognostic groups. Keenan and Brassell were interested in predicting improvement in verbal performance. They observed that auditory comprehension and verbal performance could be used to forecast a patient's future behavior. Initial reading and writing performance had little predictive use. If a patient can be classified, the behavioral profile is useful for stating prognosis. However, even if a patient can be classified, the prognostic statement is limited to an adjective and may not indicate prognosis for what.

Statistical prediction is promising but not, as yet, practical. Multiple regression analysis and two-group discriminant analysis have been used in medicine to predict mortality from coronary and from shock. Meehl (1965) believes that statistical techniques result in more precise prediction than that obtained from clinical judgment. Porch and his colleagues (1973, 1974, 1980) have used a step-wise multiple regression analysis to predict change in aphasia as measured by the PICA. Patients were tested at various times postonset, followed, and retested at a later date. A retrospective analysis was done using performance in the early test to determine whether performance on the later test could have been predicted. When predicted performance was correlated with performance actually obtained, correlations ranged from 0.74 to 0.94. All were significant, indicating the multiple regression formula was a reasonably accurate means of predicting change in aphasia. Deal et al. (1979) used the multiple regression formula developed by Porch, Collins, Wertz, and Friden (1980) to test its clinical application. The group results were significant, indicating that patients obtained PICA scores close to those predicted. However, analysis of individual data indicated less than two thirds of the sample obtained scores that fell within a -5 to $+5$ percentile range of the score predicted. Thus, the Deal et al. results lend credence to the caution counselled by Porch et al. (1980). The multiple regression formula they generated is not ready for clinical application.

So, while there has been a good deal of activity in developing prognostic tools for predicting the aphasic patient's future, we are yet to devise methods that permit us to tell the patient and his or her family, with any precision, how much improvement can be expected, when that improvement will occur, and what it will permit the patient to do.

The State of the Art

We know far less than we need to know about predicting change in the language disorders being discussed here. Whether the communicative deficit suffered by the normal aged in a communication-impairing environment will improve, remain the same, or get worse is unknown. Heuristically, we might expect change if the environment is manipulated to foster communication rather than impede it. But, we do not know if things are that simple. Can what has been depressed be elevated? We do not know. Clinical experience indicates that the patient with the language of confusion will improve. But, we play a questionable game. If he or she does improve, we assume our diagnosis was correct. If the patient does not, we may change the diagnosis, typically to dementia. There is little to tell us about the schizophrenic patient's future. Age, duration of symptoms, and social milieu are believed to influence improvement or the lack of it. But, what we know does not permit us to predict with much precision. The patient with the right hemisphere lesion may not demonstrate the severe language deficits seen in other brain-injured patients, but his or her communicative ability may be severely impaired and remain so. The meager data to date indicate that the right hemisphere patient does not make the gains made by left hemisphere patients in self-care abilities or communicative efficiency. The demented patient has a poor prognosis. The course is downhill unless he or she suffers one of the few cases that respond to treatment, and these make up less than 20% of the demented propulation. We know more about predicting change in aphasia than we do about predicting change for the other language disorders. But, our abilities are not very precise, or they are limited to predicting change on a specific language measure.

Because prognosis is so important to the patient and his or her family, and because it may justify whether to intervene with treatment, emphasis on improving our predictive ability should rise to the top of a need hierarchy in the management of language disorders in adults. To date, we have employed retrospective approaches that seek predictive variables, performance profiles on measures early postonset, and statistical prediction to forecast the future.

Perhaps the methods we have been using require ablution, or perhaps they require rejection. A possible alternative to what we have done includes looking at the patient's ability to learn. For example, regardless of our philosphy of therapy, we expect our patients to learn to do whatever it is they could not do when they came to our attention. Perhaps a brief battery of learning tasks, administered early postonset, would tell us which patient will learn and which will not. Those who do learn may have a brighter future than those who do not. Finally, we need to focus on predicting prognosis for what. For example, improved PICA performance may or may not relate to potential for returning to work, for participation in a dinner conversation, for finding enjoyable activities to fill the day.

Unfortunately, the path to improving our ability to prognose wanders through the land of the natural history study. We need to identify and follow large samples of patients over a long period of time to determine what they have to tell us about their problems and how those problems change. At the end of the path, we can take a retrospective view of what we missed along the way. Utilization of these data should assist us in predicting for future patients. The natural history study appears to be the tool for doing the task, but the natural history study has the lowest probability of attracting funding.

Treatment

LaPointe (1983) observed that the idea of shattered language being mended (that is, it can be darned instead of damned) is all too recent. He was talking about aphasia where, today, treatments abound. For many disorders—environmental influence on the normal aged, the language of confusion, schizophrenia, right hemisphere involvement—we continue to search for the proper egg, the right gauge needle, the proficient seamstress. And, frequently, we continue to fill the air with vituperative maledictions rather than proficient patches.

Two points of view have developed about treating language disorders in adults. In one, there is a leap to treat. If a problem exists, it must be treated. In the other, there is a reluctance to intervene. Because a problem exists does not mean there is a treatment for it. The former attempts to assuage symptoms. The latter awaits knowledge of the cause and evidence that a treatment is efficacious. Probably, more of the former exists than the latter. Certainly, successful treatments have not always awaited finding a cause. Quinine was given for malaria prior to the malarial parasite being identified. The cause of Parkinson's disease remains obscure, but observation of a deficit in dopamine has resulted in administration of L-dopa. In aphasia, we know the cause, but that knowledge does not assist, greatly, in treating the symptoms.

Today, many treatments exist, but many have not been demonstrated to be efficacious. In fact, the existence of a treatment often prevents research designed to test its efficacy. Because it exists, some believe it is unethical to withhold it in a treatment trial. In what follows, I will discuss what has been, is being, and is not being done to treat language disorders in adults.

Environmental Influence
on the Normal Aged

Elimination of environmentally influenced deficits in the normal aged has taken two approaches. One is modification of the environment to remove the suspected cause of the problem. The second is direct treatment through individual or group therapy. The latter is, typically, reality orientation therapy which, in a sense, is a manipulation of the environment.

Manipulation of the environment begins with the premise that normal aging is normal, not pathological (Holland, 1983), however the environment may be pathology producing. Lubinski (1981) suggests that the speech pathologist has a role in refurbishing a communication impairing environment that transcends staff education and appraisal, diagnosis, and treatment of individual patients. She suggests that the speech pathologist become a patient advocate. Her intensive (Lubinski, Morrison, & Rigrodsky, 1981) interviews with aged residents in an institutional setting lead her to suggest avoidance of individual treatment in favor of treating the patient and the environment as a single unit. Labouvice-Vief, Hoyer, Baltes, and Baltes (1974), Rebok and Hoyer (1977), and Solomon (1982) also advocate combining behavioral treatment and behavioral ecology techniques to produce behavior change. MacDonald (1976) reports that this approach will increase the rate of verbalization in elderly nursing home patients, and that it is not necessary to add new resources, but simply to rearrange existing resources.

Lubinski's (1981) specific techniques include: creating a need for residents to communicate, providing places where communication can occur, teaching staff and patients that the act of communicating is in itself treatment, reducing rules that inhibit communication, showing staff and patients what they can do and how to do it, identifying and matching communication partners, and supplementing enviromental changes with sensory training and reality orientation. Solomon (1982) adds the need to demythologize concepts about aging for staff members, use model staff members to train others by precept, and give residents autonomy by teaching them to master their environment.

Adelson, Nasti, Sprafkin, Marinelli, Primavera, and Gorman (1982) have developed a behavioral rating scale to quantify health professional's interaction with geriatric patients. They took 15 traits from the literature that are believed to affect staff and patient relationships. These were tested with two groups of staff, one group supervisors judged to have good relatioships with patients and one group supervisors judged to have poor relationships with patients. Ten of the traits correlated significantly with the supervisors' ratings. These are listed in Table 1-6. The traits that were most predictive of good relationships were banter, engaging patients in

TABLE 1-6
Behavioral traits for rating health professional's interaction with geriatric patients. (After Adelson, Nasti, Sprafkin, Marinelli, & Primavera, 1982)

* Uses patient's name by whatever title patient wishes to be called.
* Banter: Engages patient in conversation.
* Asks for feedback: Gives choices, develops options for the patient, asks if something hurts or how it feels.
* Gives procedural information: Warns patient of upcoming sensation, touch, taste, or smell.
* Compensates for disabilities: Adapts to patient's impairment, for example, loss of hearing, sight, or other physical disabilities.
* Social touches: Uses physical contact that is an expression of affection, comfort, reassurance, or concern, and not considered procedural.
* Attends to patient comfort: Expresses concern for the patient's ease and is sensitive to the patient's needs.

  Amount of appropriate smiling: Too little, adequate, very good.

  Pacing of procedure: Poor, adequate, very good; if poor, too slow or too fast.

  Pacing of speech: Poor, adequate, very good; if poor, too slow or too fast.

NOTE: * Rated in total number of occurrences and whether occurred or not.

conversation, giving procedural information; smiling appropriately; asking for feedback; and using the patient's name. The value of the Adelson et al. scale is that it permits rating what staff do and do not do and provides specific behaviors to be developed and modified in staff members. Thus, it is a means for rating how the patient's environment is influenced by staff, what to change, and how to change.

Several suggest individual and group reality orientation for the normal aged in an institutional setting. Brandt, Rose, and Lucas (in press) used the terms "remotivation and resocialization" and "reality orientation." These imply involving the patient in social activities, including group discussion, and bombarding the patient with who he or she is, who the staff are, the date, the place, his or her schedule, etc. And, they require participation by everyone in the environment, from custodians to administrators. Individual and group sessions are supplemented with a reality orientation board which is individualized for the patient. Citrin and

Dixon (1977) have reported results from a clinical trial with treated and untreated groups. The treated patients received "24-hour" reality orientation supplemented by group sessions. Change was measured by a reality orientation sheet. Their treated group displayed significantly better orientation than their untreated group at the end of the program.

Some have offered an alternative to institutionalization. The premise is that if an institutional environment erodes abilities, keeping the patient out of an institution should be attempted. Rathbone-McCuan (1976) reported the positive effects of a geriatric day care center. The service lessened the family's physical burden of daily care by providing a daily supervised environment for the aged person, psychological support for the aged person and his or her family, and gave the aged person some interaction with peers. Rathbone-McCuan suggested that the day care center permits the family to keep the aged individual at home for as long as possible and is a "last ditch" effort to avoid an institutionalized environment. Steinhauer (1982) has discussed the use of geriatric foster care as an alternative to institutionalization for the elderly who have no family. Private family residences are found to house and care for those without relatives.

Direct treatment with the normal aged in an institutional environment shows mixed results. O'Connell and O'Connell (1978) reported that overall change from direct treatment was slight. Thirty percent of their sample failed to profit from direct treatment, 50% were discharged before they reached maximum gains, and 20% made significant improvement. Hudson (1960), focusing on communication problems in the aged, reports positive results from treatment. Finlayson and Martin (1982) suggest that increased social stimulation and emotional support reduced depression in the elderly. And Hoyer, Kafer, Simpson, and Hoyer (1974) increased verbal performance in aged individuals by using operant procedures that involved administration of tokens.

Obler and Albert (1981) suggest teaching the normal elderly in an institution to use language strategies employed by the normal elderly who are not in an institution. The process, of course, requires training staff in what the strategies are and how to prompt their use by patients. A variety of techniques have been used in attempts to improve cognitive skills in the aged. The most successful are: modeling, watching use of cognitive strategies used by younger persons, and feedback of information about the correctness of a response. Direct instruction, noncognitive intervention, attempts to change response speed, attempts to motivate by giving money, and praise are not effective. Practice improves some skills, but not others.

Treatment for the normal aged in a communication-impairing environment has focused on the environment and the individual. Apparently, manipulation of both are necessary. And, as is true with most disorders, what should be done must flow from the patient—what the patient can tell us about his or her problem and what he or she can tell us about what should be done for it.

Language of Confusion

Because we expect confusional state to change, and because it usually does, few treatments have been developed for it. Probably, medical management that removes the cause of the confusion is the most appropriate treatment. Chedru and Geschwind's (1972) patients improved after the effects of alcoholic intoxication, barbituate intoxication, electro-convulsive therapy, and general anesthesia passed. In cases of trauma or surgical intervention, perhaps the time necessary for edema to subside is the appropriate treatment.

Reality orientation has been used with confused patients. Whether it is an efficacious treatment is debatable. It is employed during the confusional state and dropped when confusion is resolved. Whether reality orientation improves confusion or whether the patient becomes oriented because whatever caused the confusion has subsided in unknown. No controlled studies have been conducted.

I (1978) have suggested speech and language-specific treatment for the language of confusion. The principles involve finding appropriate stimulus and response modes that result in less confabulation and irrelevancy, using a hierarchy of tasks that permits more open-ended responses when the patient demonstrates that he or she is ready to roam verbally without confabulating, and confronting the patient with the veracity of the confabulation and the appropriateness of his or her irrelevance. Most of the confused patients I have seen improve when given this type of treatment. Whether they would have improved if I had left them alone, I do not know.

We offer the confused patient medical management if medicine has a treatment for what brings the patient to our hospital, in addition to reality orientation and speech and language specific therapy. Whether the latter two have any influence on the improvement we typically see, we do not know.

Schizophrenia

Because few schizophrenic patients are seen by speech pathologists, speech and language treatments are few. But others see these patients and they manage them. Finkel and Cohen (1982) relate that psychotherapy, behavioral modification, family psychotherapy, and pharmacotherapy are all useful approaches for managing the schizophrenic patient under the proper circumstances. Geschwind (1975) cautions that one must be certain the patient considered for these treatments is schizophrenic—and is only schizophrenic. He estimates that neurologic disorders account for 30% of all first admissions to mental hospitals, and some of these neurologic causes of psychiatric disorders respond to a neurologic treatment.

Speech and language deficits in a schizophrenic patient have been viewed in two contexts. By a few, they are considered symptoms requiring specific speech and language treatment. By most, they are considered symptoms that will indicate whether other treatment—drugs, psychotherapy—is working. Feldstein and Weingartner (1981) review the use of speech and language behavior to determine the efficacy of drug therapy with schizophrenic patients. Improvement in speech and language implies medication is working. Lack of improvement implies the need for a change in medicinal management.

Halpern (1980) is among those who advocate treating the schizophrenic patient's speech and language deficits. The techniques he suggests do not differ markedly from those used with other language disorders. He cautions that most schizophrenic patients are not concerned with their communication problems. Some need a highly structured treatment, and others require more informal approaches. Halpern advocates the use of reinforcements—food, coffee—to achieve change. He notes that progress is slow, but speech and language therapy is beneficial. Enlisting the aid of other staff, he believes, is essential to achieve carry-over outside the treatment session.

Some have used operant techniques to combat muteness in the schizophrenic patient. Isaacs, Thomas, and Goldiamond (1960) used operant techniques to reinstate verbal behavior in two patients. And, Sherman (1963) reports success in restoring speech in a mute schizophrenic patient. Operant conditioning in a 16-session treatment trial resulted in the patient's using his intact language, displayed in writing, orally.

We lack empirical evidence to demonstrate the efficacy of language therapy with the schizophrenic patient. Language deficit in schizophrenia may be like a patient's inability to run with a broken leg. Set the bone, immobilize it, wait, and, eventually, the patient will run. For schizophrenia, find the correct medicinal management and treat with psychotherapy, and the patient's language deficit may resolve. Whether this is the appropriate procedure for managing communicative deficit in schizophrenia, we do not know.

Right Hemisphere Involvement

The patient with right hemisphere involvement has been treated as interesting—and seldom treated. Myers (1981) suggests it is time for speech pathologists to relinquish this wallflower role in relation to the right hemisphere patient; it is time to dance the dance. She cautions that, prior to stepping onto the floor, we must remember what we are treating is not aphasia.

A variety of disciplines have intervened with the right hemisphere patient, and they have obtained mixed results. Taylor, Schaeffer, Blumenthal, and Grissel (1969) report no difference between treated and untreated right hemisphere patients following a program designed to improve perceptual and motor skills. LaPointe and Culton (1969) report success in remediating left neglect in a patient with a right hemisphere lesion. Diller and Weinberg (1977) were successful in training right hemisphere patients with hemi-inattention to compensate for their deficits.

Myers and West (1978) have listed the right hemisphere patient's specific deficits that may respond to rehabilitation. These include: lack of sensitivity, inappropriate behavior, denial of cognitive deficits, lack of motivation, lability, visual hallucinations, and dissociation between what is said and what is experienced. The few who have attempted to treat these problems differ in their rationale and their techniques.

Myers (1981) emphasizes that the problem of right hemisphere patients is not just perceptual, but perceptual in a broad sense. They need more than training designed to get them to look to the left or to match stimuli. Perceptual deficit impairs simultaneous discrimination and interpretation. Treatment tasks should emphasize context and its use to search for meaning. Myers advocates having right hemisphere patients use their good verbal ability to reverbalize what they experience. They will not use nonverbal cues to find meaning the way patients with a left hemisphere lesion do. Because of the right hemisphere patient's irrelevance and the inability to cope with open-ended tasks, Myers (1979) suggests maintaining rigid stimulus control in highly structured tasks and, gradually, permitting the patients more freedom on open-ended tasks when they demonstrate they are ready to deal with less structure.

Adamovich (1981) uses a more comprehensive approach in treating right hemisphere patients. She advocates treating perception, sequencing ability, auditory comprehension, verbal expression, reading, writing, organizational ability, problem solving, and auditory and visual memory. Her methodology employs developing task continua, from easy to difficult, according to cognitive and linguistic developmental hierachies.

Yorkston (1981) suggests using the right hemisphere patient's learning style to dictate how he or she is treated. Because the patient has poor generalization ability, she suggests using functional tasks; for example reading rather than canceling letters. And, because the patient can talk, she advocates having him or her provide verbal cues by talking his or her way through tasks. Because the patient tends to forget, she suggests massed practice to promote generalization. Next, because the right hemisphere patient is not very good at recognizing his or her errors and because the patient is impulsive, Yorkston uses sequential tasks that cannot continue unless errors are recognized and corrected. Finally, because the right hemisphere patient is not very good at reasoning and problem solving, she suggests breaking tasks down into numerous small steps, and if the patient fails to advance from one step to the next, adding additional steps. She asks her patients, constantly, "Have you finished this step?"

Many right hemisphere patients tend to ignore their left visual world, and because they do, they may have difficulty reading. Thus, some have focused on treating the right hemisphere patient's reading deficits. Collins (1976) has summarized the traditional techniques—encouraging oral reading and analyzing whether what is heard makes sense, using a brightly colored cardboard guide shaped like a carpenter's square to force attention to the left margin and focus on the line being read. Stanton, Yorkston, Kenyon, and Beukelman (1981) have developed a language-based reading program for right hemisphere patients with left neglect. They eschew the Diller, Ben-Yishay, Gerstman, Goodkin, and Gordon (1974) suggestion to use perceptual cues and employ Fordyce and Jones' (1966) observation that right hemisphere patients do better with verbal than with pantomime instructions. The Stanton et al. reading program requires overt verbalization—the patient cues himself or herself by talking aloud. When he fails to do so, the clinician intervenes and says, "Tell yourself." The program includes numerous small steps and employs intensive repetition. It is data based, in that the patient does not progress until he or she has reached criterion on each step. Stanton et al. provide data to demonstrate its efficacy with a sample of right hemisphere patients.

So, we are beginning to dance the dance with the right hemisphere patient. Presently, we are awkward, lack rhythm, step on toes, and know only a few steps. We are not ready to attend the cotillion, but we are looking in that direction.

Dementia

Miller (1977) has observed that dementia is usually diagnosed, but not treated. Except for those who have a treatable cause of dementia, behavioral therapy is employed in an attempt to slow dementia's progression. Mueller and Atlas (1972) report that the few gains resulting from behavioral treatment are lost when treatment stops. There have been a few efforts to find a drug or nutritional treatment for Alzheimer's patients. None has been successful. Thus, treatment for most demented patients is confined to reality orientation, or modification of demands made on the patient to permit him or her function as best he or she can.

Ratusnik, Lascoe, Herbon, and Wolfe (1979) used group sessions in an attempt to improve demented patients' awareness of themselves and others, awareness of time and place, word-finding and vocabulary usage, gestural communication, and to decrease verbal perseveration and inappropriate behaviors. The techniques included traditional stimulus-response activities and group discussion. Following approximately 2 months of treatment in 40-minute sessions 4 days a week, over half of their 16 patients improved in receptive and expressive language and in awareness of self and others. Less than half improved in memory and in orientation for time and place. Harris and Ivory (1976) used reality orientation in a 5-month treatment trial. They noted treated patients were significantly better than nontreated patients in six of nine verbal behaviors: spontaneous verbal interaction; using their own, the therapist's, and other patient's names correctly; compliance with simple requests; and correct verbalization of information pertaining to time. Schwartz et al. (1979) were unsuccessful in their attempt to teach demented patients to use their unimpaired syntax to cue semantic deficits.

General techniques for managing dementia have included attempting to keep the patient at home for as long as possible; providing proper nutrition and hydration; managing other medical problems immediately; and manipulating the environment to reduce emotional lability, promote cognition and memory, and regulate sleep and wake cycles. Bayles (1982b) has offered specific techniques for managing the demented patient. These include frequent family counselling; establishing and adhering to a fixed daily schedule; simplifying the environment but loading it with orientation materials—calendars, clocks, pictures; not arguing with the patient; using physical contact to provide support; and emphasizing health and diet. She suggests avoiding the use of verbal analogies, fragmented discourse, humor, sarcasm, indefinite referents, conversations with more than two persons, and open-ended questions. Finally, Bayles recommends periodic evaluations of the patient to detect and cope with changes in his behavior.

Thus, unless the cause of the dementia is treatable, what we have to offer is designed to slow deterioration of behavior or lessen demand as behavior deteriorates. Those of us who work with demented patients are aware of what we have to learn from the patient's family. They have lived with the disorder before it was brought to our attention. We need to set ourselves on "receive" rather than "send" when we talk with family members. We want to know what they have done that helps. We can assist them by arranging group sessions where families can gather to share.

Aphasia

Treatments for aphasia abound. A recent book (Chapey, 1981) contains at least 13 different types of aphasia therapy, and these barely scratch the literature's surface. Three chapters in this book discuss treatment of aphasic patients at various levels of severity. To avoid redundancy, I will summarize the general types of treatment used with aphasic patients and, then, consider treatment we may not call treatment, but which should be part of every aphasic patient's management.

How speech pathologists treat—and have treated—aphasic patients is influenced by their philosophy of aphasia therapy. There are probably as many philosophies of aphasia therapy as there are therapists. However, these can be organized into four broad groups. First, some treatment is "traditional." It incorporates proven methods of the past, most of which utilize a stimulus-response approach. Emphasis is placed on language content. Second, there has been a move to develop specific treatments for specific problems. Benson (1979b) suggested that speech pathologists look in this direction, and some have. These types of treatment are usually identified by easily remembered acronyms; Melodic Intonation Therapy (MIT) (Sparks, Helm, & Albert, 1974); Visual Action Therapy (VAT) (Helm & Benson, 1978); Voluntary Control of Involuntary Utterances (VCIU) (Helm & Barresi, 1980). Typically, they are applied with patients demonstrating a specific type of aphasia—MIT for the Broca's patient, VAT for the global patient. Third, some clinicians have extended the trend toward testing "functional" communication to administering "functional" treatment. The treatment developed by Davis and Wilcox (1981), Promoting Aphasics' Communicative Effectiveness (PACE), is an example of "functional" treatment. It emphasizes language context rather than language content. Fourth, larger caseloads have motivated busy clinicians to combine clients and conduct group therapy. Some (Aten, Kushner-Vogel, Haire, & Fitch-West, 1981; Bloom, 1962) believe that when three or more gather, more improvement occurs than when just two—patient and therapist—meet. Group treatments follow a variety of philosophies of aphasia therapy. Some are designed to create a social setting, and nothing more. Some are rigidly structured to lead group members, in unison, through what they might do if they were in individual treatment.

While an unassailable study on the efficacy of aphasia therapy has not been conducted, Darley's (1972) conclusion that it helps has received empirical support in recent clinical trails reports (Basso et al., 1979; Wertz et al., 1981) and numerous single-case studies. Of course, every clinician can tell tales of patients he has not helped, and some who were helped only a little. And, we continue to seek solutions to questions about when to treat, how much, where, and how. But, Benson's (1976b) conclusion that language therapy for the aphasic patient is, without a doubt, efficacious is an appropriate statement on the state of the art.

I believe there is a portion of the aphasic patient's management that we have ignored. We tend to treat language deficit, and when improvement in language slows or stops, we consider terminating treatment or moving the patient into a maintenance group. Perhaps we owe our patients more than just an attempt to improve their language skills. Perhaps we need to assist them in coping with the language deficit that remains after direct language therapy has done what it can. Figure 1-5 implies that two values may be emphasized in the management of aphasic patients. At one point, usually early postonset, we value the quality of language, and we seek its restoration through the treatment we administer. But, at some point, our value may change because improvement in the patient's language slows or stops. We change our value to the quality of the patient's life and emphasize coping with the language deficit that remains. We seek ways for the patient to live the best he or she can with his or her residual language deficits. We look for meaningful ways to help the patient fill his or her days, for family members to find freedom from constant care and attention. We do a lot of the first—attempts to restore language—but I am not certain we do much of the latter—assist in coping with disability. And, because aphasia goes on a long time, and language therapy fills only a small portion of that time, the most important thing we can do for our patients is what we probably do the least.

So the treatment of aphasia has blossomed in the last decade. It has been watered by numerous techniques and fed by alternatives to tradition. The clinician is no longer buffeted by storms that question whether treatment's soil is arable. Empirical evidence indicates it is. But, we continue to seek means for improving the product, and we need to consider treatment that may be necessary after the treatment we have demonstrated we do well has done what it can.

The State of the Art

Treatment implies we have something to do and that that something is, in fact, treatment—it improves whatever is being treated. There are

FIGURE 1-5
How the value emphasized in aphasia therapy may change over time (After Wertz, 1983b)

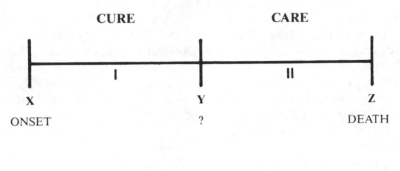

TREATMENT: A CURE-CARE CONUNDRUM

TIME

CURE   CARE

| I | II |

X   Y   Z

ONSET   ?   DEATH

VALUES   EMPHASIS
I = QUALITY OF LANGUAGE   X - Y = RESTORATION OF
II - QUALITY OF LIFE   LANGUAGE

Y - Z = COPING WITH DISABILITY

many treatments for the aphasic patient, and the treatments administered appear to improve the patient's language. Such is not the case for the other language disorders being discussed here. For the normal aged in a communication-impairing environment, there appear to be several things we can do, both with the patient and with his or her environment. Whether what we can do will improve communication, we do not know. For the patient who suffers the language of confusion, there are fewer available techniques. While we could develop more, it is not clear that they are necessary. Confusion appears to clear in these patients. Whether treatment is the cause of this improvement or whether it speeds the course, we do not know. Language deficit in schizophrenia is seldom treated by the speech pathologist. Whether it should be, or could be, is not certain. We are beginning to see the patient with right hemisphere involvement for therapy. The patient's language, usually, is fairly intact. We are beginning to treat his or her failure to use this language to communicate. Fair enough! These patients have a problem, and it deserves remediation. Whether it is capable of being remediated awaits evidence. Finally, most demented patients are not expected to improve. The treatments we offer are designed to slow loss of communicative ability and to reduce demands to a level where the patient can use what he or she retains. This is treatment if it works. We seek evidence to support our belief that it does.

Some treatment techniques stand out by their resistance to classification. I have suggested a need for techniques that assist the patient to cope with residual deficits remaining after we have worked as much magic as we can. While this was discussed for aphasia, it is appropriate to consider it for the other language disorders. Our experience with assisting patients to cope is limited. Many of us are confined by our clinics and have little knowledge of need—let alone solutions—that exist beyond the setting in which we usually see patients. We need to learn from patients by seeing what they can do and cannot do in their natural habitats. Simply, we need to learn from patients. Linge (1980), a clinical psychologist who suffered head trauma in an automobile accident and made sufficient recovery to return to work, has told us about some things that hinder, and some that help. He suggests eliminating distractions (one thing at a time); developing a highly structured routine, imposing order and developing habit; creating a serene environment, removing emotional tension; keeping situations one-on-one (avoiding groups); if the patient is capable, encouraging excessive note taking; and using all possible sensory channels. Of course, what was best for Linge will not be best for all. But, many of our patients who have walked at least a portion of the road back may verify some of his suggestions, and they probably have others to offer. If we can compile a list, we can cull from it those things appropriate for today's patient.

Finally, we must remember that not all patients want, need, or can gain from treatment. Again, the presence of a problem does not indicate that there is a means for solving it. Too often, I believe, we put patients into treatment when they do not want to be nor should be there. Perhaps there is a message for us in the following AP wire bulletin.

> FT. WORTH, TEXAS (AP). The telephone rang as Mrs. F. A. Farnum was vacuuming her canary's cage. She wheeled to pick up the phone and—whoosh—up the vacuum cleaner nozzle went Joey Boy with one desperate "cheep!" Mrs. Farnum jerked the bag open, grabbed out her canary, and desperately shook off a little dust. Joey Boy was still unrecognizable, so she put him under the faucet. Then, to be sure the bird did not catch cold, she put him under her electric hair dryer. "He has not been singing since then," Mrs. Farnum said, "he just sits hunched over and stares a lot. But he is eating well."

How like many of our patients after they have been probed with PICAs, pelted with PACE, and massaged with MIT. Eating well. Not much singing, but a lot of staring. Sometimes, what follows a traumatic event transcends the trauma.

The State of The Clinical Art

What follows is repetitious, but that is what summaries tend to be. Pride will usually prevent a retreat even in some unimportant matter like doing the dishes before sitting down to dessert. Therefore, this is not a retreat but a reiteration.

The Disorders

I have listed and explored what I think we know about six language disorders that may be present in adults. Are there others? Perhaps. I continue to see patients I cannot classify. Are there too many? Some do not classify communicative deficit in schizophrenia as a language disorder. Some report the right hemisphere patient's language as not impaired; it is his failure to use his good language to communicate effectively that concerns us. Should the disorders listed be subdivided into subgroups? Some do this in aphasia. Some do not.

Little attention has been given to the possibility of coexisting disorders. I have argued against talking about the presence of one disorder *in* another. However, it is possible for a schizophrenic patient to suffer a left hemisphere CVA and demonstrate subsequent aphasia. Similarly, the demented patient who is undergoing gradual cortical atrophy may suffer a left hemisphere CVA and display, in addition to his generalized language deficit, signs of focal aphasia. Therefore, I have no reservations about one disorder coexisting *with* another.

I have not discussed the language of patients who suffer bilateral head trauma, or those who suffer a focal right hemisphere CVA and, later, a focal left hemisphere CVA. Many of these do not fit into the aphasic or demented bins. Where do we put what Eisenson (1947) has called an "inconsistent and unconventional lot?"

Six disorders have been discussed. The proof that aphasia and dementia should be on a list of language disorders has been demonstrated in the clinic and in the literature. Whether environmental influence on the communication of the normal aged, the language of confusion, schizophrenia, and right hemisphere involvement should reside on the list, awaits data and resolution of debate.

Appraisal

The purposes of appraisal, I believe, are to permit diagnosis, determine severity, state a prognosis, and, if appropriate, focus therapy. We do not have a single, economic measure that will accomplish these purposes for all of the language disorders discussed here. In fact, we do not have a battery of several, uneconomical measures that meets our purposes. We have measures for some of the disorders that will meet some of our purposes. Perhaps it is futile to seek the all-purpose appraisal measure. We may have to settle for developing one that tells us who is who, and once that question is answered, branch into appropriate batteries designed to meet the additional needs.

Our experience dictates that we should avoid using measures developed for one disorder to appraise another. Administer a test for aphasia and there is a high probability of observing aphasia in the normal aged, the confused patient, the schizophrenic patient, the patient with a right hemisphere lesion, the demented patient, and, sometimes, small appliances. There is a need to do what Bayles (1982b) has done: develop measures for the disorder being appraised.

Technology offers some hope. LaPointe (1983) has observed that neurology has undergone a technological revolution. PET and CT have contributed mightily to answer the riddle of "lesion, lesion, where is the lesion?" In fact, a new publication, *Journal of Cerebral Blood Flow and Metabolism*, has resulted from technological advance. The influence of technology on speech pathology, LaPointe observes, is nil. "We remain a Model A in a space shuttle world." When technology reaches us, and it will, we must remember it is the product, not the process, that will be productive.

So, we continue to seek the means to meet appraisal's purposes. In aphasia, we refine. In the other disorders, we develop. We attempt to change Mosher and Feinsilver's (1971) summary on schizophrenia: "Despite decades of effort, schizophrenia continues to defy adequate description and classification"—not only for schizophrenia, but also for other language disorders one sees in adults.

Diagnosis

Diagnosis should be more than a system for organizing our files. I have argued that what you call it makes a difference; a difference in prognosis, a difference in management. Aphasia, for example, has a different future and requires a different management than does dementia.

The labels we use and the arguements we have about them are more than exercises in semantics. What we call something is, increasingly, dictating whether there are funds available to pay for its treatment. Second-, third-, and, probably, 15th-party payers provide dollars to care for some disorders, but not others. The war continues to be waged to find funds to pay for aphasia therapy. Try finding support for treating communication deficit in the normal aged resulting from a communication-impairing environment. A physician friend has told me of a dilemma he experienced during World War II, and his solution for it. Regulations restricted the use of penicillin to treat venereal disease in fighter pilots. This "keep them in the air" philosophy shunned many who needed the drug. His solution was a simple, but effective one. His medical unit experienced an epidemic of "gonorrhetic pneumonia." There may be a need, therefore, to relax rigidity and accept "Alzheimer's aphasia" or "environmental aphasia."

It is necessary for us to argue our diagnostic differences to agreement. We need a list of labels that are applied correctly and uniformly. The implications in the diagnosis of one clinician should not require inferences by another.

Treatment

I continue to stress, here and elsewhere (Wertz, 1983a), the need to determine whether our treatment is treatment; that we have something to do for language disorders in adults and that that something works. Some—usually speech and language clinicians—tell me what we do is efficacious. Others—usually physicians and biostatisticians—tell me there is no unassailable evidence that treatment works. I can agree with both, specifically, for the treatment of aphasia. Those I cannot agree with are the ones who suggest we should stop asking the question. The test of repair is whether the broken gets fixed. We ask this of our mechanics, and our patients ask it of us. And, we have some answers for the treatment of aphasia. But, we have little data to back the need for our deeds with other language disorders in adults.

Changes in the treatment of language disorders have come in Toffleresque profusion and have led, in some cases, to Kafkaesque confusion. We seem eager to change our treatments, but we have lost the art of preservation. Rosenbek (1979) has listed some of our cherished treatments that may be abandoned for the new. He suggests looking both ways, to the past and to the future, in the search for methods to mend broken language. The true have not, necessarily, been tried. Neither have the new. Rosenbek advises clinicians to plant their feet in the stream of clinical change and not emerge until they find a few facts about what does, and what does not, work in the management of language-impaired adults.

Along with my suggestion to avoid appraising one disorder with a measure designed for another, I believe we should be wary about administering treatment methods demonstrated to be effective for one disorder to rehabilitate another. We need to refine and to define, to determine what works for whom. Reality orientation cannot be a panacea for all language deficits. The meager literature implies it is. Some have failed to tell us who got oriented, except that they were old. Helm (1978) developed and tested careful selection criteria for patients who profit from MIT. Similar efforts are necessary for the methods we develop and administer to combat the other langauge disorders suffered by adults. In addition, we want to know more than just what works for whom. There is a need to know when, where, and for how long. Should we intervene early postonset or later? Is treatment for a specific disorder done best in the individual treatment session or in a group session, or, perhaps, in the patient's home? How long should treatment go on? Often, it is easier to get a patient into treatment than to get him or her out of it. Often patients have only so many dollars to spend on treatment. Should these be spent early postonset or later; in an intensive, short treatment trial or spaced less intensively over a longer period? I do not think we know.

Finally, there is a need to assist patients beyond treatment's duration. We have focused our efforts on mending language and have done little to assist patients in living with the deficits that cannot be mended. Only recently have we focused our therapy on function. I suggest we extend this to function after therapy has ended. Our source for developing this assistance is a simple one, the patient. The human brain is designed to enable us to accept someone else's experience, celebrate that acceptance, and be someone else for at least an hour. Much of what I know about successful treatment of language disorders in adults I learned by accepting the experience of patients, celebrating that acceptance, and *being* a patient for as long as it took to plan appropriate treatment. Suffering a language disorder, for some, is the straw that breaks. For others, it is the tie that binds. Many we see in treatment leave it to fill their days as best they can, but fill them they do. We can learn from them to save others from emptiness.

The State of This
State of the Clinical Art

Most state-of-the-art statements end with "Perhaps in the next 10 years. . . ?" Many of the questions and several of the needs posed here are answered and met in the other chapters in this book. Rosenbek (1983) has written an appropriate ending. He acknowledges that we are developing a data base, but we need not fear that all of the questions will soon be answered. As we learn more and more, we learn we need to learn more and more. We have been active. The sparks spread in this chapter have not been stolen from the ashes of inertia. This has represented my view of the state of the art—what it is and what I hope it will become. You, with different biases and more knowledge, will have a different view. That is as it should be, and that is good.

References

Adamovich, B.L. Language versus cognition: The speech-language pathologist's role. In R. H. Brookshire (Ed.), *Clinical Aphasiology: Proceedings of the Conference.* Minneapolis: BRK Publishers, 1981, 277-281.

Adamovich, B. L., & Brooks, R. L. A diagnostic protocol to assess the communication deficits of patients with right hemisphere damage. In R. H. Brookshire (Ed.), *Clinical Aphasiology: Proceedings of the Conference.* Minneapolis: BRK Publishers, 1981, 244-253.

Adelson, R., Nasti, A., Sprafkin, J. N., Marinelli, R., Primavera, L. H., & Gorman, B. S. Behavioral ratings of health professional's interactions with the geriatric patient. *The Gerontologist,* 1982, *22,* 277-281.

Alajouanine, T., Castaigne, P., Lhermitte, F., Escourolle, R., & Ribancourt, B. Etude de 43 cas d'aphasie post traumatique. *Encephale,* 1957, *46,* 1-45.

Alexander, M. P. & Lo Verme, S. R. Aphasia after left hemispheric intracerebral hemorrhage. *Neurology, 30,* 1980, 1193-1202.

Anderson, T., Bourestom, N., & Greenberg, R. Rehabilitation predictors in completed stroke. Final Report. *American Rehabilitation Foundation,* Minneapolis, 1970.

Appell, J., Kertesz A., & Fishman, M. Language in Alzheimer patients. Paper presented to the Academy of Aphasia, London, Ontario, 1981.

Archibald, Y. M., & Wepman, J. M. Language disturbance and nonverbal cognitive performance in eight patients following injury to the right hemisphere. *Brain,* 1968, *91,* 117-127.

Aten, J., Kushner-Vogel, D., Haire, A., & Fitch-West, J. Group treatment for aphasia: A panel discussion. In R. H. Brookshire (Ed.), *Clinical Aphasiology: Proceedings of the Conference.* Minneapolis: BRK Publishers, 1981, 141-154.

Baker, H., & Leland, B. *Detroit Test of Learning Aptitude.* Indianapolis: Bobbs-Merrill, 1967.

Basso, A., Capitani, E., & Vignolo, L. Influence of rehabilitation on language skills in aphasic patients. A controlled study. *Archives of Neurology,* 1979, *36,* 190-196.

Bayles, K. A. Language function in senile dementia. *Brain and Language,* 1982, *16,* 265-280. (a)

Bayles, K. A. Language and dementia producing diseases. *Communicative Disorders: A Journal for Continuing Education,* 1982, *7,*131-146. (b)

Bayles, K. A., & Boone, D. R. The potential of language tasks for identifying senile dementia. *Journal of Speech and Hearing Research,* 1982, *47,* 210-217.

Beasley, D. S., & Davis, G. A. *Aging: Communication processes and disorders.* New York: Grune & Stratton, 1981.

Benson, D. F. Psychiatric aspects of aphasia. *British Journal of Psychiatry*, 1973, *123*, 555–556.

Benson, D. F. Disorders of verbal expression. In D. F. Benson & D. Blumer (Eds.), *Psychiatric aspects of neurologic disease*. New York: Grune & Stratton, 1975, 121–137.

Benson, D. F. *Aphasia, alexia, and agraphia*. New York: Churchill Livingstone, 1979. (a)

Benson, D. F. Aphasia rehabilitation. *Archives of Neurology*, 1979, *36*, 187–189. (b)

Benton, A. L., Van Allen, M. W., & Fogel, M. L. Temporal orientation in cerebral disease. *Journal of Nervous and Mental Disorders*, 1964, *139*, 110–119.

Blazer, D., & Williams, C. D. Epidemiology of dysphoria and depression in an elderly population. *American Journal of Psychiatry*, 1980, *137*, 439–444.

Bloom, L. M. A rationale for group treatment of aphasic patients. *Journal of Speech and Hearing Disorders*, 1962, *27*, 11–16.

Bollinger, R. L. Communication disorders of "chronic brain injured" patients. Unpublished doctoral dissertation, University of Washington, 1970.

Borkowski, J. G., Benton, A. L., & Spreen, O. Word fluency and brain damage. *Neuropsychologia*, 1967, *5*, 135–140.

Branch, C., Milner, B., & Rasmussen, T. Intercarotid sodium amytal for the lateralization of cerebral dominance. *Journal of Neurosurgery*, 1964, *21*, 399–405.

Brandt, S. D., Rose, P., & Lucas, R. Speech-language consultation as part of a multidisciplinary team in long-care facilities. *Communicative Disorders: A Journal for Continuing Education*, in press.

Brosin, H. Acute and chronic brain syndromes. In A. Friedman & H. Kaplan (Eds.), *Comprehensive textbook of psychiatry. Baltimore: Williams & Wilkins*, 1967, 708–711.

Brown, R. Schizophrenia, language, and reality. *American Psychologist*, 1972, *28*, 395–403.

Buschke, H. Method for evaluating language competence in neurological patients. *Transactions of the American Neurological Association*, 1975, *100*, 169–171.

Caton, C. L. M. Effect of length of inpatient treatment for chronic schizophrenia. *American Journal of Psychiatry*, 1982, *139*, 856–861.

Chaika, E. A linguist looks at schizophrenic language. *Brain and Language*, 1974, *1*, 257–276.

Chapey, R. (Ed.). *Language intervention strategies in adult aphasia*. Baltimore: Williams & Wilkins, 1981.

Chapman, J. The early symptoms of schizophrenia. *British Journal of Psychiatry*, 1966, *112*, 225–251.

Chedru, F. & Geschwind, N. Disorders of higher cortical functions in acute confusional states. *Cortex*, 1972, *8*, 395–411.

Citrin, R. & Dixon, D. Reality orientation: A milieu therapy used in an institution for the aged. *The Gerontologist*, 1977, *17*, 39–43.

Collins, M. J. The minor hemisphere (A discussion session). In R. H. Brookshire (Ed.), *Clinical Aphasiology: Proceedings of the Conference*. Minneapolis: BRK Publishers, 1976, 339–352.

Critchley, M. Speech and speech-loss in relation to the duality of the brain. In V. B. Mountcastle (Ed.), *Interhemispheric relations and cerebral dominance*. Baltimore: The Johns Hopkins Press, 1962. 208–213.

Crosson. B., & Warren, R. L. Use of the Luria-Nebraska Neuropsychological Battery in aphasia: A conceptual critique. *Journal of Consulting and Clinical Psychology*, 1982, *50*, 22–31.

Damasio, A. The nature of aphasia: Signs and syndromes. In M. T. Sarno (Ed.), *Acquired aphasia*. New York: Academic Press, 1981, 51–65.

Darby, J. K. (Ed.). *Speech evaluation in psychiatry*. New York: Grune & Stratton, 1981.

Darley, F. L. *Aphasia*. Philadelphia: W. B. Saunders, 1982.

Darley, F. L. (Ed.). *Evaluation of appraisal techniques in speech and language pathology.* Reading, Massachusetts: Addison-Wesley, 1979. (a)

Darley, F. L. The differential diagnosis of aphasia. In R. H. Brookshire (Ed.), *Clinical Aphasiology: Proceedings of the Conference.* Minneapolis: BRK Publishers, 1979, 23–29. (b)

Darley, F. L. The efficacy of language rehabilitation in aphasia. *Journal of Speech and Hearing Disorders,* 1972, *37,* 3–21.

Darley, F. L. Aphasia: Input and output disturbances in speech and language processing. Paper presented to the American Speech and Hearing Association, Chicago, 1969.

Darley, F. L. *Diagnosis and appraisal of communication disorders.* Englewood Cliffs, NJ: Prentice-Hall, 1964.

Davis, G. A., & Wilcox, J. M. Incorporating parameters of natural conversation in aphasia treatment. In R. Chapey (Ed.), *Language intervention strategies in adult aphasia.* Baltimore: Williams & Wilkins, 1981. 169–194.

Deal, J. L., & Deal, L. A. Efficacy of aphasia rehabilitation: Preliminary results. In R. H. Brookshire (Ed.), *Clinical Aphasiology: Proceedings of the Conference.* Minneapolis: BRK Publishers, 1978, 66–77.

Deal, J. L., Deal, L. A., Wertz, R. T., Kitselman, K., & Dwyer, C. Right hemisphere PICA percentiles: Some speculations about aphasia. In R. H. Brookshire (Ed.), *Clinical Aphasiology: Proceedings of the Conference.* Minneapolis: BRK Publishers, 1979, 30–37.

Deal, L. A., Deal, J. L., Wertz, R. T., Kitselman, K., & Dwyer, C. Statistical prediction of change in aphasia: Clinical application of multiple regression analysis. In R. H. Brookshire (Ed.), *Clinical Aphasiology: Proceedings of the Conference.* Minneapolis: BRK Publishers, 1979, 95–100.

Deal, J. L., Wertz, R. T., & Spring, C. Differentiating aphasia and the language of generalized intellectual impairment. In R. H. Brookshire (Ed.), *Clinical Aphasiology: Proceedings of the Conference,* Minneapolis: BRK Publishers, 1981. 166–173.

Delis, D. C., & Kaplan, E. The assessment of aphasia with the Luria-Nebraska Neuropsychological Battery: A case critique. *Journal of Consulting and Clinical Psychology,* 1982, *50,* 32–39.

Denny-Brown, D., Meyer, J. S., & Horenstein, S. The significance of perceptual rivalry resulting from a parietal lesion. *Brain,* 1952, *75,* 433–471.

DeRenzi, E. & Vignolo, L. A. The Token Test: A sensitive test to detect receptive disturbances in aphasia. *Brain,* 1962, *85,* 665–678.

Diller, L., Ben-Yishay, Y., Gerstman, L., Goodkin, R., Gordon, W., & Weinberg, J. Studies in cognition and rehabilitation in hemiplegia. *Rehabilitation Monograph,* 1974, *50.*

Diller, L., & Weinberg, J. Hemi-inattention in rehabilitation: The evolution of a rational remediation program. In E. A. Weinstein & R. P. Friedland (Eds.), *Advances in Neurology, volume 18, Hemi-inattention and hemisphere specialization.* New York: Raven Press, 1977, 63–82.

Di Simoni, F. G., Darley, F. L., & Aronson, A. E. Patterns of dysfunction in schizophrenic patients on an aphasia test battery. *Journal of Speech and Hearing Disorders,* 1977, *42,* 498–513.

Dresser, A. C., Meirowsky, A. M., Weiss, G. H., Mc Neel., M. L., Simon, G. A., & Caveness, W. F. Gainful employment following head injury: Prognostic factors. *Archives of Neurology,* 1973, *29,* 111–116.

Duffy, J. R. What is aphasia? (A discussion session). In R. H. Brookshire (Ed.), *Clinical Aphasiology: Proceedings of the Conference.* Minneapolis: BRK Publishers, 1981, 327–329.

Duffy, J. R. & Keith, R. Performance of non brain-injured adults on the PICA: Descriptive data and comparison to patients with aphasia. *Aphasia Apraxia Agnosia,* 1980, *2,* 1–30.

Eisenson, J. Aphasics: Observations and tentative conclusions. *Journal of Speech and Hearing Disorders*, 1947, *12*, 290–292.

Eisenson, J. Prognostic factors relating to language rehabilitation in aphasic patients. *Journal of Speech and Hearing Disorders*, 1949, *14*, 262–264.

Eisenson, J. *Examining for Aphasia*. New York: The Psychological Corp., 1954.

Eisenson, J. Language and intellectual modifications associated with right cerebral damage. *Language and Speech*, 1962, *5*, 49–53.

Eisenson, J. Aphasia: A point of view as to the nature of the disorder and factors that determine prognosis for recovery. *International Journal of Neurology*, 1964, *4*, 287–295.

Elmore, C. M., & Gorham, D. R. Measuring the impairment of the abstracting function with the proverbs test. *Journal of Clinical Psychology*, 1957, *13*, 263–266.

Emerick, L. *Appraisal of language disturbance*. Marquette, MI: Northern Michigan University Press, 1971.

Ernst, B., Dalby, M. A., & Dalby, A. Aphasic disturbances in presenile dementia. *Acta Neurologica Scandinavia*, 1970, *46*, 99–100.

Fairbanks, H. Studies in language behavior. II. The quantitative differentiation of samples of spoken language. *Psychological Monographs*, 1944, *56*, 19–38.

Farber, R., & Reichstein, M. B. Language dysfunction in schizophrenia. *British Journal of Psychiatry*, 1981, *139*, 519–522.

Feldstein, S., & Jaffee, J. Vocabulary diversity of schizophrenics and normals. *Journal of Speech and Hearing Research*, 1962, *5*, 76–78.

Feldstein, S., & Weingartner, H. Speech and psychopharmacology. In J. K. Darby (Ed.), *Speech evaluation in psychiatry*. New York: Grune & Stratton, 1981, 369–396.

Finkel, S. I., & Cohen, G. Guest editorial: The mental health of the aging. *The Gerontologist*, 1982, *22*, 227–228.

Finlayson, R. E., & Martin, L. M. Recognition and management of depression in the elderly. *Mayo Clinic Proceedings*, 1982, *57*, 115–120.

Foley, J.M. Differential diagnosis of the organic mental disorders in elderly patients. In C.M. Gaitz (Ed.), *Aging and the brain*. New York: Plenum Press, 1972, 153–161.

Folsom, J. Reality orientation for the elderly mental patient. *Journal of Geriatric Psychiatry*, 1968, *1*, 291–307.

Fordyce, W., & Jones, R. The efficacy of oral and pantomine instructions for hemiplegic patients. *Archives of Physical Medicine and Rehabilitation*, 1966, *61*, 359–365.

Forer, S., & Miller, L. Rehabilitation outcome: Comparative analysis of different patient types. *Archives of Physical Medicine and Rehabilitation*, 1980, *61*, 359–365.

Freeman, F. R., & Rudd, S. M. Clinical features that predict potentially reverseable progressive intellectual deterioration. *Journal of the American Geriatrics Society*, 1982, *30*, 449–451.

Friedland, R. Cerebral metabolic indices of dementia pathophysiology. Paper presented to the Veterans Administration Audiology and Speech Pathology Educational Conference, Martinez, CA, October, 1982.

Fromkin, V.A., A linguist looks at "A linguist looks at 'schizophrenic language.' " *Brain and Language*, 1975, *2*, 498–503.

Gardner, H. *The shattered mind*. New York: Knopf, 1975.

Gerson, S. N., Benson, D. F., & Frazier, S. H. Diagnosis: Schizophrenia versus posterior aphasia. *American Journal of Psychiatry*, 1977, *134*, 966–969.

Geschwind, N. Writing disturbances in acute confusional states. In N. Geschwind (Ed.), *Selected papers on language and the brain*. Dordrecht, Holland: D. Reidel Publishing Co., 1974. 482–497. (a)

Geschwind, N. *Selected papers on language and the brain*. Dordrecht, Holland: D. Reidel Publishing Co., 1974. (b)

Geschwind, N. The borderland of neurology and psychiatry: Some common misconceptions. In D. F. Benson & D. Blumer (Eds.), *Psychiatric aspects of neurologic disease*. New York: Grune & Stratton, 1975, 1–9.

Golden, C. J., Hammeke, T. A., & Purisch, A. D. *The Luria-Nebraska Neuropsychological Battery: Manual*. Los Angeles: Western Psychological Services, 1980.

Golper, L. A. A study of verbal behavior in recovery of aphasic and nonaphasic persons. In R. H. Brookshire (Ed.), *Clinical Aphasiology: Proceedings of the Conference*. Minneapolis: BRK Publishers, 1980, 28–38.

Goodglass, H, & Kaplan, E. *The assessment of aphasia and related disorders*. Philadelphia: Lea & Febiger, 1972.

Gordon, E., Drenth, V., Jarvis, L., Johnson, J., & Wright, V. Neuropsychologic syndromes in stroke as predictors of outcome. *Archives of Physical Medicine and Rehabilitation*, 1978, *59*, 339–403.

Halpern H. The differential diagnosis of speech and language impairment in the adult neuropsychiatric patient. *Communicative Disorders: An Audio Journal for Continuing Education*, 1980, *5*.

Halpern, H., Darley, F. L., & Brown, J. Differential language and neurological characteristics in cerebral involvement. *Journal of Speech and Hearing Disorders*, 1973, *38*, 162–173.

Halstead, W. C., Wepman, J. M., Reitan, R. M., & Heimburger, R. F. *Halstead Aphasia Test, Form M*. Chicago: University of Chicago Industrial Relations Center, 1949.

Harris, C. & Ivory, P. An outcome evaluation of reality orientation therapy with geriatric patients in a state mental hospital. *The Gerontologist*, 1976, *16*, 496–503.

Harrison, R. J., & Holmes, R. L. (Eds.), *Progress in anatomy* (Vol. 1). London: Cambridge University Press, 1981.

Hartman, J. Measurement of early spontaneous recovery from aphasia with stroke. *Annals of Neurology*, 1981, *9*, 89–91.

Hecaen, H., & Albert M. L. *Human neuropsychology*. New York: John Wiley & Sons, 1978.

Hecaen, H., MaGurs, G., Remier, A., et al. Aphasic croisée chez un sujet droitier bilingue. *Revue Neurologique*, 1971, *124*, 319–323.

Hecaen, H. and Marcie, P. Disorders of written language following right hemisphere lesions: Spatial dysgraphia. In S. Diamond & L. Beaumont (Eds.), *Hemisphere function in the human brain*. London: Paul Elek, 1974, 345–366.

Helm, N. Criteria for selecting aphasia patients for melodic intonation therapy. Paper presented to the American Academy for the Advancement of Science, Washington, DC, 1978.

Helm, N, & Barresi, B. Voluntary control of involuntary utterances: A treatment approach for severe aphasia. In R. H. Brookshire (Ed.), *Clinical Aphasiology: Proceedings of the Conference*. Minneapolis: BRK Publishers, 1980, 308–315.

Helm, N., & Benson, D. G. Visual action therapy for global aphasia. Paper presented to the Academy of Aphasia, Chicago, IL, 1978.

Holland, A. L. Factors affecting functional communication skills of aphasic and nonaphasic individuals. Paper presented to the American Speech and Hearing Association, San Francisco, 1978.

Holland, A. L. *Communicative Abilities in Daily Living*. Baltimore: University Park Press, 1980.

Holland, A. L. Aphasia in head injury. Paper presented to the Clinical Aphasiology Conference, Oshkosh, Wisconsin, 1982. (a)

Holland, A. L. A criticism of the language of the Luria—Nebraska Battery. A paper presented to the Veterans Administration Regional Medical Education Conference on Neuropsychology, Northport, NY, 1982. (b)

Holland, A.L. Observing functional communication of aphasia adults. *Journal of Speech and Hearing Disorders*, 1982, *47*, 50–56. (c)

Holland, A. L. Language intervention in adults: What is it? In J. Miller, D. Yoder, & R. Schiefelbusch (Eds.), *Contemporary Issuses In Language Intervention, ASHA Reports 12.* Rockville, MD: The American Speech-Language-Hearing Association, 1983, 3-14.

Hooper, E. *The Hooper Visual Organization Test.* Los Angeles: Western Psychological Services, 1958.

Horner, J., & Heyman, A. Aphasia associated with Alzheimer's dementia. Paper presented to the International Neuropsychological Society, Pittsburgh, 1982.

Horsfall, G. H. An investigation of selected language performance in adult schizophrenic subjects. Unpublished doctoral dissertation, University of Florida, 1972.

Hoyer, W. J., Kafer, R. A., Simpson, S. C., & Hoyer, F. W. Reinstatement of verbal behavior in elderly mental patients using operant procedures. *The Gerontologist*, 1974, *14*, 149-152.

Hudson, A. Communication problems of the geriatric patient. *Journal of Speech and Hearing Disorders*, 1960, *25*, 238-248.

Hughes, C. P., Berg, L., Danziger, W. L., Coben, L. A., & Martin, R. L. A new clinical scale for the staging of dementia. *The British Journal of Psychiatry*, 1982, *140*, 566-572.

Issacs, W., Thomas, J., & Goldiamond, I. Application of operant conditioning to reinstate verbal behavior in psychotics. *Journal of Speech and Hearing Disorders*, 1960, *25*, 8-12.

Jaffe, J. The psychiatrist's approach to managing the aphasic patient. In R. T. Wertz (Ed.), Aphasia: Interdisciplinary approach, *Seminars, Speech, Language, Hearing*, 1981, *2*, 249-258.

Jellinek, H. M., & Harvey, R. F. Vocational/educational services in a medical rehabilitation facility: Outcomes in spinal cord and brain injured patients. *Archives of Physical Medicine and Rehabilitation*, 1982, *63*, 87-88.

Joynt, R.J., & Goldstein, M. N. The minor cerebral hemisphere. In W. J. Friedlander (Ed.), *Advances in neurology, volume 7: Current reviews of higher nervous system dysfunction.* New York: Raven Press, 1975, 147-183.

Kahn, R., Goldfarb, A., Pollack, M., & Peck, A. Brief objective measures for the determination of mental status in the aged. *American Journal of Psychiatry*, 1960, *117*, 326-328.

Kaplan, E., Goodglass, H., & Weintraub, S. *Boston Naming Test.* Experimental edition, 1976.

Keenan, J. S. Communicative disorders and institutionalized geriatric patients. *Communicative Disorders: An Audio Journal for Continuing Education*, 1979, *4*.

Keenan, J. S., & Brassell, E. G. A study of factors related to prognosis for individual aphasic patients. *Journal of Speech and Hearing Disorders*, 1974, *39*, 257-269.

Keenan, J. S., & Brassell, E. G. *Aphasia Language Performance Scales.* Murfeesborough, TN: Pinnacle Press, 1975.

Kertesz, A. *Aphasia and associated disorders: Taxonomy, localization , and recovery.* New York: Grune & Stratton, 1979.

Kertesz, A. *Western Aphasia Battery.* New York: Grune & Stratton, 1982.

Kertesz, A., & McCabe, P. Recovery patterns and prognosis in aphasia. *Brain*, 1977, *100*, 1-18.

Kitselman, K. Language impairment in aphasia, delirium, dementia, and schizophrenia. In J. K. Darby (Ed.), *Speech evaluation in medicine.* New York: Grune & Stratton, 1981, 199-214.

Kleist, K. Schizophrenic symptoms and cerebral pathology. *Journal of Mental Science*, 1960, *106*, 246-255.

Klonoff, H., Fibiger, C. H., & Hutton, G. H. Neuropsychological patterns in chronic schizophrenia. *Journal of Nervous and Mental Disease*, 1970, *150*, 291-300.

Labouvice-Vief, G., Hoyer, W. J., Baltes, M. M., & Baltes, P. B. Operant analysis of intellectual behavior in old age. *Human Development*, 1974, *17*, 259-272.

LaPointe, L. L. Aphasia intervention with adults: Historical, present, and future approaches: In J. Miller, D. Yoder, & R. Schiefelbusch (Eds.), *Contemporary Issues In Language Intervention, ASHA Reports 12.* Rockville, MD: The American Speech-Language-Hearing Association, 1983, 127-136.

LaPointe, L. L., & Culton, G. L. Visual-spatial neglect subsequent to brain injury. *Journal of Speech and Hearing Disorders*, 1969, *34*, 82-86.

LaPointe, L. L. & Horner, J. *Reading Comprehension Battery for Aphasia.* Tigard, OR: C. C. Publications, 1979.

Linge, F. R. What does it feel like to be brain damaged? *Canadian Mental Health*, 1980, 4-7.

Lomas, J., & Kertesz, A. Patterns of spontaneous recovery in aphasic groups: A study of adult stroke patients. *Brain and Language*, 1978, *5*, 388-401.

Lorenze, E., & Canero, P. Dysfunction in visual perception with hemiplegia: Its relation to activities of daily living. *Archives of Physical Medicine and Rehabilitation* , 1962, *43*, 514-517.

Lubinski, R. Speech language and audiology programs in home health care agencies and nursing homes. In D. S. Beasley & G. A. Davis (Eds.), *Aging: Communication processes and disorders*. New York: Grune & Stratton, 1981, 339-356.

Lubinski, R., Morrison, E. B., & Rigrodsky, S. Perception of spoken communication by elderly chronically ill patients in an institutional setting. *Journal of Speech and Hearing Disorders*, 1981, *46*, 405-412.

Ludlow, C. L. Identification and assessment of aphasic patients for language intervention. In J. Miller, D. Yoder, & R. Schiefelbusch (Eds.), *Contemporary Issues In Language Intervention, ASHA Reports 12.* Rockville MD: The American Speech-Language-Hearing Association, 1983, 75-91.

Luria, A. R. *Restoration of function after brain injury.* New York: Macmillan, 1963.

Luria, A. R. *Traumatic aphasia.* The Hague: Mouton, 1970.

MacDonald, M. L. Environmental programming for the socially isolated aging. Paper presented to the 2nd Annual Convention of the Midwestern Association of Behavior Analysis, Chicago, IL, 1976.

McNeil, M. R., & Prescott, T. E. *Revised Token Test.* Baltimore: University Park Press, 1978.

Mayo Clinic, *Clinical examinations in neurology* (4th Ed.). Philadelphia: W. B. Saunders, 1976.

Meehl, P. E. Seer over sign: The first good example. *Journal of Experimental Research In Personality*, 1965, *1*, 27-32.

Metzler, N. G., & Jelinek, J. E. Writing disturbances in patients with right cerebral hemisphere lesions. In R. H. Brookshire (Ed.), *Clinical Aphasiology: Proceedings of the Conference.* Minneapolis: BRK Publishers, 1977, 214-225.

Miller, E. The management of dementia: A review of some possibilities. *British Journal of Social and Clinical Psychology*, 1977, *16*, 77-83.

Mills, R. H. & Drummond, S. S. Analysis of impaired naming in language of confusion. Paper presented to the American Speech-Language-Hearing Association, Detroit, 1980.

Mosher, L. R., & Feinsilver, D. *Special report on schizophrenia.* Publication (HSM) 72-9042. Bethesda, MD: U.S. Department of Health, Education and Welfare, National Institute of Mental Health, 1971.

Moss, C. S. *Recovery With aphasia: The aftermath of my stroke.* Urbana: University of Illinois Press, 1972.

Mueller, D., & Atlas, L. Resocialization of regressed elderly residents: A behavioral management approach. *Journal of Gerontology*, 1972, *27*, 361-363.

Mueller, P. B. Communicative disorders in a geriatric population. Paper presented to the American Speech and Hearing Association, San Francisco, 1978.

Mueller, P. B., & Peters, T. J. Needs and services in geriatric speech-language pathology and audiology. *Asha*, 1981, *23*, 627–632.

Myers, P. S. Analysis of right hemisphere communication deficits: Implications for speech pathology. In R. H. Brookshire (Ed.), *Clinical Aphasiology: Proceedings of the Conference*. Minneapolis: BRK Publishers, 1978, 49–57.

Myers, P. S. Profiles of communication deficits in patients with right cerebral hemisphere damage. In R. H. Brookshire (Ed.), *Clinical Aphasiology: Proceedings of the Conference*. Minneapolis: BRK Publishers, 1979, 38–46.

Myers, P. S. Treatment of right hemisphere damaged patients: A panel presentation and discussion. In R. H. Brookshire (Ed.), *Clinical Aphasiology: Proceedings of the Conference*. Minneapolis: BRK Publishers, 1981, 272–276.

Myers, P. S., & Linebaugh, C. W. Comprehension of ideomatic expressions by right-hemisphere-damaged adults. In R. H. Brookshire (Ed.), *Clinical Aphasiology: Proceedings of the Conference*. Minneapolis: BRK Publishers, 1981, 254–261.

Myers, P. S. & West, J. F. The speech pathologist's role with right hemisphere damaged patients. In R. H. Brookshire (Ed.), *Clinical Aphasiology: Proceedings of the Conference*. Minneapolis: BRK Publishers, 1978, 364–365.

Nelson, H. E., & O'Connell, A. Dementia: The estimation of premorbid intelligence levels using the New Adult Reading Test. *Cortex*, 1978, *14*, 234–244.

Obler, L. K, & Albert, M. L. Language and aging: A neurobehavioral analysis. In D. S. Beasley & G. A. Davis (Eds.), *Aging: Communication processes and disorders*. New York: Grune & Stratton, 1981, 107–122.

O'Connell, P., & O'Connell, E. Speech-language pathology services in a skilled nursing facility. Paper presented to the American Speech and Hearing Association, San Francisco, 1978.

Ojemann, G. A. Subcortical language mechanisms. In H. Whitaker & H. A. Whitaker (Eds.), *Studies in neurolinguistics, volume 2*. New York: Academic Press, 1975, 103–138.

Orzeck, A. Z. *Orzeck Aphasia Evaluation*. Los Angeles: Western Psychological Services, 1964.

Osler, W. The Gulstonian Lectures on malignant endocarditis. *British Medical Journal*, 1885, *1*, 467–470, 522–526, 577–579.

Ostwald, P. F. *Soundmaking: The acoustic communication of emotion*. Springfield, IL: Charles C. Thomas, 1963.

Parsons, O. Current perspectives in neuropsychology. Paper presented to the Veterans Administration Conference on Multidisciplinary Approaches to the Brain Impaired Patient, Topeka, KN, 1982.

Pollack, M., Levenstein, D. S. W., & Klein, D. F. A three-year posthospital follow up of adolescent and adult schizophrenics. *American Journal of Orthopsychiatry*, 1968, *38*, 94–110.

Porch, B. E. *Porch Index of Communicative Ability*. Palo Alto, CA: Consulting Psychologists Press, 1973.

Porch, B. E., Collins, M. J., Wertz, R. T., & Friden, T. Statistical prediction of change in aphasia. *Journal of Speech and Hearing Research*, 1980, *23*, 312–322.

Porch, B. E., Friden, T., & Porec, J. Objective differentiation of aphasic versus nonorganic patients. Paper presented to the International Neuropsychological Society, Santa Fe, NM, 1976.

Porch, B. E., Wertz, R. T., & Collins, M. J. Recovery of communicative ability: Patterns and prediction. Paper presented to the Academy of Aphasia, Albuquerque, NM, 1973.

Porch, B. E., Wertz, R. T., & Collins, M. J. A statistical procedure for predicting recovery from aphasia. In B. E. Porch (Ed.), *Clinical Aphasiology: Proceedings of the Conference*. Albuquerque, NM: Veterans Administration, 1974, 27–37.

Prins, R., Snow, C., & Wagenaar, E. Recovery from aphasia: Spontaneous speech versus language comprehension. *Brain and Language*, 1978, *6*, 192–211.

Rathbone-McCuan, E. Geriatric day care: A family perspective. *The Gerontologist*, 1976, *16*, 517–521.

Ratusnik, D., Lascoe, D., Herbon, M., & Wolfe, V. Group language stimulation for patients with senile dementia, a pilot project. *Aphasia Apraxia Agnosia*, 1979, *1*, 14–29.

Rausch, M. A., Prescott, T. E., & De Wolfe, A. S. Schizophrenic and aphasic language: Discriminable or not? *Journal of Consulting and Clinical Psychology*, 1980, *48*, 63–70.

Raven, J. C. *Coloured Progressive Matrices*. London: H. K. Lewis & Co., 1962.

Rebok, G. W., & Hoyer, W. J. The functional context of elderly behavior. *The Gerontologist*, 1977, *17*, 27–34.

Rioch, M. J., & Lubin, A. Prognosis of social adjustment for mental hospital patients under psychotherapy. *Journal of Consulting Psychology*, 1959, *23*, 313–318.

Rochester, S. R., Martin, J. R., & Thurston, S. Thought process disorder in schizophrenia: The listener's task. *Brain and Language*, 1977, *4*, 95–114.

Rochford, G. A study of naming errors in dysphasic and in demented patients. *Neuropsychologia*, 1971, *9*, 437–443.

Rosenbek, J. C. Wrinkled feet. In R. H. Brookshire (Ed.), *Clinical Aphasiology: Proceedings of the Conference*. Minneapolis: BRK Publishers, 1979, 163–176.

Rosenbek, J. C. Some challenges for clinical aphasiologists. In J. Miller, D. Yoder, & R. Schiefelbusch (Eds.), *Contemporary Issues In Language Intervention, ASHA Reports 12*. Rockville, MD: The American Speech-Language-Hearing Association, 1983, 317–325.

Rubens, A. B. Aphasia with infarction in the territory of the anterior cerebral artery. *Cortex*, 1975, *11*, 239–250.

Sarno, M. T. *Functional Communication Profile*. New York: Institute of Rehabilitation Medicine, New York University Medical Center, 1969.

Sarno, M. T., & Levita, E. Recovery in aphasia during the first year post stroke. *Stroke*, 1979, *10*, 663–670.

Schuell, H. A short examination for aphasia. *Neurology*, 1957, *7*, 625–634.

Schuell, H. *The Minnesota Test for Differential Diagnosis of Aphasia*. Minneapolis: University of Minnesota Press, 1965. (a)

Schuell, H. *Differential diagnosis of aphasia with the Minnesota Test*. Minneapolis: University of Minnesota Press, 1965. (b)

Schuell, H., Jenkins, J. J., & Carroll J. B. A factor analysis of the Minnesota Test for Differential Diagnosis of Aphasia. *Journal of Speech and Hearing Research*, 1962, *5*, 349–369.

Schuell, H., Jenkins, J. J., & Jimenez-Pabon, E. *Aphasia in adults: Diagnosis, prognosis, and treatment*. New York: Hoeber Medical Division, Harper, 1964.

Schwartz, M. F., Marin, O. S. M., & Saffran, E. M. Disassociation of language function in dementia: A case study. *Brain and Language*, 1979, *7*, 277–306.

Sherman, J. A. Reinstatement of verbal behavior in a psychotic by reinforcement methods. *Journal of Speech and Hearing Disorders*, 1963, *28*, 398–401.

Sklar, M. *Sklar Aphasia Scale*. Los Angeles: Western Psychological Services, 1966.

Snyder, L. H., Pyrek, J., & Smith, K. C. Vision and mental function of the elderly. *The Gerontologist*, 1976, *16*, 491–495.

Solomon, K. Social antecedents of learned helplessness in the health care setting. *The Gerontologist*, 1982, *22*, 282–287.

Sparks, R., Helm, N., & Albert, M. Aphasia rehabilitation resulting from melodic intonation therapy. *Cortex*, 1974, *10*, 303–316.

Spiers, P. A. Have they come to praise Luria or bury him?: The Luria-Nebraska Battery controversy. *Journal of Consulting and Clinical Psychology*, 1981, *49*, 331–341.

Spreen, O., & Benton, A. L. *Neurosensory Center Comprehensive Examination for Aphasia.* Victoria B.C.: University of Victoria Neuropsychology Laboratory, 1969.

Stanton, K. M., Yorkston, K. M., Kenyon, V. T., & Beukelman, D. R. Language utilization in teaching reading to left neglect patients. In R. H. Brookshire (Ed.), *Clinical Aphasiology: Proceedings of the Conference.* Minneapolis: BRK Publishers, 1981, 262–271.

Steinhauer, M. B. Geriatric foster care: A prototype design and implementation issues. *The Gerontologist*, 1982, *22*, 293–300.

Strohner, H., Cohen, R., Kelter, S., & Woll, G. "Semantic" and "acoustic" errors of aphasic and schizophrenic patients in a sound-picture matching task. *Cortex*, 1978, *14*, 391–403.

Swisher, L. P., & Sarno, M. T. Token test scores of three matched patient groups: Left brain-damaged with aphasia, right brain-damaged without aphasia, nonbrain damaged. *Cortex*, 1969, *5*, 264–273.

Taylor, M. A., Greenspan, B., & Abrams, R. Lateralized neuropsychological dysfunction in affective disorder and schizophrenia. *American Journal of Psychiatry*, 1979, *136*, 1031–1034.

Taylor, M. M., Schaeffer, J. N., Blumenthal, F. S., & Grissel, J. L. Controlled evaluation of perceptual and motor training therapy after stroke resulting in left hemiplegia. Final Report, Social and Rehabilitation Service, RD 2215-M. Department of Health, Education and Welfare, Washington, DC, 1969.

Todt, E. H., & Howell, R. J. Vocal cues as indices of schizophrenia. *Journal of Speech and Hearing Research*, 1980, *23*, 517–526.

Vignolo, L. A. Evolution of aphasia and language rehabilitation: A retrospective study. *Cortex*, 1964, *1*, 344–367.

Watson, R. T., & Heilman, K. M. The differential diagnosis of dementia. *Geriatrics*, 1974, *29*, 145–154.

Watson, J. M. & Records, L. E. The effectiveness of the Porch Index of Communicative Ability as a diagnostic tool in assessing specific behaviors of senile dementia. In R. H. Brookshire (Ed.), *Clinical Aphasiology: Proceedings of the Conference.* Minneapolis: BRK Publishers, 1978, 93–105.

Weinstein, E. A. Affections of speech with lesions of the non-dominant hemisphere. *Research Publication Association for Research of Nervous and Mental Disorders*, 1964, *42*, 220–225.

Weisbroth, S., Esibill, N., & Zuger, R. R. Factors in the vocational success of hemiplegic patients. *Archives of Physical Medicine and Rehabilitation*, 1971, *52*, 441–446, 486.

Wells, C. E. Refinements in the diagnosis of dementia. *American Journal of Psychiatry*, 1982, *139*, 621–622.

Wepman, J. M, & Jones, L. V. *The Language Modalities Test for Aphasia.* Chicago: Education-Industry Service, 1961.

Wertz, R. T. Neuropathologies of speech and language: An introduction to patient management. In D. F. Johns (Ed.), *Clinical management of neurogenic communicative disorders.* Boston: Little, Brown & Company, 1978, 1–101.

Wertz, R. T. Language deficit in aphasia and dementia: The same as, different from, or both. Paper presented to the Clinical Aphasiology Conference, Oshkosh, WI, 1982.

Wertz, R. T. Language intervention context and setting for the aphasic adult: When? In J. Miller, D. Yoder, & R. Schiefelbusch (Eds.), *Contemporary Issues In Language Intervention, ASHA Reports 12.* Rockville, MD: The American Speech-Language-Hearing Association, 1983, 196–220. (a)

Wertz, R. T. A philosophy of aphasia therapy: Some things patients have not said but you can see if you listen. *Communication Disorders: A Journal for Continuing Education*, 1983, *8*, 1-17. (b)

Wertz, R. T., Collins, M. J., Weiss, D., Kurtzke, J. F., Friden, T., Brookshire, R. H., Pierce, J., et al. Veterans Administration cooperative study on aphasia: A comparison of individual and group treatment. *Journal of Speech and Hearing Research*, 1981, *24*, 580-594.

Wertz, R. T., Kitselman, K. P., & Deal, L. A. Classifying the aphasias: Contributions to patient management. Paper presented to the Academy of Aphasia, London, Ontario, 1981.

Wertz, R. T., & Rosenbek, J. C. Appraising apraxia of speech. *Journal of the Colorado Speech and Hearing Association*, 1971, *5*, 18-36.

Yarnell, P., Monroe, P., & Sobel, L. Aphasia outcome in stroke: A clinical neuroradiological correlation. *Stroke*, 1976, 514-522.

Yorkston, K. M. Treatment of right hemisphere damaged patients: A panel presentation and discussion. In R. H. Brookshire (Ed.), *Clinical Aphasiology: Proceedings of the Conference*. Minneapolis: BRK Publishers, 1981, 281-283.

Yorkston, K. M., & Beukelman, D. R. A system for quantifying verbal output of high-level aphasic patients. In R. H. Brookshire (Ed.), *Clinical Aphasiology: Proceedings of the Conference*. Minneapolis: BRK Publishers, 1977, 175-180.

G. Albyn Davis

Effects of Aging on Normal Language

Aphasia usually arises in persons who already have been undergoing gradual and hardly perceptible changes in their cognitive systems. These changes continue relentlessly throughout the rest of an aphasic individual's life. The changes of aging, a combination of development and decline, reflect the genetically programmed predisposition of the human species to have a limited life span of around 100 years. Diseases, accidents, bad habits, and pollution contribute to a longevity or life expectancy in the United States of around 74 years. Aging of the language function is of particular interest to the speech-language pathologist because of its potential contribution to language behaviors in aphasic clients. It poses a special problem of differential diagnosis within a patient, namely, between the deficits of aphasia and the normal "deficits" which arise from simply being old. Unfortunately, we have little information with which to make this differentiation. As Cohen (1979) observed recently, "Geriatric psycholinguistics is virtually an unexplored territory" (p. 412).

Few investigators have set out intentionally to study the effect of aging on the language behaviors involved in diagnosis and assessment of aphasia. However, several have explored the relationship between aging and language functions indirectly, while answering questions about verbal learning, memory, or problem solving skill. Because language processing is a cognitive function, constrained by short-term memory and involving long-term memory, the study of cognitive changes has some relevance for the study of language changes. Language research with middle-aged and elderly adults is at a level that is similar to psycholinguistic research of the early 1960s; issues about sentence processing are raised more often with respect to memory than with respect to comprehension. This chapter shows that a few indications are available concerning the effect of aging on the language behaviors impaired in aphasia, such as digit memory span, sentence comprehension, picture naming, and word fluency.

What is Meant By Aging?

There is a fuzzy distinction between normal aging and the pathologies of aging. The physiological changes of each are similar. Certain changes underlying Alzheimer's dementia, for example, simply are exaggerations of the changes associated with normal aging. Also, the heightened prevalence of disease processes in old age makes it difficult to separate the effects of disease from the effects of species-specific programmed decline and simple wear-and-tear on the neurophysiological systems supporting cognitive function. To some extent, we may have to accept susceptibility to disease as part of the normal dynamics of aging. One way of making a distinction between normal and pathological aging is to consider whether cognitive changes are either not significant enough to prohibit independent functioning or, on the other hand, are serious enough to impair independent living sometimes to an extent that requires insitutionalization. Still, there is overlap with this criterion, as "the ability to live independently in the community does not by itself rule out the early stages of dementia" (Jacoby, Levy, & Dawson, 1980, p. 249). Some changes of language function in normal aging may be considered to represent a *decline* of function, while pathological changes such as in dementia may be thought of as *deficits* of function.

Many factors contributing to variations of cognitive function are independent of chronological age per se but, nevertheless, often accumulate with increasing age. Living environment, depression, and medications can contribute to the appearance of decline or deficit in cognitive function. In an instructive lesson on medication in the elderly, Salzman (1982) noted that 22% of drug prescriptions in the United States are received by persons of age 65 and older. Almost two-thirds of these involve five to 12 medications every day. Chronological age is not a good predictor of a person's cognitive status, because cognitive status is influenced by so many other factors. One consistent result in research on aging is an increase in variability of performance with increasing age. It is difficult to describe a typical 70-year-old, an age at which one could be a physically fit president of the United States or a legally incompetent resident of a nursing home. The most trustworthy depiction of aging cognition may require (1) identifying functions that develop, remain stable, or decline throughout the life span, (2) comparing the relative rates of development or decline among some functions, and (3) not counting on being able to identify the changes with chronological age per se.

Because of the number of factors that contribute to changes associated with aging, subjects for studying cognitive change should be carefully selected. The typical design for investigating cognitive functions is called a *cross-sectional design*, in which groups of different ages are compared. Different subjects are selected for each group, and so all ages are tested during the same time period. Sometimes only two groups are compared: a young adult group of college age and an elderly group of subjects at least 60 or 65 years of age. Frequently, three groups are used, identified as young, middle-aged, and old. A middle-aged group usually averages around 45 to 50 years of age. As Schaie (1980) noted, it is difficult to obtain data on normal aging beyond the late 60s, because it is more difficult to find old subjects with a health status that is reasonably comparable to young and middle-aged adults.

The principal confounding factor in a cross-sectional design is the *cohort effect* in which certain inherent differences between age-defined populations are present because they were born at different times. A factor such as education level can contribute to differences on cognitive tasks shown by different age groups. The population born between 1915 and 1925 has received less formal education than the population born between 1955 and 1965. Education has been a difficult variable to control, and some investigators have had to settle for reporting educational as well as age differences in describing their subjects. In Borod, Goodglass, and Kaplan's (1980a) norms for the *Boston Diagnostic Aphasia Examination* (Goodglass & Kaplan, 1972), variability of performance was shown to be influenced by age and education. Sometimes different age groups are equated on one measure before being compared with another measure (Feier & Gerstman, 1980). The education variable may be factored out in the statistical analysis of cross-sectional data (Botwinick, West, & Storandt, 1975), or groups are made comparable by creating two young and two old groups of high- and low-education levels (Cohen, 1979).

A basic question in this chapter is how much of an aphasic patient's deficit, if any, can be attributed to aging? A comparison between aphasic subjects and an age-matched normal control group may answer this question in part, but the language function in question may be one that maintains at a constant level across the life span, or one that declines. Therefore, the question cannot be answered confidently until the language function is measured across the life span. Furthermore, generalizations about the intrusion of a naturally declining language function on a deficit of aphasia should be considered with respect to the average age of a peacetime aphasic population. The average aphasic patient is around 55 years of age (Davis & Holland, 1981) and some age-related cognitive changes do not seem to occur until after 60 years. Therefore, aphasia is likely to occur before any significant interaction with aging is possible.

The Classic Aging Pattern

A broad range of cognitive functions is measured with intelligence tests such as the *Wechsler Adult Intelligence Scale* (WAIS). These tests often are divided into verbal and nonverbal (performance) skills, and the effects of aging on these general categories have been studied frequently (for an excellent review, see Schaie, 1980). The classic aging pattern is for verbal measures to maintain a constant level or even increase, and for nonverbal measures to decline gradually, especially in speed of performance. Verbal skills sometimes are referred to as "hold" functions while nonverbal skills are functions that "don't hold." When young adults and old adults are matched in overall score on the WAIS, elderly subjects are better than the young on verbal scores, while young subjects are better than the elderly on nonverbal scores. In longitudinal studies, in which a single group is tested repeatedly over many years, overall IQ is maintained until the decade of the 70s.

Further suggestion of decline in nonverbal functions comes from the norms for Raven's *Coloured Progressive Matrices*. This measure of visuospatial thinking is often given to aphasic adults (see Kertesz & McCabe, 1975). Peak performance of normal adults is reached in the early 20s; and then a decline begins at about age 30, and continues gradually to 85 years (Raven, Court, & Raven, 1976). Johnson, Cole, Bowers, et al. (1979) found age-related decline in music recognition. Because visuospatial and musical abilities are managed primarily by the right cerebral hemisphere, Johnson et al. concluded that the aging process includes a decline of right hemisphere function. In dichotic listening, older subjects were shown to be poorer than younger subjects in recalling digits presented to the left ear, presumably to the right hemisphere (Clark & Knowles, 1973). Kocel (1980) proposed that aging is accompanied by an increased reliance on the left hemisphere as reflected in maintained or improving verbal abilities.

One verbal behavior commonly cited as being maintained, or even increasing, is vocabulary tested by having the examinee define several words.

Suspecting that qualitative scoring of such tests might better capture changes than simple quantitative scoring, Botwinick et al. (1974, 1975) developed a scoring system that was more descriptive of nuances in definitional responses. Their qualitative scoring included attention to the "superior synonym" as the best response, with explanations and descriptions receiving lower scores. First, they compared a younger group ($\overline{X}$ = 18.4, 17–20 years) and an older group ($\overline{X}$ = 70.6, 62–83 years) matched for quantitative level of vocabulary performance. The elderly group gave significantly fewer superior synonyms. Later, Botwinick et al. (1975) investigated qualitative responses over the life span with groups representing each decade from the 20s throught the 70s. A gradual decline in use of superior synonyms did not appear; instead, quantitative and qualitative scores were maintained at the same level until the 70s, when a sharp decline did occur. These studies demonstrate the value of obtaining data across the life span rather than only from young and old groups. We cannot assume that all changes between young and old age are characterized by gradual decline. Expressing nuances of word meaning appears to hold until rather late in life.

As indicated by nonverbal performance scores across the life span, the most consistent behavioral change seen with advanced age is a decline in success with fast-paced tasks and a "generalized slowness of behavior" (Birren, 1964; Crook, 1979). Regarding intellectual and problem-solving abilities, Schaie (1980) concluded:

> When all is said and done, we conclude . . . [that there is] little change until midlife, except for the need to take somewhat more time to achieve equal levels of accuracy. Slowing sensory and perceptual processes may make it likely that older people, particularly those beyond the early seventies, will tend to make mistakes by simplifying their conceptual frameworks even when this is maladaptive and by failing to spend as much time as their central nervous sytem requires to obtain adequate solutions because of real or perceived pressures "to get on with it. " (p. 279)

The Possibility Of An Aging Language Function

If cognitive processes simply slow down in late adulthood, the prospect for an interesting discussion of aging and language function appears to be somewhat restrained. The processes of language comprehension and production may simply be caught up in the generalized slow down.

However, it would be of interest to determine the regions of linguistic performance in which central slowing has an impact on linguistic accuracy and style. Furthermore, we should not rely on the extensive results from intelligence testing as the final word on aging and language function. Such verbal tests are often confounded by demands on general knowledge and problem solving, and they are not aimed at subtle linguistic dimensions of syntax and semantics. Cohen (1979) argued that the verbal subtests of IQ batteries, especially the vocabulary subtest "yield very little insight into the vastly more complex process involved in ordinary language functions such as the comprehension of discourse and written texts" (p. 412). However, the well-established findings on the aging of sensory systems, the central nervous system, and memory are suggestive of the possibility that language function changes with advancing age.

Sensory Functions

Reductions of auditory and visual sensitivity are a common feature of aging. Hearing loss due to aging is called *presbycusis*, and visual acuity decline, similarly, is called *presbyopia*. Elderly people often benefit from hearing aids, lipreading, and special auditory training. They also may require more lighting in a room, and large-print or magnifiers for reading. A gradual decline of color perception begins between ages 30 and 40 with loss of blue-green discrimination and, then, red-green deterioration, beginning around age 55-60 (Voke, 1982).

Much has been written on hearing loss as a function of aging (Beasley & Davis, 1981; Bergman, 1980; Henoch, 1979; Maurer & Rupp, 1979). Such changes certainly affect ability to comprehend. Obler and Albert (1981) relied on hearing loss in the elderly in order to conclude that "language comprehension appears both to deteriorate and to change with aging" (p. 110). However, change in language comprehension was not demonstrated in normally hearing older subjects in Obler and Albert's review. Adequate hearing sensitivity and speech perception are prerequisites for auditory language comprehension, but are not the processes of auditory language comprehension. In order to analyze the linguistic mechanisms of comprehension, processses common to auditory comprehension and reading should be considered.

The Central Nervous System

Slowing of cognitive processes in aging may be attributed to changes in the central nervous system. Valenstein (1981) described certain gross morphological changes. Brain weight increases rapidly until three years, and then increases slowly until 18 years; it remains stable for three decades and "then slowly declines, so that the average brain weight in persons over 86 is 11% less than the mean brain weight of younger adults" (p. 88). Ventricular size is larger in elderly adults, and the cerebral cortex atrophies. Atrophy begins to reach statistically significant proportions around age 50 (Yamaura, Ito, Kubota, & Matsuzana, 1980). The appearance of these changes on CT scans (computed tomography) is important because of the continuing need for age-related normative CT data (Jacoby, Levy, & Dawson, 1980). Certain microscopic changes have also been recorded (Adams, 1980; Valenstein, 1981). Schulz and Hunziker (1980) found atrophy of neurons in the precentral gyrus for subjects aged 85 to 94, but not in subjects aged 65 to 74. Gross morphological atrophy may be attributed, in part, to neuronal dropout or loss of neurons. However, dropout occurs only in certain areas including prefrontal cortex and the hippocampus. The temporal lobe has not been shown to lose neurons in the normally aging brain. In addition, lipofuscin, a yellow-brown pigment, accumulates in nerve and glial cells; neurofibrillary tangles appear in the hippocampus of the normally aging brain; and neuritic or "senile" plaques are seen in the amygdala of the corpus striatum deep within the brain.

Adams (1980) advised: "Aging affects all parts of the body and, in view of the interdependency of organs, there is a certain artificiality in discussing the changes in the nervous system in isolation. Aging in the pituitary and endocrine glands, the liver, heart, and lungs are all capable of altering function and structure of the brain" (p. 149).

Physiological changes have been measured from the aging brain (Michalewski, Thompson, & Saul, 1980; Valenstein, 1981). In the healthy old person, little relationship has been demonstrated between intellect and EEG. Alpha activity decreases over the life span; and in 30% to 70% of the normal elderly, episodic abnormalities of EEG occur over the temporal region. Other changes in EEG are associated with dementia. Several changes in evoked potentials have been observed. The clearest changes are in passive response to visual stimuli; amplitude of early components of the cortical measure increase, and later components decrease. Response latencies are longer. During active processing of stimuli, more latency than amplitude changes are seen. Valenstein (1981) noted that changes in cerebral blood flow occur primarily in adults with dementia.

Memory

The literature on aging contains many vague and sometimes erroneous statements about changes in memory. The normal aging of memory carries important implications for the possibility of aging language function, because this function is supported by the different components of the memory system. An accurate portrayal of aging memory involves attention to its different components. However, memory has been portrayed in two slightly different ways. Thorough reviews of aging memory include one based on a *multistore* memory model (Smith & Fullerton, 1981) and another based on *depth of processing* in primary and secondary memory (Craik, 1977). The multistore model divides memory into sensory memory, short-term memory, and long-term memory. The attention mechanism selects information from sensory memory to be processed in the limited capacity short-term memory. The active processes of language comprehension and expression are carried out within the constraints of short-term memory. The depth of processing orientation, on the other hand, states that variations of capacity and time in memory are related to the extent to which material is processed. Memory is seen to be more of a continuum than a segmentation of qualitatively distinct components.

Attention

Only a portion of information in sensory memory is selected for the depth of processing occurring in short-term memory. Investigators have been interested in the level of processing applied to relatively unattended stimuli. One research paradigm is the dichotic presentation of word lists or messages (see Craik, 1977). Subjects are instructed to recall the stimulus to one ear first, and the other ear second. Stimuli to the second ear are not attended to as well as those to the first ear. The elderly are equal to young adults in recall from the first ear, but show a decline of recall from the second ear. Craik emphasized that the elderly have immediate recall problems under conditions of divided attention. Parkinson, Lindholm, and Urell (1980) found that when the young and old are equated in digit span, the age difference in dichotic listening is eliminated. They concluded that immediate recall of digits, and dichotic memory, are mediated by a common storage mechanism which may decline somewhat with age.

Short-Term Memory

In multistore models, short-term memory (STM) is considered to represent active or working memory which has a limited capacity and in which traces are retained no longer than 30 seconds (Norman, 1976). In the depth of processing orientation, time of storage is seen as continuum; primary memory, which is similar to STM, is considered to represent information that is "in mind," still being rehearsed, and the focus of attention (Craik, 1977).

The possibility of STM deficit has been seized upon as a basis for predicting declines of auditory language comprehension (Cohen, 1979; Feier & Gerstman, 1980). In an article on comprehension, Nash and Wepman (1973) stated: "One aspect of auditory functioning which has been well documented is auditory memory. Short-term memory declines with age" (p. 244). Cohen (1979) cited a common notion that STM in the elderly is more vulnerable to interference than in younger subjects, but Craik (1977) stressed that there is no empirical evidence for this view.

Capacity traditionally has been measured with a test of immediate memory span for digits. Digit span does not change much with age. Craik (1977) cited Botwinick and Storandt's (1974) findings regarding digit spans across several decades: 6.7 (20s), 6.2 (30s), 6.5 (40s), 6.5 (50s), 5.5 (60s), and 5.4 (70s). These findings are fairly consistent. More recently, college students averaged 6.4 digits, and elderly subjects averaged 5.8 digits, a difference which lacked statistical significance (Parkinson, Lindholm, & Urell, 1980). Also, in immediate recall of supraspan word lists, the recency effect, which indicates recall from STM or primary memory, remains unchanged by normal aging (Smith & Fullerton, 1981). Digit span backwards, on the other hand, does decline with advanced age. A consistent conclusion is that significant changes in STM capacity occur only in conditions of divided attention or when reorganization of the material is required.

Scanning of sequences in STM is one process of working memory which may be involved in sentence comprehension. In studies of this process, the subject is presented a set of subspan digits and then must decide whether a particular digit was contained in the set. Scanning is assumed to be the process by which the subject mentally compares the test digit with each item in the remembered set. Response time is taken as a measure of rate of scanning and also to determine whether each set is scanned exhaustively, or only partially. Aging has been shown to decrease the rate of scanning (Anders, Fozard, & Lillyquist, 1972; Madden & Nebes, 1980). A significant decrease is evident by middle-age (Anders et al., 1972). Search time in the elderly is double that of college-age adults. The mode of process, however, does not change with increasing age. Scanning has been studied with aphasic adults, also (Swinney & Taylor, 1971; Warren, Hubbard, & Knox, 1977). Aphasic subjects scan items in STM at a slower rate than age-matched normal controls. Scanning speed in aphasia, therefore, may be a result of focal brain injury and the aging process.

Long-Term Memory

Aging with respect to long-term memory (also, secondary memory) involves several issues. Proponents of multistore and depth-of-processing models agree that we should consider acquisition of information (learning), storage, and retrieval from storage. Smith and Fullerton (1981) made an additional distinction between episodic and semantic memory. Episodic memory pertains to remembering specific events, and is observed in the laboratory with verbal learning tasks of word list recall and paired-associate recall. Semantic memory refers to our general knowledge of the world, and investigators are most interested in how concepts are organized in relatively permanent storage. Semantic memory is studied with respect to recognition and recall of sentence and word meanings.

In general, experimental paradigms require either *recognition* (identification of to-be-remembered material from some choices) or *recall* (production of to-be-remembered material). Recognition has been considered to reflect acquisition, while recall requires acquisition, search for the item in LTM, and retrieval. Recognition usually produces more accurate memory scores. For some time, aging was believed to affect recall but not recognition, because recall is a more demanding function requiring search and retrieval processes. However, in a thorough and forceful critique of research on aging of long-term memory, Burke and Light (1981) cited evidence that recognition memory also declines during adulthood, but to a lesser degree than recall. These reviewers argued that recognition is more complex than it may seem, because it also involves search and retrieval during the initial encoding of information.

Aging appears to affect *acquisition* of new information for long-term storage. Acquisition is facilitated by the application of encoding[1] strategies to stimuli. We may memorize lists with the help of mnemonic devices, such as visual imagery; and when experimental subjects are asked to learn word lists, they recall the most words when they can use visual imagery or their semantic knowledge to organize the words during the acquisition process. It has been suggested that organization and mnemonics are not utilized as spontaneously by the elderly as they are by younger adults (Craik, 1977). That is, the elderly are able to use encoding strategies, but they must often be instructed to do so. Smith and Fullerton (1981) suggested that reduced encoding occurs primarily in acquisition for episodic memory.

While the decline of spontaneous encoding for LTM acquisition has been proposed frequently as a specific characteristic of aging, Burke and Light's (1981) examination of the relevant research produced a different conclusion. The elderly still do not recall as well as the young when instructed to encode word lists. Therefore, aging may reduce the ability to organize new information, even when this ability is not applied spontaneously. Burke and Light suggested that this reduced ability can be thought of as a retrieval problem, namely, in the retrieval of organizational cues from semantic memory that are used to encode information during acquisition.

Aphasic adults fail to use organizational cues from word lists to facilitate recall (Tillman & Gerstman, 1977). Aging acquisition strategies may contribute to the aphasic impairment, but language-disordered patients still are much more impoverished in this mental ability than age-matched controls. Many of Tillman and Gerstman's aphasic subjects ($\overline{X}$ = 56.6, 32–82 years) were younger than the elderly groups in many studies of normal aging. Aphasia may eliminate encoding for memory acquisition at any age, while aging simply reduces its efficiency or frequency of use. Also, aphasic subjects failed to benefit from training in the use of organizational cues, while elderly normal adults sometimes did better with such training, but still not as well as younger adults.

Storage of episodic memories has been studied with respect to the susceptibility of memory traces to interference in LTM. As with STM, there is no evidence to support the idea that aging increases vulnerability to interference. Regarding semantic memory, Smith and Fullerton (1981) suggested that amount of information stored probably increases with advancing age. Vocabulary size probably increases, for example (Riegel, 1968). However, organization of semantic memory has not been studied directly with adults of different age groups.

Although the free word association paradigm may be an indicator of semantic organization, the nature of associates given by different subjects is also likely to reflect a preference for using certain aspects of semantic organization. Age differences have been observed with respect to tendencies in providing paradigmatic (in-class) and syntagmatic (other class) responses (Riegel, 1968). The age-related changes include an increase in variability of word associates given by older individuals. Young adults tend to give fairly standard paradigmatic responses, but with advancing age there is a shift to idiosyncratic and more syntagmatic responses. The elderly still use more paradigmatic than syntagmatic responses; the change occurs in the proportion of use of syntagmatic responses. The elderly tend to provide more verbs in response to concrete nouns and to provide more concrete nouns in response to adjectives. They also give more subjective responses, including personal statements and expressions of feelings, attitudes, and stereotypes. Such changes have been interpreted as a response to changing needs and environmental demands as a person proceeds through adulthood. Paradigmatic responses come more readily from young adults who are still influenced by formal education's organization of information according to within-class hierarchical category relationships. The elderly may be more oriented to adapting to real-life situations and, therefore, tend to prefer concrete functional relationships. Smith and

Fullerton (1981) suggested that slight changes in semantic organization may occur, partly due to increases in vocabulary size.

Acquisition and retention of semantic information from complex sentences was studied by Walsh and Baldwin (1977). One sentence was *The rock which rolled down the mountain crushed the tiny hut at the edge of the woods.* An elderly group ($\overline{X} = 67.3$ years) performed as well as young adults ($\overline{X} = 18.7$ years) in acquisition and retention of the semantic content in such sentences, in spite of the older group's inferior performance on the primacy portion of a free recall task. The investigators felt that tests of semantic memory are more valid than tests of episodic memory as measures of memory in one's everyday environment. Therefore, memory may function better for the elderly in real life than in the laboratory, with respect to word lists.

Retrieval from episodic memory involves recall of specific events from the past, and the elderly often appear to recall from the remote past more readily than from the recent past. As Craik (1977) explained, such anecdotal evidence is suspect, because remote events may have been rehearsed more; and so, retrieval comes from the most recent rehearsal. Craik reviewed a few studies in which subjects of various ages were asked to recall either names of high school teachers or news events. Older subjects recalled fewer episodes than younger subjects; and, in the study of news events, recall declined with increasing remoteness of the event dating from one month to two years prior to testing. Smith and Fullerton (1981) suggested that a decline in retrieval reflects the decline of encoding during acquisition of information. Craik (1977) concluded that aging does involve a decline of retrieval from episodic memory.

Retrieval from general knowledge (semantic memory) was studied by Lachman, Lachman, and Thronesbery (1979) who asked subjects to answer 190 questions about history, geography, the Bible, literature, sports, mythology, famous people, news events, and general information. There was no difference in accuracy of recall among young, middle-aged, and elderly adults. This type of investigation leads us into investigations of language function as it is commonly assessed with aphasic patients. Studies of picture naming have been considered to represent retrieval from semantic memory (Burke & Light, 1981; Smith & Fullerton, 1981). These investigations will be reviewed later in this chapter.

Conceptual Style

. As was suggested in regard to free word association, experimental behaviors based on the static organization of semantic memory may also be indicative of how one chooses to use semantic memory. Organization of concepts may be structured according to their paradigmatic and syntagmatic relationships to each other, and yet a subject's use of these relationships may be based on other considerations such as their pragmatic value. In addition, investigation of an aphasic's semantic memory is limited because of the language disorder; it is difficult for an experimenter to present words to represent concepts, when the aphasic subject may have trouble comprehending the words. This, in turn, prohibits the investigator's inferences about semantic memory in aphasia. Therefore, studies of semantic organization in aphasia have included pictures to represent concepts, instead of words. Pictures also have been used to study semantic organization styles in young and old normal adults.

Young adults (males, 21.8 years; females, 20.3 years) were compared with old adults (males, 71.3 years; females, 71.6 years) by Kogan (1974) who administered an object-sorting task. Fifty cards with black-and-white line drawings of common objects were used. Subjects were asked to group the pictures however they wished, and results were analyzed with reference to three possible conceptual styles. The elderly subjects formed fewer groups, which Kogan interpreted as indicative of low concept differentiation. The higher differentiations by adults were considered to be suggestive of literalness and weaker imagination. Young adults had a strong inclination toward using one style, namely, *categorical-inferential*, in which each group member is an example of a concept, such as grouping pots and knives as kitchen utensils. The relationship among the members of such groups is often referred to as a class relationship. Around 13% of the young adults' groupings were *relational-thematic*, in which group membership was defined according to functional relationship, such as a match goes with a pipe. Even fewer groupings were *analytic-descriptive*, in which members were defined according to an attribute, such as shape. Like the young adults, the elderly subjects had a strong preference for categorical-inferential groups, but there was a significant shift in the use of relational-thematic strategy to around 25% by the elderly subjects. Kogan's interpretation was similar to interpretation regarding shifts in free word association. The categorical-inferential style was similar to paradigmatic word association, and the relational-thematic style was similar to syntagmatic word pairs. Kogan suggested that the elderly had become more adventuresome in organizing concepts.

Cicirelli (1976) repeated the object-sorting task and compared children (5–7 years), young adults (19–21 years), and three groups of elderly adults (60–69, 70–79, 80–89 years). His results indicated that the shift to more thematic conceptualization is not a gradual one, but occurs during the period of old age. The 60-year-old subjects maintained the same level of thematic organization as the young adults. The increase in thematic classification (and reciprocal decrease in categorical classification) occurred between the 60s and 80s. Also, the elderly left more objects ungrouped; and this characteristic, as well as their style preference, were similar to the children's groupings. Cicirelli suggested that, perhaps, the elderly's strategy represents a decline during old age to an early stage of cognitive development rather than a preference because of needs and demands typical of old age.

Whichever is the case, normal aging does seem to result in a change of conceptual organization style. This consideration might be applied to interpreting aphasic performance in tasks involving the classification and pairing of objects. There has been interest in whether the word retrieval deficit of, at least, certain types of aphasia is related to disorganization of semantic memory (Goodglass & Baker, 1976). Grober, Perceman, Kellar, and Brown (1980) compared anterior and posterior aphasias by asking subjects to decide whether a pictured object belongs to a particular category presented by the experimenter. Aphasic subjects took longer to decide than two normal controls; however, age-related shifts in conceptual style were not considered in design and interpretation. Age of the subjects was not reported. Categorical-inferential and relational-thematic classifications were addressed by Semenza, Denes, Lucchese, and Bisiacchi (1980) with Broca's and Wernicke's aphasics and age-matched controls. Again, ages of the subjects were not reported. A picture-matching task was employed in which one of two choices was matched with a target picture. The relationship of objects within the picture triads was based on either class membership (categorical-inferential) or theme membership (relational-thematic). Broca's aphasics had more difficulty with thematic relationships; Wernicke's aphasics had difficulty with both, but much more so with class relationships. Therefore, a pronounced double dissociation occurred with respect to conceptual style. One is left to wonder whether the normal elderly's tendency to use thematic style has anything to do with these results. The problem may be worth considering, especially because Broca's aphasics tend to be at least a decade younger than Wernicke's aphasics (Harasymiw, Halper, & Sutherland, 1981; Holland, 1980; Kertesz & Sheppard, 1981; Obler, Albert, Goodglass, & Benson 1978).

Studies Of Language Function

Investigations of memory and aging present different prospects as to whether language functions change through adulthood. The effect of aging on language may vary, depending on which language function is being considered, and on the complexity of that function. Certainly with adequate compensation for hearing loss, the elderly should have enough STM capacity to process language, although slowed scanning speed may affect comprehension at some level and in certain situations. Increased vocabulary size and subtle reshaping of semantic organization may enhance flexibility of language use as we become older. Retrieval from semantic memory, as observed in verbal responses, may change primarily with respect to the kind of information a person is retrieving. Changes in language behavior may be due to declining perceptual-motor processes, instead of declining comprehension and retrieval processes. Finally, changes may be due to changing real-life demands as an individual retires, adjusts goals, and moves to a different living environment.

Aphasia Test Norms

A few comprehensive aphasia tests are accompanied by information regarding the performance of age-matched normal adults in order to permit comparison with aphasic performance. For example, Schuell's diagnostic battery was administered to 50 normal adults, and their scores are contained in the test manual (Schuell, 1973). Age was depicted in terms of percentages, with 50% age 60 or older, and 38% below and 62% above age 50 (Schuell, Jenkins & Jimenez-Pabon, 1964). Many tests were performed without error, but tendencies to make mistakes occurred primarily on subtests which are related to formal education, including paragraph reading, oral and written spelling, and writing sentences. Aphasia test norms tell us only about the basic language abilities of a general population of adults representing a wide age range. In order to make them comparable in age to the aphasic population, ages of the normal subjects are skewed in the direction of older adulthood with an average age around the late 50s. As they are generally presented, these data tell us little about whether the language skills on these tests change with increasing age.

On the *Porch Index of Communicative Ability* (Porch, 1967), normal adults with an average age of 56.8 achieve an overall score of 14.46 and a small standard deviation of .33 (Duffy, Keith, Shane, & Podraza, 1976). This score represents performance on a scale from 1 to 16 (15 is the best typical performance) averaged from 18 subtests which cover auditory comprehension, reading, speaking, and writing. Relative to the traditional subtest categories, average performance on gestural subtests is 14.66 (SD = .31); verbal subtests, 14.55 (SD = .33); and graphic subtests, 14.12 (SD = .71). The lowest subtest score is for writing sentences, a 12.57 (SD = 1.78); the only other scores below 14.00 are on verbal description of object function (13.72, SD = 1.01) and demonstrating object function (13.68, SD = 1.31). Therefore, adults generally appear to hold at a high level of performance with the language skills measured by the PICA. The lowest score could be based on varying education levels, as was indicated with Schuell's norms. Because the scoring system is rather rigid, verbal description variation is likely to result from variations of style.

Nevertheless, Duffy et al. (1976) found significant negative correlations between age and PICA scores. The correlations were small, however, with a − .34 for the overall score being typical. The interaction between age and education probably was strong, because education also was correlated significantly with the overall score and was relatively strong for the writing category (r = .53).

Normal adult performance on the *Boston Diagnostic Aphasia Examination* (BDAE) was reported by Borod, Goodglass, and Kaplan (1980a). Age and education contributed to scores on several subtests, and age alone was related only to repeating low probability sentences, word fluency measured by animal naming, narrative writing, and most of the primarily visuospatial parietal lobe tests. The result with parietal tests is consistent with the "don't hold" status of nonverbal intelligence tests. In an unpublished report, these norms were presented according to five age groups: 25–39 years, 40–49 years, 50–59 years, 60–69 years, and 70–85 years (Borod, Goodglass, & Kaplan, 1980b).

If a few basic language functions change as a person ages, then we might want our clinical assessment manuals to include normal adult performance differentiated according to age. Perhaps, scores for young, middle, and late adulthood would be sufficient. Whether this is warranted depends on the susceptibility of language functions to change with aging.

Comprehension

Except for the barriers created by auditory and visual sensory declines, comprehension of words and basic sentences appears to be unaffected by the aging process. Comprehension of sentences by adults is indicated in the norms for the *Auditory Comprehension Test for Sentences* (Shewan, 1979). Over a broad age range of 21 to 76 years (median = 61) adults scored 20.07 of 21 points with little variability (SD = 1.17). In Borod and associates' (1980b) BDAE norms, there was no significant change from the 30s through the 70s in the auditory comprehension subtests. A slight drop can be seen in the 70s for "complex ideational material," which in cludes yes/no questions about short paragraphs, but this change was not statistically significant. Age and education had a significant impact on the subtest for reading sentences and paragraphs; the age effect occurred again as a drop in the 70s, as opposed to a gradual decline over the life span. This is the same pattern across the decades shown with superior synonym definitions.

Studies of Memory

It is tempting to infer an aging effect on comprehension from certain studies of semantic memory. Equal accuracy among young, middle-aged, and elderly adults in answering questions indicates that there is no change in understanding them (Lachman et al., 1979). Camp (1981) studied ability to answer visually presented "direct-access" questions such as *What man's wife was turned into a pillar of salt?* (answer: Lot) and "inferential" questions such as *What U.S. President was the first to see an airplane fly?* (answer: T. Roosevelt). Access to semantic memory was tested in two recognition paradigms. Subjects included members of MENSA and emeritus professors. Elderly and young adult groups did not differ in accuracy of response for both types of questions, but the elderly group was slower in responding when yes/no answers were required. Camp interpreted slower responses as slower processing of the problem in addition to slower perceptual-motor speed. In such a task, comprehension is not observed as purely as the psycholinguist would like; the subject's task involves dealing with one's fund of knowledge, known to be highly variable among individuals.

Ability to encode inferences from sentences was examined in a study of sentence list recall (Till & Walsh, 1980). Young ($\overline{X} = 20.4$ years) and old ($\overline{X} = 68.4$ years) subjects were compared in free and cued recall of 16 sentences, such as (1) *The pupil carefully positioned the thumbtack on the chair* and (2) *The chauffeur drove on the left side*. In the condition of cued recall, the subject was given a cue to the sentence to be produced. Cues were based on information that could be inferred from the sentence, such as *prank* from (1) and *England* from (2). Young adults recalled more sentences in the cued condition than in the free recall condition, indicating that they encoded inferences from the sentences. However, the old adults recalled fewer sentences in the cued condition than in the free recall condition, indicating some difficulty in detecting inferences from sentences.

It is not clear whether Till and Walsh's finding can be generalized to drawing inferences during sentence comprehension. In a subsequent experiment, these investigators had their subjects engage in a "comprehension" task during sentence list acquisition (Till & Walsh, 1980). Subjects were asked to produce written responses that might reflect sentence meanings. Then, in cued recall of these sentences, the previous age difference was eliminated as the old adults equalled recall by the young adults. Comprehension abilities during list presentations were not compared; however, we might infer that aging does not affect comprehension of inferences as much as it affects the use of encoding in the learning and recall process.

Sentence Comprehension

We begin to get a look at comprehension directly in an investigation of recoding with a verbal-pictorial verification task. Nebes (1976) was concerned about the elderly's tendency not to use imagery or elaborative encoding strategies in acquisition of information for episodic memory. Would the elderly exhibit a similar decline in simply recoding a verbal stimulus into a pictorial code during a verification task? Models of the mental processes underlying sentence verification have included two stages: (1) encoding the stimuli into mental representations, and (2) comparing the mental codes of the two stimuli. Response times have been assumed to include time to carry out each of these stages. In Nebes's study, elderly adults ($\overline{X}=69$ years) took longer than young adults ($\overline{X}=19$ years) in determining a match between a phrase *(square outside circle)* and a picture, and in matching two pictures. The verbal-picture condition took longer than the picture-picture condition, and this additional time was assumed to consist of the formulation of a mental pictorial image from the phrase. This time difference between conditions was the same for the young and old adults, indicating that aging does not affect encoding in this task. Nebes's analysis indicated that the mental process of comparing the two pictorial cues was the locus of slower processing by the elderly.

Sentence verification has been of some interest in the study of comprehension in aphasia (Brookshire & Nicholas, 1980; Just, Davis, & Carpenter, 1977), and effect of aging on this function might be worth exploring further. We might anticipate that aging will affect latency but not accuracy, while aphasia affects latency and accuracy.

Walsh and Baldwin's (1977) previously cited study involved recalling meaning derived from some fairly complex sentences such as *The warm breeze blowing from the sea stirred the heavy evening air*. In a measure of comprehension accuracy, no differences were found between old adults ($\overline{X}=68$ years) and young adults ($\overline{X}=19$ years). A similarly complex comprehension level was tested by Feier and Gerstman (1980). Adult subjects heard sentences with center-embedded and right branching relative clauses about animals doing a variety of unusual things. Each type of clause was either subject relative or object relative:

1. *The giraffe that bumped into the cow kicked the hippo.*
2. *The lion that the elephant pushed jumped over the horse.*

3. The giraffe kicked the hippo that bumped into the cow.

4. The lion jumped over the horse that the elephant pushed.

Young adults (18–25 years) and older adults (52–58) years, 63–69 years, 74–80 years) indicated comprehension by manipulating small animal or human figures. Comprehension accuracy held between the young adult period and the 50s; it dropped in the 60s, and dropped further in the 70s. There was no interaction between sentence type and age. Feier and Gerstman's study was the first indication of an effect of aging on comprehension accuracy. Lack of pragmatic reality in these sentences may combine with their complexity to produce this aging effect.

One might predict that a similar effect would occur with the Token Test (DeRenzi & Vignolo, 1962), especially with the complex instructions of Part V. This test of auditory comprehension also possesses little pragmatic reality in instructions to manipulate tokens of different color, size, and shape. When this test was given to nonbrain-injured adults, age was found not to be a factor in test performance (DeRenzi, 1979; Orgass & Poeck, 1966; Swisher & Sarno, 1969). Instead, DeRenzi (1979) found that years of schooling had a greater effect. Noll and Randolph (1978) gave the test to 25 normal adults ($\overline{X} = 54$, 29–76 years), and these subjects averaged only 2.2 errors on Part V. They averaged 59.7 of 62 points on the whole test with a standard deviation of 2.2 (range 52–62). There is little evidence of age-related decline in Token Test performance. We could be suspicious of the decline in color discrimination cited earlier as possibly influencing Token Tests scores after age 60.

An age effect on reading comprehension occurred with lengthy sentences describing an event and containing one date and one country name. Such sentences were used in a study of recall, but a test of comprehension was included (Gordon, 1975). Four multiple choice questions were asked about each of five sentences, such as *In the year 1958 a crisis in Denmark occurred when rural lobbyists tried to persuade the parliament to increase duties on man-made textiles.* Elderly adults ($\overline{X} = 71$ years) were less accurate than young adults ($\overline{X} = 21$ years).

Cohen (1979) asked subjects to detect semantic anomalies in sentences such as *Mary had lost weight—her dress was too small.* Subjects were grouped according to age and education level: old and highly educated ($\overline{X} = 68$, 65–79 years), old with low education ($\overline{X} = 79$, 70–95 years), young and highly educated ($\overline{X} = 24$, 20–29 years), and young with low education ($\overline{X} = 24$, 18–29 years). Both elderly groups made significantly more errors than their respective young adult groups, with the difference being greater between the less-educated age groups. Cohen added that the most striking aspect of the less-educated elderly's performance was "the large number of value judgements which were based on irrelevant moral grounds rather than on semantic or logical considerations . . . it seems as if personal values are more salient than semantic coherence for this group" (p. 423). Whether the moral grounds were irrelevant may be a judgment by the experimenter. Nevertheless, there are some similarities here with the findings with free word association, namely, the tendency to give idiosyncratic and evaluative responses.

Paragraph Comprehension

A few investigators have found aging effects at the discourse level of comprehension. As in some aphasia tests, this level is tested by having subjects listen to, or read, a short paragraph, and then answer questions about the content in the paragraph. A few specific issues were addressed in the studies: (1) Does aging have a differential effect on comprehension of explicit and implicit meaning in a text (Belmore, 1981; Cohen, 1979)? The previously cited difficulty in detecting inferences for cued recall indicates that aging may impinge upon comprehension of implicit information more than explicit information. (2) Aging may affect task performance, especially when a paragraph is read to subjects, because of a decline in recall of the paragraph, rather than because of a decline in comprehension (Belmore, 1981; Taub, 1979). (3) As indicated by Cohen's study on detecting semantic anomalies in sentences, aging may be a factor, depending on the education level or basic lifelong language ability of the subject (Taub, 1979). (4) Does aging affect the ability to comprehend jokes (Schaier & Cicirelli, 1976)?

In studies of inferencing, subjects are asked two types of questions about a paragraph. One type asks about facts or information explicitly stated in the paragraph. The other type asks about inferences or information implied by a paragraph. Explicit and implicit questions are used in the *Reading Comprehension Battery for Aphasia* (LaPointe & Horner, 1979). Cohen's (1979) normal subjects were divided according to education level, described in the previous section. He found an age-related reduction in accuracy for implicit questions but not for explicit questions in high- and low-educated groups.

While Cohen's study involved listening to paragraphs, Belmore (1981) examined inferencing with a reading task in which subjects verified true and false statements about a paragraph. Here is one example (p. 318):

STIMULUS PARAGRAPH: Everyone sat down for dinner.
There was a crystal vase on the long

table. The guests all admired the lovely
roses.

TRUE PARAPHRASE: There was a vase on the table.

TRUE INFERENCE: There were roses in the vase.

Belmore measured accuracy and response latency for an old ($\overline{X} = 67$ years)
and young ($\overline{X} = 18$ years) group. With respect to accuracy, the dependent
variable in Cohen's study, there was no age effect when statements were
verified immediately after reading the paragraph. However, when only
the statements were presented again, requiring a much greater demand
on paragraph retention, the old group was less accurate than the young
group. Unexpectedly, the age-related reduction occurred more for explicit
information (the paraphrase) than for implicit information (inference).
The older subjects took significantly longer than the younger subjects to
verify both types of statements. Belmore concluded that the general decline
in speed was not specific to explicit or implicit meaning. In the condition
of immediate comprehension testing, whether there is an age effect on
inferencing is equivocal. This effect may depend on how paragraph comprehension is tested. "clearly, such an impairment is not an inevitable result
of the aging process" (Belmore, 1981 p. 321).

Belmore's study points to the conclusion that age effects in paragraph
comprehension are related more to recall demands than to comprehension per se. An investigator may look for changes in comprehension as
evidence that the age effect in a recall task occurs at the acquisition (encoding) stage. Taub (1979) studied paragraph comprehension in three conditions: (1) questions were presented with the paragraph, and unlimited
time was given to read and answer; (2) unlimited time for paragraph
reading was provided, but questions were presented after the paragraph
was removed, and (3) after the first condition, the same questions were
presented, placing an even greater demand on paragraph retention.
Without demands on retention, called the "comprehension" condition,
there was greater accuracy than with (2) and (3). Old subjects ($\overline{X} = 70$ years)
were less accurate than young subjects ($\overline{X} = 27$ years) in comprehension
and in the recall conditions (2) and (3). Also, the elderly were less reliable
in their answers. That is, they tended to change their answers in condition (3), which involved the same questions as condition (1). Taub concluded that the age effect in discourse comprehension requiring recall can
be attributed to inadequate acquisition of the paragraph when presented.

Furthermore, Taub (1979) found that the age-related reduction in
paragraph comprehension occurred with subjects classified as low and mid-

dle in giving definitions on the WAIS vocabulary test. The subjects classified as high in vocabulary did not show an age effect. This is similar to Cohen's finding that recognition of anomalous sentences produced an age effect for the less educated subjects. Therefore, aging may influence language comprehension only in individuals with lower verbal abilities throughout adulthood. However, this is not necessarily so, because Belmore's (1981) subjects were relatively well educated.

A person may have to do some inferencing in order to get the point of a joke. Schaier and Cicirelli (1976) compared three older groups in their 50s, 60s, and 70s as to their ability to comprehend paragraph-length jokes. Twelve jokes were based on Piagetian concepts of conservation of mass, weight, or volume; and these were compared with 12 "noncognitive"jokes. Here are two of the conservation jokes:

> MASS: Mr. Jones went in to a pizza parlor and ordered a whole pizza for his dinner. When the waiter asked if he wanted it cut into 6 or 8 pieces, Mr. Jones said: "Oh, you'd better make it 6! I could never eat 8 pieces."

> WEIGHT: George and Bob had a raft they made out of old logs. One day they took the raft out into the middle of the lake for a picnic lunch. As soon as they finished their lunch the raft began to sink. George said, "Oh, no! We've eaten too much" (p. 579).

Schaier and Cicirelli measured appreciation of the jokes with a rating scale for funniness. Comprehension was determined by asking subjects to explain what was funny about each joke.

What was funny about the results was that with less comprehension of humor, there was more appreciation. In comparing the two types of jokes, conservation jokes were comprehended better, but appreciated less. The following age effects were found: (1) the group aged 50–59 appreciated the jokes less than the older groups, (2) there was an age-related decline in comprehension, and (3) gender interacted with the comprehension results, as the reduction in females occurred between the 60s and 70s, while the reduction in males occurred sooner, between the 50s and 60s. Schaier and Cicirelli concluded that decline in humor comprehension accompanies a decline in cognitive ability, while appreciation increases until the cognitive demands of the joke are too great and the joke is not understood at all.

Summary

Compared with the voluminous research on adult psycholinguistics with college students as subjects, very little has been done to study aging and comprehension of language. It appears that comprehension accuracy for sentences holds throughout the life span, except for semantically unusual and syntactically complex sentences. With these special sentences, decline may begin in the 60s. Depth of comprehension, especially for discourse, may be reduced with old age in the derivation of inferences from statements and paragraphs. In tasks of discourse comprehension, when new information must be acquired for answering questions, retention may be more of a factor than comprehension per se. However, there is some evidence that comprehension at this level declines, a conclusion sometimes phrased in terms of encoding at the acquisition stage of a recall task.

The term "decline" should be used carefully, especially to depict results from the usual comparison of only a young and an old group. This comparison does not tell us whether the change is gradual from early adulthood, begins at middle age, or begins even later in adulthood. Many of the studies already done need to be replicated with groups between youth and old age, and with elderly groups divided into decades, as in the study of joke comprehension. Changes did not occur until the 60s or 70s for object sorting, giving definitions, and sentence comprehension. Also, education and/or intelligence may interact with aging of the language function, another variable leading to qualification of any age effect.

Word Retrieval

The response form in previously mentioned studies of semantic memory has been word retrieval. The paradigms included free word association and question answering. Aging is accompanied by a shift to more syntagmatic and idiosyncratic word associations than in young adulthood. Retrieving answers about stored knowledge does not appear to change, but accuracy when inferencing is involved appears to drop beginning in the 60s. There is some slowing of response time. Aging of word retrieval per se has been investigated with respect to picture naming and word fluency, usually in order to examine retrieval from semantic memory.

Convergent Retrieval

Word retrieval is often assessed by having subjects converge on one lexical item. The most common clinical paradigm is object naming, called *confrontation naming*. There was no effect of age on the BDAE subtests of responsive naming (answering questions) and body part naming (Borod et al., 1980a, 1980b). Age-related norms were determined for the *Boston Naming Test* (Kaplan, Goodglass, & Weintraub (1976) consisting of 85 line drawings for words of varied frequency of use. In terms of number correct, the following average scores were obtained: 72.8 (under 40 years),

76.5 (40–49), 75.6 (50–59), 70.8 (60–69), and 63.2 (over 70). Again we see a decline beginning in the 60s. However, the authors warned that education could have been a factor, because the oldest groups had fewer years of schooling. Education was a significant factor: 57.0 (0 -8 years), 71.3 (9-12 years), and 75.9 (13-16 years). Furthermore, only six subjects were in the group over age 70, while 30 subjects were in the 60–69 age group. Nevertheless, Borod, et al. (1980a) suggested that the cut-off score for diagnosing aphasia be lowered for adults age 60 and older.

Thomas, Fozard, and Waugh (1977) analyzed the few errors made by their subjects on a picture-naming task. Five age groups were studied: 25–35, 36–45, 46–55, 56–65, and over 65. In the four groups from age 25 to 65, 76% of the errors were semantic confusions, errors in the same semantic category as the correct word. Only 12% of the errors were perceptual, a name of an object that was perceptually similar to the pictured object. In the oldest group, over age 65, there was an increase in perceptual errors to 35%. Therefore, in this age group, confrontation naming may be influenced by the visual decline common in the elderly.

Distinguishing between perceptual-motor processing and the central process of interest has been an important consideration in aging research. Anatomical and physiological aging definitely produce changes in perceptual-motor processing, and the status of a central psycholinguistic process must be extracted from tasks that include perceptual-motor functions. Thomas et al. (1977) attempted this distinction in measuring picture-naming latency. They had found that naming latency increases with age. Picture-naming latency was assumed to consist of perceptual-motor time (picture recognition + word formulation) and lexical search and retrieval time. Presenting the word with the picture to be named was assumed to generate perceptual-motor time only. This assumption was reinforced by the finding that word frequency did not affect naming latency in this condition, but did affect latency in naming the picture only. The age effect on confrontation naming latency was greater for picture naming than for picture + word naming. Thomas et al. concluded that while an age-related decline of perceptual-motor speed is a component of decreased speed in picture naming, aging also affects speed of lexical search and retrieval. In addition, practice in naming the same pictures reduced the diferences among age groups.

Eysenck (1975) analyzed word retrieval time by comparing naming of a category and letter, such as "fruit-A," with recognition of correct category-instance pairs, such as "fruit-apple." The recognition condition was assumed to represent a "decision" component of the retrieval process, namely, deciding whether the lexical search process was successful. Older subjects (55–65 years) took longer than the younger subjects (18–30 years) in the recognition task but not in the retrieval task. Eysenck concluded that the decision process is affected by aging, but not the search process. However, if we are to assume that decision is included in the process of naming to category + letters, then decrease in decision time should be reflected in this condition, also. Therefore, either the recognition condition did not truly assess a decision process, or a decision process is not a component of word retrieval in the category + letter-naming task.

Familiarity of objects contributes to the speed in naming them. Poon and Fozard (1978) looked into whether familiarity interacts with age to produce variation in object naming latency. They compared young (18–22 years), middle-aged (45–54 years), and older (60–70 years) adults in their naming of contemporary and dated objects. Pictures of dated objects were selected from 1910 commercial catalogues. Dated unique objects (churn, wringer) were compared with contemporary unique objects (calculator, hair dryer). Objects common to each period, in old and new versions, also were presented (razor, shoes). Young adults named contemporary unique objects faster than did the older adults, while the older adults named dated unique objects faster. Age did not affect the speed of naming common contemporary objects. Therefore, object familiarity is another variable that determines whether there will be an age effect in ease of lexical retrieval.

Divergent Retrieval

Divergent behavior involves a quantity and variety of responses instead of a convergence on one response (Chapey, Rigrodsky, & Morrison, 1977). Word fluency is a common measure of divergent word retrieval. In tests of word fluency, the subject is asked to produce as many words as possible which begin with a particular letter or belong to a particular concept category. Usually there is a brief time limit. Kamin (1957) found that elderly persons had lower word fluency scores than high schoolers when given an initial letter. Institutionalized elderly had lower scores than the elderly living in the community. Borod et al. (1980a, 1980b) found a gradual decline across the life span in animal naming, a word fluency activity which is affected by even nonspecific sites of brain damage. Adults under age 40 average 26.6 animal names in 60 seconds, while adults in their 50s produce 21.4, and adults in their 70s produce 18.6. An aging component, therefore, is likely to exist in an aphasic patient's performance on this task. This component probably is small, because aphasic persons produce an average of only 6.3 names with a standard deviation of 6.0 (Goodglass & Kaplan, 1972).

Stones (1978) used word fluency with categories and letters to study aging and semantic memory. In a unique effort to control for cohort effects, each older subject ($\overline{X} = 49$ years) was the parent of at least one subject in the younger group ($\overline{X} = 17$ years). The middle-aged group was significantly more diversified in its responses than the younger group. It is not clear from the article as to exactly what this meant with respect to the nature of word fluency responses. Nevertheless, Stones suggested that there are two sources of explanation. One is that the processes of semantic memory change. The second is that environmental influences change from the formal education period to the individual differences of experience by middle age.

Battig and Montague (1969) presented norms for the production of words from 56 categories. These norms were obtained from university undergraduate students. Howard (1980) investigated whether these norms would be applicable to middle-aged and old adults. The *dominance* of a response was of particular interest, namely, the order of frequency with which different words are produced in each category. Howard presented 21 of the 56 categories to young (20–39 years), middle-aged (40–59 years), and elderly (60–79 years) adults. The groups were comparable in education level. Many of Battig and Montague's categories were omitted partly in order to eliminate any obvious cohort effects that might occur with categories such as "A type of dance." Subjects were given 30 seconds to write their words for each category. Howard found a significant decrease in the average number of responses per category with increasing age: young, 7.05; middle-age, 7.12; and old, 6.06. This decrease was indicative of slower performance with age. However, the dominance of category members was similar among the age groups. Also, unlike free word association, variability of word fluency between subjects did not increase with age. Howard concluded that the Battig and Montague norms would be valid for research with any adult age group.

Summary

There may be some decline of accuracy in confrontation naming after age 60, especially when tested with a wide range of word frequency. Word retrieval speed certainly decreases, perhaps due to a combination of effects on peripheral and central (cognitive) processes. The decrease in speed explains the reduction in number of responses on word fluency tasks which are administered with a time limit of 60 seconds. Variables that influence performance by the elderly on tasks of word retrieval include: (1) the perceptual-motor changes of aging, (2) educational differences, and (3) familiarity with objects that are uniquely contemporary.

Sentence Production

Age did not affect the speed or grammaticality of sentence production when subjects were asked to incorporate word pairs in creating their sentences (Nebes and Andrews-Kulis, 1976). However, elderly subjects performed less well than young adults when discourse was investigated in a story-retelling task (Cohen, 1979). Again, responses depended in part on retention of experimental stimuli. The elderly provided fewer correct propositions, fewer modifiers, and fewer summary propositions representing the gist of the story. These differences were seen in Cohen's high- and low-educated groups. Also, the elderly, especially in the low-educated group, made many more "errors of anaphoric reference" such as the use of pronouns for which the referent was unclear. Buckingham (1979), by the way, had found that "indefinite anaphora" is a common occurrence in the fluent language of anomic aphasia. We should consider, nevertheless, that the reduction of encoding for episodic memory may contribute to the changes of verbal expression observed by Cohen.

With a picture-description task in a study of aphasia, Yorkston and Beukelman (1980) presented some pertinent data concerning amount of information conveyed in connected discourse and efficiency of communication. Younger normal adults ($\overline{X}$ = 31 years) were compared with older normal adults ($\overline{X}$ = 73 years) as control groups. These groups did not differ in amount of information expressed nor in number of syllables per minute. However, regarding message efficiency, the older group produced significantly fewer content units (basic ideas) per minute than the younger group.

Functional Communication

So far, aging has been considered with respect to linguistic function measured in experimental paradigms which minimize natural communicative context. With Holland's (1980) norms for *Communicative Abilities in Daily Living* (CADL), we can begin to consider whether aging affects ability to understand and convey messages by any means, including language. The CADL consists of a series of communication problems based on real-life situations in which extralinguistic context can be used to comprehend, and any communicative mode can be used to get a message across. The norms include 130 normal adults classified according to age and according to living environment (institutionalized versus noninstitutionalized). Holland found that both factors contribute to performance on the CADL. The group over 65 scored significantly below three younger age groups (below 46, 46–55, 56–65). Also, in the two oldest age groups, noninstitutionalized subjects tended to score higher than the institution-alized subjects. We might assume that institutionalized subjects are more affected by the aging process. In sum, however, it appears that aging has some influence on communicative abilities that are more general than language function per se.

Concluding Remarks

If aging has a significant impact on language function, there would be at least three conspicuous clinical implications: (1) If test scores are to be used to identify language deficit (as opposed to decline), norms and cutoff scores should be differentiated according to age. This has been done with the CADL (Holland, 1980) and has been suggested for the BDAE (Borod et al., 1980a). (2) Once aphasia has been identified in a patient, the clinician may need to identify the degrees to which aging and aphasia contribute to performances with different language functions. This review indicates that paragraph comprehension, naming, and word fluency might be targets of concern, especially for patients over 60 years old. (3) The degree to which aging is a factor may influence prognosis and decisions about emphasis in treatment.

Though there are some definite signals from the research that aging in-fluences language functions, we should be careful about searching for aging language in our patients until more data are obtained. We are on firmer ground when we consider perceptual and motor factors in language per-formances. A life-span psycholinguistics has not blossomed into a data-rich field of study. Our theories of adult language processing have been built almost exclusively from data produced by college-age subjects. In the study of aging, more effort has gone into investigations of learning and memory, instead of the immediate comprehension and production that occurs in a conversation. However, sometimes purely linguistic behaviors have been the means by which investigators have examined issues in learning and memory, and so the relevant psycholinguistic questions have to be applied to this research on a post hoc basis. Currently key-words for finding research on word retrieval, for example, include "seman-tic memory" or "recall."

A life-span psycholinguistics would focus increased attention on the possibility of hearing loss and presbyopia in elderly subjects. Just as at-tempts are made to equate age groups on education, these groups might also be equated on auditory and visual perception. Several issues can be addressed in this research. One is whether changes occur as a gradual decline over the life span or as a decline beginning in old age. A gradual decline would impact on aphasic patients of both middle and old age, while a later decline would impact primarily on elderly patients. We need to learn more about when the slowing of processing speed begins to be accompanied by reductions in accuracy. One specific question pertains to the slowing of STM scanning rate. This decline may only affect comprehension of complex sentences, such as those investigated by Feier and Gerstman. As has been found with studies of problem solving, the elderly may retain all necessary cognitive abilities to perform as younger subjects if input is slowed down and more time is available for response.

If aging does contribute meaningfully to certain clinical behaviors such as tasks involving paragraph retention and word fluency, it may be of greatest concern for mild aphasias occurring in the age span from 60 to 70. The percentage of impact is likely to be greatest in mild aphasia, and some changes appear to occur only in old age. Given the areas of research reported in this chapter, investigators of aphasia might at least begin to report age of their aphasic subjects more often. We also might heighten our desire to include age-matched normal controls in aphasia research. However, increasing variability of performance, reflecting wide individual variation in rate of normal aging, indicates that chronological age-matching may not mean a great deal. It may be more accurate, but less realistic, to match brain-injured subjects with normal subjects possessing an equivalent physiological age of the central nervous system. After all, a stroke may arise from a CNS that is "older" than the CNS of a healthy age-matched control. We should, at least, be careful about interpreting differences between aphasic subjects and a small number of age-matched normal subjects.

Age has been of greatest concern in clinical aphasiology as one indicator of prognosis. Based on CNS and cognitive changes, our intuition that increasing age has a detrimental effect on recovery seems relatively secure. Aging probably does provide a magnet which draws recovery backward to some extent. It is disconcerting that most attempts to examine the relationship between chronological age and recovery have failed to produce a significant correlation (Davis & Holland, 1981). However, it is aging and not age that makes a difference.

Note

[1]The term *encoding*, as used in cognitive psychology, can be confusing to speech-language pathologists who were weaned on a different conception of the term. In communication models, encoding has referred to production as opposed to the "decoding" of input. However, in the study

of memory and cognition, encoding refers to the mental representation of stimuli, that is, the process of developing an internal code which is a kind of "mental response" to stimuli. The term decoding is not used; and, in fact, psychologists' use of encoding is similar to the communicologist's use of decoding.

References

Adams, R. D. The morphological aspects of aging in the human nervous system. In J. E. Birren and R. B. Sloane (Eds.), *Handbook of mental health and aging*. Englewood Cliffs, NJ: Prentice-Hall, 1980.

Anders, T. R., Fozard, J. L., & Lillyquist, T. D. Effects of age upon retrieval from short-term memory. *Developmental Psychology*, 1972, *6*, 214-217.

Battig, W. F., & Montague, W. E. Category names for verbal items in 56 categories. *Journal of Experimental Psychology Monographs*, *80*, 1969.

Beasley, D. S., & Davis, G. A. (Eds.). *Aging: Communication processes and disorders*. New York: Grune & Stratton, 1981.

Belmore, S. M. Age-related changes in processing explicit and implicit language. *Journal of Gerontology*, 1981, *36*, 316-322.

Bergman, M. (Ed.). *Aging and the perception of speech*. Baltimore, MD: University Park Press, 1980.

Birren, J. E. *The psychology of aging*. Englewood Cliffs, NJ: Prentice-Hall, 1964.

Borod, J. C., Goodglass, H., & Kaplan, E. Normative data on the Boston Diagnostic Aphasia Examination, Parietal Lobe Battery, and the Boston Naming Test. *Journal of Clinical Neuropsychology*, 1980, *2*, 209-215. (a)

Borod, J. C., Goodglass, H., & Kaplan, E. Normative data on neuropsychological tests. Boston V. A. Medical Center: Unpublished manuscript 1980. (b)

Botwinick, J., & Storandt, M. Vocabulary ability in later life. *Journal of Genetic Psychology*, 1974, *125*, 303-308.

Botwinick, J., West, R., & Storandt, M. Qualitative vocabulary test responses and age. *Journal of Gerontology*, 1975, *30*, 574-577.

Brookshire, R. H., & Nicholas, L. E. Verification of active and passive sentences by aphasic and nonaphasic subjects. *Journal of Speech and Hearing Research*, 1980, *23*, 878-893.

Buckingham, H. W. Linguistic aspects of lexical retrieval disturbances in the posterior fluent aphasias. In H. Whitaker & H. A. Whitaker (Eds.), *Studies in neurolinguistics* (Vol. 4). New York: Academic Press, 1979.

Burke, D. M., & Light, L. L. Memory and aging: The role of retrieval processes. *Psychological Bulletin*, 1981, *90*, 513-546.

Camp, C. J. The use of fact retrieval vs. inference in young and elderly adults. *Journal of Gerontology*, 1981, *36*, 715-721.

Chapey, R., Rigrodsky, S., & Morrison, E. B. Aphasia: A divergent semantic interpretation. *Journal of Speech and Hearing Disorders*, 1977, *42*, 287-295.

Cicirelli, V. G. Categorization behavior in aging subjects. *Journal of Gerontology*, 1976, *31*, 676-680.

Clark, L., & Knowles J., Age differences in dichotic listening performance. *Journal of Gerontology*, 1973, *28*, 173-178.

Cohen, G. Language comprehension in old age. *Cognitive Psychology*, 1979, *11*, 412-429.

Craik, F. I. M. Age differences in human memory. In J. E. Birren & K. W. Schaie (Eds.), *Handbook of the psychology of aging*. New York: Van Nostrand Reinhold, 1977.

Crook, T. H. Psychometric assessment in the elderly. In A. Raskin & L. F. Jarvik (Eds.), *Psychiatric symptoms and cognitive loss in the elderly*. Washington: Hemisphere, 1979.

Davis, G. A., & Holland, A. L. Age in understanding and treating aphasia. In D. S. Beasley & G. A. Davis (Eds.), *Aging: Communication processes and disorders*. New York: Grune & Stratton, 1981.

DeRenzi, E. A shortened version of the Token Test. In F. Boller & M. Dennis (Eds.), *Auditory comprehension : Clinical and experimental studies with the Token Test*. New York: Academic Press, 1979.

DeRenzi, E. & Vignolo, L. A. The Token Test: A sensitive test to detect receptive disturbances in aphasics. *Brain*, 1962, *85*, 665–678.

Duffy, J. R., Keith, R. L., Shane, H., & Podraza, B. L. Performance of normal (non-brain-injured) adults on the Porch Index of Communicative Ability. In R. H. Brookshire (Ed.), *Clinical Aphasiology Conference Proceedings*. Minneapolis: BRK, 1976.

Eysenck, M. W. Retrieval from semantic memory as a function of age. *Journal of Gerontology*, 1975, *30*, 174–180.

Feier, C. & Gerstman, L. Sentence comprehension abilities throughout the adult life span. *Journal of Gerontology*, 1980, *35*, 722–728.

Goodglass, H., & Baker, E. Semantic field, naming, and auditory comprehension in aphasia. *Brain and Language*, 1976, *3*, 359–374.

Goodglass, H., & Kaplan, E. *The assessment of aphasia and related disorders*. Philadelphia: Lea & Febiger, 1972.

Gordon, S. K. Organization and recall of related sentences by elderly and young adults. *Experimental Aging Research*, 1975, *1*, 71–80.

Grober, E., Perecman, E., Kellar, L., & Brown, J. Lexical knowledge in anterior and posterior aphasics. *Brain and Language*, 1980, *10*, 318–330.

Harasymiw, S. J., Halper, A., & Sutherland, B. Sex, age, and aphasia type *Brain and Language*, 1981, *12*, 190–198.

Henoch, M. A. (Ed.) *Aural rehabilitation for the elderly*. New York: Grune & Stratton, 1979.

Holland, A. L. *Communicative abilities in daily living*. Baltimore: University Park Press, 1980.

Howard, D. V. Category norms: A comparison of the Battig and Montague (1969) norms with the responses of adults between the ages of 20 and 80. *Journal of Gerontology*, 1980, *35*, 225–231.

Jacoby, R. J., Levy, R. & Dawson, J. M. Computed tomography in the elderly: I. The normal population. *American Journal of Psychiatry*, 1980, *136*, 249–255.

Johnson, R. C., Cole, R. E., Bowers, J. K., Foiles, S. V., Nikaido, A. M., Patrick, J. W., & Woliver, R. E. Hemispheric efficiency in middle and later adulthood. *Cortex*, 1979, *15*, 109–119.

Just, M. A., Davis, G. A., & Carpenter, P. A. A comparison of aphasic and normal adults in a sentence-verification task. *Cortex*, 1977, *13*, 402–423.

Kamin, L. J. Differential changes in mental abilities in old age. *Journal of Gerontology*, 1957, *12*, 66–70.

Kaplan, E., Goodglass, H., & Weintraub, S. *Boston Naming Test* (experimental edition). Boston: Veterans Administration Medical Center, 1976.

Kertesz, A., & McCabe, P. Intelligence and aphasia: Performance of aphasics on *Raven's Coloured Progressive Matrices* (RCPM). *Brain and Language*, 1975, *2*, 387–395.

Kertesz, A., & Sheppard, A. The epidemiology of aphasic and cognitive impairment in stroke: Age, sex, aphasia type and laterality differences. *Brain*, 1981, *104*, 117–128.

Kocel, K. M. Age-related changes in cognitive abilities and hemispheric specialization. In J. Herron (Ed.), *Neuropschology of left-handedness.* New York: Academic Press, 1980.

Kogan, N. Categorizing and conceptualizing styles in younger and older adults. *Human Development,* 1974, *17,* 218-230.

Lachman, J. L., Lachman, R., & Thronesbery, C. Metamemory through the adult life span. *Developmental Psychology,* 1979, *15,* 543-551.

LaPointe, L. L., & Horner, J. *Reading Comprehension Battery for Aphasia.* Tigard, OR: C. C. Publications, 1979.

Madden, D. J., & Nebes, R. D. Aging and the development of automaticity in visual search. *Developmental Psychology,* 1980, *16,* 377-384.

Maurer, J. F., & Rupp, R. R. *Hearing and aging: A guide to rehabilitation.* New York: Grune & Stratton, 1979.

Michalewski, H. J., Thompson, L. W., & Saul, R. E. Use of the EEG and evoked potentials in the investigation of age-related clinical disorders. In J. E. Birren & R. B. Sloane (Eds.) *Handbook of mental health and aging.* Englewood Cliffs, NJ: Prentice-Hall, 1980.

Nash, M., & Wepman, J. M. Auditory comprehension and age. *The Gerontologist,* 1973, Summer, 243-247.

Nebes, R. D. Verbal-pictorial recoding in the elderly. *Journal of Gerontology,* 1976, *31,* 421-427.

Nebes, R. D., & Andrews-Kulis, M. S. The effect of age on the speed of sentence formation and incidental learning. *Experimental Aging Research,* 1976, *2,* 315-331.

Noll, J. D., & Randolph, S. R. Auditory semantic, syntactic, and retention errors made by aphasic subjects on the Token Test. *Journal of Communication Disorders,* 1978, *11,* 543-553.

Norman, D. A. *Memory and attention: An introduction to human information processing* (2nd Ed.). New York: John Wiley & Sons, 1976.

Obler, L. K., & Albert, M. L. Language and aging: A neurobehavioral analysis. In D. S. Beasley & G. A. Davis (Eds.), *Aging: Communication processes and disorders.* New York: Grune & Stratton, 1981.

Obler, L. K., Albert, M. L., Goodglass, H., & Benson, D. F. Aging and aphasia type. *Brain and Language,* 1978, *6,* 318-322.

Orgass, B., & Poeck, K. Clinical validation of a new test for aphasia: An experimental study of the Token Test. *Cortex,* 1966, *2,* 222-243.

Parkinson, S. R., Lindholm, J. M., & Urell, T. Aging, dichotic memory and digit span. *Journal of Gerontology,* 1980, *35,* 87-95.

Poon, L. W., & Fozard, J. L. Speed of retrieval from long-term memory in relation to age, familiarity, and datedness of information. *Journal of Gerontology,* 1978, *33,* 711-717.

Porch, B. E. *Porch Index of Communicative Ability, Volume I: Theory and development.* Palo Alto, CA: Consulting Psychologists Press, 1967.

Raven, J. C., Court, J. H., & Raven, J. *Manual for Raven's Progressive Matrices and Vocabulary Scales, Section 1: General overview.* London: H. K. Lewis, 1976.

Riegel, K. F. Changes in psycholinguistic performances with age. In G. A. Talland (Ed.), *Human aging and behavior.* New York: Academic Press, 1968.

Salzman, C. A primer on geriatric psychopharmacology. *American Journal of Psychiatry,* 1982, *139,* 67-74.

Schaie, K. W. Intelligence and problem solving. In J. E. Birren & R. B. Sloane (Eds.), *Handbook of Mental Health and Aging.* Englewood Cliffs, NJ: Prentice-Hall, 1980.

Schaier, A. H., & Cicirelli, V. G. Age differences in humor comprehension and appreciation in old age. *Journal of Gerontology,* 1976, *31,* 577-582.

Schuell, H. M. *Differential diagnosis of aphasia with the Minnesota Test* (2nd Ed., rev. by J. W. Sefer). Minneapolis: University of Minnesota Press, 1973.

Schuell, H. M., Jenkins, J. J., & Jiménez-Pabón, E. *Aphasia in adults*. New York: Harper & Row, 1964.

Schulz, U., & Hunziker, O. Comparative studies of neuronal perikaryon size and shape in the aging cerebral cortex. *Journal of Gerontology*, 1980, *35*, 483–491.

Semenza, C., Denes, G., Lucchese, D., & Bisiacchi, P. Selective deficit of conceptual structures in aphasia: Class versus thematic relations. *Brain and Language*, 1980, *10*, 243–248.

Shewan, C. M. *Auditory Comprehension Test for Sentences*. Chicago: Biolinguistics Clinical Institutes, 1979.

Smith, A., & Fullerton, A. M. Age differences in episodic and semantic memory: Implications for language and cognition. In D. S. Beasley & G. A. Davis (Eds.), *Aging: Communication processes and disorders*. New York: Grune & Stratton, 1981.

Stones, M. J. Aging and semantic memory: Structural age differences. *Experimental Aging Research*, 1978, *4*, 125–132.

Swinney, D. A., & Taylor, O. L. Short-term memory recognition search in aphasics. *Journal of Speech and Hearing Research*, 1971, *14*, 578–588.

Swisher, L. P., & Sarno, M. T. Token Test scores of three matched patient groups: Left brain-damaged with aphasia; right brain-damaged without aphasia; non-brain damaged. *Cortex*, 1969, *5*, 264–273.

Taub, H. Comprehension and memory of prose material by young and old adults. *Experimental Aging Research*, 1979, *5*, 3–13.

Thomas, J. C. Fozard, J. L., & Waugh, N. C. Age-related differences in naming latency. *American Journal of Psychology*, 1977, *90*, 499–509.

Till, R. E. & Walsh, D. A. Encoding and retrieval factors in adult memory for implicational sentences. *Journal of Verbal Learning and Verbal Behavior*, 1980, *19*, 1–16.

Tillman, D., & Gerstman, L. J. Clustering by aphasics in free recall. *Brain and Language*, 1977, *4*, 355–364.

Valenstein, E. Age-related changes in the human central nervous system. In D. S. Beasley & G. A. Davis (Eds.), *Aging: Communication processes and disorders*. New York: Grune & Stratton, 1981.

Voke, J. A brief review of age changes in colour discrimination. *The Optician*, 1982, January 18.

Walsh, D. A., & Baldwin, M. Age differences in integrated semantic memory. *Developmental Psychology*, 1977, *13*, 509–514.

Warren, R. L., Hubbard, D. J., & Knox, A. W. Short-term memory scan in normal individuals and individuals with aphasia. *Journal of Speech and Hearing Research*, 1977, *20*, 497–509.

Yamaura, H., Ito, M., Kubota, K., & Matsuzana, T. Brain atrophy during aging: A quantitative study with computed tomography. *Journal of Gerontology*, 1980, *35*, 494–498.

Yorkston, K. M., & Beukelman, D. R. An analysis of connected speech samples of aphasic and normal speakers. *Journal of Speech and Hearing Disorders*, 1980, *45*, 27–36.

Craig W. Linebaugh

Mild Aphasia

An Opening Dilemma

As one begins reading a chapter on *mild* aphasia, he or she ought to ask—and legitimately so—What is *mild* aphasia? Who among my patients is *mildly* aphasic? Is it those whose PICA (Porch, 1967) overall performance is above the 90th percentile? Or should it be the 80th percentile? Is it the patient who responds in the negative when asked if a hammer is good for cutting wood, but fails to recognize why the bugler had trouble finding friends (from the *Boston Diagnostic Aphasia Examination,* Goodglass & Kaplan, 1972)? Is it a 62-year-old, noninstitutionalized male with a *CADL* (Holland, 1980) score above 112 but below 124? Is it those my standard aphasia battery proclaims to be "within normal limits," but my communicative experience with them tells me otherwise?

Please excuse the hyperbole, for it is born of the desire to emphasize a dilemma we share as clinicians and researchers. The dilemma is this: The "mildness" of the mildly aphasic person's aphasia depends not on his or her score on some standardized test. Rather, it depends on the degree to which the aphasia impairs his or her ability to communicate at the level demanded by personal, social, vocational, educational, and recreational needs. The degree to which we can quantify a patient's aphasia in absolute terms, using some standardized measure, is reduced to a person-by-person relativism in the realm of functional communication. Language performance which is "unimpaired" for a person with few verbal needs may be a "mild" impairment for one with somewhat greater needs. What is a "mild" impairment for that one may be a "moderate," even disabling, impairment for the lawyer, teacher, or politician.

This was the conclusion of the participants in a round-table discussion at the 1978 Clinical Aphasiology Conference (Wertz, 1978) when confronted with the same question: What is mild aphasia? It was valid then, and it is valid as you read this chapter. Indeed, its validity is eternal.

A second conclusion reached by the participants in that round-table discussion was that we had far to go in our understanding, assessment, and treatment of mildly aphasic persons. This chapter represents a tour of the ground that has been covered in the four years which have since elapsed. The section on Phenomenology is intended to draw clinical implications from the recent data regarding the performance of mildly aphasic patients. The Assessment and Treatment sections are intended to familiarize the reader with recently developed procedures. All three sections are intended to provide sufficient information to allow the reader to decide whether or not a study or procedure has applications to his or her own clinical and research endeavors.

Phenomenology

Auditory Comprehension

Recent studies of auditory comprehension in mildly aphasic patients have dealt with two areas. The first has been that of context. In a 1978 study, Wilcox, Davis, and Leonard investigated aphasic subjects' comprehension of indirect requests presented via a videotape depicting a natural communicative situation. The indirect requests used were of the type "Can you move the table?" or "Will you close the door?" The context in which the requests were made was such that the conveyed intention was indeed a request for some action, rather than the literally interpreted request for information. In addition, the investigators assessed the influence of affirmative versus negative surface forms of the request.

This study included 10 aphasic subjects described as having a high level of auditory comprehension. This designation was based on their having scored 60% or above "on a battery of standard comprehension tests requiring literal interpretation" (Wilcox et al., 1978, p. 366). Results showed significantly better performance by the high level aphasic subjects than the low level subjects. This difference was attributed to the low level group's generally depressed comprehension abilities. In a second experiment in which the effects of positive versus negative intent of the requests was studied, the results were similar. Here, too, the high level subjects performed significantly better than the low level subjects. These results essentially mirror the differences between high and low level aphasic patients on standard tests and, as such, are less than startling. What is of particular significance, however, is the degree to which context appeared to facilitate comprehension. On the standard tests, the high level group performed at a mean accuracy level of approximately 76%. In comprehending contextually supported requests, the mean accuracy level was nearly 95%. For the record, the low level group showed an even more impressive gain when contextual support was available. What may be inferred from these findings is that aphasic persons can successfully employ the extralinguistic cues available in natural communicative situations to enhance their auditory comprehension. Particular to this discussion, even mildly aphasic persons appear to benefit significantly from contextual information.

A second series of experiments concerning the role of context in the auditory comprehension of mildly impaired aphasic patients was conducted by Waller and Darley (1978a, 1978b, 1979). These investigators assessed the effects of pictorial, verbal, and combined pictorial and verbal prestimulation on sentence and paragraph comprehension. The prestimulation served to establish a context appropriate to the stimulus which followed. Results of this study indicated that verbal prestimulation significantly enhanced paragraph comprehension by aphasic individuals. No facilitative effects were observed for sentence comprehension. Also of note is the deleterious effect of pictorial prestimulation as compared to a control condition (no prestimulation). The authors speculate that this seemingly incongruous finding may have resulted from difficulty encountered by the aphasic subjects in attempting to recode the pictures verbally, using their disrupted language systems. Normal controls performed equally well in the picture and control conditions. That interference was exerted by pictorial prestimulation is at odds with recent findings of Elmore-Nicholas and Brookshire (1981). These investigators reported a facilitating effect for the presence of a sentence-relevant picture on a sentence verification task. The differences in these two studies may be related to the greater complexity of the pictures used by Waller and Darley, and to their having removed the picture prior to presentation of the stimulus. Under Waller and Darley's conditions, the need for verbal recoding of the picture would have been substantially greater than in the conditions employed by Elmore-Nicholas and Brookshire.

The second area of recent activity has been studies of the effects of extraneous factors on the auditory comprehension of the mildly aphasic. In particular, the effects of a distractor task and those of competing auditory signals have been investigated. The former were assessed in a study by DeRenzi, Faglioni, and Previdi (1978). These researchers investigated the ability of mildly aphasic subjects to carry out commands under three conditions: no delay, with a 20-second unfilled delay, and with a 20-second delay during which the subject was counting backwards by ones, twos, or threes. No significant differences were found among normal control, brain-damaged nonaphasic, and aphasic subjects' ability to carry out the commands in the no-delay and unfilled-delay conditions. All subjects, however, experienced significant performance decrements in the filled-delay condition. Here, the normal and brain-damaged nonaphasic subjects experienced mean decrements of 24% and 27%, respectively. Aphasic subjects showed a mean decrement of 48%, indicating their greater susceptibility to a distractor task.

In a study of the effects of competing auditory signals on Token Test performance, Basili, Diggs, and Rao (1980) assessed the relative effects of white noise and speech babble. Normal controls, right cerebral hemisphere-damaged, and left hemisphere-damaged aphasic subjects were administered the Token Test in quiet, in the presence of white noise, and in the presence of speech babble. As expected, the aphasic subjects performed at a lower level than either of the other two groups in all conditions. Regarding the three conditions, the aphasic subjects performed at comparable levels in quiet and in the presence of white noise, but experienced a decrease in performance in the presence of speech babble. The authors suggest that the differential effects exerted by white noise and speech babble may be related to difficulty in separating the acoustically more complex babble from the primary speech stimulus, or to difficulty in ignoring the linguistic nature of the babble.

Verbal Expression

Among the most frequently observed deviations in the verbal output of mildly aphasic individuals are residual word retrieval difficulties and disruptions of the flow of speech. Most clinicians who work with aphasic patients have at one time or another suspected that the two were somehow related, but until recently this relationship had not been examined empirically. A 1981 study by Brown and Cullinan begins to fill this void. Brown and Cullinan examined the performance of 24 anomic aphasic patients, 21 of whom were described as having mild or minimal speech deficits, on three tasks. The tasks were (1) naming 38 objects, 15 actions, and 9 colors, (2) describing pictures, and (3) engaging in a conversation, usually with one of the experimenters. The latter two tasks were employed to obtain samples of connected speech which were subsequently analyzed for the presence of various types of dysfluency. Two categories of dysfluency were analyzed, the first consisting of dysfluencies likely to be considered as "stuttering" (e.g., vocal-segregate repetitions, part-word repetitions, prolongations), and the second consisting of types likely to be considered "normal dysfluencies" (e.g., revisions, word and phrase repetitions, parenthetic remarks). Hesitations were considered separately.

The subjects' performances on the naming task were examined for both accuracy and latency of response. These variables were then correlated with various measures of the frequency of occurrence of the dysfluency types. These analyses revealed a significant relationship between word retrieval difficulty and dysfluency. That is, as the number of correct naming responses decreased and latency increased, the number of dysfluencies increased. In addition, the proportion of stuttering-like dysfluencies increased as both word-retrieval difficulty and the total number of dysfluencies increased. These findings led the authors to suggest that the aphasic individual is reacting to both word-retrieval difficulty and the incidence of dysfluencies, thereby casting himself into a whirlpool of increasing disruption of speech flow.

A second area of investigation has dealt with the ability of mildly aphasic persons to produce connected discourse. Ulatowska and her colleagues (1980, 1981) have reported an elaborate study investigating the ability of 10 aphasic subjects to produce narrative and procedural discourse. Narratives were elicited by asking the subjects to recount a memorable experience, tell a story concerning a sequence of pictures, and to retell a story following an examiner's reading of it. Procedural descriptions concerned routine, frequently performed tasks, such as brushing teeth or combing hair, and procedures learned by special instruction and possibly never performed (bowling, changing a tire).

Variables related to the complexity of the language produced, and to discourse length and structure, were analyzed for both narratives and descriptions. The primary findings of this study may be summarized as follows: The subjects produced well-formed narrative and procedural discourse, including all the elements essential to discourse superstructure. Discourse errors produced by the aphasic subjects differed from those of normal controls in number, but not in kind. The aphasic subjects produced language that was both less copious and less complex than was the language of normal controls. Reduced complexity was made particularly evident by less embedding. The reduction in quantity of language appeared to be, at least in part, selectively distributed. This is particularly apparent for the narratives, where the reduction in language was primarily displayed on nonessential, elaborative portions of the narrative. In procedural descriptions, however, language reduction resulted in the omission of essential, as well as ancillary, steps. For a full elaboration of the findings of this study, the reader is referred to Ulatowska, North and Macaluso-Haynes (1981).

In a separate study of 11 mildly aphasic subjects, Ulatowska, Hildebrand, and Haynes (1978) compared spoken and written language in both isolated sentences and connected discourse. The results of this study are consistent with the study just discussed. Here, too, aphasic subjects were observed to produce less complex language than normal controls, especially in writing. The aphasic subjects in this study were also observed to produce more preposition and semantic errors than the controls, the greater difference again being in written language. Overall, the aphasic subjects produced fewer errorless word sequences of the type being analyzed in writing than they did in spoken language. (The unit of linguistic analysis in this and the preceding study was the T-unit. A T-unit is defined as one independent clause and its dependent modifiers.) Nevertheless, on ratings of communicative adequacy, which focused on the intelligibility and specificity of the message apart from any disruptions of form, a majority of aphasic individuals were rated better or equal in written, as compared to spoken, language. Moreover, the aphasic subjects' communicative adequacy for both written and spoken language was substantially higher than their overall level of linguistic function as measured on the *Boston Diagnostic Aphasia Examination* (BDAE) (Goodglass & Kaplan, 1972). What is critical to note, however, is that the high level of communicative adequacy achieved by the mildly aphasic subjects was done so only at the expense of considerable time. In one example cited by the investigators, two samples of written discourse, rated equally for communicative adequacy, required of their normal and aphasic authors 3 and 30 minutes, respectively.

Studies of discourse thus provide us with several bits of important information regarding mild aphasia. First, both the spoken and written discourse of mildly aphasic persons is reduced in amount and complexity of language. In addition, substantial percentages of word sequences (T-units) produced contain some form of linguistic error. In spite of these disruptions of language, however, mildly aphasic subjects tend to preserve the discourse superstructure necessary to provide information in a coherent manner. Indeed, they are able to achieve a high degree of communicative adequacy. To do so, however, they must be allowed substantially longer amounts of time to accomplish communicative tasks than is required by their nonaphasic counterparts.

Coverbal Behavior

Katz, LaPointe, and Markel (1978) have reported a study in which they assessed the integrity of the coverbal behavior of aphasic patients. Coverbal behaviors are those such as head nodding, shaking, or tilting, and eyebrow raising, which are produced in association with speech. Katz et al. made video-tape recordings of aphasic and control subjects as they alternately told what they thought about 20 common words (e.g., "What do you think about laughing/black/friend?"). Several of the 10 aphasic subjects studied had relatively mild language deficits. Coverbal behaviors selected for study included eye contact, eyebrow raising, smiling, head nodding, head shaking, and head tilting. No significant differences in frequency of occurrence of these behaviors separated the aphasic and control subjects. The aphasic subjects, however, did tend to engage in a given coverbal behavior for a longer time period than did the controls.

Regarding mildly aphasic patients, the data on eye contact is particularly interesting. Those aphasic subjects who had milder verbal expressive deficits maintained eye contact for shorter durations than did those subjects with greater degrees of verbal involvement. The authors suggest that this may indicate that the subjects with milder impairments were less dependent on eye contact to maintain their speaking turn than were those with more severe deficits. For aphasic persons, in general, it was suggested that the preservation of coverbal behavior contributes to their being better communicators than language users.

Communicative Burden

It is generally recognized that successful communication by an aphasic speaker is to some extent dependent on his listeners' assuming a greater share of the burden of communication than might have been necessary prior to the onset of aphasia. In a recent study, Linebaugh, Kryzer, Oden, and Myers (1982) sought to objectively assess this reapportionment of communicative burden. As a measure of communicative burden, these investigators used the percentage of communicative exchanges initiated by the aphasic speaker as compared to his nonaphasic listener. A communicative exchange was operationally defined as an "utterance (in any modality or combination of modalities) produced by one participant in a communicative interaction, and the other's response to it." Percentages of exchanges initiated by the aphasic speakers were obtained from communicative interactions that were essentially narrative in form. Five different topics were discussed by the aphasic speakers. Several of the 12 subjects could be described as mildly aphasic.

The percentage of communicative exchanges initiated by the aphasic speakers ranged from 42 to 91%. These percentages were correlated to a significant degree with the subjects' scores on the *CADL* (Holland, 1980). This indicated that the amount of communicative burden which the aphasic individual was able to assume was directly related to his functional communicative abilities, as measured by the *CADL*. Specific to this discussion, the mildly aphasic subjects were able to carry the bulk of the communicative burden in the type of interaction assessed. Nevertheless, the listener occasionally had to probe for essential bits of information, indicating his need to assume at least a slightly greater amount of the communicative burden.

Implications

The following implications can be drawn from the recent reasearch on mild aphasia:

1.   Mildly aphasic individuals benefit from the context provided in natural communicative situations and through verbal prestimulation. The effectiveness with which a patient can utilize contextual information should be assessed. The patient can be taught strategies by which he or she can derive maximum benefit from contextual information. Those with whom the patient routinely communicates can be trained to provide additional contextual information when appropriate.

2.   Mildly aphasic individuals are highly susceptible to distractor tasks and competing signals. The effects of these deterrents to optimal performance should be assessed for the individual patient. He or she should be prepared to deal with them as they are encountered in natural communicative situations.

3.   The dysfluency experienced by some mildly aphasic patients may be related both to word retrieval difficulty and to the occurrence of dysfluencies. To minimize dysfluency, patients should learn to deal productively with instances of anomia. For example, one can use a delay to search for the desired, or synonymous, word or to formulate a circumlocution. The patient should also try to control any negative emotional reactions to his dysfluencies which may exacerbate the disruption of his flow of speech.

4.   Mildly aphasic patients preserve the essential elements of discourse, in spite of using language that is reduced in amount and complexity. This contributes to their ability to communicate more effectively than might be inferred from their linguistic performance alone.

5.   Mildly aphasic patients, as a group, appear able to communicate with a high degree of adequacy, but they require substantially more time to do so than do their normal counterparts. Patients with mild aphasia must, therefore, be trained to indicate their need for more time, and those with whom they communicate should be encouraged to provide it.

6.   That aphasic patients' communicative skills exceed their language skills may be attributable in part to the preservation of coverbal behaviors.

Clinicians should seek to develop their patients' purposeful use of these behaviors to enhance communication.

7.   While able to carry the bulk of the burden of communication in some interactions, mildly aphasic speakers must nevertheless rely on their communication partners to assume an additional share of the burden in other interactions. This depends on several factors, including the type of interaction, the subject matter, and the familiarity of the partner with both the aphasic speaker and the topic. The aphasic speaker should be trained in recognizing the need to shift some portion of the burden, and in acceptable ways of doing so.

Assessment

Assessment of the language and communication skills of mildly aphasic patients has long been a major problem for clinicians. Traditionally, we have relied on measures such as the Token Test (DeRenzi & Vignolo, 1962) or the Word Fluency Measure (Borkowski, Benton, & Spreen, 1967), or "home-made" measures, such as answering questions about a reading passage or retelling a story. The former are limited by the wide range of normal performance on such measures and their questionable relevance to functional communication. The latter are suspect because of their obvious lack of standardization. In this section, we shall consider several recent attempts to provide more sensitive measures of mild aphasia, as well as the applicability of some recently published tests to this population.

Auditory Comprehension

The Token Test was designed to be, and has long been, a standard measure of mild auditory comprehension deficits. Perhaps no other test of aphasia has undergone closer scrutiny or more revisions. Two recent efforts to enhance the Token Test bear particular mention.

The first was undertaken by Brookshire (1978). He developed a "Token Test Battery," which consisted of six versions of the standard Token Test (DeRenzi & Vignolo, 1962). These included three basic test conditions using two response modes. The three test conditions were (1) the standard version of the Token Test, (2) a configurational condition in which the subject pointed to the one of four groupings of the tokens shown on a card which best fit a command, and (3) a visual condition in which the subject matched a configuration of tokens representing a command to one of four choices. The two response modes were immediate and delayed, in which the tokens were covered during presentation of the command, and for 10 seconds thereafter.

Brookshire administered this battery to 25 aphasic, 10 right hemisphere-damaged, and 10 normal subjects. The normal subjects responded accurately and promptly on essentially all test items. The aphasic subjects performed worst in the standard condition, followed by the configurational and, then, the visual conditions. The right hemisphere-damaged group reversed this order of difficulty. Both groups of brain-damaged subjects had greater difficulty in the delayed response mode. Brookshire developed "order-of-difficulty matrices" which permit an individual patient's performance on the six subtests to be compared with that of the group. He suggested that marked deviations from the group pattern are indicative of the presence of associated problems. For example, if an aphasic patient showed greater-than-expected difficulty in all the delayed response conditions, one might suspect a more general memory deficit. To date, no additional studies using this Token Test Battery have been reported, and one can only speculate on its true clinical utility.

A second attempt to enhance the power and usefulness of the Token Test has received much wider attention and study. Recognizing the psychometric shortcomings of the original Token Test, McNeil and Prescott (1978) undertook development of the *Revised Token Test* (RTT). Among the RTT's improvements are standardized administration procedures, a multidimensional scoring system, percentile scores based on large samples of normal, left brain-damaged, and right brain-damaged subjects, and guidelines for test interpretation. If not familiar with the RTT, the reader is encouraged to study the test manual carefully, and determine the usefulness of the RTT in his or her clinical practice.

A second recently published test which this clinician has found useful with mildly aphasic patients is the *Auditory Comprehension Test for Sentences* (ACTS) (Shewan, 1980). This test is based on the work of Shewan and Canter (1971), who examined the relative influence of length, vocabulary, and syntax on the auditory comprehension of aphasic subjects. Two aspects of the ACTS, in particular, provide useful information regarding mildly aphasic persons. First, the most difficult sentences for each of the three factors represent a rather severe test of the aphasic patient's auditory comprehension in the absence of contextual support. Regrettably, the test includes only three items at the most complex level of each factor (length, vocabulary, and syntax), and there are no stimulus sentences by which the cumulative effects of increased difficulty in two or three factors can be assessed. While the author is to be commended for the economy of her test, one cannot help but wish for more items of greater difficulty so that different patterns of auditory processing deficits at the most complex levels could be identified.

The second aspect of the ACTS, which is particularly revealing, is not a part of the test per se. For each test item, a picture accurately depicting the content of the stimulus is presented along with three foils. Each foil differs from the correct response by a single element. This configuration allows the examiner to determine which stimulus element the subject apparently failed to comprehend. In many instances, the difference between the correct picture and a foil is rather obscure in the context of the whole picture. (Indeed, these minor differences may limit the applicability to certain, particularly visually impaired, patients.) As a result, the patient must carefully scan each response alternative, paying close attention to detail. Whether serendipitously or by design, Shewan has given us a convenient vehicle to observe patients' ability to organize their analysis of a group of alternative responses, while they maintain a high degree of attention to detail over a series of stimuli of varying complexity.

Another instrument which may be employed to assess the auditory comprehension of mildly aphasic patients in the Advanced Auditory Battery (AAB) proposed by Berry (1976). Designed as a supplement to the *Porch Index of Communicative Ability* (PICA) (Porch, 1967), the AAB includes 10 tasks, each comprising items, which sample a subject's comprehension of auditory stimuli of various levels of complexity. The battery uses the objects from the PICA, and a scoring system based on the PICA's 16-point multidimensional scale, but tailored to each of the 10 subtests. Berry (1976) provides a description of the test items and the scoring system in sufficient detail to allow accurate replication.

Recently Tompkins, Rau, Marshall, Lambrecht, Golper, and Phillips, (1980) investigated a number of considerations regarding the AAB. These investigators compared the performances of 24 aphasic subjects with mild auditory comprehension deficits with those of three nonbrain-damaged controls. They found that the two groups differed significantly on four of the subtests. These included subtests involving (1) three nouns, a verb, a locative preposition, and a temporal preposition denoting sequence; (2) three nouns to be responded to in sequence; (3) two nouns, two verbs, and a temporal preposition denoting sequence; and (4) two nouns and a locative preposition. Five subtests yielded scores different from those obtained on PICA subtests VI (pointing by function) and X (pointing by name). These included the four subtests listed above, plus one involving two nouns and a temporal adverb. These five subtests, therefore, were found to provide information not available from the PICA. Tompkins et al. concluded that, with appropriate revisions, the AAB could be a useful clinical tool for assessing mild auditory comprehension deficits. Specifically they called for further research on an abbreviated form of the battery using the most discriminating subtests, and also suggested refinement of the scoring system.

Verbal Expression

Two potentially useful tools for the assessment of the verbal expression of mildly aphasic patients have appeared recently. One is the Reporter's Test developed by DeRenzi and Ferrari (1978). At its most basic level, the Reporter's Test can be described as the Token Test in reverse. The subject's task is to describe what the examiner has done with a configuration of tokens in sufficient detail so that a person who could not see the tokens would be able to replicate the maneuver. There are five parts to the Reporter's Test. The first four parallel the first four parts of the standard Token Test. Part V required substantial revision of Part V of the Token Test because the commands did not lend themselves to the reporter format. Seven standard Token Test items were retained and three new items added. Scoring is done on a pass/fail basis for the entire response and in Parts I–IV a weighted score is also derived based on the patient's response to each critical element in the stimulus (e.g. color, size, shape).

DeRenzi and Ferrari reported data from the administration of the Reporter's Test to 70 nonbrain-damaged hospital patients, 60 left brain-damaged adults with mild to moderate expressive deficits, 20 nonaphasic, left brain-damaged adults, and 20 right brain-damaged adults. The scores of all subjects were corrected for the influence of educational background. Comparison of the Reporter's Test with various other measures of verbal expression, including visual confrontation, naming, and word fluency, revealed it to be a powerful discriminator between aphasic and nonaphasic subjects.

The second measure to be developed recently, of use in assessing mild expressive impairments, has perhaps greater functional relevance than does the Reporter's Test. Yorkston and Beukelman (1977, 1980) have developed a means for quantifying subjects' descriptions of the "Cookie Theft" picture from the BDAE. Using transcripts of Cookie Theft descriptions from 78 normal speakers, these investigators compiled a list of 57 content units expressed by at least one of the normal speakers. A content unit was defined as a "grouping of information that was always expressed as a unit by normal speakers."

Three measures were generated from the descriptions. These were (1) number of content units that indicated the amount of information conveyed, (2) syllables per minute, and (3) content units per minute that served as a measure of rate of information transfer. These measures were calculated for five groups of subjects: (1) 48 normal adult speakers rangeing in age from 19 to 49 years, (2) 30 normal geriatric speakers ranging in age from 58 to 93 years, (3) 17 mildly aphasic speakers with PICA verbal percentiles ranging from the 81st to 99th percentile, (4) 16 highmoderate aphasic speakers with PICA verbal percentiles ranging from the 66th to 80th percentile, and (5) 17 low-moderate aphasic speakers with PICA verbal percentiles ranging from the 50th to 65th percentile. The mildly aphasic group did not differ from the two normal groups in terms of the number of content units produced. The mildly aphasic subjects did, however, produce significantly fewer syllables and content units per minute than either of the normal groups. These findings indicate that while the mildly aphasic subjects conveyed as much information as did the normals, they did so much less efficiently. Again we see, as we did earlier in the work of Ulatowska and her colleagues (1980, 1981), that the mildly aphasic individual communicates at an essentially normal level of adequacy, but needs substantially more time than do normal speakers.

I employ an additional count of syllables per content unit. Approximate means of 4.8, 5.7, and 6.3 syllables per content unit for the normal, geriatric, and mildly aphasic groups, respectively, can be derived from Yorkston and Beukelman's data. This measure has proven especially useful for documenting increasing communicative efficiency over time for patients who used excessive amounts of verbalization. For such patients, the goal of treatment was to move their inflated number of syllables per content unit in the direction of the mean of the age-appropriate normal group. These values can likewise serve as goals for nonfluent patients whose mean length of utterance needs expansion.

In addition to their content-based analysis, Yorkston and Beukelman (1978) have developed a system for assessing the grammaticality of connected speech samples. This analysis was based on the mean length of uninterrupted grammatical strings. A *string* was defined as a "series of words which have a grammatical relationship to each other." An elaborate set of rules for determining mean string length is provided by the authors.

Analyzing the Cookie Theft descriptions from their previous study, Yorkston and Beukelman found that mildly aphasic subjects fell below normals for mean length of grammatical string. Review of the transcripts, however, suggested that in several instances, strings were broken by errors which were not necessarily due to a failure to apply grammatical rules. As a result, the mean length of grammatical string was reduced by factors other than faulty syntax. The normal and mildly aphasic subjects were then compared on a second measure, "mean of the three longest strings." On this measure there was no significant difference between the mildly aphasic and normal subjects. These findings suggest that while mildly aphasic patients are similar to normals in their ability to produce long grammatical strings, their overall performance is reduced in efficiency. Whether this is because of a loss of syntactic knowledge, faulty application of this knowledge, or other nongrammatical problems remains unclear.

In a 1980 study, Golper, Thorpe, Tompkins, Marshall, and Rau also sought to extend the types of information that could be extracted from descriptions of the Cookie Theft picture. In addition to the content and grammaticality analyses of Yorkston and Beukelman, these investigators used five measures intended to assess the flow of verbal propositions. Golper et al. used the performance deviations employed by Loban (1967) for describing language development for this analysis. The measures included word and phrase interruptions or revisions, sequence interrupters in words and phrases (noncontentive utterances such as "uh" or "I mean"), and morpho/syntactic deviations. They also included a category of "phonetic error" which encompassed phonemic substitutions, omissions, and any unintelligible phonemes.

Transcripts of Cookie Theft picture descriptions obtained from 10 mildly aphasic subjects (PICA overall percentiles between 79th and 95th percentile), five of whom were fluent and five nonfluent, 10 right hemisphere-damaged subjects, and 10 normal geriatric subjects were analyzed. These analyses revealed that the aphasic subjects produced significantly more of each type of deviation than did either of the other two groups. Fluent and nonfluent aphasic subjects differed only in their incidence of word and phrase interrupters, with the nonfluent aphasic subjects producing more. The authors suggested that these additional measures may be useful for assessing mildly aphasic patients and for documenting their improvement over time.

Communicative Efficiency

In the preceding discussion it has been stated that mildly aphasic speakers generally are able to convey amounts of information comparable to those conveyed by normal speakers, but that they do so with reduced efficiency. Yorkston, Beukelman, and Flowers sought to address the matter of communicative efficiency more directly in a 1980 study. These investigators video tape-recorded aphasic speakers answering specific questions asked by a listener who was not able to see a series of stimulus pictures. After the listener had asked the designated question, he and the aphasic individual were free to use any means they chose to achieve the transfer of information. When the listener thought he had the desired information, or when a time limit had expired, he wrote his answer on a response sheet.

The listener's written answer was scored for accuracy, and the duration of the interaction was timed separately for each picture in the series. The investigators developed a method for comparing the relative efficiency of two communication samples based on a rank ordering procedure. This readily replicated method is described by Yorkston et al. (1980). The authors also provide case illustrations by which they demonstrate the usefulness of their method in assessing differences in a given patient's communicative efficiency over time and with different communication partners. This procedure appears to have considerable potential for both documenting improvement and identifying successful communication strategies.

Treatment

The literature of recent years contains little in the way of treatment procedures targeted on the mildly aphasic patient. One source rich in treatment approaches for the mildly aphasic was a panel discussion held at the 1980 Clinical Aphasiology Conference (Darley, Helm, Holland, & Linebaugh, 1980). Among the suggestions offered were (1) having the aphasic patient "teach" the clinician about his area of expertise, (2) retelling and summarizing stories of increasing length, (3) writing letters and keeping a diary, (4) forming sentences using designated words, (5) performing multiple-step verbal cognitive tasks such as giving directions, (6) writing captions for cartoons, (7) interpreting metaphors and idioms, (8) various divergent semantic tasks (Chapey, 1977), and (9) working on specific job-related tasks. In addition to these suggestions, three more elaborate descriptions of specific treatment approaches have also appeared recently.

The first of these is a program designed to improve word retrieval called SORRT (Logue & Dixon, 1979). SORRT is an acronym for semantic, oppositional, and rhyming retrieval training. As part of their program, Logue and Dixon provide a set of probes consisting of four single-word response tasks and one conversational analysis procedure. From these probes, the clinician is able to determine the primary types of response and retrieval strategies used by the patient, as well as those that are rarely or inaccurately used. The focus of the SORRT program is to expand the patient's repertoire of retrieval strategies. This is done through three levels of training. The first level is "discrimination training." Here the patient is presented pairs of words auditorily. At various stages in this training procedure, the patient is asked to respond "yes" or "no" as to whether the words in a given pair rhyme, are synonyms, or are antonyms. The second level of training is "selective matching." At this level, the patient is required to select from among three alternatives the word that rhymes or is a synonym or antonym of a stimulus word. The third level, "expressive-generative training," requires the patient to produce a word that rhymes or is a synonym or antonym of a stimulus word. Logue and Dixon provide a detailed description of the SORRT program, along with data on the performance of fluent and nonfluent subjects, and three case reports demonstrating the program's effectiveness. What remain to be developed are criteria identifying those patients who are appropriate candidates for this program.

Another approach to facilitating word retrieval by mildly aphasic patients has been described by Linebaugh (1983). This approach, known as Lexical Focus, is predicated on the observation that many of the word retrieval errors of mildly aphasic persons represent verbal paraphasias. That is, the word produced in error is related to the desired word, the two frequently being members of a common superordinate category. The assumption is made, therefore, that the aphasic speaker was able to access the appropriate superordinate category (one of many factors involved in the organization of one's lexicon), but was unable to retrieve the specific lexical item desired. Lexical Focus is thus described by Linebaugh as designed to improve the aphasic patient's "lexical dexterity" (Darley et al., 1980).

In this approach, patients are asked to name as many items in a designated superordinate category as they can. To facilitate performance, patients are encouraged to employ "search strategies." For example, if they are to name as many fruits and vegetables as they can, the patients may be instructed to imagine they are walking through the produce section of a supermarket or looking in their refrigerator. When the patients' performances reach criterion on a broad superordinate category, they are asked to name as many items as they can in a narrower subcategory (e.g., fruits *and* vegetables/fruits *or* vegetables; sports/sports played with a ball). A third, yet narrower, subcategory (e.g., fruits/citrus fruits, berries; sports played with a ball/sports played with a ball and a stick) may be presented upon reaching criterion for the second level category. Linebaugh (1983) has provided a detailed description of the Lexical Focus procedure along with suggested categories and criteria.

The third approach derives from a 1979 study by Cooper and Rigrodsky that assessed the effects of verbal training on aphasic patients' explanations of conservation, i.e., the preservation of equivalent volume or weight despite irrelevant perceptual changes. The specific conservation tasks employed were (1) a liquid conservation task where two equivalent amounts of water in identical containers remain equivalent when the contents of one container are poured into a taller, thinner container, and (2) a weight conservation task where two identical balls of clay remain equivalent in weight when one is elongated.

For both tasks, nine aphasic subjects were required to explain verbally the continued equivalence of the two amounts of water or clay. The subjects' responses were judged for the inclusion of various concepts by which the continued equivalence could be explained, rather than linguistic accuracy or complexity. Following pretesting, the nine subjects underwent an experimental protocol, part of which included listening to possible explanations for the weight conservation task. These explanations were intended to serve as verbal models for the subjects. Comparisons of pre- and post-training explanations of conservation revealed significant improvement in the explanations for the weight task for which training had been provided, and a nonsignificant trend toward improvement in the liquid task. Cooper and Rigrodsky interpreted these findings as indicating that verbal modeling had a facilitating effect on the task which received training, with some generalization to the untrained task.

A Closing Admonition

Patients with mild aphasia frequently require intensive treatment to enable them to return successfully to their work. These patients are sometimes dismissed too casually because their needs are less obvious. The difference between success and failure can be tragic when the potential is so high.

Schuell, Jenkins, and Jiménez Pabón
(*Aphasia in Adults*, 1964, p. 368)

As you conclude your reading of this chapter, it would be my desire that your interest in the mildly aphasic patient would be increased. Overall, the interest of aphasiologists in mild aphasia has grown since 1978, but it remains low as compared with other aspects of this disorder. As you read this chapter, did you notice the decrease in the number of relevant sources as you progressed from the section on Phenomenology to that on Treatment? Surely this disparity exists in all aspects of aphasiology, for description must precede application. But as clinicians, can we afford to be complacent in applying our available information? More to the point, can our mildly aphasic patients afford this complacency? As clinical scientists, we have the ability and responsibility to develop new treatment approaches and assess their efficacy. Would that we all might be challenged by the above words of Schuell and her colleagues, rather than haunted by them.

References

Basili, A. G., Diggs, C. C., & Rao, P. R. Auditory processing of brain-damaged adults under competitive listening conditions. *Brain and Language*, 1980, *9*, 362–371.

Berry, W. R. Testing auditory comprehension in aphasia: Clinical alternatives to the Token Test. In Brookshire, R. H. (Ed.), *Clinical Aphasiology: Conference Proceedings*. Minneapolis: BRK Publishers, 1976.

Borkowski, J. G., Benton, A. L., & Spreen, O. Word fluency and brain damage. *Neuropsychologia*, 1967, *5*, 135–140.

Brookshire, R. H. A token test battery for testing auditory comprehension in brain-damaged adults. *Brain and Language*, 1978, *6*, 149–157.

Brown, C. S., & Cullinan, W. L. Word-retrieval difficulty and disfluent speech in adult anomic speakers. *Journal of Speech and Hearing Research*, 1981, *24*, 358–365.

Chapey, R. A divergent semantic model of intervention in adult aphasia. In Brookshire, R. H. (Ed.), *Clinical Aphasiology: Conference Proceedings*. Minneapolis: BRK Publishers, 1977.

Cooper, L. D., & Rigrodsky, S. Verbal training to improve explanations of conservation with aphasic adults. *Journal of Speech and Hearing Research*, 1979, *22*, 818–828.

Darley, F. L., Helm, N. A., Holland, A., & Linebaugh, C. W. Techniques in treating mild or high-level aphasic impairment. In Brookshire, R. H. (Ed.), *Clinical Aphasiology: Conference Proceedings*. Minneapolis, BRK Publishers, 1980.

DeRenzi, E., Faglioni, P., & Previdi. Increased susceptibility of aphasics to a distractor task in the recall of verbal commands. *Brain and Language*, 1978, *6*, 14–21.

DeRenzi, E., & Ferrari, C. The Reporter's Test: A sensitive test to detect expressive disturbances in aphasics. *Cortex*, 1978, *14*, 279–293.

DeRenzi, E., & Vignolo, L. A. The Token Test: A sensitive test to detect receptive disturbances in aphasics. *Brain*, 1962, *85*, 665–678.

Elmore-Nicholas, L., & Brookshire, R. H. Effects of pictures and picturability on sentence verification by aphasic and nonaphasic subjects. *Journal of Speech and Hearing Research*, 1981, *24*, 292–298.

Golper, L. A. C., Thorpe, P., Tompkins, C., Marshall, R. C., & Rau, M. T. Connected language sampling: An expanded index of aphasic language behavior. In Brookshire, R. H. (Ed.), *Clinical Aphasiology: Conference Proceedings*. Minneapolis: BRK Publishers, 1980.

Goodglass, H., & Kaplan, E. *Boston Diagnostic Aphasia Examination*. Philadelphia: Lea & Febiger, 1972.

Holland, A. *Communicative Abilities in Daily Living*. Baltimore: University Park Press, 1980.

Katz, R. C., LaPointe, L. L., & Markel, N. N. Coverbal behavior and aphasic speakers. In Brookshire, R. H. (Ed.), *Clinical Aphasiology: Conference Proceedings*. Minneapolis: BRK Publishers, 1978.

Linebaugh, C. W. Treatment of anomic aphasia. In Perkins, W. H. (ed.), *Current therapy of communication disorders: Language handicaps in adults*. New York: Thieme-Stratton, 1983.

Linebaugh, C. W., Kryzer, K. M., Oden, S. E., & Myers, P. S. Reapportionment of communicative burden in aphasia. In Brookshire, R. H. (Ed.), *Clinical Aphasiology: Conference Proceedings*. Minneapolis: BRK Publishers, 1982.

Loban, W. *Language development: K through 12*. National Council of Teachers of English Report #18. Champaign, IL, 1967.

Logue, R. D., & Dixon, M. M. Word association and the anomic response: Analysis and treatment. In Brookshire, R. H. (Ed.), *Clinical Aphasiology: Conference Proceedings*. Minneapolis: BRK Publishers, 1979.

McNeil, M. R., & Prescott, T. E. *Revised Token Test*. Baltimore: University Park Press, 1978.

Porch, B. E. *Porch Index of Communicative Ability*. Palo Alto, CA: Consulting Psychologists Press, 1967.

Schuell, H., Jenkins, J. J., & Jiménez-Pabón, E. *Aphasia in adults*. New York: Harper & Row, 1964.

Shewan, C. M. *Auditory Comprehension Test for Sentences*. Chicago: Biolinguistics Clinical Institutes, 1980.

Shewan, C. M., & Canter, G. J. Effects of vocabulary, syntax, and sentence length on auditory comprehension in aphasic patients. *Cortex*, 1971, *7*, 209–226.

Tompkins, C. A., Rau, M. T., Marshall, R. C., Lambrecht, K. J., Golper, L. A. C., & Phillips, D. S. Analysis of a battery assessing mild auditory comprehension involvement in aphasia. In Brookshire, R. H. (Ed.), *Clinical Aphasiology: Conference Proceedings*. Minneapolis: BRK Publishers, 1980.

Ulatowska, H. K., Hildebrand, B. H., & Haynes, S. M. A comparison of written and spoken language in aphasia. In Brookshire, R. H. (Ed.), *Clinical Aphasiology: Conference Proceedings*. Minneapolis: BRK Publishers, 1978.

Ulatowska, H. K., Macaluso-Haynes, S., & North, A. J. Production of narrative and procedural discourse in aphasia. In Brookshire, R. H. (Ed.), *Clinical Aphasiology: Conference Proceedings*. Minneapolis: BRK Publishers, 1980.

Ulatowska, H. K., North, A. J., & Macaluso-Haynes, S. Production of narrative and procedural discourse in aphasia. *Brain and Language*, 1981, *13*, 345–371.

Waller, M. R., & Darley, F. L. Effect of prestimulation on sentence comprehension by aphasic subjects. *Journal of Communication Disorders*, 1979, *12*, 461–479.

Waller, M. R., & Darley, F. L. The influence of context on the auditory comprehension of aphasic subjects. In Brookshire, R. H. (Ed.), *Clinical Aphasiology: Conference Proceedings*. Minneapolis: BRK Publishers, 1978. (a)

Waller, M. R., & Darley, F. L. The influence of context on the auditory comprehension of paragraphs by aphasic subjects. *Journal of Speech and Hearing Research*, 1978, *21*, 732–745. (b)

Wertz, R. T. Treating mildly aphasic patients. In Brookshire, R. H. (Ed.), *Clinical Aphasiology: Conference Proceedings*. Minneapolis: BRK Publishers, 1978.

Wilcox, M. J., Davis, G. A., & Leonard, L. B. Aphasics' comprehension of contextually conveyed meaning. *Brain and Language*, 1978, *6*, 362–377.

Yorkston, K. M., & Beukelman, D. R. A system for assessing grammaticality in connected speech of mildly aphasic individuals. In Brookshire, R. H. (Ed.), *Clinical Aphasiology: Conference Proceedings*. Minneapolis: BRK Publishers, 1978.

Yorkston, K. M., & Beukelman, D. R. A system for quantifying verbal output of high-level aphasics. In Brookshire, R. H. (Ed.), *Clinical Aphasiology: Conference Proceedings*. Minneapolis: BRK Publishers, 1977.

Yorkston, K. M., & Beukelman, D. R. An analysis of connected speech samples of aphasic and normal speakers. *Journal of Speech and Hearing Disorders*, 1980, *45*, 27–36.

Yorkston, K. M., Beukelman, D. R., & Flowers, C. R. Efficiency of information exchange between aphasic speakers and communication partners. In Brookshire, R. H. (Ed.), *Clinical Aphasiology: Conference Proceedings*. Minneapolis: BRK Publishers, 1980.

Jennifer Horner

Moderate Aphasia

Treatment of the aphasic individual has, in past years, been governed by concepts of auditory stimulation (Duffy, 1981; Schuell, Jenkins, & Jiménez-Pabón, 1964), intermodality deblocking (Weigl & Bierwich, 1970), task continua facilitation (Rosenbek, Lemme, Ahern, Harris, & Wertz, 1973), cognitive retraining (Martin, 1981; Wepman, 1972) and operant methodology (Holland, 1972; LaPointe, 1977). With these models as background, the purpose of this chapter is to review recent studies describing deficits of the moderately impaired aphasic individual from a psycholinguistic perspective. Clinical implications of these descriptive investigations will be highlighted. Psycholinguistic treatment studies, though sparsely represented in recent literature, will be described.

Assessing Moderate
Aphasic Impairment

A current view of diagnosis is: "Diagnosis in [a]phasia implies the effort to identify the configuration of deficits in a particular case with one of the dozen or so recognized syndromes. Secondarily, it implies the identification of the probable site of lesion, on the basis of established correlations between syndromes and their most frequent lesion sites" (Albert, Goodglass, Helm, Rubens, & Alexander, 1981, p. 17). Identifying "the configuration of deficits" requires both quantitative and qualitative description. To achieve a quantitative description, one must define the degree of impairment in a variety of language behaviors. To achieve a qualitative description, one must interpret the resultant profile with regard to the recognized aphasia syndromes (and with regard to normal language performance). Quantifying an aphasic deficit involves defining the deficit as mild, moderate, or severe. Qualifying an aphasic deficit involves making inferences about the mechanisms underlying the aphasia, and it is for this purpose that the psycholinguistic model is particularly helpful.

Moderate aphasia can be operationally distinguished from mild and severe aphasia as follows. *Mild aphasia* is usually characterized by a language pattern that shares more features with normal language than deviates from it. Anomia is usually a predominant feature. Communicative competence is usually well preserved in the sense that the individual is aware of his or her deficits and uses compensatory strategies (e.g., delay, circumlocution) to deliberately compensate for aphasic performance difficulties (see Linebaugh's chapter). *Severe aphasia* is characterized by a marked reduction in the repertoire of language forms, such as a reduced lexical dictionary or simplified syntactic rules. A patient with severe aphasia is no longer able to use language for successful communicative interchange (see Helm-Estabrooks' chapter). The language performance in *moderate aphasia* falls on standardized tests in defined ranges: e.g., 40 to 70th percentile on the *Porch Index of Communicative Ability* (Porch, 1967); 40.0 to 70.0 aphasia quotient on the *Western Aphasia Battery* (Kertesz, 1980), or rating of "2" or "3" on the 5-point severity scale of the *Boston Diagnostic Aphasia Exam* (Goodglass & Kaplan, 1972a). The moderately aphasic individual has a broad language repertoire, which argues against a "loss" of linguistic forms and rules. On the other hand, *language is fundamentally altered from normal with regard to its specificity, complexity, and organization.* In addition, the language of the moderately aphasic individual is affected by memory and vigilance limitations (Brookshire, 1978), and reduced awareness of response accuracy (Martin, 1974; Porch, 1981).

With this definition in mind, the purpose of this chapter is to review psycholinguistic studies regarding the lexical-semantic, morphosyntactic, phonologic, and pragmatic abilities of moderately aphasic individuals. This chapter will attempt to show why a qualitative psycholinguistic assessment —above and beyond a quantitative assessment—is imperative to a clinically adequate description of aphasic language.

Psycholinguistics

By way of introduction to the psycholinguistic literature, a general understanding of the goals of linguistics is in order. Simply, *linguistics* involves the study of the regularities of language structure. The branch of linguistics known as *psycholinguistics* involves the study of the psychological processes underlying language performance. The primary contribution of psycholinguistic research to aphasiology has been to enhance our understanding of the mechanisms underlying aphasic language disruption. While many of the findings of this research may apply to mild aphasia and severe aphasia, moderate aphasia has been most widely studied in this regard. According to Ulatowska (1979), recent contributions of linguistics to aphasiology are empirical, procedural, and theoretical in nature. Among the *empirical* contributions are the ideas that aphasic error types and patterns are uniform across aphasia types (e.g., Blumstein, 1973) and that aphasic deficits can be selective (Geschwind, 1965a), two points that speak to the regularity of language organization in the brain. From a *procedural* perspective, linguistics has contributed new approaches for analysis of aphasic speech and language. Recent applications include: transformational grammar (Myerson & Goodglass, 1972), case grammar (Tonkovich, 1979), phonological process analysis (Kearns, 1980), metalinguistic tasks (von Stockert, 1972), sentence verification procedures (Brookshire & Nicholas, 1980a, 1980b, 1981). From a *theoretical* perspective, models of markedness theory (Ulatowska & Baker, 1975), lexical-semantic organization (Caramazza & Berndt, 1978), phonology (Kean, 1977), and pragmatics (Davis & Wilcox, 1981; Holland, 1980) are representative of the breadth of the contribution of linguistics to aphasiology. Thus, evolving theories of linguistics have contributed significantly to our understanding of the psycholinguistic mechanisms underlying historically recognized aphasia syndromes. (See Berndt & Caramazza, 1981; Blumstein, 1981; Buckingham, 1981 for exemplary reviews.) Psycholinguistic principles can also be used to identify idiosyncratic compensatory aphasic behaviors as shown in a case study by Hand, Tonkovich, and Aitchison (1979).

Thus, diagnosis in aphasia requires both quantitative and qualitative assessment. The challenge to the clinician is to go beyond quantitative analyses that yield overall percentiles, quotients, and severity ratings within specific performance areas. The challenge to the clinician is to ferret out the systematic nature of language errors, and to develop a qualitative description of aphasic symptoms. The challenge to the clinician is to describe not only *what* is wrong and *how much* the behavior deviates from normal, but also to describe *why particular errors occur.*

Dissociation of Functions in Aphasia

Dissociation of functions is a basic concept underlying recent psycholinguistic research. Dissociation refers to the phenomenon of functional disconnection of higher cortical functions. On the one hand, a function (code, modality, process) may be *preserved but functionally disconnected* from related subsystems that normally contribute to the realization of a behavior. Weigl and Fradis (1977) called this a "transcoding deficit." On the other hand, a function may be *selectively impaired and thereby functionally disconnected* from its parent system. In short, two functions may be intact but noninteractive because of an impairment in the connecting pathway, or a function may be selectively impaired and therefore noncontributory to related systemic functions. The degree to which an intact dissociated function can be assessed by intact pathways, or the degree to which an impaired dissociated function can be facilitated through the process of pairing intact with impaired functions ("deblocking," Weigl & Bierwisch, 1970) may affect recovery of the impaired function. The recovered function (the reorganized behavior) may differ qualitatively from the original behavior, but if treatment is successful, the reorganized or substituted behavior will be adequate to its purpose. In this chapter, the functions of interest are purposeful oral-verbal communication behaviors.

The concept of dissociation of functions helps the student of aphasia understand how the varieties of aphasia are defined in terms of the relative preservation or impairment of behaviors such as naming, fluency, comprehension, and repetition (Albert et al., 1981; Benson, 1979a, 1979b; Kertesz, 1979). Furthermore, the concept of dissociation of functions provides a thread that ties together the psycholinguistic studies described in this chapter. The reader is advised to keep in mind the concept of dissociation and related assumptions. First, the lexical-semantic (or syntactic, or phonologic) system can be selectively impaired. Second, processes underlying lexical-semantic (or morphosyntactic, or phonologic) performance may be selectively impaired within each system. Third, the quality of aphasic errors reflects the pattern of dissociation among language functions. Fourth, by analyzing the relative impairment or sparing of performance intersystemically (e.g., by comparing lexical-semantic with morphosyntactic performances) or intrasystemically (e.g., by analyzing lexical-semantic ability in spontaneous speech versus confrontation naming), one can infer the nature of the psycholinguistic process disruption.

Marin, Saffran, and Schwartz (1976) suggest three clinical implications emanating from the dissociation of functions model. First, the brain-damaged individual is adaptive and will strive to accomplish his or her functions as best as he or she can. Second, the functional impairment can alter the ways in which intact processes emerge in behavior. Third, recovery of language does not represent the creation of new subsystems; rather, recovery of language implies a reorganization that emphasizes intact subsystems (p. 869).

To summarize, the dissociation model suggests that focal brain damage may selectively impair a language function and/or may selectively impair the various pathways of access to specific functions. Once a qualitative analysis is completed, the clinician can develop rationale for task selection. The clinician may choose to pair intact and impaired functions using deblocking procedures with the goal of improving the impaired function *per se*. The clinician may choose to train the patient to use intact functions to circumvent the deficient function. Or, the clinician may choose to train the patient to use intact functions to deliberately access an intact but behaviorally disconnected function.

Lexical-Semantic Disruption

The moderately impaired aphasic individual invariably presents some degree of word-finding difficulty. The recent literature suggests that lexical-semantic errors reflect one (or more) of the following problems: (1) incomplete *access* to the semantic properties of the intended word, (2) *impoverishment* of semantic associations within a semantic field, or (3) *lexical* disorganization (e.g., broadening or misalignment of semantic features or boundaries). The research has shown that lexical-semantic performance is affected by: (1) spontaneous (nonconstrained) versus semantically- or syntactically-constrained contexts, (2) by the semantic feature composition or markedness value of words, and (3) by lexical dimensions such as semantic category, word frequency and form class. The major conclusion of recent studies is that naming ability is not an all-or-none phenomenon but rather represents the end result of a variety of processes that may be impaired alone or in combination depending on the locus and/or extent of the aphasia-producing lesion. Some representative studies will be described.

Benson (1979c) has presented an excellent overview of the anomias and their neurologic correlates. By integrating past research (Geschwind, 1965b; Goodglass & Baker, 1976; Goodglass, Barton, & Kaplan, 1968; Goodglass, Kaplan, Weintraub, & Ackerman, 1976; Luria, 1966), Benson identified nine varieties of anomia. He identified "word production anomia," "semantic (nominal) anomia," "word selection (word dictionary) anomia," "category-specific anomia," "modality-specific anomia," and others. For the purpose of illustration, *word selection anomia* will be briefly contrasted with *semantic anomia*. Word selection anomia is described by Benson as a "pure anomic aphasia," i.e., with no other disturbance of production, comprehension, repetition, reading or writing. According to Benson, this patient fails to name objects on confrontation but readily demonstrates their use, proving that the individual recognizes the object but cannot produce the name (Benson, 1979c, p. 303). This is a one-way defect in that the patient is unable to select the correct word from the lexicon despite the ability to recognize it when spoken by another person. *Semantic anomia,* in contrast, occurs when the patient is both unable to retrieve the name and unable to recognize the word when it is either spoken or written. The patient with a word selection deficit is more likely to respond to phonetic and contextual cues than the patient with semantic anomia.

Benson describes the neurologic correlates of each clinical variety of anomia. He describes how visual, auditory, and tactile association areas converge on the angular gyrus, and, as such, the angular gyrus represents a polymodal "semantic field." Interference with polymodal association by damage to the angular gyrus is likely to cause semantic anomia. In contrast, word selection anomia is more likely to occur after a more specific lesion in the temporal-occipital function areas, wherein the "concept" is preserved but access to the lexical dictionary is impeded. Thus the distinction between a loss of words versus a problem of access appears to be clinically valid and lesion-specific.

Many factors influence the way in which words are represented (associated or organized) in the brain and subsequently how words are retrieved. Some influencing factors are: word frequency and picturability (Goodglass, Hyde, & Blumstein, 1969), grammatical class (Goodglass, Gleason, Bernholtz, & Hyde, 1972), and operativity (Gardner, 1973). Concept arousal and word retrieval depend not only on number and type of associations (Goodglass & Baker, 1976), but also on the ability of the individual to access intact representations (Milberg & Blumstein, 1981).

An innovative approach to the study of semantic disorganization is the "semantic features" model. In this model, certain features comprising a word are considered "defining features" (i.e., essential properties of a concept), and others are considered "characteristic features" (i.e., accidental properties, often referential or affective). Using a semantic categorization paradigm, Grober, Perceman, Kellar, and Brown (1980) noted that patients with anterior lesions observed semantic category boundaries defined by both "defining" and "characteristic" features, while patients with posterior lesions did not. The latter group based their categorization decisions on "characteristic" features only. (See also Zurif, Caramazza, Myerson, & Calvin, 1974.)

Also using a semantic features paradigm, Buckingham and Rekart (1979) analyzed types of anomic errors in light of their component features. Their findings suggested three possible reasons for the occurrence of semantic paraphasias: (1) unshared features of the target word and the paraphasic error are missing from the repertoire of semantic features; (2) shared features are more important than unshared features, causing the latter to lose their discriminatory effect, and/or (3) during an individual's search for an intended word, unshared features may be erroneously activated (Buckingham & Rekart, 1979, p. 206).

The effects of cues and contextual factors on naming performance have also been explored in recent psycholinguistic studies. Weigl and Bierwisch (1970) suggest that aphasic individuals do not have restricted access to a particular semantic field (category) but lack precision in selecting words within the chosen field. Marshall and Ewanowski (1976) confirmed this idea, finding that contextual information enhanced naming ability *if* the information unequivocally directed the aphasic individual to a particular semantic field. If the semantic field was correctly accessed, selection of a specific word within that field was enhanced. If the contextual information was nonspecific or ambiguous the likelihood of either a related or unrelated semantic error was increased. Wales and Kinsella (1981) further suggested that syntactic constraints can influence word retrieval, with content words more easily retrieved than functors. Pease and Goodglass (1978) studied the effect of six types of cues on naming, and discovered that regardless of type of aphasia, initial phoneme and context completion cues were most helpful, a finding supported by Podraza and Darley (1977). Looking at the influence of contextualization in a somewhat different way, Williams and Canter (1981) compared noun recall in response to pictures in isolation to noun recall in response to identical stimuli presented in composite pictorial form. In this study, Broca's aphasic patients were able to name pictures more readily when they were presented in isolation, while Wernicke's aphasic patients had greater success in the composite pictorial condition.

The markedness[1] value of words also affects accessibility of nouns. Drummond, Gallagher, and Mills (1981) compared word retrieval ability for adjectives controlled for semantic feature complexity and markedness. Marked adjectives were more easily retrieved on a sentence completion task than unmarked adjectives (though unmarked adjectives proved to be easier than marked adjectives on a recognition task). Adjectives defined as "less complex" in terms of the types of features comprising them—

TABLE 4-1
Semantic Disruption in the Adult: An Organization and Retrieval
Model (Fedor, 1981).

MODEL:

The mature semantic system organizes vocabulary on at least two levels; according to word meaning (Level I) and word sound (Level II). Organization mechanisms act with retrieval mechanisms at both levels when the system is functioning normally. In anomia, impairment may occur in either organization or retrieval mechanisms, at either level in the system.

ASSESSMENT:

 I. First Decision: Is the problem one of *organization* or *retrieval*?
 II. Second Decision: Is the problem at Level I (meaning) or Level II (sound)?

TREATMENT:

 A. **Disorganization, Level I Tasks**

   1. Categorization according to semantic relationships, e.g.,

    (a) Grouping contrast coordinates with target (*knife,* fork, spoon)
    (b) Grouping functional associates with target (*knife,* cut, spread)
    (c) Grouping superordinates with target (*knife,* utensils, silverware)

   2. Pair modalities, e.g.,

    Patient gestures while verbalizing target words.

 B. **Disorganization, Level II Tasks**

   1. Categorization according to phonologic relationships, e.g.,

    (a) Grouping words having same initial phoneme
    (b) Grouping words that rhyme

 Disorganization, Levels I or II Tasks (Compensatory)

   Teach use of *circumlocution, pause* and *indefinites* to replace neologisms and paraphasias.

C. Retrieval, Level I Tasks. Cues are Facilitative.

1. Sentence completion tasks
   High Probability, e.g., "Eat soup with a _____."
   Low Probability, e.g., "There are many _____."
2. Paired associate tasks

D. Retrieval, Level II Tasks. Cues are Facilitative.

1. Produce target after initial sound/syllable cue.
2. Produce target after initial letter name, written, and/or spoken.
3. Produce target after cued with word that rhymes.

Retrieval, Levels I or II Tasks

1. Oral reading
2. Writing to dictation
3. Writing to picture-object confrontation

---

and corresponding perceptual dimensions coded by these features—were found to be easier than adjectives defined as "more complex." These findings suggest that semantic properties of words interact with task type, perceptual factors, and type of aphasia on word retrieval tasks. Findings regarding word retrieval at the sentence level are also of interest. Buckley and Noll (1981) evaluated the ability of aphasic adults to recall sentences. They found that operative nouns were more easily recalled than figurative nouns, dynamic verbs were more easily recalled than stative verbs, and high-probability words were more easily recalled than low-probability words.

While disruption of lexical-semantic abilities in aphasia is unquestionably a complex issue, the recent literature has contributed to our understanding of psycholinguistic dimensions relevant to the act of naming. Clinically, it is possible to control stimuli and stimulus contexts along these relevant dimensions to assess the type of anomia and to maximize a patient's success in using his or her lexical repertoire. Fedor (1981), for example, outlined a treatment approach based on organization and retrieval concepts described above and by others (Buckingham & Kertesz, 1974; Goodglass & Baker, 1976; Zurif et al., 1974). As outlined in Table 4-1, Fedor suggests specific treatment tasks depending on two decisions: (1) Is the naming problem one of organization or retrieval? and (2) Does the naming problem occur at the level of meaning (i.e., selecting from the lexical dictionary), or sound (i.e., mapping phonologic representations onto lexical choices)? (A discussion of the interaction of lexical and phonologic disorders is presented later.) When treating anomia, controlling the modality of performance, the intensity of stimulation, and the hierachical presentation of cues is important, as illustrated by Linebaugh and Lehner (1977) and Rosenbek, Green, Flynn, Wertz, and Collins (1977).

Returning to the idea of dissociation, a patient described by Hier and Mohr (1977) is of interest. In this patient, written naming was superior to oral naming—an oral-graphic dissociation. When treating such a patient, one would hope for, but not necessarily observe, generalization from the relatively spared ability (written naming) to the relatively deficient ability (oral naming). A methodology is available for identifying generalization effects, either across behaviors, across modalities, or across stimuli (LaPointe, 1978a). Rosenbek, Becher, Shaughnessy, and Collins (1979) recommend the use of single-case designs for identifying dissociations among behaviors and corresponding generalization effects in treatment. For example, Thompson and Kearns (1981) evaluated acquisition, generalization, and maintenance by an anomic patient for homogeneous lexical sets. In their patient, improvement in recall of treated lexical items did not generalize to untreated semantically related lexemes. In a study of an individual with conduction aphasia, Sanders, Davis, and Hubler (1979) studied generalization across modalities. Specifically, they treated naming ability and measured the effect on repetition ability. Similar performance in both areas during treatment led the authors to tentatively conclude that naming and repetition were not dissociated in their patient, but rather that naming and repetition were governed by interdependent mechanisms. Treatment generalization effects may be related to the form class of the stimuli. For example, retrieval of prepositions was a treatment goal for a chronic Broca's aphasic patient described by Fedor, Schafer, and Horner (1981). This patient was able to learn prepositions in three modalities treated in succession (gesture, oral-verbal, and graphic), but intermodality generalization was minimal, suggesting a three-way dissociation. It is clear that more single-subject studies are needed to identify dissociations of functions and to assess treatment generalization effects.

In summary, recent descriptions of lexical-semantic disruption suggest several clinical implications. Regarding definition of anomia, it is possible to differentiate at least three major types of lexical-semantic difficulty: (1) a problem of access to the semantic properties of words, (2) an impoverishment within a semantic field, or (3) a problem of lexical organization *per se*. The literature also suggests several relevant psycholinguistic dimensions a clinician may control when developing treatment tasks and cueing hierarchies: types of cues and contexts, semantic feature and markedness value, semantic category, word frequency, form class, imageability, and operativity and dynamicity of lexical items. Identification of dissociated functions may be critical to the success of treatment in terms of improvement on the criterion behavior as well as generalization across behaviors, modalities, and stimuli.

Morphosyntactic Disruption

The moderately aphasic individual often has difficulty expressing ideas at the sentence level. Recent research has shown that morphosyntactic performance by aphasic adults is affected by (1) spontaneous (non-constrained) versus constrained task formats, (2) modality of performance, and (3) the length, complexity, and grammatical topography of sentences. Recent advances in the study of morphosyntactic abilities are several. First, the definition of "sentence meaning" has been refined. Second, the concept of syntactic processing is broadened to include syntactic comprehension as well as syntactic production. Third, syntactic processing abilities in different types of aphasia have been distinguished. Fourth, the influence of phonology on syntactic realization is better understood. Finally, the idea that the abilities of the intact minor hemisphere may be used to restore functional language has been proposed. Representative literature will be cited to illustrate these advances.

Recent literature suggests that aphasia-producing lesions may selectively impair the syntactic system independently of the lexical system. To clarify this issue of lexical-syntactic dissociation, Caramazza and Berndt (1978) describe the essential differences between lexical and sentence meaning. They state that lexical meaning and sentence meaning differ in the way they are represented semantically. Three distinctions can be made. First, lexical meaning is fixed, while sentence meaning is novel. Second, the lexicon is acquired through several separate dimensions: phonologic, syntactic, semantic, and (in literate adults) graphemic, while sentence meaning is usually acquired primarily through the auditory modality. Third, words have meaning in isolation, while sentences have meaning only by virtue of word combinations, i.e., sentence meaning involves a "combinatorial operation" wherein a finite set of rules is applied recursively to produce an unlimited number of sentence types. Thus, novelty, the mode of acquisition, and combination rules distinguish sentence meaning from word meaning and help explain why lexical-syntactic dissociations can occur.

Several studies confirm the concept of lexical-syntactic dissociation. Using an anagram "sentence ordering task" von Stockert (1972) observed that an individual with Broca's aphasia performed well when sentence construction depended on major lexical items. Individuals with Wernicke's aphasia, in contrast, performed well when sentence construction (via constituent ordering) depended on the syntactic relations conveyed by grammatical morphemes. It appears from this and subsequent studies (e.g., Gallagher, 1981; Heilman & Scholes, 1976; Rothi, McFarling, & Heilman, 1982) that lexical knowledge is spared and syntactic knowledge is impaired in nonfluent aphasia while the reverse is true in fluent aphasia. This lexical-syntactic processing dissociation has been identified in the comprehension as well as in the production abilities of Broca's and Wernicke's aphasic patients (Gallagher, 1981; Saffran, Schwartz, & Marin, 1980; Zurif & Caramazza, 1976). The idea that lexical-syntactic processing strategies are similar in receptive and expressive modalities supports the psychological reality of a syntactic processing mechanism. Our understanding of "agrammatism" has been enhanced by these recent notions.

The idea that prosodic-phonologic factors influence syntactic processing is another concept that has been recently described. The importance of prosodic features to nonfluent (Broca's) aphasic language was recognized by Goodglass (1968). He proposed a "stress-saliency" hypothesis to explain the preservation or loss of functors in sentences. The term "saliency" refers to informational load, affective tone, and increased intonational emphasis. Goodglass suggested that "...a basic feature of Broca's aphasia is the increased difficulty mobilizing the speech output system which requires a stressed element to put it into action" (1976, p. 252). The stress-saliency hypothesis accounts in part for the telegraphic form of Broca's aphasic speech as well as the effortful and interrupted delivery of speech, notably at phrase boundaries.

Kean (1977) extended this phonologic interpretation of agrammatism. She defined a "phonologic word" as: ". . . the strings of segments marked by boundaries which function in the assignment of stress to a word" (p. 22). As such, the realization of segmental (phoneme) and suprasegmental (stress and intonation) features are inseparable during speech. In Kean's model, affixes and functors are deemed not to be "phonologic words" because, by definition, ". . . they do not carry stress or affect the stress pattern of the sentence" (p. 23). In short, Kean interprets agrammatism to be a phonologic disorder primarily characterized by *phonological simplification of sentences.* The findings of Swinney, Zurif, and Cutler (1980) support Kean's model. They suggest that normal adults use stress in sentence comprehension and production for two purposes: (1) to distinguish among word classes, and (2) to locate high information words.

They suggest that in Broca's aphasia, a deficiency in the assignment of stress accounts for an impaired ability to distinguish substantive (open class) words from function (closed class) words. Because functors are unstressed, difficulties for this class of words ensue in Broca's aphasia. For example, processing of prepositions by agrammatic aphasic individuals is impaired as described in both historical and more recent literature (Friederici, 1981; Mack, 1981; Seron & Deloche, 1981). This current view of the interaction of phonologic-prosodic form with syntactic form represents a significant departure from more traditional models that represent grammatical rules and phonological rules as distinct psycholinguistic entities.

Recent literature also contributes to treatment of aphasic syntactic deficits. In 1972, Goodglass, Green, Bernholtz, and Hyde developed a "Story Completion Task," whereby a variety of increasingly complex phrase and sentence types, as defined by transformational rules, are elicited. Helm-Estabrooks, Fitzpatrick, and Barresi (1981) recently developed a *Syntax Stimulation Program (SSP)* for eight sentence types using this story completion paradigm. Briefly, this approach involves presentation of stories designed to elicit sentences in a hierarchy of difficulty. Two levels of response difficulty are addressed: the first requires the patient to produce a delayed repetition of the target response; the second requires the patient to complete the given story with a self-retrieved target response. All stories are accompanied by line drawings depicting the associated story. Measureable gains in sentence formulation by a chronically agrammatic individual suggest the *SSP* to be an efficacious syntax program.

In 1979, Tonkovich studied the language of a Broca's aphasic individual using Fillmore's case grammar. Fillmore's conception of syntax is that the verb is the core of a sentence and that nouns in sentences assume specific "case relations" to the verb depending on their functions in sentences. For example, the word *table* in the following sentences assumes different cases depending on the context: (1) The *table* fell (objective case); (2) The vase fell from the *table* (source case); (3) She put flowers on the *table* (locative case), etc. (Tonkovich, 1979, p. 245). Tonkovich found that in Broca's aphasia agentive and objective cases were more robust than instrumental, source, or goal cases; semantically similar cases such as source and goal were likely to be confused; and semantically redundant forms were likely to be omitted or in error. As an extension of Fillmore's model, Loverso, Selinger, and Prescott (1979) developed a "verb as core" treatment for aphasic syntactic deficits. In this approach, verbs are used as the pivot-stimuli and wh-questions are provided as cues to elicit sentences of the "actor-action-object" type, both graphically and verbally. Standardized test-retest measures showed this "verbing strategy" to be an effective approach to remediation of sentence formulation deficits.

Finally, a "minor-hemispheric mediation" approach to aphasia treatment has recently been proposed (Horner, 1983; Horner and Fedor, 1983). The underlying assumptions of this model are: (1) under appropriate stimulus conditions, the minor hemisphere can be tapped to mediate language recovery, and (2) the potential for aphasia recovery can be enhanced through systematic pairing of linguistic behaviors with ideographic stimuli, subserved by the domimant and minor hemispheres, respectively. Specific treatment tasks for moderately impaired aphasic individuals presenting either Broca's or Wernicke's aphasia are outlined using three general types of ideographic stimuli: prosodic-affective, visual-spatial-holistic, and rudimentary linguistic behaviors.

In summary, current psycholinguistic notions about syntactic disruption in aphasia were presented. First, syntactic processing may be selectively impaired, suggesting a dissociation from other psycholinguistic functions. Second, syntactic comprehension appears to parallel syntactic production. Third, phonology interacts with syntactic disruption in nonfluent aphasia. Treatment approaches have been described, or suggested, by recent advances. Among these, a "minor hemispheric mediation" approach to treatment of moderate aphasia has been proposed.

Phonologic Disruption

The moderately aphasic individual often suffers an impairment in the phonologic realization of utterances. Phonology encompasses not only the selection and sequencing of phonemes in the creation of words, but also the prosodic ("stress-saliency") dimensions of speech operating at the sentence level. Recent studies of aphasic phonologic disorders suggest that phonologic realization varies as a function of (1) propositional-automatic-imitative constraints, (2) phoneme type, (3) prosodic features, (4) overall speech fluency, and (5) lexical and syntactic features. Representative studies will be reviewed.

Selection and sequencing of sounds is no longer viewed as merely a surface manifestation of language. Phonology is recognized as a rule-governed linguistic system in its own right. Analyses of phonologic errors in aphasia suggest that the psycholinguistic mechanisms governing selection and sequencing of sounds interact in a dynamic if not predictable fashion with lexical-semantic and syntactic subsystems. Furthermore, traditional substitution, omission and distortion analyses are being replaced by distinctive feature, markedness and phonological process analyses of aphasic phonologic disruption.

Kellar and Roch Lecours (1980) and Shewan (1980) discussed two aspects of phonologic production. The first aspect is the internal representation that constitutes the plan for phoneme realization; errors at this level are "phonemic" errors. The second aspect is the internal monitor for speech, which involves organizing the motor commands for sound production *per se*; failures at this level are "phonetic" errors. Conceived as such, aphasic speech sound errors may result from a defect of the "phonological-articulatory" process, i.e., at either the phonemic level, the phonetic level, or both. The important point here is that *common linguistic principles* are likely to influence *both* phonemic and phonetic errors (Goodglass, 1975). This conclusion is drawn in part from Blumstein's early study (1973) in which she found that phonologic error patterns in Broca's, Wernicke's, and Conduction aphasia were *qualitatively* similar. For all three subject groups, two-thirds of phoneme errors differed from the target by one distinctive feature and unmarked-for-marked substitutions outnumbered marked-for-unmarked substitutions 2 to 1. Further analyses revealed differences among the aphasia types: In Broca's aphasia, phonologic processing appeared to operate at the syllabic level, while in Wernicke's and Conduction aphasia, phonologic processing appeared to operate at the level of phrases and sentences. To discern error patterns researchers suggest it is necessary to use stimuli controlled for type of phoneme and phoneme word-position, and to elicit speech in a variety of contexts: self-initiated, automatic, and imitative speech (Burns & Canter, 1977). Furthermore, it is essential that analyses account for the fluent or nonfluent nature of the presenting aphasia (Roch Lecours & Rouillon, 1976).

Recent studies document the interaction of phonology with syntax (see Kean, 1977) and phonology with lexicon. The latter is addressed in recent studies of neologistic jargon aphasia. O'Connell (1981) suggests that neologisms have several sources. A neologism may be: (1) a complex phonemically paraphasic distortion of a correctly retrieved word, (2) a two-stage error where faulty semantic retrieval undergoes phonological disruption, or (3) the product of recombinations of units from surrounding utterances to "fill in" for intended words (O'Connell, 1981, p. 301). O'Connell's first explanation is consistent with a "conduction theory" (Kertesz & Benson, 1970) which suggests that neologisms result from an excessive accumulation of phonemic paraphasias, such that the intended utterance is no longer recognizable. O'Connell's second and third explanations derive from a "masking theory" (Buckingham, 1979) wherein phonologic distortions appear to "fill anomic gaps." A "level of activity notion" proposed by Farmer and O'Connell (1979) suggests that phonemic paraphasias and neologisms reflect an overaroused language system in which selection of both lexical and phonemic units are compromised.

The coincidence of phonologic and lexical-semantic disruption appears to be related to site and extent of lesion. Cappa, Cavallotti, and Vignolo (1981) correlated lesion sites identified by CT scan with prevalence of lexical versus phonemic errors in fluent aphasia. Phonemic errors (phonemic paraphasias, phonemic groping [conduites d'approche], neologisms, and phonemic jargon) correlated with lesions near the sylvian fissure. Lexical errors (circumlocution, verbal paraphasia, semantic jargon) correlated with lesions distant from the sylvian fissure.

Of special interest in recent literature is an innovative application of "phonological process" analysis to description of acquired neurogenic phonologic disorders. Kearns (1980) defines this approach: "Phonological analysis procedures attempt to generate rules which relate phonetic errors to underlying forms and to intended sounds. An important component of the analysis procedure is the incorporation of environmental (contextual) considerations into the rule derivation" (Kearns, 1980, p. 187). Kearns evaluated a moderately aphasic-apraxic adult and identified several general error trends using the "phonological process" analysis. In terms of *syllable structure processes,* final consonant deletion and cluster reduction were observed. In terms of *phonemic substitution processes,* stopping and fronting occurred frequently. The third process, *assimilation,* was also observed. Kearn's study recommends the phonological process approach to the study of phonologic disruption and, potentially, to the development of treatment rationale.

In summary, it is now recognized that phonology is governed by psycholinguistic rules, and that phonology interacts in aphasia syndromes with syntactic and lexical-semantic performance. Although phonologic errors manifest somewhat differently in fluent and nonfluent aphasia syndromes, the commonalities and differences are not yet fully understood. As psycholinguistic principles governing phonologic disruption evolve, it is hoped that corresponding treatment approaches can be developed. Current research suggests that phonologic treatment rationale will necessarily include considerations of prosodic contour, fluency of speech, phonologic contextual influences, and lexical and syntactic constraints as well as the distinctive feature and markedness composition of phonologic error profiles.

Pragmatic Disruption

The final area of concern in this chapter is the area of pragmatic abilities of the moderately impaired aphasic individual. Recent literature emphasizes the need for evaluation of communicative competence as a function complementary to linguistic competence and the importance of incorporating pragmatic considerations in the treatment of aphasic individuals. Representative literature will be reviewed.

By way of introduction to pragmatics, it is necessary to understand the various ways in which meaning is conveyed through language. Meaning can be conveyed by (1) word in isolation (conveying both referential and descriptive meaning), (2) words in relation to other words (semantic fields, features, and networks), (3) words in sentences, and (4) relations among sentences (Lesser, 1978; Schachter, 1976). In the broader perspective of "language pragmatics," the study of meaning involves investigations into how one's communicative intentions are mapped onto linguistic form. Pragmatic rules govern how language is used in social contexts (Bates, 1976) to convey a variety of intentions: requesting, asserting, questioning, ordering, arguing, advising, and warning (Searle, 1969). An individual's use of language based on an understanding of how language works in social interactions is termed "communicative competence" (Holland, 1977, p. 171). Major advances have been made in recent years in the study of pragmatics and communicative competence in aphasia.

One premise of these studies is that functional communication by aphasic adults is not related to the accuracy of utterances but rather to "getting a message across" through the use of both linguistic and paralinguistic behaviors. Studies have found that aphasic adults are limited in the variety of speech acts which they use (Wilcox & Davis, 1977), and are below normal in the proportion of communicative attempts to communicative successes (Holland, 1978). Holland (1977) and Ulatowska, Haynes, Hildebrand, and Richardson (1977) agree that some moderately aphasic individuals are extremely "functional" depending on their use of compensatory strategies. It appears that linguistic competence and communicative competence interact in ways not completely predictable by the overall severity of aphasia.

Studies of comprehension suggest that aphasic individuals who are able to use extralinguistic cues such as contextually conveyed meaning tend to perform better in "real-life situations" than one might expect from their performance on standard aphasia batteries (Stachowiak, Huber, Poeck, & Kerschensteiner, 1977; Wilcox, Davis, & Leonard, 1978). Studies of expression suggest that patients who use a variety of compensatory strategies (e.g., nonverbal signs) are able to convey their intentions, despite linguistic failures (Prinz, 1980).

Chapey and her associates have contributed to our understanding of aphasic communicative competence by studying divergent semantic behavior. Chapey (1977) suggests that aphasic patients may have both convergent and divergent linguistic difficulties. She suggests that many aphasic individuals are functionally deficient in situations that require the use of divergent semantic strategies, i.e., information-getting, problem solving, and persuasion. Chapey, Rigrodsky, and Morrison (1977) further suggest that aphasic individuals are unable to "proliferate" ideas on a topic both in terms of the number and the variety of relevant ideas. Divergent language also involves a "judgment ability," i.e., the ability to evaluate the adequacy of messages and revise them depending on the pragmatic intentions and the demands of the situation. Chapey and Lubinski (1979) found aphasic patients to be below normal in overall semantic judgment scores and suggest that divergent and convergent behaviors are distinct abilities for aphasic individuals. The rationale, principles, and stages of divergent semantic therapy are described by Chapey (1981).

The most notable advances in the area of pragmatics include the development of a test, *Communicative Abilities in Daily Living (CADL)* by Holland (1980) and the development of a treatment approach, *Promoting Aphasics Communicative Effectiveness (PACE)* by Davis and Wilcox (1981). Holland's test has the unique purpose of assessing the "functional communication" of aphasic adults. It provides the clinician with a valuable means of measuring communicative behavior in natural contexts, which may then be compared with the patient's language impairment. Ten functional categories are evaluated using the *CADL* (See Table 4-2).

Regarding treatment, Prinz (1980) advised: "It is incumbent on the clinician to emphasize the patient's communicative assets by providing a conversational setting designed to elicit a variety of pragmatic intentions and the appropriate use of strategies to realize these intentions" (p. 71). Davis (1980) and Davis and Wilcox (1981) attempt to incorporate parameters of natural conversation in aphasia treatment. This treatment approach: (a) emphasizes the use of language in context, (b) controls structural aspects of face-to-face conversation and (c) stimulates the use of nonverbal as well as verbal channels to convey messages. The main goal of the *PACE* approach is the communication of messages, not linguistic accuracy or complexity. Four interdependent principles of *PACE* are:

1. There is an exchange of new information between the clinician and the patient.
2. The patient has a free choice as to which communicative channels he or she may use to convey new information.
3. The clinician and the patient participate equally as senders and receivers of messages.
4. Feedback is provided by the clinician in response to the patient's success in conveying a message. (Davis & Wilcox, 1981, p. 180).

TABLE 4-2
Ten Categories of Performance on the CADL (Holland, 1980).

1. Reading, writing, and using numbers to estimate, calculate, and judge time
2. Speech acts
3. Utilizing verbal and nonverbal context
4. Role playing
5. Sequenced and relationship-dependent communicative behavior
6. Social conventions
7. Divergencies
8. Nonverbal symbolic communication
9. Deixis
10. Humor, absurdity, metaphor

Thus, recent studies of pragmatics and divergent semantic behavior have served to broaden our view of aphasic communicative impairments. Several conclusions from the literature are: (1) the variety of speech acts used by aphasic individuals may be depressed; (2) the contexts in which language is used may be restricted; (3) the adequacy of conveying intentions reflects the interaction of both linguistic competence (divergent and convergent aspects) and communicative competence and (4) communicative competence in part reflects the patient's ability to use alternate (i.e., non-linguistic) communication channels. In general, studies suggest that communicative competence and linguistic competence are not synonymous functions. In an aphasic individual, overall language competence may not always predict his "communicative competence."

In summary, several clinical guidelines from the study of pragmatics are: (1) evaluate communicative competence in a variety of communicative contexts (e.g., *CADL*); (2) control the variety of pragmatic functions (intentions) of speech acts; (3) emphasize communication adequacy over linguistic accuracy; (4) use spontaneous compensatory strategies to enhance communicative effectiveness and/or train the patient in the use of alternate behaviors; (5) train flexibility in the choice of communicative channels (verbal and/or nonverbal); and (6) treat both convergent and divergent semantic abilities.

Summary

Treatment of aphasic individuals requires an appreciation for the nature of language disorganization following focal brain damage. Descriptive psycholinguistic studies have enhanced our appreciation for how linguistic subsystems can be disrupted and/or dissociated, how linguistic subsystems interact with one another, and how aphasic deficits influence the way intact functions emerge in behavior. The clinician's task is not only to describe the degree of language impairment but also to assess the qualitative features of language impairment. The prevalent theme expressed in this chapter is that the psycholinguistic approach to aphasia is particularly well-suited to this qualitative diagnostic purpose. The literature reviewed in this chapter focused on lexical-semantic, morphosyntactic, phonologic, and pragmatic studies of the moderately aphasic individual. From this review it became apparent that an understanding of psycholinguistic mechanisms operating in aphasic language, notably "dissociation of functions," is necessary if aphasia clinicians are to render well-reasoned and effective treatment. Perhaps through a heightened appreciation for the psycholinguistic intricacies of aphasic language we may help our patients realize their full communicative potential.

Note

[1] "Among related categories which differ in markedness, we define the unmarked member as compared to the marked member as: 1) conceptually and/or formally simpler, and therefore more natural, 2) usually statistically more frequent, 3) usually acquired earlier in the process of language development." (Ulatowska & Baker, 1975, p. 153).

Acknowledgment

Funded, in part, by the Axe-Houghton Foundation, New York, NY. My appreciation to Dr. Craig Linebaugh for his review of this chapter.

References

Albert, M. L., Goodglass, H., Helm, N. A., Rubens, A. B., & Alexander, M. P. *Clinical aspects of dysphasia*. New York: Springer-Verlag Wien, 1981.

Bates, E. Pragmatics and sociolinguistics in child language. In D. Morehead & A. Morehead (Eds.), *Directions in normal and deficient child language*. Baltimore: University Park Press, 1976.

Benson, D. F. *Aphasia, alexia, and agraphia*. New York: Churchill Livingstone, 1979. (a)

Benson, D. F. Aphasia. In K. M. Heilman & E. Valenstein (Eds.), *Clinical neuropsychology*. New York: Oxford University Press, 1979, 22–58. (b)

Benson, D. F. Neurologic correlates of anomia. In H. Whitaker & H. A. Whitaker (Eds.), *Studies in neurolinguistics* (Vol. 4). New York: Academic Press, 1979, 293–328. (c)

Berndt, R. S., & Caramazza, A. Syntactic aspects of aphasia. In M. T. Sarno (Ed.), *Acquired aphasia*. New York: Academic Press, 1981, 157–182.

Blumstein, S. E. *A phonological investigation of aphasic speech*. Hague: Mouton, 1973.

Blumstein, S. Phonological aspects of aphasia. In M. T. Sarno (Ed.), *Acquired aphasia*. New York: Academic Press, 1981, 129–156.

Brookshire, R. H. Auditory comprehension and aphasia. In D. F. Johns (Ed.), *Clinical management of neurogenic communicative disorders*. Boston: Little, Brown & Company, 1978, 103–128.

Brookshire, R. H., & Nicholas, L. E. Verification of active and passive sentences by aphasic and nonaphasic subjects. *Journal of Speech and Hearing Research*, 1980, *23*, 878–893. (a)

Brookshire, R. H., & Nicholas, L. E. Sentence verification and language comprehension of aphasic persons. In R. H. Brookshire (Ed.), *Clinical Aphasiology: Conference Proceedings, 1980*. Minneapolis: BRK Publishers, 1980, 53–63. (b)

Brookshire, R. H., & Nicholas, L. E. Comprehension of spoken active and passive sentences by aphasic and nonaphasic subjects. In R. H. Brookshire (Ed.), *Clinical aphasiology: Conference Proceedings, 1981*. Minneapolis: BRK Publishers, 1981, 108–114.

Buckingham, H. W. Linguistic aspects of lexical retrieval disturbances in the posterior fluent aphasias. In H. Whitaker & H. A. Whitaker (Eds.), *Studies in neurolinguistics*, (Vol. 4). New York: Academic Press, 1979, 269–292.

Buckingham, H. W. Lexical and semantic aspects of aphasia. In M. T. Sarno (Ed.), *Acquired aphasia*. New York: Academic Press, 1981, 183–214.

Buckingham, H. W., & Kertesz, A. A linguistic analysis of fluent aphasia. *Brain and Language*, 1974, *1*, 43–62.

Buckingham, H. W., & Rekart, D. M. Semantic paraphasia. *Journal of Communication Disorders*, 1979, *12*, 197–209.

Buckley, C. E., & Noll, J. D. Lexical parameters affecting sentence recall by aphasic adults. In R. H. Brookshire (Ed.), *Clinical aphasiology: Conference proceedings, 1981*. Minneapolis: BRK Publishers, 1981, 96–104.

Burns, M. S., & Canter, G. J. Phonemic behavior of aphasic patients with posterior cerebral lesions. *Brain and Language*, 1977, *4*, 492–507.

Cappa, S., Cavallotti, G., & Vignolo, L. A. Phonemic and lexical errors in fluent aphasia: Correlation with lesion site. *Neuropsychologia*, 1981, *19*, 171–178.

Caramazza, A., & Berndt, R. S. Semantic and syntactic processes in aphasia: A review of the literature, *Psychological Bulletin*, 1978, *85*, 898–918.

Chapey, R. A divergent semantic model of intervention in adult aphasia. In R. H. Brookshire (Ed.), *Clinical Aphasiology: Conference Proceedings, 1977*. Minneapolis: BRK Publishers, 1977, 257–264.

Chapey, R. Divergent semantic intervention. In R. Chapey (Ed.), *Language intervention strategies in adult aphasia*. Baltimore: Williams & Wilkins, 1981.

Chapey, R., & Lubinski, R. Semantic judgment ability in adult aphasia. *Cortex*, 1979, *15*, 247–256.

Chapey, R., Rigrodsky, S., & Morrison, E. M. Aphasia: A divergent semantic interpretation. *Journal of Speech and Hearing Disorders*, 1977, *42*, 287–295.

Davis, G. A. A critical look at PACE therapy. In R. H. Brookshire (Ed.), *Clinical Aphasiology: Conference Proceedings, 1980*. Minneapolis: BRK Publishers, 1980, 248–257.

Davis, G. A., & Wilcox, M. J. Incorporating parameters of natural conversation in aphasia treatment. In R. Chapey (Ed.), *Language intervention strategies in adult aphasia*. Baltimore: Williams & Wilkins, 1981, 169–193.

Drummond, S. S., Gallagher, T. M., & Mills, R. H. Word retrieval in aphasia: An investigation of semantic complexity. *Cortex*, 1981, *17*, 63–82.

Duffy, J. R. Schuell's stimulation approach to rehabilitation. In R. Chapey (Ed.), *Language intervention strategies in adult aphasia*. Baltimore: Williams & Wilkins, 1981, 105–140.

Farmer, A., & O'Connell, P. Neuropsychological processes in adult aphasia: Rationale for treatment. *British Journal of Disorders of Communication*, 1979, *14*, 39–49.

Fedor, K. H. *Semantic disruption in the adult: An organization and retrieval model*. Paper presented to the North Carolina Speech-Language-Hearing Association. Asheville, 1981.

Fedor, K. H., Schafer, N., & Horner, J. *Transcoding across three modalities in Broca's aphasia*. Paper presented to the American Speech-Language-Hearing Association. Los Angeles, 1981.

Friederici, A. D. Production and comprehension of prepositions in aphasia. *Neuropsychologia*, 1981, *19*, 191–200.

Gallagher, A. J. Syntactic versus semantic performance of agrammatic Broca's aphasics on tests of constituent-element-ordering. *Journal of Speech and Hearing Research*, 1981, *24*, 217–223.

Gardner, H. The contribution of operativity to naming capacity in aphasic patients. *Neuropsychologia*, 1973, *11*, 213–220.

Geschwind, N. Disconnexion syndromes in animals and man. *Brain*, 1965, *88*, 237–294, 585–644. (a)

Geschwind, N. The varieties of naming errors. *Cortex*, 1965, *3*, 97–112. (b)

Goodglass, H. Studies on the grammar of aphasics. In S. Rosenberg & J. Koplin (Eds.), *Developments in applied psycholinguistic research*. New York: Macmillan, 1968.

Goodglass, H. Phonological factors in aphasia. In R. H. Brookshire (Ed.), *Clinical Aphasiology: Conference Proceedings, 1975*. Minneapolis: BRK Publishers, 1975, 28–44.

Goodglass, H. Agrammatism. In H. Whitaker & H. A. Whitaker (Eds.), *Studies in neurolinguistics* (Vol. 1). New York: Academic Press, 1976, 237–260.

Goodglass, H., & Baker, E. Semantic field, naming and auditory comprehension in aphasia. *Brain and Language*, 1976, *3*, 359–374.

Goodglass, H., & Kaplan, E. *The Boston Diagnostic Aphasia Exam*. Philadelphia: Lea & Febiger, 1972. (a)

Goodglass, H., & Kaplan, E. *Assessment of aphasia and related disorders*. Philadelphia: Lea & Febiger, 1972. (b)

Goodglass, H., Barton, M. I., & Kaplan, E. Sensory modality and object-naming in aphasia. *Journal of Speech and Hearing Research*, 1968, *3*, 257–267.

Goodglass, H., Hyde, M. R., & Blumstein, S. Frequency, picturability and availability of nouns in aphasia. *Cortex*, 1969, *5*, 104–119.

Goodglass, H., Kaplan, E., Weintraub, S., & Ackerman, N. The tip-of-the-tongue phenomenon in aphasia. *Cortex*, 1976, *12*, 145–153.

Goodglass, H., Gleason, J. B., Bernholtz, N. A., & Hyde, M. R. Some linguistic structures in the speech of a Broca's aphasic. *Cortex*, 1972, *8*, 191–212.

Grober, E., Perceman, E., Kellar, L., & Brown, J. Lexical knowledge in anterior and posterior aphasics. *Brain and Language*, 1980, *10*, 318–330.

Hand, C. R., Tonkovich, J. D., & Aitchison, J. Some idiosyncratic strategies utilized by a chronic Broca's aphasic. *Linguistics*, 1979, *17*, 729–761.

Helm-Estabrooks, N., Fitzpatrick, P. M., & Barresi, B. Response of an agrammatic patient to a syntax stimulation program for aphasia. *Journal of Speech and Hearing Disorders*, 1981, *46*, 422–427.

Heilman, K. M., & Scholes, R. J. The nature of comprehension errors in Broca's conduction and Wernicke's aphasics. *Cortex*, 1976, *12*, 258–265.

Hier, D. B., & Mohr, J. P. Incongruous oral and written naming. Evidence for a subdivision of Wernicke's aphasia. *Brain and Language*, 1977, *4*, 115–126.

Holland, A. L.   Case studies in aphasia rehabilitation using programmed instruction. *Journal of Speech and Hearing Disorders*, 1972, *37*, 3–21.

Holland, A. L.   Some practical considerations in aphasia rehabilitation. In M. Sullivan & M. S. Kommers (Eds.), *Rationale for adult aphasia therapy*. Omaha: University of Nebraska, 1977, 167–180.

Holland, A. L.   Functional communication in the treatment of aphasia. In L. J. Bradford (Ed.), *Communication disorders: An audio journal for continuing education* (Vol. 3). New York: Grune & Stratton, 1978.

Holland, A. L.   *CADL: Communicative abilities in daily living*. Baltimore: University Park Press, 1980.

Horner, J.   Broca's aphasia: Facilitation and reorganization. In W. H. Perkins (Ed.), *Current therapy of communication disorders*. New York: Thieme-Stratton, 1983.

Horner, J., & Fedor, K. H.   Minor hemisphere mediation in aphasia treatment. In H. Winitz (Ed.), *Treating language disorders: For clinicians by clinicians*. Baltimore: University Park Press, 1983.

Kean, M. L.   The linguistic interpretation of aphasic syndromes: Agrammatism in Broca's aphasia, an example. *Cognition*, 1977, *5*, 9–46.

Kearns, K. P.   The application of phonological process analysis to adult neuropathologies In R. H. Brookshire (Ed.), *Clinical Aphasiology: Conference Proceedings, 1980*. Minneapolis: BRK Publishers, 1980, 187–195.

Kellar, E., & Roch Lecours, A.   Sequences of phonemic approximations in aphasia. *Brain and Language*, 1980, *11*, 30–44.

Kertesz, A.   *Aphasia and associated disorders: Taxonomy, localization, and recovery*. New York: Grune & Stratton, 1979.

Kertesz, A.   *Western Aphasia Battery*. London, Canada: University of Western Ontario, 1980.

Kertesz, A., & Benson, D.   Neologistic jargon: A clinicopathological study. *Cortex*, 1970, *6*, 362–386.

LaPointe, L. L.   Base-10 programmed-stimulation: Task specification, scoring and plotting performance in aphasia therapy. *Journal of Speech and Hearing Disorders*, 1977, *42*, 90–105.

LaPointe, L. L.   Aphasia therapy: Some principles and strategies for treatment. In D. F. Johns (Ed.), *Clinical management of neurogenic communicative disorders*. Boston: Little, Brown & Co., 1978, 129–190. (a)

LaPointe, L. L.   Multiple baseline designs. In R. H. Brookshire (Ed.), *Clinical Aphasiology: Conference Proceedings, 1978*. Minneapolis: BRK Publishers, 1978, 20–39. (b)

Lesser, R.   *Linguistic investigations of aphasia*. New York: Elsevier, 1978.

Linebaugh, C., & Lehner, L.   Cueing hierarchies and word retrieval: A therapy program. In R. H. Brookshire (Ed.), *Clinical Aphasiology: Conference Proceedings, 1977*. Minneapolis: BRK Publishers, 1977, 19–31.

Loverso, F. L., Selinger, M., & Prescott, T. E.   Applications of verbing strategies to aphasia treatment. In R. H. Brookshire (Ed.), *Clinical Aphasiology: Conference Proceedings, 1979*. Minneapolis: BRK Publishers, 1979, 229–238.

Luria, A. R.   *Higher cortical functions in man*. New York: Basic Books, 1966.

Mack, J. L.   The comprehension of locative prepositions in nonfluent and fluent aphasia. *Brain and Language*, 1981, *14*, 81–92.

Marin, O. S. M., Saffran, E. M., & Schwartz, M. F.   Dissociations of language in aphasia: Implications for normal function. *Annals of the New York Academy of Science*, 1976, *280*, 868–884.

Martin, A. D.   A proposed rationale for aphasia therapy. In B. Porch (Ed.), *Clinical Aphasiology: Conference Proceedings, 1974*. Albuquerque, NM, 1974, 79–94.

Martin, A. D. An examination of Wepman's thought centered therapy. In R. Chapey (Ed.), *Language intervention strategies in adult aphasia*. Baltimore: Williams & Wilkins, 1981, 141–154.

Marshall, T. D., & Ewanowski, S. J. *The effects of linguistic context on the word finding abilities of aphasic adults*. Paper presented to the American Speech-Language-Hearing Association, Houston, 1976.

Milberg, W., & Blumstein, S. E. Lexical decision and aphasia: Evidence for semantic processing. *Brain and Language*, 1981, *14*, 371–385.

Myerson, R., & Goodglass, H. Transformational grammars of aphasic patients. *Language and Speech*, 1972, *15*, 40–50.

O'Connell, P. F. Neologistic jargon aphasia: A case report. *Brain and Language*, 1981, *12*, 292–302.

Pease, D. M., & Goodglass, H. The effects of cueing on picture naming in aphasia. *Cortex*, 1978, *14*, 178–189.

Podraza, B.L., & Darley, F. L. Effect of auditory prestimulation on naming in aphasia. *Journal of Speech and Hearing Research*, 1977, *20*, 669–683.

Porch, B. *The Porch Index of Communicative Ability*. Palo Alto, CA: Consulting Psychologists Press, 1967.

Porch, B. E. Therapy subsequent to the *PICA*. In R. Chapey (Ed.), *Language intervention strategies in adult aphasia*. Baltimore: Williams & Wilkins, 1981, 283–296.

Prinz, P. M. A note on requesting strategies in adult aphasics. *Journal of Communication Disorders*, 1980, *13*, 65–73.

Roch Lecours, A., & Rouillon, F. Neurolinguistic analysis of jargonaphasia and jargonagraphia. In H. Whitaker & H. A. Whitaker (Eds.), *Studies in neurolinguistics* (Vol. 2). New York: Academic Press, 1976, 95–144.

Rosenbek, J., Becher, B., Shaughnessy, A., & Collins, M. Other uses of single-case designs. In R. H. Brookshire (Ed.), *Clinical Aphasiology: Conference Proceedings, 1979*. Minneapolis: BRK Publishers, 1979, 311–316.

Rosenbek, J., Green, E., Flynn, M., Wertz, R. T., & Collins, M. Anomia: A clinical experiment. In R. H. Brookshire (Ed.), *Clinical Aphasiology: Conference Proceedings, 1977*. Minneapolis: BRK Publishers, 1977, 103–111.

Rosenbek, J. C., Lemme, M. L., Ahern, M. B., Harris, E. H., & Wertz, R. T. A treatment for apraxia of speech in adults. *Journal of Speech and Hearing Disorders*, 1973, *38*, 462–472.

Rothi, L. J., McFarling, D., & Heilman, K. M. Conduction aphasia, syntactic alexia, and the anatomy of syntactic comprehension. *Archives of Neurology*, 1982, *39*, 272–275.

Saffran, E. M, Schwartz, M. F., & Marin, O. S. M. The word order problem in agrammatism. II. Production. *Brain and Language*, 1980, *10*, 263–280.

Sanders, S. B., Davis, G. A., & Hubler, V. A study of the interdependence of word retrieval and repetition in conduction aphasia. In R. H. Brookshire (Ed.), *Clinical Aphasiology: Conference Proceedings, 1979*. Minneapolis: BRK Publishers, 1979, 270-277.

Schachter, J. Some semantic prerequisites for a model of language. *Brian and Language*, 1976, *3*, 292–304.

Schuell, H., Jenkins, J., & Jiménez-Pabón, E. *Aphasia in adults*. New York: Harper & Row, 1964.

Searle, J. R. *Speech acts*. London: Cambridge University Press, 1969.

Seron, X., & Deloche, G. Processing of locatives "in," "on," and "under" by aphasic patients: An analysis of the regression hypothesis. *Brain and Language*, 1981, *14*, 70–80.

Shewan, C. M. Phonological processing in Broca's aphasics. *Brain and Language*, 1980, *10*, 71–88.

Stachowiak, F. J., Huber, W., Poeck, K., & Kerschensteiner. Comprehension in aphasia. *Brain and Language*, 1977, *4*, 177–195.

Swinney, D. A., Zurif, E. B., & Cutler, A. Effects of sentential stress and word class upon comprehension in Broca's aphasics. *Brain and Language*, 1980, *10*, 132–144.

Thompson, C. K., & Kearns, K. An experimental analysis of acquisition, generalization and maintenance of naming behavior in a patient with anomic aphasia. In R. H. Brookshire (Ed.), *Clinical Aphasiology: Conference Proceedings, 1981.* Minneapolis: BRK Publishers, 1981, 35–45.

Tonkovich, J. D. Case relations in Broca's aphasia: Some considerations regarding treatment. In R. H. Brookshire (Ed.), *Clinical Aphasiology: Conference Proceedings. 1979.* Minneapolis: BRK Publishers, 1979, 239–247.

Ulatowska, H. K. Application of linguistics to treatment of aphasia. In R. H. Brookshire (Ed.), *Clinical Aphasiology: Conference Proceedings. 1979.* Minneapolis: BRK Publishers, 1979, 317–323.

Ulatowska, H. K., & Baker W. D. On a notion of markedness in linguistic systems: Application to aphasia. In R. H. Brookshire (Ed.), *Clinical Aphasiology: Conference Proceedings. 1975.* Minneapolis: BRK Publishers, 1975, 153–164.

Ulatowska, H. K., Haynes, S. M., Hildebrand, D. H., & Richardson, S. M. The aphasic individual: A speaker and listner, not a patient. In R. H. Brookshire (Ed.), *Clinical Aphasiology: Conference Proceedings. 1977.* Minneapolis: BRK Publishers, 1977, 198–213.

von Stockert, T. R. Recognition of syntactic structure in aphasic patients. *Cortex*, 1972, *8*, 323–334.

Wales, R., & Kinsella, G. Syntactic effects in sentence completion by Broca's aphasics. *Brain and Language*, 1981, *13*, 301–307.

Weigl, E., & Bierwisch, M. Neuropsychology and linguistics: Topics of common research. *Foundations of language*, 1970, *6*, 1–18.

Weigl, E., & Fradis, A. The transcoding processes in patients with agraphia to dictation. *Brain and Language*, 1977, *4*, 11–22.

Wepman, J. Aphasia therapy: A new look. *Journal of Speech and Hearing Disorders*, 1972, *37*, 203–214.

Wilcox, M. J., & Davis, G. A. Speech act analysis of aphasic communication in individual and group settings. In R. H. Brookshire (Ed.), *Clinical Aphasiology: Conference Proceedings. 1977.* Minneapolis: BRK Publishers, 1977, 166–174.

Wilcox, M. J., Davis, G. A., & Leonard, L. B. Aphasics' comprehension of contextually conveyed meaning. *Brain and Language*, 1978, *6*, 362–377.

Williams, S. E., & Canter, G. On the assessment of naming disturbances in adult aphasia. In R. H. Brookshire (Ed.), *Clinical Aphasiology: Conference Proceedings. 1981.* Minneapolis: BRK Publishers, 1981, 155–165.

Zurif, E. G., & Caramazza, A. Psycholinguistic structures in aphasia: Studies in syntax and semantics. In H. Whitaker & H. A. Whitaker (Eds.), *Studies in neurolinguistics* (Vol. 1). New York: Academic Press, 1976, 261–292.

Zurif, E., Caramazza, A., Myerson, R., & Calvin, J. Semantic feature representation for normal and aphasic language. *Brain and Language*, 1974, *1*, 167–187.

Nancy Helm-Estabrooks

Severe Aphasia

Severe Aphasia Defined

The diagnosis of severe acquired aphasia indicates that an individual no longer is able to use the primary (verbal expression and comprehension) and secondary (writing and reading comprehension) language modalities for successful communicative interchange. Such an individual may earn an aphasia severity rating of 0 or 1 on the Boston Diagnostic Aphasia Examination (Goodglass & Kaplan, 1972a, 1972b) with a score of 0 indicating "no usable speech or auditory comprehension" and a score of 1 indicating "all communication is through fragmentary expression, great need for inference, questioning, and guessing by the listener. The range of information which can be exchanged is limited, and the listener carries the burden of communication."

An aphasia severity rating should be based on both conversational and expository speech samples, and the patient's ability to produce or comprehend written messages. The reason for this is that certain syndromes may affect only verbal production or auditory comprehension while other language areas and pathways remain intact. The patient with aphemia, for example, may be unable to communicate verbally, but have normal writing, auditory, and reading comprehension skills (Albert, Goodglass, Helm, Rubens, & Alexander, 1981). Aphemia and pure word deafness, a syndrome which affects only auditory process, are not truly aphasic syndromes because language per se is not impaired. Patients with these disorders may be misdiagnosed as having severe aphasia if reading and writing skills are not considered.

Encompassing Syndromes

The term severe aphasia is a quantitative one insofar as it refers to a significant degree of language impairment. Although this term most typically is associated with the syndrome called *global aphasia*, other aphasic syndromes and conditions can quantitatively be classified as severe. Among these are: severe *Broca's aphasia*, *severe Wernicke's aphasia*, and mixed *transcortical aphasia*. Added to these distinct syndromes are the cases of nonclassifiable severe aphasia, that is, patients whose language profiles do not coincide with those of specific aphasia syndromes. All such classes of patients may earn similar low scores on the BDAE aphasia severity rating. Qualitatively, however, they may be quite distinguishable both in terms of behavior and site of brain lesions. Likewise, although the common clinical goal for these patients is to regain functional communication skills, the treatments will vary qualitatively among patients, so that a prescriptive approach cannot be followed. Instead, the clinician must approach each severely aphasic patient as an individual who brings to language tasks a unique set of spared and impaired skills. These assets and deficits can be identified, described, and understood in such a way that the spared neurobehavioral features serve as a means for regaining or circumventing those which *appear* lost.

This chapter addresses the treatment of severe aphasia. It does not offer prescriptions. Rather, it suggests a *qualitative* approach to the most devastating of human social problems. This approach will be illustrated through case studies of patients, all of whom were diagnosed quantitatively as having severe aphasia, but who were qualitatively quite different and thus were treated according to their individual neurobehavioral profiles and not according to a diagnostic label.

The Qualitative Approach To Severe Aphasia

Perhaps no other aphasic condition requires quite so careful a diagnostic evaluation as severe aphasia. This statement may appear incongruous to clinicians who would point out that severely aphasic patients will perform poorly in all language modalities and, therefore, will earn poor scores on many of the standardized measures of aphasia. The rhetorical question for them becomes, "What's to test?" "They can't do *anything*." It may *never* be the case, however, that severely aphasic patients can do "nothing," but only careful assessment will reveal the exact nature of the patient's retained skills. In addition to standardized testing, assessment will require nonstandardized administration of standardized assessment tools and administration of informal tests. Above all, it will require that the clinician describe the patients' response to each test item, rather than simply scoring those responses. As noted above, the severely aphasic patient, by definition, will have low scores on language tests. Merely confirming that fact is not only uninteresting, it contributes nothing to the treatment plan, particularly if one is to use retained skills as a rehabilitative springboard.

It is axiomatic that aphasia therapy should begin where the patient has the greatest chance of success. With severely aphasic patients, identification of the patients' strengths presents a significant challenge. To meet that challenge, we may have to call upon colleagues, such as neuropsychologists, and other allied health and medical personnel, as well as family members.

Examples of all of the above will serve to clarify the qualitative approach to severe aphasia.

Noting the Nature
of the Response

With the possible exception of the Porch Index of Communicative Abilities multidimensional scoring system (Porch, 1971), a simple score earned on a test is not particularly informative and contributes little to the treatment plan. In the case of severe aphasia, it is important to know *what* the patient did when he or she failed to perform correctly. For example, a hypothetical patient may have given the following responses during administration of the Boston Diagnostic Aphasia Exam (BDAE): Instead of repeating the word "chair" correctly, he said "I don't know." When asked to point to the picture *cactus*, he pointed to *hammock*. Instead of writing his whole name, he wrote the first three letters then began to perseverate on the third. Realizing his errors, he threw down the pen. When asked to match the written word *circle* to its geometric representation, he matched it instead to *square*.

Rather than assigning scores of zero to each of these responses, the clinician should record or describe each unique response, because these and similiar pieces of information are crucial to understanding the patient's assets and deficits. In the above example, the first response tells us that the patient has some capacity for meaningful speech (he said "I don't know"). The second response tells us that he knows or appreciates that "cactus" is an object and not a letter or color (semantic categories also represented on the test card). The third response indicates that he recognizes when he is writing inappropriate letters and is appropriately frustrated (he threw down his pen when he began to perseverate), and the final one, wherein he matched the word *circle* with a square, suggests that he may have a form of "deep dyslexia," in which a close semantic reading error is made (Marshall & Newcombe, 1973).

Given this and similiar pieces of qualitative information regarding the patient's performance, the clinician is ready to explore the effects of a nonstandardized administration of the same tasks.

Non-Standardized Administration of Standardized Tests

While the patient described above earned low scores on a standard administration of the BDAE, nonetheless he offered a rich variety of responses. The clinical question now becomes, "What will happen to the patient's performance if I change X?" Some examples of the way one might approach this question are offered below.

Auditory Comprehension

Instead of pointing to the BDAE picture of the *cactus*, the patient pointed to *hammock*. If an audiogram has already established an adequate level of speech reception, the BDAE task itself can be altered to investigate auditory comprehension further. In the standardized format, word discrimination is tested with two cards (7" x 10") with 18 items each, offered one at a time. These items are divided into three semantic categories (card 1 = objects, letters, colors; card 2 = actions, geometric forms, and numbers). It is possible, given this array, that visual scanning, visual discrimination, or figure/ground problems may complicate the assessment of auditory comprehension for single words. If, however, the individual components of the pictures are cut out and placed farther apart on a dark background, the patient's performance on this task may change. This point was demonstrated quite dramatically with a 63-year-old patient. At the time of hospital discharge, four months following onset of a stroke, he earned a score of 46/72 on the BDAE word-discrimination subtest. Approximately three months later, he was readmitted after a second stroke and found to have a score of 27/72, indicating that his auditory comprehension problems were now in the severe range. When this BDAE subtest was readministered using the cut-up stimuli, however, he earned a score of 47/72, indicating that the new stroke had not exacerbated his previously moderate auditory comprehension deficit. Instead, it appeared to have caused visual-spatial or visual discrimination problems which interfered with his ability to select pictured stimuli from a composite card. Thus, a nontraditional administration of this standardized auditory comprehension test contributed valuable information which could be used in designing a treatment plan.

Writing

The hypothetical patient described earlier was unable to write his name because of perseveration problems. Typically, writing skills are tested with the BDAE by offering the patient an unlined 8½" x 11" piece of paper placed lengthwise. This allows us to assess visual field neglect and inability to maintain the horizontal plane. Perseveration after the first few correctly formed letters is not an uncommon phenomenon. If such a patient is allowed to "window-write," however, this phenomenon may cease to occur. In "window-writing," the clinician cuts a small square opening in an index card, places the card on unlined paper, and instructs the patient to write the first letter of the target word in the opening, or window. The card is then moved to allow for the next letter. The patient is unable to see the previous letter and, thus, is not "pulled" to that letter. In the case of a long word, the clinician may have to remind or show the patient what letter(s) he or she has already written, as the "window-writing" process is a somewhat slow and laborious one, and the patient may forget what has gone before. This approach does allow us, however, to sort out what may be a visual "pull" form of perseveration from a spelling problem or motor perseveration, an important distinction when planning treatment.

Reading

The BDAE tests the comprehension of printed words by asking patients to look at a word and then point to its pictured representation on one of the two composite cards described above. Our hypothetical patient pointed to *square* after reading "circle," thus showing a semantic appreciation of the target word. Given that the BDAE pictures are black line drawings on a white background, figure/ground problems rather than "deep dyslexia" possibly underlie such an error. The visual problem may be circumvented by coloring in the line drawing and thus allowing a fairer assessment of the ability to comprehend written words. We recently saw a patient who could not match unshaded line drawings to real objects at better than chance level. Once the drawings were shaded in, his performance was 100%, and he went on to successfully complete a program of Visual Action Therapy (Helm-Estabrooks, Fitzpatrick, & Barresi, 1982).

These examples serve to illustrate how nonstandardized administration of standardized tests may provide the clinician with valuable diagnostic and treatment-planning information. Another important source of information comes from the administration of nonstandardized or informal tests.

Informal Tests

Severely aphasic patients sometimes have retained ability to understand and execute "whole body" commands, that is, commands carried out using axial pathways (Geschwind, 1967; Johnson, Sahoske, Grembowski, & Rubens, 1976), yet few, if any, formal aphasia tests assess this ability. Any clinician who is expected to treat a patient with severely impaired auditory comprehension, therefore, must construct an informal test of whole-body commands such as "stand up," "turn around," "bend over," "stand like a boxer," "take a bow." As Johnson et al. have suggested, the preserved ability to follow axial commands may serve as basis for treating severe aphasia.

Similarly, clinicians are advised to test both limb and facial praxis skills in severely aphasic patients. Degradation of these skills often co-occurs with severe language problems (DeRenzi, Pieczuro, & Vignolo, 1966; Liepman, 1905). Just as facial apraxia may interfere with speech production, limb apraxia may interfere with the execution of symbolic gestures and/or writing. Thus, severe apraxia may effectively block outgoing communication pathways and require specific therapeutic intervention.

Another valuable source of information not assessed by standardized tests relates to the patient's ability to communicate *nonvocally* in a natural setting. Experienced clinicians know that some patients can earn poor scores on formal tests of aphasia but seem to interact quite successfully in their daily environments. Realizing how important this information is for both planning and assessing the effects of therapy, our staff developed a simple nonvocal communication scale to be rated by family members, nursing staff, and other members of the rehabilitation team. It meets none of the requirements for a standardized test, but it does meet a clinical need.

Finally, informal tests can be used to delineate further a skill already evaluated by a standardized test. For example, the hypothetical patient described above earned a score of 0/10 on the BDAE subtest of word repetition, but he clearly said "I don't know" for *chair*. Can he now repeat the phrase "I don't know"? Our ongoing study of a treatment approach called Voluntary Control of Involuntary Utterances (Helm & Barresi, 1980), shows that severely aphasic patients, indeed, may repeat their real word stereotypes and involuntary verbalizations. Furthermore, patients can often correctly read these utterances aloud, despite failure to read BDAE subtest words aloud. This preserved ability can serve as a basis for treatment, as will be demonstrated in a case study to follow.

Obtaining Critical Information from Others

The nonvocal communication scale mentioned above is rated by a variety of people who interact with the severely aphasic patient. These people also may serve as a good source of information regarding the patient's verbal successes and failures. Holland (1982) has shown that even severely aphasic patients (according to standardized test results) may communicate successfully, using a variety of verbal strategies in settings outside the language-therapy room. This kind of information can be incorporated into the treatment plan. For example, we treated a globally aphasic patient who, according to the nursing staff, drew a toilet and a bottle of milk of magnesia when they failed to understand his verbal and gestural attempts to tell them he was constipated. We then discovered that when this patient was allowed to depict target messages graphically, his ability to verbalize these messages improved dramatically. Perhaps the best example of the use of drawing for rehabilitation of severe aphasia is seen in the work of Van Eeckhout, Pillon, Signoret, and Lhermitte (1981). By encouraging a former cartoonist with a right hemiplegia and global aphasia to express himself through left-hand drawing, these investigators were able to develop a rehabilitation program which has resulted in two published books for aphasic patients (Lorant, Van Eeckhout, & Sabadel, 1980; Van Eeckhout & Sabadel, 1982). It should be noted that during the process of working on left-handed drawing the patient began to show recovery of verbal skills.

While informal observations made by our colleagues may offer valuable cues as to the patient's capacity for and mode of communication, their formal observations may prove even more valuable. For example, we used Visual Action Therapy in an attempt to treat one nonglobal, but severely aphasic patient, who failed to respond to any of several verbal/auditory treatment methods. With Visual Action Therapy he progressed rapidly to the final step of Level I. This step requires the patient to look at two objects, and watch while both are hidden for a few seconds. The clinician then returns one object to the patient's view and the patient must gesturally represent the object which remains hidden. This particular patient was unable to remember which item remained hidden. We conferred with the neuropsychologist, who informed us that the patient had performed poorly on tests of both verbal and nonverbal short-term memory. A check of his CT (computerized tomographical) scan showed two left-hemisphere lesions, one of which involved the middle temporal gyrus extending into the inferior temporal gyrus. Horel (1978) suggests that this area may play a role in human memory. These neuropsychological and CT scan findings appeared sufficient to explain the patient's failure to respond to any of our treatment approaches and he was discharged.

As this case demonstrates, knowledge of lesion localization is of more than academic interest to the speech/language pathologist. The site and extent of the brain lesion may be crucial to planning the treatment approach. Another example of the value of CT scan information for aphasia rehabilitation is a study which retrospectively examined the relationship between lesion sites and response to Melodic Intonation Therapy (Helm, Naeser, & Kleefield, 1980). Two of the four patients who responded poorly to MIT had small right hemisphere lesions in addition to a significant left hemisphere lesion. Although they were able to complete the Melodic Intonation Therapy program, their conversational speech did not improve. This information can be used to help determine whether future patients are candidates for this particular treatment approach. Furthermore, this finding lends some credence to the notion that Melodic Intonation Therapy exploits intact right hemisphere functions such as appreciation of melody (Kimura, 1964) and intonation (Blumstein & Cooper, 1974) for purposes of aphasia rehabilitation (Helm-Estabrooks, 1983b).

Thus, lesion localization is an important part of the diagnostic evaluation and treatment plan and, whenever possible, the speech-language pathologist should request and receive this or other neurological information. Just as it is necessary to identify preserved areas of performance, it is necessary, when treating severely aphasic patients, to identify preserved areas of the brain.

Treating Severe Aphasia: Five Case Studies

Global Syndromes

Individuals with global aphasia are severely impaired in their ability to perform through any language modality. In addition, global aphasic patients may have oral/facial and limb apraxia as part of their symptom complex. Classically, global aphasia is associated with a large left hemisphere lesion which destroys the cortical frontotemporo parietal language zones and extends deeply into the white matter (Albert, Goodglass, Helm, Rubens, & Alexander, 1981). Recent research using CT scan localization techniques and BDAE test results, however, show that a relatively smaller, and mostly subcortical, lesion involving the internal capsule and putamen may undercut the primary language zones and produce a global aphasia (Naeser, Alexander, Helm-Estabrooks, Levine, Laughlin, & Geschwind, 1982).

Case I: Global Aphasia

Neurobehavioral Characteristics. Patient A was a 56-year-old right-hemiparetic male, 3-months post onset of a left hemisphere stroke when we first saw him. Administration of the Boston Diagnostic Aphasia Examination showed him to have a severe aphasia, earning a severity rating of .5 for his ability to converse and describe the "Cookie Theft" picture. His verbalizations were restricted to "good," "no," "I don't know," and "okay." His overall auditory comprehension Z score was −1.0 standard deviation away from the norm for aphasic patients. Of the four BDAE auditory comprehension subtests, his relatively worse performance was on word discrimination, earning only 17 out of 72 points. He had no ability to name items verbally, or to produce automatized verbal sequences. He repeated 3/10 words, but could not repeat sentences. By contrast, he wrote 20 numbers, 9 letters, and the words "key" and "chair" in a written confrontation naming task. His symbol discrimination was excellent. He matched all 10-letter/word stimuli to their differently written counterparts, e.g., matching block printing to cursive script. Reading comprehension was less spared, with earned scores of 4/10 on word/picture matching and 3/10 on sentences and paragraphs.

A's overall PICA score was 7.07. He earned 7.41 on gestural subtests, 4.25 on verbal subtests, and 7.23 on graphic subtests. He refused to produce pantomimes for subtests II and III, and his comprehension of verbs and nouns was 6.9 and 5.5, respectively.

Praxis examination showed him to have severe facial, but only moderate limb apraxia. Neuropsychological testing indicated relatively good visual skills. On the "parietal lobe" battery, he earned 9.5/13 for drawing, 8/10 for constructing block designs, and 12/12 for reproducing stick designs. CT scanning showed a subcortical, putaminal lesion. A was concerned, cooperative, alert, and motivated.

Course of Treatment. A's test results indicated good visual and matching skills (10/10 word discrimination, 15 on PICA subtest VIII, and good block and stick designs) and only moderate limb apraxia. On the basis of these preserved skills, A was entered into a course of Visual Action Therapy (VAT). This method trains patients to produce symbolic hand gestures for hidden items. VAT has been described elsewhere (Helm-Estabrooks, 1983 (a); Helm-Estabrooks, Fitzpatrick, & Barresi, 1982).

Following a one-month, completed course of VAT (approximately 20 sessions), A earned an overall PICA score of 9.25, with 10.6 gestural, 6.68 verbal, and 9.16 graphic scores.

Because he was now producing more spontaneous speech, A was entered into a course of Voluntary Control of Involuntary Utterances described below in association with another case.

Unclassifiable
Severe Aphasia

Perhaps 60% of the aphasic population can be classified into specific aphasia syndromes (M. Alexander, personal communication). For example, the syndrome known as global aphasia is associated with severe impairment of all language modalities, yet some patients have severely restricted verbal and written output but relatively more intact auditory and reading comprehension skills. While not truly *globally* aphasic, nonetheless, these patients are *severely* aphasic. Because the clinician often is called upon to rehabilitate such patients, two cases will be described here.

Case II: Unclassifiable
Severe Aphasia

Neurobehavioral Characteristics. Patient B was a 55-year-old, right-hemiplegic male who was two months beyond a left hemisphere stroke when we first saw him. On the basis of conversational and expository speech, he was assigned an aphasia severity rating of .5. He had no "running" speech but, instead, produced occasional utterances such as "oh," "yes," "no," and the nonsense-stereotype "oh-win-ee-oh." His overall auditory comprehension score was − .25 standard deviation from the mean for aphasic individuals. He had marked oral/facial, and limb apraxia. He produced no verbal naming, repetition, automatized speech, oral reading, singing, or rhythms.

Islands of preserved language ability were: good auditory comprehension of nouns, verbs, and one- and two-stage commands; good comprehension of written language (8/10 for word/picture matching, 8/10 for sentences and paragraphs); ability to write the names of 9/10 items in a written confrontation-naming task. Examination of his incorrect verbal responses showed that he said "who" when asked to blow, and "I go" when asked to repeat "I got home." He also said "mama" and "thanks" during the test for verbal agility.

His untimed Wechsler Adult Intelligence Scale performance IQ was 108. CT scanning showed a patchy cortical lesion in Wernicke's area with a more complete lesion in the white matter deep to Wernicke's area. The largest portion of the lesion involved the anterior supramarginal gyrus, corona radiata, and periventricular white matter lateral to the body of the lateral ventricle. There was no lesion in or deep to Broca's area. He was alert, cooperative, appropriately concerned, frustrated, and eager to work.

Course of Treatment. Although B was unable to read any BDAE words aloud, clinical experience with other patients suggested that B might be able to read words orally that he had produced spontaneously in other contexts. This proved to be the case. When presented with *oh*, *mama*, *thanks*, *I go*, *you*, *no*, and *who*, he read these aloud. Importantly, we knew from his good BDAE reading comprehension scores that this oral reading was not an automatic, meaningless exercise for him. To the original list, we then added words with emotional value, such as *love* and *die*. In keeping with the findings of Landis, Graves, and Goodglass (1982), we have found that some severely aphasic patients are able to read such words far better than emotionally neutral words. B was no exception. He easily read "love" and "die." Each word then was printed separately on 3" x 5" cards for self-practice. His reading list soon consisted of many emotion-laden words, including *fun*, *hit*, *lucky*, *ouch*, *shame*, *bull*, and *kiss*. Some of these were chosen by the clinician and some were spontaneous words newly uttered by B. This treatment approach, which we call Voluntary Control of Involuntary Utterances (VCIU), has been described elsewhere (Helm-Estabrooks, 1983a). Briefly, the patient determines the practice lexicon in VCIU, although the clinician begins the treatment process of offering words which the patient has been heard to say or is thought to be capable of reading aloud. If, instead of producing the target word, the patient says another real word, then the original stimulus word is set aside and the "error" word is offered for oral reading. In order to qualify as a practice word (the 3" x 5" word cards are given to the patient for self-practice), the patient must have read the target word aloud correctly and with ease, that is, without articulatory or paraphasic struggle. In addition to oral reading, responsive naming or exercises for the target words are incorporated into the treatment session. For example, to elicit the word "love," the clinician may ask "what is the opposite of hate?"

Within approximately four months, B had a list of 267 words and short phrases which he could read aloud and use in conversation. Most were highly functional, for example, *buddy, care, dime, beer, dirty, more, nice, warm, Dottie, sis, where is it? I'm hot, I don't care, I love you, I'm cold.*

Although his BDAE verbal scores rose significantly during this period, they did not reflect the extent of his functional communication. And, interestingly enough, although he could read 267 of his self-determined words and phrases, he read aloud only one of the BDAE words and none of the sentences upon retesting.

Case III: Unclassifiable
Severe Aphasia

Neurobehavioral Characteristics. Patient C was a 55-year-old male referred to us two months following onset of a left hemisphere stroke which left him with right hemiplegia and severe aphasia. His conversation and expository speech output consisted of the nonsense-stereotype "dee-oh-ah." Although he appeared to have good comprehension for personally relevant conversational material, he earned an overall BDAE score of −1.0 standard deviation for auditory comprehension. A score lower than this would be consistent with a diagnosis of global aphasia, given his other language deficits. He had no ability to name or produce automatized verbal sequences. He repeated two words but no sentences and orally read only one word. He wrote his name and a few numbers and letters. All reading skills were severely compromised. His best BDAE performance was to sing popular songs with good melody and word approximations and to perform rhythmic tapping.

He had severe oral/facial apraxia earning 0/30 points on our praxis exam. Gestural limb praxis skills were moderately intact with an earned score of 32/60.

C's WAIS performance IQ was 83, while his "parietal lobe" drawings were assigned 9/13 points. He lost only one point on a test of his ability to copy stick designs.

A CT scan showed a lesion in the anterior limb of the left internal capsule which extended forward beyond the frontal horn, and anteriorly and superiorly to involve white matter. He was alert and cooperative but very frustrated by his speech problems.

Course of Treatment. A summary of C's preserved skills showed that he could break out of his verbal stereotype and produce real words when

he sang familiar songs such as "I've Been Working on the Railroad."
He had good visual/spatial skills and fair ability to produce representational gestures to command and upon imitation.

We decided upon a combined treatment approach which would capitalize
on all of his intact skills. During a trial of Melodic Intonation Therapy,
he was asked, first, to listen to the intoned phrase "I am fine" and then
slowly sing it in unison with the clinician, who helped him tap it out syllable
by syllable. He then repeated it correctly, and finally was able to produce
this phrase in response to a probe question. Because this was the first time
in 2 months that C had produced meaningful speech, he began to cry
after hearing himself intone "I am fine." His family was equally emotional when his performance was repeated at bedside during visiting hours.
C was enrolled in a simultaneous course of Melodic Intonation Therapy
(Sparks, Helm, & Albert, 1974; Sparks & Holland, 1976) and Visual Action
Therapy for improving limb gestures. He completed Limb/VAT in 15 sessions and was evaluated with the PICA. (At the same time he also had
received 15 sessions of Melodic Intonation Therapy). His overall PICA
score was 8.11, with a gesture score of 10.9, a verbal score of 4.47, and
a graphic score of 6.83. On the ward he had been heard to utter
multisyllable words such as "tomorrow" spontaneously, and phrases such
as "I did" and "this morning." Because of his persistent oral/facial
apraxia, he was entered into a course of Facial/VAT which was developed
for training oral/facial praxis items (Helm-Estabrooks & Albert, 1980).
Following along the same task hierarchy used for Limb/VAT, the
oral/facial program trains patients to represent hidden items, (flower,
whistle, cup, razor, chapstick, kaleidoscope, straw, and lollipop) with
gestures which involve the face or oral apparatus.

C completed the Facial/VAT program in 31 sessions. PICA
re-evaluation showed an overall score of 10.25, with a gestural score of
12.4, a verbal score of 11.4, and a graphic score of 6.6. Significantly, his
verbal score had improved 6.93 points with a combination of Face/VAT
and MIT.

Four months after admission, C's overall BDAE auditory comprehension Z score was at nearly zero, an improvement of one standard deviation. Furthermore, he now showed some verbal naming skills, improving
these scores by more than one full standard deviation.

Severe Wernicke's Aphasia

Unlike global or other nonfluent aphasias, Wernicke's aphasia is
characterized broadly as fluent, that is, the patient's speech output has

good prosody, good articulation, normal or greater than normal phrase length, and a full range of grammatical forms. The presence of literal, verbal, and neologistic paraphasias, however, make this output difficult or impossible to understand. Furthermore, the patient with Wernicke's aphasia may have several auditory-comprehension problems so that communication through the auditory/verbal mode is drastically compromised. In addition, the written output of Wernicke's patients often mirrors their verbal output, while reading may or may not be as impaired as auditory comprehension (Heilman, Rothi, Campanella, & Wolfson, 1979).

Case IV: Severe Wernicke's Aphasia

Neurobehavioral Characteristics. Patient D was a 51-year-old non-hemiparetic male who was admitted to our service two months following a stroke. He was alert and cooperative, but apparently unconcerned about his fluent paraphasic speech output. His conversation and BDAE "Cookie Theft" description were rated .5 on the Aphasia Severity Rating Scale. His speech had normal prosody, phrase length, and articulation, but was very paraphasic. His speech contained verbal, literal, and neologistic errors and thus was fluent but without information. In addition, he had obviously severe auditory comprehension problems and earned an overall auditory comprehension Z score of − 1.5. He earned no points for oral naming, reading, automatized speech, or repetition. His best oral reading performance was the word "class" for *chair*. Examples of his repetition errors are as follows: *chair* was repeated as "chess," *You know how* was repeated as "Let us doubt him," *hammock* was "To may who it were." Singing and rhythmic tapping were impaired. He often appeared confused by the tasks and required special care in establishing "set."

He demonstrated good comprehension of "whole body" commands.

D's WAIS performance IQ was 77. He reproduced 9/10 stick designs to memory on the Boston "parietal lobe" test. It was noted that D was unable to supplement his impaired verbal output with meaningful gestures. Despite the absence of hemiparesis, he used vague, nonrepresentational gestures. The CT scan showed a left-hemisphere lesion which had almost completely isolated Wernicke's area.

Course of Treatment. Despite his severe Wernicke's aphasia, D had good visual memory (he recalled 9/10 stick designs) and moderately intact visual recognition (7/10 scored on BDAE symbol/word recognition). He produced *real word* approximations for *chair* in repetition ("class") and oral reading ("chess").

Based on the findings, we chose to enroll him in a course of Visual Action Therapy to improve his ability to establish "set" for structure tasks, to become aware of task expectations, to increase his critical skills, and to encourage production and use of representational gestures. (The tendency of Wernicke's patients to use copious, but nonspecific gestures was described by Cicone, Wapner, Foldi, Zurif, & Gardner, 1979). Furthermore, it was thought that the use of this silent method might lead to better self control of D's "press of speech."

D completed Limb/VAT in 10 sessions and Face/VAT in 6 sessions. By this time, he was producing closer verbal approximations in naming, e.g., "hand" for *glove*. He now orally read 5/10 BDAE words. Repetition still was severely impaired.

It was decided that a modified VCIU approach now might offer him better control of his verbal output. Beginning with the BDAE words which he had correctly read aloud and adding others, we employed the following procedure: (1) D read the word aloud; (2) D repeated the word after the clinician without seeing the printed word; (3) D chose the target word upon hearing it from an array; (4) D used the word in a confrontation of responsive naming task.

Approximately 3½ months following admission, D left the hospital to resume management of his own small neighborhood grocery store after several 3-day weekend passes showed him capable of carrying out the tasks necessary for that job.

Case V: Severe
Wernicke's Aphasia

Neurobehavioral Characteristics. Patient E was a 55-year-old nonhemiparetic male transferred to our medical center 2 months after sustaining a left temporal/parietal contusion with significant intracerebral hemorrhaging. Administration of the Boston Diagnostic Aphasia Examination showed that E was alert but not well oriented and had great difficulty attending to tasks. He demonstrated great "press" of neologistic fluent speech, and his auditory comprehension deficits immediately became obvious in conversation. He seemed aware of his difficulty with language tasks, quickly becoming annoyed and obstinate about testing. Despite this, he remained polite, using phrases like "thank you" and "excuse me." Perseveration was prominent on those tasks which were attempted.

Due to his reluctance and the severity of his problem, he earned no points on BDAE subtests beyond 3/8 points for automatized speech, 2/10 for word repetition, and 2 points for good ability to produce a familiar tune.

He also could produce correct runs of words in song and showed an obvious fondness for music.

Within the first 2 weeks of evaluation, he became preoccupied with hospital discharge and showed increased paranoid tendencies. By the 3rd week he refused both testing and treatment.

When presented at Aphasia Round one month after admission, he showed improved conversational turn-taking, good use of nonvocal communication skills such as gestures and facial expressions, some runs of clear speech, and a tendency to get the first few items correct when a new task was introduced.

Course of Treatment. Following Aphasia Rounds, E's case was reviewed for possible re-introduction of treatment. Because he now refused to enter the treatment room, we decided instead to sit down with him in the hall, TV room, or bedside in a casual and friendly way. Because he was able to respond to the first few items correctly when new tasks were introduced, we decided to employ four different tasks during short (10-15 minute sessions) several times a day. Because he associated the BDAE tester with his frustration and failure, two other speech-language pathologists were designated as his therapists.

Based on his performance strengths, the treatment tasks were (1) repetition of words he used correctly in speech, (2) verbal identification of popular taped songs, (3) verbal identification of photographed faces associated with music, particularly jazz, and (4) singing songs while reading the lyrics.

Within 2 weeks of this approach, E had experienced sufficient success to participate willingly in more typical 30-minute therapy sessions carried out in a treatment room. He also began attending the twice-weekly, hour-long aphasic group meetings. Two months later, re-evaluation showed that his overall BDAE auditory comprehension score had improved by nearly 2 standard deviations and that his aphasia severity rating for conversation was 2, indicating that he shared the burden of communication with the examiner. At that time, he was introduced to the Helm-Elicited Language Program for Syntax Stimulation (Helm-Estabrooks, 1981), originally developed for use with agrammatic patients (Helm-Estabrooks, Fitzpatrick, & Barresi, 1981). This program, which uses a story-completion format to elicit examples of eleven syntactic constructions, has subsequently proven useful with paragrammatic patients. After a brief introduction to HELPSS, E was discharged from the hospital with pictured stimuli. This allows the program to be carried out via daily calls in which the verbal story stimuli are presented by the clinician. Several other patients have been treated successfully in this way, thereby allowing early hospital discharges for patients who are unable to attend clinic-based outpatient therapy sessions. This format particularly favors nonhemiparetic patients who have no need for physical and occupational therapy.

Summary

This chapter has addressed the treatment of severe aphasia defined here as a disorder of both primary (verbal expression and comprehension) and secondary (writing and reading comprehension) language skills. Several classifiable aphasic syndromes, including global aphasia and Wernicke's aphasia, as well as nonclassifiable syndromes, may generally be labelled as forms of severe aphasia because they seriously compromise the patient's ability to communicate effectively. It is proposed, however, that successful management of these patients will be based upon a careful qualitative analysis of the individual's performance on standardized and experimental language and neuropsychological tests, as well as neurological findings.

An understanding of the qualitative approach to treatment will enable the clinician to determine which method(s) make the best use of an individual patient's retained skills for purposes of re-integrating or circumventing his or her areas of communication deficits.

This qualitative approach, illustrated through five case studies of patients with differing forms of severe aphasia, has shown how the unique language, neuropsychological, and neurological findings of each case led to individualized rehabilitation programs which incorporated both established and custom-made treatment methods.

References

Albert, M., Goodglass, H., Helm, N., Rubens, A., & Alexander, M. *Clinical aspects of dysphasia*. New York: Springer-Verlag, 1981.

Blumstein, S., & Cooper, W. Hemispheric processing of intonation contours. *Cortex*, 1974, *10*, 146-150.

Cicone, M., Wapner, W. Foldi, N., Zurif, E., & Gardner, H. The relationship between gesture and language in aphasic communication. *Brain and Language*, 1979, *8*, 324-439.

DeRenzi, E., Pieczuro, A., & Vignolo, L. Oral apraxia and aphasia. *Cortex*, 1966, *2*, 50-73.

Geschwind, N. The apraxias. In E. W. Straus & R. M. Griffith (Eds.), *Phenomenology of will and action*, pp. 91-102. Pittsburgh: Duquesne University Press, 1967.

Goodglass, H., & Kaplan, E. *Assessment of aphasia and related disorders*. Philadelphia: Lea & Febiger, 1972. (a)

Goodglass, H., & Kaplan, E. *Boston Diagnostic Aphasia Examination*. Philadelphia: Lea & Febiger, 1972. (b)

Heilman, K., Rothi, N., Campanella, D., & Wolfson, S. Wernicke's and global aphasia without alexia. *Archives of Neurology*, 1979, *36*, 129–133.

Helm, N., & Barresi, B. Voluntary Control of Involuntary Utterances: A treatment approach for severe aphasia. In R. H. Brookshire (Ed.), *Clinical Aphasiology: Conference Proceedings*. Minneapolis: BRK Publishers, 1980.

Helm, N., Naeser, M., & Kleefield, J. CT scan localization and response to melodic intonation therapy. Academy of Aphasia Annual Meeting, South Yarmouth, MA, October, 1980.

Helm-Estabrooks, N. *Helm Elicited Language Program for Syntax Stimulation.* Austin, TX: Exceptional Resources, 1981.

Helm-Estabrooks, N. Approaches to testing subcortical aphasias. In W. H. Perkins (Ed.), *Current therapy of communication disorders*. New York: Thieme-Stratton, 1983. (a)

Helm-Estabrooks, N. Exploiting the right hemisphere fore language rehabilitation: Melodic intonation therapy. In E. Perceman (Ed.), *Cognitive processing in the right hemisphere*. New York: Academic Press, Inc., 1983. (b)

Helm-Estabrooks, N., & Albert, M. *Visual Action Therapy for Global Aphasia*, Veterans Administration Merit Review Grant, 1980.

Helm-Estabrooks, N., Fitzpatrick, P., & Barresi, B. Response of an agrammatic patient to a syntax stimulation program for aphasia. *Journal of Speech and Hearing Disorders*, 1982, *46*, 422–427.

Holland, A. L. Observing functional communication of aphasic adults. *Journal of Speech and Hearing Disorders*, 1982, *47*, 50–56.

Horel, J. A. The neuroanatomy of amnesia. *Brain*, 1978, *101*, 403–445.

Johnson, M., Sahoske, P., Grembowski, C., & Rubens, A. Preservation of responses requiring whole body movements in severe aphasia. Paper presented to American Speech and Hearing Association Convention, Houston, 1976.

Kimura, D. Left-right differences in the perception of melodies, *Quarterly Journal of Experimental Psychology*, 1964, *15*, 335–358.

Landis, J., Graves, R., & Goodglass, H. Aphasic reading and writing: Possible evidence for right hemisphere participation. *Cortex*, 1982, *18*, 105–112.

Liepmann, H. Die lenke Hemisphare und das Handeln, *Munch. Med. Wschr.*, 1905, *2*, 2375–2378.

Lorant, G., Van Eeckhout, P., & Sabadel. *L'Homme qui ne savant plus parler*. Paris: Nouvelles Editions Baudinière, 1980.

Marshall, R. C., & Newcombe, F. Patterns of paralexia: A psycholinguistic approach. *Journal of Psycholinguistic Research*, 1973, *2*, 175–199.

Naeser, M., Alexander, M., Helm-Estabrooks, N., Levine, H., Laughlin, S., & Geschwind, N. Aphasia with predominately subcortical lesion sites, *Archives of Neurology*, 1982, *39*, 2–14.

Porch, B. E. *Porch Index of Communicative Ability*. Palo Alto, CA: Consulting Psychologist Press, 1971.

Sparks, R., Helm, N., & Albert, M. Aphasia rehabilitation resulting from melodic intonation therapy. *Cortex*, 1974, *10*, 303–316.

Sparks, R., Holland, A. Method: Melodic intonation therapy for aphasia, *Journal of Speech and Hearing Disorders*, 1976, *41*, 287–297.

Van Eeckhout, P., Pillon, B., Signoret, J., & Lhermitte, F. The application of drawings to the rehabilitation of an aphasic patient. Paper presented at Symposium on Aphasia Therapy, Eramus University, Rotterdam, The Netherlands, October 1981.

Van Eeckhout, P., & Sabadel. *Histoires Insolites Pour Faire Parler*. Paris: Medecine et Sciences Internationales, 1982.

Penelope Starratt Myers

Right Hemisphere Impairment

Introduction

There has long existed an intuitive knowledge among speech-language pathologists that right hemisphere-damaged patients do not communicate adequately. Clinicians working with this population on motor-speech disorders or on reading and writing deficits have observed that their patients appear to manage well on a superficial level, but experience problems with more sophisticated communication demands. Yet, the precise nature of their problems remained elusive, and the idea of treating the disorders was not seriously entertained until very recently. In the last 5 to 10 years, research with brain-damaged, split-brain, and normal subjects using new and sophisticated techniques has generated enough data to shed new light on the role of the right hemisphere (RH) in the fully functioning brain. Clearly, the most significant advance in RH communication disorders has been a more precise delineation of the deficits themselves. Rather than merely drawing inferences from the well-known litany of RH perceptual deficits, it has now become possible to extract some of the unifying themes that carry through from a basic perceptual level to the higher order cognitive one. Clinically, this knowledge has helped refine intuition and anecdotal evidence into systematic data-based judgement.

This chapter will explore the nature of the perceptual and cognitive deficits associated with RH damage, and the ways in which they relate to each other to create communication impairments. Read the following discussion with several notes of caution in mind. First, this area of study is in its infancy and, despite significant advances, much less is known about the operations of the right than the left hemisphere. Second, in some aspects, the RH is more diffusely organized and is not as neatly packaged as the left (Goldberg & Costa, 1981; Semmes, 1968). Very few localization studies on RH communication disorders have been done, and many more are needed to account for variables such as site, size, and depth of lesion, degree of handedness, age, sex, and education level of the patient. Not all RH patients will experience all of the problems described below.

Finally, adequate diagnostic tools and therapy materials do not exist in published form at this time. Guidelines for assessment and treatment are provided throughout this chapter (for more detail, see Myers, 1982). Research bearing directly on the efficacy of specific techniques has yet to be done, so the therapist is cautioned accordingly.

The long list of impairments associated with RH disease can be broken down into four major categories: (1) lower-order perceptual problems, which include left-sided neglect and various visuospatial deficits; (2) problems with affect and prosody; (3) linguistic disorders; and (4) higher-order perceptual and cognitive deficits, including those impairments that result in general communicative inefficiency.

Many of the disorders in each category are related to those in other areas and can exert a cumulative effect on communication. For speech pathology, the advances in knowledge about the last two areas holds special significance. Most of the lower-order perceptual disorders in the first category have been well known for the past 40 years, but new work in this area has had an impact on our understanding of the communication deficits experienced by RH patients. Although therapy procedures have not been developed for working on prosodic impairments and affect, there has been a heightened interest in their effect on communication in RH patients. Each of the four categories will be discussed separately below.

Section I: Lower-Order Perceptual Deficits

The act of perception incorporates several simultaneous processes. At its most basic level, it involves the recognition or discrimination of a stimulus. On a higher level, perception involves certain associative operations so that the stimulus is not only recognized, but understood. Extracting meaning from sensory information on this higher level requires that the perceiver take into account the external context in which the stimulus is embedded, and that he integrate it with certain internal associations. The notion of "pure perception" is too simplistic to explain this nonverbal or preverbal process. There probably is no such thing as "pure perception," since no stimulus is truly isolated or truly neutral. Perception is thus both a discriminatory and an interpretive act. Breaking it down into lower and higher order operations is somewhat artificial, but serves as a useful organizational tool for purposes of discussion. The disorders discussed in this section, then, reflect deficits in basic perceptual processes, but have an effect on higher-order perception as well. They are grouped together here as lower-order perceptual disorders to lay the foundation for a discussion of their impact on communication in Section IV.

The lengthy list of visuospatial disorders associated with RH disease usually includes deficits in the following abilities: (1) visual discrimination; (2) visual memory; (3) visual integration; (4) visual imagery; (5) facial recognition (prosopagnosia); (6) topological and geographic orientation; (7) visuoconstructive deficits (constructional apraxia); (8) spatial orientation; and (9) neglect of the left half of space (see Joynt & Goldstein, 1975 for an excellent review). Many of these deficits affect the patient's ability to regain independence and care for himself. In the early months post onset he may, for example, forget how to get back to his room, have difficulty remembering familiar faces, or be unable to groom himself properly.

Neglect

Almost all of these disorders will be significantly heightened if the patient also suffers from neglect of the left half of space. Unlike homonymous hemianopsia, which prevents the patient from seeing the left side, left-sided neglect inhibits his ability to conceive of and, therefore, act on or respond to input from the left. It is usually seen in cancellation tasks, in which the patient is asked to cross out randomly spaced figures on a page, or in copy drawing, as well as from behavioral observation. The left-neglect patient will draw objects, such as a flower, with extraneous detail on the right and omissions on the left. In copying a clock face, the patient may include all the numbers on the right and leave the left side blank. Sometimes neglect is accompanied by denial of illness or the patient's refusal to recognize his or her paretic extremities as his or her own (anosognosia). In addition, the patient may appear inattentive and unresponsive. Although spatial neglect has been found in lesions of the left hemisphere (LH), it has been most closely associated with lesions in the right temperoparietal and occipitoparietal areas (Critchley, 1953; Fredericks, 1963; Heilman, 1979; Heilman & Watson, 1977; LeDoux, 1978).

The exact nature of the disorder is unclear and numerous theories have been proposed to explain it. (See Bisiach, Luzzatti, & Perani, 1979; Heilman, 1979, for more detail and further references.) In the early 20th century, the notion of an internal representation of the body or "body schema" was introduced by H. Head (1920), and was later invoked by a number of researchers to explain unilateral neglect (Brain, 1941; Critchley, 1953; Gerstman, 1942). The main problem with this explanation is that it fails to account for the full range of symptoms associated with neglect, including the fact that it extends to the entire left half of space. Another early theory proposed that neglect was caused by a lack of synthesis in the flow of information to one hemisphere (Denny-Brown, Myers & Horenstein, 1952).

More recently, Heilman and his associates have proposed that neglect is a deficit in attention and a breakdown in the orienting response (Heilman, 1979; Heilman & Valenstein, 1972; Watson, Heilman, Cauthen, & King, 1973). Their theories are based on work done with animals (Watson, Miller, & Heilman, 1977; Watson et al., 1978) and with RH patients. As Heilman explains it, the orienting response is an alerting mechanism that prepares or alerts the organism to sensory stimulation and reduces the threshold to incoming stimuli. Heilman (1979) states that "Lesions which induce the unilateral neglect syndrome produce a unilateral reduction of arousal. Because one hemisphere is hypoaroused, it cannot prepare for action and it is therefore akinetic" (p. 284). In a detailed account of the anatomical and physiologic basis of the theory, he designates three cortical regions (inferior parietal lobule, dorsilateral frontal lobe, and the cingulate gyrus), their interconnections, and their connections to the brain stem reticular formation as the critical areas involved in orienting, attention, and trimodal association.

Other researchers take issue with the purely physiologic approach. Bisiach and his colleagues (1979, 1981) see neglect as a disorder affecting the internal representation of the spatial schema of all incoming stimuli. In one study, for example, they found their RH subjects made errors of omission in their verbal descriptions of the left half of a familiar scene— in this case, the cathedral square in Milan—regardless of the orientation they were asked to assume in recalling the image. Their results indicated that the patients' internal concept of, or representation of, the scene was as flawed as their response to real, externally presented stimuli.

It may seem superfluous for speech pathologists to become involved in the theoretical debate over the causes of neglect. Yet, there are several reasons why they should. First, patients with neglect usually present the most severe disorders in visuospatial perception and communication. Second, speech pathologists are called on to treat reading and writing disturbances that are a direct result of neglect (Collins, 1976; LaPointe & Culton, 1969; Metzler & Jelinek, 1976; Stanton et al., 1979, 1981). Finally, since neglect has a very definite impact on the recovery of independence in daily activities, speech pathologists may be consulted by other members of a rehabilitation team about ways to overcome the effects of neglect in a number of tasks. Yorkston (1981), for example, reports a fairly typical request for intervention in helping a left-neglect patient learn to transfer from wheelchair to bed. In such cases, she suggests breaking tasks into small steps and orienting the patient through a series of verbal cues. Each of the steps in the transfer was preceded by an anticipatory question ("How well did you do on this step?") and followed by a review question ("How well did you do?"). Although the task had to be broken down initially into 27 steps, the number was eventually reduced, and the patient was able to transfer successfully. Diller and Weinberg (1977) suggest that retraining of this type is possible with neglect patients via awareness training, small steps, and intensive repetition. Stanton et al. (1981) advocate a verbal cueing strategy accompanied by mass practice for retraining reading skills. It appears that such a strategy can be successful, though not necessarily generalizable.

The implicit assumption in verbal cueing strategies is that the language system can be used to help the patient orient and attend to the left half of space. the degree to which one supports such a strategy partly reflects one's concept of neglect. If one believes it is the result of inattention, one would anticipate that verbal cues, vigilance training, and constant repetition first by the clinician, then by the patient, would be successful. If, on the other hand, one subscribes to a more representational theory, one might want to make more use of other modalities and tasks (such as tactile exploration) as a means of helping the patient refine his internal concept of space. Most of the work on neglect, of course, is aimed at compensation rather than recovery, and most speech pathologists use a combination of strategies. Other professionals (physical and occupational therapists) work on neglect as well, so it is wise to coordinate efforts and program type with them.

Although some of the more disruptive aspects of the syndrome (denial of illness and hemispatial neglect) abate somewhat, flatness of affect and attenuated responsiveness may persist over time (Heilman, 1979). Flat affect and impaired prosody will be discussed in Section II. Neglect is a collection of symptoms and is not really a lower-order perceptual deficit, but because it is implicated in a number of the visuospatial disorders explored below, an understanding of its course and behavioral manifestations is critical at the outset to any discussion of RH patients.

Visuospatial Deficits

Although visual discrimination disorders are often associated with RH disease, the discrimination of such attributes as size or curvature has not been found to be significantly impaired in any brain damaged group (Benton, 1979). Bisiach, Nichelli, and Spinnler (1976) did find significant deficits in the perception of length, and figure-ground disorders have been found in both aphasic and right parietal populations (Russo & Vignolo, 1967; Weinstein, 1964).

Spatial orientation deficits have also been found in patients with RH lesions. For example, Ratcliff (1979) found right posterior patients significantly impaired compared to left posterior subjects in performing a mental rotation task. Benton, Hannay, and Varney (1975) found severe impairments in the ability to determine the directional orientation of visually presented lines. In addition, RH patients are often impaired in the ability to orient to geography, either in map reading, maze solving, or in describing familiar routes (Benton, 1979). Neglect of the left side may make a significant contribution to failure in such tasks. It has also been suggested that impaired topological orientation is affected by the ability to maintain an internal spatial representation. Butters and Barton (1970) found parietal lobe patients, especially those with RH damage, were impaired in three tasks requiring them to shift or reverse perspective in thought, and they suggested that the ability to perform reversible operations in space (i.e. dressing) is associated with a deficit in imaging processes.

Although the ability to read a map or find one's way home does not impact directly on communication skills, the idea that these disorders reflect a deficit in internal visuospatial representation does. The list of visual processing deficits associated with RH disease almost always includes a reference to impaired "visual imagery" or "visual image making." The implications of such deficits for communication are far reaching, but for the practitioner, the problem with these terms is, what do they mean? What exactly is a visual image, and why has it become associated with RH damage?

In part, the connection between the two is based on the idea that thinking involves more than words, and since the LH is dominant for language, the RH must be dominant for nonverbal thought. Visual images have been conceived as a construct for nonverbal thought by many people thoughout history. Much of the recent work in visual imagery has been undertaken in psychological experiments using a paired-associate learning (PAL) paradigm (Bugeleski, 1968, 1970; Bower, 1970; Paivio, 1969, 1971; Rowher, 1970). In such experiments, subjects learn lists of word pairs and are then asked to report the second word of a pair in a recall experiment. The investigators look at the mnemonic power of various types of words (abstract vs. concrete, for example) and various strategies used in the recall task. It has been found that the generation of an internal picture or image is an effective strategy, and that the more concrete a word, the more "highly imageable" it is. Based on work of this type, proponents of the Dual Coding Theory (Paivio, 1971) claim that there is a dual coding system in which verbal processes and nonverbal imagery represent the two alternate systems. Extending these results to the area of hemisphere asymmetry, some researchers have suggested that the RH, specialized for visuospatial input, is dominant for visual imagery coding. And, because concrete words are more readily imaged in a PAL task, some assume that the RH is more adept with concrete input and visual imagery (West, 1977, 1978). Hence, speech pathologists are cautioned in lecture halls, symposia, and workshops that the RH patient may have a deficit in visual imagery, without a clear understanding of what this means in the abstract, or what it means for the patient.

The work done in PAL tasks envisions images as a sort of "mental picture" in the "mind's eye" or as a "sensory-like datum" (Paivio, 1969; Weber & Bach, 1979). It is important to note, however, that many researchers take issue with this view (see Pylyshn, 1973, for an excellent review and counterpoint). It would be a mistake to extrapolate this rather narrow view of images as tools in a PAL task to represent the sum total of our experience of images. As Myers (1980) points out, "The assumption that images are mental pictures specialized to depict concrete events denies the essential complexity and multidimensional aspects of imagery" (p. 69). She goes on to say:

> Rather than a picture or recording that bears some structural relation to raw sensory data, an image is a non-verbal confluence of emotion, intellect and sensation. An image is a simultaneous integration of multiple dimensions and levels of perceived (i.e. interpreted) experience. It represents a synthesis of internal (to the perceiver) and external events free of time and space limitations. Thus the word "home" may evoke a single image which in one instant of time captures knowledge of multiple and possibly conflicting aspects of all the homes one has known across temporal boundaries. These qualities make possible the feeling that one has recalled the essence of an experience. It is these same qualities that make it difficult to transfer complex images directly into words. (p. 69).

It is also these same qualities that suggest a more powerful connection between the RH and imagery, but that makes its discussion out of place in a section on lower-order perception. The issue will be raised again, but the reader is cautioned to remember that there is no direct evidence to indicate that RH patients actually do suffer from a deficit in image making. Most of the claims are based on inference and, when they are made, the reference is usually to images in the most narrow sense of the word—i.e., as ideographic reconstructions.

Facial recognition disorders (prosopagnosia) have sometimes been linked to a deficit in visual recall or the recall of images. Many people, however, think of prosopagnosia as less of a defect in matching external stimuli to internal images or in discrimination of discrete attributes than as the inability to integrate them simultaneously. Prosopagnosia is often found in patients with bilateral lesions, but it has been associated specifically with RH lesions as well (Benton & Van Allen, 1968; DeRenzi, Faglioni, & Spinnler, 1968; DeRenzi & Spinnler, 1966; Warrington & James, 1967). Isolated case reports in the literature are often arresting. Among the most dramatic was Charcot's patient who could not recognize his own face in the mirror. Myers (1978) discusses a patient, 20 years post onset, who had trained himself to use specific visual and auditory cues (hair color, vocal features, etc.) to recognize his clients at work, members of his own family, and the characters in a television drama. The disorder may be socially embarrassing or isolating for the patient. Family and friends unaware of prosopagnosia as a distinct deficit may assume that the patient is suffering from general confusion. Current treatment in our profession is generally restricted to increasing family and patient awareness, and providing suggestions for using analytic cues as a means of compensation.

Benton and Van Allen (1968) refer to prosopagnosia as a form of "simultagnosia" or a deficit in synthesizing disparate elements into a meaningful composite. Other visual integration deficits have been found in RH patients. Newcombe and Russell (1969), for example, found RH subjects significantly impaired in visual closure tasks, and Warrington and James (1967) found that their performance on a task involving the perception of incomplete figures was significantly worse than that of their LH subjects. In fact, many of the visuospatial skills in the intact RH are thought to reflect a facility for synthesizing sensory input (Bogen, 1969; Galin, 1974, Ornstein, 1977; Sperry, 1968; Zaidel, 1978). Myers (1979) and Myers and Linebaugh (1980) found RH patients severely impaired on a test specifically designed to assess visual integration, *The Hooper Visual Organization Test* (Hooper, 1958). Out of a possible 30 points the mean for the RH subjects in the latter study was 9.88, compared to 23.2 for the normal controls.

Finally, various visuoconstructive deficits have been found in RH patients, though they have also been reported frequently in LH patients. Performance, of course, depends on task demands (block design, visual sequential memory, copy drawing, spontaneous graphic production) and the degree to which the subject relies on, or can rely on, verbal strategies in task execution. In RH patients the collection of constructive disorders is usually referred to as constructional apraxia, and will often impair graphic performance.

Reading and Writing Deficits

Reading and writing disturbances in this population are often noted clinically. Treatment for these deficits has a longer history in our profession than does treatment for any other type of RH communication disorder (motor speech problems excepted). Before providing treatment, it is obviously important to distinguish between perceptually based deficits and those that are linguistic in nature. The perceptual deficits in reading may reflect impaired scanning and tracking as well as left-sided neglect. La-Pointe and Culton (1969) have described a treatment program they used with a single neglect case. Their program included copy-drawing drills, drawing from memory, and tactile tracing. As previously mentioned, Stanton et al. (1981) advocate a verbal cueing strategy, and had success using it with two RH neglect patients. In addition, clinicians have used standard cues such as a red line drawn down the left side of the page to help remind the patient to attend to the left. Myers (in press) has outlined a systematic series of tasks for both reading and writing deficits that are perceptually based.

Writing disturbances in RH patients generally include omission of strokes and graphemes as well as perseveration. Metzler and Jelinek (1976), for example, found that their 20 subjects were significantly impaired compared to normal controls on a number of graphic tests. The writing deficits in their experimental group included: spelling errors (usually due to perseverated or omitted graphemes); perseveration of strokes, graphemes, syllables, and words; omissions of words and strokes; failure to dot *i's* and cross *t's*; and extra capitalization. Treatment involving drills in copying and tactile exploration may be effective. Increasing the patient's awareness of errors is almost always a necessary first step.

This concludes the section on lower-order perceptual disorders. As stated earlier, many of these deficits will be affected by, and have an effect on, higher-order processing and production in the complex process of communication.

Section II: Affect and Prosody

Among the disorders most commonly ascribed to RH damage are deficits in affect and prosody. RH patients may lack the normal range of facial expression (flat affect), and speak in a monotone because the prosodic features of their speech are attenuated. Unlike anterior aphasic patients, who can be painfully aware of and depressed by their disorder, many RH patients evince little or no response to their impairments. Some RH patients with neglect may even deny illness altogether, making it difficult to motivate them in the rehabilitation process. Their minimization of their problems led Hecaen (1962) to use the term "indifference reaction" to characterize this constellation of symptoms, and led others to investigate the possible connection between the RH and the mediation of emotion. This is one of the most important and difficult questions in this area. Does the flat affect found in some RH patients reflect an underlying emotional attenuation? Or is it simply a superficial deficit in the ability to adequately express experienced affective states? The answer has far-reaching implications for the rehabilitation of this population, and much of the research reported in this section addresses the issue directly or indirectly. The solution to the puzzle has not been found, but recent research has helped link some of the pieces together.

Experimental evidence of the flat emotional responses in RH patients is well documented. Gianotti (1972), for example, found that the response to failure among 160 left- and right-hemisphere patients differed significantly. Left hemisphere (LH) patients tended to display catastrophic reactions (heightened anxiety, tears, refusal to complete the task), while RH patients either joked about, or appeared relatively unaffected by, the stress of failure. Furthermore, physiologic measurements of RH patients demonstrate hypoarousal to pain and to emotionally laden stimuli. Using a measure of a galvanic skin response (GSR), Heilman, Schwartz, and Watson (1978) found that RH subjects with left neglect demonstrated significantly lower GSR's to pain than did either the LH or non-neurologically impaired control group. Recently, Morrow, Vrtunsk, Kim, and Boller (1981) discovered a difference in GSR's in response to emotional and neutral slides. Their LH and RH groups had significantly smaller GSR's than normal controls, and GSR's in the RH subjects were significantly smaller than those in the LH group. The LH and control group had a significantly larger response to emotional (vs. neutral)slides, while the RH group produced almost no GSR at all to either type of slide.

RH superiority in reacting to emotionally laden auditory and visual stimuli has been found in normal subjects. Various dichotic studies have shown a left ear (RH) advantage in evaluating the emotional tone of recorded voices (Carmon & Nachson, 1973; Haggard & Parkinson, 1971; King & Kimura, 1972). In a review of dichotic studies investigating prosodic features, particularly intonational contour, Zurif (1974) concluded that "the ear advantage is determined less by the acoustic correlates of a linguistic property than by the use to which those correlates must be put. Thus, when the acoustic parameters of intonational contour...must be processed or matched independently of their linguistic medium, they become tied to the right hemisphere. In contrast, when these same parameters are used in the service of linguistic decisions, they are focused upon and utilized by the language mechanisms of the left hemisphere" (p. 395). Among the problems posed in dichotic studies investigating asymmetry for affective and prosodic elements is the difficulty in separating out the various features which are present as a result of the linguistic nature of the stimuli.

Visual studies with normal subjects using tachistoscopic presentation pose different limitations. The stimuli are presented to one visual half-field while the subject fixates on a central point. Thus, the input goes to only one hemisphere. Stimulus duration is circumscribed by normal lateral eye movement and generally can only be displayed for approximately 40 to 60 msec. Despite this limitation, tachistoscopic studies have advanced our knowledge about the role of the RH in responding to affective input. Numerous studies have tested asymmetry for facial recognition and, in recent years, have looked at the perception and discrimination of faces with emotional expressions. Generally, the results of these experiments have supported the view that facial recognition is faster or more accurate with a left visual-field (RH) presentation (Geffin, Bradshaw, & Wallace, 1971; Hilliard, 1973; Jones, 1979; Klein, Muscovitch, & Vigna, 1976; Leehey & Cahn, 1979; Rizzolatti, Umilita, & Berlucchi, 1971). Galper and Costa (1980), however, offer a good argument against what they term the "simplistic view" that the RH is the "sole mediator" of facial recognition. Numerous variables, such as the field dependence or independence of the subject, the sex of the subject, or the sex of the depicted face can play a role (Rapaczynski & Ehrlichman, 1979; Strauss & Muscovitch, 1981). A right visual-field (LH) superiority has been found, for example, in the recognition of the faces of famous people (Marzi & Berlucchi, 1977).

In an effort to better understand the role of the RH in both face recognition and the mediation of emotion, several people have used emotional faces as a variable (Hansch & Priozzollo, 1980; Strauss & Moscovitch, 1981; Suberi & McKeever, 1977). In general, the results of these studies have been consistent with a RH superiority in face and expression recognition, and in the recall of affective visual input.

Diamond and his colleagues (1976) were able to overcome the time limitation imposed on stimuli in tachistoscopic methods by using opaque contact lenses with off center slits which are designed to send visual input to a single half-field. Thus, they were able to show three films (a Tom and Jerry cartoon, a travelogue, and a surgical operation) to 14 right-handed normal subjects. The subjects rated the films on a nine-point scale as humourous, pleasant, unpleasant, or "horrific." No significant differences were found between the hemispheres on the first two ratings, but differences were found for the judgment of "unpleasant" on all films. In the left visual-field condition, the subjects tended to find more unpleasant features than in either the right visual-field or free vision conditions. The authors suggest that "each hemisphere has its own distinct emotional vision of the world" and that "each makes a unique contribution to the whole" (p. 692). They add that the right visual-field condition and free vision condition so closely resembled each other that it appears the RH response is more latent, or is perhaps suppressed in the intact brain by the LH.

Dekosky, Heilman, Bowers, and Valenstein (1980) looked at the ability of unilaterally brain damaged patients to discriminate emotional input in free vision. In six different tasks, their 27 subjects were required either to name the emotion depicted in a scene or face, or to discriminate between two faces or emotions (same or different). The RH subjects were significantly worse than the LH and normal control group in naming the emotional scenes, discriminating between neutral faces, and discriminating between emotions depicted in facial expressions. All nine of the RH subjects had neglect. The authors also report a tendency for the RH patients to be more impaired than the LH group in tasks where they had to either name or choose the accurate facial emotion.

Facial recognition, facial expression, detection of commonality of emotion between pictured emotional scenes and verbally described emotional situations were all investigated in a study by Cicone, Wapner, and Gardner (1980). Aphasic, RH, frontal leucotomy, and normal controls served as subjects. The RH group demonstrated reduced emotional sensitivity with verbal as well as visual stimuli. In discussing the quality of the RH responses, the authors explain that while many RH subjects were able to infer emotions correctly, they had difficulty applying this "inferential process" to the task. They state, "These observations suggest, at least in the case of some right hemisphere patients, a general impairment of the ability to apply inferential processes realistically to the external environment" (p. 156).

The degree to which recognizing a facial expression or emotion depends on facial recognition skills remains unclear. The results of the Dekosky study did not demonstrate them as separate abilities in brain damaged subjects. In the Cicone et al. study, only the RH and frontal leucotomy subjects had trouble in the facial recognition task. However, the correlation between scores on that test and those on the emotional expressions test was very low. And, some studies using normal subjects have indicated an independence between facial recognition skills and the recall of emotional faces (Ley & Bryden, 1979).

Another source of inquiry into the nature of emotional representation and its possible alteration as a result of RH disease has been in the area of auditory processing using right brain damaged subjects. Heilman, Scholes, and Watson (1975) have used the term "auditory affective agnosia" to describe the impaired ability to right parietal patients with neglect to discriminate and comprehend affectively toned sentences. Using a group of LH patients with lesions corresponding to those in the RH group, they found that neither group was impaired in comprehending the meaning of the tape-recorded stimulus sentences. The RH group, however, was significantly worse than the LH group in comprehending the mood (happy, sad, angry, or indifferent) of the speaker. In 1977, Tucker, Watson, and Heilman extended the study to further clarify the findings. In one task, subjects had to determine whether or not two identical neutral sentences were said with the same or different emotion (in 16 trials) and had to judge the mood of the speaker in an additional 16 trials. Their RH subjects, performing at a level no better than chance, were significantly more impaired on these tasks than the LH group. These results are at odds with the findings of Schlanger, Schlanger, and Gerstman (1976), although only three of their 20 subjects had temporoparietal lesions and it is uncertain whether or not they had neglect.

To find out if discrimination of affect extended to production of emotional tone, Tucker et al. (1977) designed a second experiment in which they asked their subjects to listen to tape-recorded sentences in which the speaker's tone was neutral. The sentences were followed by a mood marker (happy, sad, angry, or indifferent) and subjects were asked to repeat the sentence with the indicated emotional overlay. Their sentences were taped and evaluated for mood by three judges. Again, the RH group did not perform above the level of chance.

Rather than looking at deliberate emotional expression produced on command, Buck and Duffy (1981) designed a study investigating the production of spontaneous expression among four groups of subjects: aphasic, RH, parkinsonian, and normal controls. The subjects were shown affective slides that were divided into four categories including landscapes, unusual configurations, people familiar to the patient, and unpleasant scenes. The subjects' reactions were videotaped as they watched the slides. Naive judges were asked to: (a) guess the nature of the slide by categorizing the facial expression of the subject, and (b) rate the overall expressiveness of the subject. The judges gave significantly lower expressiveness ratings to RH and parkinsonian subjects, compared with aphasic and control patients. There were no significant differences in ability to categorize facial expression (and, hence determine the nature of the slide) between the aphasic and control groups. But the judges were significantly less accurate in judging the emotional reactions of the RH and parkinsonian groups.

In fact, no significant differences were found between the last two groups. The authors concluded that the power of a nonverbal message "arising spontaneously" from the affective state of the patient may not be disrupted by LH damage, but may be impaired by RH damage.

The prosodic features on nonaffective messages can also be disturbed in RH damage (Weintraub, Mesulam, & Kramer 1981; Ross & Mesulam, 1979). More precise documentation and analysis of prosodic deficits have been undertaken recently. Kent and Rosenbek (in press) used spectographic analysis to study the prosodic disturbances associated with various sites of lesion. In the RH group, their results revealed a reduction in acoustic energy in higher and midfrequency regions, and nasalization occurring with inadequate oral articulation. Like parkinsonian dysarthria, the RH subjects had a normal (or faster) rate, less than normal energy in frequencies above 500 Hz, and reduced acoustic contrast, so that they were perceived as speaking in a monotone with indistinct articulation and a mild to moderate hypernasality. Ross (1981) proposed a model of prosodic production and comprehension in which the anterior RH subserves the production of prosody, and the posterior RH is crucial to the comprehension of prosodic and affective speech. Damage to the anterior area, he suggests, creates a motor "aprosodia" characterized by poor expression, but good comprehension of affective speech. Damage to the posterior region, on the other hand, would lead to a more severe defect in receptive prosodic disturbances. His findings regarding the posterior RH are at odds with those of Tucker et al. (1977), who found their posterior patients impaired in production, as well as in comprehension of intonation pattern. More localization studies investigating the possible dissociation between prosodic expression and reception are needed.

The experimental evidence to date suggests a strong RH involvement in processing and producing prosodic and affective features of messages. It is interesting to note that exaggerated intonational contour has been used successfully in the treatment of anterior aphasia utilizing a technique called melodic intonation therapy (Sparks, Helm, & Albert, 1974). Research has also supported clinical reports of flat affect, impaired comprehension of emotional tone, and disturbed or attenuated prosody in some RH patients. Therapy for these disorders, beyond counselling the patient and family, is almost nonexistent. There is good reason for this. We still do not know if the patient's flat affect reflects a deeper emotional deficit or if it is an impairment superimposed over an intact emotional structure. Ferreting out the patient's internal emotional state from its outward projection is tricky business. One of the few investigations that has attempted to look at the subjective experience of emotion in RH patients is an unpublished study by Enders (1979). She gave the Lorr Feeling and Mood

Scale to RH, LH, and non-neurologically impaired controls and did not find significant differences among the groups on self-ratings of anger, energy, cheerfulness, anxiety, depression, or friendliness. She points out, however, that the results of the study did not always correspond to some of the subjective reports of attenuated feelings of anger from the RH patients.

More work investigating emotional responsiveness in RH patients is needed. Research with normal subjects suggests a significant role for the RH, not only with prosody and emotional expressiveness, but also in the internal affective state. We must be careful, however, about making automatic assumptions regarding the effect of cortical brain damage on what appear to be functions of the same area in the intact brain. The lack of responsiveness noted in RH patients may be caused by other factors besides emotion. These will be explored in Section IV. Still, we must beware of treating the symptoms without a more thorough grasp of the cause. It may be possible to retrain patients to express affect by improving prosodic and nonverbal features of their messages, for example, or by training them to recognize and comprehend the meaning of affective material. The latter poses less risk, and would probably be helpful to the overall receptive skills of patients. But the former task, while helping patients communicate better on one level, may mask a deeper deficit with which we are not equipped to deal.

Section III:
Linguistic Deficits

Right hemisphere communication disorders clearly fall outside the continuum of aphasic-like behaviors. However, some RH patients do demonstrate deficits on pure linguistic tasks. Auditory and visual processing demands, and syntactic complexity appear to play a role in the linguistic problems discussed below. Performance on more sophisticated communication tasks can be attributed to the higher-order cognitive and perceptual problems covered in Section IV.

Because standardized diagnostic batteries designed specifically for RH patients have not yet been developed, many clinicians use aphasia tests as part of their assessment. These tests may serve as useful tools, but should be administered with caution. The test stimuli are not generally sophisticated or divergent enough to reveal higher-level deficits. Scoring systems are generally inadequate in accounting for the full range of RH communication behavior. Often, for example, the patient's extraneous comments noted by the clinician in the margin of the test will be more revealing than the scores themselves. Depressed scores may be less a result of linguistic problems than of impaired visuospatial skills or neglect (see Section I). A complex visual array of target and foils may result in delayed responses as the patient searches for an adequately understood target item.

With these cautionary notes in mind, several researchers have used aphasia batteries to look at RH performance on linguistic tasks. Deal, Deal, Wertz, Kitselman, and Dwyer (1979) compared the performance of RH subjects with that of aphasic subjects on the *Porch Index of Communicative Abilities* (PICA) (Porch, 1967) to see if there were similarities. Their retrospective study of 111 RH subjects revealed that while the RH subjects did make errors, the PICA was probably not the best instrument to use with this population. Some subjects, for example, had more difficulty on tasks considered easier for aphasic patients, and had less difficulty on subtests considered harder for aphasic patients.

Subtests of the *Boston Diagnostic Aphasia Examination* (BDAE) (Goodglass & Kaplan, 1967) have been used by a number of researchers. Myers (1978) found that the mean scores of her 8 subjects on the 18 subtests of the BDAE were above the cut-off level for aphasia. However, the range of reported scores demonstrated that some patients fell below the norm in word discrimination, comprehension of complex ideational material, animal naming (word fluency), oral sentence reading, word recognition and word-picture matching. Using the same test, Adamovich and Brooks (1981) found significant differences between their 5 RH subjects and 5 normal controls on several BDAE subtests. Scores on word discrimination, body part identification, and complex ideational material were lower in the experimental group. The authors point out that errors on numbers and letters made a significant contribution to the low scores on the word discrimination test. Complex ideational errors were thought to be a function of linguistic complexity and length. Body part identification errors may have been less the result of comprehension deficits than of impaired right-left discrimination, or of anosognosia, though the authors do not comment on this.

In the verbal expression subtests of the BDAE, Adamovich and Brooks's subjects were significantly impaired compared with controls on automatic sequencing and in responsive naming. The authors point out that the errors on the visual confrontation-naming subtest tended to be on naming items that were visually similar to the target items. They suggest that visual integration deficits as revealed by the *Hooper Visual Organization Test* (Hooper, 1958) in their experimental group may have been a contributing factor. It is interesting to note, however, that in a study using both the latter tests, Myers and Linebaugh (1980) found their 12 RH subjects were significantly impaired on the Hooper test, but had near perfect scores in the visual confrontation-naming subtest of the BDAE. Out of a possible 105 points, the mean for the RH subjects on this test was 97.

To further investigate naming, Adamovich and Brooks used the *Boston Naming Test* (Kaplan, Goodglass, & Weintraub, 1976) and found significantly lower scores in their RH group compared with controls. On the Word Fluency Measure (Borkowski, Benton, & Spreen, 1967), they also found their RH group had consistently lower scores than controls. Milner (1974) also found that word fluency tasks reveal RH deficits. Such an impairment in this population may partly reflect impaired control over available linguistic information. The animal-naming subtest of the BDAE in the Myers (1978) study showed that the RH subjects tended to use random strategies reflecting impaired use of associations.

Auditory comprehension disorders have been noted in tests other than the BDAE. McNeil and Prescott found that linguistic complexity was a factor in the impaired RH performance on the *Revised Token Test (RTT)* (McNeil & Prescott, 1978). Their results are consistent with those found by Adamovich and Brooks on the same test. In the latter study, the authors did not find significant differences between normal control and RH groups on two auditory memory tasks, and they concluded that complexity (embedding), rather than length, was the major factor in the impaired performance of the RH group on the RTT.

Factors other than linguistic complexity or verbal memory may play a role in the impaired performance of RH patients on the auditory comprehension tests listed above. In a study investigating recognition memory for verbal and nonverbal material, Riege, Metter, and Hanson (1980) found a double dissociation in stroke patients by task demands. Test stimuli in the auditory portion of the experiment included words (verbal) and bird calls (nonverbal). Subjects were asked to signal recognition of 10 previously presented test items which were randomly embedded in a list of 40 items. On the verbal portion of the test, they found that aphasic subjects were significantly impaired, but RH subjects performed as well as controls. However, the reverse was true on the nonverbal tasks. RH subjects were significantly impaired and aphasic subjects were not. These results were consistent across the long-term and the short-term memory conditions.

While this finding suggests that RH patients do not have deficits in word recognition and recall, it further demonstrates that auditory memory is not a unilateral function. The bird calls in this study were patterns of notes, and it is thought that the RH may be more adept with pattern recognition. Only a few years ago it was popular to associate the RH with musical abilities. Now it is recognized that musical performance and recognition, like language, is a complex behavior. Variables include intensity, duration, pitch, temporal sequencing, rhythm, and more. Generally, results of various studies have shown that the LH is more specialized for detecting temporal order (Carmon & Nachson, 1971; Halperin, Nachson, & Carmon, 1973; Mills & Rollman, 1980), duration and rhythm (Gordon, 1978). (See Gates & Bradshaw (1977) for a thorough review.) The RH has been associated with the detection of pitch. Milner (1962), for example, found that right temporal lobectomy patients were impaired in timbre and melody recognition. Shapiro, Grossman, and Gardner, (1981) found subjects with lesions in the right anterior, right central areas, and left central areas were significantly impaired in detecting phrasing and rhythm errors, while right anterior and right central patients were impaired in pitch recognition.

Sidtis (1980) states that the perception of pitch, timbre, and interval relationships between chords is partly determined by the harmonic composition of the tone. Reviewing the sometimes conflicting results of dichotic studies with normal subjects, he observes: "their results suggest that auditory function of the right hemisphere is specialized for the analysis of harmonic information" (p. 322). Sidtis sees harmonic information as the unifying factor in pitch perception. His study was designed to examine its role in eliciting hemisphere asymmetries for pitch discrimination in normal subjects. His results with the 96 right-handed subjects supported his hypothesis and he concludes: "It should also be noted that while complex pitch perception is an important expression of the right hemisphere's capacity for harmonic information processing, this function is likely to play a role in a wide range of auditory perception" (p. 328).

These findings are consistent with the studies demonstrating RH deficits in the detection of prosodic features and mood (see Section II). On complex and lengthy material, it may be that the examiner's phrasing and intonation patterns are not detected by the subject, or that the effort to discriminate them may interfere with overall comprehension of lengthy and complex test items. Thus, overall acoustic dimensions of the test stimuli may be as much a factor as linguistic embedding.

Phonemic discrimination, on the other hand, does not appear to play a role in linguistic comprehension tasks in RH patients. In a recent study Gianotti, Caltagirone, Miceli, and Masullo (1981) gave tests of semantic and phonemic discrimination to 50 RH and 39 control subjects. The performance of the RH group on word-to-picture matching (semantic) was significantly worse than that of controls, while there were no significant differences on the phonemic discrimination test.

In the same study, RH subjects were found not to be impaired in the ability to match printed words to pictures. These findings are consistent with those of Rivers and Love (1980) on a similar task, and with the findings in the Adamovich and Brooks (1980) study. In the latter, the authors report that, while single word reading was not impaired, their RH group was significantly worse than controls in the Sentence and Paragraph subtest of the BDAE. Performance deteriorated as stimulus length increased.

Other comprehension and expression deficits on tasks involving complex material are probably less a function of disorders in linguistic processing per se, than in extralinguistic and higher cognitive operations. These problems will be addressed in Section IV. When deficits are found that are thought to be purely linguistic in nature, most clinicians use the standard stimulation techniques used in aphasia therapy (Adamovich, 1981; Myers, 1982).

Section IV: Higher Cognitive Impairments

Although RH patients may demonstrate some language impairments as measured by aphasia tests, these deficits tell only a small part of the story. The true extent of RH communication disorders is apparent only when the patient is engaged in more sophisticated and open-ended communication tasks. The less concrete and the more complex the task, the more likely the patient will manifest the following deficits: (1) difficulty in organizing information in an efficient, meaningful way; (2) a tendency to produce impulsive answers that are rife with tangential and related, but unnecessary, detail; (3) difficulty in distinguishing between what is important and what is not; (4) problems in assimilating and using contextual cues; (5) a tendency to overpersonalize external events; (6) a tendency to lend a literal interpretation to figurative language; and (7) a reduced sensitivity to the communicative situation and to the pragmatic or extralinguistic aspects of communication (Myers, 1982).

Less than 10 years ago, the best we could do in describing these symptoms was to characterize RH speech as bizarre, inappropriate, confused, or confabulatory. While we recognized that the term "aphasic-like behavior" was wholly inadequate in describing what we observed, we were not able to be very specific in explaining why. Research in this area has sought a more precise delineation of the disorders and, in the last 5 or 6 years, has significantly advanced our understanding of the nature of RH communication impairments on this higher level. As a result, some unifying themes are beginning to emerge. Two of the most prominent are that RH patients appear to have difficulty in organizing information, and a deficit in relating to contextual cues.

In extensive interviews with 20 RH patients, Myers (1979) noted that when responding to open-ended questions, many patients could address, but not answer, the question. They seemed unable to structure the information at hand in a meaningful way. It appeared that they were not able to isolate and integrate relevant items and, that they catalogued random facts, rather than providing the interpretation of events called for by the question. Noting this same tendency, Gardner and Hamby (1979) designed a pilot study looking at the role of the RH in organizing information for communication. Their work was later refined into a more extensive investigation into the ability of RH subjects to manage complex linquistic material (Wapner, Hamby & Gardner, 1981). In both studies, RH subjects and controls were presented with several tasks, one of which was to retell auditorily presented stories which emphasized either spatial, emotional, or noncanonical (unexpected or nonsensical) elements. The retold stories of the RH group, particularly in those with noncanonical endings, demonstrated that the RH subjects seemed to be uncertain about what was important and what was incidental. Gardner and Hamby explained that their patients seemed "unable to isolate, and to appreciate the relations among, the key points of the story. The basic schema—the major episodes organized in an hierarchically-appropriate manner—seems disturbed." They suggested that "the basic scaffolding of the story has not been satisfactorily assimilated. And, without this organizing principle, patients cannot even judge which details, or parts, matter."

Delis, Wapner, Gardner, and Moses (in press) studied this organizing principle directly by asking 10 RH and 10 intact controls to arrange mixed-up sentences into meaningful paragraphs. The paragraphs fell into three categories conveying primarily spatial, temporal, or categorical components. The RH group was significantly impaired relative to controls on all three paragraph types. Further analysis revealed that the RH subjects organized the temporal paragraphs with significantly more accuracy than the spatial ones, and arranged the latter with significantly more accuracy than the categorical ones. The effects of fatigue, memory, and attention were ruled out in the experiment. It is interesting to note that one of their subjects who achieved a verbal IQ of 148 (99.9th percentile) on the *Wechsler Adult Intelligence Scale* scored a mean of only 38.12% in this study, compared to an overall mean for all RH subjects of 49.82%. This fact lends further support to the notion that even when linguistic information is readily available, RH patients may still have difficulty organizing it into a meaningful pattern. This may partly account for the rambling inclusion of tangential detail so characteristic of RH responses to divergent questions.

In the Wapner et al. (1981) study, it was noted by the authors that their RH subjects had no difficulty using phonology and syntax in retelling narratives. But they also point out that while normal controls usually paraphrased the stories, 10 of the 15 RH subjects repeated segments verbatim without recoding them—another sign of difficulty in interpreting events.

Two studies (Myers, 1979, Myers & Linebaugh, 1980) looked at this deficit in interpreting events by asking subjects to reach conclusions about pictured material. In the latter study 12 RH subjects and 12 normal controls (age and education matched) were asked not to describe—but to explain—what was happening in the Cookie Theft picture from the *Boston Diagnostic Aphasia Examination.* Subject responses were analyzed for content in the following manner: a list of concepts used by normal speakers in describing the picture was obtained from a study by Yorkston and Beukelman (1980). The list was then divided into interpretive and literal concepts. Literal concepts were operationally defined as those that had meaning separate from the context of the depicted events. Interpretive concepts were defined as those whose meaning was derived from the context of events in the picture. Thus, "woman" was considered literal, while "mother" was considered interpretive. Three judges rated the response transcripts and the results demonstrated that the RH subjects had significantly fewer interpretive concepts, compared with controls. The experimental group tended to itemize isolated bits of information—such things as cups and saucers, curtains, and so on—which did not further a description of the action. Where a control subject might explain that the little girl was reaching up for a cookie, the typical RH patient might say that she had her arm up. The connection between her arm, the boy reaching into the jar, and handing a cookie to her went unnoticed. Thus, the RH group often missed the relationships among the elements of the picture, and, consequently, failed to infer meaning from those relationships.

As was noted in Section I, the subjects in this study were also significantly impaired relative to controls in a test of visual integration. The authors suggested that this deficit in visual synthesis on a low order perceptual level may extend to a deficit in integration on a higher level. Their subjects had difficulty in extracting the critical bits of information, and in apprehending the relationships among them. Thus, they failed to make the best use of contextual cues in deriving the meaning of the depicted events.

Rivers and Love (1980) found the same pattern on a series of visual processing tasks presented to normal controls, LH and RH groups. Their RH subjects had no significant difficulty in giving word definitions, or in a word-reading test, but were significantly worse than controls in utilizing sentence clues to substitute a real for a nonsense word. In another one of the seven tasks in their study, subjects were asked to make up a story based on the events depicted in a series of three sequential pictures. According to the authors, the RH responses in this task indicated "a reduced ability to use fully the information contained in the sequences of three pictures to tell complete stories." (p. 360)

That this deficit in responding appropriately to contextual clues extends beyond visually presented stimuli is evident from both the Gardner and Hamby and the Wapner et al. studies, since their subjects were required to listen to auditorily presented narratives. In addition, Metzler and Jelinek (1976) found their RH subjects had problems in retelling the auditorily presented quicksand paragraph from *The Minnesota Test for Differential Diagnosis of Aphasia* (Schuell, 1957). Their subjects had significantly more irrelevancies than controls.

Impaired use of contextual clues may have been an indirect factor in another study. Wapner and Gardner (1980) looked at the ability of 47 brain-damaged patients and 10 normal controls to process various types of linguistic and nonlinguistic symbols. The symbols included such things as trademarks, traffic signs, and symbols associated with numbers. The subjects had to choose one of four pictures in which the target symbol was correctly displayed. That is, they had to demonstrate an understanding of the symbol by finding the picture that showed it in its correct context. The results demonstrated that both the RH and LH groups were significantly impaired relative to controls, but that the two brain-damaged groups did not differ significantly from each other in overall success rate. However, the RH group relied more heavily on linguistic cues, and their performance deteriorated as these cues were faded. Their performance was inferior to the LH group, for example, in the pictorial trademarks test—they tended to choose the "unrelated" foil more often. The results of this study suggest that, without linguistic cues, RH subjects may have more difficulty than LH ones in determining what sort of traffic sign is most appropriately displayed in front of a school, or where the Playboy bunny belongs. The RH group may have had problems not only in understanding the symbols, but in processing the contextual cues that were intended to help them in the task.

Nonlinguistic symbols have presented problems for RH patients in other studies. Gardner and Denes (1973) looked at aphasic patients' responses to connotative versus denotative material and included six RH subjects in the experimental population. The denotative section of the study required subjects to match a spoken target word to one of four pictures. The connotative task was derived from an adaptation of Osgood's pictorial semantic differential test (Osgood, 1960). Subjects had to point to one of two sets of geometric forms or expressive lines drawn in such a way as to "capture an aspect of connotation of the particular word" (p. 186). The authors noted that the behavior of the RH group on the connotative task was very different from that of the aphasic subjects. In general, the RH subjects protested against the task. Two of the six refused several times to take this part of the test. The scores of the three who did take it were lower than that of the average anterior aphasic patient. It may be that the difficulty in the RH group stemmed directly from a problem in handling connotative material, as the authors suggest. Or it may be that the novelty of the task disrupted their performance, just as other RH subjects found it difficult to relate to the unexpected or noncanonical elements in the previously reported research.

Clinical observations that RH patients tend to be literal-minded, to miss nuance and subtlety, to overlook intended and connotative meanings has been supported in several studies. Winner and Gardner (1977) asked aphasic and RH subjects to match a metaphoric sentence to its appropriate interpretation depicted in one of four pictures. Aphasic subjects chose significantly more metaphoric (correct) pictures than the RH subjects. The most frequent error choice in the RH group was a literal depiction of the metaphor. When asked to explain the meaning of the metaphors, most RH subjects gave an accurate interpretation and appeared unaffected by the dissociation between their verbal explanations and their picture choices.

Myers and Linebaugh (1981) investigated patients' comprehension of connotative language by looking at their understanding of common idiomatic expressions. RH, LH, and control subjects were presented with two-sentence stories, each of which ended with a common idiom. The outcome of the story could only be determined through an accurate interpretation of the idiom. The five response categories varied according to literal vs. accurate depiction of the idiom, and according to correct or incorrect context or setting of the story events. A final foil depicted the opposite outcome of the story. The results showed that the RH group made significantly more errors than either controls or aphasic subjects, and that, while they selected the correct context significantly more often than the wrong one, they selected the literal depiction of the idiom significantly more often than the appropriate one.

These findings appear, at first, to be at odds with the findings of Stachowiak, Huber, Poeck, and Kerschensteiner 1977),who looked at text comprehension in aphasic, RH, and normal controls. Subjects were asked to choose one of five pictures that most closely matched a six-sentence story read aloud to them. The story stimuli contained an idiom, and one of the foil pictures showed a literal depiction of the idiom. However, the idiom was used only as a means of making the material redundant, since it was itself defined in the third sentence of each story. Thus, the thrust of the study was comprehension of text, rather than of metaphoric language, and RH and control subjects performed without significant differences on the task.

Gardner, King, Flamm, and Silverman (1975) suggested that humorous material fuses both the cognitive and affective aspects of communication. With this in mind, they designed a study in which RH, LH, and control subjects had to pick out the most humorous picture from a set of four. Both right and left brain-damaged populations were significantly impaired in their ability to pick out the cartoon pictures, and there were no significant differences in their performances relative to one another. More recently, Wapner et al. (1981) looked at subjects' ability to choose the correct punchline from a set of four, after listening to the body of the joke. The four choices included endings that were: (1) appropriate and funny; (2) appropriate and straightforward, but not funny; (3) sad; and (4) a nonsequitur that did not flow from the body of the joke. The RH subjects chose endings in the fourth category three times as often as controls. In addition, they often confabulated, as they had in other parts of the study, to explain a link between their choice of a nonsequitur and the joke. And, when these same subjects were presented with a cartoon picture series, they responded in a serious, rather than amused way, to the cartoons, demanding explanations for what other subject groups found funny.

Taken together, this research adds to data-based evidence to support several clinical observations, such as the oft-noted failure of RH patients to appreciate humor (their own or other peoples'), as well as failure to appreciate the connotative aspects of communication. RH patients often appear unresponsive to intended meaning and to extralinguistic cues, while the opposite pattern has been found in aphasic patients (see Wilcox, Davis & Leonard, 1978). Their overall impairment in apprehending and using contextual information to derive meaning may partly explain their insensitivity to the pragmatic aspects of communication—they seem unable to fully appreciate the speaker's intentions, purpose of the exchange, or their listener's needs. In addition, the results reported in this section suggest RH patients have difficulty in tasks that require them to extract and isolate key elements, see the relationships among them, integrate them into an overall structure, and draw inferences based on those relationships.

How should we treat these disorders? Should we attempt to treat them at all? Clearly, treatment of communication deficits of any type is within the purview of speech and language pathologists. But we must be cautious. The research reported in this setion represents only a beginning. From trial treatment we can continue to expand our knowledge base. Myers (1982) offers specific suggestions for presenting the patient with material that requires him to associate, interpret, and derive meaning from context. Adamovich (1981) has suggested another approach based on theories of cognitive development. And there will doubtless be others. Those working directly with this population should be religious in keeping data, and should recognize the obligation they have to share that information in the form of single-case or group studies.

Speech pathologists have been well trained to work with communicatively impaired people, but few have had formal training in working with the symptoms described here. Only by educating ourselves through clinical experience and by keeping abreast of the rapidly expanding literature on the RH will we be able to apply our formal training to the needs of this population.

Summary

We have travelled what may seem like a long journey across several landscapes, exploring lower-order perceptual impairments, neglect, prosodic and affective deficits, and higher-order language impairments, and the effect of each on RH communication. These disorders may appear to be discrete entities, but, for several reasons, it would be a mistake to assume they are wholly distinct from one another. First, many patients, particularly those with extensive lesions, will be impaired to some extent in each area. Second, while aphasia disrupts a certain system or class of behaviors (language), RH damage appears to disturb a less specific, more generalized response to experience itself. If perception is understood as involving the ability to both discriminate and interpret at the same time, then the link between lower-order perception and the management of complex material is apparent. At no stage of perception does man act as a mere sensory recorder. He constantly weighs and relates the fragments of external and internal experience into a personal unique whole. He derives meaning from events by filtering out the irrelevant, extracting what seems critical, and by relating those chosen elements into a pattern. Thus, experience is interpreted through an almost instantaneous operation which is performed prior to verbalization. To perceive is to know something directly, without subjecting it to analysis. The perceiver is not passive, but is an active participant allowing his internal associations and knowledge to guide him. An impairment in perception, as it is described here, would impair the ability to grasp the essense of events, or to experience a sense of connectedness with the outside world. It is not surprising that RH patients, then, have difficulty utilizing and responding to all the extralinguistic or pragmatic aspects of communication, or that the linguistic system itself is inadequate in helping them derive meaning from on-going events. To understand and accurately communicate experience clearly requires the participation of both sides of the brain.

Much has been made of the differing processing styles of the two intact hemispheres. Originally, they were thought to differ according to stimulus type-linguistic versus nonlinguistic. Research with brain-damaged, split-brain (in particular), and normal subjects refined this notion. Currently, it is popular to assign propositional, linear, sequential, and analytic or feature detection capabilities to the LH. The RH is thought to be more adept at apprehending the gestalt, in detecting patterns without feature analysis, and in appropositional, simultaneous, synthetic, integrative processing (Bogen, 1969; Gazzaniga, 1970; Ornstein, 1977; Zaidel, 1978; Patterson & Bradshaw, 1975; Cohen, 1973). Experimental data support this hypothesis, though not definitively. And it can be related to some extent to some of the deficits described in this chapter.

New evidence, however, constantly refines our understanding of the roles of the two hemispheres and their cooperation in complex tasks. Recent neuroanatomical and cytoarchitectural data support the view that the RH is more adept with complex input. Reviewing the evidence, Goldberg and Costa (1981) suggest that the RH has greater neuronal capacity to deal with informational complexity, has more associative cortex, has more intraregional connections, and has a greater ability to process many modes of representation within a single cognitive task. The LH, they explain, has more sensory and motor representation, has more interregional connections, and is superior in tasks which require fixation upon a single mode of representation (p. 148).

The thrust of their argument is that the LH is adept with descriptive systems (language, mathematics, and other coded behaviors), while the RH is pivotal in managing novel tasks for which no descriptive system exists. A descriptive system, as they define it, is one which "implies any set of discrete units of encoding or rules of transformation that can be successfully applied to the processing of a certain class of stimuli" (p. 151). Reliance on a routinized descriptive system, they explain, puts demands on the LH, while the RH appears to have more facility for utilizing associative areas of the cortex and for cross-modal integration.

This hypothesis, based on evidence too extensive to cite here, supports, but also extends and enriches, our earlier understanding of how the two hemispheres operate alone and in concert. It also helps us conceive of what may occur with unilateral brain damage.

Many of the deficits outlined in this chapter appear to affect experiential processing or operations that do not rely on routinized codes—i.e. assimilating contextual cues, distinguishing what is important from what is not, perceiving relationships, interpreting events. RH patients appear impaired on tasks in which they cannot rely on language or any other descriptive system to provide clues about their experience. They do not deal well with novel or unexpected situations or stimuli. The rules that operate on the pragmatic aspects of communication are not as neatly defined or coded as are the rules governing language itself. And so it may be that the inappropriate behaviors of the RH patient represent, in part, difficulty in managing situations in which he cannot apply an objective routine or code, or may represent an excessive reliance on descriptive systems that do not apply to the situation at hand.

This speculation is offered as a way of helping to conceptualize and weave together the multiple aspects of RH communication disorders. The differing capacities of the two hemispheres is of interest to people in a wide range of fields. The clinician working with this population should read widely, and be cautious in accepting any simple notion of hemisphere asymmetry. The capacities of the RH, and the impact of damage in that hemisphere on communication, is a story that is just beginning to unfold.

References

Adamovich, B. L. Treatment of right hemisphere damaged patients: A panel presentation. A. Davis (Moderator), In R. H. Brookshire (Ed.), *Clinical Aphasiology: Conference Proceedings.* Minneapolis: BRK Publishers, 1981.

Adamovich, B. L., & Brooks, R. L. A diagnostic protocol to assess the communication deficits in patients with right hemisphere damage. In R. H. Brookshire (Ed.), *Clinical Aphasiology: Conference Proceedings.* Minneapolis: BRK Publishers, 1981.

Benton, A. L. Visuoperceptive, visuospatial, and visuoconstructive disorders. In K. M. Heilman & E. Valenstein (Eds.), *Clinical neuropsychology.* New York: Oxford University Press, 1979.

Benton, A. L., Hannay, J., & Varney, N. R. Visual perception of line direction in patients with unilateral brain disease. *Neurology, 1975 25,* 907–910.

Benton, A. L., & Van Allen, M. W. Facial recognition in patients with cerebral disease. *Cortex, 1968, 4,* 344–358.

Bisiach, E. Capitani, E., Luzzatti, C., & Perani, D. Brain and conscious representation of outside reality. *Neuropsychologia, 1981, 19,* 543–551.

Bisiach, E., Luzzatti, C., & Perani, D. Unilateral neglect, representational schema and consciousness. *Brain, 1979, 102,* 609–618.

Bisiach, E., Nichelli, P., & Spinnler, H. Hemispheric functional asymmetry in visual discrimination between univariate stimuli: An analysis of sensitivity and response criterion. *Neuropsychologia, 1976, 14,* 335–342.

Bogen, J. The other side of the brain. II. *Bulletin of the Los Angeles Neurological Society, 34,* 1969.

Borkowski, J. G., Benton, A. L., & Spreen, O. Word fluency and brain damage. *Neuropsychologia, 1967, 5,* 135–140.

Bower, J. H. Imagery as a relational organizer in associative learning. *Journal of Verbal Learning and Verbal Behavior, 1970, 9,* 529–533.

Brain, W. R. Visual disorientation with special reference to lesions of the right cerebral hemisphere. *Brain, 1941, 64,* 244–272.

Bugeleski, B. R. Images as mediators in one-trail paired-associate learning, II. *Journal of Experimental Psychology,* 1968, *77,* 328–334.

Bugeleski, B. R. Words and things and images. *American Psychologist, 25,* 1970.

Buck, R., & Duffy, R. J. Non-verbal communication of affect in brain-damaged patients. *Cortex,* 1981, *6,* 351–362.

Butters, N., & Barton, M. Effect of parietal lobe damage on the performance of reversible operations in space. *Neuropsychologia,* 1970, *8,* 205–214.

Carmon, A., & Nachson, I. Ear asymmetry in perception of emotional and non-verbal stimuli. *Acta Psychologia,* 1973, *37,* 351–357.

Cicone, M., Wapner, W., & Gardner H. Sensitivity to emotional expressions and situations in organic patients. *Cortex,* 1980, *16,* 145–158.

Cohen, G. Hemispheric differences in serial verses parallel processing. *Journal of Experimental Psychology,* 1973, *97,* 349–356.

Collins, M. The minor hemisphere. In R. H. Brookshire (Ed.), *Clinical Aphasiology: Conference Proceedings.* Minneapolis: BRK Publishers, 1976.

Critchley, M. *The parietal lobes.* London: Edward Arnold, 1953.

Deal, J., Deal, L., Wertz, R., Kitselman, K., & Dwyer, C. Right hemisphere PICA percentiles: Some speculations about aphasia. In R.H. Brookshire (Ed.), *Clinical Aphasiology: Conference Proceedings.* Minneapolis: BRK Publishers, 1979.

Delis, D.C., Wapner, W., Gardner, H., & Moses, J. The contribution of the right hemisphere to the organization of paragraphs. *Cortex,* in press.

Dekosky, S., Heilman, K., Bowers, D., & Valenstein, E. Recognition and discrimination of emotional faces and pictures. *Brain and Language,* 1981, *9,* 206–214.

Denny-Brown, D., Myers, J. S., & Horenstein, S. The significance of perceptual rivalry resulting from parietal lesion, *Brain,* 1952, *75,* 443–471.

DeRenzi, E., & Spinnler, H. Facial recognition in brain damaged patients, *Neurology,* 1966, *16,* 145–152.

DeRenzi, E., Faglioni, P., & Spinnler, H. Performance of patients with unilateral brain damage on face recognition tasks. *Cortex,* 1968, *4,* 17–34.

Diamond, S. J. Differing emotional responses from right and left hemispheres. *Nature,* June, 1976, 261.

Diller, L., & Weinberg, J. Hemi-inattention in rehabilitation: The evolution of a rational remedial program. In E. A. Weinstein & R. P. Friedland (Eds.), *Advances in neurology* (Vol. 18). New York: Raven Press, 1977.

Enders, M. Emotional responses in subjects with cerebral hemisphere damage. Rehabilitation Research and Training Center Grant #16-P-56803/3, The George Washington University Medical Center, Washington, D.C., unpublished study, 1979.

Fredericks, J. A. M. Constructional apraxia and cerebral dominance. *Psychiatria, Neurologia, Neurochirurgia,* 1963, *66,* 522–530.

Galin, D. Implications for psychiatry of left and right cerebral specialization, *Archives of General Psychiatry,* 1974, *31,* 572–583.

Galper, R. E., & Costa, L. Hemispheric superiority for faces depends on how they are learned. *Cortex,* 1980, *16,* 21–38.

Gardner, H., & Denes, G. Connotative judgements by aphasic patients on a pictorial adaptation of the semantic differential. *Cortex,* 1973, *9,* 183–96.

Gardner, H., King, P., Flamm, L., & Silverman, J. Comprehension and appreciation of humorous material following brain damage. *Brain,* 1975, *98,* 399–412.

Gardner, H., & Hamby, S. The role of the right hemisphere in the organization of linguistic materials. Paper presented to the International Neuropsychology Symposium, Dubrovnik, Yugoslavia, June, 1979.

Gates, A., & Bradshaw, J. L. The role of the cerebral hemispheres in music. *Brain and Language,* 1977, *4,* 403–31.

Gazzaniga, M. *The bisected brain.* New York: Appleton-Century-Crofts, 1970.

Geffin, G., Bradshaw, J. L., & Wallace, G. Interhemispheric effects on reaction time to verbal and non-verbal visual stimuli. *Journal of Experimental Psychology,* 1971, *87,* 415–422.

Gerstman, J. The problem of imperception of disease and of impaired body territories with organic lesions. *Archives of Neurology and Psychiatry,* 1942, *48,* 890–913.

Gianotti, G. Emotional behavior and hemispheric side of lesion. *Cortex,* 1972, *8,* 41–55.

Gianotti, G., Caltagirone, C., Miceli, G., & Masullo, C. Selective semantic-lexical impairment of language comprehension in right-brain-damaged patients. *Brain and Language,* 1981, *13,* 201–211.

Goodglass, H., & Kaplan, E. *The Boston Diagnostic Aphasia Examination.* Philadelphia: Lea & Febiger, 1967.

Goldberg, E., & Costa, L. Hemispheric differences in the acquisition and use of descriptive systems. *Brain and Language,* 1981, *14,* 144–173.

Gordon, H. Left hemisphere dominance for rhythmic elements in dichotically-presented melodies. *Cortex,* 1978, *14,* 58–69.

Haggard, P., & Parkinson, A. M. Stimulus and task factors as determinants of ear advantages. *Quarterly Journal of Experimental Psychology,* 1971, *23,* 168–177.

Halperin, Y., Nachson, I., & Carmon, A. Shift of ear superiority in dichotic listening to temporally patterned nonverbal stimuli. *Journal of the Acoustical Society of America,* 1973, *53,* 46–50.

Hansch, E. C., & Priozollo, F. J. Task relevant effects on the assessment of cerebral specialization for facial emotion. *Brain and Language,* 1980, *10,* 51–59.

Head, H. *Studies in neurology.* London: Oxford University Press, 1920.

Hecaen, H. Clinical symptomatolgy in right and left hemisphere lesions. In V. B. Mountcastle (Ed.), *Interhemispheric relations and cerebral dominance.* Baltimore: Johns Hopkins University Press, 1962.

Heilman, K. M., & Valenstein, E. Frontal lobe neglect in man. *Neurology,* 1979, *22,* 660–664.

Heilman, K.M., Scholes, R., & Watson, R. T. Auditory affective agnosia. *Journal of Neurology, Neurosurgery, and Psychiatry,* 1975, *38,* 69–72.

Heilman, K. M., & Watson, R. T. The neglect syndrome: A unilateral defect in the orienting response. In S. Harnad (Ed.), *Lateralization in the nervous system.* New York: Academic Press, 1977.

Heilman, K. M., Schwartz, H. D., & Watson, R. T. Hypoarousal in patients with neglect and emotional indifference. *Neurology,* 1978, *28,* 229–232.

Heilman, K. M. Neglect and related disorders. In K. M. Heilman & E. Valenstein (Eds.), *Clinical neuropsychology.* New York: Oxford Univ. Press, 1979.

Hilliard, R. D. Hemispheric laterality effects in facial recognition tasks in normal subjects. *Cortex,* 1973, *9,* 246–258.

Hooper, E. *The Hooper Visual Organization Test.* Los Angeles: Western Psychological Services, 1958.

Jones, B. Lateral asymmetry in testing long term memory for faces. *Cortex,* 1979, *15,* 183–186.

Joynt, R., & Goldstein, M. The minor hemisphere. *Advances in Neurology,* 1975, *7,* 147–183.

Kaplan, E., Goodglass, H., & Weintraub, S. *The Boston Naming Test,* experimental edition, 1976.

Kent, R. D., & Rosenbek, J. C. Prosodic disturbance and neurologic site of lesion. *Brain and Language,* in press.

King, F. L., & Kimura, D. Left ear superiority in dichotic perception of vocal non-verbal sounds. *Canadian Journal of Psychology,* 1972, *26,* 111–116.

Klein, D., Muscovitch, J., & Vigna, C. Attentional mechanisms and perceptual asymmetries in recognition of words and faces. *Neuropsychologia*, 1976, *14*, 55–66.

LaPointe, L., & Culton, G. Visual-spatial neglect subsequent to brain injury. *Journal of Speech and Hearing Disorders*, 1969, *34*, 82–86.

LeDoux, J. E. Parietooccipital symptomatology: The split brain perspective. In M. Gazzaniga (Ed.), *Handbook of neuropsychology*. New York: Plenum Press, 1978.

Leehey, S. C., & Cahn, A. Lateral asymmetries in the recognition of words, familiar faces and unfamiliar faces. *Neuropsychologia*, 1979, *17*, 619–635.

Ley, R. G., & Bryden, M. P. Hemispheric differences in processing emotions and faces. *Brain and Language*, 1979, *7*, 127–138.

Marzi, C. A., & Berlucchi, G. Right visual field superiority for accuracy of recognition of famous faces in normals. *Neuropsychologia*, 1977, *15*, 751–756.

Metzler, N., & Jelinek, J. Writing disturbances in patients with right cerebral hemisphere lesions. In R. H. Brookshire (Ed.), *Clinical Aphasiology: Conference Proceedings*. Minneapolis: BRK Publishers, 1976.

McNeil, M. R., & Prescott, T. E. *Revised Token Test*. Baltimore: University Park Press, 1978.

Mills, L., & Rollman, G. Hemispheric asymmetry for auditory perception of temporal order. *Neuropsychologia*, 1980, *18*, 41–47.

Milner, B. Laterality effects in audition. In V. B. Mountcastle (Ed.) *Interhemispheric relations and cerebral dominance*. Baltimore: Johns Hopkins University Press, 1962.

Milner, B. Hemispheric specialiation: Scope and limits. In F. Schmitt & F. Worden (Eds.), *Neurosciences third study program*. Cambridge: MIT Press, 1974.

Morrow, L., Vrtunsk, P. B., Kim, Y., & Boller, F. Arousal responses to emotional stimuli and laterality of lesion. *Neuropsychologia*, 1981, *19*, 65–71.

Myers, P. S. Analysis of right hemisphere communication deficits: Implications for speech pathology. In R. H. Brookshire (Ed.), *Clinical Aphasiology: Conference Proceedings*. Minneapolis: BRK Publishers, 1978.

Myers, P. S. Profiles of communication deficits in patients with right cerebral hemisphere damage. In R. H. Brookshire (Ed.), *Clinical Aphasiology: Conference Proceedings*. Minneapolis: BRK Publishers, 1979.

Myers, P. S. Visual imagery in aphasia treatment: A new look. In R. H. Brookshire (Ed.), *Clinical Aphasiology: Conference Proceedings*. Minneapolis: BRK Publishers, 1980.

Myers, P. S. Right hemisphere communication disorders. In W. H. Perkins (Ed.), *Current therapy in communication disorders*. New York: Thieme-Stratton, in press.

Myers, P. S., & Linebaugh, C. W. The perception of contextually conveyed relationships by right brain damaged patients. Paper presented to the American Speech-Lauguage-Hearing Association Convention, Detroit, 1980.

Myers, P. S., & Linebaugh, C. W. Comprehension of idiomatic expressions by right-hemisphere-damaged adults. In R. H. Brookshire (Ed.), *Clinical Aphasiology: Conference Proceedings*. Minneapolis: BRK Publishers, 1981.

Newcombe, F., & Russell, W. R. Dissociated visual perceptual and spatial deficits in focal lesions of the right hemisphere. *Journal of Neurology, Neurosurgery, and Psychiatry*, 1969, *32*, 78–81.

Ornstein, R. *The psychology of human consciousness*. New York: Harcourt, Brace, Jovanovich, 1977.

Osgood, C. The cross cultural generality of visual-verbal synesthetic tendencies. *Behavioral Science*, 1960, *5*, 146–169.

Paivio, A. Mental imagery in associative learning and memory. *Psychological Review*, 1969, *76*, 241–263.

Paivio, A. *Imagery and verbal processes*. New York: Holt, Rinehart, & Winston, 1971.

Patterson, K., & Bradshaw, J. Differential hemispheric mediation of nonverbal visual stimuli. *Journal of Experimental Psychology*, 1975, *1*, 246–252.

Porch, B. *The Porch Index of Communicative Abilities*. Palo Alto: Consulting Psychologist Press, 1967.

Pylyshn, Z. What the mind's eye tells the mind's brain: A critique of mental imagery. *Psychological Bulletin*, 1973, *80*, 1–24.

Rapaczynski, W., & Ehrlichman, H. Opposite visual hemifield superiorities in face recognition as a function of cognitive style. *Neuropsychologia*, 1979, *17*, 645–652.

Ratcliff, G. Spatial thought, mental rotation, and the right cerebral hemisphere. *Neuropsychologia*, 1979, *17*, 49–53.

Riege, W., Metter, E. J., & Hanson, W. R. Verbal and nonverbal recognition memory in aphasic and non-aphasic stroke patients. *Brain and Language*, 1980, *10*, 60–70.

Rivers, D. L., & Love, R. J. Language performance on visual processing tasks in right hemisphere lesion cases. *Brain and Language*, 1980, *10*, 348–366.

Rizzolatti, C., Umilita, C., & Berlucchi, G. Opposite superiorities of the right and left cerebral hemispheres in a discriminative reaction time to physiognimical and alphabetical materials. *Brain*, 1971, *94*, 431–442.

Ross, E. D. The aprosodias. *Archives of Neurology*, 1981, *38*, 561–569.

Ross, E. D., and Mesulam, M. Dominant language functions of the right hemisphere? *Archives of Neurology*, 1979, *36*, 144–148.

Rowher, W. D. Images and pictures in children's learning: Research results and educational implications. *Psychological Bulletin*, 1970, *72*, 399–403.

Russo, M., & Vignolo, L. A. Visual figure-ground discrimination in patients with unilateral cerebral disease. *Cortex*, 1967, *3*, 113–127.

Schlanger, B. B., Schlanger, P., & Gerstman, L. J. The perception of emotionally toned sentences by right-hemisphere damaged and aphasic subjects. *Brain and Language*, 1976, *3*, 396–403.

Schuell, H. *The Minnesota Test for Differential Diagnosis of Aphasia*. Minneapolis: University of Minnesota Press, 1957.

Semmes, J. Hemispheric specialization: A possible clue to mechanism. *Neuropsychologia*, 1968, *6*, 11–26.

Shapiro, B., Grossman, M., & Gardner, H. Selective musical processing deficits in brain damaged populations. *Neuropsychologia*, 1981, *19*, 161–168.

Sidtis, J. On the nature of the cortical function underlying right hemisphere auditory perception. *Neuropsychologia*, 1980, *18*, 321–330.

Sparks, R., Helm, N., & Albert, M. Aphasia rehabilitation resulting from melodic intonation therapy. *Cortex*, 1974, *10*, 303–316.

Sperry, R. W. Hemispheric disconnection and unity in conscious awareness. *American Psychologist*, 1968, *23*, 723–733.

Stachowiak, F. F., Huber, W., Poeck, K., & Kerschensteiner, M. Text comprehension in aphasia. *Brain and Language*, 1977, *4*, 177–195.

Stanton, K., Flowers, C., Kuhl, P., Miller, R., & Smith, C. Teaching compensation of left neglect through a language-oriented program. Paper presented to the American Speech-Language-Hearing Association Convention, Atlanta, 1979.

Stanton, K., Yorkston, K. M., Talley-Kenyon, V. T., & Beukelman, D. R. Language utilization in teaching reading to left neglect patients. In R. H. Brookshire (Ed.), *Clinical Aphasiology: Conference Proceedings*. Minneapolis: BRK Publishers, 1981.

Strauss, E., & Muscovitch, M., Perception of facial emotion. *Brain and Language*, 1981, *13*, 308–332.

Suberi, M., & McKeever, W. Differential right hemisphere memory for storage of emotional and non-emotional faces. *Neuropsychologia*, 1977, *15*, 757–768.

Tucker, D. M., Watson, R. T., & Heilman, K. M. Discrimination and evocation of affectively intoned speech in patients with right parietal disease. *Neurology*, 1977, *27*, 947–950.

Wapner, W., & Gardner, H. Profiles of symbol-reading skills in organic patients. *Brian and Language*, 1980, *12*, 303–312.

Wapner, W., Hamby, S., & Gardner, H. The role of the right hemisphere in the appreciation of complex linguistic material. *Brain and Language*, 1981, *14*, 15–33.

Warrington, E. K., & James, M. An experimental investigation of facial recognition in patients with unilateral cerebral lesions. *Cortex*, 1967, *3*, 317–326.

Watson, R. T., Heilman, K. M., Cauthen, J. C., & King, F. A. Neglect after cingulectomy. *Neurology*, 1973, *23*, 1003–1007.

Watson, R. T., Miller, B., & Heilman, K. Nonsensory neglect. *Annals of Neurology*, 1978, *3*, 505–508.

Watson, R. T., Miller, B., & Heilman, K. M. Evoked potentials in neglect. *Archives of Neurology*, 1977, *34*, 224–227.

Weber, R. J., & Bach, M. Visual and speech imagery. *British Journal of Psychology*, 1969, *60*, 199–202.

Weinstein, S. Deficits concomitant with aphasia or lesions of either cerebral hemisphere. *Cortex*, 1964, *1*, 151–169.

Weintraub, S., Mesulam, M., & Kramer, L. Disturbances in prosody: A right-hemisphere contribution to language. *Archives of Neurology*, 1981, *38*, 742–744.

West, J. Imaging and aphasia. In R. H. Brookshire (Ed.), *Clinical Aphasiology: Conference Proceedings*. Minneapolis: BRK Publishers, 1977.

West, J. Heightening the action imagery of materials used in aphasia treatment. In R. H. Brookshire (Ed.), *Clinical Aphasiology: Conference Proceedings*. Minneapolis: BRK Publishers, 1978.

Wilcox, M. J., Davis, G. A., & Leonard, L. B. Aphasic's comprehension of contextually conveyed meaning. *Brain and Language*, 1978, *6*, 362–377.

Winner, E., & Garnder, H. The comprehension of metaphor in brain-damaged patients. *Brain*, 1977, *100*, 719–727.

Yorkston, K. M., & Beukelman, D. R. An analysis of connected speech samples of aphasic and normal speakers. *Journal of Speech and Hearing Disorders*, 1980, *45*, 27–36.

Yorkston, K. M. Treatment of right hemisphere damaged patients: A panel presentation. A. Davis (Moderator), In R. H. Brookshire (Ed.), Clinical Aphasiology: Conference Proceedings. Minneapolis: BRK Publishers, 1981.

Zaidel, E. The elusive right hemisphere of the brain. *Engineering and Science*, 1978, Sept.-Oct., 10–32.

Zurif, E. Auditory lateralization: Prosodic and syntactic features. *Brain and Language*, 1974, *1*, 391–404.

Kathryn A. Bayles

Language and Dementia

Dementia

Dementia is a condition of chronic progressive deterioration of intellect, memory, and communicative function resulting from organic brain disease. In early dementia the behavioral manifestations may be subtle and apparent only to family members and close acquaintances. Eventually intellect, personality, and language become so impaired that the individual is unable to function socially or occupationally.

The term dementia denotes a constellation of behavioral abnormalities. Aretaeus of Cappadocia introduced the term in the second century B.C., to refer to a chronic degenerative mental disease associated with old age. Since then, dementia has been applied to a variety of disorders and often used synonymously with insanity. Emil Kraepelin (1919) redefined dementia in the late 1800s as a mental disorder characterized by memory disturbance and loss of the ability to reason. Kraepelin specified two types, senile and presenile dementia. The presenile form of the disease was described by Alois Alzheimer (1907), a neuropathologist who had observed the progressive deterioration of intellect, memory, and orientation in a 51-year-old woman. After her death, Alzheimer examined the brain and discovered cerebral atrophy and the presence of senile plaques and neurofibrillary tangles in the neocortex.

The disease Dr. Alzheimer described was thought to occur only in the presenium, prior to the age of 65, and a variety of other terms became popular for Alzheimer's disease when it occurred in the senium. The term "chronic brain syndrome" became popular after its use was recommended in the 1952 edition of the *Diagnostic and Statistical Manual on Mental Disorders* (DSM-I). In this edition, a distinction was introduced between the terms "acute" and "chronic" brain syndrome, and dementia became "chronic brain syndrome associated with senile brain disease." The terms "chronic" and "acute" proved confusing because their application involved a clinical judgment about disease onset and progress. Authors of the second edition of the *Diagnostic and Statistical Manual* (DSM-II) (1968), seeking to eliminate confusion, made the use of "acute" or "chronic" optional.

The Committee on Organic Mental Disorders of the American Psychiatry Association reviewed the definition of organic mental disorders preparatory to publishing *DSM-III* (1980). Additional revisions were made in the terminology applied to mental disorders. Dementia was recognized as being caused by several different diseases which were categorized as "primary degenerative" and "secondary degenerative." For the first time, senile, presenile, and circulatory dementias were classified together as "primary degenerative dementias" and senile brain disease was referred to as Alzheimer's disease (AD).

In addition to revising the terminology used to refer to degenerative brain disorders, the Committee on Organic Mental Disorders established a set of diagnostic criteria for differentiating dementia from other disorders. Some of the conditions *must* be present, while others *may* be present. Aphasia, described as a loss of language due to brain dysfunction, is a condition noted to be sometimes present. However, research of the last decade suggests that language impairment is present in all stages of dementia (Bayles, 1982; Irigaray, 1973; Obler & Albert, 1981a). In the early stages, cognitive changes are subtle and it is only with tests of much subtlety that language changes are also detected. Often these language changes are well concealed by patients in everyday interactions. To believe that language is not affected when intellect, memory, attention, and other higher cortical functions are deteriorating is not consistent with what is known about the relationship of thought to language.

Use of the term aphasia to describe language dysfunction associated with dementia is likely to be confusing to speech-language pathologists, because it denotes a loss in the ability to manipulate linguistic symbols as a result of focal brain damage, usually of sudden onset, as a result of cerebral vascular accident. Since none of these conditions apply to dementia, the term "aphasia" seems inappropriate for denoting the language deficits in such patients.

TABLE 7-1.
Types of Dementia. (Foley's taxonomy with modifications noted by *)

Remedial Nonvascular Causes

Intoxications
Infections
Metabolic Disorders
Nutritional Defects (Korsakoff's Syndrome)*
Subdural Hematoma
Benign Intracranial Tumors
Occult Hydrocephalus (Normal Pressure Hydrocephalus [NPH])
Sensory Deprivation
Depression*

Irreversible Nonvascular Dementia with Movement Disorder

Parkinson's Disease*
Huntington's Chorea
Creutzfeldt-Jacob Disease
Progressive Supranuclear Palsy
Progressive Subcortical Gliosis

Irreversible Nonvascular Dementia without Movement Disorder

Alzheimer's Disease
Pick's Disease
Senile Brain Atrophy

Vascular Dementia

Multiple Infarctions

Classification of Dementia-Producing Diseases

Although all dementia-producing diseases are associated with neural degeneration, they can be differentiated from each other in many respects. One classification system that identifies many of the differentiating characteristics is that of Foley's (1972), shown in Table 7-1. Foley distinguishes among the dementing illnesses on the bases of being reversible, associated with movement disorder, or vascular in origin.

Albert (1978) has proposed a classification system in which dementias are designated as cortical or subcortical. This classification appears to the author to be perplexing and premature because it implies that the brain damage causing dementia is solely cortical or subcortical, an implication that remains to be documented. For example, Albert classifies Parkinson's disease as a subcortical dementia, yet degenerative changes, similar to those found in Alzheimer's patients, occur in the neocortex of some Parkinson's disease patients. If intellectual and memory deterioration can be shown to occur in subcortical dementia without observable cortical changes, then Albert's distinction may be useful. While it is true that the majority of neurological changes in Parkinson's disease or Huntington's disease may be subcortical, the changes that result in dementia may not be subcortical.

Prevalence and Incidence of Dementia

One in every 100 persons 65 years or older suffers from severe dementia and 10 from mild dementia (Wang, 1981). In the absence of effective treatment, it has been estimated that the prevalence of dementia should double within the lifetime of our children and triple within the lifetime of our grandchildren (Katzman, 1981). Dementia-producing diseases primarily affect the 65-plus age group, the fastest growing segment of this country's population. There are currently 24.7 million Americans 65 years and older, and by the year 2000 the 65-plus population is expected to rise 32% to 32 million people, or 1 out of every 8 persons. That ratio will change to 1 of every 6 persons by the year 2020.

Because dementia patients are eventually incapable of self-care, many are placed in nursing homes. According to a report of the National Center of Health Statistics (1978), dementia afflicts 58% of the more than 1 million Americans in nursing homes, and is the most common syndrome among nursing home residents. The cost of caring for dementia patients represents 30% of the health care costs of the country (Frederickson, 1981), a figure that will increase with the imminent, dramatic growth of the elderly population.

Incidence

The incidence of dementia diseases, as well as their sex distribution, was studied by Malamud (1972), whose data are presented in Table 7-2.

TABLE 7-2
Distribution of Types of Degenerative Disorders among 1,225 Cases (Malamud, 1972).

	Age range	# Cases	%	Male/female ratio
Senile Brain Disease	65– 98	416	(34)	3:2
Alzheimer's Disease	40– 64	103	(8.4)	2:3
Pick's Disease	35– 72	35	(2.8)	1:1
Creutzfeldt-Jacob Disease	43– 86	32	(2.7)	2:1
Multi-infarct Dementia	42–100	356	(29)	2:1
Mixed: Senile Brain Disease and Multi-infarct Dementia	62– 94	283	(23)	4:3

Senile brain-disease patients comprised the largest category, accounting for 34%. However, Malamud distinguished between senile brain disease and Alzheimer's disease by age of onset. If they are grouped together as they are in many incidence reports, the incidence rate is 42%, only slightly lower than the 50% reported by Tomlinson (1977) in his study of 50 dementia patients. Multi-infarct dementia, a term introduced by Hachinski, Lassen, and Marshall (1974) for dementia resulting from frequent small vascular lesions, is the second most frequently occurring such disease. This finding is consistent with Tomlinson's (1977) report that multi-infarct disease occurs alone in 20% of the cases and with Alzheimer's disease in 18% of the cases.

Incidence figures for dementia do not include dementia patients with Parkinson's disease. Parkinson's disease affects approximately 100 individuals in every 100,000 (Pollock & Hornabrook, 1966) although incidence rises sharply with advancing age as shown in Table 7-3. Presently, in the United States, approximately 375,000 individuals have Parkinson's disease (Reisberg, 1981).

Although dementia is not an inevitable consequence of Parkinson's, it occurs in a significant percentage of cases, a fact that is becoming more widely recognized (Diamond, Markham, & Treciokas, 1976; Martin,

TABLE 7-3
Incidence Rates by Age for Parkinson's disease

Age	Number of affected individuals per 100,000
50–59	239
60–69	758
70–84	1,407

TABLE 7-4
Incidence of Dementia in Parkinson's disease

Year	Author	Percentage
1923	Lewy	77
1949	Mjönes	40
1951	Monroe	33
1966	Pollock & Hornabrook	20
1972	Loranger et al.	36.5 to 57.1
1979	Boller et al.	33
1979	Lieberman et al.	32
1982	Pirozzolo et al.	93

Loewenson, & Resch, 1973; Selby, 1968; Sweet, McDowell, & Feigenson, 1976). The percentage of Parkinson's disease patients who become demented is uncertain, but is probably between 30 and 39%, as can be seen in Table 7-4.

The explanation is still being sought for why some Parkinson's patients develop an associated dementia while others do not. It may be that Alzheimer's disease is co-occurring with Parkinson's disease in patients with dementia because Alzheimer's-like morphological changes have been found in many Parkinson's disease patients with dementia (Hakim & Mathieson, 1979; Selby, 1968). Several investigators suggest there may be two forms of the disease (Boller, Mitzutani, Roessmann, & Gambetti,

1979; Garron, Klawans, & Narin, 1972; Hirano & Zimmerman, 1962; Lieberman, Dziatolowski, Kupersmith, Serby, Goodgold, Korein, & Goldstein, 1979), a motor disorder without dementia in which degenerative changes are limited to subcortical structures, and a second form in which dementia is associated with motor dysfunction and cortical as well as subcortical changes.

Dementia is a certainty in Huntington's disease, a rare autosomal dominant genetic disorder characterized by abnormal involuntary movements, intellectual deterioration, and affective disorders. Four to seven individuals per 100,000 are stricken with Huntington's disease, and at least twice this number are at risk because it is a genetically transmitted disease. Prevalence estimates are scarce because the disease is rare and may often be misdiagnosed or concealed.

Characteristics of Major Dementia-Producing Illness

Alzheimer's Disease (AD): Senile Brain Disease (SBD)

Alzheimer's disease and senile brain disease are neuropathologically indistinguishable and differ only in age of onset. AD occurs in the presenium, and SBD after the age of 65. Because age of onset appears to be the only difference between AD and SBD, there has been an increasing tendency to consider them as a single disease entity. The 1980 edition of the Diagnostic and Statistical Manual eliminated the age of onset as a criterion for AD. AD was defined as a primary degenerative brain disorder which reduces life span and produces dementia.

Morphological changes. The classic neuropathological changes associated with AD are the formation of senile plaques (SP), neurofibrillary tangles (NFT), and granulovacuolar degeneration (GVD) in the neocortex, particularly the temporal lobe and hippocampus. Senile plaques, also called neuritic plaques, consist of an amyloid core surrounded by an outer ring of granular filamentous material (Corsellis, 1962) and are thought to interfere with the transmission of nerve impulses.

Neurofibrillary tangles, the most characteristic change of AD, typically consist of multitudes of twisted intraneuronal fibers, or pairs of helically wound filaments (Kidd, 1963). The fibers making up NFTs have a marked twist unlike normal neurofibers. The nucleus of cells with NFT is essentially normal, except for twisted tubules coursing through the cytoplasm of the cell body, displacing and replacing the organelles normally found in this location (Terry & Wisniewski, 1975). NFT occur throughout the cortical mantle, the hippocampal formation, and the amygdala, but seem to prefer the hippocampus, an area of brain associated with recent memory. When bilateral damage occurs to the hippocampus, recent memory is permanently impaired. The amygdala is a series of nuclei in the temporal lobe that are thought to affect emotion. Degenerative changes in the amygdala may cause the flat affect and passivity characteristic of many dementia patients.

Granulovacuolar degeneration, GVD, the third type of morphological change associated with AD, is a descriptive term for changes occurring inside the cell, namely the accumulation of fluid-filled vacuoles and granular debris. These intracytoplasmic granules are sensitive to silver staining and are seen in the hippocampus (Malamud, 1972).

Particularly intriguing to scientists is the finding that morphological changes characteristic of Alzheimer's disease occur in the brains of the healthy elderly, but to a lesser degree. Tomlinson and Henderson (1976) studied postmortem brain samples and found small numbers of senile plaques in the brains of 15% of people in the 5th decade, in 50% of the people in the 7th decade and 75% of people in the 9th decade. Small concentrations of NFT were found in 10 to 20% of healthy older people, while 40% of dementia patients had numerous, widely scattered tangles. Granulovacuolar degeneration was unusual in 70% of the normal elderly. Tomlinson and Henderson believed the differences between SP, NFT, and GVD in normal and demented were quantitative, not qualitative, and indicated that their presence in the "healthy elderly person" suggests that AD many be an exaggeration of normal aging. Demented individuals had 14 or more plaques per low power field of standard size, and a total volume of 50 ml or more of macroscopically evident softening.

Symptomatology. Memory impairment, mood changes, and personality disturbances are among the first symptoms of AD. Intellectual deterioration is insidious and inexorable. As the disease progresses, impairment in both recent and long-term memory becomes noticeable and the person becomes disoriented for time, place, and self. Eventually, there is global failure of all memory, as well as apathy and incontinence.

Cause(s). Recent research which documents a malfunction in the cholinergic system among Alzheimer's patients may provide a clue to its cause or causes. The cholinergic system is a group of neurons that transmit nerve impulses through acetylcholine. The enzymes CAT (choline acetyltransferase) and ACT (acetylcholinesterase) are necessary for the manufacture of acetylcholine, and the degree to which enzymatic activity is present in the cells reveals the ability of those cells to manufacture acetylcholine. Both CAT and ACT have been found to be reduced by 80% in AD patients (CAT: Davies & Mahoney, 1976; Perry, Perry, Blessed, & Tomlinson, 1977; Reisine, Yamamura, Bird, Spokes, & Enna, 1978; White, Hiley, Goodhardt, Carrasco, Keet, Williams, & Bowen, 1977; ACT: Perry, Perry, Blessed, & Tomlinson, 1978). The brain areas associated with CAT and ACT reduction are the hippocampus, septum, and temporal lobe, precisely those anatomic areas suffering the most extensive degenerative changes in Alzheimer's disease.

Because AD appears to selectively destroy acetylcholine producing neurons, researchers have theorized that raising body levels of acetylcholine might arrest the disease. Because the nervous system is incapable of synthesizing choline (Sparf, 1973; Yavin, 1976), there has been much interest in administering choline derivatives or lecithin, the body's natural source of choline. As yet, results of such treatments are quite nuclear.

Some researches are investigating the possibility that excessive accumulation of environmental toxins and trace metals, most notably aluminum, may cause AD. Crapper, Krishnan, and Quittkat (1976), reported increased levels of aluminum in the brain cells of AD patients. However, McDermott, Smith, Iqbal, and Wisniewski (1977) could not replicate this finding and reported elevated levels of aluminum in both AD patients and age-matched controls. They concluded that intracellular aluminum concentration, particularly in the hippocampus, increases with age. The data of Caster and Wang (1981) suggest that dietary aluminum is neither an essential nutrient nor a toxic element, and tends to accumulate in the membrane tangles in AD. Perl and Brody (1980) examined aluminum levels in hippocampal neurons of three AD patients with scanning electron microscopy and x-ray spectrometry, and found concentrations in the nuclear regions of neurons containing neurofibrillary tangles in both controls and AD patients. Normal-appearing neurons were free of aluminum. Excessive concentrations of aluminum are of concern because their presence is thought to disrupt intracellular protein synthesis (McDermott et al., 1977). As yet, it is unclear whether aluminum concentration may contribute to the neuropathological changes associated with AD or whether it merely increases in the neurons after they have degenerated.

Also under investigation is the possibility that AD results from a slow virus similar to those that result in Creutzfeldt-Jacob disease or Kuru, both of which also are accompanied by dementia. Kuru is a disease once prevalent among the cannibalistic Fore tribe of New Guinea, and is transmitted through ingestion of brain tissue from an affected individual. In 1965, Gajdusek and Gibbs found that when monkeys and chimps were innoculated with brain tissue extracts from Kuru or Creutzfeldt-Jacob disease, they developed degenerative brain disease. Recently, a factor taken from the brains of AD patients was injected into cell cultures of neurons from aborted human fetuses. Neurofilaments with the paired helical pattern typical of AD were produced (Crapper & De Boni, 1979).

Genetics of Alzheimer's Disease. A predisposition to AD may be genetically transmitted; individuals with a first-order relative have a four times greater chance of having the disease than people without such familial relationship (Larsson, Sjörgren, & Jacobson, 1963). This finding has led some researchers to suggest an autosomal dominant mode of inheritance. Others suggest a multifactorial mode (Slater & Cowie, 1970).

Alzheimer's disease is also associated with Down's syndrome (mongolism), a defect characterized by the presence of an extra chromosome, and, like Down's syndrome, may be the consequence of chromosomal abnormality (Reisberg, 1981). The morphological changes characteristic of Alzheimer's disease are found in individuals with Down's syndrome in numbers disproportionate to the normal population. Additionally, there is evidence of an increased incidence of Down's syndrome in families with a history of Alzheimer's disease (Heston & Mastri, 1977; Wisniewski, Howe, Williams, & Wisniewski, 1978).

Malamud (1972) examined the frequency of occurrence of dementia in 347 Down's syndrome cases and 813 cases representing other forms of mental retardation. Of the 347 cases with Down's syndrome, 40 patients (12%), ranging in age from 20 to 69 at the time of death, showed pathologic changes characteristic of senile brain disease, and 60% of these (7% of the total) had severe atrophy. This finding dramatically contrasted with the virtual absence of cortical atrophy among the 813 other retardates. There were no patients with Down's syndrome past the age of 40 in whom such changes were not found. Elam and Blumenthal (1970) suggested the high incidence of cortical atrophy in Down's syndrome cases represented a predisposition toward premature aging, and when associated with signs of delayed maturation, also typical of Down's syndrome, indicated a more rapid aging process. Ball and Nuttal (1980) studied the degree of neurofibrillary tangle formation, granulovacuolar degeneration, and nerve cell loss in serial sections of the hippocampal formation of the brains of five adults with Down's syndrome who were dying. They observed neurofibrillary tangle formation in hippocampal neurons to be more extensive than that occurring in normal elderly subjects. In only one of their subjects were morphological changes within normal limits. Granulovacuolar degeneration, however, fell within the normal range for the three youngest of the five patients, which led Ball and Nuttal to suspect granulovacuolar degeneration may be influenced as much by age as the presence of Down's syndrome. Neuronal density in the hippocampal cortex averaged 60% of that in the control population, and was of the same magnitude as that found in Alzheimer's disease patients. Ball and Nuttal thus hypothesized that a pathogenetic aging mechanism may be the key to understanding Alzheimer's disease.

Multi-infarct
Dementia (MID)

Multi-infarct dementia is a term for vascular dementia caused by the accumulation of brain damage resulting from multiple small infarctions. In the majority of cases, one or more large areas of infarction exist and involve the middle and posterior cerebral arteries more often than the anterior. Like stroke, MID is most likely to occur between the ages of 40 and 60 years, and males are more likely to be affected than females. There is usually a history of hypertension or extracerebral vascular disease (Hachinski, et al., 1974), and individuals with MID often also have diabetes, hyperlipidemia, or arteriosclerotic heart disease. Unlike Alzheimer's disease, changes in mental status occur suddenly as a result of stroke and the course is fluctuating due to the occurrence of mild cerebral ischemic episodes. Intellectual functions gradually deteriorate and the exact nature of the person's cognitive and language deficits depends on the site, location, and extent of cerebral infarctions.

Morphological Changes. Diffuse subintimal hyperplasia, a build-up of cells in the inner wall of blood vessels, and multiple small infarctions are common throughout the carotid and vertebrobasilar systems. Often there is evidence of bilateral corticobulbar or corticospinal tract disease manifested as a gait disturbance, or pseudobulbar palsy (Scheinberg, 1978). Focal neurological signs, pathology associated with a specific brain area, appear when more than 50 grams of brain tissue have been destroyed. Destruction of more than 100 grams of tissue throughout the cerebral hemispheres uniformly results in dementia.

Pick's Disease

Pick's disease is a rare primary degenerative dementia usually occurring between the ages of 40 and 60. Its frequent occurrence within a family suggests a dominant autosomal mode of inheritance.

Pick's disease resembles Alzheimer's disease clinically, and many American neurologists do not differentiate them. The hippocampal formation is more preserved in Pick's disease, which may explain why memory is less impaired than in AD. Microscopically, nonspecific degeneration of the cortex particularly in the frontal and temporal lobes, is associated with silver sensitive inclusions called Pick bodies, as well as cell loss, and extensive gliosis (Malamud & Hirano, 1974).

Parkinson's Disease (PD)

There are two basic types of Parkinson's disease, idiopathic (accounting for 85% of the cases), and postencephalitic (accounting for 15%). The idiopathic, or major form, typically occurs in the late 50s (Pollock & Hornabrook, 1966) and has three principal symptoms: rigidity, rest tremor, and bradykinesia. Patients have flexed posture, a slow shuffling gait and are incoordinated. Dementia is often present (Boller et al., 1979) and is manifested as memory impairment, disorientation, impaired concept formation, and expressive-receptive language deficits.

Morphological Changes. Parkinson's disease results from a loss of cells in the substantia nigra, a subcortical structure in the basal ganglia responsible for the production of the neurotransmitter dopamine. The histopathology of the disease is somewhat controversial. Alzheimer-like changes are frequently found in the neurons of the substantia nigra in post-encephalitic PD patients (Wisniewski, Terry, & Hirano, 1970). Whether or not they are a consequence of PD or the result of the co-occurrence of AD and PD is unknown.

Huntington's Disease (HD)

Huntington's disease is a primary degenerative dementia inherited as a Mendelian single-dominant autosomal gene. Autosomal means that it strikes men and women equally, and dominant means that each child of an affected parent has a 50% chance of inheriting the disease. Symptoms usually appear between the ages of 35 and 45, but can occur later; 10% of the cases become apparent before the age of 20. The disease is chronic, progressive, and terminal. Although akinetic forms exist, choreoathetoid involuntary movements are typical and appear first as clumsiness, but eventually involve all body parts. Initial mental changes involve forgetfulness, irritability, depression, and withdrawal. During the disease course there are major reasoning, memory, and linguistic deficits (Fedio, Cox, Neophytides, Canal-Frederick, & Chase, 1979).

Morphological Changes. There is neuronal loss particularly in the striatum, and cerebral atrophy, particularly in the frontal lobes. The constant movements of HD patients are related to the loss of gamma aminobutyric acid and acetylcholine, brain chemicals which inhibit nerve action (Bird, 1980).

Korsakoff's Disease (KD)

In the late 1800s, S. S. Korsakoff, a Russian physician, described a syndrome of polyneuritis and psychological impairment that accompanied alcoholism. The syndrome became known as Korsakoff's psychosis, but, under the new classification system of the DSM-III, was termed Korsakoff's disease (KD). It is a secondary dementia developing after long-term alcohol abuse and vitamin B deficiency (Butters & Cermak, 1976). Vitamin B deficiency is thought to produce atrophy of diencephalic and limbic structures causing the classic symptom of KD amnesia for recent events. Other symptoms include disorientation to time and place, inattentiveness, and misperception.

The most-studied aspect of KD is memory deficit. Research suggests that Korsakoff's patients require more time than normals to process and form durable memories (Butters & Cermak, 1976). Affected individuals do not seem to employ the same memory-encoding strategies, and appear to rely more heavily on phonemic than semantic analysis. Verbal memory is more impaired than nonverbal. With proper diet and thiamine, KD patients may become more alert but memory problems persist.

Morphological Changes. Brain lesions occur in the thalamus (particularly the mammillary bodies which receive strong hippocampal input), hypothalamus, and the frontal and associative areas of the neocortex.

The aforementioned dementia-producing diseases are those most commonly seen by the speech-language pathologist. However, there are several other illnesses associated with dementia, such as progressive supranuclear palsy, progressive subcortical gliosis, Wilson's disease, and Creutzfeldt-Jacob disease.

Literature Review

Language impairment is present in all stages of dementia (Bayles, 1982; Obler & Albert, 1981). Impairment is subtle in the early stages, because cognition is only subtly affected. Speech articulation, or the mechanical production of words, usually is spared in dementing diseases not associated with movement disorders. The mechanics of language production are not reliant on higher-order cognitive processes, but the rules of language are, although our semantic, syntactic, phonologic, and pragmatic competencies are not uniformly affected in dementia. Research has demonstrated that semantic knowledge is more reliant on cognition than phonologic and syntactic knowledge (Bayles, 1982; Irigaray, 1973; Obler, 1977), and clinical observations suggest the same is true of pragmatics, our knowledge of how to use language in social interactions.

The bulk of our information about the effects of dementing illness on language has come from clinical observations of dementia patients, rather than controlled studies of disease effects. Of the studies completed, many have serious methodological limitations, most notably heterogeneous patient samples. Historically, dementia patients have been grouped together with little regard for etiology or severity, which makes interpretation of reported findings difficult.

Naming Research

The most widely studied dementia-associated language deficit is naming. Word finding difficulties and a reduction in functional vocabulary have been reported by Critchley, 1964; Ernst, Dalby, and Dalby, 1970; Stengel, 1964. As dementia worsens, naming errors increase (Bayles & Tomoeda, in press; Overman, 1979).

A popular explanation for the naming errors of dementia patients is impaired perception (Lawson & Barker, 1968; Rochford, 1971). Lawson and Barker compared the performance of 100 dementia patients to that of 40 normal elderly on a 24-item naming task. Dementia patients were found to have longer latencies, particularly for naming less common objects. When object function was demonstrated, naming was facilitated, a finding which motivated the authors to hypothesize that dementia patients are perceptually impaired. Like Lawson and Barker, Rochford (1971) concluded that dementia patients are perceptually deficient. He administered an eight-item naming test to 23 dementia patients, and classified their responses as correct, misrecognized, unclassifiable, or no response. Because the most frequent response was misrecognition, occurring 55% of the time, and because 35% of the responses were visually similar to the stimulus, Rochford concluded dementia patients may be "perceptually off course."

More recent research has failed to substantiate the perceptual impairment hypothesis and has motivated another explanation of the misnamings of dementia patients, that of erosion of referential boundaries in the mental lexicon (Bayles & Tomoeda, in press; Schwartz, Marin, & Saffran, 1979; Warrington, 1975; Wilson, Kaszniak, Fox, Garron, & Ratusnik, 1981). Schwartz, Marin, and Saffran described a woman with senile dementia,

WLP, who was able to name only one object on a 70-item naming test, but who could, nevertheless, demonstrate object recognition through intricate gestures. The authors asked WLP to select the name of stimulus items she could not name from the following five choices: two unrelated object names, a phonologically and orthographically similar name, the name of an item in the same semantic category, and the target name. At the time of initial testing, the patient selected the semantic distractor 85% of the time. Twenty-one months later, the semantic distractor was chosen only 61% of the time, leading the authors to suggest erosion of the associative network that exists between words. A specific example of such semantic erosion was WLP's gradual overextension of the word "dog." Initially "dog" was used to refer to "dogs," then "dogs and cats," and eventually was extended to "squirrels" and "rabbits."

Wilson et al. (1981), who studied the naming ability of 32 dementia patients and 32 age-matched controls, observed a phenomenon similar to that reported by Schwartz and associates. The majority of their subjects' naming errors were words semantically related to the stimulus items or perseverations of previous responses. Bayles and Tomoeda (in press) studied naming errors in four groups of dementia patients for whom dementia etiology and severity were specified, and found the most common response of moderately impaired dementia patients was the name of a semantically associated object (Alzheimer's disease 60%; Huntington's disease 67%; and Parkingson's disease 50%). Bayles and Tomoeda argued that linguistic impairment, rather than perceptual impairment, better accounts for the majority of misnamings of dementia patients. This argument is intuitively appealing because research has shown the semantic aspects of language are most vulnerable to dementia disease effects.

Semantic System More Impaired Than Syntactic and Phonologic

A number of researchers have reported the differential vulnerability of linguistic subsystems to dementia (Bayles & Boone, 1982; de Ajuriaguerra & Tissot, 1975; Irigaray, 1973; Schwartz et al., 1979; H. A. Whitaker, 1976). Irigaray studied the performance of 32 dementia patients on a variety of language tasks and discovered that their semantic and pragmatic subsystems were disturbed, while their morphosyntactic and phonologic subsystems were preserved. Haiganoosh Whitaker described an advanced AD patient who had been silent for years and was incapable of self-care, but who would echo sentences if eye contact was established. An intriguing aspect of her echolalia was her propensity to correct errors of syntax and phonology, but not semantics. Similarly, WLP, the patient of

Schwartz, Marin, and Saffran (1979) described earlier, could disambiguate spoken homophones (i.e., weak/week) with syntactic but not semantic cues. Bayles and Boone (1982) found the inability to perceive semantic errors in sentences to be the most discriminating of five language tasks for identifying senile brain-disease patients. Like Whitaker's patient, the seven severely demented subjects in the Bayles and Boone study frequently made spontaneous corrections of phonologically and syntactically anomalous sentences.

A variety of explanations have been offered for the vulnerabilty of semantic and pragmatic language subsystems in dementia. De Ajuriaguerra suggested that as dementia worsens, affected individuals regress to earlier stages of cognitive development, similar to those specified by Piaget (1923) in his description of the development of higher cognitive functions in children. Dementia patients become less able to perceive that which is illogical, are more likely to talk when performing an action, and become more egocentric.

Whitaker hypothesized the existence of a grammatical filter that operates independently of cognition, and is capable of analyzing syntactic and phonologic features of linguistic stimuli. According to Bayles (1982), intellectually deteriorated individuals retain their ability to analyze phonologic and syntactic features of linguistic stimuli, because the rules of phonology and syntax are finite, learned early, and quite well practiced. Conversely, meaning analysis relies on higher mental operations, because the number of sentences any language can generate is infinite and contextual effects must be analyzed to extract a speaker's communicative intention.

Language Profiles of Etiologically Different Dementia Patients

As we become more knowledgeable about the neurology of dementing illness, it is of clinical and theoretical value to explore the possibility that dementias of different etiologies may be associated with different language performance profiles reflecting their unique patterns of neural degeneration. Halpern, Darley, and Brown (1973) compared patients with aphasia, apraxia, confused language, and general intellectual impairment on ten language tasks. Because the groups were not controlled for severity, intergroup comparisons could not be made. Instead, individual language functions were compared against the group mean, and when a language function retained a fairly constant relation to the mean in all groups, that relation was designated as insignificant for intergroup differentiation. Patients who suffered general intellectual impairment (presumably from dementing disease) were distinguished by impaired reading comprehension, with verbal fluency, writing to dictation, and relevance relatively unaffected. These results are surprising and difficult to interpret because the cause and severity of general intellectual impairment were not specified, and other researchers have reported fluency and relevancy to be impaired in dementia patients (Albert, 1981, Bayles, 1982; Borkowski, Benton, & Spreen, 1967; Irigaray, 1973).

In his previously described dichotomy of dementia, Albert (1978) also argued that, while both cortical and subcortical dementias share some language impairments, each also has a unique profile. The shared deficits of these patients include lack of initiative to speak, perseveration, and naming impairment. Characteristics associated with subcortical dementia patients are slow rate, low volume, disturbances in rhythm, pitch, articulation, decreased output in verbal fluency tests, agraphia, and impaired ability to make verbal abstractions.

Cortical dementia patients, of which AD is the main type, exhibit logorrhea, empty speech, verbal paraphasias, impaired naming, impaired comprehension, preserved repetition, and topic digression. Cortical dementia patients are described as having all the language problems of subcortical patients plus agnosias, apraxias, and aphasias (Obler & Albert, 1981), and were likened to Wernicke's and anomic aphasics. Albert's profiles appear to be based on extensive clinical observation rather than formal studies in which the language behaviors of etiologically different dementia patients controlled for severity were compared.

Mildworf (1978) compared the performance of patients with Huntington's disease, Parkinson's disease, and normals on several language tasks. No significant intergroup differences were found on the confrontation and generative naming tasks for PD and normals. HD patients were, however, significantly more impaired on these tasks. Reading, writing, and oral naming of spelled words were all significantly harder for HD than for PD patients or normal subjects. HD subjects wrote telegrammatic versions of the Cookie Theft picture (Goodglass & Kaplan, 1972) while Parkinsonians used more words than normals to describe the same number of themes. Mildworf was not explicit about whether the PD patients had dementia. Therefore random selection of nondemented PD patients could have accounted for the superior performance of PD patients on some tasks.

Bayles et al. (in progress) compared the performance of patients with AD, HD, PD, and normal elderly on neuropsychological tests and language tasks. The dementia patients, whose average age, IQ, and years of education are presented in Table 7-5, were given a severity rating based on neurological evidence of brain damage and neurobehavioral criteria.

TABLE 7-5
Age, IQ, Years of Education of Dementia Subjects and Normals

Group	Total N	$\overline{X}$ Age	$\overline{X}$ Yrs. Ed.	$\overline{X}$ IQ
AD	22	72	12	113
PD	14	69	14	118
HD	8	45	13	116
Normals	33	70	13	115

Alzheimer's patients were the most impaired of the dementia groups, differing significantly from normals on all 21 variables except the Digit Span subtest of the *Wechsler Adult Intelligence Scale* Wechsler (1955). PD patients ranked second, performing significantly more poorly than normals on 17 tasks. No significant differences were found between PD patients and normals on judgment of syntactic and semantic errors, digit span, and naming. HD patients were least impaired of the disordered groups, a finding which should be interpreted cautiously both because of the small number in the group of subjects and because the HD patients were substantially younger than subjects in other groups. They differed from normals on 7 of the 21 variables: verbal description, *Peabody Picture Vocabulary Test* (PPVT), lexical disambiguation, surface structure disambiguation, selecting speaker intention from context, judging syntax errors, and naming.

When compared to neuropsychological tests, language tasks were found to be of equal or greater sensitivity for detecting dementia. The tasks on which all groups differed from normals were sentence disambiguation (lexical, surface structure, deep structure), verbal description, PPVT, and a pragmatic task of selecting speaker intent given utterance context.

Differences among dementia groups were fewer than those between dementia groups and normals. It must be mentioned that there is great intersubject variability between dementia patients. However, when scores are averaged across a group, AD and PD patients differed significantly only on the confrontation-naming task, although most test scores of AD patients were generally slightly lower. AD patients performed significantly more poorly than HD patients on three tasks: Block Design, *Mental Status Questionnaire*, and naming. HD patients were significantly inferior to PD patients on two sections of the pragmatics test, the ability to select the most appropriate utterance for a particular context from among four choices and the ability to judge the literality of utterances.

Whereas Obler and Albert found naming to be impaired in both subcortical and cortical dementias, a significant naming impairment was not observed in either moderate HD or PD patients (Bayles & Tomoeda, in press). If HD and PD patients are categorized as subcortical dementia patients and AD patients are categorized as cortical, then our data show the groups' common characteristics to include impaired receptive vocabulary, difficulty comprehending the meanings of ambiguous sentences, impaired ability to describe common objects verbally, and impaired ability to identify a speaker's intention in producing a particular utterance.

Language Disturbance During the Progression of Dementing Disease

Longitudinal studies of etiologically specific dementia patients have not been done. Consequently, we cannot specify an order in which language behaviors deteriorate. Nevertheless, numerous researchers have provided descriptions of language impairment at different stages of dementing illness, which enabled us to summarize their common observations (Bayles, 1982; de Ajuriaguerra & Tissot, 1975; Irigaray, 1973; Obler, 1977; H. Whitaker, 1976).

Early Stages

In the early or "forgetful" stage of dementia (Reisberg, 1981), when patients are disoriented for time but generally not for place or person, both short- and long-term memory deficits exist. These deficits are likely to be dismissed as benign forgetfulness. Thus, language impairment is likely to be imperceptible in casual conversation. Affected individuals know that something deleterious is happening to them and may attempt to conceal their shortcomings by avoiding challenging situations, dismissing a task as trivial, or refusing to perform it. In conversation, they are apt to digress from the topic and ramble at length, a behavior that Irigaray (1973) and Obler (1977) called disinhibition. Although the content of such discourse may be somewhat inappropriate due to word boundary erosion, dementia patients adhere to the rules of syntax and phonology. The combined effects of slight cognitive deterioration and semantic-pragmatic impairment may result in an inability to detect humor and sarcasm. As the ability to produce and comprehend language deteriorates, there is greater reliance on clichés.

EXAMPLES

1. Mild

Example 1:   Patient was describing a common object.

   Examiner: Tell me everything you can about this (a gray button).

   Patient: This is a button. This button is grayish in color, and, uh, it is useful. And, uh, I'd say it's grayish in color. (Pause) It's flat. I've already said it's gray. I think. I can't think of anything else.

Example 2:   Patient was told an anecdote and had difficulty recognizing contextual effects on speaker intent.

   Anecdote: A mother and her son arrive home from shopping with a car full of groceries. The young son rushes from the car empty-handed. The mother says to him: "What's the matter, have you broken your arms ?"

   Examiner: Why did the mother say, "What's the matter, have you broken your arms?"

   Patient: Well, I suppose she's putting over a point that he would understand that he should be careful where he puts his hands and arms.

Middle Stages of Dementia

By now an affected individual is disoriented for time and place, but orientation to self is maintained. Short and long-term memory problems are obvious, and the person is no longer capable of managing personal finances, a job, or his or her medication. Language impairment is apparent, and discourse is vague, empty, and often irrelevant. Terms like "thing" and "this one" are substituted for substantive nouns. Utterances are phonologically wellformed, but syntactic terms affecting meaning are likely to be misused, whereas purely syntactic forms still present little difficulty. Semantic paraphasias are more common than phonemic, and there is an obvious loss of the more specific and abstract semantic features of words. Individuals are no longer able to generate verbal sequences of meaningfully related ideas, and become increasingly apathetic towards other individuals and their environment. Language becomes egocentric, and there is less adherence to the conversational maxims that govern normal conversations. Affected individuals neither ask questions of their conversational partners nor comment on their utterances. Verbal perseverations are frequent, particularly ideational repetition, the repetition of an idea after another idea has been expressed. Self-correction of linguistic errors is rare. The language problems apparent in oral discourse are mirrored in what is written. Just as the mechanics of speech may be spared, so may be the mechanics of reading and writing.

EXAMPLES

2. Moderate

Example 1:   Patient was describing a common object.

> *Examiner:*   Tell me everything you can about this (a gray button)
>
> *Patient:*   Oh, that's a needle. But...buttonhole scissors. And they go ahead the put buttons or they put, that's how they put buttons on your coat with it. I guess.

Example 2:   Patient was asked to explain what it means to describe and guarantee.

> *Examiner:*   What does it mean to describe?
>
> *Patient:*   Well, like you're a buttoning your blouse would be an example.
>
> *Examiner:*   What does it mean to guarantee?
>
> *Patient:*   Guarantee you're gonna get it. I guess we're gonna have company or something. That would be a guarantee, wouldn't it?

Late Stages of Dementia

In the late stages of dementing illness, an individual is disoriented for time, place, and person, and frequently does not recognize family members. No longer can the person care for himself, and assistance with dressing, washing, feeding, and toileting is needed. Many severe dementia patients wander aimlessly and require placement in a protective environment. Life may seem to become a continuously fading dream, as one is unable to form new, lasting memories. Persons may be mute, echolalic, palilalic, use only jargon, or produce bizarre nonsensical utterances. Symptom variations probably reflect differences in the distribution of neural lesions. Pragmatic competencies of language may be so devastated that eye contact must be established before these dementia patients recognize that they are being spoken to. Syntax and phonology are grossly disrupted, particularly among jargon and palilalic patients.

EXAMPLES

3. Severe

Example 1:   Conversation with a severe dementia patient.

   Examiner: Where did you get these flowers?

   Patient: Just a little bit, this place is always smoky.

   Examiner: Are these flowers yours?

   Patient: It's supposed to be Jesus.

Example 2:   Conversation with a severe dementia patient.

   Examiner: Where are we now?

   Patient: Just like, like a n-normal person. And guy, guys, guys, girls in the class. They all pay attention, pay attention. You don't pay attention. Don't say, don't say, don't say...

Example 3:   Severe dementia patient was asked to describe a marble.

   Examiner: Tell me about this (marble).

   Patient: Well, that's pretty darn good.

   Examiner: It is. What can you tell me about it?

   Patient: Well, he was standing there looking you know, so I. It's not mine. I didn't have it.

Diagnosing Dementia

Language-speech evaluations have not been conducted routinely as part of the examination of dementia patients. Only recently has there been evidence of language impairment in all stages of dementia (Bayles, 1982; Obler, 1977), a finding that may be important in making differential diagnoses and patient management decisions.

Unfortunately a battery of language tests for evaluating dementia patients with different etiologies does not exist. Further, speech-language pathologists do not have normative data on the performance of dementia patients on individual language tasks. Clinicians must plan evaluations based on literature reports about the nature of such patients' intellectual and linguistic deterioration. Bayles and Boone (1982) studied the efficacy of certain language tasks for diagnosing dementia, and recommended evaluating receptive and expressive skills in patients' phonologic, syntactic, semantic, and pragmatic domains. They used a discriminant-function analysis to analyze the performance of AD, PD, HD, and MID patients on the following tests: For neuropsychological evaluation, Block Design, Digit span, and Similarities subtests of the *Wechsler Adult Intelligence Scale* (Wechsler, 1955), the Nonsense Syllable Learning Task (Alexander, 1973) and the *Mental Status Questionnaire* (MSQ) (Goldfarb & Antin, 1975); for language evaluation, Naming Task, Lexical, Surface and Deep Structure Disambiguation Task, Judgment and Correction of Phonologic, Syntactic, and Semantic Errors, *Peabody Picture Vocabulary Test*, Pragmatics Task (Five parts: P1, P2, P3, P4A, P4B), Verbal Description Task, and Story-retelling Task. Table 7–6 lists the results of the discriminant function analysis, in order of most to least discriminative tests. The discriminant-function equation was found to classify subjects with 75% accuracy. Reliability and validity data are being amassed on these measures and, while they show promise for differentiating among dementia patients and normals, they are unstandardized.

Particularly in its early stages, the diagnosis of a dementia-producing disease frequently requires neurological, physical, and psychological examinations. Of the major dementing illnesses, AD is the most difficult to diagnose and usually becomes diagnosis by exclusion. A thorough case history is needed to identify the associated behavioral and personality changes characteristic of the diagnosis. In addition to the case history, the physician may rely on information from CT Scan, pneumoencephalography, regional cerebral blood flow, and electroencephalography.

CT Scan

The CT scan has become an important tool in the diagnosis of dementia. CT is an acronym for computerized axial tomography, a technique in which a narrow x-ray beam is passed through a succession of axial slices

TABLE 7-6
Measures Included in the Discriminant Function Equation (F ratio significant beyond .01 level).

Measure	Wilk's Lambda	Equivalent r
P3: Choosing best utterance for a particular context	.41	18.2
Block Design (WAIS)	.27	11.8
P2: Selection of speaker intent	.17	10.1
Verbal Description	.12	9.2
Naming	.09	7.8
Peabody Picture Vocabulary Test	.08	6.9
Similarities (WAIS)	.06	6.3
Mental Status Questionnaire	.05	5.8
P4A: Judging literality of utterance	.047	5.3
SCSJ: Ability to make syntactic judgments	.04	4.9
Lexical Disambiguation	.04	4.6
Digit Span (WAIS)	.03	4.3

Measures not included in the Discriminant Function Equation

P1:	Defining illocutionary speech acts
P4B:	Explaining speaker intent
SCPJ:	Ability to judge phonologic errors
SCPC:	Ability to correct phonologic errors
SCSC:	Ability to correct syntactic errors
SCSEJ:	Ability to judge semantic errors
SCSEC:	Ability to correct semantic errors

Nonsense Syllable Learning Task
Story Retelling
Surface Structure Disambiguation
Deep Structure Disambiguation

of the cranium (Pear, 1977). The resulting image varies with the density of the substance visualized. A CT scan may not distinguish dementia, because it is not uncommon to see dementia in patients showing no evidence of cortical atrophy on the scan; nor is it unusual to see prominent atrophy without clinical manifestations of dementia. Early attempts to correlate intellectual deterioration with brain atrophy were disappointing (Fox, Kaszniak, & Huckman, 1979; Roberts & Laird, 1976), but recent correlational studies using new generation CT scanners have been more encouraging (deLeon, Ferris, George, Reisberg, Kricheff, & Gershon, 1980).

Pneumoencephalography

Before the development of the CT technique, pneumoencephalography was commonly used. In this procedure, air is injected into the ventricles enabling physicians to look at ventricular enlargment.

Regional Cerebral Blood Flow

Another promising diagnostic procedure is regional cerebral blood flow measurement, rCBF. Patients inhale an inert radiolabeled gas, usually xenon 133. Its dispersion is then measured by skull sensors which detect the precise location of the radioactive gas. Information from the skull detectors is sent to a computer which provides a display of the brain regions to which blood is flowing.

In dementia, the parameters of rCBF have shown a flow decrease when there is intellectual degeneration (Freyhan, Woodford, & Kety, 1951; Hagberg & Ingvar, 1976) and the areas of diminished flow correspond to areas in which brain decay is most pronounced in dementia patients at autopsy (Ingvar, Brun, Hagberg, & Gustafson, 1978). Gustafson, Hagberg, and Ingvar (1978) studied flow patterns in presenile dementia patients during speech and found that verbal ability fails only when there is a marked general flow reduction in the dominant hemisphere. Further, a relation was found between the type of language-speech defect and the distribution of rCBF abnormalities in the dominant hemisphere. Receptive language disturbances were associated with marked flow reduction in postcentral regions, particularly in the temporoparietal area, whereas expressive language disturbances were associated with marked frontal and anterior temporal flow reductions. Depending on its ultimate availability, regional cerebral blood flow measurement might be valuable for differentiating between depression and AD, because the general and regional CBF are routinely normal in depressive states (Silfverskiold, Gustafson, Johanson, & Risberg, 1979).

Electroencephalography

Since Berger's report in 1931 of a pathological electroencephalogram (EEG) in an AD patient, there have been many EEG studies of dementia patients. The most commonly reported EEG pattern in AD is a diminution of the alpha rhythm (8-12 Hz in normals) into theta (5-7 Hz) and, eventually, delta ranges (4 or less Hz) (Obrist & Henry, 1958; Short & Wilson, 1971). Slowing of patients' alpha rhythm has been significantly correlated with the number of senile plaques (Deisenhammer & Jellinger, 1974), degree of cognitive deterioration (Mundy-Castle, Hurst, Beerstecker, & Prinsloo, 1954), and vocabulary impairment (Johannesson, Hagberg, Gustafson, & Ingvar, 1979).

Although EEG records provide insufficient evidence for specifying dementia etiology, they are suggestive. For example, diffuse slowing is seen in multi-infarct disease (Muller & Schwartz, 1978), while in Pick's disease, EEG's are often normal (Johannesson et al., 1977). In Huntington's disease a low voltage EEG is not uncommon (Scott, Healthfield, Toone, & Margerison, 1972), and in the advanced stages of Creutzfeldt-Jacob's disease, EEG's are characterized by bilateral rhythmic polyphasic complexes (Burger, Rowan, & Goldensohn, 1972).

Distinguishing the Effects of Normal Aging

In normal aging, changes in the brain and body result in sensory impairments as well as in memory, intelligence, and speed of responding. Familiarity with normal, age-related changes is a prerequisite for evaluating the behavior of mildly demented elderly patients. What follows is a brief review. A more comprehensive description of language in normal aging is provided by Davis's chapter in this volume.

In addition to the relatively well-known changes in the visual and auditory systems, there are age-related changes in the brain. Brain weight and volume decrease with age (Dekaban & Sadowsky, 1978; Pearl, 1922), the ventricles enlarge (Barron, Jacobs, & Kinkel, 1976), and the fissures widen and deepen (Wright, Spink, & Andrew, 1974). Microscopic histological studies of the cortex show the formation of senile plaques, neurofibrillary tangles, and sites of granulovacuolar degeneration (Blessed, Tomlinson, & Roth, 1968).

Age primarily affects long-term memory that requires the synthesis of new information (Craik, 1977). Senescents appear to employ less effective strategies for organizing new information (Craik & Masani, 1967; Mandler, 1967). Short-term memory store, typically 7 ± 2 items (Miller,

1956), is modestly reduced, usually by one item (Botwinick & Storandt, 1974; Freidman, 1974).

Intellectual functions most susceptible to age are those related to physiological abilities such as speed printing, perceptual speed, associative memory, and figural and inductive reasoning (Horn, 1972). Intellectual functions likely to be maintained are those dependent on culturally transmitted information and skills, such as verbal comprehension and general information (Horn, 1972).

Reaction time slows with age (Welford, 1958), and individuals become more cautious in responding (Botwinick, 1971), making many older people reluctant to guess on confusing test items.

Language and Aging

Language skills appear to be more resistant to age effects than some other areas of cognitive functioning. Botwinick (1973) called the maintenance of verbal functions and the decline in performance on adult intelligence tests the "classic aging pattern." This is not to say there are no age effects on langue skills. Comprehension appears to be disturbed in many senescents as a result of loss of hearing acuity (Corso, 1977), the ability to perceive and discriminate speech (Bergman, 1971; Feldman & Roger, 1967; Glorig, 1977), and reduced attention span (Rabbitt, 1965).

Studies of expressive language skills showed discourse patterns of the elderly to be different from younger subjects, but not necessarily inferior. Obler, Mildworf, and Albert (1977) analyzed the written discourse of elderly subjects who wrote descriptions of the Cookie Theft Picture of the Boston Diagnostic Aphasia Examination (Goodglass & Kaplan, 1972). Elderly subjects used more elaborate syntax, more embedded constructions, and more words, but did not express more themes. If fluency is considered, the elderly tend to use more filler words and interjections, and evidence more incomplete phrases (Yairi & Clifton, 1972). This finding may be a consequence of the more cautious demeanor of the elderly, rather than of linguistic impairment (Botwinick, 1971).

Management of Dementia Patients

The first step in patient management should be consultation with the patient's physician to learn the etiology and severity of the dementing illness. When the physician is unsure about the diagnosis, a follow-up medical, psychological, and language-speech evaluation should be rescheduled within

6 to 8 months. In most cases of dementing illness, language functions will have worsened in this period.

The care of an individual with a dementing disease can be an overwhelming experience for an individual or family. In addition to the personal sorrow of watching intellect and personality deteriorate in a loved one, there are usually burgeoning expenses and care-taking responsibilities. Spouses typically become depressed over the loss of their marital partner. As the dementia worsens, the dementia patient requires more and more personal care and eventually needs continuous supervision. It is important to meet with the family members and advise them of what to expect, and discuss how they can cope with the changes they observe in the affected family member. The following list is a modified version of a list of management strategies published in *Family Handbook: A Guide for the Families of Persons with Declining Intellectual Functions, Alzheimer's Disease, and Other Dementias* (Mace & Rabins, 1980).

DO:

Establish a routine

Make the routine simple

Forecast deviations from the routine

Minimize distractions

Keep household objects in the same place

Provide indirect orientation to place and time

Display pictures of family members

Have an identification bracelet made for the affected individual

Dispense the patient's medication

Expect the patient to deny the problem

Expect the patient to blame others for his or her problems

Expect the behavior of the affected individual to worsen with fatigue

Avoid arguing with the dementia patient

Expect to lose your temper

Try not to solve disagreements with the affected individual, but change the subject

Expect a change in the patient's condition when there is a major change in his or her lifestyle

Use more concrete and familiar terms when talking to the patient

Avoid sarcasm

Avoid long complex explanations and anecdotes

Arrange to have frequent relief from care-taking responsibilities

Expect to feel a sense of loss

Therapy

Comparative studies of therapy techniques with dementia patients have not been done. The most widely promoted technique has been "Reality Orientation," in which patients are repeatedly oriented. Reality therapy does not result in lasting change, nor does any other known technique. The outlook for finding a behavioral therapy technique that will arrest the progressive deterioration of language function is poor. More promising may be discovery of techniques by which we can better communicate with persons in the various stages of dementing illness. HD patients for example may live for 15 to 25 years after the onset of the disease. If we know the course of language dissolution and the best way of modifying our verbal input to patients, we may greatly improve their comprehension and ability to function.

More appropriate than therapy for the dementia patient may be therapy for the family. Reisberg and colleagues (1981) have established a therapy program for relatives of dementia patients at New York University. It is reported to be well received, particularly by men. Reisberg (1981) suggested that the reason more men seek counseling is that they have greater difficulty assuming a supportive and care-taking role than women. The frustration they feel in coping with a dementing spouse is manifested most often as anger. Children of dementia patients also have participated in the program. They are primarily concerned over the fate of their sick parent and the possibility they themselves might be affected in their later years. The clinician-counselor should be prepared to answer questions about the cause, treatments, disease course, and current research on dementing illnesses as well as questions about the diagnostic process and its accuracy for a particular individual. If counseling is not available for family members, help can be sought from the following national organizations, which provide information and supportive services:

Alzheimer's disease

Alzheimer's Disease and Related Disorders Association
292 Madison Avenue
8th Floor
New York, NY 10017
(212) 683-2868

Huntington's disease

National Huntington's Disease Association
128A East 74th Street
New York, NY 10021
(212) 744-0302

Parkinson's disease

Parkinson's Disease Foundation
William Black Medical Research Building
Columbia Presbyterian Medical Center
640 West 168th Street
New York, NY 10032
(212) 923-4700

National Parkinson's Foundation
1501 N. W. 9th Avenue
Miami, FL 33136
(305) 324-0156

United Parkinson's Foundation
220 S. State Street
Chicago, IL 60604
(312) 922-9734

Acknowledgment

The author wishes to express her gratitude to Karen K. Eagans and Cheryl K. Tomoeda for their assistance in the preparation of this chapter, and to Richard F. Curlee, PhD, and Daniel R. Boone, PhD, of the University of Arizona for their critical comments in reviewing the manuscript. This work was supported by grant number 5R21 AGO2154-02 CMS from the National Institute of Aging.

References

Albert, M. L. Subcortical dementia. In R. Katzman, R. D. Terry, & K. L. Bick (Eds.), *Alzheimer's disease: Senile dementia and related disorders* (*Aging*, Vol. 7), 173–180. New York: Raven Press, 1978.
Albert, M. L. Changes in language with aging. *Seminars in Neurology*, 1981, *1*, 43–46.
Alexander, D. A. Some tests of intelligence and learning for elderly psychiatric patients: A validation study. *Brit. J. Soc. Clin. Psych.*, 1973, *12*, 188–193.
Alzheimer, A. *Allg. Z. Psychiat.*, 1907, *64*, 146–8.
Aretaeus. In F. Adams (Ed.), *The extant works of Aretaeus, the cappadocian*, 1861, 103.

Ball, M. J., & Nuttall, K. Neurofibrillary tangles, granulovacuolar degeneration and neuron loss in Down's syndrome: Quantitative comparison with Alzheimer dementia. *Annals of Neurology*, 1980, *7*, 462–465.

Barron, S. A., Jacobs, L., & Kinkel, W. R. Changes in the size of normal lateral ventricles during aging determined by computerized tomography. *Neurology*, 1976, *26*, 1011–1013.

Bayles, K. A. Language function in senile dementia. *Brain and Language*, 1982, *16*, 265–280.

Bayles, K. A., & Boone, D. R. The potential of language tasks for identifying senile dementia. *Journal of Speech and Hearing Disorders*, 1982, *47*, 210–217.

Bayles, K. A., & Tomoeda, C. K. Confrontation naming impairment in dementia, *Brain and Language*, 1983, *19*, 98-114.

Berger, H. Uber das Elektrenkephalogramm des Menschen. Dritte Mitteilung. *Archiv Fur Psychiatrie und Nervenkrankheiten*, (Berlin) 1931, *94*, 16–60.

Bergman, M. Hearing and aging. *Audiology*, 1971, *10*, 164 171.

Bird, E. D. Chemical pathology of Huntington's disease. *Annual Review of Pharmacology and Toxicology*, 1980, *20*, 533–551.

Blessed, G., Tomlinson, B. E., & Roth, M. The association between quantitative measures of dementia and of senile change in the cerebral grey matter of elderly subjects. *British Journal of Psychiatry*, 1968, *114*, 797–811.

Boller, F., Mitzutani, T., Roessmann, V., & Gambetti, P. Parkinson disease, dementia and Alzheimer disease: Clinicopathological correlations. *Annals of Neurology*, 1980, *7*, 329–335.

Borkowski, J. G., Benton, A. L., & Spreen, O. Word fluency and brain damage. *Neuropsychologia*, 1967, *5*, 135-140.

Botwinick, J. Sensory-set factors in age difference in reaction time. *Journal of Genetic Psychology*, 1971, *119*, 241–249.

Botwinick, J. *Aging and behavior*. New York: Springer Publishing, 1973.

Botwinick, J., & Storandt, M. *Memory, related function and age*. Springfield, IL: Charles C. Thomas, 1974.

Burger, L. J., Rowan, A. J., & Goldensohn, E. S. Creutzfeldt-Jacob disease, an electroencephalographic study. *Archives of Neurology*, 1972, *26*, 428–433.

Butters, N., & Cermak, L. Neuropsychological studies of alcoholic Korsakoff patients. In G. Goldstein & C. Neuringer (Eds.), *Empirical studies of alcoholism*. Cambridge: Ballinger Publishing, 1976.

Caster, W. O., & Wang, M. Dietary aluminum and Alzheimer's disease—a review. *Science of the Total Environment*, 1981, *17*, 31–36.

Corsellis, J. A. N. *Mental illness and the aging brain*. London: Oxford University Press, 1962.

Corso, J. Presbycusis, hearing aids and aging. *Audiology*, 1977, *16*, 146–163.

Craik, F. I. M. Age differences in human memory. In J. E. Birren & K. W. Schaie (Eds.), *Handbook of the psychology of aging*. New York: Van Nostrand Reinhold, 1977, 384–420.

Craik, F. I. M., & Masani, P. A. Age differences in the temporal integration of language. *British Journal of Psychology*, 1967, *58*, 291-299.

Crapper, D. R., & DeBoni U. Etiological factors in dementia. International Society for Neurochemistry Satellite Meeting on Aging of the Brain and Dementia, Florence, Italy, Aug. 27-29, 1979, *Abstracts*.

Crapper, D. R., Krishnan, S. S., & Quittkat, S. Aluminum, neurofibrillary degeneration and Alzheimer's disease. *Brain*, 1976, *99*, 67-80.

Critchley, M. The neurology of psychotic speech. *British Journal of Psychiatry*, 1964, *110*, 353-364.

Davies, P., & Mahoney, A. J. F. Selective loss of cholinergic neurons in Alzheimer's disease. *Lancet*, 1976, *2*, 1403.

de Ajuriaguerra, J., & Tissot, R. Some aspects of language in various forms of senile dementia. In E. H. Lenneberg & E. Lenneberg (Eds.), *Foundations of Language Development* (Vol. 1). New York: Academic Press, 1975, 323–339.

de Leon, M. J., Ferris, S. H., George, A. E., Reisberg, B., Kricheff, I. I., & Gershon, S. Computed tomography evaluations of brain behavior relationships in senile dementia of the Alzheimer's type. *Neurobiology of Aging, Experimental and Clinical Research*, 1980, *1*, 69–79.

Deisenhammer, E., & Jellinger, K. EEG in senile dementia. *Electroencephalography and Clinical Neurophysiology*, 1974, *36*, 91.

Dekaban, A. S., & Sadowsky, D. Changes in brain weights during the span of human life: Relation of brain weights to body heights and body weights. *Annals of Neurology*, 1978, *4*, 345–356.

Diagnostic & statistical manual of mental disorders. American Psychiatric Association, Washington, DC, 1952.

Diagnostic & statistical manual of mental disorders. American Psychiatric Association. 2nd Edition, 1968.

Diagnostic & statistical manual of mental disorders. American Psychiatric Association, 3rd Edition, 1980.

Diamond, S. G., Markham, C. H., & Treciokas, L. J. Long term experience with L-dopa: Efficacy, progression and mortality. In W. Birkmayer & O. Hornykeiwicz, (Eds.), *Advances in parkinsonism*, Basel: Roche, 1976, 444–455.

Elam, L. H., & Blumenthal, H. T. Aging in the mentally retarded. In H. T. Blumenthal (Ed.), *Interdisciplinary topics in gerontology*. New York: S. Karger, 1970, 7, 87.

Ernst, B., Dalby, M. A., & Dalby, A. Aphasic disturbances in presenile dementia. *Acta Neurologica Scandinavica Supplementum* 1970, *43*, 99–100.

Fedio, P., Cox, C. S., Neophytides, A., Canal-Frederick, G., & Chase, T. N. Neuropsychological profile of Huntington's disease: Patients and those at risk. In T. N. Chase, N. S. Wexler, & A. Barbeau (Eds.), *Advances in neurology, Vol. 23, Huntington's disease*. New York: Raven Press, 1979, 239–255.

Feldman, R. M., & Roger, S. N. Relations among hearing, reaction time and age. *Journal of Speech and Hearing Research*, 1967, *10*, 479–495.

Foley, J. M. Differential diagnosis of the organic mental disorders in elderly patients. In C. M. Gaitz (Ed.) *Aging and the brain*, New York: Plenum Press, 1972, 153–161.

Fox, J. H., Kaszniak, A. W., & Huckman, M. Computerized tomographic scanning not very helpful in dementia—nor in craniopharyngiomia. *New England Journal of Medicine*, 1979, 300.

Frederickson, D. S. Introductory statement: A view from National Institutes of Health. In N. E. Miller & G. D. Cohen (Eds.) *Clinical aspects of Alzheimer's disease and senile dementia (Aging, Vol. 15)*. New York: Raven Press, 1981.

Freidman, H. Interrelation of two types of immediate memory in the aged. *Journal of Psychology*, 1974, *87*, 177–181.

Freyhan, F. A., Woodford, R. B., & Kety, S. S. Cerebral blood flow and metabolism in psychosis of senility. *Journal of Nervous and Mental Disease*, 1951, *113*, 449–456.

Gajdusek, D. C., & Gibbs, J. C., Jr. Slow, latent, and temperate virus infections of the central nervous system. *Research Publications-Association for Research in Nervous and Mental Disease*, 1968, *44*, 254–280.

Garron, D. C., Klawans, H. L., & Narin, F. Intellectual functioning of persons with idiopathic Parkinsonism. *Journal of Nervous and Mental Disease*, 1972, *154*, 445–452.

Glorig, A. Auditory processing and age. In H. Shore & M. Ernst (Eds.), *Sensory processes and aging*, 39–60. Denton, TX: University Center for Community Services, 1977.

Goldfarb, A. I., & Antin, S. Unpublished data. In R. Goldman & M. Rockstein (Eds.), *The physiology and pathology of human aging.* New York: Academic Press, 1975.

Goodglass, H., & Kaplan, E. *The assessment of aphasia and related disorders.* Philadelphia: Lea & Febiger, 1972.

Gustafson, L., Hagberg, B., & Ingvar, D. H. Speech disturbance in presenile dementia related to local blood flow abnormalities in the brain. *Brain and Language,* 1978, *5,* 103-118.

Hachinski, V. C., Lassen, N. A., & Marshall, J. Multi-infarct dementia: A cause of mental deterioration in the elderly. *Lancet,* 1974, *2,* 207-210.

Hagberg, B., & Ingvar, D. H. Cognitive reduction in presenile dementia related to regional abnormalities of the cerebral blood flow. *British Journal of Psychiatry,* 1976, *128,* 209-222.

Hakim, A. M., & Mathieson, G. Dementia in Parkinson's disease: A neuropathologic study. *Neurology,* 1979, *29,* 1209-1214.

Halpern, H., Darley, F. L., & Brown, J. R. Differential language and neurological characteristics in cerebral involvement. *Journal of Speech and Hearing Disorders,* 1973, *38,* 162-173.

Heston, L. L. & Mastri, A. R. The genetics of Alzheimer's disease. *Archives of General Psychiatry,* 1977, *34,* 976-981.

Hirano, A., & Zimmerman, H. M. Alzheimer's neurofibrillary changes. *Archives of Neurology,* 1962, *7,* 227-242.

Horn, J. L. Intelligence: Why it grows, why it declines. In J. M. Hunt (Ed.), *Human intelligence,* 53-74. New Brunswick, NJ: Transaction Books, 1972.

Ingvar, D. H., Brun, A., Hagberg, B., & Gustafson, L. Regional cerebral blood flow in the dominant hemisphere in confirmed cases of Alzheimer's disease, Pick's disease, and multi-infarct dementia: Relationship to clinical symptomatology and neuropathological findings. In R. Katzman, R. D. Terry, & K. L. Bick (Eds.), *Alzheimer's disease: Senile dementia and related disorders,* (*Aging,* Vol. 7). New York: Raven Press, 1978.

Irigaray, L. *Le langage des déments.* The Hague: Mouton, 1973.

Johannesson, G., Brun, A., Gustafson, L., & Ingvar, D. H. EEG in presenile dementia related to cerebral blood flow and autopsy findings. *Acta Neurologica Scandinavica,* 1977, *56,* 89-103.

Johannesson, G., Hagberg, B., Gustafson, L., & Ingvar, D. H. EEG and cognitive impairment in presenile dementia. *Acta Neurologica Scandinavica,* 1979, *59,* 225-240.

Katzman, R. Early detection of senile dementia. *Hospital Practice,* June, 1981, 61-76.

Kidd, M. Paired helical filaments in electron microscopy in Alzheimer's disease. *Journal of Neuropathology and Experimental Neurology,* 1963, *22,* 629-642.

Kraepelin, E. *Dementia praecox and paraphrenia.* Krieger: Huntington, NY, 1919.

Larsson, T., Sjögren, T., & Jacobson, G. Senile dementia. *Acta Psychiatrica Scandinavica Supplementum,* 1963, *167,* 39.

Lawson, J. S., & Barker, M. G. The assessment of nominal dysphasia in dementia: The use of reaction time measures. *British Journal of Medical Psychology,* 1968, *41,* 411-414.

Lewy, F. H. *Monographs of Neurological Psychiatry,* 1923, *34,* 32.

Lieberman, A., Dziatolowski, M., Kupersmith, M., Serby, M., Goodgold, A., Korein, J., & Goldstein, M. Dementia in Parkinson disease. *Annals of Neurology,* 1979, *6,* 355-359.

Loranger, A. W., Goodell, H., & McDowell, F. Intellectual impairment in Parkinson's syndrome. *Brain,* 1972, *95,* 402-412.

Mace, L., & Rabins, P. V. *Family handbook: A guide for the families of persons with declining intellectual functions, Alzheimer's disease and other dementias.* Baltimore: Johns Hopkins University, 1980.

Malamud, N. Neuropathology of organic brain syndromes associated with aging. In C. M. Gaitz (Ed.), *Aging and the brain.* New York: Plenum Press, 1972, 63-87.

Malamud, N., & Hiraṇo, A. *Atlas of neuropathology.* Berkeley: University of California Press, 1974.

Mandler, G. Organization and Memory. In K. W. Spence & J. T. Spence (Eds.), *The psychology of learning and motivation: Advances in research and theory* (Vol. 1), 327–372. New York: Academic Press, 1967.

Martin, W. E., Loewenson, R. B., & Resch, J. A. Parkinson's disease: Clinical analysis of 100 patients. *Neurology*, 1973, *23*, 783–790.

McDermott, J. R., Smith, A. J., Iqbal, K., & Wisniewski, H. M. Aluminum and Alzheimer's disease. *Lancet*, 1977, *2*, 710–711.

Mildworf, B. Cognitive function in elderly patients. Unpublished master's thesis, Hebrew University, 1978.

Miller, G. A. The magical number seven, plus or minus two: Some limits on our capacity for processing information. *Psychological Review*, 1956, *63*, 81–97.

Mjönes, H. *Acta Psychiatrica Neurologica, Supplement 54*, 1949.

Monroe, R. T. *Diseases in old age.* Cambridge, MA: Harvard University Press, 1951.

Muller, H. F., & Schwartz, G. Electroencephalograms and autopsy findings in geropsychiatry. *Journal of Gerontology*, 1978, *33*, 504–513.

Mundy-Castel, A. C., Hurst, L. A., Beerstecker, D. M., & Prinsloo, T. The electroencophalogram in the senile psychoses. *Electroencephalography and Clinical Neurophysiology*, 1954, *6*, 245–252.

National Center of Health Statistics, survey conducted 1973–74, reported 1978.

Obler, L. K. Language and brain dysfunction in dementia. In S. Segalowitz (Ed.), *Language functions and brain organization.* New York: Academic Press, 1977.

Obler, L. K., & Albert, M. L. Language in the elderly aphasic and the dementing patient. In M. T. Sarno (Ed.), *Acquired aphasia.* New York: Academic Press, 1981, 385–398. (a)

Obler, L. K., & Albert, M. L. Language and aging: A neurobehavioral analysis. In D. S. Beasley & G. A. Davis (Eds.), *Aging communication processes and disorders*, New York: Grune & Stratton, Inc., 1981, 107–121. (b)

Obler, L. K., Mildworf, B., & Albert, M. L. Writing style in the elderly. Montreal: *Academy of Aphasia Abstracts*, 1977.

Obrist, W. D., & Henry, C. E. Electroencephalographic findings in aged psychiatric patients. *Journal of Nervous and Mental Disorders*, 1958, *126*, 254–267.

Overman, C. A. Naming performance in geriatric patients with chronic brain syndrome. Paper presented at the Annual Convention of the American Speech-Language-Hearing Association, Atlanta, 1979.

Pear, B. L. The radiographic morphology of cerebral atrophy. In W. L. Smith & M. Kinsbourne (Eds.), *Aging and dementia.* New York: Spectrum Publications, 1977, 57–76.

Pearl, R. *The Biology of death.* Philadelphia: J. B. Lippincott, 1922.

Perl, D. P., & Brody, A. R. Alzheimer's disease: X-ray spectometric evidence of aluminum accumulation in neurofibrillary tangle-bearing neurons. *Science*, 1980, *208*, 297–299.

Perry, E. K., Perry, R. H., Blessed, G., & Tomlinson, B. E. Necropsy evidence of central cholinergic deficits in senile dementia. *Lancet*, 1977, *1*, 189.

Perry, E. K., Perry, R. H., Blessed, G., & Tomlinson, B. E. Changes in brain cholinesterases in senile dementia of the Alzheimer type. *Neuropathology and Applied Neurobiology*, 1978, *4*, 273–277.

Piaget, J. *Le language et la pensée chez l'enfant.* Neuchâtel: De la Chaux & Niestlé, 1923.

Pirozzolo, F. J., Hansch, E. C., Mortimer, J. A., Webster, D. D., & Kuskowski, M. A. Dementia in Parkinson disease: A Neuropsychological analysis. *Brain and Cognition*, 1982, *1*, 71–83.

Pollock, M., & Hornabrook, R. W. The prevalence, natural history and dementia of Parkinson's disease. *Brain*, 1966, *89*, 429–448.

Rabbitt, P. An age decrement in the ability to ignore irrelevant information. *Journal of Gerontology*, 1965, *20*, 233–238.

Reisberg, B. *Brain failure*. New York: The Free Press, 1981.

Reisine, T. D., Yamamura, H. I., Bird, E. D., Spokes, E., & Enna, S. J. Pre- and post-synaptic neurochemical alterations in Alzheimer's disease. *Brain Research*, 1978, *159*, 477–480.

Roberts, M. A., & Laird, F. I. Computerized tomography and intellectual impairment in the elderly. *Journal of Neurology, Neurosurgery and Psychiatry*, 1976, *39*, 986–989.

Rochford, G. A study of naming errors in dysphasic and demented patients. *Neuropsychologia*, 1971, *9*, 437–445.

Scheinberg, P. Multi-infarct dementia. In R. Katzman, R. D. Terry, & K. L. Bick (Eds.), *Alzheimer's disease: Senile dementia and related disorders* (*Aging*, Vol. 7). New York: Raven Press, 1978.

Schwartz, M. F., Marin, O. S. M., & Saffran, E. M. Dissociations of language function in dementia: A case study. *Brain and Language*, 1979, *7*, 277–306.

Scott, D. F., Healthfield, K. G. W., Toone, B., & Margerison, J. H. EEG in Huntington's chorea: A clinical and neuropathological study. *Journal of Neurology, Neurosurgery and Psychiatry*, 1972, *35*, 97–102.

Selby, G. Parkinson's disease. In P. J. Vinken & G. W. Bruyn (Eds.), *Handbook of clinical neurology*. Amsterdam: North Holland, 1968, *6*, 173–211.

Short, M. J., & Wilson, W. P. The electroencephalogram in dementia. In C.E.Wells (Ed.), *Dementia*. Philadelphia: F. A. Davis, 1971, 81–89.

Silfverskiold, P., Gustafson, L., Johanson, M., & Risberg, J. Regional cerebral blood flow related to the effect of electroconvulsive therapy in depression. In Ballus (Ed.), *Proceedings from the Second World Congress of Biological Psychiatry*. Amsterdam: Elsevier/North Holland Biomedical Press, 1979.

Slater, E., & Cowie, V. Senescence, senile and presenile dementias. In *Genetics of mental disorders*. London: Oxford University Press, 1970.

Sparf, B. On the turnover of acetylcholine in the brain. *Acta Physiologica Scandinavica Supplement*, 1973, *397*, 1–47.

Stengel, E. Speech disorders and mental disorders. In A. De Reuch & M. O'Connor (Eds.), *Symposium on disorders of language*. Boston: Little Brown and Co., 1964.

Sweet, R. D., McDowell, H., & Feigenson, J. S. Mental symptoms in Parkinson's disease during treatment with levodopa. *Neurology*, 1976, *26*, 305–310.

Terry, R. D., & Wisniewski, H. M. Structural and chemical changes in the aged human brain. In S. Gershon & A. Raskin (Eds.), *Aging: Genesis and treatment of psychologic disorders in the elderly* (Vol. 2). New York: Raven Press, 1975, 127–142.

Tomlinson, B. E. Morphological changes in dementia in old age. In W. L. Smith & M. Kinsbourne (Eds.), *Aging and dementia*. New York: Spectrum Publications, 1977. 25–56.

Tomlinson, B. E., & Henderson, G. Some quantitative cerebral findings in normal and demented old people. In R. D. Terry & S. Gershon (Eds.), *Neurobiology of aging*. New York. Raven Press, 1976, 183–204.

Wang, H. S. Neuropsychiatric procedures for the assessment of Alzheimer's disease, senile dementia and related disorders. In N. E. Miller & G. D. Cohen (Eds.), *Clinical aspects of Alzheimer's disease and senile dementia*, (*Aging*, Vol. 15). New York: Raven Press, 1981.

Warrington, E. K. The selective impairment of semantic memory. *Quarterly Journal of Experimental Psychology*, 1975, *27*, 635–657.

Wechsler, D. *Manual for the Wechsler Adult Intelligence Scale*. New York: Psychological Corporation, 1955.

Welford, A. T. *Aging and human skill*. London: Oxford University Press, 1958.

Whitaker, H. A. A case of isolation of the language function. In H. Whitaker & H. A. Whitaker (Eds.), *Studies in neurolinguistics.* (2). New York: Academic Press, 1976.

White, P., Hiley, C. R., Goodhardt, M. J., Carrasco, L. H., Keet, J. P., Williams, I. E. I., & Bowen, D. M. Neocortical cholinergic neurons in elderly people. *Lancet,* 1977, *1,* 668.

Wilson, R. S., Kaszniak, A. W., Fox, J. H., Garron, D. C., & Ratusnik, D. L.Language deterioration in dementia. Paper presented at the 9th Annual Meeting of the International Neuropsychological Society, Atlanta, 1981.

Wisniewski, H. M., Terry, R. D., & Hirano A. Neurofibrillary pathology. *Journal of Neuropathology and Experimental Neurology,* 1970, *29,* 163–176.

Wisniewski, K., Howe, J., Williams, G. D., & Wisniewski, H. M. Precocious aging and dementia in patients with Down's syndrome. *Biological Psychiatry,* 1978, *18,* 619–627.

Wright, E. A., Spink, J. M., & Andrew, W. *Brain structure and aging.* New York: M.S.S. Information, 1974.

Yairi, E., & Clifton, N. Dysfluent speech behavior of preschool children, high school seniors and geriatric persons. *Journal of Speech and Hearing Research,* 1972, *15,* 714–719.

Yavin, E. Regulation of phospholoid metabolism in differentiating cells from rat brain cerebral hemispheres in culture. *Journal of Biological Chemistry,* 1976, *251,* 1392–1397.

Chris Hagen

Language Disorders in Head Trauma

Post-closed-head-injury (CHI) dysfunction presents the speech-language pathologist with a unique and complex diagnostic, prognostic, and treatment challenge. The CHI patient demonstrates a breakdown in communication abilities that is in certain respects similar to, but in many ways quite different from, those language disturbances caused by vascular, penetrating, or space-occupying lesions. While these patients manifest impaired receptive and expressive abilities, they do not seem to be "aphasic" in the same way that a stroke patient is "aphasic." The uniqueness of this population is not only evident in our daily clinical endeavors with them, but also can be seen in the studies that have been conducted with this population.

Language Dysfunction

Early studies (Arseni, Constantinovici, & Iliesca, 1970; Caveness, 1969; Fahy, Irving, & Millac, 1967; Hooper, 1969; Lewin, 1966, Russell, 1932) reported that head-injured patients experienced an initial period of complete dissolution of language abilities, but then gradually and spontaneously recapitulated the ontogeny of language, and eventually attained "normal speech." The most frequent behavioral residuals reported were cognitive problems of impaired concentration and short-term memory. However, these studies were directed toward the broader issues of charting and identifying the natural course of general recovery from head trauma. Language dysfunction was not a specific area of focus. As a consequence, the evaluation of patients' abilities in this area was quite general and cursory. Heilman, Safron, and Geschwind (1971) also present evidence of specific and isolated post CHI language impairments; they classified their subjects as having anomic disturbances or as having Wernicke's aphasia. Levin, Grossman, Sarwar, and Meyers (1981) found half of their language-impaired subjects to have specific linguistic deficits and half to have generalized receptive and expressive impairments.

The results of several studies suggest that CHI causes multiple language disturbances. Thomsen's (1976) subjects shifted from global to sensory aphasia and eventually stabilized as "amnestic aphasics." Although these subjects demonstrated anomic errors as a predominant feature, the majority of the subjects also had impaired auditory and reading comprehension, verbal paraphasia, and agraphia. This same pattern of deficits has also been reported in other studies. Sarno (1980) found her subjects to have either aphasia, "subclinical" aphasia, or "subclinical" aphasia with dysarthria. For aphasic subjects, Sarno further categorized 39% as fluent aphasics, 38% as nonfluent aphasics, 11% as anomic, and 11% as global aphasics. All groups, those with aphasia, subclinical aphasia, and subclinical aphasia with dysarthria, exhibited a wide range of language impairments. Of significance is the finding that, when compared with the test responses of a normal population, even those with the mildest impairments (subclinical aphasia with and without dysarthria) had significant impairments. Although subjects in the Levin, Grossman, and Kelly study (1976) had predominantly anomic errors and word-finding difficulties, they, too, exhibited a wide range of impairment.

In addition to the types of specific language impairments, other investigators find "confused language" to be a common characteristic of CHI. In general, confused language can be described as receptive/expressive language that may be intact phonologically, semantically, and syntactically, yet is lacking in meaning because the behavioral responses are irrelevant, confabulatory, circumlocutory, or tangential in relation to a given topic, and lacking a logicosequential relationship between thoughts.

Levin, Grossman, Rose, and Teasdale's (1979) subjects had specific aphasic language disorders, as well as conversational language that was frequently fragmented, tangential, and "often drifted to irrelevant topics." Thomsen (1975) found that half of his subjects had symptoms of aphasia and impaired language organization. Groher (1977) found that "confused language" was the primary residual symptom 4 months post onset. All of Groher's subjects initially had anomia as well as other language deficits.

At the end of 4 months, the anomic symptomatology had remitted, but test scores still indicated reduced expressive and receptive language abilities. Many subjects carried on conversations in which their "thought content was confused, seldom relevant to the discussion, and inappropriate in length." Groher concluded that the major post-CHI deficit is the discrepancy between the seemingly normal ability to communicate and impaired organizational and retention skills. Halpern, Darley, and Brown (1973) also found confused language to be characteristic of CHI patients. They investigated the language characteristics of patients with various neurologic etiologies, including head trauma. They measured the subjects' "relevance of responses" as well as more typical language skills. While all patients in the confused-language group manifested some degree of impairment in all areas measured, it was the category of "relevance" that clearly differentiated subjects with head trauma from the other etiologic categories.

Not only is there variability within and between CHI patients, but the literature is not unanimous with respect to the nature and temporal course of post-CHI-language dysfunction. On the basis of the literature, one could respond in at least four different ways to the question: What type of language disorder follows CHI? It could be said that such individuals regain "normal" linguistic abilities. Some may hold that specific and isolated language impairments occur across patients with no single type of disorder common to the population as a whole. Others might contend that such patients are characterized by the presence of multiple language impairments with anomia being a feature common to all. Finally, it might be said that CHI results in either specific or multiple language disorders and a coexisting presence of confused language.

To a certain extent the variability and findings are a reflection of the fact that complete homogeneity does not exist within any of the neurologic etiology categories. However, the variability may also be related, in part, to such factors as the lack of an agreed-upon taxonomy for language disorders, the use of language assessment instruments that do not evaluate the more complex levels of language utilization, or the lack of common agreement as to what constitutes a language disorder. All of these factors influence the manner in which data, either clinical or research, are analyzed and interpreted. For example, it is entirely possible that the separate findings of anomia, word-finding problems, auditory and reading comprehension deficits, and paraphasic responses are all symptoms of an underlying, more common, linguistic dysfunction, rather than five discrete disorders. The majority of language-assessment instruments focus on presence and degrees of absence of specific language abilities. As such, they yield considerable data about language power, but little about process and quality.

In the case of the CHI patient, the critical data are often found in organization of the linguistic data base, rather than in the degree to which the data base is impaired. A CHI patient will often appear to have minimal to no language impairment on the basis of available test instruments, yet manifest significant functional communication difficulties in real-life situations.

The definition of what constitutes a language disorder also heavily influences data interpretation. If one is oriented toward the more classical categorical disturbances such as aphasia and apraxia, Wernicke's and Broca's, or fluent and nonfluent aphasia, then it is entirely possible that patients with confused language, but without these symptoms, would not be considered to have a language disorder. Yet, in my experience, language disorganization is a more frequent cause of impaired ability to communicate than is the presence of a categorical linguistic deficit. For example, when asked to describe what was absurd or wrong about a picture of a man standing in the rain holding a closed umbrella, one patient stated, "First off, he's wearing slippers out in the rain and then, no I guess that's it, ya, he should wear his jacket, he's got his coat off and umbrella off and he's standing in the rain." When asked to describe what was absurd about a picture showing a bride and groom coming out of a barber shop to an awaiting car, with rice being thrown over their heads, another patient stated, "The guy should have gotten his hair cut before he picked up the bride for the wedding. Anyway, that's not the kind of costume to wear into a barber shop." While both patients scored quite well on a frequently used test battery, and while they did not manifest frank symptoms of what is often considered to be aphasia, neither could use language as an effective tool in communication situations above the level of meeting basic needs. Thus, while not aphasic or apraxic, they were nonetheless language-impaired.

The great variability of findings is not solely a reflection of the heterogeneity found within our profession's approach to language disorders. To a considerable extent, it represents the uniqueness and reality of this clinical population. In a sense, variability is their commonality. As such, it is as important to understand the source of variation as it is to identify the areas of similarity. At this time, the most observable sources appear to arise from the cognitive sequelae, as well as the neurological dynamics and pathological consequences of CHI.

Cognitive Dysfunction

Cognitive impairments have been found to be a major residual of CHI. Initially the most frequently reported problems were inability to sustain concentration and impaired memory (Brock, 1960; Hooper, 1969; Jacobsen, 1963; Lewin, 1966; Russell, 1932; Walker, 1969). The primary memory deficits reported were retrograde and anterograde amnesia (Brock, 1960; Lewin, 1966; Russell & Smith, 1961). As early as 1932, Russell (1932) suggested that the memory impairment might be a factor underlying the language dysfunction. The amnesic types of memory loss are not the only memory disturbances caused by CHI. Such patients also experience long-term deficits in immediate and recent memory as well (Brooks, 1972, 1976; Brooks, Aughton, Bond, Jones, & Rizvi, 1980; Jacobsen, 1963; Levin et al., 1979; Schilder, 1934; Smith, 1974). CHI has also been found to produce other cognitive impairments. The Levin et al. (1979) finding that subjects were inefficient in filtering extraneous material suggests possible selective-attention problems. Miller (1970) interpreted his findings of slower reaction time in relation to task complexity as reflecting reduced speed of information processing and decision making. Several investigators (Cronholm, 1972; Miller & Stern, 1965; Thomsen, 1975) have found abstract thought to be impaired. The findings of Schilder (1934), Mandleberg (1976); Mandleberg and Brooks (1975); Dye, Milby and Saxon (1979), Hallgrim and Cleeland (1972) suggest that CHI subjects have particular difficulty with the integration and synthesis of elemental parts of a whole perception. Perhaps these attention impairments of memory, analysis, and synthesis are related to Levin, Grossman, Rose and Teasdale, (1979) finding that their more severe CHI subjects had conceptual disorganization and unusual thought content.

In general, then, the literature indicates that the CHI patient incurs impairments in concentration, attention, memory, nonverbal problem solving, part/whole analysis and synthesis, conceptual organization, abstract thought, and speed of processing. Because these cognitive abilities are inextricably involved in language formulation and processing, it would seem reasonable to assume that post-CHI-language dysfunction is heavily influenced, and in some instances created, by cognitive dysfunction. Consequently, it is conceivable that some of the language variability found within and between CHI patients arises from a dynamic and reciprocal interaction between linguistic and nonlinguistic cognitive dysfunction. It has been my clinical observation that many of the previously noted specific language-disorder symptoms, such as anomia, paraphasia, and impaired auditory comprehension fluctuate considerably in relation to cognitive factors. These fluctuations appear to occur either in relation to the congitive demands inherent in a given linguistic task (test or real-life interactions) or to the intrinsic status of a patient's cognitive functions at any point in time, regardless of task demands. Both of these factors are influenced by the type, nature, and severity of cognitive dysfunction. Depending upon these cognitive factors, a previously observed specific language impairment may become worse, spread, and contaminate more functional language abilities. On the other hand, patients who do not have specific language impairments but do have confused language often demonstrate specific language impairments when their cognitive abilities are challenged.

Neurological Dysfunction

The very nature and dynamics of CHI is another source of the variability of language dysfunction found within this population. CHI is a term used to indicate those cases in which the primary source of brain injury is one of blunt trauma to the skull. There may or may not be a concurrent fracture of the skull and/or discontinuity of neural substance. The use of this term, then, excludes brain injury that is secondary to penetrating head wounds, cerebral vascular insults, and space-occupying lesions.

The force of a blow to the skull is distributed to all parts of the brain. Thus, all parts of the brain suffer to a greater or lesser degree (Brain & Walton, 1969). At the moment of impact, the brain accelerates, rotates, compresses, and expands within the skull. The dynamics of these motions produce pressure waves within the brain substance (Brain & Walton, 1969; Field, 1970). All of these effects function to damage cerebral tissue through the dynamics of compression, tension, and shearing. (Brain & Walton, 1969; Greenfield & Russell, 1963; Tomlinson, 1964; Walker, 1969) Compression forces tissue together; tension pulls it apart; and shearing, which produces contusions and lacerations, develops at the points where the brain impinges upon bony or ligamentous ridges within the cranial vault. Cerebral edema, which produces increased intracranial pressure, occurs shortly after this mechanical displacement and disruption of the brain substance (Meyer & Denny-Brown, 1955). In view of the magnitude and multiplicity of these negative forces, Russell's, (1932) and Adams and Sidman's (1968) descriptions of the effects of CHI as being a "molecular commotion" would appear quite appropriate. The very molecular structure of the brain is disrupted, disorganized, bruised, and/or lacerated. These gross neuropathological effects of CHI have been found to produce permanent microscopic alterations of both white and gray matter. Brain and Walton (1969) report widely scattered punctate hemorrhages throughout the brain associated with CHI. Severe localized demyelination was found by Greenfield (1938), and others (Stritch, 1956; Tomlinson, 1964) have reported wide-spread white-matter degeneration. Nerve cell damage after CHI has been reported both by Courville and Amyes (1952) and Horowitz and Rizzoli (1966). Other permanent neurological impairments result from the contusions, lacerations, and hemorrhages (Brain & Walton, 1969; Courville, 1942) that occur when the brain substance rotates against the bony shelves of the skull, from direct trauma at the site of the blow to the skull, or contra-coup trauma that occurs when the brain strikes the skull on the side opposite the point of trauma. Lesions of the corpus callosum have also been reported (Lindberg, Fisher, & Durlacher, 1955; Rowbotham, 1949; Rubens, Geschwind, Mahowald, & Mastri, 1977; Stritch, 1969).

The variety of the possible neuropathological consequences of CHI suggests that the initial generalized impairment of language/cognitive processes is a manifestation of the massive, yet, to a degree, reversible disruption and disorganization of neurophysiological activity. Conversely, the irreversible neurologic damage could, subsequently, produce a potentially wide variety of cognitive/language impairments that would not be expected to remit spontaneously.

Clinically, there appear to be at least three general phases of post-CHI neurologic-communicative-cognitive dysfunction. During the initial phase the patient is in a state of "cerebral paralysis" (Russell, 1932). At this time there is a global suppression of all communicative and cognitive functions. In the intermediate phase, a mixture of reversible and irreversible neurologic impairments coexist. Consequently, at this time it is not unusual to observe wide swings in the presence or absence, as well as types of, cognitive/communicative impairment. However, one may also begin to find certain symptoms persisting across time during this phase. The irreversible neurologic impairments and their concommitant communicative and cognitive sequelae become evident during the long-term phase.

Thus, the variability of post-CHI-language dysfunction characterizes the dynamic interactions between the natural course of neurological recovery, the type, extent, and location of residual neurologic impairment, and the degree to which cognitive abilities are disturbed. It has been my experience that three general types of patients ultimately emerge from the diffuse symptomatology of the first two phases: (1) those with disorganized language secondary to cognitive disorganization, who may or may not have a coexisting specific language disorder; (2) those with the predominant feature of a specific language disorder and coexisting minimal cognitive impairment; and (3) those with attentional, retentional, and recent memory impairments, but without language dysfunction. The remainder of this chapter will focus on the assessment and treatment of those patients who fall into the first two categories.

The speech-language pathologist who treats the CHI patient must answer the same critical questions related to clinical management as they do with other disorders, namely to whom, when, what, and how care should be rendered. One cannot reason solely from experience and information related to language disorders secondary to other types of neurological impairments. Head trauma patients cannot be successfully understood, diagnosed, and treated within the framework of our traditional approaches to language disorders. The communicative dysfunction of the CHI patient is quite dynamic. Consequently, our clinical approach must also be dynamic. Ongoing assessment and subsequent modification of the treatment approach is a primary requisite for the appropriate management of this population.

The purpose of this chapter is to present an approach to evaluation and treatment that has been drawn from my clinical experience with more than 2,500 CHI patients over the past 18 years. Other work that broadens the scope in this field may include Adamovich (1981), Adamovich and Brooks (1981), Adamovich and Henderson (1982), Adamovich and Henderson (1983), Ben-Yishay (1978, 1979, 1980), Buschke and Fuld (1974), Butler (1981), Glick and Holyoak (1980), Hedberg-Davis and Bookman (1979), Ledwon-Robinson and Beh-Arendshorst (1980), Lezak (1979), Ligne, Sinatra, and Kimbarow (1979), and Yorkston, Stanton and Beukelman (1981). This approach is based on the premise that the majority of the post-CHI-language dysfunction is a secondary consequence of an underlying impairment, suppression, and/or disorganization of the nonlinguistic cognitive processes that support language processes. This is not to suggest that the CHI patient does not have a language disorder but rather indicates that the observed language disorder is the sum of both linguistic and nonlinguistic cognitive dysfunctions.

Characterictics of Cognitive-Language Disorganization

Typically, our internal and external environment is fluctuating, fluid, and random. Under normal circumstances we bring stability, structure, and organization to this otherwise chaotic world by automatically yet willfully focusing only on those things that we deem necessary and relevant to our needs. At a minimum, this ability to focus our awareness on only certain aspects of our environment is derived from the following seven cognitive processes:

1. Attentional abilities (alertness, awareness, attention, attention span, and selective attention);
2. Discrimination;

3. Sequential ordering of sensory stimuli and internal thoughts;
4. Memory abilities (retention span, immediate, recent, and remote memory);
5. Categorization of sensory stimuli and internal thoughts;
6. Association /integration of sensory stimuli and internal thoughts;
7. Analysis/synthesis of sensory stimuli and internal thoughts.

These seven cognitive processes become disrputed as a result of CHI. The patient is unable to exert the influence of these processes on the internal and external environment. As a result, the patient has difficulty organizing, structuring, and predicting the sequential order of thoughts. This leads to a breakdown in the patient's ability to structure mental processes volitionally to deal differentially with stimuli, to mentally structure ongoing events, to shift cognitive sets, and to modify/dampen emotional reactions. As a result, such individuals become disoriented, disorganized, confused, stimulus bound, and reduced in both initiation and inhibition. As a consequence, the patient's receptive, integrative, and expressive language can also become

1. *Disoriented*—not appropriate to the situation, question, statement or discussion.
2. *Disorganized*—fragmented and incomplete understanding of what has been heard or expressed by the patient.
3. *Confused*—confabulatory, circumlocutory, tangential in relation to the content of the situation, question, statement, or discussion.
4. *Stimulus bound*—relevant to a part, but not the whole idea of a statement, question, or discussion.
5. *Reduced in initiation*—reliant upon others to stimulate the occurence and structure of language responses.
6. *Reduced in inhibition*—Once language response is initiated, it is lacking in specificity and precision in relationship to the original question or statement.

Typically, these six consequences of cognitive disorganization appear in the patient's receptive and expressive language in the form of combinations of the following symptoms:

1. Decreased auditory comprehension;
2. Decreased visual and reading comprehension;
3. Expressive language that does not make sense;
4. Language expressions that are grammatically correct but not relevant to the question, statement, or discussion;

5. Lack of ability to inhibit verbal expressions;

6. Inappropriate ordering of words in sentences and/or inappropriate grammar;

7. Inability to recall specific words.

Many of these symptoms are characteristic of the aphasic disorders found in patients with vascular or space-occupying lesions. A CHI patient may, in fact, have a specific language disorder caused by a focal lesion. However, while many of these receptive and expressive language problems are like aphasia, the majority are symptomatic of the language confusion that results from the underlying disorganization of the seven cognitive processes listed above. Because of this, a major part of the patient's communication rehabilitation program must be directed toward cognitive reorganization. Typically, as cognitive processes become reorganized, there will be a major decrease in the patient's language disorganization.

Assessment

The following variables must be addressed when evaluating the CHI patient: the patient's ability to cooperate with testing, the rapid and random fluctuations in symptoms, clinically apparent language dysfunction with little or no impairment reflected in test scores, and the dynamic interaction between cognitive and language impairments. In the early phases of recovery, patients are confused, disoriented, and unable to deal purposefully with internal and external stimuli. Consequently, assessment should not be completely dependent upon a patient's ability to cooperate volitionally in the more typical stimulus-response test-taking procedures. Structured, systematic, and consistent clinical observation and evaluation of spontaneous behavior will be needed. The rapid and random fluctuations in the type and severity of symptoms necessitate frequent re-evaluation. During the first 4 to 8 weeks of recovery, a patient's communication disorder usually results from the combined effects of the temporary global interruption of neural activity, the language and cognitive disorganization secondary to irreversible diffuse structural damage and, possibly, a specific language disorder secondary to a focal lesion. Fluctuations in symptomatology are reflective of the interplay between the subsidence of reversible neurological dysfunction and the emergence of the long-term neurologic impairments. It is neither practical nor instructive to repeat standardized tests on a daily to weekly basis; however, clinical direction depends upon some form of frequent reassessment. Consequently, during the early phases of recovery the evaluation approach should include a means of describing, categorizing, and scaling the type and nature of language/cognitive behavior at very frequent intervals. Standardized tests should be employed when the more global cognitive disorganization begins to remit.

During the later phases of recovery, it is not unusual to find that patients who demonstrate minimal to no impairment on standard aphasia test instruments will experience difficulty with language in their natural environment. Because of this, one must assess those language abilities that are not evaluated by most aphasia tests, such as the verbal reasoning and thought organization that lie behind the use of language.

The assessment approach that I have found to be the most helpful consists of four evaluation methods: (1) categorizing the patient's spontaneous behavioral responses to randomly occurring environmental stimuli; (2) scaling responses to nontest stimuli that are presented and controlled by someone other than the patient, as in the daily nursing routine; (3) administering a standard aphasia test battery; and (4) administering higher-level cognitive and verbal tests. Depending on the patient's level of functioning, these four assessment approaches may be applied sequentially in steps that parallel the longitudinal course of recovery or, when appropriate, combinations of all four methods may be applied simultaneously.

Categorizing Spontaneous Behavior

Clinical observation is the primary method of identifying and categorizing behavioral manifestations of cognitive/linguistic dysfunction during the early phases of recovery. When present, the symptoms will be readily apparent in the patient's manner of handling daily activities, interacting with others, using familiar objects, and the manner and content of the patient's responses to language tests. Some of the more common behavioral characteristics are the following:

1. *Disorientation*—behavior that is not appropriate to prevailing stimuli; lack of awareness of time, space and place;
2. *Confusion*—behavioral responses that randomly fluctuate between appropriate and inappropriate; difficulty in discriminating between animate and inanimate objects; confabulatory, circumlocutory, tangential, or completely inappropriate language responses;
3. *Distractability and impulsivity*—decreased attention and attention span;

4. *Reduced initiation*—reliant upon external stimuli for the occurrence and structure of responses;

5. *Reduced inhibition*—once responses are initiated, they continue beyond logical point of cessation and usually lack specificity in relation to the stimulus;

6. *Concreteness*—deals with stimuli in their literal sense, responses are relevant to a part of a stimulus, but not the implied whole concept;

7. *Reduced cognitive flexibility*—either does not shift cognitively or carries part of a previous thought/response into a succeeding response, or needs an abnormal length of time to shift from one stimulus condition to another;

8. *Disorganization*—behavioral responses generally appropriate to stimulus, but are organized in an illogical sequential manner and display periodic intrusion of extraneous responses not relevant to stimulus;

9. *Reduction in judgment*—does not grasp cause-effect relationships.

The purpose of categorizing patient's behavior is not simply to generate a diagnostic label. Rather, this information provides a very general statement about the broad area of dysfunction that must be addressed, as well as the general goal of treatment. Categorizing patients is the first step in discerning the differences among patients whose behavior may appear superficially similar. For example, the knowledge that one must decrease confusion in one patient, increase cognitive flexibility in another, and decrease distractibility and impulsiveness in a third will, when combined with other assessment data, assist in the development of a treatment plan that focuses on individual patient needs.

Scaling of Behavioral Responses

Historically, head-trauma patients have been classified according to such categories as coma, stupor, delirium, and confusion (Hooper, 1969; Lewin, 1966). In recent years the Glasgow Coma Scale (Jennett & Teasdale, 1981; Teasdale & Jennett, 1974) has also been extensively used. While the major purpose of the Glasgow Scale is the early prediction of mortality and morbidity, it also provides some very useful general descriptive categories of patient responses which are characteristic of different levels of coma. This scale is particularly useful during the acute phase of treatment. The Levels of Cognitive Functioning (Hagen & Malkmus, 1979) described in abbreviated form in Table 8-1 has been found to be quite helpful in identifying a patient's most intact level of cognitive functioning throughout the entire course of rehabilitation. The Glasgow Coma Scale is used for prognosis.

TABLE 8-1
Levels of Cognitive Functioning.

    I. *No Response:* Patient appears to be in a deep sleep and is completely unresponsive to any stimuli.

   II. *Generalized Response:* Patient reacts inconsistently and nonpurposefully to stimuli in a nonspecific manner. Responses are limited and often the same, regardless of stimulus presented. Responses may be physiological changes, gross body movements, and/or vocalization.

  III. *Localized Response:* Patient reacts specifically, but inconsistently, to stimuli. Responses are directly related to the type of stimulus presented. May follow simple commands such as, "Close your eyes" or "Squeeze my hand" in an inconsistent, delayed manner.

  IV. *Confused-Agitated:* Behavior is bizarre and nonpurposeful relative to immediate environment. Does not discriminate among persons or objects, is unable to co-operate directly with treatment efforts, verbalizations are frequently incoherent and/or inappropriate to the environment, confabulation may be present. Gross attention to environment is very short, and selective attention is often nonexistent. Patient lacks short term recall.

   V. *Confused, Inappropriate, Non-Agitated:* Patient is able to respond to simple commands fairly consistently. However, with increased complexity of commands, or lack of any external structure, responses are nonpurposeful, random, or fragmented. Has gross attention to the environment, but is highly distractible, and lacks ability to focus attention on a specific task; with structure, may be able to converse on a social-automatic level for short periods of time; verbalization is often inappropriate and confabulatory; memory is severely impaired, often shows inappropriate use of subjects; may perform previously learned tasks with structure, but is unable to learn new information.

  VI. *Confused-Appropriate:* Patient shows goal-directed behavior, but is dependent on external input for direction; follows simple directions consistently and shows carry-over for relearned tasks with little or no carry-over for new tasks; responses may be incorrect due to memory problems, but appropriate to the situation; past memories show more depth and detail than recent memory.

 VII. *Automatic-Appropriate:* Patient appears appropriate and oriented within hospital and home settings, goes through daily routine automatically, but is frequently robot-like, with minimal-to-absent

**TABLE 8-1 (Continued)
Levels of Cognitive Functioning.**

confusion; has shallow recall of activities; shows carry-over for new learning, but at a decreased rate; with structure, is able to initiate social or recreational activities; judgment remains impaired.

VIII. *Purposeful and Appropriate:* Patient is able to recall and integrate past and recent events, and is aware of and responsive to the environment, shows carry-over for new learning and needs no supervision once activities are learned; may continue to show a decreased ability, relative to premorbid abilities in language, abstract reasoning, tolerance for stress and judgment in emergencies or unusual circumstances.

The Levels of Cognitive Functioning, in contrast, is used to identify a patient's best level of functioning, and, thereby, to indicate the best way to approach the patient during the course of treatment.

The purpose of this type of evaluation is to establish the presence and pattern of change in such basic neurobehavioral dichotomies as:

1. Response to external stimuli versus no responses;
2. Gross undifferentiated response to stimuli versus differentiated response to stimuli;
3. Differentiated response to stimuli, but no continued response after withdrawal of stimuli, versus differentiated and sustained response after withdrawal of stimuli;
4. Sustained response to stimuli only if stimuli brought to patient, versus sustained response on basis of patient's self-directed behavior;
5. Inappropriate versus appropriate responses to stimuli, whether externally presented or self-initiated.

These behavioral responses represent the manner in which the Levels of Cognitive Functioning Scale should be interpreted with respect to levels of information processing. In this regard, Item 1 represents reception of sensory stimuli versus no reception; Item 2 represents reception of stimuli, but with minimal to no relation to specific sensory modalities; Item 3 represents response to specific sensory modalities, but inability to retain the response for purposes of processing; Item 4 represents ability to process information, if information is continually presented, versus ability to process information on a self-initiated basis; and Item 5 represents a qualitative evaluation of the patient's behavioral responses on Items 2 through 4. We have found that, for patients at and between Levels II and VII, the rating scale is most useful when all disciplines interacting with the patient rate him or her.

Such a behavioral-scaling technique is a means for systematically describing and categorizing the patient's level of cognitive/language functioning across time, be it a day, week, or month. In the early phases of recovery, it provides an immediate and sensitive picture of the dynamics of the course of change. This type of assessment has several benefits. Systematic observation and assessment of the type, nature, and quality of a patient's behavioral responses assists in estimating the level at which the patient is functioning in the hierarchy of cognitive processes. Behavioral scaling also allows one, as early as possible, to differentiate between those language-impairment characteristics secondary to temporary interruption of cognitive/language processes, those that reflect potential long-term cognitive/language disorganization, and those that may indicate the presence of a language disorder secondary to a focal lesion. Clear patterns of change emerge through daily-to-weekly charting. Through these patterns, one is able to differentiate between the rapidly resolving, and, therefore, most probably temporary and reversible, symptoms and the more slowly remitting symptoms characteristic of the irreversible diffuse and/or focal damage. By observing the type and nature of the patients' responses to the environment, and, then, to purposefully introduce stimuli that are contextually relevant to the patient's total treatment program, one will find that behavioral responses characteristic of a particular level occur more frequently than others. Most patients have a characteristic range of cognitive function, showing a preponderance of behavior at one level and a scatter of behavioral responses below and above that level. Determining the patient's range of cognitive/communicative behavior provides three types of information important to planning and maintaining an appropriate treatment plan: (1) Knowledge of the patient's most typical cognitive level identifies the highest level of functioning we can expect from a patient at a given point in time. Knowing this, the stimuli we present and the way in which we present them will be consonant with his or her capabilities. A program that presents stimuli in a manner that matches the patient's most stable level of functioning, and that slightly challenges the next highest level simultaneously is optimal. Such treatment decreases the behavioral swings below the most intact level and increases the swings above. In time, the next highest level becomes the patient's most typical level, with a scatter of responses remaining from the previous level, but now the emergence of abilities at the next highest level are observed. (2) Responses below the patient's most consistent level of functioning are extremely important signs. They indicate that the environment should be altered to maintain the patient's highest level of cognitive/communicative organization for the longest period of time.

Responses characteristic of a lower level of function signal regression, and, as such, tell us to alter the way in which we interact with the patient or what we request from the patient. (3) Similarly, the emergence and stabilization of behavioral responses characteristic of the next highest level indicate that it is safe to alter the treatment plan in a manner that challenges the patient to move toward this next level of function. It is on the basis of these three types of information, i.e., the patient's most typical cognitive level, responses below, and above, that level, that one is able to construct the type of treatment plan that will maintain cognitive organization.

Direct Assessment of Cognitive Functioning

Evaluation of language processes should occur concurrently with assessment of the patient's cognitive abilities. Because of the interrelationship and reciprocal interplay between linguistic and cognitive processes, it is necessary to have information regarding type and level of nonlinguistic cognitive dysfunction to interpret the dynamic nature of the linguistic disturbance. The type and nature of cognitive dysfunction will provide information as to why and how the patient is experiencing a breakdown in language organization. At a minimum, one should assess the general cognitive processes of (1) attentional abilities (alertness, awareness, attention, attention span, and selective attention); (2) discrimination; (3) temporal ordering; (4) memory abilities (retention span, immediate, recent, and remote memory); (5) categorization; (6) association/integration; (7) analysis/synthesis; (8) maintenance of sequential goal-directed behavior. At the phonemenological level, language disorganization (i.e., confused language) may appear similar across patients at different points in time. However, the source of the cognitive disorganization that underlies the language disorganization is often different for each patient. Appropriate and effective treatment is heavily dependent on treatment of the specific impaired-cognitive abilities.

All eight cognitive abilities are assessed during the previously described processes of categorizing and scaling spontaneous behavior. But, they cannot be directly assessed until the patient reaches Level VII. Following are examples of tests that can be used to assess these various abilities.

To measure attention, discrimination, temporal sequencing, and retention span abilities, the following tests are used: Visual Sequential Memory subtest of the ITPA (Kirk, McCarthy, & Kirk, 1968); the WAIS Digit Span subtest (Wechsler, 1955); the Auditory Attention Span for Unrelated Words and Related Syllables and the Visual Attention Span for Objects and Letters subtests of the DTLA (Baker & Leland, 1959); the Developmental Test of Visual Perception (Frostig, 1963); the Southern California Figure-Ground Visual

Perception Test (Ayres, 1966); Luria's tests for Perception and Reproduction of Pitch Relationships and Perception and Reproduction of Rhythmic Structures (Christensen, 1975); The G-F-W Sound-Symbol Tests (Goldman, Fristoe, & Woodcock 1974b); and the G-F-W Test of Auditory Discrimination (Goldman, Fristoe, & Woodcock, 1970).

To measure immediate and recent memory abilities, the following tests are used: The Wechsler Memory Scale (Wechsler & Stone, 1945); the Digit Symbol subtest of the WAIS (Wechsler, 1955); The Goldstein-Scheerer Stick Test (Goldstein & Scheerer, 1945); the Benton Revised Visual Retention Test (Benton, 1963); Luria's mnestic tests (Christensen, 1975); and the G-F-W Auditory Memory Tests (Goldman, Fristoe, & Woodcock, 1974a).

To measure categorization, association, integration, and synthesis abilities, we use the Weigle-Goldstein-Scheerer Color Form Sorting Test (1945); the Disarranged Pictures subtest of the DTLA (Baker & Leland, 1959); the Block Design, Object Assembly, and Picture Arrangement subtests of the WAIS (Wechsler, 1955); The Ross Test of Higher Cognitive Processes (Ross & Ross, 1976), and the tests of higher level language organization listed in the section on language, following the section on language assessment. Finally, the Nonverbal Test of Cognitive Skills (Johnson & Boyd, 1981) provides a means of evaluating a number of the various cognitive abilities within the context of a single test battery.

The various tests which have been described do not constitute a "test battery." The list represents tests that can be drawn upon relative-to-specific types and levels of language impairments known to exist in a particular patient. For example, to assess attention, selective attention, or retention span in patients with significant language impairments, one would not use those tests that were dependent upon auditory comprehension or highly intact speech production abilities. Instead, one would select those tests not dependent on these abilities. Because of the need to control for confounding variables such as these, as well as the effect of fatigue, one should use those few tests that focus with the greatest precision on the areas of breakdown.

The various cognitive abilities have been placed in clusters because of the close interaction between them. However, from the standpoint of actual cognitive processing, there is a functional interaction both within and between these clusters of cognitive abilities. Consequently it is not solely the presence or absence of an error that is of significance. It is this *plus* the dynamic nature of the dysfunction. In this regard, the interpretation of the pattern of deficits leads to the determination of cognitive/language dysfunction. This determination is not based on the scores on specific tests. For example, one could not infer the presence of a problem with categorization, association, and synthesis if a patient exhibits severe impairments of attention and memory, even though the patient did very poorly on tests related to those higher level skills. Here, one is undoubtedly observing a cause-effect relationship rather than areas of discrete impairment.

Comparison of behavioral responses under different conditions and analysis of variations in behavioral responses under the same condition provides two means of interpreting the pattern of response errors. For example, a comparison of the type and level of dysfunction that is identified through clinical observation (e.g., categorizing and scaling spontaneous behavior) with the type and level of dysfunction found during direct assessment could lead to one of the following interpretations: Better performance in spontaneous activities requiring cognitive abilities similar to those directly tested would suggest that the patient is able to maintain better cognitive stability and organization when provided with familiarity, contextual cues, and the structure of an actual event. The individual cannot internally evoke and organize these same attributes independently. Conversely, the patient who does better on test tasks than on tasks using environmental stimuli is a person who is more cognitively organized by the structure of tasks, and who has trouble spontaneously and independently organizing the random and fluctuating stimuli of the environment. Table 8-2 presents possible interpretations of variations in the pattern of errors that occur under similar task conditions.

Finally, the interpretation of the quality and pattern of both language and cognitive organization impairments is considerably aided by gathering information relative to factors that are not implicit in the tests themselves. Specifically, it is important to assess and identify the manner in which the patient approaches a given problem. I have found that each patient has an optimal and stable level of performance in relationship to the rate, amount, duration, and complexity of stimulus input. Variations either above or below a patient's optimal level of receiving and processing stimuli act to intensify his or her already impaired ability to remain organized. With respect to the patient's problem-solving approach, I have found it helpful to watch for the following characteristics: immediately recognizes a solution, studies task before attempting solution, is organized and systematic, approaches task in an impulsive or trial-and-error manner, develops alternate strategies when unsuccessful, over-attends to details, must be prompted to start, as well as continue, task, perseverates approach across tasks, benefits from cues and correction, and independently carries cues or corrections over to next task. Knowing the optimal manner for presenting stimuli, as well as the patient's problem-solving approach, is critical diagnostic information. The behavioral-rating scale and the tests yield information that tells us what the level of the problem is, and what should and should not be treated. Knowledge about stimulus presentation and task approach tells how to treat the problem.

TABLE 8-2
Variations in Pattern of Errors Within Similar Task Conditions.

A. Random and fluctuating errors across time—suggests attention span and/or selective attention problems;

B. Errors that occur on the first several stimuli of tasks, but not later in the task, across test tasks—suggestive of attentional/selective attention impairments;

C. Errors that consistently occur during the last several stimuli of tasks, but not earlier—suggestive of attentional, selective attention, or retention span fatigue;

D. Clustering of errors at relatively similar time intervals during a task—suggests problems with amount and duration of stimuli, and gives insight into what would be optimal for a given patient relative to these parameters during treatment;

E. Errors decrease relative to certain types of cues: auditory, visual, visualmotor, contextual, breaking up stimulus into its parts, providing whole idea, etc.—suggestive of problems with categorization, association, and/or analysis/synthesis;

F. Errors increase/decrease with rate, amount, and duration of stimuli—affects all cognitive abilities;

G. Errors increase in relation to complexity—suggestive of impaired memory abilities, including retention span and/or weakened categorization, association, and analysis/synthesis problems;

H. Responds appropriately to parts of stimulus, but not whole or vice versa—suggestive of associative, integrative, analysis/synthesis impairment;

I. Carry-over of responses to previous tasks to succeeding ones—suggestive of cognitive shift problems.

Language Assessment

The previously described approaches to behavioral categorization and scaling also provide a means of on-going language assessment. Charting and describing a patient's behavior across time provides information that is most useful in determining the presence of a specific language disorder, and, if it exists, distinguishing between it and communication impairment secondary to language disorganization. The presence of specific language disorders, such as apraxia or aphasic syndromes, will rapidly become apparent through the persistence of their characteristic symptoms across time, even though their severity levels might vary. Similarly, the presence of language disorganization will also become apparent through the observed persistence of the characteristics noted in Table 8-3.

A high degree of confusion and disorientation decreases the validity of standardized test results prior and up to Level V of cognitive functioning. However, even though validity with respect to isolating specific language disorders is diminished, it is important to present patients with stimuli relative to various communication skills in a categorical and systematic fashion as early as possible. A patient's failure to respond or to give a response that is completely without form and/or meaning is as significant as a response that fits into a more recognizable speech- or language-disturbance category. Tests administered to such severely involved patients will generate very important information regarding language functioning under controlled, identifiable, and systematic conditions; this performance may contrast significantly with performance under spontaneous conditions. The delineation of the difference between responses to structured versus unstructured stimulus conditions generates very important base-line data. For example, the type and quality of responses of a confused and disoriented patient to auditory subtests should be interpreted in relation to the patient's ability to focus attention on a task and remember the instructions, rather than to the auditory tasks themselves. In essence, the purpose of this level of evaluation is to determine the stimulus conditions under which the patient becomes less confused and more oriented, rather than to attempt to determine whether the problem is one of aphasia or apraxia. Diagnosis of specific language impairments become clearer as the patient moves from Level V towards Level VIII.

As patients approach Level VII it is not unusual to find that they have minimal to no deficits in the majority of the categorical language abilities, but, at the same time, observe that they have difficulty using language to understand and convey the meaning of thoughts. This disparity between apparent linguistic competence on tests and poor performance in a natural communication environment is typically the result of two factors. First, the temporary disruption of neural activity that produced the global disturbances of language has, by now, remitted almost completely. Second, since most aphasia tests are oriented primarily toward the assessment of the categorical elements (i.e., phonology, semantic, and syntactic) of language, test results now accurately portray the patient's improvement in these areas of language. This does not necessarily mean that the patient has normal functional language abilities. Our tests do not assess in depth the organizational structure of expressed discursive thought, the use of language as a verbal reasoning tool, or the auditory processing counterpart of these

TABLE 8-3
Language Disorganization.

Language expressions that are

    I. Inappropriate

    II. Irrelevant

    III. Confabulatory

    IV. Fragmented

    V. Have no logical sequential relationship

    VI. Circumlocutious

    VII. Tangential

   VIII. Concrete

    IX. Intermittent and random auditory confusion

---

expressive functions. Thus, it is entirely possible for a patient to do well on discrete identification, naming, sentence completion/understanding, and short-answer tasks within the structured context of a test, but to be unable to organize these same language processes across time.

In many instances, then, good test performance only reflects the fact that the patient has reached the upper limits of those factors that a particular test was designed to assess. It is the quality of the language behavior that now becomes of diagnostic and therapeutic significance. One must now evaluate to determine whether the language-disorganization characteristics shown in Table 8-3 are present. This usually becomes necessary after a patient has reached Level VI. The following are a number of the tests that can be used to assess the higher levels of language integrity: The Wechsler Adult Intelligence Scale (WAIS)(Wechsler, 1955); subtests of the Detroit Test of Learning Aptitude (DTLA)(Baker & Leland, 1959); the Goldstein-Scheerer Object Sorting Test (Goldstein & Scheerer, 1951); subtests of the Illinois Test of Psycholinguistic Abilities (ITPA)(Kirk, McCarthy, & Kirk, 1968); and Luria's tests of understanding both logical grammatical structures and thematic pictures and texts (Christensen, 1975). Although some of these tests were developed for and standardized on a children's population, the intention in using them is not to derive an age-comparable score, but, rather, to assess the manner in which the patient responds to the tasks.

Treatment

The treatment approach discussed here is based on the following postulates:

1. Treatment should be directed toward the reorganization of the cognitive processes, rather than modification of the abnormal language consequences of the cognitive disorganization.

2. As cognitive processes become reorganized, there will be a commensurate reorganization of phonological, semantic, syntactic, andverbal-reasoning abilities.

3. The reorganization of cognitive abilities follows a predictable and systematic hierarchical sequence, in which the reacquisition and stabilization of lower level processes is necessary for the emergence and stabilization of higher level activities.

4. Cognitive structure is maximized and behavioral responses become more organized when the treatment program progresses sequentially from the patient's highest level of cognitive abilities through all of the necessary steps following that level.

5. Treatment stimuli should be presented through the patient's single-most intact sensory modality, and generalized to other modalities only as increasing cognitive abilities support the ability to deal with multiple stimuli.

6. Regardless of the level of cognitive abilities toward which treatment is directed, the manner of stimulus input is critical to the elicitation of structured and appropriate behavioral responses. Consequently, one must manipulate the rate, amount, duration, and complexity of stimulus input in a manner consistent with the patient's cognitive abilities at any given time.

The goal of treatment is to promote the conscious processing of language stimuli in an orderly, sequential manner. This is accomplished through the appropriate manipulation of the patient's environment, as well as through direct treatment of cognitive-linguistic disorganization.

Environmental Manipulation

The rate, quality, and ultimate level of recovery is critically dependent upon the degree to which the patient's environment allows him or her to function at the threshold of his most intact level of cognitive abilities. Maintaining a balance between the type and manner of stimulus input and the patient's most intact level of cognitive functioning is the single-most critical factor in the successful reorganization of cognitive/communicative abilities. A patient is able to process internal and/or external stimuli in the most organized manner, and, consequently, to function at his or her optimum level when the demands of the environment match existing cognitive abilities. Environmental stimulation that is below the patient's most functional level will not challenge recovery in a structured, controlled, and predictable manner. Stimulation above a patient's optimum level of functioning will be overwhelming, and, as a result, will suppress and impede recovery. The speech-language pathologist can provide guidance to other members of the rehabilitation team regarding the manner in which a patient's environment can be optimally structured. In addition to the usual recommendations relative to increasing awareness of a patient's most functional receptive and expressive modes of communication, the recommendations that follow are pertinent.

LEVELS I, II, AND III:
NO, GENERALIZED, AND LOCALIZED RESPONSE

The goal of treatment for Levels I and II is to activate a behavioral response and, thereby, initiate the patient's movement toward the early phases of awareness of his or her environment.

Activation of behavioral responses will occur within the context of routine patient care. Special efforts outside this routine are unnecessary. Stimulating the patient toward Level III will, however, be enhanced by giving special consideration to the manner in which the nursing routine is carried out. The following ways of interacting with patients have good potential for stimulating awareness of the environment:

1. Be calm and soothing in manner of speech and physical manipulation of the patient;

2. Do not talk to others when working with the patient;

3. Assume that the patient can understand all that is said. While the degree to which patients can actually understand will be unknown at this time, it is wiser not to risk his or her hearing comments about themselves or other patients. Hearing and understanding such conversations can be traumatizing and create emotions that potentially affect the course of future recovery. Consequently, all comments or discussions of medical status, behavior, prognosis, and family concerns, as well as discussions about other patients, should be avoided in the patient's presence.

4. Talk to the patient. It is quite difficult to carry on a conversation with an unresponsive patient; however, one should try to avoid

concluding that since the patient cannot answer, there is not much point in talking to him or her. Talking is a natural form of stimulation. Use appropriate greetings such as, "Good morning Mr. or Mrs. Smith." Describe what you are going to do with the patient before you do it, describe such occurrences as family visits, upcoming occupational therapy treatment, etc., talk about the weather conditions, or even things or events that are of personal interest to you. Try to learn about the patient's family and/or friends so that you can talk about them by name and describe some of the things they are doing. However, it is important not to overwhelm the patient with talking. Talk slowly and calmly. Describe what you are about to do with the patient; then, without talking, do it and then describe the next event. It will be important to leave moments of silence between verbal stimuli.

5. Manage environmental stimuli. While activation of the patient's behavioral responses at these lower levels is dependent on the presence of external stimulation, too much stimulation can suppress an increasing awareness of environment. A TV or radio is a very useful source of stimulation. However, it is important to use them sporadically and for short durations. The patient will rapidly get habituated and fail to respond to such stimuli when they are on continuously. Only one source of stimulation should occur in the environment at a time. For example, if talking is occurring, then the radio or TV should be off.

6. Determine which type of stimuli seems to cause the patient to respond. Certain topics, statements, TVprograms, music, etc. may elicit a response. Often family voices or the voice of a particular staff member seem to stimulate a response. In the case of these latter two, tape recordings can be made of those to whom the patient reacts, and these can be played intermittently. Identify key stimuli and present them to the patient on a routine basis. The patient, however, will become fatigued and overwhelmed if such stimuli are allowed to continue for long periods of time. To a large extent, arousal and awareness depend on the novelty of the stimulus. In this regard, all activities should be kept very brief. Present several different types of stimuli rather than a single lengthy stimulus.

7. Encourage the family to follow the above pattern of interaction. Special caution should be taken to describe the problems of presenting simultaneous multiple stimuli and stimulating the patient for too long a period of time. If family members do not understand the problems, they can unknowingly overwhelm the patient.

LEVEL IV:
CONFUSED-AGITATED

The goals for this level are to increase the patient's awareness of, and attention to, the environment, to minimize the frequency of occurrence of agitated behavior, and to decrease the duration of agitated behavior when it occurs.

One's physical handling and moving of patients, as well as one's manner of interacting with them, is most important at this stage. Patients are beginning to be aware of, and alert to, the environment and are trying to process information. Their neurological status at this time, however, is such that they often make exaggerated responses to internal and external stimuli. Thus, patients at this level are susceptible to the triggering of defensive motor reflexes and emotional reactions, such as acute fear, anxiety, and anger. Many of these behavioral responses occur spontaneously and are unavoidable, but the nurse can take steps to minimize the degree and duration of such responses. However, the degree to which one is able to keep from triggering the patient's defensive responses relates to the degree to which the patient is neurologically ready to move towards the environment rather than away from it. The following approaches can be taken with patients at this level:

1. Be calm and soothing in manner when handling the patient;

2. Move slowly around the patient and move the patient slowly when it is necessary to change his or her position or range, to bathe, or to transfer the patient;

3. Talk slowly and softly. Talking loudly may trigger a startle reflex, and speaking rapidly will be overwhelming;

4. Do not talk to others while working with the patient. Multiple stimuli—such as physical manipulation and an ongoing conversation with others—will be more than a patient can handle;

5. Always describe what you are going to do with the patient before you do it. Even if what you say is not totally understood by the patient, the patient will have time during the explanation to adjust to your presence in the room and to become aware that something is going to happen;

6. Before physically handling patients in accordance with the desired task, take time first to simply touch them, gently rub one of the extremities, head, or back, and/or gradually move an extremity. Such activities will decrease the occurrence of defensive motor reflexes and emotional reflexes—that is, the activities allow time to adjust;

7. If the patient becomes upset, allow time for self-adjustment. Do not try to talk a patient out of his or her reaction. At this time, talking will be an additional external stimulus that will only act to intensify the reactions;

8. If the patient remains upset, either remove him or her from the situation or remove the situation from him or her;

9. Watch for early signs that the patient is becoming agitated (e.g., more-than-usual motor movement activity, increase in vocal loudness, resistance to activity) and modify the environment immediately. It is far better to cease all of your activity than to launch the patient into a prolonged state of agitation. It will take far less time to wait then it will to calm the patient down.

LEVELS V AND VI: CONFUSED, INAPPROPRIATE, NON-AGITATED, AND CONFUSED-APPROPRIATE

The goal of this phase of rehabilitation is to create the environmental conditions whereby the patient can produce purposeful and appropriate responses to external and internal stimuli with greater frequency and duration. There are two approaches to creating the appropriate conditions. One involves the use of the more automatic behavioral responses found in some of the activities of daily living. Such activities can be used as a means of eliciting purposeful behavior and to provide environmental structure. Activities of daily living, such as dressing, eating, toilet and leisure time tasks provide numerous opportunities to gently challenge a patient to move toward purposeful and appropriate responses. For example, putting a pant leg or shirt sleeve partially over one extremity, but not over the other, encourages the patient to complete the task. Rather than allowing the patient to randomly attempt to organize the act of tooth brushing, someone should stay with him or her, lay out the various components of the task in the appropriate order, and help the patient to move stepwise through each component of the task sequence. Eating meals can be structured in the same way. In essence, any and all routine tasks that a patient carries out can be turned into cognitive reorganization tasks. All that is needed is to see the tasks as such, then assist the patient by breaking the tasks into subcomponents, initiate the first step or two, and maintain the patient's structure as he or she proceeds through the task. If the patient begins to become confused, the staff can intervene and assist in initiating the next appropriate behavioral response in the sequence, then withdraw, and allow the patient to continue.

The following are suggestions that will assist in turning routine unit tasks into a medium to help patients at this level of functioning to become cognitively organized:

1. Be calm and soothing in manner; move slowly, talk slowly and softly;

2. Present patients with only one task at a time, and allow them to complete the entire task or a subpart of it before presenting the next task. Multiple tasks and instructions will only confuse patients further;

3. Tell the patient what you want done several minutes before you actually start the task. Then tell the patient again just before you ask him or her to attempt it. This gives the patient time to become aware of you and the task and to begin to think about how to complete it. Having sufficient time to process and organize the request and response is essential to helping the patient remain cognitively organized;

4. If the patient becomes confused and resists you and your request, do not continue the activity or begin talking. Wait until the patient appears relaxed and is attending to you and then explain the activity again and continue with it;

5. Give instructions at a time or in a place that is the most quiet and least distracting;

6. Before giving an instruction, place yourself in a postion where you can be seen. Be sure the patient is paying attention to you and then touch the patient before you begin talking;

7. First, tell the patient what you want done and why it should be done, then demonstrate what you want done, and give the instruction;

8. When giving instructions, use gestures, demonstrations, and only a few of the most necessary and important words;

9. Once the sequence of routine unit activities has been established, do not change it, and, whenever possible, do not change the staff person who carries it out. Any such changes produce a completely new task. Enhancing the predictability of a routine is a major means of assisting the patient to remain cognitively organized.

Maintaining a structured environment is critical to patients at Levels V and VI. The environment includes the physical setting, the particular activity at hand, and the verbal and nonverbal interactions between the patient and others. The purpose of providing environmental structure is to keep the patient's environment as unconfusing as possible. If the activities are random, chaotic, and confusing, they will match—thereby indirectly reinforce—the patient's own inner confusion.

Because patients at Levels V and VI are experiencing internal confusion, one of the best ways to treat the confusion is to make the environment less confusing. It is easier to modify the external confusion than to request patients to modify their internal confusion. An orderly, predictable, and structured environment will help patients remain at their highest level of functioning. The following are ways in which the environment can be modified so as to engender congitive organization rather than to precipitate disorganization:

1. Continue to employ suggestions 1 through 9 from the approaches to the previous level.

2. Describe the unit routine on a daily basis. This will help patients to understand why certain things are being done to, and around, them. Relate the description of the various unit routines to the different points in time in which they occur. In this way patients can gradually be helped to predict what is most likely to occur next in their environment. The nurse can describe schedules for meals, medication, OT and PT, time to get up, time to go to bed, bathroom activities, visiting hours, etc., in relation to past and future events. For example: "It is 12:00, and you have finished lunch, next you will go to O.T." Activities which do not occur on a predictable basis should be described to the patient several times before the patient engages in them. These might be such things as special appointments, rounds and conferences, special tests, any changes in schedule, etc.;

3. Provide a constant verbal description of what the patient was doing, is now doing, and will be doing. While it might be somewhat boring to the staff, verbal description of what has occurred, is occurring, and will occur will help the patient to structure his or her behavior and relate the activity to things occuring in the environment;

4. Present all requests or instructions slowly and concisely. The patient should be given a few moments to think about what has been said before responding. Do not talk during these few moments because the added speech will be confusing. If the patient does not respond appropriately, the request should be repeated. When it is repeated, attempt to use the same vocabulary and word order you originally used. Any slight change in either of these often causes the patient to think that you are asking something entirely different;

5. Keep the patient mentally challenged. Since CHI patients have difficulty structuring their environment, it will help if they are purposefully

presented with structured tasks. Often, if patients are allowed to remain alone, they attend only to their fleeting and disjointed perceptions and thoughts. It is quite possible that this is one of the factors that eventually causes a patient to become agitated, combative, and even further confused.

Some of the following things might be done to challenge patients mentally during their free time:

1. Encourage them to watch television;

2. Ask another patient to either talk with them or go with them around the unit area and talk with people they meet;

3. Ask another patient or volunteer to read to the CHI patient, or play checkers, or some similar game, that will focus his thoughts on a task.

LEVELS VII AND VIII: AUTOMATIC-APPROPRIATE, AND PURPOSEFUL APPROPRIATE

The goal for this level is to assist patients to carry out daily unit routines with minimal-to-no supervision. One must be careful not to withdraw structured assistance too early from Level VII patients. A this point, they seem to look and act "normal," and, as a result, one may assume they can carry out their daily tasks in an appropriate manner. However, the appearance of normal functioning is only superficial. Underneath, the patient is still somewhat disorganized cognitively, and retention span and short memory impairments are beginning to surface as significant problems. While it may not be apparent, the major reason a patient is able to function with the appearance of normalcy is because of the structure provided by the environment. If the structure is removed prematurely, the patient will begin to fluctuate between Levels VI and VII. Consequently, the approach should be to continue with the suggestions for Level VI but to alternate the way in which they are used. Specifically, one should continue to supply the type of structure implicit in all of the suggestions given for Levels V and VI, but now only assist the patient to initiate the activity and help the patient with each task component. Now, verbal instructions need not be given several moments before a task, nor must they be repeated when it is initiated. However, it will still be important to present only one task and one instruction at a time. Providing structure and predictability of behavior through verbal descriptions can be substantially decreased at this point, but not eliminated. Verbal structure should be used only for those activities or times when the patient is becoming confused.

At this time, reduced retention span and short-term memory are beginning to emerge as the patient's more significant cognitive/communicative impairments. The staff should find the following suggestions helpful in assisting the patient:

1. Have the patient's schedule located where he or she can easily read it. Be sure it is clearly marked with respect to morning and afternoon, as well as the individual hours of the day. Be sure that it is up to date. The patient should be requested to refer to the schedule before and after each activity. If a staff member is with the patient, the patient should be encouraged to discuss the activity just completed and the one that is to be done next;

2. Have a clock and large calendar located in a place to which the patient has easy visual access. Have the date of the given day indicated on the calendar. When a patient is away from the schedule, he or she should be asked to use the calendar and clock to determine what is next in the routine. If difficulty occurs he should be asked to review the schedule. You should not give the information. However, if the patient becomes confused, then go together to the schedule board and review it until the patient is reoriented to what is to be done next;

3. Patients in this phase of recovery are prone to becoming lost. This is a manifestation of the short-term memory problem. Because of this, it can be helpful to review with the patient how to go to and return from activities. The patient should be the one to supply most of the information, with the staff intervening only to supply correct information. It will be helpful to have a floor-plan drawing available with key areas, such as the patient's room, the nursing station and other treatment areas clearly marked, for use if there is difficulty with verbally describing the route. The patient should trace and simultaneously describe where he or she is expected to go;

4. Have the patient keep a written daily log of activities. Depending on length of the patient's short-term memory, he or she may need to fill out the log after each activity, at the end of a small block of time, or at the end of the day.

Direct Treatment of Cognitive-Linguistic Disorganization

Treatment is the process of causing the patient to re-establish an equilibrium between the linguistic, cognitive, and psychosocial spheres of communicative behavior. Typically, the patients's nonlinguistic cognitive abilities provide the greatest residuals for achieving this balance. Maximizing cognitive abilities increases the patient's conscious ability to:

1. Deal differentially with impinging internal and external stimuli;
2. Structure inner mental processes;
3. Mentally structure ongoing environmental events;
4. Predict most probable and appropriate responses on the basis of previous information; and
5. Shift cognitive sets fluidly and appropriately in relation to an ever fluctuating and random environment.

Regardless of the level of dysfunction, these five cognitive abilities are central to a patient's ability to deal with and benefit from treatment. In addition they form the basic structure within which the patient can continue to maintain the necessary equilibrium independent of the structured treatment setting.

Treatment serves to challenge and channel spontaneous recovery, maximize residual function, and compensate for lost abilities. The critical therapeutic factor in all three of these phases of language rehabilitation is the creation of the critical balance between the patient's most appropriate level of cognitive functioning and type and manner of stimulus input. When the balance is maintained, the patient is able to process internal and/or external stimuli in the most organized manner and, consequently, utilize language processes at a more organized level. To this end the speech-language pathologist uses treatment tasks specifically designed to cause the patient to (1) attend to the stimulus (attention); (2) attend for a sufficient length of time to grasp its form and quality (attention span); (3) suppress irrelevant stimuli (selective attention); (4) recognize the differences between stimuli (discrimination); (5) analyze groups of stimuli and determine the whole on the basis of the parts (temporal ordering, retention span, categorization); (6) relate this information to similar past learned information (association/memory); (7) associate and integrate this information with information from other areas of stimulus analysis (association/integration/memory); (8) determine the most appropriate sequence of behavioral events by analyzing and synthesizing information derived from steps (6) and (7) (analysis/synthesis/memory); (9) transmit the sequence; (10) attend to the output; (11) compare the actual with the intended output; (12) determine whether change is necessary; and (13), if necessary, produce a modified response.

Depending upon level of severity, some patients must begin at the level of first stabilizing attending abilities, and sequentially work their way through each subsequent cognitive skill. Others may already possess a number of the lower level abilities. Consequently, their treatment begins at a higher level and progresses sequentially from that point. Still others may exhibit marginally functional abilities at all of these levels, but the abilities rapidly disintegrate under stress. Thus, for some, this treatment process is carried out as a series of separate goals over a period of months. For others, the progression through these thirteen steps occurs within a given treatment session, while, for others, the goal may be to cause the patient to apply the steps consciously as a strategy for dealing with and solving a treatment task, or, possibly, identifying a discrete stimulus with a task. However, we have found that for patients whose lower level cognitive skills (e.g., attention, discrimination, temporal ordering, categorization) are functional, we must still use treatment tasks that cause them to consciously begin with attending abilities and progress to the level that is the focus of treatment. If treatment commences only at the level of deficit, the patient often experiences a weakening of the lower level skills because of the increased cognitive demands. Under such conditions, the patient then must rapidly solve two cognitive tasks. Simultaneously, he or she must try to deal with the original stimulus and attempt to maintain the weakening subskills. By beginning with the lower level skills, the patient is provided with the external structure that will be necessary to deal with the tasks that are at the level of dysfunction.

The therapeutic value of this approach does not lie in proceeding repetitively through these steps (though mass practice is extremely necessary) or in the stimuli that are used to elicit a response, or in the response itself. These three factors are simply the media through which the patient is taught cognitive strategies for processing language information. The general strategy is that he or she now must do something consciously that the brain previously did automatically. The secondary strategies arise because the patient must learn to evaluate his or her cognitive/language behavior in any given situation, consciously to determine at what point in this hierarchy of thirteen steps the breakdown is experienced and then to focus attention on consciously manipulating the information through that particular stage. Within this context, treatment tasks are oriented towards both strengthening weakened abilities and learning compensatory mechanisms. Treatment for any of these cognitive abilities must first be directed toward increasing the power of the ability, and, then, once power is established, moved toward increasing the quality of the skill. Power is improved by increasing the rate, amount, and duration of stimulus input that a patient can handle while holding complexity constant. Quality of ability is enhanced by increasing complexity while holding rate, amount, and duration constant.

Manipulation of
Treatment Stimuli

Several parameters are critical to the success of treatment, regardless of cognitive/linguistic level. One should present stimuli at the rate, amount, duration, and complexity that is optimal for the patient. The task solutions should not require a level of problem solving above the patient's ability. Treatment tasks should initially require nonverbal congitive skills, and move toward their linguistic counterparts when proficiency at the nonverbal level is demonstrated. For example, the ability to selectively attend to nonlinguistic stimuli should be fairly stable prior to presenting tasks such as identifying embedded target words. Tasks that require nonlinguistic analysis and synthesis, such as block designs, should be presented prior to tasks that require the patient to synthesize part-whole language concepts, such as those that occur in story-telling.

I have found the following sequence of tasks to be quite helpful: visual-visual (e.g., pointing to pictures that are similar to stimulus pictures), visual-motor (e.g., tracing, copying, or supplying the missing parts of a visual stimulus), visual-auditory (e.g., identifying the visual response to an auditory stimulus), auditory motor (e.g., producing a motor response to an auditory stimulus); and auditory-verbal (e.g., producing a verbal response to an auditory stimulus).

A given patient's movement from nonlinguistic to linguistic tasks and visual-visual to auditory-verbal analysis and response modalities will be dependent on the severity of the dysfunction. For some, these treatment parameters will represent the various sequential steps they will take over a period of months, whereas others will progress through them within a given treatment session or treatment task. The treatment value does not exist in the stimulus per se but rather in the increase in the patient's ability to handle higher and higher levels of rate, amount, duration, and complexity of stimulus processing. A treatment program that requires a higher level of cognitive functioning than the patient is capable of producing, that appeals to all sense modalities simultaneously, and that attempts to elicit and modify language before the lower level cognitive abilities necessary to support it have been stabilized will impede progress. Initially, the speech-language pathologist creates the balance between the patient's most functional level of cognitive functioning and the type and manner of presenting stimuli. The goal of treatment should be to transfer the responsibility for maintaining this critical balance to the patient.

References

Adamovich, B. B. Language vs. cognition: The speech-language pathologist's role. *Clinical Aphasiology Conference Proceedings, 1981*. Minneapolis: BRK Publishers, 1981.

Adamovich, B. B., & Brooks, R. A diagnostic protocol to assess the communication deficit of patients with hemispheric damage. *Clinical Aphasiology Conference Proceedings, 1981*. Minneapolis: BRK Publishers, 1981.

Adamovich, B. B., & Henderson, J. Cognitive changes in head trauma patients following a treatment period. Presented at the American Speech-Language-Hearing Association convention, Toronto, 1982.

Adamovich, B. B., & Henderson, J. Treatment of communication deficits resulting from traumatic head injury. In W. H. Perkins (Ed.), *Current therapy of communication disorders*. New York: Thieme-Stratton, 1983.

Adams, R., & Sidman, R. L. *Introduction to neuropathology*. New York: McGraw-Hill, 1968.

Arseni, C., Constantinovici, A., & Iliesca, D. Considerations of post traumatic aphasia in peacetime. *Psychiatrica, Neurologica, Neurochirurgica*, 1970, *73*, 105–112.

Ayres, A. J. *Southern California Figure-Ground Visual Perception Test*. Los Angeles: Western Psychological Services, 1966.

Baker, H. J., & Leland, B. *Detroit Test of Learning Aptitude*. Indianapolis: Bobbs-Merrill, 1959.

Benton, A. L. *The Revised Visual Retention Test*. New York: Psychological Corp., 1963.

Ben-Yishay Working approaches to remediation of cognitive deficits in brain damaged patients. Institute of Rehabilitation Medicine, New York University Medical Center, Department of Behavioral Sciences. Supplements for June 1978, May 1979, May 1980. (Studies for grant 13-P-556 23 and RT-93.)

Brain, L., & Walton, J. N. *Brain's diseases of the nervous system* (7th ed.). New York: Oxford University Press, 1969.

Brock, S. *Injuries of the brain and spinal cord* (4th ed.). New York: Springer, 1960.

Brooks, D. N. Memory and head injury. *Journal of Nervous and Mental Disease*, 1972, *155*, 350–355.

Brooks, D. N. Wechsler memory scale performance and its relationship to brain damage after severe closed head injury. *Journal of Neurology, Neurosurgery and Psychiatry*, 1976, *39*, 593–601.

Brooks, D. D., Aughton, M. E., Bond, M. R., Jones, P., & Rizvi, S. Cognitive sequelae in relationship to early indicies of severity of brain damage after severe blunt head injury. *Journal of Neurology, Neurosurgery and Psychiatry*, 1980, *43*, 529–534.

Buscke, H., & Fuld, P. Evaluation, storage, retention and retrieval in disordered memory and learning. *Neurology*, 1974, *24*, 1019–1025.

Butler, K.G. Mnemonic and retrieval strategies for language disordered adolescents. Paper presented at American Speech-Language-Hearing Association convention, Los Angeles, 1981.

Caveness, W. F. Introduction to head injuries. In E. Walker, W. Caveness, & M. Cutchley (Eds.), *The late effects of head injury*. Springfield, IL: Charles C. Thomas, 1969.

Christensen, A. L. *Luria's neuropsychological investigation*. New York: Spectrum, 1975.

Courville, C. B. Coup, contre-coup mechanisms of craniocerebral injuries: some observations. *Archives of Surgery*, 1942, *45*, 19–43.

Courville, C. B., & Amyes, E. W. Late residual lesions of the brain consequent to dural hemorrhage. *Bulletin of the Los Angeles Neurology Society*, 1952, *17*, 163.

Cronholm, B. Evaluation of mental disturbances after acute head injury. *Scandinavian Journal of Rehabilitation Medicine*, 1972, *4*, 35–38.

Dye, O. A., Milby, J. B., & Saxon, S. A. Effects of early neurological problems following head trauma on subsequent neuropsychological performance. *Acta Neurologica Scandinavia*, 1979, *59*, 10–14.

Fahy, T. J., Irving, M. H., & Millac, P. Severe head injuries. *Lancet*, 1967, 7514.

Field, J. R. Head injuries pathophysiology. *Journal of the Arkansas Medical Association*, 1970, *66*, 340–347.

Frostig, M. *Developmental Test of Visual Perception*. Chicago: Follett, 1963.

Glick, M. L., & Holyoak, K. J. Analogical problem solving. *Cognitive Psychology*, 1980, *12*, 306–355.

Goldman, R., Fristoe, M., & Woodcock, R. W. *G-F-W Test of Auditory Discrimination*. Circle Pines, MN: American Guidance Service, 1970.

Goldman, R., Fristoe, M., & Woodcock, R. W. *G-F-W Auditory Memory Tests*. Circle Pines, MN: American Guidance Service, 1974. (a)

Goldman, R., Fristoe, M., & Woodcock, R. W. *G-F-W Sound-Symbol Tests*. Circle Pines, MN: American Guidance Service, 1974. (b)

Goldstein, K., & Scheerer, M. *Goldstein-Scheerer Stick Test*. New York: Psychological Corp., 1945.

Greenfield, J. G. Some observations on cerebral injuries. *Proceedings of the Royal Society of Medicine*, 1938 1939, *32*, 15.

Greenfield, J. G., & Russell, D. S. Traumatic lesions of the central and peripheral nervous systems. In W. Blackwood (Ed.), *Greenfield's neuropathology*. Chicago: Year Book Medical Publishers, 1963.

Groher, M. Language and memory disorders following closed head trauma. *Journal of Speech and Hearing Research*, 1977, *20*, 212–223.

Hagen, C., & Malkmus, D. Intervention strategies for language disorders secondary to head trauma. American Speech-Language-Hearing Association Convention Short Course, Atlanta, 1979.

Hallgrim, K. & Cleeland, C. S. The relationship of neuropsychological impairment to other indicies of severity of head injury. *Scandinavian Journal of Rehabilitation Medicine*, 1972, *4*, 55–60.

Halpern, H., Darley, F. L., & Brown, J. R. Differential language and neurologic characteristics in cerebral involvement. *Journal of Speech and Hearing Disorders*, 1973, *38*, 162–173.

Hedberg-Davis, N., & Bookman, M. An information processing approach to language and learning disabilities appraisal. Presented at the American Speech-Language-Hearing Association convention, Atlanta, 1979.

Heilman, K. M., Safron, A., & Geschwind, N. Closed head trauma and aphasia. *Journal of Neurology, Neurosurgery, and Psychiatry*, 1971, *34*, 265–269.

Hooper, R. *Patterns of acute head injury*. Baltimore: Williams & Wilkins, 1969.

Horowitz, N., & Rizzoli, H. V. Complications following the surgical treatment of head injuries: Clinical neurosurgery. *Proceedings of the Congress of Neurological Surgeons*, 1966, 277–287.

Jacobsen, S. A. Disturbances of mental function: Effects of head trauma on mental function. In S. A. Jacobsen (Ed.), *The post-traumatic syndrome following head injuries: Mechanisms and techniques*. Springfield, IL: Charles C. Thomas, 1963.

Jennett, B., & Teasdale, G. Management of head injuries. Philadelphia: F. A. Davis, 1981.

Johnson, G. O., & Boyd, H. F. *Nonverbal Test of Cognitive Skills*. Columbus: Charles E. Merrill, 1981.

Kirk, S. A., McCarthy, J., & Kirk, W. D. *Illinois Test of Psycholinguistic Abilities*. Champaign: University of Illinois, 1968.

Ledwon-Robinson, E., & Beh-Arendshorst, M. University of Michigan Cognitive protocol: Pragmatically assessing verbal-nonverbal communication. Presented at the American Speech-Language-Hearing Association Convention, Houston, 1980.

Levin, H. S., Grossman, R. G., & Kelly, P. J. Aphasic disorder in patients with closed head injury. *Journal of Neurology, Neurosurgery, and Psychiatry*, 1976, *39*, 1062–1070.

Levin, H. S., Grossman, R. G., Rose, J. E., & Teasdale, J. Long term neuropsychological outcome of closed head injury. *Journal of Neurosurgery*, 1979, *50*, 412–422.

Levin, H. S., Grossman, R. G., Sarwar, M., & Meyers, C. A. Linguistic recovery after closed head injury. *Brain and Language*, 1981, *12*, 360–374.

Lewin, W. *The management of head injuries*. Baltimore: Williams & Wilkins, 1966.

Lezak, M. D. Recovery of memory and learning functions following traumatic brain injury, *Cortex*, 1979, *15*, (1), 63–72.

Ligne, M. E., Sinatra, K. S., & Kimbarow, M. L. Language assessment battery for evaluation of closed head trauma patients. Paper presented at the American Speech-Language-Hearing Association convention, Atlanta, 1979.

Lindberg, R., Fisher, R. S., & Durlacher, S. H. Lesions of the corpus callosum following blunt mechanical trauma to the head. *American Journal of Pathology*, 1955, *31*, 297–317.

Mandleberg, I. A. Cognitive recovery after severe head injury. *Journal of Neurology, Neurosurgery and Psychiatry*, 1976, *39*, 1001–1007.

Mandleberg, I. A., & Brooks, D. N. Cognitive recovery after severe head injury. *Journal of Neurology, Neurosurgery, and Psychiatry*, 1975, *38*, 1121–1126.

Meyer, J. S., & Denny-Brown, D. Studies of cerebral circulation in brain injury: II. Cerebral concussion. *Neurophysiology*, 1955, *7*, 529–544.

Miller, E. Simple and choice reaction time following severe head injury. *Cortex*, 1970, *6*, 121–127.

Miller, H., & Stern, G. The long term prognosis of severe head injury. *Lancet*, 1965, 225–229.

Ross, J. D., & Ross, C. M. *Ross Test of Higher Cognitive Processes*. Novato, CA: Academic Therapy Publications, 1976.

Rowbotham, G. F. *Acute injuries of the head*. Baltimore: Williams & Wilkins, 1949.

Rubens, A. B., Geschwind, N., Mahowald, M. W., & Mastri, A. Post traumatic cerebral hemispheric disconnection syndrome. *Archives of Neurology*, 1977, *34*, 750–755.

Russell, R. W. Cerebral involvement in head injury. *Brain*, 1932, *55*, 549–603.

Russell, W. R., & Smith, A. Post-traumatic amnesia in closed head injury. *Archives of Neurology*, 1961, *5*, 4–17.

Sarno, M. T. The nature of verbal impairment after closed head injury. *The Journal of Nervous and Mental Disease*, 1980, *168* 11, 685–692.

Schilder, P. Psychic disturbance after head injuries. *American Journal of Psychiatry*, 1934, *91*, 155–188.

Smith, E. Influence of site of impact on cognitive impairment persisting long after severe closed head injury. *Journal of Neurology, Neurosurgery, and Psychiatry*, 1974, *37*, 719–726.

Stritch, S. J. Diffuse degeneration of the cerebral white matter in severe dementia following head injury. *Journal of Neurology and Psychiatry*, 1956, *19*, 163.

Stritch, S. J. The pathology of brain damage due to blunt head injuries. In A. E. Walker, W. F. Caveness, & M. Critchley (Eds.), *The late effects of head injury*. Springfield, IL: Charles C. Thomas, 1969.

Teasdale, G., & Jennett, B. Assessment of coma and impaired consciousness. *Lancet*, 1974, *2*.

Thomsen, I. V. Evaluation and outcome of aphasia in patients with severe closed head trauma. *Journal of Neurology, Neurosurgery, and Psychiatry*, 1975, *38*, 713–718.

Thomsen, I. V. Evaluation and outcome of traumatic aphasia in patients with severe verified focal lesions. *Folia Phoniatrica*, 1976, *28*, 362–377.

Tomlinson, B. E. Pathology. In G. F. Rowbotham (Ed.), *Acute injuries of the head* (4th ed.). Edinburgh: Livingstone, 1964.

Walker, E., Caveness, W., & Critchley, M. (Eds.). *The late effects of head injury*. Springfield, IL: Charles C. Thomas, 1969.

Wechsler, D. *Wechsler Adult Intelligence Scale*. New York: Psychological Corp., 1955.

Wechsler, D., & Stone, C. P. *Wechsler Memory Scale*. New York: Psychological Corp., 1945.

Weigle, E., Goldstein, K., & Scheerer, M. *Color Form Sorting Test*. New York: Psychological Corp., 1945.

Yorkston, K. M., Stanton, K. M., & Beukelman, D. R. Language-based compensatory for closed head injured patients. *Clinical Aphasiology Conference Proceedings, 1981*. Minneapolis: BRK Publishers, 1981.

Kathryn M. Yorkston
Patricia A. Dowden

Nonspeech Language and Communication Systems

Normal speech is an extremely rapid, efficient and concise means of communication. It requires so little physical effort and preplanning that it comes almost automatically for the normal speaker. Often the complexity of speech is not fully appreciated until one is confronted with the task of developing a functional alternative communication system for an adult who has lost the ability to communicate verbally, as a result of a brain injury or a degenerative neurological disorder. Watching these individuals interact in natural communicative situations confirms an observation made by Holland (1977) that severely speech-impaired adults "communicate better than they talk." (p. 173) Wertz (1978) states the same idea in an eloquent way when he writes:

> Somewhere behind the insolvable ejaculations of neurologically impaired patients is a music awaiting lyrics. Putting words to the music is the primary task in patient management, and the variety of songs eventually sung is the primary test of its effectiveness. (p. 17)

The "words" which we are able to provide adults who are not independent verbal communicators may take a number of forms. The systems may be divided into two broad categories (ASHA Ad Hoc Committee on Communication Processes and Nonspeaking Persons, 1980). "Unaided" communication augmentation systems are those that do not require physical aids, for example, gestural techniques. "Aided" communication systems are those that require a physical board or chart, or a mechanical or electronic device. These systems may serve three functions: (1) as a replacement when no verbal communication is possible, (2) as a supplement when verbal communication is not sufficiently understandable, or inefficient in certain situations, or (3) as a facilitator when speech flows more easily when accompanied by gestures. In some cases, the nonspeech communication systems described here are permanent in that they provide a long-term alternative to verbal communication. With progressive neurological deterioration, however, the communication systems change in order to meet the increasing demands of the nonspeaking individual. In other cases, the systems are used temporarily to provide a means of communication during the early stages of recovery and are eliminated when speech becomes functional once again.

The task of selecting and training an individual to use an appropriate nonspeech communication system, whether aided or unaided, is a challenging one. It requires the clinician's thorough familiarity with systems available and the demands each system would place on a user. It also requires that, in serving a nonspeaking individual, a clinician make at least three decisions in parallel. One, the clinician must decide if an individual is a candidate for a communication augmentation system. This requires a thorough knowledge of the nonspeaking individual's capabilities in such diverse areas as speech, language, cognition, and motor control. Two, the clinician must identify the communication needs of the individual so that an appropriate match can be made between the abilities and needs of the patient, and the communication system. Three, the clinician must decide which of the many alternative communication systems are appropriate for the individual, and consider making modifications based on performance trial results.

The nonvocal adults described in this chapter are individuals who are not independent verbal communicators, and may be labelled as nonvocal, nonoral, nonspeaking, or anathric (Harris & Vanderheiden, 1980). This population is diverse in the etiology and the nature of their communication disorders, as well as in their needs as communicators. The course of the disorder may vary depending on the etiology. Some disorders, such as amyotrophic lateral sclerosis, are degenerative. Others, such as brain stem stroke or traumatic head injury, are characterized by sudden onset followed by a period of recovery and later stabilization. Nonspeaking adults may be diagnosed as having aphasia, apraxia of speech, and dysarthria, or a combination of these disorders. For our purposes, *aphasia* is defined as a disorder of the central language process which underlies the various language modalities, including listening, speaking, reading, and writing (Darley, 1964). It is an impairment in the ability to interpret and formulate language symbols as a result of brain damage. Most typically, the etiology of aphasia is left-cerebral vascular accident, but other common etiologies include arteriovenous malformations, tumor, and focal head injury. *Apraxia of speech* is a sensory motor disorder of articulation and prosody. Although apraxia may exist as an entity, it frequently accompanies aphasia, and may also coexist with dysarthria (Rosenbek, 1978). The apraxic individual does not exhibit significant weakness or incoordination when performing reflexive or automatic movements. There is, instead, an impaired ability to program the positioning of the speech mechanism and to sequence the movements for volitional speech. In its most severe form, apraxia can render expressive verbal communication impossible, while leaving the patient's auditory comprehension relatively intact. *Dysarthria* refers to a disorder of motor control of the speech mechanism resulting from damage to the central or peripheral nervous system, and is characterized by weakness, slowness, and incoordination of the speech mechanism musculature (Darley, Aronson, & Brown, 1975). Dysarthric speakers usually have normal auditory comprehension, can select words correctly, and order them into grammatical strings without difficulty. They usually possess intact reading and spelling skills. The damage to the nervous system may be a consequence of a number of adult onset disorders, including closed head injury, anoxia, brain stem stroke, amyotrophic lateral sclerosis, multiple sclerosis, or Parkinson's disease. The speech disorder may or may not be part of more general motor control disorder, which may limit ambulation and restrict use of the extremities.

Although initially a group consisting of aphasic, apraxic, and dysarthric speaker may seem quite diverse, there are a number of reason for considering the group as a whole. First, a clinical case load in an adult rehabilitation center typically includes patients from each of these diagnostic categories. Second, these disorders often coexist in a single patient. The overlap in communication diagnosis is especially characteristic of the closed head-injured population, where the cerebral damage is diffuse rather than focal. Third, these individuals share one overriding characteristic—the severity of their impairment. Nonspeech systems, whether aided or unaided, should be considered only when an individual cannot communicate independently via speech. Even marginally functional speakers with poor speech intelligibility and speaking rates of 15 to 20 words per minute often find it quicker to communicate verbally with those who are familiar with them than to use a communication augmentation system. However, when interacting with unfamiliar partners, communication may break down more often and a communication augmentation system may be more effective and less frustrating than verbal communication. Fourth, this population is similar in that their language skills developed in a normal manner prior to the onset of the communication disorder. This implies that they have int_rnalized many "rules" of normal communicative interaction such as turn taking, attention getting, or leave taking.

The focus of this chapter will be a clinical one. The authors hope to provide the readers with information that will help them make certain clinical management decisions. First, we will focus on the aided and unaided systems available, analyzing each system in terms of its components and the demands placed on the user. We will also discuss the implications of research and case study literature regarding these systems. For the aided systems, we will touch on the structure of service delivery and future trends. The end of the chapter will be devoted to the needs assessment, which must be completed prior to any system selection, whether aided or unaided systems are under consideration.

Gestural Systems

Gestural communication systems have long been appealing to clinicians working with nonspeaking adults. Indeed, there are a number of clinical case reports which suggest that gestural communication can serve as an acceptable alternative to speech for some individuals. However, there is a growing body of research literature which indicates that gestures should not be considered a panacea for the nonspeaking individual. This literature documents the nearly universal presence of gestural deficits in nonspeaking adults with language-based or motor speech impairments. This discussion will focus on the clinical implications of the theoretical studies and the clinical case reports. First, however, it is necessary to analyze the demands that the different gestural systems place on the user.

Components of Gestural Systems

A number of gestural systems are available and are reviewed in detail by Silverman (1980). Appropriate selection of these systems is dependent upon the clinician's understanding of the characteristics of each system, specifically the symbolic load, motoric complexity, and communicative function of the system. Before electing to teach any gestural system, the clinician must decide if the patient's skills are commensurate with the requirements of that system, and if the system has the potential for meeting the patient's communication needs.

Symbolic Load

Each system of gestural communication carries a different symbolic load, that is, the systems vary in the extent to which a gesture is an arbitrary symbol for the concept it conveys. According to Peterson and Kirshner (1981), the most symbolic gestures "bear a codified or arbitrary relationship to their referent" (p. 335). Listeners must be familiar with the particular code, as in American Sign Language, in order to understand the letter, word, morpheme, or phoneme intended.

Gestures that do not have an arbitrary or symbolic relationship with a referent are typically placed in three other categories: iconic, referential, or coverbal. Iconic gestures are those in which the meaning is expressed in the form of the movement, or where there is a widely accepted interpretation. American Indian Sign Language (Amerind) comprises both types of iconic gestures. For example, "baby" is conveyed by crossed arms swaying cradle-style, and "bad" is conveyed by the widely understood movement, "thumbs down." Amerind is not a language, but a signal system with simple, but vivid concrete representation of the dominant characteristics of objects, actions, or persons. (Skelly, 1979) There is theoretically nothing arbitrary in the gesture-referent relationship and there is no true syntactic structure. Amerind is considered by Skelly to be highly intelligible to the untrained viewer.

Referential, or indicative, gestures are less symbolic than iconic gestures in that meaning is conveyed in the presence of the object itself, for example, pointing to or showing the function of an object in its presence. Perhaps the least symbolic types of gestures are the paraverbal or coverbal movement. According to Katz, LaPointe, and Markel (1978), these nonverbal behaviors "communicate information such as emotional states, attitudes, relative status, turn taking during conversations and other affective and regulatory information fundamental to dyadic interaction" (p. 164-165). These more or less universal gestures, including eye contact, eyebrow raising, smiles, and head movements carry no specific proportional content, but play a significant role in conversational interactions.

It is important to assess the symbolic load of a gestural system for a number of reasons. First, the symbolic load has an impact on the language-impaired patient's ability to learn the gestural system (Griffith, Robinson, & Panagos, 1981). One could predict that a severely language-impaired individual is not likely to learn the large number of symbolic gestures necessary for functional communication. If, for this reason, a less symbolic system is selected for a patient, the potential messages that can be conveyed are limited. For example, referential gestures can only be used in relationship to an object, and coverbal gestures are only meaningful when accompanied by speech. Second, highly symbolic gestural systems are limited in their usefulness for individuals who need to communicate with listeners unfamiliar with the system. The less symbolic systems may be understood without training, as in the case of iconic gestures, or do not need to be understood by the communication partner, as in the case of the gestures used for facilitation of speech.

Motoric Complexity

The second dimension along which gestures vary is motoric complexity. A single gesture may involve only a fairly simple movement, or entail a highly complex sequence of movements. Similarly, some gestural systems consist of simple repetitive movements, such as the "finger tapping" suggested by Simmons (1978). Other systems comprise a large number of unique gestures, such as the 250 concept labels included in Amerind (Skelly, 1979). Furthermore, some gestures are more or less automatic and are paired with other activities, for example, coverbal behaviors associated with speech. Other gestures are clearly volitional movements requiring complex planning and execution of sequential movements.

Motoric complexity is an important consideration in system selection because successful use of some gestural systems may be precluded by problems in motor learning or motor control. Individuals with apraxia of speech often have motor sequencing problems, with movements of their hands similar to the motor-planning problems seen in the speech mechanism. Individuals with severe dysarthria are often unable to make rapid or precise movements with their hands. Several authors are systematically assessing the motor control requirements of signing and its impact in learning (Kohl, 1981; Shane & Wilbur, 1980).

Communicative Function

Gestures may serve a number of communicative functions. At times, they are a replacement for speech when verbal expression is not functional. A number of authors (Eagleson, Vaughn, & Knudson, 1970; Simmons & Zorthian, 1979; Skelly, Schinsky, Smith, Donaldson, & Griffin, 1975) reported favorable results in training adults with aphasia and/or apraxia to use gestures to express basic self-care needs. Others use gestures to facilitate or "deblock" verbal expression. Rosenbek, Collins, and Wertz (1976), for example, suggested that gestures can be used as a form of "intersystemic organization," in which gestures accompany the speech act in a unique form with unique regularity. These gestures are then faded as verbal communication improves. Rao and Horner (1978) described the use of gesture to deblock receptive and expressive skills in an adult aphasic. Skelly, Schinsky, Smith, and Fust (1974) reported increased verbal performance for patients trained in Amerind gestural code.

Davis and Wilcox (1981) suggested that gestures can supplement speech as one of the multiple channels of communication. In their treatment approach, Promoting Aphasics Communicative Effectiveness (PACE), they proposed that gestures be used to supplement verbal expression, writing, communication aids, and other possible means of expression. Selection of a communication mode is based on its effectiveness, and the aphasic individual is encouraged to use any modality or combination of modalities, as long as the message is conveyed successfully. Coverbal behaviors can be described as serving a supplementary function, since they convey certain information necessary for conversational interaction, but do not carry the primary content of the communication.

It is obvious that the three components of gestural systems—symbolic load, motoric complexity, and function—are interrelated. Typically, the most symbolic gestures are relatively independent of speech, and are capable of expressing a large repertoire of unique ideas. These symbolic gestures also require complex sequences of movements. On the other hand, the less symbolic gestures, i.e. referential or coverbal behaviors, require less complex movements, but are more limited in terms of the concepts which can be expressed. An understanding of each of these components is critical in making appropriate decisions about the selection of a gestural system. Figure 9-1 is a schematic representation of the components of gestural communication systems and illustrates the characteristics of two gestural systems. A simple deblocking gesture uses nonmeaningful, repetitive movements to facilitate speech, while Amerind uses the moderately symbolic, iconic gestures and simple unilateral movements to replace speech.

Studies in the Nature of Gestural Deficits

The observation that nonspeaking individuals often do not attempt to communicate gesturally has spurred research into the nature of gestural deficits and the consequences of damage to the left hemisphere. Although much of the research addresses theoretical issues, the results have implications for the clinical management of aphasic or apraxic individuals and must be taken into account in attempting to select a gestural communication system for a nonspeaking individual. Peterson and Kirshner (1981), in their review of gestural impairment, suggested that there are two broad schools of thought regarding the basis of gestural deficits. The first holds that the deficits are related to motor apraxic impairments; the second maintains that the deficits are a manifestation of underlying linguistic deficits.

FIGURE 9-1
A Schematic Representation of the Components of a Gestural Communication System. Illustrated are the components of "deblocking" gestural system and Amerind sign.

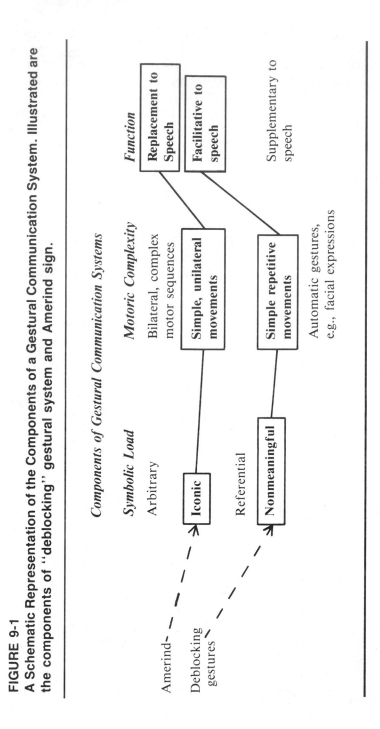

Apraxic Motor Theory

Goodglass and Kaplan, in their 1963 study, proposed that gestural deficits in aphasia are correlated with deficits in motor programming. Their subjects included 20 "mixed, predominantly expressive" aphasic patients ranging from mild to moderately severe, matched for age and "intellectual efficiency" to a group of nonaphasic controls from the neurological ward. The subjects were asked to perform a series of gestural tasks including the following: naturally expressive gestures, conventional gestures, simple pantomime, action with objects, and object description. The results led the authors to conclude that aphasics have a gestural deficiency which is best understood as an apraxic disorder. Goodglass and Kaplan concluded, further, that gestural deficits could not be considered a "central communication disorder" for two primary reasons. First, there was no strong correlation in their study between the severity of the aphasia and gestural deficit. There was, in fact, a "relative independence of severity of aphasia and gestural deficiency" (p. 715), making it difficult to maintain a common underlying cause. Second, their results suggested that the gestural disturbance was related specifically to deficits in the execution of movements, since the aphasic group was disproportionately poor in the ability to imitate gestures.

Kimura and her colleagues (Kimura, 1976; Kimura & Archibald, 1974; Kimura, Battison, & Lubert, 1976) provided additional evidence that the gestural deficits which appear in aphasia may be related to certain motor dysfunctions. In her 1976 review, Kimura stated that the cortical areas important in symbolic language processing may also play an important role in the production of motor sequences. She provided four lines of evidence for this theory:

1. The association between hand preference and speech lateralization;
2. The frequent association of hand movements with speaking in normals, and of vocal utterances with hand signing in the deaf;
3. The frequent association of ideomotor or ideational limb apraxia with aphasia in left hemisphere lesions; and
4. The fact that disorders of manual communication in the deaf occur from left hemisphere lesions, as do disorders of vocal communication. (p. 146)

Kimura suggested an overlap in the neural control of symbolic motor sequences in both the gestural and vocal modalities.

DeRenzi, Motti, and Nichelli (1980) examined gestural imitation ability in an interesting extension of Kimura's theory. Specifically, they studied three dimensions: (1) independent finger movement versus whole hand movement, (2) holding of position versus carrying out motor sequences, and (3) symbolic versus nonsymbolic gestures. Their experimental groups included 80 patients with history of right hemisphere damage, 100 patients with left hemisphere damage, and 100 patients with no evidence of brain damage. Their finding that the left hemisphere-damaged group performed more poorly on nonsymbolic than symbolic gestures led them to conclude that the gestural deficits are not directly related to the "symbolic value" of the gesture. Furthermore, there were no critical differences in whether the movements involved fingers or whole-hand movements, or entailed holding a position or carrying out sequences of movement. Their conclusion was, "what seems to be critical was whether the patient has to organize a sequentially ordered motor program on verbal or visual command, in the absence of contextual or inner motivation, or if the gesture meets a real need" (p. 10). It appears, then, that the motor patterns still exist in these patients, but they are somehow inaccessible without a particularly strong flow of stimulation.

Language-Based Theory

A number of researchers have suggested that gestural deficits are not due to apraxia, but are a consequence of underlying language-based deficits. Several of the authors have come to this conclusion after studying aphasic subjects' productions of propositional and subpropositional gestures. Duffy and Buck (1979) studied both pantomime and facial expression abilities in groups of aphasic, right hemisphere-damaged patients and control subjects. Their results indicated that the aphasic subjects performed poorly, compared to the patients with right hemisphere damage and controls, on tasks including pantomime expression and recognition. However, there were no differences among the groups in the performance of facial expressions, their measure of subpropositional behavior. It was concluded that aphasic patients are impaired in their ability to produce propositional gestures, but not in their ability to make subpropositional, coverbal movements appropriately. Similar results were reported by Katz et al. (1978) who found that coverbal behaviors of a group of 10 mild and moderate aphasic subjects did not differ from normal. No significant differences were found in the mean rate, duration, and average length of these nonpropositional behaviors of the control and aphasic groups. It was concluded that mild and moderate aphasic subjects are not impaired in their use of coverbal behaviors.

Other studies examined the relationship between receptive and expressive language deficits and gestural ability. Gainotti and Lemmo (1976), in their study of 128 patients with unilateral hemisphere damage, found that "within the aphasic group, the inability to understand the meaning of symbolic gestures is highly related to verbal semantic impairment" (p. 457). The authors stressed the link between semantic disintegration in the verbal and nonverbal modalities. Pickett (1978) studied gestural deficits in 28 brain-injured adults and 25 control subjects on eight experimental verbal and gestural tasks, as well as on the *Porch Index of Communicative Ability* (PICA), (Porch, 1967). Of interest in his results is the conclusion that gestural deficits appeared to be "part of the total communicative involvement of the aphasic patient and not a function of apraxia. (p. 102)

Cicone, Wapner, Foldi, Zurif, and Gardner (1979) studied two anterior and two posterior aphasic subjects and their use of gestures in spontaneous speech. Results indicated that gestures closely paralleled speech; that is, the Broca's aphasic subject used simple unelaborated units, whereas the Wernicke's subject produced elaborate and complex gestures which were often vague and unfocused. These findings led the authors to suggest that speech and gestures are either dependent upon language or that there may be a central organizer directing both. Similar results were reported by Duffy, Duffy, and Mercaitis (1979). These investigators studied pantomime performance of two chronic aphasic subjects who showed equivalent overall severity, but distinctive subtypes of aphasia. The subjects' gestures were analyzed in terms of the number of pauses, the numbers of total arm movements and different arm movements, ratings of effort and smoothness, and the average number of seconds per response. All measures were analogous to those used to describe motor speech performance. Results indicated that both subjects exhibited deficits in their ability to convey information through gestures, but their gestural patterns were quite distinctive and paralleled their speech pattern. Specifically, the gestural performance of the Broca's patient was characterized as "constricted," with brief, sparse and unelaborated movements of the hand; the gestures of the Wernicke's patient was termed "excessive," with elaborate arm, head, and torso movements which seemed irrelevant and tangential.

Duffy and Duffy (1981) took a statistical approach in examining the causal relationship between language and gestural deficits. In the first of the three studies cited, these authors examined pantomime recognition in groups of aphasic patients, right hemisphere-damaged patients (N = 27), and a control group. Significant deficits in pantomime recognition were found in the aphasic group. Further, a strong relationship existed between deficits in verbal and nonverbal behavior. In their second study, they examined the relationship among deficits in pantomime expression, pantomime recognition, and three verbal measures. Duffy and Duffy concluded that: (1) there was a strong relationship between pantomime recognition and expression, and (2) expressive and receptive pantomime deficits correlated highly with verbal deficits. In the third study, the causal theories of pantomime deficits were examined. From the results of zero order correlations, partial correlations, and multiple regression analyses, the authors concluded that neither limb apraxia nor intellectual deficits were the cause of pantomimic deficits in the aphasic population. Instead, the results supported two possible theories: (1) that deficits in pantomime are due to central symbolic deficits which are also responsible for the language deficit, or (2) that the pantomime impairments are due to the verbal deficits, because nonverbal behaviors may be dependent on verbal modality. According to Duffy and Duffy, aphasia is not primarily, or solely, a verbal impairment, but a communication deficit in the verbal and nonverbal modalities. They maintain that to understand the nature of aphasia, one must also understand the nature of the nonverbal deficits, which are a fundamental component of the communication deficit.

Clinical Implications

Regardless of the differences among these theoretical studies in terms of the conclusions and the models postulated, all the findings are similar in one respect. All researchers agree that individuals with left hemisphere damage and communication impairment exhibit some deficits in the expression of propositional gestures. This finding is not surprising in light of the fundamental similarities between verbal and gestural communication. Both modes of expression have a symbolic component, relying on some arbitrary relationship between words or gestures and the meaning expressed. Both rely on complex sequences of movement which require a combination of volitional and automatic movements, possibly governed by a single neuromechanism. The existence of gestural deficits in the aphasic population comes as no surprise to the experienced clinician who has seen severely apraxic patients who cannot imitate gestures, or severely aphasic patients who do not use either iconic or referential gestures spontaneously.

This review of theoretical literature has been presented here not as part of a critical review of the related models of aphasia, but in order to draw the clinician's attention to the wide range of possible deficits which may limit a patient's use of gestures. It is clear that there is a need for more precise diagnostic protocols that would assess both motor control/motor learning abilities and symbolic/language ability as they relate to gestures. Research has been based on widely varying sampling techniques (Daniloff, Noll, Fristoe, & Lloyd, 1982; Duffy & Duffy, 1981; Koller & Schlanger, 1975; Pickett, 1974). Some tasks sample understanding of gestural communications; others sample gestural expression. Some of the tasks provide instructions verbally; while others base their instructions solely on gestural input. Some of the tasks use pictorial depictions of gestures; some use examiner-presented gestures; still others use video-taped presentations. Some tasks are based on recall and others are based on recognition. In short, the tasks which sample gestural performance are a mixed bag of instruction modes, task types, and levels of difficulty. With the possible exception of Pickett (1974), none appears to provide the broad representation needed to sample gestural performance in the clinical settings.

The "ideal" diagnostic tool would sample gestural performance along several dimensions, including symbolic load and motoric complexity. This diagnostic protocol would also sample the use of gestures in a variety of functions, including the replacement, supplementation, and facilitation of speech. Further, a complete diagnostic protocol would allow the clinician to compare the relative effectiveness of gestural and verbal communication. Some research has suggested such differential effectiveness. For example, Davis, Artes, and Hoops, (1979) found that some aphasic patients used expressive pantomime more effectively than verbal expression. Beukelman, Yorkston, and Waugh (1980) found that severely involved individuals followed single-stage directions given in a combined verbal and pantomime mode as accurately, or more accurately, than when given in either the verbal or pantomime mode alone. It would seem that whether or not gestures are useful for a given patient needs to be assessed empirically with standard clinical protocols. However, complete understanding of a nonspeaking individual's gestural ability is probably not possible solely from an "in-clinic" stimulus-response task format—no matter how complete the task sampling. Clearly, there is a need to supplement this direct testing with observational data obtained in natural communication settings (Holland, 1982). The observation of spontaneous expression and understanding of gestures is especially important in the assessment of severely impaired individuals who may not accurately demonstrate their potential in direct-testing situations.

Clinical Reports

Despite these words of caution found throughout the literature relating to gestural deficits, it would be misleading to conclude that all tasks and approaches in the nonverbal modality should be abandoned for patients with gestural deficits. It is no more appropriate to abandon the gestural mode on the basis of gestural deficits than it is to abandon the verbal modality because of speech or language deficits. According to Duffy (in press), the presence of a deficit does not mean "the absence of a communication skill" in the area of the deficit. Duffy suggested that the best approach is to determine which communication system, or combination of systems, is most functional for a given patient for short or long term communication needs, and then to direct treatment accordingly. Duffy suggested further that gestures have a place in the clinical setting because they may be more "primitive" than verbal communication and, therefore, may require less of the patients' symbolic abilities than speech. This would apply, of course, to the less symbolic gestures as defined above, such as coverbal, referential, or some iconic gestures. From his point of view, gestures may also circumvent some "non-aphasic" communication problems. There are some apraxic or dysarthric patients for whom gestures may be the most appropriate means of communication.

Successful application of gestural systems for nonspeaking individuals has been reported and reviewed in the clinical literature (Peterson & Kirshner, 1981; Silverman, 1980). This literature has important implications for the clinical management of these patients. The selection of an appropriate communication mode requires that the clinician be familiar with factors that have contributed to a successful match between systems and users for other clinicians.

The clinical and research literature contains reports describing the training of a number of gestural systems which differ in symbolic load. Glass, Gazzaniga, and Premack (1973) used a highly symbolic system to study the ability of global aphasic patients to learn symbols. They trained seven global aphasic patients to use an "artificial language," in which paper symbols of various colors, sizes, and shapes were associated with words. Although learning varied from patient to patient, some learned to express simple action statements using symbols.

A number of authors have described the use of iconic systems, such as Amerind gestural code, for training aphasic and/or apraxic individuals (Dowden, Marshall, & Tompkins, 1981; Rao & Horner, 1978; Skelly, 1979; Skelly, Schinsky, Smith, Donaldson, & Griffin, 1975; Skelly, Schinsky, Smith & Fust, 1974). Amerind signs in combination with signs derived from Ameslan (Kirshner & Webb, 1981) or modified Amerind signs (Simmons & Zorthian, 1979) have also been employed. Schlanger (1976) and her colleagues (Schlanger & Freiman, 1979; Schlanger, Geffner, & DiCarrado, 1974; Schlanger & Schlanger, 1970) have written extensively on the application of pantomime training for aphasic individuals.

Iconic signs or nonpropositional limb movements have been used as facilitators of verbal output. Rosenbek, Collins, and Wertz (1976) suggested the use of emblems, a form of iconic gestures, in an intersystemic reorganization program. Simmons (1978) used a finger-counting system to facilitate verbal output for an aphasic/apraxic patient. The author attributed an increased verbal score on the PICA to the "systematic and exaggerated use of this simple and nonmeaningful gesture in a facilitory task hierarchy" (p. 177). Sparks and Holland (1976) used finger-tapping and melody to facilitate speech in their Melodic Intonation Therapy program.

The literature does not provide any clearly defined rules that allow the clinician to predict which patients will benefit from training in gestural communication. However, some trends emerge when one reviews case reports of success with gestural communication. The pattern of these cases suggests that the usefulness of gestural systems, or the extent of the training required, can be predicted by the nature and pattern of the patient's communication deficits. Gestural training has been most successful with patients with predominantly "expressive" disorders, such as nonfluent aphasia, apraxia of speech, and dysarthria. For example, the patient in Eagleson et al. (1970) was described as "right hemiplegic and predominantly expressive" in aphasia type. Schlanger's group of patients (1976) included the following: one patient with hemiparesis, one with apraxia, one with dysarthria, one with "halting, inarticulate" speech and one with "perserverative jargon and good auditory comprehension." Skelly et al.'s patients in 1974 included six apraxic patients, one glossectomee, one dysphonic, one laryngectomee, and one dysarthric patient. Reports of success with patients who exhibit auditory comprehension impairment also appear, although it seems that the training programs must be prolonged. Simmons and Zorthian (1979) report that a fluent aphasic began using trained gestures spontaneously after the seventh month of training, and self-generated signs after the ninth month.

Rao and Horner (1978) listed some possible prerequisite abilities for the use of gestures as verbal facilitators. According to these authors, six skills are positive prognostically for the use of subpropositional gestures to facilitate speech. These include (1) gestural recognition ability, (2) gesture production, including object use, imitation of gestures and spontaneous use of pantomime, (3) facilitation of auditory and visual comprehension when paired with gesture, (4) verbal imitation of single words, (5) good scores on the Raven's Progressive Matrices Test, and (6) motivation to communicate.

Aided Systems

The term *aided communication* refers to a broad group of communication augmentation systems including boards, books, and mechanical or electronic devices, which serve functions similar to those described above for the gestural systems. These aids are designed to replace, supplement, or facilitate the verbal communication of individuals who are not independent verbal communicators in all situations. In contrast to the gestural communication, the area of aided communication is a relatively new one characterized by an ever-changing computer-based technology. During the past several years, an increasing number of systems have become commercially available. These systems, ranging from a modified electric typewriter to computer-based systems with synthesis and rapid printing output, have joined the simple communication boards and books in the clinical management of some patients. Undeniably, communication augmentation devices have enhanced the communication speed, flexibility, and independence of the nonvocal adult for whom appropriate aids have been selected. It has become possible to serve many individuals who had been unable to communicate due to severe physical, linguistic, and cognitive limitations.

Users of Communication Devices

The extent to which communication aids are being used clinically is well beyond the number of reports which have become published literature. Perhaps the best source of personal accounts of devices by their users and descriptions of one-of-a-kind systems is *Communication Outlook*, a newsletter which focuses on communication aids and techniques. (*Communication Outlook* is edited and published jointly by the Artificial Language Laboratory, Michigan State University, and the TRACE Center for the Severely Communicatively Handicapped, University of Wisconsin.) Preliminary descriptions of successful users of communication aids are beginning to appear in the literature. Beukelman, Yorkston, Gorhoff, Mitsuda, and Kenyon (1981) described a series of 13 adults for whom Canon Communicators (distributed by Telesensory Systems, Inc., 3408 Hillview Ave., P. O. Box 10099, Palo Alto, CA 94304) were recommended. This group varied in many respects including age, etiology, funding source, and communication environments. The decision-making process which led to a recommendation of a communication augmentation system also varied from patient to patient. On the basis of this preliminary work, the population appears to be diverse. Disorders may be either degenerative, stable, or improving; they may be adult onset or congenital. The use of devices may be temporary or long term.

Communication aids may serve a variety of functions. They most typically serve as a replacement for speech for chronic severely impaired patients, (Beukelman et al. 1981), for patients who are respirator-dependent, or for patients with acute neurological disease (Henry, 1981).

Some aids also serve to supplement speech. Picture and alphabet boards may be used as a means to re-establish early communication for the recovering brain stem-injured patient (Beukelman & Yorkston, 1978). Alphabet boards have also been used as a means of making the transition from dependence upon a communication aid to independent speech. Beukelman and Yorkston (1977) describe a system in which the individual is taught to point to the first letter of words on an alphabet board as each word is spoken. By providing the listener with additional information, this system permits the patient to attempt functional speech at a point earlier in the treatment program than the level of intelligibility would permit without assistance. Although this system is clearly serving a supplementary function, it may also be facilitating the recovery of speech, since the severely dysarthric patient is able to practice speaking in a functional context. Warren and Datta (1981) reported a case in which a communication aid may have facilitated the recovery of speech. Their patient was a severely head-injured individual with a diagnosis of severe nonfluent aphasia, who was trained to use a communication device with speech synthesized output (Handivoice 110, distributed by H C Electronics, 250 Camino Alto, Mill Valley, CA 94941). Although the patient was considered stable when the aid was introduced, verbal communication began to appear after only a short period of system use.

Despite the diversity existing in the population of nonspeaking adults, these users of communication aids share a number of characteristics that distinguish them from severely physically handicapped nonspeaking children. Often in the adult, severe physical deficits are combined with intact language skills. Unlike nonvocal children, many adults who use communication aids exhibit good reading comprehension, spelling proficiency, and extensive vocabularies. Together, these skills provide the language base which may allow the use of complex communication devices. Further, nonvocal adults, especially those who have a history of normal language development prior to onset, are able to use devices functionally because they do not need to be taught the underlying principles of communication interaction, such as turn taking, attention getting, leave taking, etc. The communication interaction patterns of nonvocal adults are discussed by Beukelman and Yorkston (1982).

Nonvocal adults who use communication aids may also be distinguished from nonvocal children in terms of their communication needs. Because of their intact language skills, nonvocal adults often prefer to communicate subtle differences in meaning with unique vocabulary selection and grammatical constructions. Often these adults are not satisfied with the relatively restricted vocabulary that may be appropriate for use with children who are acquiring language skills, as well as learning to operate the communication augmentation device. In addition to their need to produce unique messages, adults often need to be independent communicators, and may require multiple communication systems, each of which meet specific needs. For example, nonspeaking adults may use one system for preparation of printed output and another for face-to-face conversational interactions. In short, the communication needs of the adult are dictated by a number of social, residential, educational and vocational requirements.

Device Components

It is beyond the scope of this chapter to present a detailed discussion of all possible communication aids. Vanderheiden's *Nonvocal Communication Resource Book* (1978) provides a yearly update of systems and devices. The 1978 version contained over 60 commercial, precommercial, and experimental communication aids. The variety of systems available may initially be somewhat confusing for the clinician who is attempting to select a communication aid. However, like the gestural systems, aided systems may be evaluated in terms of their basic components. For aided systems, these components are control, process, and output.

Control

The control component of a communication aid is the means by which the user operates the system, involving a display and an interface. The *display* refers to the means by which selections are presented to the user. For example, the display for a conventional typewriter is the keyboard containing the complete alphabet and digits. A second type of display consists of a panel or grid containing a number of locations which may be illuminated to offer selections to the user. Some systems contain no control display. For example, in some systems the selections are presented auditorily, and in others, the user memorizes codes, such as Morse Code, in order to operate the system.

The *interface* refers to the means by which the user actually operates the device. Interfaces may involve single or multiple control switches activated by displacement, touch, light intensity, temperature, moisture, or EMG control (Preston, 1980). The selection of an interface for a communication aid depends primarily upon the physical control ability of the user. Minimal physical control may require a single-switch interface in which the user is presented with a series of options that can be either accepted or rejected by means of that switch. Such a system is typically described as a "scanning system." Users with greater motor control can make selections by directly activating a large number of switches. A conventional typewriter is a familiar example of a multiple-switch, direct-selection interface.

The choice of the control option is perhaps the most critical step in the selection of a communication aid for a severely physically handicapped adult. Without an appropriate display and interface, even the most elaborate of aids cannot be used effectively. The display or presentation mode is selected on the basis of the user's visual abilities, cognitive, and language skills. For example, an individual with reduced visual acuity may need an enlarged display in order to make reliable selections, or an individual with poor reading skills, either pre-or postmorbidly, may be unable to use systems with extensive written messages in their display.

The selection of the interface requires the greatest team effort. For adults with severe motor control deficits, the team must develop proper seating and head control before interface selection can be considered. The selection of the most appropriate interface must be made on the basis of specific motor capacity. Specifically, it is necessary to assess the nature of the most reliable voluntary movement, the speed and accuracy of that response, and the effects of fatigue, positioning, and communicative pressure upon the reliability of those movements. The selection of an interface has important implications for the ultimate efficiency that can be expected from a given communication aid. The selection of single switches, although it may be appealing from the perspective of motor control, may be undesirable when one considers the severely slow communication rate which is a characteristic of single-switch scanning systems. On the other hand, the selection of a direct-selection interface, which is relatively rapid but quite fatiguing, may be less appropriate than the selection of a slower, but more reliable single-switch scanning system. In short, a number of important factors must be weighed in making any decision about the most appropriate interface for a severely impaired nonspeaking individual. For adults with less severe motor control deficits, several interface options may be available. In such cases, selection of an interface may be secondary to other considerations, such as the processes or output potential of the aid.

Systems Processes

The processes that can be performed by a communication aid vary considerably in sophistication, from those systems which only transmit messages without enhancing, storing, or decoding them (for example, a conventional typewriter) to systems with complex microprocessing computer-based processes. The general goal of any of these processes is to improve the user's communication efficiency. For the language-intact, but severely physically impaired adult, this is typically an attempt to increase the communication rate beyond the extremely slow rate produced in letter-by-letter selection.

Memory storage and retrieval is a process available in a number of commercial systems. This process allows the user to prepare a message, store it, and retrieve the message by activating a single "memory read" or "recall" switch. For example, the Handivoice 110 contains two memory storage units which can be programmed by the user. The chief benefit of this process is the reduction of the communication partners' time commitment. Using such a system, nonspeaking individuals take as much time as they need to prepare a message correctly; the message can then be delivered to the partner at a relatively rapid rate.

Encoding is a process by which words, phrases, and sentences may be stored in specific locations on a device and called up by the selection of a relatively short code. Communication aids which have encoding capability differ in flexibility. Some are programmed at the factory and cannot be changed without modifying the hardware of the system. Others can be programmed by the manufacturer to meet specific vocabulary needs of the users. Other units are programmable in the field by the user, an attendant, or any adult who has knowledge of the particular system. The field-programmable units offer the most flexibility because their vocabulary or selection options can be altered or enhanced at any time when new communication demands are placed on the user. The Express I (distributed by Prentke Romich Co., Shreve, OH) is an example of a field-programmable unit in which a number of locations can be programmed, and messages called up with the selection of a single entry.

Another process available in some microprocessor-based systems is prediction. Here, the computer predicts the completion of the message on the basis of the first units entered. A language-based prediction system which is currently operating is a Morse Code-based communication device (Wilson, 1981). After the first letter of a word is selected, the device offers the user (on a control display) the most probable completion of the word. If the computer has "guessed" correctly, the user selects a space and the complete word is selected. If the prediction is incorrect, the user simply selects the next letter of the word, and with this additional information, another prediction is made. This continues until the prediction is accepted or until the word is spelled correctly, letter by letter. Linguistic information, as well as the user's most frequently occurring vocabulary, have been programmed into the system to assist the accuracy of the computer guessing. Still another process available in most microprocessor-based systems is that of text editing. Here, the user is able to make corrections in the text, insert or delete portions, or shift the order of elements before the text is printed in its final form.

Selection of the most appropriate process depends to a great extent on the communication needs, along with the user's ability to learn to operate the system correctly. Some individuals require a system to express only basic needs, concerns, and self-care requests to persons who are familiar with them. Others require a system that can be used to express complex messages in educational, vocational settings to strangers. Individuals who must use single switches with scanning displays, or who are extremely slow as they press keys on the keyboard, need communication aids which are capable of speeding up communication. A system with code retrieval, encoding, or predictive capability has this potential.

System Output

Output choices available in communication aids can be divided into these three broad categories—visual, auditory, and electronic. Some visual, and all auditory, output are transient in nature. For example, the output of a communication board is visually transient; the communication partner observes as letters or words are indicated by the user, and no permanent record is left. Visual output systems such as television screens and marquee-type displays are semitransient in that the output is displayed only temporarily. Many communication aids such as a typewriter, strip printer, or computer-driven printer produce permanent visual output. The output of some communication aids is electronic in that the output controls the operation of another system or device. For example, the Prentke-Romich Lapboard Strip Printer (distributed by Prentke Romich Co., Shreve, OH) may operate a TTY computer.

As in the case of the selection of the system processes, output selection depends heavily on the communication needs of the individual. For example, when the communication environment demands that the nonvocal individual interact either with people out of visual contact or several partners at a time, as in a classroom, synthesized speech might be a useful output option. On the other hand, for patients in nursing homes, systems are selected so that messages can be prepared in advance and transmitted rapidly. This requires the selection of systems with either hard copy output or systems which have memory or storage capacities.

Figure 9-2 is a schematic representation of the components of communication aids. The components of some communication aids are simple. For example, the Canon Communicator is a portable tape typewriter, in which the control display contains the letters of the alphabet, and the interface consists of multiple switches or keys which the user depresses as selections are made. The Canon is capable of one-system process, that of direct conversion of the keys selected to letters, and the output is printed

FIGURE 9-2
A Schematic Representation of Communication Augmentation Devices, Including Control, Process, and Output. The Components for Canon Communicator are illustrated.

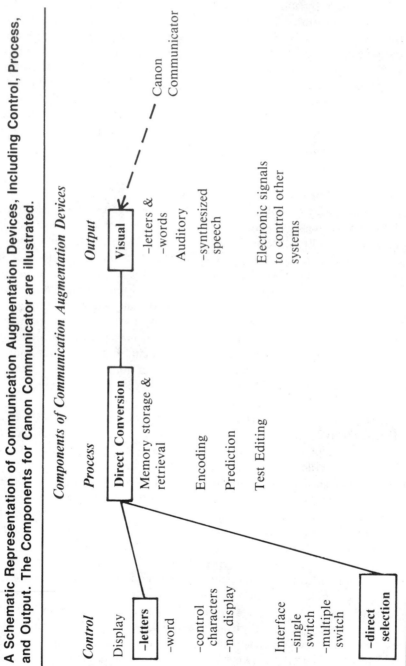

Components of Communication Augmentation Devices

letters on a strip of thermal-sensitive tape. Other communication aids have multiple component options. For example, the Express III system (Prentke Romich) uses a display that contains letters, words, and control characters. A number of single- and multiple-switch interfaces may be used to control the system. The processes include direct conversion of letters into print, memory, and encoding to call up entire preprogrammed messages. The output of such a system may be the printed word, synthesized speech, or electronic output to control other devices.

Service Delivery Systems

An interdisciplinary approach to the selection process is now required in light of the extensive skills and knowledge necessary as part of the service delivery process. Often the selection and customization of communication aids is carried out in large centers where family members together with professionals in communication, engineering, physical control, and adaptation of devices can cooperate. Their efforts are supplemented by the expertise of individuals in the area of medicine, psychology, social services, and vision. Shane and Bashir (1980) suggested that the evaluation process involves two phases—election and selection. The election phase leads to a decision about whether or not a nonvocal individual is a candidate for a communication aid. This process requires both formal and informal assessment of intelligence, language, memory, motor control, reflex pattern, vision, and hearing. Once the election process has been completed and the decision about candidacy made, selection may begin. Selection involves the careful review of the capabilities and communication needs of the nonspeaking individual. Components of the communication aid are then matched to these capabilities and needs.

A third phase of the evaluation process, called performance evaluation, may also be added. The performance evaluation typically involves a period of training followed by a period of trial use of the aid. These trials can be carried out in the clinical setting by obtaining information about the rate and accuracy with which the individual is able to perform a series of message-preparation tasks. Performance evaluation may also be carried out in natural communication settings (Beukelman & Yorkston, 1980). Assessment of performance in natural settings is especially useful in addressing such issues as the frequency of communication exchanges, patterns of communicator initiation, patterns and frequency of communication breakdown and message types.

Future Trends

Communicative efficiency is clearly one of the greatest limitations in the use of communication aids by adults in natural interactions. Even the most optimistic rate of 20 words per minute is nearly 10 times slower than a normal verbal communication rate. Beukelman and Yorkston (1982) reviewed a number of approaches being developed to increase the efficiency of communication aids. Some of these enhancement approaches have been described earlier, including encoding, memory storage, retrieval systems, and prediction.

Other systems designed to maximize communication efficiency use the retrieval of phoneme or letter sequences rather than individual sounds or letters. Goodenough-Trepagnier (1980) and Goodenough-Trepagnier and Prather (1981) have suggested two such approaches for increasing the message preparation. SPEEC, or Sequence of Phonemes for an Efficient English Communication, contains frequently occurring sequences of sounds; WRITE contains frequently occurring sequences of letters. These sound or letter sequences can be combined by the user to form a message.

Another approach to enhancing efficiency is through the optimization of entry locations. Goodenough-Trepagnier and Rosen (1981) have suggested a computer-based model for retrieving the "best key set" for a nonspeaking individual. Three factors included in this model are the number of language units per word, the average number of acts required to encode each unit, and the average time for each act. Beukelman and Poblette (1981) have developed a computer simulation of a row-column scanning system in an effort to identify the optimum location of entries in a scanning system. The relative time to communicate a message can be computed for a variety of display arrangements in a 10 x 10 matrix. The most efficient systems were found to be those in which the most frequently occuring letters were located in the upper left quadrant of the display.

Speculations about future trends in the field of communication augmentation often revolve around the application of computer technology to aid the handicapped. Clearly there has been a trend toward customization in the recent past. This has often taken the form of interface customization. Commercially available devices are often adapted to unique motor needs by customizing switches to allow the user to control the device. As low-cost microprocessing computers become widely available, there is also a trend toward customization of the processes available in communication aids. For example, specific vocabulary and messages can be entered and stored, or any number of output options—including printed output and synthesized speech—may be selected by the user. Microprocessing computers may also function in areas other than communication

(Vanderheiden, 1981). These applications may include recreation and educational activities, as well as systems for management of information, or for control systems for work or home environments.

Needs Assessment

To say that needs assessment is important in the selection of communication augmentation systems seems at first to be a statement of the obvious. However, a thorough understanding of the communication needs of the individual is not a trivial matter. Clinicians often do a better job of assessing the capabilities of their patients, and matching these capabilities with the demands of the systems, than they do in identifying specific communication needs of their patients. Failure to understand and account for these needs often results in selection of a system which is inappropriate, not because it is too demanding, either linguistically or motorically, but because it does not allow the user to perform needed communication functions.

Inappropriate system selection may be avoided by making a needs assessment an integral part of every phase of the selection and customization process. Although no formal evaluation format is available, a needs assessment may be thought of as a listing of a series of specific "needs statements." Many of these needs statements revolve around the messages which the patient needs to communicate. For example, a partial list of needs statements for a patient who is confined to bed may include:

> This man needs to call the nurse.
> This man needs to ask for his glasses.
> This man needs to ask for the bedpan.
> etc.

Other needs statements specify listener requirements. For example, a list of needs statements for a handicapped individual who lives in a residential center might include:

> This woman needs to communicate with nonreaders.
> This woman needs to communicate with people who are not familiar with her.
> This woman needs to deliver her message to listeners rapidly.
> This woman needs to communicate with people who are not sufficiently mobile to come to her.

Finally, needs statements may reflect environmental requirements:

> This woman needs to communicate when she is in her wheelchair.
>
> This woman needs to communicate when she is in her bed.
>
> This woman needs to communicate when she is outdoors.

Once a complete list of needs statements is made, it will have a bearing on both the selection and the customization process. There are patients for whom the selection of a device is made on the basis of their specific communication needs rather than on their capabilities. Consider the patient who is able to use an alphabet board, an electric typewriter, and a Canon Communication with equal proficiency, but who resides in a nursing home where staff time is limited and portability is necessary. The needs statements would dictate the selection of the Canon Communicator because it clearly would meet more communication needs than the other systems.

Needs assessment is also an important part of the customization process, in which systems are individualized for specific motor control requirements and vocabulary needs. Severely aphasic/apraxic individuals may not need to communicate many of the "standard" messages that are easily picturable in communication books, or easily understood with simple iconic gestures. For example, most commercially available picture communication boards contain a picture representing the notion "drink." Patients who have independent mobility would be more likely simply to get the drink than to ask for it. Some sampling of the patient communication needs in a natural environment may be required in order to select messages appropriately. Often the patient's spouse or nurse will be able to supply this type of information by keeping a diary for several consecutive days. This diary would contain all messages that the patient is expressing—either independently via spontaneous gestures, or with the assistance of a communication partner who leads the patient through a series of questions and answers. From this raw material a relatively small corpus of messages can be developed. Some of these messages are more easily pictured through a communication book. For example, a calender may be used for communication of time-related messages. Other messages may be more easily gestured. An example of such a message is the universally understood signal for "come here." Working from a relatively small corpus of "needed messages" allows the clinician to train specific messages, as well as to select the most appropriate communication vehicle to transmit those messages. Often, for severely impaired adults, multiple communication systems are appropriate. Perhaps the patient may use highly codified gestures with familiar partners and a communication book with others.

In closing, we will reiterate that nonspeech language and communication systems cannot be as efficient or as flexible as speech. However, they may be the only alternative for individuals who are severely limited verbally as the result of motor-control, motor-planning, or language deficits. There are no hard and fast rules dictating system selection. Of course, the capabilities of the patient and the demands of the system must be taken into account. It is clear that communication needs must also be considered in order to select the most effective system possible. Systematic observation of nonspeaking individuals in natural communication situations would appear to be essential for understanding their needs. This in turn would help us to select appropriate systems, as well as to develop new systems to better meet the needs of our patients.

References

ASHA Ad hoc Committee on Communication Processes in Nonspeaking Persons. "Nonspeech Communication: A position paper." *Asha*, 1980, *22*: (4). 267–272.

Beukelman, D. R., & Poblette, M. Maximizing communication rates of row column scanning communication systems. A paper presented at the annual convention of the American Speech-Language-Hearing Association, Los Angeles, November, 1981.

Beukelman, D. R., & Yorkston, K. M. A communication system for the severely dysarthric speaker with an intact language system. *Journal of Speech and Hearing Disorders*, 1977, *42*, 265–270.

Beukelman, D. R., & Yorkston, K. M. A series of communication options for individuals with brain stem lesions. *Archives of Physical Medicine and Rehabilitation*, 1978, *59*, 337–342.

Beukelman, D. R., & Yorkston, K. M. Non-vocal communication: Performance evaluation. *Archives of Physical Medicine and Rehabilitation*, 1980, *61*, 272–275.

Beukelman, D. R., & Yorkston, K. M. Communication interaction strategies for severely speech impaired adults. *Topics in Language Disorders*, 1982, *2*(2), 39–54.

Beukelman, D. R., Yorkston, K. M., Gorhoff, S. C., Mitsuda, P. M., & Kenyon, V. T. Canon Communicator use by adults: A retrospective study. *Journal of Speech and Hearing Disorders*, 1981, *46*, 374–378.

Beukelman, D. R., Yorkston, K. M., & Waugh, P. F. Communication in severe aphasia: Effectiveness of three instruction modalities. *Archives of Physical Medicine and Rehabilitation*, 1980, *61*, 248–252.

Cicone, M., Wapner, W., Foldi, N., Zurif, E., & Gardner, H. The relationship between gesture and language in aphasic communication. *Brain and Language*, 1979, *8*, 324–349.

Daniloff, J. K., Noll, J. D., Fristoe, M., & Lloyd, L. L. Gesture recognition in patients with aphasia. *Journal of Speech and Hearing Disorders*, 1982, *47*, 43–47.

Darley, F. L. *Diagnosis and appraisal of communication disorders*. Englewood Cliffs, NJ: Prentice-Hall, 1964.

Darley, F. L., Aronson, A. E., & Brown, J. R. *Motor speech disorders*. Philadelphia: W. B. Saunders, 1975.

Davis, G. A., & Wilcox, M. J. Incorporating parameters of natural conversation in aphasia treatment: PACE therapy. In R. Chapey (Ed.), *Language intervention strategies in adult aphasia*. Baltimore: Williams & Wilkins, 1981.

Davis, S., Artes, R., & Hoops, R. Verbal expression and expressive pantomime in aphasic patients. In Lebrun & Hoope (Eds.), Problems of Aphasia, a volume in Series *Neurolinguistics.* Swets & Zeitliyer B. V., Lisse: 1979.

DeRenzi, E., Motti, F., & Nichelli, P. Imitating gestures: A quantitative approach to ideomotor apraxia. *Archives of Neurology*, 1980, *37*, 6–10.

Dowden, P. A., Marshall, R. C., & Tompkins, C. A. Amer-Ind sign as a communicative facilitator for aphasic and apraxic patients. *Proceeding of the Clinical Aphasiology Conference*, Minneapolis: BRK Publishers, 1981, 133–140.

Duffy, J. F. Comment on Baratz's Case study. *Aphasia, Apraxia and Agnosia* (in press).

Duffy, R. J., & Buck, R. A. A study of the relationship between propositional (pantomime) and subpropositional (facial expression) extraverbal behaviors in aphasics. *Folio Phoniatrica*, 1979, *31*, 129–136.

Duffy, R. J., & Duffy, J. R. Three studies of deficits in pantomimic expression and pantomimic recognition in aphasia. *Journal of Speech and Hearing Research*, 1981, *24* (1), 70–34.

Duffy, R. J., Duffy, J. R., & Mercaitis, P. A. Pantomimic Motor Behaviors of a Broca's and a Wernicke's Aphasic. A paper presented at the Annual Convention of the American Speech-Language-Hearing Association, Atlanta, GA, November 1979.

Eagleson, H. M., Vaughn, G. R., & Knudson, A. B. C. Hand signals for dysphasia. *Archives of Physical Medicine and Rehabilitation*, 1970, *51*, 111–113.

Gainotti, G., & Lemmo, M. A. Comprehension of symbolic gestures in aphasia. *Brain and Language*, 1976, *3*, 451–460.

Glass, A. V., Gazzaniga, M. S., & Premack, D. Artificial language training in global aphasics. *Neuropsychologia*, 1973, *11*, 95–103.

Goodenough-Trepagnier, C. Rate of Language Production with SPEEC Nonvocal Communication System. *Proceedings of International Conference on Rehabilitation Engineering.* Ottawa: Canadian Medical Biological Engineering Society, 1980.

Goodenough-Trepagnier, C., & Prather, P. Communication systems for the nonvocal based on frequent phoneme sequences. *Journal of Speech and Hearing Research*, 1981, *24*, 322–330.

Goodenough-Trepagnier, C., & Rosen, M. J. Model for computer based procedure to prescribe optimal "keyboard." Paper presented at the 4th Annual Conference in Rehabilitation Engineering, Washington, DC, September, 1981.

Goodglass, H., & Kaplan, E. Disturbances of Gesture and Pantomime in Aphasia. *Brain*, 1963, *86*, 703–720.

Griffith, P. L., Robinson, J. H., & Panagos, J. M., Perception of iconicity in American Sign Language by hearing and deaf subjects. *Journal of Speech and Hearing Disorders*, 1981, *46*, 388–397.

Harris, D., & Vanderheiden, G. C. Enhancing the development of communication interaction. In R. L. Schiefelbusch (Ed.), *Nonspeech language and communication: Analysis and intervention.* Baltimore: University Park Press, 1980, 227–259.

Henry, C. Communication for hospital patients acutely deprived of speech. Paper presented at the annual convention of the American Speech-Language-Hearing Association, Los Angeles, 1981.

Holland, A. L. Some practical considerations in aphasia rehabilitation. In M. Sullivan & M. S. Kansmers (Eds.), *Rationale for adult aphasia therapy.* Lincoln: University of Nebraska Medical Center, 1977.

Holland, A. L. Observing functional communication of aphasic adults. *Journal of Speech and Hearing Disorders*, 1982, *47*, 50–56.

Katz, R., LaPointe, L., & Markel, N. Coverbal behavior and aphasic speakers. *Clinical Aphasiology Conference Proceedings.* Minneapolis: BRK Publishers, 1978, 164–173.

Kimura, D. The neurological basis of language qua gesture. In H. Whitaker & H. A. Whitaker (Eds.), *Studies in neurolinguistics* (Vol. 2). New York: Academic Press, 1976.

Kimura, D., & Archibald, Y. Motor functions of the left hemisphere. *Brain*, 1974, *97*, 337–350.

Kimura, D., Battison, R., & Lubert, B. Impairment of nonlinguistic hand movements in a deaf aphasic. *Brain and Language*, 1976, *3*, 566–571.

Kirshner, H., & Webb, W. Selective involvement of the auditory - verbal modality in an acquired communication disorder: Benefit from sign language therapy. *Brain and Language*, 1981, *13*, 161–170.

Kohl, F. Effects of motoric requirements on the acquisition of manual sign responses by severely handicapped students. *American Journal of Mental Deficiency*, 1981, *85* (4), 396–403.

Koller, J., & Sclanger, P. Identification of action words and activity pantomimes by aphasics. Paper presented at the annual convention of the American Speech and Hearing Association, Washington, DC, 1975.

Pickett, L. An assessment of gestural and pantomime deficits in aphasic populations. *Acta Symbolica*, 1974, *5* (3), 69–86.

Pickett, L. Assessment of gestural and pantomimic deficit in aphasia patients. In R. Brookshire (Ed.), *Clinical Aphasiology: Collected Proceedings, 1972-1976*. Minneapolis: BRK Publishers, 1978, 86–103.

Peterson, L., & Kirshner, H. Gestural impairment and gestural ability in aphasia: A review. *Brain and Language*, 1981, *14*, 333–348.

Porch, P. E. *Porch Index of Communicative Ability*. Palo Alto, CA: Consulting Psychologists Press, 1967.

Preston, J. *Controls: Reference catalog to aid physically limited people in operation of assistive devices*. Palo Alto, CA: Rehabilitiation Engineering Center, Children's Hospital at Stanford, 1980.

Rao, P. R. & Horner, J. Gesture as a deblocking modality in a severe aphasic patient. In R. Brookshire (Ed.), *Proceedings of Clinical Aphasiology Conference*. Minneapolis: BRK Publishers, 1978, 180–187.

Rosenbek, J. C. Treating apraxia of speech. In D. F. Johns, (Ed.), *Clinical management of neurogenic communication disorders*. Boston: Little, Brown & Company, 1978.

Rosenbek, J. C., Collins, M. J., & Wertz, R. T. Intersystemic reorganization for apraxia of speech. In R. Brookshire (Ed.), *Proceedings of the Clinical Aphasiology Conference*. Minneapolis: BRK Publishers, 1976, 255–260.

Schlanger, P. H. Training the adult aphasic to pantomime. Paper presented at the annual convention of the American Speech-Language-Hearing Association, Houston, November, 1976.

Schlanger, P., & Frieman, R. Pantomime therapy with aphasics. *Aphasia-Apraxia-Agnosia*, 1979, *1* (2), 34–39.

Schlanger, P., Geffner, D., & DiCarrado, C. A comparison of gestural communication with aphasics: Pre- and post-therapy. Paper presented at the annual convention of the American Speech and Hearing Association, Las Vegas, 1974.

Schlanger, P., & Schlanger, B. Adapting role-playing activities with aphasic patients. *Journal of Speech and Hearing Disorders*, 1970, *35*, 229–235.

Shane, H. C., & Bashir, A. S. Election criteria for the adaption of an augmentative communication system: Preliminary considerations. *Journal of Speech and Hearing Disorders*, 1980, *45*, 408.

Shane, H. D., & Wilbur, R. B. Prediction of experience sign potential based on motor control. *Sign Language Studies*, 1980, Winter, 331–348.

Silverman, F. H. *Communication for the speechless*. Englewood Cliffs, NJ: Prentice-Hall, Inc., 1980.

Simmons, N. Finger counting as an intersystemic reorganizer in apraxia of speech. In R. Brookshire (Ed.), *The Proceedings of the Clinical Aphasiology Conference*, Minneapolis: BRK Publishers, 1978, 174–179.

Simmons, N., & Zorthian, A. Use of symbolic gestures in a case of fluent aphasia. In R. Brookshire (Ed.), *The Proceedings of the Clinical Aphasiology Conference*, Minneapolis: BRK Publishers, 1979, 278–285.

Skelly, M. *Amerind gestural code based on universal American Indian hand talk*. New York: Elsevier North Holland, 1979.

Skelly, M., Schinsky, L., Smith, R. W., Donaldson, R. C., & Griffin, J. M. American Indian sign: A gestural communication system for the speechless. *Archives of Physical Medicine and Rehabilitation*, 1975, *56*, 156–160.

Skelly, M., Schinsky, L., Smith, R. W., & Fust, R. S. American Indian sign (Amerind) as a facilitator of verbalization for the oral verbal apraxic. *Journal of Speech and Hearing Disorders*, 1974, *39* (4), 445–455.

Sparks, R., & Holland, A. Method: Melodic intonation therapy for aphasia. *Journal of Speech and Hearing Disorders*, 1976, *41*, 287–297.

Vanderhieden, G. *Nonvocal communication resource book*. Baltimore: University Park Press, 1978.

Vanderheiden, G. C. Practical application of microcomputers to aid the handicapped. *Computer*, 1981, 54–61.

Warren, R. L., & Datta, K. D. The return of speech 4½ years post head injury: A case report. In R. Brookshire (Ed.), *Proceedings of the Clinical Aphasiology Conference*, Minneapolis: BRK Publishers, 1981, 301–308.

Wertz, R. T. Neuropathologies of speech and language: An introduction to patient management. In D. F. Johns (Ed.), *Clinical management of neurogenic communication disorders*. Boston: Little, Brown & Company, 1978.

Wilson, W. R. A alternative communication system for the severely physically handicapped. Grant to Handicapped Media Services and Captioned Films Program. Department of Education, 1981.

AUTHOR INDEX

A

Abbs, J., 356, 357, 379, 380, 382, 387, 389, 391, 392, 394, 395, 396, 397, 399, 400
Abelson, R., 571
Abelson, R. P., 683
Abrams, R., 775
Ackerman, N., 895
Adams, J. A., 133, 135, 136, 141, 149, 150
Adams, M., 234, 239, 248, 262, 264, 265, 271
Adams, M. R., 509, 520, 529
Adams, R., 1010
Adams, R. D., 843
Adams, R. E., 98
Adamovich, B. B., 814, 952
Adamovich, B. L., 778, 950, 952, 953, 958, 1010
Adelson, R., 809, 810
Ahern, M. B., 891
Ahlsten-Taylor, J., 588
Ahmed, M., 449
Ainsworth, S., 293, 301
Aitchison, J., 893
Alajouanine, T., 804
Albert, M., 176, 817, 929, 948
Alber, M. L., 761, 791, 793, 795, 811, 842, 850, 891, 894, 917, 925, 968, 970, 979, 983, 993
Aldes, M., 447
Alexander, D. A., 989
Alexander, M. P., 767, 891, 894, 917, 925
Alexander, R. M., 372
Alfrey, A. C., 246
Allen, G., 55, 56, 57
Alper, J., 238
Alzheimer, A., 967
Aman, L. A., 169
American Speech-Language-Hearing Association, 93
Ames, S., 317, 328, 543, 554

Aminoff, M., 437, 438
Amyes, E. W., 1008
Anders, T. R., 845
Andersen, E., 689
Anderson, K. E., 743
Anderson, M. C., 683, 686
Anderson, R. C., 683, 686
Anderson, S., 62
Anderson, T., 804
Andrew, W., 992
Andrews, A., 435
Andrews, G., 234, 239, 240, 241, 242, 244, 245, 248, 249, 250, 267, 300, 314, 315, 316, 319, 321, 335, 336, 339, 395, 397, 513, 514, 517, 522, 523, 524, 527, 528, 531, 540, 541, 542, 545, 548, 562, 565
Andrews-Kulis, M. S., 863
Angle, E. H., 204
Ansberry, M., 4, 507
Antin, S., 989
Appell, J., 768, 779, 793, 795
Appenteng, K., 397
Aram, D. M., 167, 168, 169, 171, 173, 181, 586
Archambault, P., 98
Archer, L., 725
Archibald, Y. M., 764, 791, 1049
Aretaeus, 967
Armour, R., 362
Arndt, W., 6, 16, 139, 140, 142, 143, 144, 151
Aronson, A., 353, 355, 356, 392, 394, 407, 408, 478
Aronson, A. E., 763, 775, 776, 787, 788, 793, 798, 799, 801, 1043
Arseni, C., 1003
Arter, J., 574
Artes, R., 1053
Askenfelt, A., 436

1071

SUBJECT INDEX

A

Ablation, of vocal tract structures,
360–362
Acetylocholinesterase (ACT), 974–975
Achievement tests
adolescent problems, 709
California Achievement Test, 705
Metropolitan Achievement Tests, 705
*Peabody Individualized Achievement
Tests*, 705
Wide Range Achievement Tests, 705
Acquired aphasia, convulsive disorders
assessment protocol, 613–614
audiological characteristics, 606
auditory verbal agnosia, 616–618
behavioral characteristics, 606
cognitive characteristics, 606
communication breakdowns, 625,
634–639
comparative data, *622–623*
defined, 599
EEG disturbances, 600, 609–611
etiologies, 599
evaluation, 613
filled pauses, 625, 634 635
grammatical marker usage, 635
intervention, 600, 639
language characteristics, *70–71, 607,
612–613*
language samples, 621
learning-disabled data, 624
male vs. female, 601–603
mean length of utterance (MLU),
621, 626–629
muteness, 607
narrative vs. conversational samples,
625
neurological characteristics, 601
onset, 600–603

pathogeneses, 609–611
pilot data, 614–619
prognosis, 600, 611–612
research, 600–601, 612, 639
similarities to learning-disabled, 635
syntactic reformations, 635
*Systematic Analysis of Language
Transcripts (SALT),* 620
utterance types, 625, 630–633
vs. developmental, 615–616
vs. learning-disabled, 619 639
voice quality, 607
word / phrase revision, 625, 635
word retrieval problems, 635
Acquisition, normal language
adult-child interaction, 647 650 (*see
also* Maternal speech)
age norms, 50–51, 592–593
& cognitive abilities, *594, 693–694*
assessment, 591 595, 695 (*see also*
Assessment)
Brown's stages, 592–593
causal relations, 566–567
cohesive devices, 569–571
communicative competence, 644,
650
communicative functions, 547–549,
550–552, 553, 568–569
complex sentences, 565–568
comprehension, 544–546, 553–554,
571–572
contingent speech, 559–561
conversational turn-taking, 562–563
environmental influences, 589, 656
(*see also* Environmental influences)
feedback, effects of, 647–650 (*see
also* Maternal speech)

1101